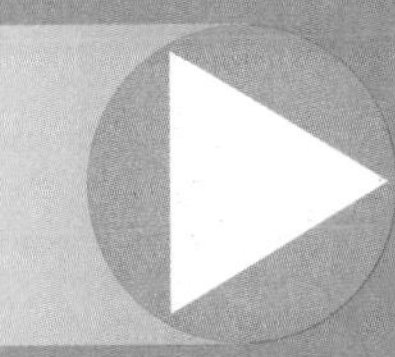

THERAPYED'S

National Physical Therapy Examination Review & Study Guide

25th Edition

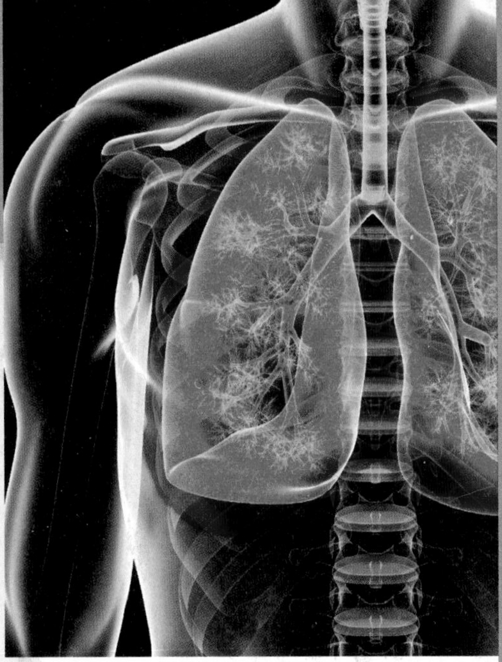

SUSAN B. O'SULLIVAN, PT, EdD
Professor Emerita
Department of Physical Therapy
College of Health Sciences
University of Massachusetts Lowell
Lowell, Massachusetts

RAYMOND P. SIEGELMAN, PT, DPT, MS
President Emeritus
TherapyEd
Boston, Massachusetts

SCOTT SHAFFER, PT, PhD, ECS
Professor
School of Physical Therapy
University of the Incarnate Word
San Antonio, Texas

THOMAS SUTLIVE, PT, PhD
Professor
Doctoral Program in Physical Therapy
Army-Baylor University
Joint Base San Antonio
Fort Sam Houston, Texas

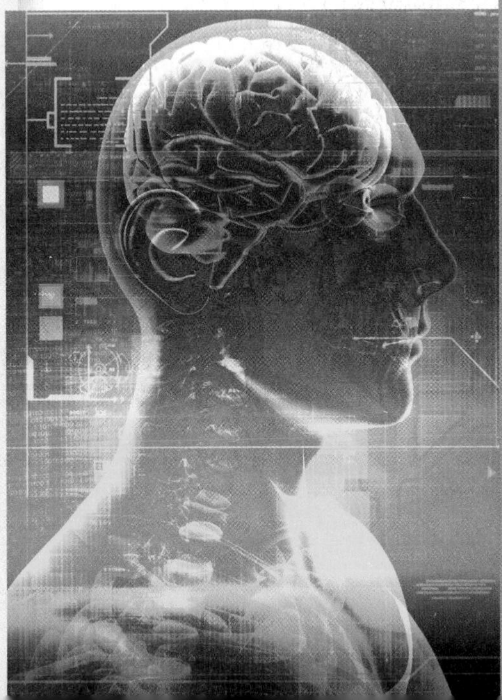

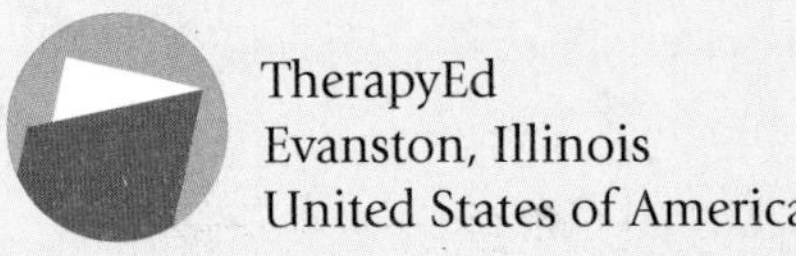

TherapyEd
Evanston, Illinois
United States of America

ISBN: 978-1-73384776-6

The authors and contributors have made a faithful attempt to include relevant summaries of current physical therapy practice and other information at the time of publication. It is recognized that recommended practices, drug therapies, equipment, devices, governmental regulations, administrative procedures and other protocols and factors may change or be open to other interpretations. Therapists should take responsibility for updating their knowledge of technological advances, new information or conclusions available through publications, research, new regulations or guidelines.

The publisher disclaims any liability or loss incurred as a result of direct or indirect use of this book. Use of this book does not guarantee successful passage of the National Physical Therapy Examination.

Copies of this book may be obtained from:
TherapyEd
3023 N. Clark St., Suite 119
Chicago, IL 60657
Telephone (888) 369-0743 or (847) 328-5361
Fax (847) 328-5049
www.TherapyEd.com

25th Edition of the TherapyEd Review and Study Guide!

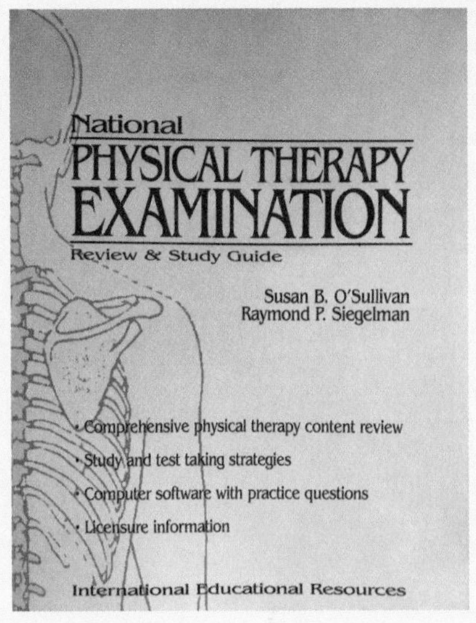

1st Edition of the Review and Study Guide (1997)

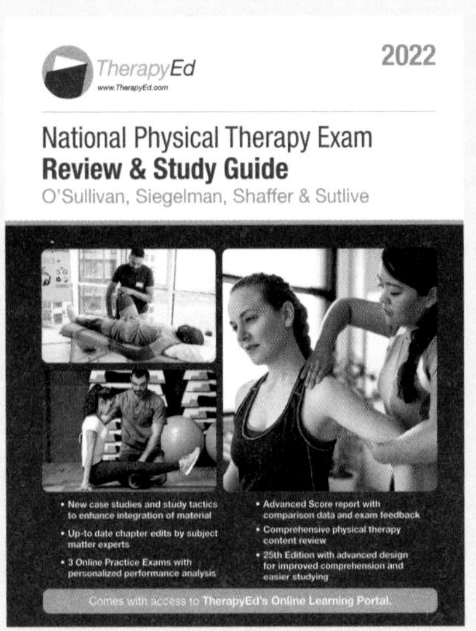

25th Edition of the Review and Study Guide (2021)

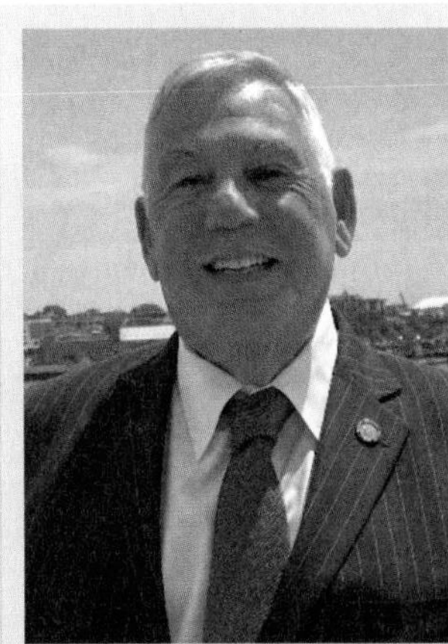

Dr. Raymond Siegelman

The 25th edition of TherapyEd's National Physical Therapy Exam Review and Study Guide is dedicated to Dr. Raymond Siegelman and Dr. Susan O'Sullivan. Ray and Susan's vision, ingenuity, and commitment have enhanced physical therapy education and clinical practice for more than 100,000 physical therapy graduates and profoundly impacted the care of an immeasurable number of grateful patients.

Dr. Siegelman is the founding President and President Emeritus of TherapyEd. He has been a physical therapist and physical therapy educator for more than 50 years, including serving on the faculty of the Boston and Northeastern University physical therapy programs. **Dr. O'Sullivan** is the author of the renowned text *Physical Rehabilitation*, the most widely adopted book in physical therapy education. She is Professor Emerita of the University of Massachusetts–Lowell DPT program and also served on the faculty at Boston University where she and Dr. Siegelman were colleagues.

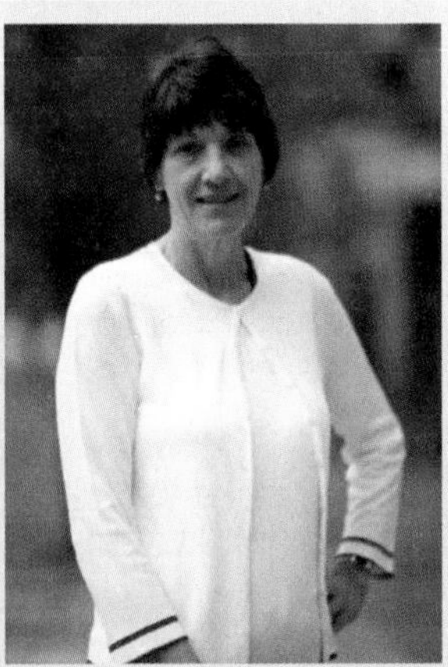

Dr. Susan O'Sullivan

Thank you, Ray and Susan, for your outstanding leadership in the profession, your unparalleled contributions to physical therapy education, and your invaluable mentorship to countless physical therapy students, physical therapists, and educators!

With our sincere gratitude, The TherapyEd Family

How We Can Help You Pass the NPTE

One of the final hurdles for physical therapists to become licensed to practice in the United States is successful completion of the National Physical Therapy Examination (NPTE). This exam requires candidates to combine basic physical therapy knowledge with clinical reasoning skills in order to process information, reach decisions, and determine actions. Clinical decisions are the outcomes of the clinical reasoning process and form the basis of patient/client management and success on the NPTE. In order to protect the public, state licensing boards use NPTE results along with graduation from an accredited institution as the main resources to determine whether a candidate has demonstrated minimal standards necessary for *safe, professional, and effective practice.*

Founded in 1988, TherapyEd offers an Examination Preparatory Course and the National Physical Therapy Examination Review & Study Guide (PT-R&SG). The PT-R&SG and the preparatory course help exam candidates assess their strengths and weaknesses and focus preparation based on exam criteria (the exam blueprint) published by the Federation of State Boards of Physical Therapy (FSBPT). The PT-R&SG provides a comprehensive content review and incorporates current Clinical Practice Guidelines (CPGs). It provides three online practice exams and includes a detailed analysis (teaching points) of the online exam questions in the book, including rationale for correct answer, discussion of the incorrect choices, and type of reasoning required for success on the question. The practice exams help familiarize therapists with the format and type of questions to expect on the NPTE.

The PT-R&SG is an ongoing work that is updated every year. It is organized into 16 content chapters, a chapter summarizing review questions/answers, and the online simulated examination questions with answers and rationales. A central element of the book is a strong pedagogical format designed to facilitate content review. This includes information on licensure, strategies for study, and content review organized by outline format with figures, summary tables, and boxes. Relevant examination, differential diagnosis, and intervention strategies are summarized.

Our greatest asset is the outstanding group of contributing authors and item writers, all recognized experts in their fields. This group of distinguished individuals has graciously shared their knowledge and clinical practice expertise by providing relevant, up-to-date, and practical information within their respective content areas.

There have been numerous updates made to several chapters in this 2022 edition, including:

- Chapter 2, Musculoskeletal
- Chapter 3, Neuromuscular
- Chapter 4, Cardiovascular and Lymphatics
- Chapter 5, Pulmonary
- Chapter 6, Therapeutic Interventions
- Chapter 7, Integumentary
- Chapter 8, Other Systems
- Chapter 9, Pediatrics
- Chapter 10, Geriatrics
- Chapter 11, Therapeutic Modalities

The 2022 R&SG also includes extensive review of the practice exams with the addition of more than 40 new simulated examination questions. Finally, authors have included case studies to Chapters 6 through 10 to enhance learning.

The National Physical Therapy Examination Review & Study Guide is designed to help physical therapist candidates prepare for the National Physical Therapy Examination (NPTE). Each chapter is presented in an easy-to-read outline format. Specific chapters focus on musculoskeletal, neuromuscular, cardiovascular, pulmonary, lymphatic, integumentary, metabolic, endocrine, gastrointestinal, and genitourinary systems as well as other aspects of physical therapy practice. Relevant anatomy, kinesiology, and pathophysiology of different diagnostic categories are briefly reviewed. Important medical, pharmacological, and surgical interventions are also identified. Each chapter reviews the elements of physical therapy practice, including examination, evaluation of data, determination of an appropriate diagnosis, prognosis, plan of care, interventions and reevaluation of interventions selected. Additional chapters focus on the professional roles assumed by the physical therapist: consultant, administrator, educator, and researcher. Chapters on pediatrics, geriatrics, therapeutic interventions, research and evidence-based practice, therapeutic modalities, technologies and functional devices, safety, and protection are also included.

It is vital for candidates to master the elements of physical therapy practice in order to apply the information to clinical situations. This book was developed to help you organize and focus your review efficiently and effectively. However, you may elect to pursue a more in-depth review of topics, terms, or procedures as needed by referring to our recommended references.

The online practice exams will help you assess your understanding of particular content areas and your ability to apply this knowledge to real-world situations. The practice exam format simulates the actual NPTE format, with a question counter and running clock on the top of the screen to help you keep track of your progress. The programming also allows you to go back to questions you would like to review. When you are finished, the program will analyze your results and provide feedback to help you focus on areas for additional study.

At the back of the text are the question explanations along with critical reasoning rationales to help you understand how the answers were derived. Reading and interpreting these practice questions will also help prepare you for the various forms of multiple-choice questions you may encounter on the actual NPTE.

It is important to note that although these challenging practice tests are designed to help you diagnose the strengths and weaknesses of your academic and clinical preparation, they should not be used as sole criteria to measure minimal entry-level competency or predict your score on the NPTE.

We encourage and appreciate feedback from our many readers. It is our hope that all exam candidates who use this book receive good news about their results and go on to a successful career in physical therapy. We acknowledge the important contributions that physical therapists make in the lives of their patients and in the health of society as a whole.

Table of Contents

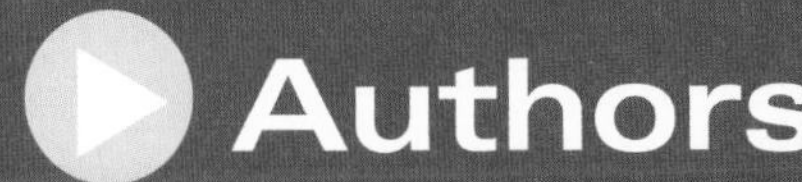

Authors

Thomas Bianco, PT, MSPT
President
Sensible Ergonomic Solutions
Wilbraham, Massachusetts

Michael Crowell, PT, DPT, DSc, OCS, SCS, FAAOMPT
Associate Professor
Baylor University-Keller Army Community Hospital
Division 1 Sports Physical Therapy Fellowship
West Point, New York

Jodi B. Cusack, MHS, PA-C
Gastrointestinal Medical Associates
Cranston, Rhode Island

Rita P. Fleming-Castaldy, PhD, OTL, FAOTA
Professor
Occupational Therapy Program
University of Scranton
Scranton, Pennsylvania

Suzanne M. Giuffre, PT, EdD
Associate Professor/Program Director
Doctor of Physical Therapy Program
Cleveland State University
Cleveland, Ohio

Stephen L. Goffar, PT, DPT, PhD, OCS
Associate Dean for Academic Affairs
Professor
School of Physical Therapy
University of the Incarnate Word
San Antonio, Texas

Anne Harrison, PT, PhD
Professor Emerita
Department of Physical Therapy
University of Kentucky
Lexington, KY

Carrie Hoppes, PT, PhD, NCS, OCS, ATC, CSCS
Associate Professor/Program Director
Doctoral Program in Physical Therapy
Army-Baylor University
JBSA-Fort Sam Houston, TX

Kari Inda, OTR, PhD, CEAS
Professor
Occupational Therapy Department Chairperson
Mount Mary University
Milwaukee, Wisconsin

Chad Jackson, PT, DPT, EdD
Associate Professor and Program Director
School of Physical Therapy
University of the Incarnate Word
San Antonio, Texas

Edward Kane, PT, PhD, SCS, ATC
Professor
University of Saint Augustine for Health Sciences
San Marcos, California

Jennifer Kish, PT, DPT, SCS, COMT
Assistant Professor
Academic Coordinator
School of Physical Therapy
University of the Incarnate Word
San Antonio, Texas

L. Vincent Lepak III, PT, DPT, MPH, CWS, CES
Associate Professor
Division of Rehabilitation Sciences
University of Oklahoma Health Sciences Center
Tulsa, Oklahoma

Mark Lester, PT, DPT, PhD, OCS
Associate Professor
Texas State University
Department of Physical Therapy
Round Rock, Texas

Kelly Macauley, PT, EdD, DPT, CCS, GCS
Interprofessional Faculty
School of Physical Therapy
Husson University
Bangor, Maine

Susan B. O'Sullivan, PT, EdD
Professor Emerita
Department of Physical Therapy
College of Health Sciences
University of Massachusetts Lowell
Lowell, Massachusetts

Todd C. Sander, PT, PhD, ATC
Associate Professor
Department Chair and Director
Department of Physical Therapy
Grand Valley State University
Grand Rapids, MI

Kelly Sass, PT, PhD
Clinical Assistant Professor
Academic Coordinator of Clinical Education
Department of Physical Therapy & Rehabilitation Science
University of Iowa
Iowa City, Iowa

Scott Shaffer, PT, PhD, ECS
Professor
School of Physical Therapy
University of the Incarnate Word
San Antonio, Texas

Raymond P. Siegelman, PT, DPT, MS
President Emeritus
TherapyEd
Boston, Massachusetts

Thomas Sutlive, PT, PhD
Professor
Doctoral Program in Physical Therapy
Army-Baylor University
JBSA-Fort Sam Houston, Texas

Bradley Tragord, PT, DSc, OCS, FAAOMPT
Associate Professor
Department of Physical Therapy
University of Texas Health Science Center-San Antonio
San Antonio, Texas

Jason M. Wilken, PT, PhD
Associate Professor
Director, Collaborative Research and Development
Department of Physical Therapy & Rehabilitation Science
University of Iowa
Iowa City, Iowa

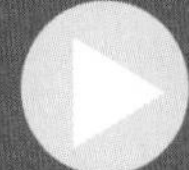 Exam Item Writers

Jaqueline Banker, PT, DPT, OCS, FAAOMPT
Institute of Higher Learning
Brooks Rehabilitation
Jacksonville, Florida

Jason Beneciuk, PT, DPT, PhD, MPH, FAAOMPT
Residency and Fellowship Scholarly Mentor
Institute of Higher Learning
Brooks Rehabilitation
Jacksonville, Florida

Nathan Brown, PT, DPT, GCS
Associate Professor
School of Physical Therapy
University of the Incarnate Word
San Antonio, TX

Tava Buck, PT, DPT, OCS, FAAOMPT
Institute of Higher Learning
Brooks Rehabilitation
Jacksonville, Florida

Lauren Clark, PT, DPT, OCS, FAAOMPT
Institute of Higher Learning
Brooks Rehabilitation
Jacksonville, Florida

Sean Collins, PT, ScD, CCS
Professor and Chair of Physical Therapy
Plymouth State University
Plymouth, New Hampshire

Brittany Comer, PT, DPT, OCS, FAAOMPT
Institute of Higher Learning
Brooks Rehabilitation
Jacksonville, Florida

Timothy Dellwo, PT, DPT, OCS, FAAOMPT
Institute of Higher Learning
Brooks Rehabilitation
Jacksonville, Florida

Christopher J. Ivey, PT, MPT, MS, OCS, SCS, ATC
Assistant Professor
University of Saint Augustine for Health Sciences
San Marcos, California

Steven M. Laslovich, PT, DPT, CPed
Assistant Professor
University of Saint Augustine for Health Sciences
San Marcos, California

Karen A. Leyva, PT, DPT, OCS
Instructor
University of Saint Augustine for Health Sciences
San Marcos, California

Monica L. Neal, PT, DPT
Director of Rehabilitation Services & Diabetes Center
New Orleans East Hospital
New Orleans, Louisiana

Raine Osborne, PT, DPT, OCS, FAAOMPT
Program Coordinator
Orthopedic Residency Program
Brooks Institute of Higher Learning
Brooks Rehabilitation
Jacksonville, Florida

Renata Salvatori, PT, DPT, OCS, SCS, FAAOMPT
Faculty Member
Orthopedic Residency Program Coordinator and OMPT Fellowship Programs
Brooks Institute of Higher Learning
Brooks Rehabilitation
Jacksonville, Florida

Laura Smith, PT, PhD, DPT, OCS, MTC, FAAOMPT
Assistant Professor
Department of Physical Therapy
Coordinator, Orthopedic Post Professional Residency and Certificate Program
University of Michigan-Flint
Flint, Michigan

James A Viti, PT, DPT, MHSc, OHC, MTC, FAAOMPT
Assistant Professor
University of Saint Augustine for Health Sciences
Saint Augustine, Florida

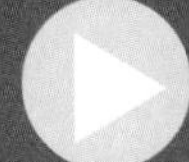

Acknowledgments

Christine Becker
Project Manager
Progressive Publishing Services
York, Pennsylvania

Lisa Noonan
LN Creative
Chelmsford, Massachusetts

Crystal Clifton
Director
Progressive Publishing Services
York, Pennsylvania

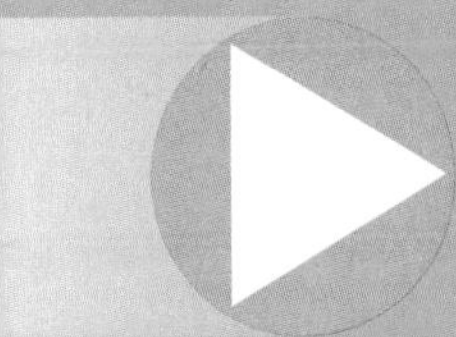

1

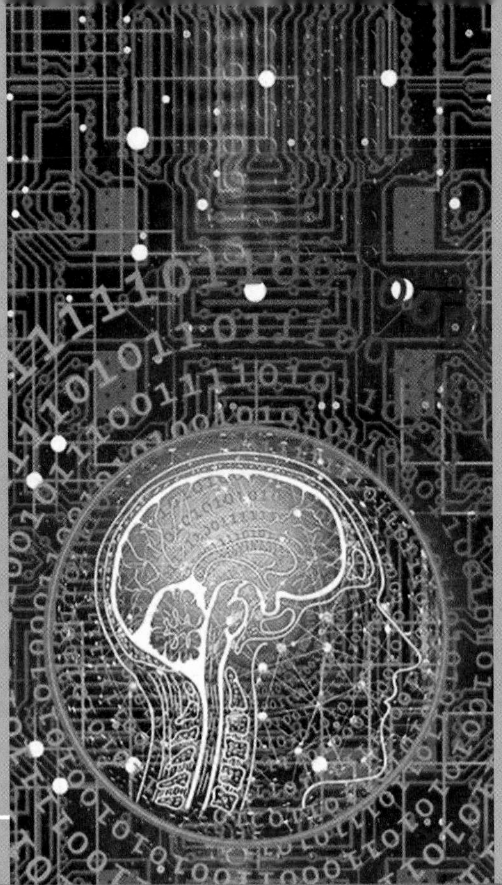

NPTE Preparation and Critical Reasoning Skills

RAYMOND P. SIEGELMAN AND KARI INDA

Review>Practice>Motivate>Analyze>Apply

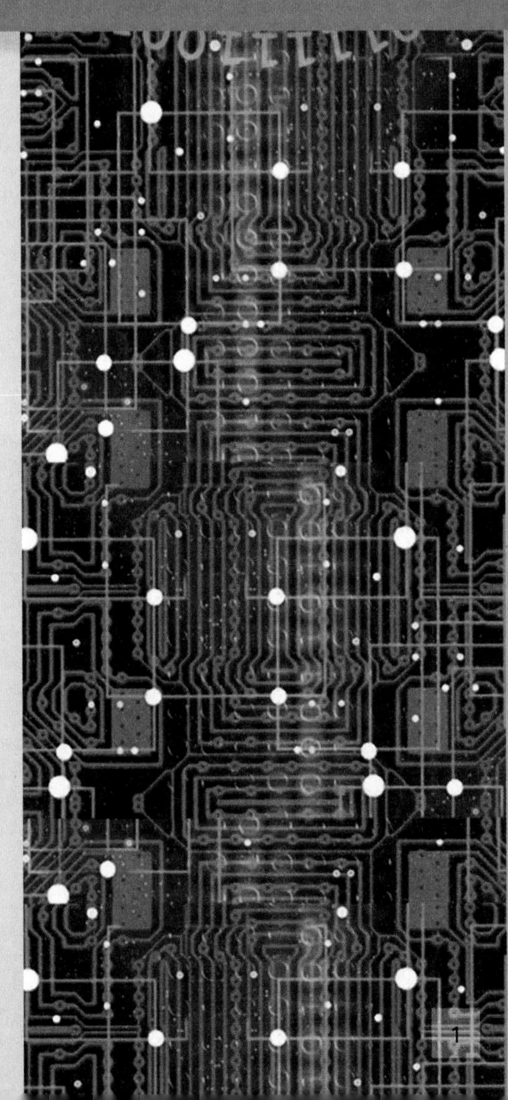

Chapter Outline

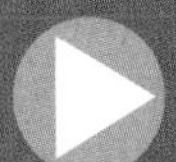

What Is the Procedure for Obtaining a License?

Licensure of health care practitioners protects the public from unsafe practices. In the United States and its territories, all physical therapists require a license to practice. Licensure is a function of state or territorial governments, not the federal government. It should be noted that physical therapist employees of the federal government are exempt from state regulation. However, a valid license in at least one state or jurisdiction is usually required by federal employers, such as the military or Public Health Service.

All jurisdictions require candidates to complete the NPTE successfully to obtain a license, but because the United States is made up of numerous states and governing entities, each state may have different requirements for you to become eligible to take the NPTE. Different states may also have different practice restrictions after you have passed the NPTE. These requirements can even differ within the same state, according to whether you graduated from a program accredited by the Commission on Accreditation in Physical Therapy Education (CAPTE). The CAPTE no longer accredits baccalaureate degree programs. In the United States, all candidates must have graduated from an entry-level master's or doctoral program or an equivalent international program. Each state has sovereignty over physical therapy licensure and regulation. Contact the individual licensing board in your jurisdiction to obtain applications and information about requirements and procedures.

Jurisprudence Examination

Some states require candidates to pass a separate examination concerning the rules, regulations, and laws governing physical therapy practice in that state. Licensed therapists who wish to obtain a license when moving to another state may have to pass a jurisprudence examination if it is required by that state. The Federation of State Boards of Physical Therapy (FSBPT) administers some, but not all, jurisprudence exams.

Fees

All states require a fee to apply for and renew a license. There are separate fees to sit for the NPTE. Fees vary widely and can change yearly.

Special Accommodation

1. Candidates with documented current disabilities can apply to their jurisdiction for special accommodation during the NPTE.
2. Medical or health conditions that may require a snack, water, medications, visual aids, a reader, extra time, wheelchair placement, and so on may be considered. Pregnancy without complications is not considered a disability by the ADA.
3. English as a second language is not considered a disability. No dictionaries or extra time will be granted.
4. Test anxiety and technophobia are not considered disabilities.
5. All accommodations must be approved at least 15 days before the exam date.
6. If special accommodation is denied, the jurisdiction may have an appeal process.

Other Requirements and Issues

Tests of English Language Proficiency. Various tests of spoken, written, or comprehended English may be required if English is not your first language. Standards and requirements differ from state to state. Personal interviews may also be required.

Fingerprinting, FBI Check, Vaccination, Malpractice Insurance. One or more of these may be required by some jurisdictions.

Credentials Evaluation. Currently, most states require physical therapists educated outside of the United States who graduated from programs not accredited by CAPTE to submit transcripts and other credentials to approved agencies for evaluation. Credentials often include course content, credit hours, grades earned, and degrees granted. This process is required to establish eligibility to take the NPTE.

Supervised Practice Period. Some states may require therapists educated outside of the United States to undergo a period of supervised practice after successfully completing the NPTE. Permanent license is not granted until this supervised practice period is successfully completed.

Temporary License. Some states grant a temporary license to candidates eligible to take the NPTE. This temporary license allows the individual to practice under the supervision of a licensed therapist before taking and passing the NPTE. In some states, this temporary license may be revoked if a candidate fails the NPTE. In some states, if a temporary license is not offered, a physical therapist may *not* practice in that state until all requirements for licensure have been satisfied. In other states without a temporary license provision, applicants who have filed to take the exam may be allowed to practice under supervision of a licensed therapist. Therefore, it is prudent for you to keep current on the rules and regulations of the state(s) in which you wish to practice.

Transfer of Scores to Other Jurisdictions. All jurisdictions use the criterion-referenced grading method, which standardizes exam scoring and allows transfer of passing scores. The Federation of State Boards of Physical Therapy (FSBPT) is responsible for score transfer (www.fsbpt.org). For a fee, you may transfer your scores online or download the Score Transfer Request Form and mail the completed form to the FSBPT. If you maintain a license, you should not have to retake the NPTE if you move to a different state. However, if you are unlicensed, let your license lapse, or never took the examination, you will have to take the NPTE when seeking a license in that jurisdiction.

Some states have joined the Physical Therapy Licensure Compact, which reduces regulatory barriers to interstate mobility and cross-state practice for physical therapists.

Retaking the Examination. Candidates may take the NPTE exam up to three times per 12-month period, which is the limit set by the FSBPT. After six attempts without passing, a lifetime ban on further testing is imposed. Candidates who incur two very low scores of 400 or less will also incur a lifetime ban. A candidate never takes the same form of an exam he or she had previously taken. Some states allow only three opportunities to take the NPTE in total. If you fail, the state may impose a stipulation that you show evidence of remedial work or study before retaking the NPTE. The state licensure board has an obligation to protect the public from practitioners who do not demonstrate competency.

License Renewal. After 1, 2, or 3 years, a license must be renewed for a physical therapist to continue practicing. Renewal notices are sent out (via post or email) by the state or territory in which the therapist is practicing. Sometimes, renewal simply involves paying the fee and returning the form. However, some states require verification of continuing education units. If you fail to notify the state of a change of address or email address and do not receive a renewal notice, fail to respond to renewal in a timely manner, or do not meet other requirements, your license could lapse. It is illegal to practice without a valid license. The state may require that a number of conditions be met to reinstate a lapsed license. One condition might include retaking the NPTE even if you had previously passed the exam. *Inform the board of any change of address or email. Do not let your license lapse!*

Continuing Education or Active Practice. Many states require the physical therapist to acquire a specific number of continuing education units (CEUs) to renew a license. Documentation, approval, and reporting of CEUs vary from state to state. Some states require evidence of continuing active practice to renew. The FSBPT and the American Physical Therapy Association (APTA) are exploring or have developed alternative means to ascertain continued competency.

Endorsement. With a valid license in one state or jurisdiction, a physical therapist may apply to another state for a "license by endorsement." All criteria established by the new state must be met. This can include taking a jurisprudence exam for that state, attending interviews, providing letters of recommendation, taking English competency exams, and accruing CEUs. Contact the licensure board in the state where licensure by endorsement is sought to get information and applications. Start the process early; it can take months.

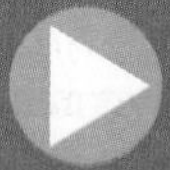

How Is the NPTE Developed?

The FSBPT is the organization that develops and owns the NPTE. The exam is based on a survey of clinical practice conducted periodically by the FSBPT, from which the "blueprint" for the exam is developed. Numerous clinicians, educators, and others contribute questions to the NPTE. Questions are designed to test knowledge and problem-solving skills that reflect current clinical practice and entry-level competency (defined as the first 6 months of practice). Various content experts and clinicians review the questions (item reviewers). Finally, the FSBPT committees and psychometricians fine-tune the questions and construct the final exam blueprint. The APTA or the individual state licensing boards do not develop, oversee, or administer the NPTE.

Each examination adheres closely to the blueprint to fairly and comprehensively assess a candidate's competency to practice. The blueprint imparts a degree of stability, consistency, and continuity between different forms of the exam. However, each exam is a unique document with its own mix of questions. Questions are referenced to physical therapy textbooks in common use (a list of textbooks is available at www.fsbpt.org) and are not derived from a specific textbook or point of view. Terminology is consistent with that used in the *Guide to Physical Therapist Practice* and other commonly used texts.

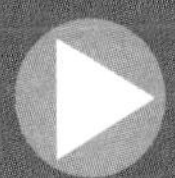

NPTE Security Agreement

Each candidate who takes the NPTE must accept the NPTE Security Agreement. In part, this agreement states that it is illegal and unethical to recall (memorize) and share NPTE questions or solicit questions from candidates who have taken the exam. The FSBPT will continue to prosecute individuals who violate the security agreement.

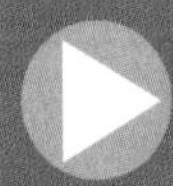

What Does the Exam Cover?

The NPTE places great emphasis on patient examination, evaluation, and plan of care for patient/client problems within a variety of systems. This includes the interactions of systems as well. About 13% of exam questions deal with nonsystem topics such as therapeutic modalities, devices, equipment, technologies, research, evidence-based practice, safety, and other supporting issues. Needless to say, the NPTE is very comprehensive. Ensure that your preparation reflects the composition of the current exam. Naturally, not every item or sub-item listed here or mentioned in the Review & Study Guide is specifically covered in every form of the examination. The NPTE consists of 250 questions, but only 200 questions count for your score. The additional 50 questions are used by the Federation of State Boards to check their validity for future use on exams. There is no way to know which questions are being used for validity purposes. The Content Outline of the NPTE is based on the 200 questions that are scored.

The information that follows has been adapted from the NPTE Content Outline of the Federation of State Boards of Physical Therapy (access at https://www.fsbpt.org/Free-Resources/NPTE-Development/NPTE-Content). It is effective for the years 2018–2022. The use of category and domain designations is specific to the TherapyEd simulated exams and is used when reporting your results on each of those exams.

Category A

Physical Therapy Examination: 44–57 Questions, or About 26% of the NPTE

- Tests and measures and their applications, including outcome measures and current best evidence
- Anatomy and physiology as related to tests and measures
- Movement analysis for most systems including such things as posture, compensatory movement, positioning for bowel movement, friction, shear, scar mobility, rib excursion, breathing patterns, and more
- Joint biomechanics and applications

Category A: Number of Questions By System

Domain I. Cardiovascular & Pulmonary	7–9 questions
Domain II. Musculoskeletal	18–21 questions
Domain III. Neuromuscular	15–17 questions
Domain IV. Integumentary	3–4 questions
Domain V. Metabolic & Endocrine	zero questions
Domain VI. Gastrointestinal	0–2 questions
Domain VII. Genitourinary	1–2 questions
Domain VIII. Lymphatic	0–2 questions
Domain IX. System Interactions	zero questions
Domain X. Nonsystem	zero questions

Category B

Foundations for Evaluation, Differential Diagnosis, and Prognosis: 58–74 Questions, or About 33% of the NPTE

- Pathophysiology related to diseases/conditions across the lifespan, and ability to establish a prognosis and carry out a plan of care including health promotion
- Differential diagnosis related to diseases/conditions
- Impact of comorbidities or multisystem involvement on patient management (for example, cancer, diabetes, pregnancy, autoimmune diseases, sarcoidosis, obesity)
- Pharmacological management
- Diagnostic imaging, medical and lab tests, medical and surgical procedures
- Psychological and psychiatric conditions such as depression, schizophrenia

Category B: Number of Questions By System

Domain I. Cardiovascular & Pulmonary	8–9 questions
Domain II. Musculoskeletal	17–20 questions
Domain III. Neuromuscular	14–16 questions

Domain IV. Integumentary	3–4 questions
Domain V. Metabolic & Endocrine	3–4 questions
Domain VI. Gastrointestinal	2–3 questions
Domain VII. Genitourinary	2–3 questions
Domain VIII. Lymphatic	1–3 questions
Domain IX. System Interactions	8–12 questions
Domain X. Nonsystem	zero questions

Category C

Interventions: 48–60 Questions, or About 28% of the NPTE

- PT interventions and their application for health promotion, rehabilitation, and performance across the lifespan according to current best evidence
- Anatomy and physiology related to PT interventions, ADLs, and environmental factors
- Adverse effects or complications based on interventions
- Motor control and motor learning
- Bladder programs, biofeedback, and pelvic floor retraining for genitourinary issues
- Bowel programs and reflux prevention for gastrointestinal issues

Category C: Number of Questions By System

Domain I. Cardiovascular & Pulmonary	8–10 questions
Domain II. Musculoskeletal	16–19 questions
Domain III. Neuromuscular	15–17 questions
Domain IV. Integumentary	3–4 questions
Domain V. Metabolic & Endocrine	2–3 questions
Domain VI. Gastrointestinal	1–2 questions
Domain VII. Genitourinary	1–2 questions
Domain VIII. Lymphatic	2–3 questions
Domain IX. System Interactions	zero questions
Domain X. Nonsystem	zero questions

Category D Nonsystem

Equipment, Devices, and Technologies: 5–6 Questions or About 2.5% of the NPTE

- Application, selection, adjustments, precautions, contraindications of various equipment, devices, and technologies across the lifespan
- Walkers, wheelchairs, adaptive seating, positioning devices, mechanical lifts, body weight support systems
- Lower and upper extremity prosthetic devices including microprocessor-controlled prostheses
- Orthotic devices including braces, helmets, taping, compression garments, serial casts, shoe inserts, splints, and robotic exoskeletons

Category E Nonsystem

Therapeutic Modalities: 6–8 Questions or About 3.5% of the NPTE

- Thermal modalities, which includes cryotherapy
- Iontophoresis
- Electrotherapy including NMES, TENS, FES, interferential and high-voltage pulsed current
- Ultrasound including phonophoresis
- Mechanical motion devices and traction
- Biofeedback
- Intermittent compression

Category F Nonsystem

Safety and Protection: 5–6 Questions or About 2.5% of the NPTE

- Safe patient handling, fall risk and prevention, guarding, equipment maintenance, environmental safety
- Function and implications for the PT regarding IV lines, catheters and collecting bags, Swan-Ganz catheter, monitoring devices such as EKG, oxygen delivery, ventilators
- CPR (adult, children, infant), first aid, and disaster response
- Infection control (standard/universal precautions, sterile technique, isolation)
- Abuse and neglect (sexual, physical, psychological)

Category G

Professional Responsibilities: 4–5 Questions or About 2% of the NPTE

- Standards of documentation including SOAP note
- Patient rights (HIPAA, ADA, IDEA, Patient Bill of Rights, Advanced Health Directives including DNR and proxy, Informed Consent)
- Human resources issues such as OSHA and sexual harassment
- Applicable state and federal laws such as CARF, state licensing board functions, Joint Commission, CMS (Medicare/Medicaid services)
- Roles and responsibilities of other health practitioners and support staff (PTA, PT aide, others)
- Ethics including reporting fraud and unprofessional behavior
- Billing, coding, reimbursement standards
- Sociocultural issues including religion, ethnicity, language differences, disability, socioeconomic, sexual preference, and gender identification
- Electronic medical records, telemedicine

Category H

Research and Evidence-Based Practice: 3–5 Questions or About 2.5% of the NPTE

- Accessing scientific proceedings, peer-reviewed publications, clinical guidelines, and prediction rules
- Research methodology (quantitative, qualitative, levels of evidence)
- Data collection such as surveys, observation
- Measurement science (variables, reliability, validity)
- Statistics (ANOVA, chi-square, T-test, correlation, likelihood ratio, effect size, confidence interval, sensitivity, specificity)

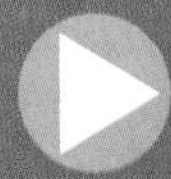

What Is the Procedure for Taking the Exam?

To start the process of preparing for the exam, contact the licensing agency in the state or jurisdiction in which you wish to apply for a license. Return or email the completed application to the appropriate agency. If you are eligible, the FSBPT will send you an "Authorization to Test" letter. Once you are eligible, you should receive information about how to contact Prometric (www.Prometric.com) to establish your test location. You may contact the FSBPT Examination Services by phone at (703)739-9420 to check on the status of your application or inquire about other general information. Note that you are *not* required to take the exam in the state where you seek a license. You may take the NPTE in a Prometric Center in the United States and territories as well as select Canadian locations. (See Box A for an outline of these steps.)

Determine the exam site for your exam. If it is necessary to travel the day before and seek lodging, make arrangements in advance. Plan to arrive at the exam site early. You *must* arrive at least 30 minutes *before* your scheduled examination. Access a map or use GPS (you can also get directions at www.2test.com), know the traffic patterns (including rush hour times), and bring money to cover possible parking fees.

Test Dates

Fixed NPTE (Physical Therapist) Dates for 2022

There are generally five testing dates per year. Dates for 2022 are:
January 26, 2022 (Wednesday)
April 27, 2022 (Wednesday)
July 27, 2022 (Wednesday)
July 28, 2022 (Thursday)
October 26, 2022 (Wednesday)
Go to www.fsbpt.org for timetable to submit application.

Candidates with documented disabilities may receive special accommodation during the exam. Special seating, extra time, a reader, use of a head covering for religious or other purposes and other considerations are possible. Any special accommodation *must be approved in advance* by the licensing board.

Prometric personnel will orient you regarding exam procedures. A tutorial before the exam should familiarize you with keyboard commands and other functions. We urge you to take the tutorial and ask for clarification of any detail before the start of the exam. If you are dissatisfied with the lighting, seating, ability to read the computer screen, noise levels or other factors, request a change to another computer cubicle *before* the exam starts. Contact Prometric personnel immediately if there is any computer malfunction.

BOX A ▷ Procedure for Registering for the Exam

1. Contact the appropriate board or agency in the jurisdiction (state, district, territory) where you seek a license once you are eligible to take the exam.
2. Complete the application materials. If you are or will soon be a new graduate, your academic program must certify your eligibility. Do this as soon as possible.
3. Register for the exam at the FSBPT website (www.fsbpt.org) as soon as you can. The registration deadline is 30 days prior to the exam date you wish to take. There is a fee.
4. If the jurisdiction approves your eligibility, they must notify the FSBPT no later than 15 days prior to the scheduled exam. If the jurisdiction does not notify the FSBPT in time, you will not get an "Authorization to Test" letter for the exam date you requested.
5. If you receive an "Authorization to Test" letter, you will be instructed to contact Prometric to schedule the site where you wish to take the NPTE.
6. You do not have to take the exam in the jurisdiction where you seek a license. You may take it at any Prometric Center in another jurisdiction. Contact Prometric at www.prometric/fsbpt.com. Do this as soon as possible after receiving the "Authorization to Test" letter. Some sites may fill up rapidly, and you may have to choose alternative sites that involve travel or overnight stays.

Test-Taking Strategies

The exam is divided into five sections of 50 questions each. The sections are balanced in terms of the content covered on the exam blueprint. Once you have completed a section and you take a break, you may not go back to any questions in that section. However, before you complete any section, you may review marked questions and change answers, if you wish. The computer screen shows a running clock of your remaining time to complete the exam. There will be a scheduled break of 15 minutes when the clock is stopped. During other breaks, the clock will run. You may also choose not to take a break. If you complete the exam before the allocated time, you may leave early.

During the exam, you may electronically mark questions you have skipped or wish to review at a later time. We do not recommend skipping questions. Answer each question to the best of your ability. Use educated guesses if you must. Guessing is not penalized. If time permits, use the computer review commands to return to previously marked items. Answers may be changed if necessary. If in doubt, stick with your original choice. Return to the marked questions before you exit each section. Once you exit a section of the exam, you cannot return to that section.

Time management is crucial. There are 250 items to answer in a 5-hour period, not counting breaks. This amounts to a time allotment of just over 1 minute (72 seconds) per question. You must complete 50 questions per hour to finish all of the examination questions. When you have completed the first 50 questions, check the running clock on the computer screen. Have you completed them in an hour or less? If not, you must increase your pace or you may not get to answer all of the questions. Check again at questions #100 and #150. Some people prefer to check the computer clock at the end of each hour and note the number of questions answered. Either way, pace yourself properly.

Also keep in mind that during the third hour of the examination, and beyond, reading skills tend to deteriorate

BOX B Test Center Procedures

1. Check in at least 30 minutes prior to the exam. When you arrive at the exam site, visit the restroom before you check in. The whole examination procedure can last up to 6 hours. You may use the restroom during breaks.
2. Remember to bring proper identification and your "Authorization to Test" letter, since you will not be allowed to take the exam without either of them. Two forms of identification are required. One must be a government-issued photo ID such as a passport or driver's license. Another can be an ID pre-printed with your name and signature, such as a credit card. Social Security cards are not accepted. We recommend that you confirm what are acceptable forms of identification with personnel at the Prometric testing center. IDs will be scanned. Your first and last names on the IDs must be the same as on the "Authorization to Test" letter. If there is any problem with the IDs, you will not be allowed to take the exam. All fees will be forfeited, and you will have to reschedule for the next fixed date. Photocopies or cell phone images of identification are not acceptable.
3. You will be fingerprinted and photographed. All testing sessions are videotaped. If you leave the testing room for any reason (e.g., to visit the restroom), you will be fingerprinted again.
4. You may request a dry erase board or scratch paper to make notes. You may not bring in your own scratch paper. The boards will be collected when you leave the testing center.
5. Personal items such as eyeglasses, contacts, and medications are allowed. Some comfort items such as tissues or mints may be allowed.
6. Earplugs are not permitted. Prometric will supply sound-dampening headphones upon request. Keep in mind that background noise may be distracting.
7. A locker will be provided for personal items. A color-coded key will be provided. The locker may or may not be accessed during the exam depending upon the key color.
8. Wear multilayer clothing to stay comfortable in various room temperatures. Jackets with pockets, "hoodie" sweatshirts, hats or scarves are not permitted. If you remove a sweater or outer shirt, you must wrap it around your waist. These items cannot be placed on the back of a chair or elsewhere in the testing room. If you must wear a head covering for health or religious reasons, you must receive approval before the testing date. Prometric personnel cannot grant approval on site.
9. No electronic devices of any kind (such as cell phones, MP3 players, or digital watches) are allowed in the testing room. They must be put in the locker.
10. Eat a good meal before taking the exam. Food or drink is officially not allowed at the computer cubicle during the examination. At some centers, water may be available in the reception area, or you may keep your own drink there.
11. You may not talk or read aloud during the exam.

and it may take longer to process each question. If English is your second language, you should think in English when answering questions. Otherwise, it may be very difficult to finish the examination on time, and this could also cause errors interpreting exam question content.

What should you do if there are only 2 minutes left and you have not answered all of the questions? Do not leave anything blank. Quickly choose answers for each question, even if you have not had a chance to read them all. Since there is no penalty for entering incorrect answers, you may be lucky and get a few correct! Over the years, many candidates have been unsuccessful on the NPTE because of failure to budget their time properly.

Once the exam has begun, communicate only with Prometric personnel. An innocent remark to a nearby test-taker or a glance at another computer screen might be mistaken for an attempt to cheat. Candidates attempting to cheat can face serious consequences. Trying to obtain a physical therapy license by fraudulent means is a crime. Don't even think about doing it.

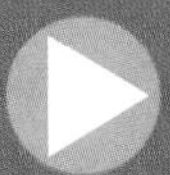

How Is the NPTE Graded, and How Are Scores Reported?

The FSBPT employs criterion-referenced performance standards. Using this system, a test score is interpreted in terms of an individual's mastery of a specified content domain. A passing criterion or standard is established by the FSBPT for each examination. A candidate must reach or exceed the designated cut score of competency to pass the exam. The cut score represents the minimal acceptable level of exam performance consistent with safe and effective practice expected of physical therapists. A panel of physical therapy content experts establishes the passing score after screening questions for performance characteristics and bias. The examinee's performance is not compared with the performance of others who took the same test. Each form of the NPTE has its own criterion-referenced passing grade, and these may vary from exam to exam. Grading on a curve, using a fixed percentage, and using the number of questions answered correctly are methods that are *NOT* used to determine passing scores.

Reporting of grades to candidates can be confusing. Scaled scores, rather than the absolute number of questions answered correctly (raw score), are reported to candidates. The scaled scoring range is from 200 to 800, with 600 always reflecting the cut score. For example, if the passing raw score is determined to be 149 out of 200 questions for an exam, this would equal a scaled score of 600. If a candidate achieved a score of 600 or better, the state licensing board would notify the candidate of his or her success and issue a license provided that all other conditions were satisfied.

Some states still convert the passing scaled score to another system based on the number 70 or 75. Your score can be reported as being above or below the number 70 or 75. This does not mean that you scored above or below 70% or 75% or correctly or incorrectly answered 70 or 75 questions. It is merely an arbitrary numbering system used to denote a pass/fail line.

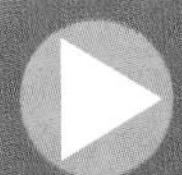

Planning Your Exam Review

After you have completed your entry-level physical therapy education, you bring all of your academic and clinical experiences to the table in preparation for the NPTE. Four to 6 weeks of structured independent review should be adequate. More time might be necessary for candidates who are not native English speakers or for candidates who were not educated through an APTA-accredited program.

Candidates with learning disabilities might require more preparation time because the processing of information may be slower. Most candidates probably do not need to take a lengthy refresher/remedial course. However, a Licensure Examination Preparatory course, such as the type offered since 1988 by TherapyEd, can be quite helpful. Extensive student feedback has indicated that this type of preparation course, when used in combination with this text, is an effective tool to provide information about current exam expectations and trends. The Course Manual and additional means of self-assessment provide even more focus and direction for exam preparation.

Please show respect for the examination process. Procrastination, skimpy review, and lack of understanding about the nature of the NPTE could lead to disappointing results. The expenses incurred to retake the examination, along with the potential loss of income because of failure to obtain a license, are significant. If you are unsuccessful, your self-esteem may take a mighty blow.

Discipline. About a month or two before your scheduled exam, establish a routine and spend 6 days per week reviewing material. Set up realistic and potentially achievable short-term goals as to what you wish to accomplish each day. Take 1 day off per week to pursue interests other than physical therapy. Give yourself a break! Life balance is important! When you are reviewing, however, allot 2 to 3 hours of uninterrupted study time each day. Study in a quiet and well-lit space. Do not study when you are tired or ill. If you work during the week, weekends may give you more flexibility and time for review.

If you break your routine, add compensatory time. Answer the on-line sample questions as a means of diagnosing strengths and weaknesses. Trying to memorize hundreds of sample questions and rationales is not a satisfactory means of preparation. Practice questions serve as templates for a multitude of item possibilities and primarily serve as diagnostic tools. You must review basic physical therapy knowledge and be able to apply that knowledge to a variety of problems, settings, circumstances, and situations. Some individuals may benefit from small group study sessions.

Although the review is for the purpose of passing the NPTE, we have received feedback through the years that this retrospective overview of one's physical therapy education has helped to sharpen and focus many aspects of clinical practice as well.

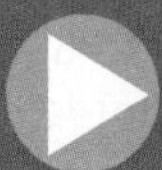

Analysis of Strengths and Weaknesses

A "shotgun" approach to exam preparation is not the best way to use your time. Try to form a composite picture of your physical therapy education and experiences.

Academic Program. Even accredited physical therapist programs can vary widely in terms of the quantity and quality of the content covered. Many programs are superb. Others may have problems with curricula or faculty. There could be a lack of emphasis on content that might be important for the NPTE. Be sure to request a copy of your school's report on performance of previous classes on the exam according to the exam blueprint. Some information is available at the FSBPT website.

Consider which content areas were presented in a comprehensive manner and which areas left something to be desired. Were there any gaps in your basic preparation that may be emphasized on the NPTE? Will this require you to spend more time gathering or reviewing information in these areas? Were academic standards poorly enforced, were grades inflated, or were some marginal students given social promotions to help enhance their self-esteem or the status of the program? Your study plan should compensate for weaknesses in your academic program, since the NPTE conforms to a standard outside the academic setting.

Classroom Performance. Generally, strong classroom performers with good English skills should fare well on the NPTE *as long as they take the time to prepare properly*. Students who performed marginally in their program, whose basic physical therapy education program lacked rigor or whose English skills are not well developed are often disappointed when they receive NPTE results.

Clinical Experiences/Affiliations. If the range of clinical experiences or internship was limited in terms of settings, patient populations, types of treatments or degree of responsibility, exam candidates may have difficulty answering questions that require the application of clinical knowledge or judgment. For example, an exam candidate with no clinical exposure in such areas as pediatrics, cardiac rehabilitation, or wound or burn care may have difficulty in reaching conclusions requiring systems review, evaluation, outcome projection, or interventions in these areas. Many NPTE questions require an amalgam of clinical experience and academic knowledge to solve problems. Selected use of the *Guide to Physical Therapist Practice* may prove helpful in areas of deficient clinical preparation. Specific examinations, goals, interventions, and outcomes may be delineated.

Analysis of Sample Question Results. At appropriate times, you should attempt to answer the practice questions in the accompanying online exams. The scoring will assist you in identifying content areas, domains, and critical reasoning categories in which your performance was sufficient and those areas that need more work. This analysis can serve as a basis for structuring further study and review. *After* taking the simulated exams, be sure to read the rationale and critical reasoning strategies for the practice exam questions in the back of the *Review & Study Guide*.

Based on your personal analysis, write down areas of weakness and try to rank order them in terms of which areas might require the most remedial work. Set priorities based on the Content Outline, *Guide to Physical Therapist Practice,* Third Edition, and expectations of the examination. Keep in mind that the NPTE emphasis is primarily on entry-level knowledge and judgment. Entry level is defined as the first 6 months of clinical practice.

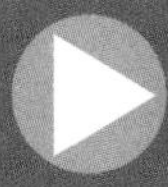

Levels of Question Difficulty

The NPTE attempts to ascertain how a candidate deals with a variety of different situations to determine how the applicant would function in the role of a physical therapist in a clinical setting. Most of the questions require problem solving at the upper levels of cognitive functioning (see Box C: Levels of NPTE Exam Questions).

BOX C Levels of NPTE Exam Questions

Question Level and Description

1. Knowledge

Recall of basic information such as characteristics of diagnoses, spinal cord level functionality, wheelchair measurements, shapes of joints, and so on.

Relevance to the NPTE

A solid knowledge foundation of all information related to entry-level PT practice is required to answer various scenarios proposed on NPTE questions.

It is highly unlikely that any NPTE questions are solely at this level. Ready recall of this information is needed in order to help solve advanced-level questions.

NPTE Exam Preparation Strategy

A strong commitment to studying is needed to remember all the relevant information acquired during PT entry-level education. This is a short-term goal of about 2 months. Fortunately, this *Review & Study Guide* (and the Course Manual, if you took a TherapyEd prep course) provides extensive information in an outline format to make your review easier.

2. Comprehension

Understanding of basic information to determine significance, consequences, or implications. For example, the impact of a tenodesis grasp on function or the possible consequences of using aquatic therapy for a group of patients with multiple sclerosis.

Relevance to the NPTE

The NPTE is not a matching test. Therefore, you must do more than recall information to succeed on the exam; you must have a firm grasp of content to understand the nuances and meaning of the questions. This may be the "who, what, where, when, and how" of the question.

NPTE Exam Preparation Strategy

When reviewing foundational knowledge, think about why this information might be important. Studying with a peer/study group and explaining to the group the relevance, significance, consequences, and implications of the study material may help you master it. Having a family member or friend quiz you on basic information may help you determine your ability to "think on your feet." Don't enter the test without strong comprehension abilities in all major areas of PT practice.

3. Application

Use of information and application of rules, procedures, or theories to new situations. For example, how to apply ergonomic principles to modify a workstation for someone with bilateral carpal tunnel syndrome.

(Continued)

BOX C Levels of NPTE Exam Questions (Continued)

Relevance to the NPTE

The NPTE requires one to integrate knowledge and comprehension as well as competencies developed during clinical experiences in order to best answer a practice scenario. Many NPTE questions should be at this level, since a main goal of the exam is to assess the candidate's ability to respond competently to different situations.

NPTE Exam Preparation Strategy

If your knowledge and comprehension are solid in all major domains of the exam as put forth in this *Review & Study Guide*, take one of the online exams that accompany this text. The challenging questions follow the format of the NPTE. Use your results to determine areas of academic, clinical, and reasoning strengths and weaknesses.

4. Analysis

Recognition of interrelationships between principles and interpretation or evaluation of data presented. For example, the most beneficial focus for discharge planning sessions for a parent and an adolescent with acquired traumatic brain injury.

Relevance to the NPTE

The NPTE assumes that test-takers have mastery and comprehension of entry-level knowledge and can apply it competently in diverse situations. Therefore, expect to analyze and respond to ambiguous situations. Direct "textbook answers" may not apply, which causes problems for some concrete thinkers. Many items are at this level, since the main objective of the exam is to determine competency in complex practice or ethical situations. In other words, practice your ability to think "outside of the box" in order to solve problems in real-world situations.

NPTE Exam Preparation Strategy

Use the analyses of the practice exams to reflect on your reasoning and judgment. Critically review the explanations for each question that you struggled with. Use peer or study groups to help determine gaps in analyses of exam questions. Ascertain what actions to take regarding deficiencies in critical reasoning skills to adequately prepare for the complexities of the NPTE.

Modified and adapted with permission from Fleming-Castaldy, R: National Occupational Therapy Certification Examination Review & Study Guide, 9th ed.

BOX D General Strategies for Answering NPTE Items

- Read the exam item carefully but quickly before selecting a response.
- Read the exam item for key words that set a priority.
- Use knowledge of medical terminology to decipher unknown words using prefixes, suffixes, and root words.
- Employ relevant clinical experience. Do not call on unusual or atypical cases to form opinions.
- Apply clinical reasoning skills to determine the relevance of the information in the question (diagnosis, setting, intervention, theoretical principles).
- Check the answer to see whether it is theoretically, diagnostically, and developmentally consistent with the item scenario.
- Choose patient/client-centered actions that focus on the emotional well-being of the person, if they are relevant to the question.
- Eliminate choices that contain contraindications (unless asked for a contraindication) or unsafe options.
- Use both your academic knowledge and clinical judgment to support your answer.
- Work rapidly but accurately. Time management is an important criterion for success.
- The NPTE is a 5-hour exam. Both mental and physical stamina are crucial for successfully completing the exam.
- Exam boredom can be a factor, especially after you have answered 200 questions, with 50 more to go. Losing interest in reading and answering questions can cost you points.

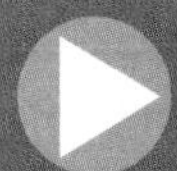

Methods of Reading Multiple-Choice Questions

Carefully read the stem of each question. What is the focus of the question? Think about the information, using your knowledge as well as your judgment. Then read each choice carefully. Begin the process by eliminating one option at a time. Every time you are able to rationalize eliminating an incorrect option, the odds of answering the question correctly increase dramatically. Be careful; sometimes options have some correct information that does not apply to the question asked. If the stem of the question is long or involved, you might wish to read the options first. This may help you focus better on the relevance of the information presented.

As the exam progresses, your reading skills may tend to deteriorate. You may have to rest your eyes for a minute. If your mind is no longer processing information properly, you may answer questions incorrectly that you normally would get right. Stop and rest for a few moments until you can refocus on the question. You might have to take a longer break after you complete a section.

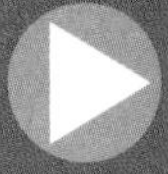

Strategies for Answering Multiple-Choice Questions

1. Look for opposites in the list of options. These are the extremes of a concept, such as positive/negative, inversion/eversion, hypoglycemia/hyperglycemia, or spasticity/flaccidity. Examine opposites first. If you cannot eliminate both of them immediately, there is a good chance that one is the correct answer. If you can eliminate both opposites right away, the chances drop to 50/50 for selecting the correct response from the remaining two choices.
2. Identify choices that are so similar that it is difficult to choose between them. These may be choices that say the same thing in slightly different ways. If you cannot discriminate between them, it is possible that both are incorrect. For example, if one option in a question is "the primary muscle of inspiration" and another choice in the same question is "the diaphragm," they both say the same thing and need to be eliminated. Sometimes a choice that is unique but not far-fetched merits greater consideration than others.
3. Identify clues in the stem that may be helpful in focusing your thoughts. For example, a question presents a recently discharged patient who can transfer independently but cannot ambulate independently for more than 20 feet. Your judgment should lead you to conclude that the patient is probably homebound. A response requiring outpatient management, use of a therapeutic pool, or elaborate therapeutic exercise equipment might be inappropriate.
4. Look for key words or phrases in the stem. If you see **BEST, MOST IMPORTANT, FIRST, OF GREATEST BENEFIT, or PRIMARY** you will need to set priorities. All of the choices could correctly answer the question; however, you must go through a process of rank ordering and elimination to reach the best option. Try to eliminate any obvious, unrealistic choices first, and work backward toward what you consider to be the top priority.
5. Look for overlapping facts in the options. If you ascertain that a fact or statement in one option is incorrect, and you see the same fact or statement in another option, both choices can be eliminated. For example, given a patient problem, two options in the question are (1) pallor and diaphoresis and (2) tachycardia and diaphoresis. If you determine that diaphoresis is never a sign of the problem, then you can automatically eliminate both choices (1) and (2).
6. Identify options that are crucial for the survival or safety of the patient. These always receive a high priority. You should give less credibility to responses that provide false reassurance to the patient, are overly optimistic, or do not address the patient's or family's feelings. Also give less credibility to responses in which the therapist gives away decision-making capability or responsibility to other health care workers. Consider abdicating responsibility only if there is a medical situation outside of the scope of practice for physical therapists, or if the therapist does not possess the skills to treat a particular type of patient problem.
7. Look for negative words or phrases in the stem. Phrases and words such as **least important, not, contraindicated,** and other negatives denote that you must search for an answer that is false, unacceptable,

BOX E Strategy Review for Answering Multiple-Choice Items

- Identify the question theme. What is the question really asking?
- Avoid "reading into" the question. Don't make up a story. Read the question, and nothing but the question.
- Identify choices that are equally plausible. If two choices say basically the same thing, eliminate both.
- Carefully consider opposites. If you cannot eliminate both right away, one may be the correct answer.
- More than one choice may correctly answer the question. Choose the one that is *most* correct.
- In most cases, select positive, active choices rather than passive, negative ones.
- When changing an answer, make sure you have a good reason to eliminate your original choice, and an even better reason to make a new choice. Don't let second-guessing talk you out of the correct answer.

Adapted from Fleming-Castaldy, R; National Occupational Therapy Review & Study Guide, 9th ed.

low priority, or contraindicated. Negative words are often in bold type. If you consider each choice as either *true* or *false* relative to the scenario presented, you should end up with three *trues* and one *false*, and therefore be able to answer the question. The false choice would be the correct answer if you categorized everything appropriately. These types of negative questions are becoming increasingly rare on the NPTE with the possible exception of questions related to contraindications.

8. Don't look for a particular pattern of answers that would cause you to alter a choice you believe to be correct. For instance, do not eliminate a correct choice because you chose the same letter or number choice as a response in the item immediately preceding the one you are currently answering. Questions are selected and randomly placed in the exam. Don't look for or think about answer patterns.
9. Don't overanalyze a question. Read the question at face value. Don't go outside of the gist of the information in the stem of the question to reach a conclusion. Sufficient information should be available in the question stem. Adding your own hypothetical conditions to the situation presented could lead you in the wrong direction.
10. Some questions may present graphic or visual representations with an accompanying question. These may include x-rays; wounds; ECG readouts; therapists performing various tests, measures, or interventions; or depictions of patients with impairments such as scoliosis or amputations. A useful strategy for these types of questions is to look at the choices first. With the choices in mind, look at the graphic representation next, and finally look at the question. Looking at the choices first may help you focus on the aspect of the graphic representation that may be most relevant to answer the question.

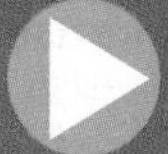

Final Review

A review consisting of *just* answering or memorizing sample questions is often unsatisfactory, since the sample questions in the accompanying online exams are not actual NPTE questions. These questions are meant to be used for diagnostic or learning purposes. Although some questions on the NPTE that you will take may seem similar to the practice questions, the NPTE questions may have entirely different answers. You, most likely, will also encounter some questions on the actual NPTE that have a different focus than the practice exam questions.

Your final review should refocus on the areas that are emphasized on the NPTE and that you have identified as areas of personal weakness. You may wish to retake the practice exams.

The Day Before the Exam

The day before the examination, make sure you have gathered all necessary documents, materials, medications, eyeglasses, and personal items you may need. It will heighten your anxiety to look for these things on the day of the exam. Do not use medications such as antihistamines or muscle relaxants, drink alcohol or use other substances that may affect your alertness. Do not "cram" or stay up late the night before, reviewing material. Do not go to a party the night before the exam. (After it's over, okay!) Try to get a good night's sleep. On the day of the test, eat a meal before the exam. You may not have the opportunity to eat again for many hours. Finally, allow extra time to arrive at the test site in case travel is delayed.

Expect to be a little nervous. Prometric personnel are trained to put you at ease and explain what will happen. However, if you are unrealistic in your expectations at the testing site, Prometric personnel may react negatively to your demands. This will not put you in the proper frame of mind to take the NPTE. Also, if you are overly anxious, your ability to process questions and recall information could be impaired. Anxiety can also lead you to dwell more on the consequences of the exam rather than the questions presented. Practice relaxation strategies you find helpful. If you have disciplined yourself to review material thoroughly, you should feel confident, and there is more likelihood of a positive outcome.

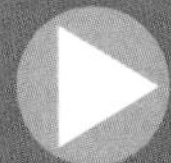

The Role of Critical Reasoning in Your Performance

Critical reasoning is an important part of NPTE preparation. At this moment, you have achieved a certain level of critical reasoning skill that has helped you succeed in academic and clinical arenas. Critical reasoning skills are the foundation for how we analyze the situations we encounter in everyday life. We often do not acknowledge how important this implicit skill is for exam success.

It is important to define critical reasoning and why you should spend time focusing your attention on this process. Critical reasoning is a decision-making process by which you use your knowledge, skills, experience, and logic to draw conclusions about everyday situations. When this process is used judiciously, it is undertaken with purpose, reflection, clarity, accuracy, and thoroughness. It is the foundation by which individuals draw conclusions about their world and what one determines to be true.

How does this relate to the NPTE, and why should you be concerned about it? The NPTE provides opportunities for you to demonstrate how well you can reason out challenging clinical, ethical, administrative, or other circumstances with the 250 questions you will need to answer for the exam. Each question will require you to draw on your knowledge, skills, and experiences to arrive at a correct conclusion. The way you arrive at a correct conclusion is primarily by using critical reasoning.

Some individuals erroneously believe that the NPTE tests only your ability to recall facts that are readily found in books. Although factual knowledge is important and provides a foundation for the exam, the NPTE also tests your ability to evaluate challenging circumstances correctly and to make prudent decisions about the situations described in each question. The exam often moves beyond simple recall of knowledge and facts to contextualized clinical information. This means that you will be given clinical scenarios in which you will need to draw conclusions about a patient's symptoms, diagnosis, response to therapy, and expected outcomes. You must draw on your knowledge to take your reasoning to the next level of application of information.

One should be aware of critical reasoning processes and skills (see Table 1-1). The following section helps you become aware of the different skills involved in the process of critical reasoning, and how NPTE success is, in part, tied to these processes.

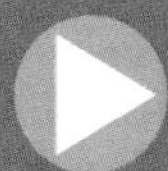

Subskills of Critical Reasoning

There are five subskills of critical reasoning that underlie the foundation for sound critical reasoning ability. They are based on expert consensus of many critical thinking experts and reported by Peter Facione (2015, 1998), who describes the skills utilized in reasoning out challenging circumstances. The five subskills of critical reasoning are **inductive**, **deductive**, **analytical**, **inferential**, and **evaluative**.

Table 1-1

Critical Reasoning Self-Assessment Questions

OBSERVED EXAM DIFFICULTY	REASONING CHALLENGE	NPTE EXAM PREPARATION STRATEGY
Do You: - Have difficulty with taking specific information and applying it to larger populations? - Selecting incorrect answers because you don't know how to generalize your knowledge?	Inductive	When studying a specific content area, think about how to apply the information you are reviewing to a diversity of situations. Use a reflective "what if" stance to think about how this information may be generalized to a broader context. This can be a fun and effective study group activity.
Do you: - Prefer to follow your instincts rather than the guidelines that a protocol may provide? - Select incorrect answers because you are unfamiliar with established practice standards or major theoretical approaches?	Deductive	When studying, be sure to master all major concepts, laws, rules, and accepted principles that guide PT practice. Carefully review all frames of reference, practice guidelines, and intervention protocols and procedures. Review the APTA Code of Ethics and Guidelines for Professional Conduct.
Do You: - Tend to misinterpret information provided and make poor judgments and apply inadequately conceived assumptions about it? - Select incorrect answers because you misjudged the effects of a clinical condition on functional performance?	Analytical	Obtain knowledge of all major clinical conditions, their symptoms, diagnostic testing and criteria, anticipated sequelae, and expected outcomes. This information is extensively reviewed in this text to help you make accurate judgments and correct assumptions about the potential impact of a clinical condition on functional performance. Review potential adverse effects (red flags in this text) and common errors associated with training.
Do You: - Have difficulty with thinking about how clinical conditions and practice situations may evolve over time? - Assume information is valid when it is not true? - Select incorrect answers because you have difficulty deciding the best course of action in a practice scenario?	Inferential	When studying clinical conditions, think about how the presentation of these conditions may sometimes vary from textbook descriptions. Use the knowledge and experience you acquired during your clinical education experiences to assess the trustworthiness of your assumptions. Study guidelines and models developed from evidence-based practice to develop a solid foundation on how to decide the best course of action.
Do you: - Feel anxious when you have questions that are ambiguous and you cannot find answers to them in a textbook? - Rely on protocols and guidelines more than gut instinct? - Select incorrect answers because you become overwhelmed by questions that present ethical dilemmas?	Evaluative	When reviewing specific content, think about the practice ambiguities and ethical dilemmas you observed during your clinical education experiences related to these areas. Review the APTA Code of Ethics and Guidelines for Professional Conduct and practice applying this information to determine a correct course of action using practice examples and case studies.

This table was adapted with permission from Dr. Kari Inda, from a table published in Fleming-Castaldy, R: National Occupational Therapy Certification Exam: Review & Study Guide, 8th ed. TherapyEd.

Inductive Reasoning

Inductive reasoning is the process of reasoning in which the assumptions of an argument are believed to endorse the conclusion but do not guarantee it. It starts with reasoning in specific situations and then moves to more generalized situations. It may start with observations about a specific situation and then require one to draw conclusions about larger circumstances.

For example, if we observe a patient who experienced a stroke demonstrating dysarthria, we might conclude that all patients with stroke have symptoms of dysarthria. We know that this is, in fact, not true. Inductive reasoning skill was used to draw this conclusion because we took observations from a specific situation and applied them to a larger, more global assumption. Recognizing that inductive reasoning can be flawed is an important part of successful exam performance. Inductive reasoning is an important skill clinically, because it helps us to examine all possible options in a clinical situation and determine the most reasonable action. It is used in diagnostic thinking, where we form assumptions about what to expect from a diagnosis as it evolves over time.

Deductive Reasoning

Deductive reasoning is the process of reasoning whereby one draws conclusions based on facts, laws, rules, or accepted principles. It is the reverse thinking process of inductive reasoning, whereby the individual starts with larger circumstances and theories and applies them to specific situations.

For example, if we read the *Physical Therapy Guide for Professional Conduct,* which states that fraudulent billing for therapy services is unethical, we could reasonably conclude that when we witness therapist A in a clinic billing for services for patient B that did not occur, therapist A is acting unethically. Here the circumstance started with a global principle and was applied to a specific circumstance.

However, deductive reasoning also has its flaws. Sometimes individuals make erroneous assumptions about the premises of a theory and then apply this error in thinking to the specific circumstance. If we start with a premise that all patients enjoy physical therapy, then patients B, C, and D all will enjoy physical therapy. Can we say this for sure? Of course not! This is a type of flawed premise that leads to a faulty conclusion. We must be sure that our deductive reasoning begins with sound theory and known principles.

Deductive reasoning is important to physical therapists because it helps them apply rules and guidelines, without necessitating independent judgment for the situation. This is especially beneficial when applying protocols for treatment approaches (e.g., functional electrical stimulation, assuming one is following a published protocol) or research guidelines (e.g., how to carry out correlational analysis of an array of data).

Analytical Reasoning

Analytical reasoning or analysis is defined as the process of interpreting the meaning of information as well as relationships within the information presented, and then making assumptions or judgments about that information. Information presented in the form of graphs, charts, tables, and pictures utilizes analytical reasoning skills, because one must interpret the information and determine what it means. Other times, information is presented in such a manner that one must make a "mental chart" of the information.

Popular questions that test one's analytical reasoning contain descriptors assigned to a group, with the key features of the group given in part. This leaves the test-taker to make assumptions about what is true about the whole group based on the information provided. Questions of this nature tend to place groups of people into categories, and the test-taker must determine the characteristics of each group, based on limited information. These questions tend to frustrate people. Nonetheless, analytical reasoning is a necessary evil!

In physical therapy practice, analytical reasoning is important because it helps one to interpret an ECG strip or determine the diagnosis when analyzing the x-ray of a patient with a "Scotty dog" fracture in the spine (necessitating the question, what is the significance?). Often, questions of this nature provide a host of symptoms, and the test-taker must determine the diagnosis (categorization of information). We also use analytical reasoning to give definitions to symptoms we are reading about (How can we describe this symptom?). Overall, analytical reasoning helps us to examine ideas and concepts and the relationships between them.

Inferential Reasoning

Inference or inferential reasoning is the process of drawing conclusions or making logical judgments based on concepts, assumptions, and evidence, rather than direct observations. Questions that ask you to determine what is **BEST, MOST IMPORTANT,** or **MOST BENEFICIAL** often test your inferential reasoning ability. Questions of this nature also ask you to determine what is believed to be true, even though you cannot be 100% sure.

Inferential reasoning skills are used in clinical situations when a physical therapist must determine what symptoms to expect from a diagnosis or what is the likely functional result from a disease process or disorder. Because we cannot be 100% sure about the nature of a disease and all its possible symptoms, we must infer this information based on our knowledge and experiences. This is an important skill for a physical therapist to possess.

Pitfalls in inferential reasoning commonly occur when we fail to consider all the information presented or use faulty logic to determine what may occur in certain situations. An example of this might be a physical therapist who determines that it is most appropriate for a patient with T12 paraplegia to focus on strengthening the upper trapezius and levator scapulae muscles in preparation for ambulation with crutches, rather than triceps and lower trapezius muscles. Here, the therapist did not consider the nature of the task at hand (ambulation with crutches) or tie the muscle functions with the use of crutches for ambulation. Hasty decisions can lead to suboptimal treatment planning with patients.

Evaluative Reasoning

Evaluation and evaluative reasoning is a process by which one weighs the merits of an argument for its validity and the inherent value of the argument itself. Here, the individual determines whether an argument "holds water," whether there is value to be found in the argument itself, and what value one can assign to it.

Individuals make value judgments all the time. We are often unaware of the thought processes involved. Every day, we evaluate ideas that are presented to us, sometimes in the form of a news story or a discussion with a friend. We tend to judge the merits and value of the information we receive. However, a good evaluative thinker listens with a skeptical ear, determining how truthful the information is and how much value one should assign to that information. Accepting information at face value can be a pitfall because we are not considering the possibility that there is more information to be heard that may complete the story or that the information could be false.

There are also times where we may have to make difficult decisions in areas that have no clear-cut answers. In physical therapy practice, we may be faced with dilemmas that pose a challenge for the correct course of action. Pay close attention to questions with the picture of the cogwheels next to them because they will help you to identify questions that pose difficult clinical and ethical situations and require evaluative reasoning.

An example of such a dilemma is a situation in which a therapist is working with a patient who becomes short of breath. The therapist must determine whether to immediately notify the physician, document the symptoms, or continue with the treatment session as planned. It is also helpful to know whether shortness of breath is an expected symptom, given the patient's medical history and past response to treatment. This information helps guide the therapist's thinking about a correct course of action. Nonetheless, these types of situations are not clear-cut and require the therapist to evaluate the circumstances, weigh the information presented, and determine a correct course of action, given his or her knowledge and experience.

Pitfalls in evaluative reasoning involve assigning great value to information that has little value to the situation, not assigning enough value to highly valuable information, and not using principles and guidelines that are put into place to help guide one's thinking (such as the Code of Ethics and *Guide to Professional Conduct*).

Summary of Reasoning Skills

You are encouraged to pay particular attention to the five types of critical reasoning listed with each practice question and accompanying explanation in the simulated examination answer section. The following five symbols have been assigned to help you key into areas that may be weaknesses:

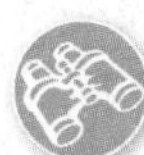 = Inductive Reasoning

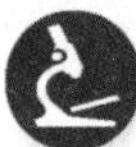 = Deductive Reasoning

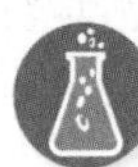 = Analytical Reasoning

 = Inferential Reasoning

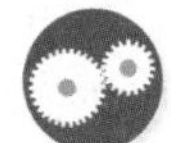 = Evaluative Reasoning

As you review the simulated examination results and print them out, pay attention to any patterns that emerge. Are you particularly weak in a certain area of reasoning? Often, individuals are stronger in certain areas of reasoning than others. Our skill in reasoning ability comes from not only our knowledge, but also our day-to-day experiences. If you notice that you have a weakness in a certain area of reasoning, do not despair. Being aware of the issue is a good first step. The next section will help you to determine your next course of action.

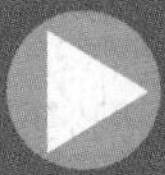

Critical Reasoning Challenge

In order to solve problems and understand the reasoning process, use the following checklist to dissect the sample questions. This training activity helps you mentally address the items in the checklist. Not all items are relevant, and a mental "not applicable" ("NA") can be inserted. The answers and explanations to the exam questions are organized in this way. Given the time constraints of the NPTE, it is not practical to use this 14-point checklist for each question on the actual exam. However, the reasoning framework will carry over. If you focus and organize your thoughts, reasoning and success will follow!

NPTE Exam Question Checklist

1. What domain and category does this question represent?
   Domains:
      Cardiovascular, Pulmonary and Lymphatic Systems

Musculoskeletal System
Neuromuscular and Nervous System
Integumentary System
Other Systems (Metabolic/Endocrine/Gastrointestinal/Genitourinary)
System Interactions
Nonsystem

Categories:
PT Examination
Evaluation, Differential Diagnosis, and Prognosis
Interventions
Equipment and Devices
Therapeutic Modalities
Safety and Protection
Professional Responsibilities
Research and Evidence-Based Practice

2. What is the diagnosis or condition of the patient/client?
3. What age is the client (if relevant)?
4. What deficit(s) or problem(s) does the client have?
5. How does the deficit or problem affect the client's function?
6. What is the setting for treatment? (e.g., inpatient, outpatient, early intervention, school)
7. What **KEY WORDS** indicate importance or priority? (e.g., **BEST, MOST, NEXT, INITIAL, GREATEST BENEFIT**)
8. What information is needed to answer the question? (e.g., type or stage of condition/disease, examination tools, treatment techniques, knowledge of statistics, lab values, type of equipment or modality)
9. Is any information in the question stem irrelevant or included only as a distracter?
10. Give a rationale for why Choice #1 is correct or why it should be eliminated.
11. Give a rationale for why Choice #2 is correct or why it should be eliminated.
12. Give a rationale for why Choice #3 is correct or why it should be eliminated.
13. Give a rationale for why Choice #4 is correct or why it should be eliminated.
14. What type of critical reasoning subtype is needed to answer this question?
Inductive
Deductive
Analysis
Inference
Evaluation

Use the checklist to solve the following challenges. Answers appear at the end of this chapter.

Critical Reasoning Challenge #1

A patient has experienced long-term lumbar pain and is diagnosed with degenerative joint disease (DJD) of the lumbar facet joints. The patient complains of numbness, paresthesias, and weakness of the bilateral lower extremities that increase with extended positions or walking greater than 100 feet. Pain persists for hours after assuming a resting position. The patient reports the ability to ride a stationary bike for 30 minutes without any problems. What is the **BEST** intervention in this case?

Choice 1 Increasing cardiovascular endurance with walking for 30 minutes, twice a day.
Choice 2 Limiting extended spinal positions and improving the dynamic control of the trunk musculature.
Choice 3 Back extension strengthening throughout the entire ROM.
Choice 4 Traction and limitation of weight-bearing positions.

Critical Reasoning Challenge #2

A patient sustained a fracture of the proximal humerus, which has healed well. Upon examination, the therapist notes limitation in active shoulder flexion. The scapula protracts, elevates, and upwardly rotates early and elevates excessively when the patient attempts to lift the arm. What should the therapist do next?

Choice 1 Passive shoulder flexion and glenohumeral accessory mobility testing.
Choice 2 Manual muscle test of serratus anterior and rhomboids.
Choice 3 Manual resistance exercises for the supraspinatus and infraspinatus.
Choice 4 Large amplitude oscillations performed at the end-range of joint play for the glenohumeral inferior and posterior capsule.

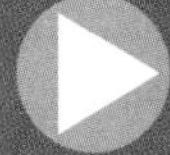

Improving Your Critical Reasoning Skills

Critical reasoning is not learned or improved in a quick lesson or by simply reading basic definitions. It requires practice with items that test these skill areas and provide feedback on your performance. The good news is that you already have this information contained in this study guide. Each practice question in this *Review and*

Study Guide has an accompanying rationale for the correct and incorrect choices. Additionally, each question has an explanation about the subskill of critical reasoning and the knowledge or skill required to arrive at a correct conclusion. Paying attention to these areas will help you to build your knowledge and experiences with critical reasoning skills and prepare you for the NPTE and all its challenges.

After you receive the results of your online practice test, refer back to your incorrect responses. This may help you uncover a pattern in the types of questions you are answering incorrectly, as related to a subskill of critical reasoning. Do you notice that you have difficulty with certain types of questions, such as those that encourage evaluative or inferential reasoning? This will help you to identify a potential area for improvement and an area to help base study strategies. Once you have identified a weakness in critical reasoning, take some time to reflect on why this is so. Look again at Table 1-1. Be sure to read not only the rationales for any questions answered incorrectly, but the correct answers as well. You want to be sure that your rationale for selecting the correct response aligns with the rationale provided for the correct answer. This extra measure further assists you in gauging your exam performance and accuracy in critical reasoning.

Enhancing Critical Reasoning Skills

What makes a person an excellent critical thinker? There are various attributes that are associated with sound critical thinking and reasoning ability. It is not just the skills one has acquired with time and practice, but also the habits of mind that provide a solid foundation for deeper thinking and reasoning about everyday life. It includes a natural curiosity about what we see and hear, truth seeking, a systematic way of thinking about life and approaches to solving problems, and the reduction of bias that can interfere with our ability to see the truth and determine a correct course of action.

Critical thinking and reasoning ability are not learned in a few quick lessons. It takes time and practice to change the way you think about the world and everyday situations. But once you begin to use these strategies, they become part of your everyday life and you may not even notice that you are asking the deeper questions that help you to get to the truth. You are more comfortable with ambiguity and uncertainty and you do not shy away from a challenge that will take some time to overcome. These are the habits that propel people toward success. Why does this matter for the NPTE? It is, in part, what helps you to succeed on high stakes examinations. What provides you with the stamina to stay focused, to minimize frustration, and to have clarity of mind as you answer each question on the NPTE. It requires you to go deeper than you may be comfortable doing right now.

If you find yourself struggling with certain practice questions or study content in this *Review & Study Guide*, take the time to go deeper. What that means is to think about the subject of the question or content at a level deeper than what you may be accustomed to doing right now. It is easy to answer a question and go immediately to the location of the correct answer. We want instant gratification. We want to know if we are on track with our studies. Avoid the immediate need to know. Instead, when you encounter a challenging question or topic area in this guide, stop and ask yourself, "What do I know about this subject? What do I remember?" Write it down—everything you can remember, symptoms, stages—without seeking out the answers. It's okay if you don't remember a lot. Be comfortable with what you do and don't know. This is the first step in thinking more deeply. Next, consider the typical evaluation and treatment approaches for that condition and how the therapy setting changes how you approach your therapy. Where might the patient be in his/her stage of recovery? How does that change your approach to care? Next, go a level deeper. Consider issues and specific situations that may alter the course of therapy, such as other disciplines that may be involved in care, patient or family concerns, the discharge plan, and environment the patient hopes to transition toward. These are the "it depends" situations. When you ask yourself, "How might I approach therapy for this patient with Parkinson's disease?" you should immediately say, "Well, it depends." It depends on the treatment setting I'm in. It depends on the stage of the patient's disease. If the patient is in an early stage, he/she is likely to be ambulatory and I can work on various mobility activities that reduce a risk of falls. If the patient is in a late stage of the disease, he/she is not likely to be ambulatory and may be confined to a bed or wheelchair. My therapy approach would be very different. These are the situations in which taking additional time to think, play out different scenarios and situations in your mind, and test your ability to develop multiple approaches to solving problems helps you to go deeper, to be comfortable solving complex problems, and in doing so without all the answers readily in front of you. This is what helps you to succeed on the NPTE.

Deeper level thinking is analogous to the layers of rock that form with weather, time, and erosion, also known as strata. With rock strata, there are typically a number of horizontal layers of soil, sand, pebbles, shells, and other material that settles with the passage of time. Some layers are more superficial and easily seen while others can be very deep and take effort to dig down toward. This is how the development of critical reasoning occurs.

Wherever you are or wherever you think you are in your comfort with critical thinking, your goal is to dig

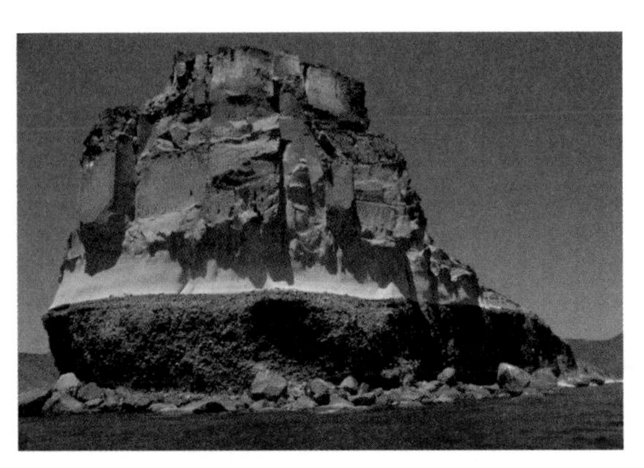

Stratified Rock near La Paz, Baja California Sur, Mexico. Author: Wonderlane. Uploaded from http://flickr.com/photo/71401718@N00/3542465243.

deeper into territories where you are less comfortable. Take opportunities to explore the "it depends" scenarios—how might this change if.... Pick topics to explore that you have identified through your studies in which you are less comfortable with the content. Taking the time to explore, to ask challenging questions, and to dig deeper will help to solidify your knowledge of this topic in a more effective and efficient way than reading, filling out or using flash cards, or memorizing facts.

Have you ever had a situation in your program where you thought you did well on an exam, only to find out that your grade was lower than expected? You may have asked yourself, "What happened? I knew this! At least I thought I did." Oftentimes, when a student receives a lower grade than expected on an exam, it can mean that they memorized the facts of the material or just used flash cards. But they failed to understand the concepts, the complexities, and how the facts change according to the circumstances at hand. For example, if a student memorizes the symptoms of left CVA and right CVA perfectly, will that serve him or her well on an exam full of questions about CVA? Yes, if the exam is only about remembering the differences between left and right CVA. This often isn't the case. What happens is that the exam asks about other types of CVA—occurring in different vessels, regions of the cortex, and physiological mechanisms of the CVA itself, such as a thrombosis or embolism. It could ask about how to approach treatment for someone who incurred a left CVA, and the hope is the test taker could extrapolate what might be effective given their memorization of left CVA symptoms. But in reality, that falls short. Facts can guide logic, but only to the extent that the facts are accurate and complete. The lower grade achieved on an exam represents how memorization alone is not enough, especially when the exam demands thinking beyond facts. As you prepare for the NPTE, keep in mind that the quantity of study is not important—it is the quality. One of the most common statements uttered by students who fail high stakes exams is, "I don't know why I failed. I read the book cover to cover three times." A statement about the quantity of study rather than the quality is a sign of insufficient studying. Your preparations should not be about how many topics you can cram into your study session. It should be about the insights you have gained from the material covered.

Think back to the rock strata and how it can be applied to a specific topic covered in this *Review and Study Guide*. Let's say you are reading content in *Chapter 4: Cardiovascular and Lymphatic Physical Therapy*. You see the topic of lymphedema and immediately think to yourself, "I don't remember a lot about this." Close the book and start at the surface: what do I remember about this diagnosis? What are the typical symptoms? Where might lymphedema be present? Which diagnoses are often associated with lymphedema? Next, go deeper. If I were in an inpatient setting, what would be the typical evaluation and treatment approaches for lymphedema? What if it were an outpatient setting? What does lymphedema look like at different stages of recovery, and how does my treatment change according to stages? What are some "red flags" or precautions and contraindications I should be aware of when working with this condition? After you have recalled as much as you can about these topics, go to a deeper level where you reach the uncertainties or the "it depends." If other disciplines or entities were involved in care, such as occupational therapy, a concerned family member, how might I work with them to ensure a successful outcome for the patient? Should I perform bandaging, and if so, how? What are the factors that indicate use of bandaging as part of treatment?

The following illustration helps you to apply the analogy of the strata to your studies for the NPTE. Find a challenging topic and then start at the top with the more superficial questions. After they have been answered, go to the next layer of depth and answer those questions. Keep going until you have reached the deepest layer and have pondered all the questions about your chosen topic. After that has been accomplished, use this *Review and Study Guide* to verify how you did. Look up the topic. What did you remember? What information did you not recall? Did you confuse any topics for a closely related diagnosis or situation? Based on this process and assessment of your knowledge, you have accomplished deeper levels of thinking and reasoning, as well as expanded your current level of knowledge about the topic area. See Figure 1-1.

Other Courses of Action. This study guide was designed to help you to identify potential weak areas

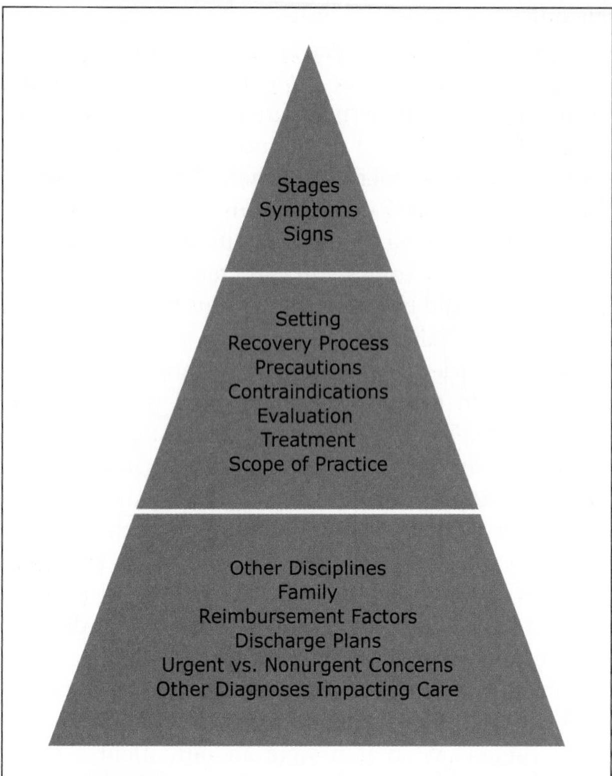

Figure 1-1 Critical reasoning strata applied to study process.

and prepare you to succeed on the NPTE. More detailed information about critical reasoning is beyond the scope and focus of this book. However, if you would like additional information about critical reasoning and practice with questions that test critical thinking and reasoning skills, the following resources may help you practice honing these skill areas:

- **Insight Assessment, Inc.** www.insightassessment.com. Offers periodic free mini-tests with rationales for correct and incorrect answers. Also offers resources that discuss the various types of reasoning.
- Burger, E. B. & Starbird, M. (2012). *The 5 elements of effective thinking*. Princeton, NJ: Princeton University Press. A helpful guide with practical strategies for implementing critical thinking at deeper levels.

Reasoning References

Facione P.A. (2015). *Critical Thinking: What It Is and Why It Counts.* Millbrae, CA: The California Academic Press.

Facione P.A. (1998). *Critical Thinking: A Statement of Expert Consensus for Purposes of Educational Assessment and Instruction: Executive Summary.* Newark, DE: The American Psychological Association. ERIC Document Reproduction Service. No. ED 315423.

Facione N.C. & Facione P.A. (2006). *The Health Sciences Reasoning Test HSRT: Test Manual 2006 Edition.* Millbrae, CA: The California Academic Press.

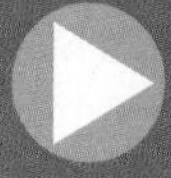

Retaking the Examination

Remember, most candidates are successful the first time! If you receive bad news about your NPTE results, life goes on, but it gets a bit more complicated. You might lose your temporary license if your state or jurisdiction has granted you one. If applicable, your visa to work as a physical therapist in the United States may be revoked. If you are working as a physical therapist, you could lose your job, or you might continue to work, albeit with a different title, responsibilities, or salary until you pass the examination. If you have accepted a future position and fail to get a license, your employer might opt not to save the position for you. Undoubtedly, you will experience various emotions, which could include frustration, anger, depression, low self-esteem and embarrassment.

What can be done? You can go online or download the Performance Feedback Request Form from the FSBPT. This report lists your score by Content area, Body Systems, and Section of the exam. The number of items correct and a percentage are given for each subsection. The current cost is $100. No personal checks are accepted. Due to examination security rules, you will not be able to access or revisit your actual examination. You may contact www.fsbpt.org, or call (703) 739-9420.

Our advice is not to dwell on past failures. Carefully evaluate your performance. Think about areas on the previous exam with which you had some difficulty. Were there any gaps in your academic or clinical knowledge? Did you find it difficult to make decisions and answer questions requiring clinical judgment or analysis? Were your English language skills inadequate?

Focus on the next exam. Reinstitute a program of disciplined study. Consider taking a preparation course if you had not previously attended one. We have found that candidates who retake the exam without adjusting their behaviors or correcting deficiencies wind up with the same disappointing results. There is no magic potion that helps you pass the exam. It is your responsibility to demonstrate competency to practice. Take a positive and determined outlook. Approach the next examination with self-confidence.

Useful Web Links

www.fsbpt.org: information on licensure, the NPTE and the role of the FSBPT, as well as addresses and links to state physical therapy boards.

www.fsbpt.net/pt: transfer of exam scores and other related information.

www.2test.com: locations of Prometric Testing Centers.

www.apta.org: information on the profession, policies regarding the role of the physical therapist, and resources in selected areas of practice.

www.TherapyEd.com: information on examination preparatory courses as well as materials for physical and occupational therapists, PTAs, OTAs, and Speech-Language Pathologists.

Answers to Critical Reasoning Challenge #1 (Answers Are in Bold)

1. What domain and category does this question represent?
   Domains:
   - Cardiovascular, Pulmonary, and Lymphatic Systems
   - **Musculoskeletal System**
   - Neuromuscular and Nervous System
   - Integumentary System
   - Other Systems (Metabolic/Endocrine/Gastrointestinal/Genitourinary)
   - System Interactions
   - Nonsystem

   Categories:
   - PT Examination
   - Evaluation, Differential Diagnosis, and Prognosis
   - **Interventions**
   - Equipment and Devices
   - Therapeutic Modalities
   - Safety and Protection
   - Professional Responsibilities
   - Research and Evidence-Based Practice
2. What is the diagnosis or condition of the patient/client?
   DJD of lumbar facet joints. Spinal stenosis?
3. What age is the client (if relevant)?
   NA
4. What deficit(s) or problem(s) does the client have?
   Pain, numbness, paresthesias both LEs.
5. How does the deficit or problem affect the client's function?
   Cannot walk >100 feet.
6. What is the setting for treatment? (e.g., inpatient, outpatient, early intervention, school)
   NA
7. What KEY WORDS indicate importance or priority? (e.g., BEST, MOST, NEXT, INITIAL, GREATEST BENEFIT)
   Intervention
8. What information is needed to answer the question? (e.g., type or stage of condition/disease, examination tools, treatment techniques, knowledge of statistics, lab values, type of equipment or modality)
   Need to limit trunk extension with spinal stenosis.
9. Is any information in the question stem irrelevant or included only as a distracter?
   No.
10. Give a rationale for why Choice #1 is correct or why it should be eliminated.
    Intervention does not deal with pain, numbness, and paresthesia. Patient cannot walk >100 feet. How could they walk for 30 minutes bid?
    ELIMINATE.
11. Give a rationale for why Choice #2 is correct or why it should be eliminated.
    Trunk extension exacerbates symptoms. Dynamic trunk control to limit extension is best intervention for spinal stenosis.
    CORRECT.
12. Give a rationale for why Choice #3 is correct or why it should be eliminated.
    Back extension exacerbates symptoms.
    ELIMINATE.
13. Give a rationale for why Choice #4 is correct or why it should be eliminated.
    Limiting weight-bearing and traction are of little help in addressing the major problems and alleviating symptoms.
    ELIMINATE.
14. What type of critical reasoning subtype is needed to answer this question?
    - **Inductive**
    - Deductive
    - Analysis
    - Inference
    - Evaluation

    This type of reasoning requires one to be a "forward thinker" and determine the best course of action for future functioning.

Answers to Critical Reasoning Challenge #2

1. What domain and category does this question represent?
   Domains:
   - Cardiovascular, Pulmonary, and Lymphatic Systems
   - **Musculoskeletal System**
   - Neuromuscular and Nervous System
   - Integumentary System
   - Other Systems (Metabolic/Endocrine/Gastrointestinal/Genitourinary)

System Interactions
Nonsystem
Categories:
PT Examination
Evaluation, Differential Diagnosis, and Prognosis
Interventions
Equipment and Devices
Therapeutic Modalities
Safety and Protection
Professional Responsibilities
Research and Evidence-Based Practice

2. What is the diagnosis or condition of the patient/client?
Proximal fracture of the humerus.
3. What age is the client (if relevant)?
NA
4. What deficit(s) or problem(s) does the client have?
Limitations in active shoulder flexion. Scapula protracts, elevates, and upwardly rotates early.
5. How does the deficit or problem affect the client's function?
Possible ADL limitations.
6. What is the setting for treatment? (e.g., inpatient, outpatient, early intervention, school)
NA
7. What KEY WORDS indicate importance or priority? (e.g., BEST, MOST, NEXT, INITIAL, GREATEST BENEFIT)
NEXT
8. What information is needed to answer the question? (e.g., type or stage of condition/disease, examination tools, treatment techniques, knowledge of statistics, lab values, type of equipment or modality)
Reasons for shoulder AROM limitations after humeral fracture. Examination approaches for shoulder AROM limitations. How to perform glenohumeral accessory mobility testing.
9. Is any information in the question stem irrelevant or included only as a distracter?
No.
10. Give a rationale for why Choice #1 is correct or why it should be eliminated.
Therapist should perform passive shoulder flexion and glenohumeral accessory mobility testing to determine the tissue at fault and proceed from this point.
CORRECT.
11. Give a rationale for why Choice #2 is correct or why it should be eliminated.
Weak serratus anterior would result in retraction of the scapula and possible winging. Rhomboids are downward rotators of the scapula, which does not match the patient presentation.
ELIMINATE.
12. Give a rationale for why Choice #3 is correct or why it should be eliminated.
This is a treatment approach for weakness of the rotator cuff. Information provided does not indicate rotator cuff weakness. There is not enough information to begin treatment. Further evaluation must be done to determine the tissue at fault.
ELIMINATE.
13. Give a rationale for why Choice #4 is correct or why it should be eliminated.
This treatment is appropriate for capsular restrictions. There is not enough information to begin treatment. Further evaluation must be done to determine the tissue at fault.
ELIMINATE.
14. What type of critical reasoning subtype is needed to answer this question?
Inductive
Deductive
Analysis
Inference
Evaluation
Based on the diagnosis, the examiner has to determine the next course of action. This requires clinical judgment, an inductive reasoning skill.

2

Musculoskeletal Physical Therapy

MICHAEL S. CROWELL AND BRADLEY S. TRAGORD

Chapter Outline

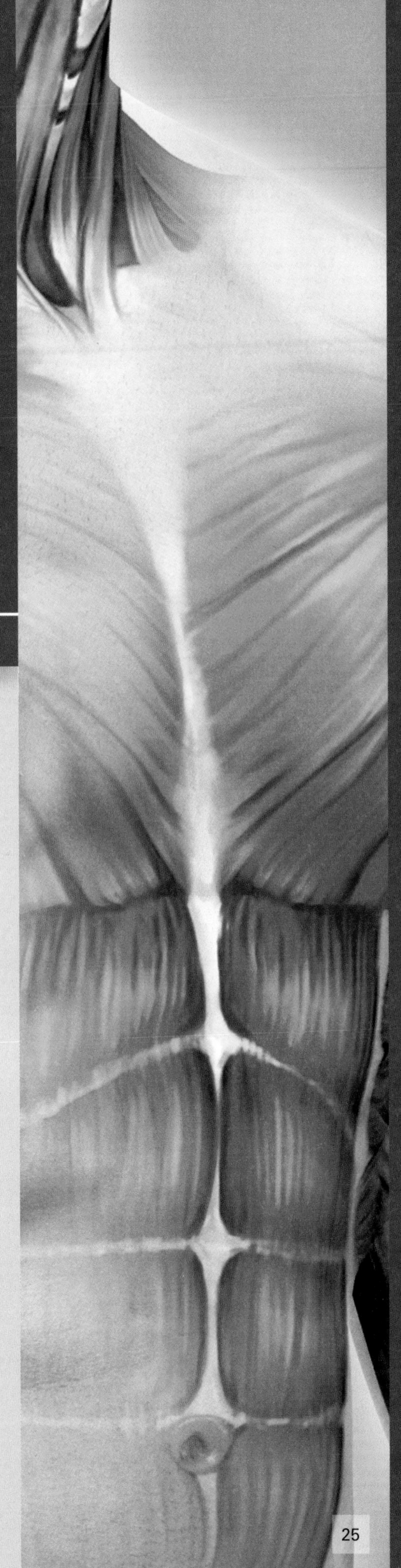

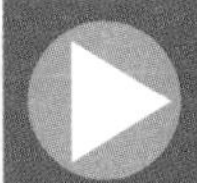

Study Tactics

Questions About the Musculoskeletal System Comprise 28% of the NPTE, or a Total of 51–60 Questions.

The Number of Questions by Category Are:

- Examination of the Patient/Client: 18–21
- Evaluation, Differential Diagnosis, Prognosis: 17–20
- Interventions: 16–19

Examination of the Patient/Client. Focus on:

- Orthopedic tests and measures, including knowledge and interpretation of special tests for a given pathology or impairment, such as ACL tears, ankle sprains, rotator cuff tears, neck instability, and so on
- Movement analysis to include range of motion assessment, mobilizations, and resisted motion testing
- Phases of the gait cycle, gait analysis, and common gait deviations
- Joint biomechanics and arthrokinematics, including aberrant movements and responses to examination techniques such as joint mobilizations or special tests (Lachman's; Sharp-Purser, etc.)
- Clinical practice guidelines and clinical prediction rules that help guide the examination process

Evaluation, Differential Diagnosis, and Prognosis. Focus on:

- The clinical features (signs and symptoms) and differential diagnosis of prevalent musculoskeletal conditions
- Musculoloskeletal disorders across the lifespan, such as congenital hip dysplasia, slipped capital femoral epiphysis, degenerative arthritis, and osteoporosis
- Connective tissue disorders to include lupus, osteogenesis imperfecta, Marfan syndrome, and Ehlers-Danlos syndrome
- Development of a plan of care to include prognosis for common musculoskeletal disorders
- Imaging techniques such as plain x-rays, MRI, CT, bone scans, and ultrasound, and the indications for the use of each technique
- Actions and side effects of pharmacological management of musculoskeletal problems

Interventions. Focus on:

- Physical therapy interventions and their applications for rehabilitation, health promotion, and performance according to current best evidence
- Principles that guide intervention strategies such as the centralization phenomenon, clinical prediction rules, FITT principle, PREs, etc.
- Clinical practice guidelines that delineate specific treatments such as mobilization or exercise prescription for a given musculoskeletal disorder based on current best evidence
- Soft tissue healing timelines that address when specific interventions should be applied for a given pathology
- Potential adverse side effects or complications on the musculoskeletal or other systems from physical therapy interventions

Anatomy and Biomechanics of the Musculoskeletal System

General Principles of Biomechanics

Levers: Rotations of a Rigid Surface About an Axis. There Are Three Types of Levers

1. First-class lever occurs when two forces are applied on either side of an axis.
   a. The effort is the force that attempts to cause movement.
   b. The resistance is the force that opposes movement.
   c. Example in human body is the contraction of triceps at elbow joint.
2. Second-class lever occurs when two forces are applied on one side of an axis.
   a. Resistance lies between the effort force and the axis of rotation.
   b. Few examples in human body (toe raises).
3. Third-class lever occurs when two forces are applied on one side of an axis.
   a. The effort force lies closer to the axis than the resistance force.
   b. Most muscles in the human body are third-class levers (elbow flexion).

Selected Kinematics

1. Arthrokinematics is defined as the movement between joint surfaces.
2. Three motions describe the movement of one joint surface on another.
   a. Roll consists of one joint surface rolling on another, such as a tire rolling on the road (e.g., movement between the femoral and tibial articular surfaces of knee).
   b. Glide consists of a pure translatory motion of one surface gliding on another, as when a braked wheel skids (e.g., movement of the joint surface of the proximal phalanx at the head of the metacarpal bone of the hand).
   c. Spin consists of a rotation of the movable component of the joint (e.g., movement between joint surfaces of radial head with humerus).
   d. Combinations of all three motions can occur at joints (e.g., between joint surfaces of humerus and scapula of shoulder).
3. Osteokinematics: movement between two bones.
4. Convex-concave rule describes relationship between arthrokinematics and osteokinematics.
   a. When a convex surface is moving on a fixed concave surface, the convex surface moves opposite to the direction of the shaft of the bony lever.
   b. When a concave surface moves on a fixed convex surface, the concave articulating surface moves in the same direction as the bony lever (see Table 2-1).
   c. In the spine, the convex rule applies at the atlanto-occipital joint. Below the second vertebra, the concave rule applies.

Capsular Positions

1. Resting or loose-packed position (see Table 2-2).
   a. Joint position where capsule and other soft tissues are in most relaxed position.
   b. Minimal joint surface contact.
   c. May perform joint play and mobilization techniques in this joint position.
2. Close-packed position (see Table 2-2).
   a. Joint position where capsule and other soft tissues are maximally tensed.
   b. Maximal contact between joint surfaces.
   c. Joint play and mobilization cannot be properly performed in this position.
3. Selected capsular patterns (see Table 2-3).
4. End-feels.
   a. Normal physiological end-feel.
      - Soft: occurs with soft tissue approximation.
      - Firm: capsular and ligamentous stretching.
      - Hard: when bone and/or cartilage meet.
   b. Pathological end-feel.
      - Boggy: edema, joint swelling.
      - Firm with decreased elasticity: fibrosis of soft tissues.
      - Rubbery: muscle spasm.
      - Empty: loose, then very hard; associated with muscle guarding or patient avoiding painful part of range.
      - Hypermobility: end-feel at a later time than on opposite side.
5. Grading of accessory joint movement.
   a. Accessory joint movement or joint play is graded to assess arthrokinematic motion of the joint and/or when it is impractical or impossible to measure joint motion with a goniometer.
      - Movement is assessed in comparison to the uninvolved extremity or adjacent vertebral joints.
      - Graded normal, hypomobile, or hypermobile.
   b. Although interrater reliability is poor, intrarater reliability is acceptable.
   c. Data gleaned provides clinician with more specific data on source of patient's problem.

Muscle Substitutions

1. Occur when muscles have become shortened/lengthened, weakened, lost endurance, developed impaired coordination, or paralyzed.
2. Stronger muscles compensate for loss of motion.

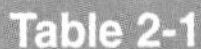

Concave-Convex Rule Application

ARTICULATION	FUNCTION	MOVING COMPONENT OF ARTICULATION	RELATIONSHIP OF CONVEX/CONCAVE RULE
Fingers	Flexion/extension	Distal phalanx	Concave moving on Convex
Metacarpal-phalangeal	Abduction/adduction	Proximal phalanx	Concave moving on Convex
Wrist	Flexion/extension	Capitate, scaphoid, lunate, triquetrum	Convex moving on Concave
		Trapezoid	Concave moving on Convex
Radioulnar			
Distal	Pronation/supination	Radius	Concave moving on Convex
Proximal	Pronation/supination	Radius	Convex moving on Concave
Humeroradial	Flexion/extension	Radius	Concave moving on Convex
Humeroulnar	Flexion/extension	Ulna	Concave moving on Convex
Glenohumeral	All movements	Humerus	Convex moving on Concave
Sternoclavicular	Elevation/depression	Clavicle	Convex moving on Concave
	Protraction/retraction	Clavicle	Concave moving on Convex
Acromioclavicular	All movements	Scapula	Concave moving on Convex
Toes	Flexion/extension	Distal phalanx	Concave moving on Convex
Metatarsal-phalangeal	Abduction/adduction	Proximal phalanx	Concave moving on Convex
Ankle/Foot			
Subtalar	All movements	Navicular, cuneiform	Concave moving on Convex
	Inversion/eversion	Cuboid, calcaneus	Convex moving on Concave
Talocrural	Dorsal/plantar flexion	Talus	Convex moving on Concave
Tibiofibular	All movements	Fibular head	Concave moving on Convex
Knee	All movements	Tibia	Concave moving on Convex
Hip	All movements	Femur	Convex moving on Concave
Temporomandibular	All movements	Mandible	Convex moving on Concave

Adapted from Kaltenborn F: Manual Mobilization of the Joints, Vol. 1: The Extremities, 8th ed. 2014.

Table 2-2

Joint Positions

ARTICULATIONS	RESTING POSITION	CLOSE-PACKED POSITION
Vertebral	Midway between flexion and extension	Maximal extension
Temporomandibular	Jaw slightly open (freeway space)	Maximal retrusion (mouth closed with teeth clenched) or maximal anterior position/mouth maximally opened/
Sternoclavicular	Arm resting by side	Arm maximally elevated
Acromioclavicular	Arm resting by side	Arm abducted 90°
Glenohumeral	40° to 55° abduction; 30° horizontal adduction (scapular plane)	Maximum abduction and ER
Elbow		
Humeroulnar	70° flexion and 10° supination	Full extension and supination
Humeroradial	Full extension and supination	90° flexion and 5° supination
Forearm		
Proximal radioulnar	70° flexion and 35° supination	5° supination
Distal radioulnar	10° supination	5° supination
Radio/ulnocarpal	Neutral with slight ulnar deviation	Full extension with radial deviation
Hand		
Midcarpal	Neutral or slight flexion with ulnar deviation	Extension with ulnar deviation
Carpometacarpal (2–5)	Midway between abduction-adduction and flexion-extension (thumb); midway between flexion and extension (fingers)	Full opposition (thumb); full flexion (fingers)
Metacarpophalangeal (MCP)	Slight flexion	Full opposition (thumb); full flexion (fingers)
Interphalangeal (IP)	Slight flexion	Full extension

(Continued)

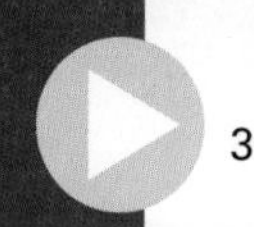

Table 2-2

Joint Positions (Continued)

ARTICULATIONS	RESTING POSITION	CLOSE-PACKED POSITION
Hip	30° flexion, 30° abduction, and slight lateral rotation	Full extension, abduction, internal rotation Bony: 90° flexion, slight abduction, and slight ER
Knee	25° flexion	Full extension and ER
Ankle/Foot		
Talocrural	Mid inversion/eversion and 10° plantar flexion	Full dorsiflexion
Subtalar	Midway between extremes of range of motion	Full inversion
Midtarsal	Midway between extremes of range of motion	Full supination
Tarsometatarsal	Midway between supination and pronation	Full supination
Toes		
Metatarsophalangeal	Neutral (extension 10°)	Full extension
Interphalangeal	Slight flexion	Full extension

Adapted from Magee DJ: Orthopedic Physical Assessment, 6th ed. 2014.

Table 2-3

Capsular Patterns

ARTICULATIONS	RELATIVE LIMITATIONS OF MOVEMENT
Temporomandibular	Limited mouth opening
Upper cervical spine (occiput–C2)	
Occipitoatlantal joint	Forward flexion limited greater than extension
Atlantoatlantal joint	Limitation with rotation
Lower cervical spine (C3–T2)	Limitation of all motions except flexion (side-bending and rotation equally limited and both greater than extension)
Glenohumeral	Greater limitation of ER, followed by abduction and internal rotation
Sternoclavicular	Full elevation limited; pain at extreme range of motion
Acromioclavicular	Full elevation limited; pain at extreme range of motion
Humeroulnar	Loss of flexion more so than extension
Humeroradial	Loss of flexion more so than extension
Proximal radioulnar	Limitation: pronation = supination
Distal radioulnar	Limitation: pronation = supination
Wrist	Limitation: flexion = extension
Midcarpal	Limitation: equal all directions
Trapeziometacarpal	Limitation: abduction more so than extension
Carpometacarpals II–V	Equally restricted all directions
Upper extremity digits	Limitation: flexion > extension
Thoracic spine	Limitation of side-bending and rotation > loss of extension > flexion
Lumbar spine	Marked and equal limitation of side-bending and rotation; loss of extension > flexion
Sacroiliac, symphysis pubis, sacrococcygeal	Pain when joints are stressed
Hip	Limited flexion/internal rotation; some limitation of abduction; no or little limitation of adduction and ER
Knee	Flexion grossly limited; slight limitation of extension
Tibiofibular (proximal & distal)	Pain when joint is stressed
Talocrural	Loss of plantarflexion greater than dorsiflexion
Talocalcaneal (subtalar)	Increasing limitations of varus; joint fixed in valgus (inversion > eversion)
Midtarsal	Supination > pronation (limited dorsiflexion, plantar flexion, adduction, and medial rotation)
First metatarsophalangeal	Marked limitation of extension; slight limitation of flexion
Metatarsophalangeal (II–V)	Variable; tend toward flexion restrictions
Interphalangeal	Tend toward extension restrictions

Adapted from Magee DJ: Orthopedic Physical Assessment, 6th ed. 2014.

3. Common muscle substitutions:
   a. Use of scapular stabilizers to initiate shoulder motion when shoulder abductors are weakened (reverse scapulothoracic rhythm).
   b. Use of lateral trunk muscles or tensor fascia latae (TFL) when hip abductors are weak.
   c. Use of passive finger flexion by contraction of wrist extensors when finger flexors are weak (tenodesis).
   d. Use of long head of biceps, coracobrachialis, and anterior deltoid when pectoralis major is weak.
   e. Use of lower back extensors, adductor magnus, and quadratus lumborum when hip extensors are weak.
   f. Use of lower abdominal, lower obliques, hip adductors, and latissimus dorsi when hip flexors are weak.

Functional Anatomy and Biomechanics

See Figures 2-1, 2-2, 2-3, and 2-4.

Shoulder Region

1. Osteology.
   a. Humerus (see Figure 2-5).
      - Proximal end of humerus is approximately half a spheroid.
      - Articular surface is covered by hyaline cartilage.
      - Head is retroverted 20°–30°.
      - Longitudinal axis of head is 135° from axis of neck.
   b. Scapula.
      - Large, flat triangular bone that sits over second to seventh ribs.
      - Costal surface and a dorsal surface.
      - Three angles: medial, superior, and lateral.
      - Lateral angle bears glenoid fossa, which faces anteriorly, laterally, and superiorly.
        - Pear shape of fossa allows for freer range of motion (ROM) in abduction and flexion.
        - Concave shape receives convex humeral head.
        - Orientation of the glenoid fossa places true abduction at 30° anterior to frontal plane.
   c. Clavicle.
      - Extends laterally and links manubrium to acromion.
      - Connects shoulder complex to axial skeleton.
2. Arthrology.
   a. Glenohumeral joint.
      - Convex humeral head articulates with concave glenoid fossa.
      - Glenoid fossa very shallow.
   b. Sternoclavicular joint.
      - Convex (superior/inferior) and concave (anterior/posterior) articulates with reciprocal shape of sternum.
      - Both articulations covered with fibrocartilage.
   c. Acromioclavicular joint.
      - A plane joint with relatively flat surfaces.
   d. Scapulothoracic joint.
      - A "clinical" articulation.
3. Muscles (depressors, elevators, protractors, retractors, internal rotators, external rotators, flexors, abductors, adductors, and extensors) (see Table 2-4).
4. Noncontractile structures.
   a. Glenohumeral joint capsule.
      - Attaches medially to glenoid margin, glenoid labrum, coracoid process.
      - Attaches laterally to humeral anatomical neck and descends approximately 1 cm on the shaft.
      - Supported by tendons of supraspinatus, infraspinatus, teres minor, subscapularis, and long head of triceps below.
      - Inferiorly capsule is least supported and most lax.
   b. Ligaments.
      - Coracohumeral ligament.
        - Base of coracoid process to greater and lesser tubercle of humerus.
        - Primary function to reinforce biceps tendon, reinforce superior capsule, and prevent caudal dislocation of humerus. Taut with external rotation (ER).
      - Coracoacromial ligament.
        - Strong triangular ligament runs from coracoid to acromion.
        - Not a "true" ligament; connects two points of same bone.
      - Glenohumeral ligaments.
        - Reinforce the glenohumeral joint capsule anteriorly and inferiorly.
        - Superior glenohumeral ligament: limits ER and inferior translation.
        - Middle glenohumeral ligament: limits ER and anterior translation.
        - Inferior glenohumeral ligament.
          - Anterior band: limits ER, anterior, and superior translation.
          - Posterior band: limits IR and anterior translation.
      - Transverse humeral ligament.
        - Broad band passing over top of bicipital groove.
        - Acts as a retinaculum for long biceps tendon.
   c. Labrum.
      - Glenoid labrum is a fibrocartilaginous ring that deepens glenoid fossa.
      - Attached to capsule superiorly and inferiorly as well as to the long head of the biceps tendon superiorly.
      - Internal surface covered with articular cartilage, which is thicker peripherally and thinner centrally.
      - Aids in lubrication, as in meniscus of knee, and serves to protect the bone.

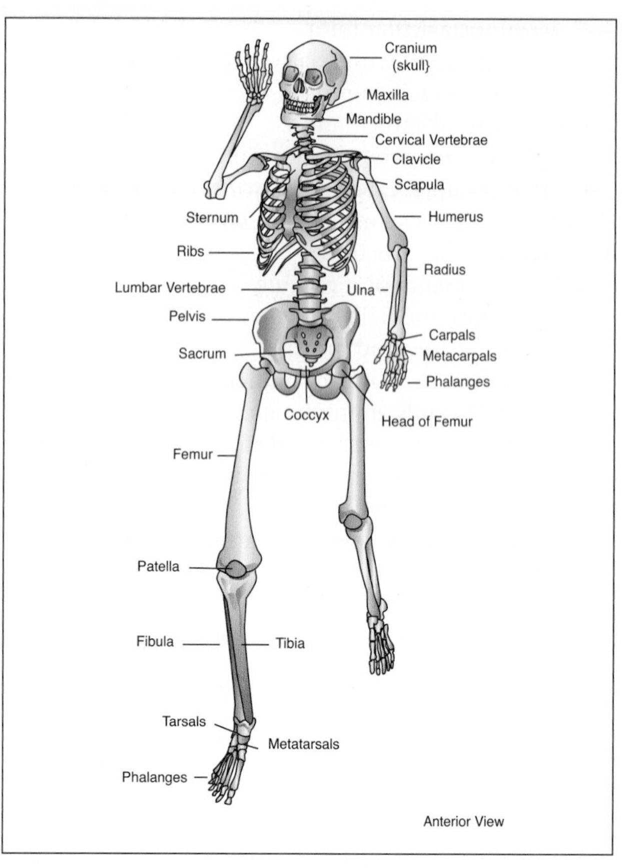

Figure 2-1 **Skeletal system—anterior view.**

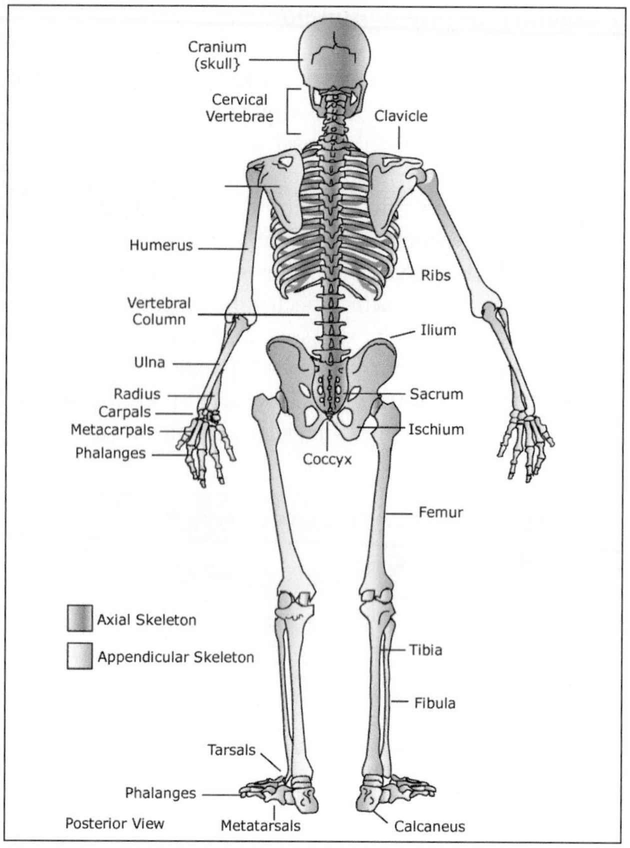

Figure 2-2 **Skeletal system—posterior view.**

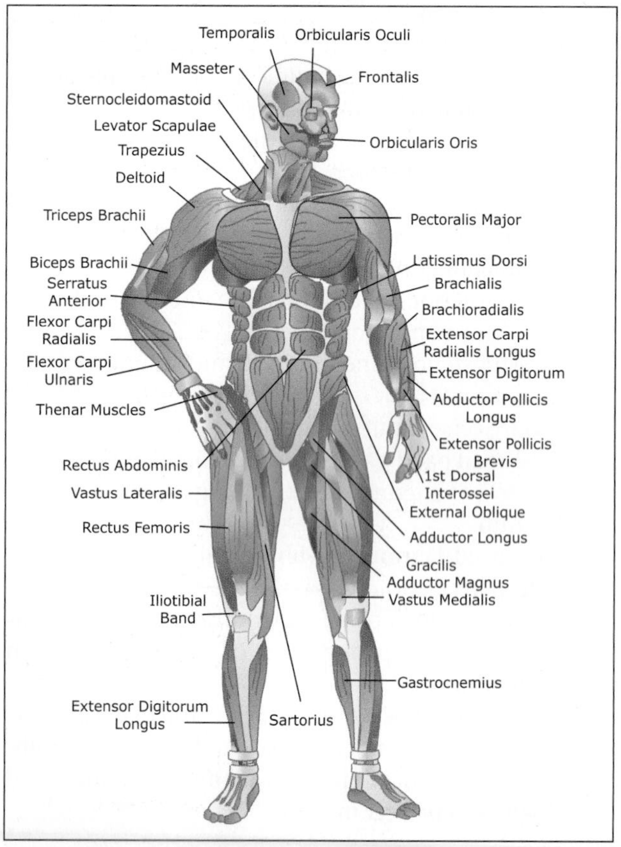

Figure 2-3 **Muscular system—anterior view.**

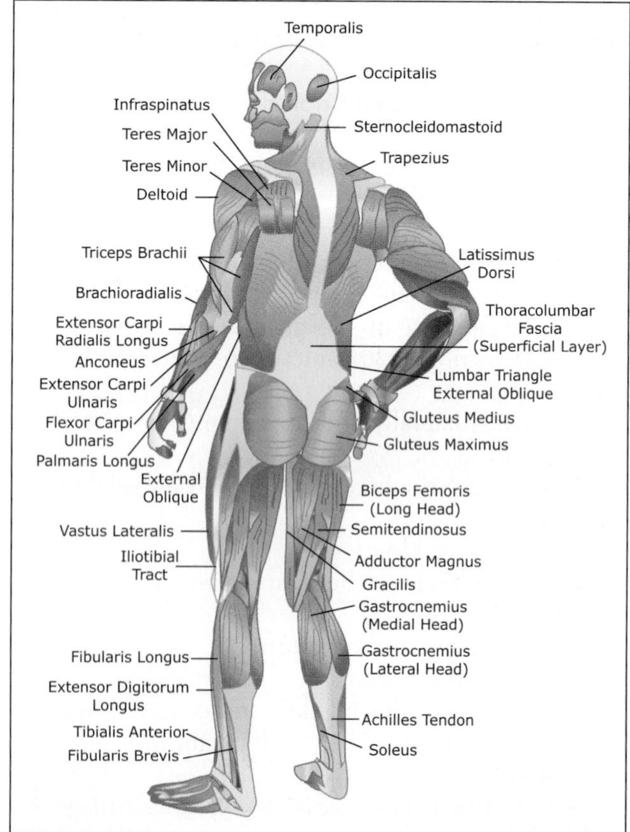

Figure 2-4 **Muscular system—posterior view.**

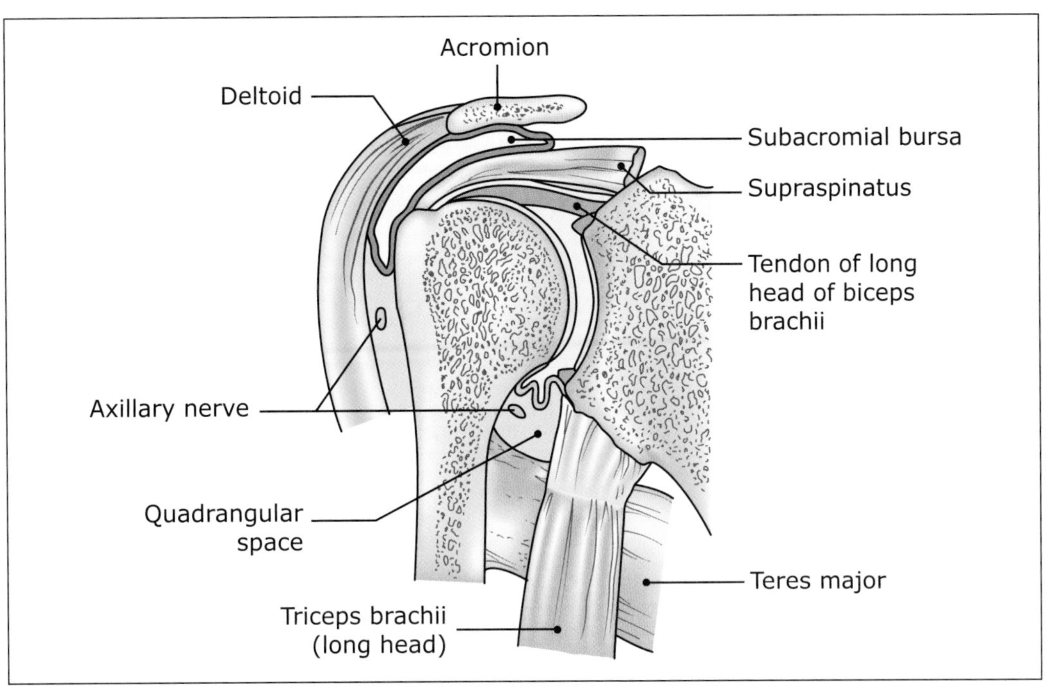

Figure 2-5 **Coronal section of shoulder.**

Table 2-4

Shoulder Girdle and Upper Extremity Muscles and Innervation

ACTION TO BE TESTED	MUSCLES	MYOTOMES	REFLEXES	CORD SEGMENT	NERVES
Neck flexion Neck extension Neck rotation Neck lateral bending	Sternocleidomastoid, trapezius, other deep neck muscles			C1–C4	C3-4 posterior rami; CN XI (spinal accessory)
Shoulder shrug, scapular upward rotation	Upper trapezius	C4		C1–C4	CN XI (spinal accessory)
Shoulder horizontal adduction	Pect. major/minor			C5–C8, T1	Medial/lateral pectoral
Scapular downward rotation	Pectoralis minor			C8–T1	Medial pectoral
Shoulder protraction, scapular upward rotation	Serratus anterior			C5–C7	Long thoracic
Scapular elevation, downward rotation	Levator scapula			C5	Dorsal scapular
Scapular adduction, elevation, downward rotation	Rhomboids			C4–C5	Dorsal scapular
Shoulder abduction	Supraspinatus			C4–C6	Suprascapular
Shoulder lateral rotation	Infraspinatus			C4–C6	Suprascapular
Shoulder medial rotation, adduction	Latissimus dorsi, teres major, subscapularis, and pectoralis major			C5–T1	Thoracodorsal, upper/lower subscapular, and medial/lateral pectoral
Shoulder abduction, flexion, extension	Deltoid	C5		C5–C6	Axillary
Shoulder lateral rotation	Teres minor			C5–6	Axillary
Elbow flexion, forearm supination	Biceps brachii	C6	C5	C5–C6	Musculocutaneous

(*Continued*)

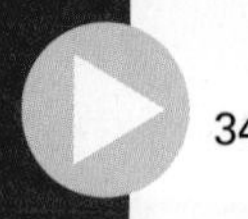

Table 2-4

Shoulder Girdle and Upper Extremity Muscles and Innervation (Continued)

ACTION TO BE TESTED	MUSCLES	MYOTOMES	REFLEXES	CORD SEGMENT	NERVES
Shoulder flexion, adduction	Coracobrachialis			C6–C7	Musculocutaneous
Elbow flexion	Brachialis, biceps brachii			C5–C6	Musculocutaneous
4th and 5th digit DIP flexion	Flexor digitorum profundus (ulnar part)			C7–T1	Ulnar
Wrist ulnar flexion	Flexor carpi ulnaris	C7		C7–T1	Ulnar
Thumb adduction	Adductor pollicis			C8–T1	Ulnar (deep ulnar)
5th digit abduction	Abductor digiti minimi			C8–T1	Ulnar (deep ulnar)
5th digit opposition	Opponens digiti minimi			C8–T1	Ulnar (deep ulnar)
5th digit MCP flexion	Flexor digiti minimi brevis			C8–T1	Ulnar (deep ulnar)
2nd–5th digit MCP flexion, adduction, abduction	Interossei	T1		C8–T1	Ulnar (deep ulnar)
Forearm pronation	Pronator teres, pronator quadratus			C6–C7	Median (anterior interosseous)
Wrist radial flexion	Flexor carpi radialis			C6–C7	Median
Wrist flexion	Palmaris longus			C7–T1	Median
2nd–5th digit proximal IP flexion	Flexor digitorum superficialis			C7–T1	Median
Thumb IP flexion	Flexor pollicis longus			C7–T1	Median (anterior interosseous)
2nd–3rd digit distal IP flexion	Flexor digitorum profundus (radial part)			C7–T1	Median (anterior interosseous)
Thumb abduction	Abductor pollicis brevis			C8–T1	Median
Thumb MCP flexion	Flexor pollicis brevis			C8–T1	Median/ulnar
Thumb opposition	Opponens pollicis			C8–T1	Median
2nd–5th digit MCP flexion, IP extension	Lumbricals			C8–T1	Median/ulnar
Elbow flexion in mid-supination/pronation	Brachioradialis		C6	C5–C6	Radial
Elbow extension	Triceps brachii		C7	C6–C8	Radial
Wrist extension/radial deviation	Extensor carpi radialis longus			C6–C7	Radial
2nd–5th digit MCP, IP extension	Extensor digitorum			C7–C8	Radial (deep radial)
Wrist ulnar extension	Extensor carpi ulnaris			C7–C8	Radial (deep radial)
Forearm supination	Supinator			C7–C8	Radial (deep radial)
Thumb MCP abduction	Abductor pollicis longus	C8		C7–C8	Radial (posterior interosseous)
Thumb extension	Extensor pollicis longus/brevis			C7–C8	Radial (posterior interosseous)
2nd digit extension	Extensor indicis			C7–C8	Radial (posterior interosseous)

Adapted from Kendall FP, et al: Muscles: Testing and Function, with Posture and Pain, 5th ed. 2005.

d. Bursae.

- Multiple bursae found within this region.
- Primary bursa involved with pathology is subacromial bursa between deltoid and capsule. Also runs under acromion and coracoacromial ligament and between the supraspinatus tendon.

5. Shoulder biomechanics.

a. Glenohumeral joint arthrokinematics/osteokinematics.

- Occurs in opposite directions. With elevation of humerus, head of humerus moves in an inferior direction because of convex moving on concave.

- Rolling-gliding occurs during elevation of the humerus, so that the instantaneous center of rotation varies considerably during the complete range.
- At approximately 75° of elevation, ER (conjunct rotation) occurs, preventing compression of greater tubercle against the acromion.

b. Scapulothoracic and glenohumeral rhythm (scapulohumeral rhythm) is the ratio of movement of the glenohumeral with the scapulothoracic joint.
- Maximum range of elevation is 150° to 180°.
- The glenohumeral joint contributes 100° to 120° of flexion and 90° to 120° of abduction.
- An overall 2:1 ratio of glenohumeral : scapulothoracic motion is described, although substantial variability exists between individuals.
- The first 30° to 60° of elevation occurs mainly in the glenohumeral joint.

c. Requirements of full elevation.
- Scapular stabilization.
- Inferior glide of humerus.
- ER of humerus.
- Rotation of the clavicle at sternoclavicular joint.
- Scapular abduction and lateral rotation of acromioclavicular joint.
- Straightening of thoracic kyphosis.

Elbow Region

1. Osteology and arthrology (ulnohumeral, radiohumeral, superior, and inferior radioulnar).
   a. Humeroulnar joint (see Figure 2-6).
   - Distal end humerus (trochlea) articulates with proximal end of ulna.
   - Trochlea and trochlear notch face anteriorly at a 45° angle, allowing space between ulna and humerus during flexion.

   b. Humeroradial joint.
   - Distal end humerus (capitulum) articulates with concave oval facet of proximal radius.

   c. Proximal radioulnar joint.
   - Radial head is ovoid and cone-shaped.
   - Medial radius articulates with radial notch (of ulna).

   d. Distal radioulnar joint.
   - Convex ulna articulates with concave radius (opposite to proximal articulation of these two bones).
2. Muscles (flexors, extensors, supinators, and pronators) (see Table 2-4).
3. Noncontractile structures (ulnar collateral ligament, radial collateral ligament, annular ligament, elbow capsule, associated bursae, nerves, and vessels).
   a. Capsule.
   - Encloses entire elbow joint complex. It is thin, both anteriorly and posteriorly. Continuous medially

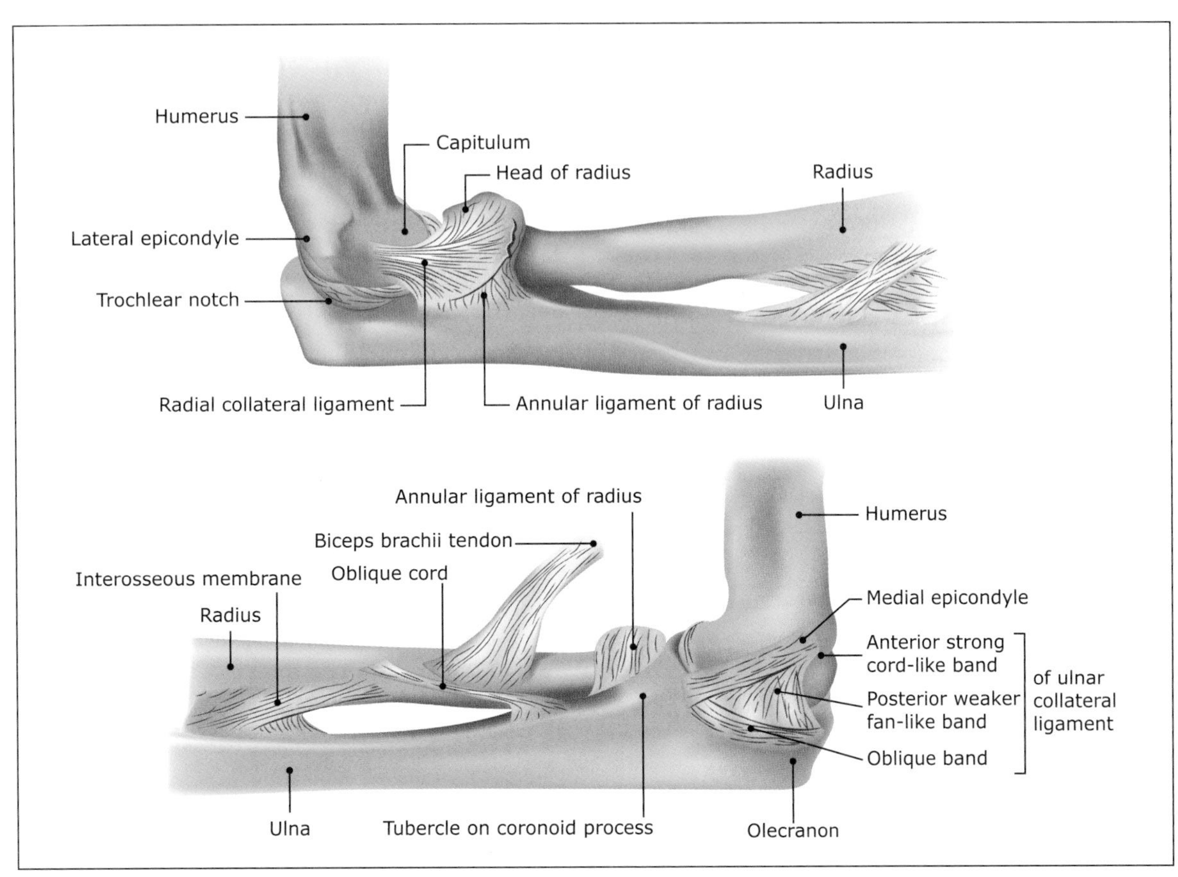

Figure 2-6 **Elbow: lateral view.**

with ulnar collateral ligament and laterally with radial collateral ligament.

b. Ligaments.
- Ulnar collateral.
  - anterior band, posterior band, oblique band
  - Ligament is triangular-shaped consisting of three parts.
  - Reinforces humeroulnar joint medially.
- Radial collateral.
  - Ligament is fan-shaped and runs from lateral epicondyle of humerus to annular ligament.
  - Reinforces humeroradial joint laterally.
- Annular.
  - An osteofibrous ring attached to medial ulna and encircles radial head.
  - Cone shaped, inner surface is lined with fibrocartilage.
  - Protects radial head, especially in semi-flexion, where it is very unstable. Taut in extremes of pronation and supination.
- Quadrate.
  - Extends from radial notch (ulna) to the neck of radius.
  - Reinforces inferior joint capsule, maintains radial head in opposition to ulna, limits amount of spin in supination and pronation.
- Distal radioulnar.
  - Anterior radioulnar ligament: primarily strengthens capsule.
  - Posterior radioulnar ligament: primarily strengthens capsule.

c. Bursa.
- Olecranon bursa located on posterior aspect of elbow over olecranon process.

d. Blood supply.
- Elbow joint receives blood supply from brachial artery, anterior ulnar recurrent artery, posterior ulnar recurrent artery, radial recurrent artery, and middle collateral branch of the deep brachial artery.

e. Elbow joint stability.
- Elbow joint complex possesses significant inherent stability.
- Main contributor to bony stability is articulation between the trochlea (humerus) and trochlear fossa (ulna).
- Ulnar collateral ligament provides strong resistance to valgus forces.
- Resistance of radial collateral ligament to varus forces is minimal, due to its attachment to another soft tissue structure (annular ligament).
- Functionally, this relationship is beneficial, since functional activities place tensile forces medially and compressive forces laterally. Therefore, the lateral ligament does not have to be as strong as the medial ligament.

4. Elbow biomechanics.

a. Conjunct rotations.
- Ulna pronates slightly with extension. Ulna supinates slightly with flexion.
- Proximal ulna glides medially during extension and laterally during flexion.
- Flexion/extension of elbow is accompanied by a screw-home mechanism with conjunct rotation of ulna. Ulna externally rotates (or supinates) during elbow flexion and internally rotates (or pronates) during elbow extension.

Wrist and Hand Region

1. Osteology (radius, ulna, carpals, metacarpals, and phalanges) (see Figure 2-7).

a. Radius is biconcave relative to carpals.

b. Ulna is convex at its distal end relative to the triquetrum.

c. Proximal aspect of proximal row is biconvex. Distal aspect of proximal row is concave at lunate/capitate

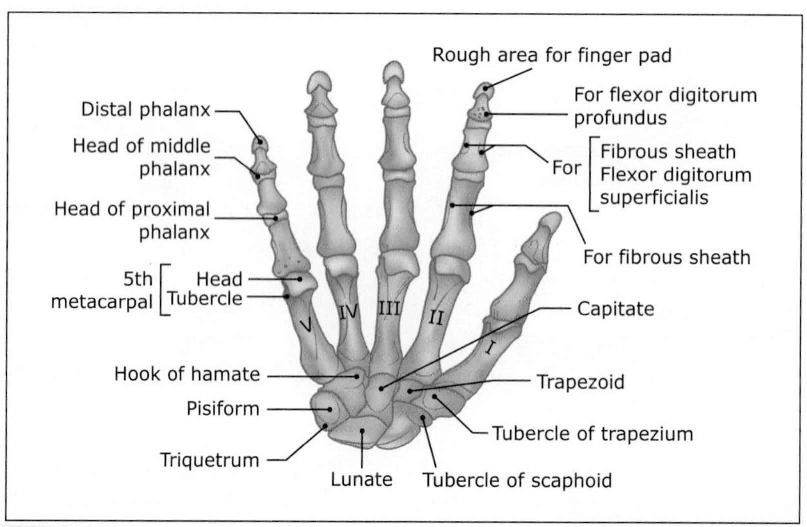

Figure 2-7 **Bones of the hand.**

and triquetrum/hamate articulations. Scaphoid is convex anterior/posterior and concave medial/lateral relative to trapezium/trapezoid. Capitate is convex and articulates with concavities of scaphoid, hamate, and trapezoid.

d. Metacarpal heads are biconvex, and bases are generally flat relative to distal row of carpals.

e. Phalanges' proximal ends are mostly biconcave, with a ridge running down the center, dividing it into two surfaces. Distal end is pulley-shaped, and mostly biconvex, with a groove running through the center.

2. Arthrology (radiocarpal, midcarpal, carpometacarpal, metacarpophalangeal [MCP], and interphalangeal [IP]).
   a. Radiocarpal joint.
      - Convex scaphoid and lunate articulate with concave radius.
   b. Midcarpal joint.
      - Articulation between four proximal and four distal carpal bones is known as midcarpal joint.
      - Functional rather than anatomical joint.
      - Can be divided into middle pillar (lunate and triquetrum with capitate and hamate) and lateral pillar (scaphoid with trapezoid and trapezium).
   c. Carpometacarpal (CMC) joint.
      - First CMC (thumb) is a saddle articulation with trapezium being convex in medial/lateral direction and concave in anterior/posterior direction.
      - First metacarpal is opposite in shape to trapezium.
      - The second through fifth CMC joints are essentially flat between bases of metacarpals and distal row of carpals.
   d. Metacarpalphalangeal (MCP) joints consist of convex metacarpals with concave proximal phalanges.
   e. Proximal interphalangeal (PIP) joints consist of convex distal aspects of proximal phalanges with concave proximal aspect of middle phalanges. Same orientation exists at distal interphalangeal (DIP) joints.
3. Muscles (wrist flexors, wrist extensors, radial deviators, ulnar deviators, extrinsic finger flexors, extrinsic finger extensors, and intrinsic finger muscles) (see Table 2-4).
4. Noncontractile structures (volar carpal, radiocarpal, collateral, and palmar ligaments; extensor hood; associated capsules; volar plate; nerves; and vessels).
   a. Ligaments.
      - Fingers (see Figure 2-8).
         - Collaterals: run separately from lateral condyle to distal phalanx and lateral volar plate at each MP, PIP, and DIP joint. All fibers tighten with flexion and volar fibers tighten with extension.
         - Accessory: run from condylar head to volar plate.
         - Transverse: present at MCP joints. Provide stability linking MCP joints and providing reinforcement to anterior capsule.
      - Wrist.
         - Dorsal radiocarpal: limits flexion, pronation, and possibly radial deviation.
         - Radiate: stabilizes hand for any impact.

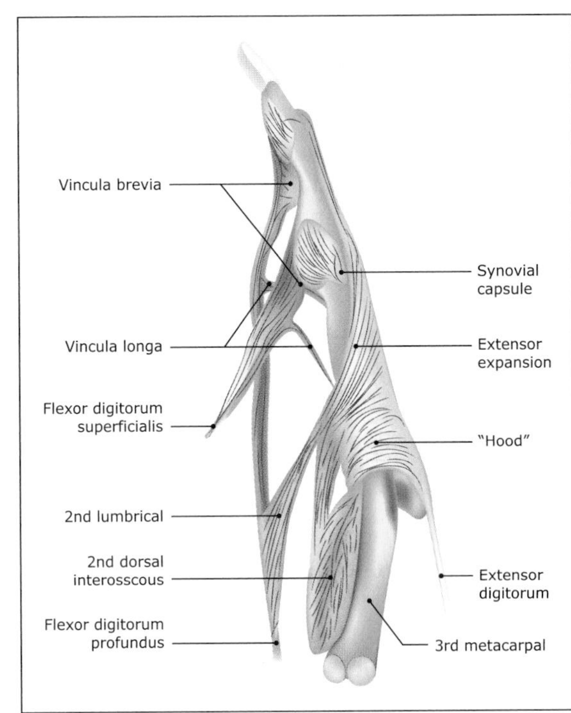

Figure 2-8 **Dissection of the third digit.**

         - Radial collateral: limits ulnar deviation.
         - Ulnar collateral: limits radial deviation.
         - Palmar ulnocarpal: limits extension and supination.
         - Palmar radiocarpal: limits extension and supination through knuckles.
   b. Extensor hood.
      - Fibrous mechanism on the dorsum of each finger that is a fibrous expansion of the extensor digitorum tendon.
      - Its purpose is to assist with extension of the PIP and DIP joints.
   c. Capsule.
      - Fingers.
         - MCP, PIP, and DIP joints all have fibrous capsules that are strong but lax and supported by ligaments.
      - Wrist.
         - Radiocarpal joint shares fibrous capsule (which is thicker palmarly and dorsally) with midcarpal joint, but usually has its own synovial membrane.
   d. Volar plate.
      - Present on palmar aspect of the MCP, PIP, and DIP joints. Thickening of capsule. Functions to increase articular surface during extension and protect joint volarly. Volar plate more mobile at MCP than at IPs.
   e. Nerves.
      - Ulnar innervates hypothenar region (palmarly and dorsally), fifth digit, and medial half of fourth digit.
      - Median nerve innervates remainder of palmar surface not innervated by ulnar nerve and

dorsal portions of second, third, and lateral half of fourth digit from DIP joint to tip of finger.
- Radial nerve innervates remainder of dorsum of hand not innervated by ulnar or median nerves.

f. Blood supply from ulna and radial arteries. Merge to form palmar arch and then send digital branches that run up medial and lateral aspects of each digit.

5. Hand and wrist biomechanics.
   a. Hand.
   - PIPs and DIPs.
     - During flexion digits rotate radially to enhance grasp and opposition.
   - MCPs.
     - During flexion digits rotate radially to enhance grasp and opposition.
   - First CMC.
     - Due to position of trapezium (anteriorly and medially rotated relative to other carpals) plane of flexion/extension is perpendicular to other digits.
     - During flexion/extension, it is concave moving on convex.
     - During abduction/adduction, it is convex moving on concave.
     - During flexion and abduction, the first metacarpal rotates ulnarly.
     - During extension and adduction, the first metacarpal rotates radially.

   b. Wrist.
   - Flexion. Proximal aspect of scaphoid/lunate glide dorsally relative to radius.
   - Extension. Proximal aspect of scaphoid/lunate glide ventrally relative to radius.
   - Radial deviation. Proximal row glides ulnarly. Proximal surface of scaphoid rotates palmarly.
   - Ulnar deviation. Proximal row glides radially as a unit.

Hip Region

1. Osteology (femur and acetabulum of pelvis) (see Figure 2-9).
   a. Femur.
   - Head is two-thirds of a sphere with a depression at its center called the fovea capitis femoris.
   - Head is oriented superiorly, anteriorly, and medially.
   - Articular cartilage covers entire head, except for fovea capitis.
   - Angle of inclination normally 115°–125°.
     - Coxa valga is angle >125°.
     - Coxa vara is angle <115°.
   - Femoral neck angles anteriorly 10°–15° from frontal plane to form anterior antetorsion angle.
     - Anteversion: considered excessive if anterior antetorsion angle >25°–30°.
     - Retroversion: considered excessive if anterior antetorsion angle <10°.

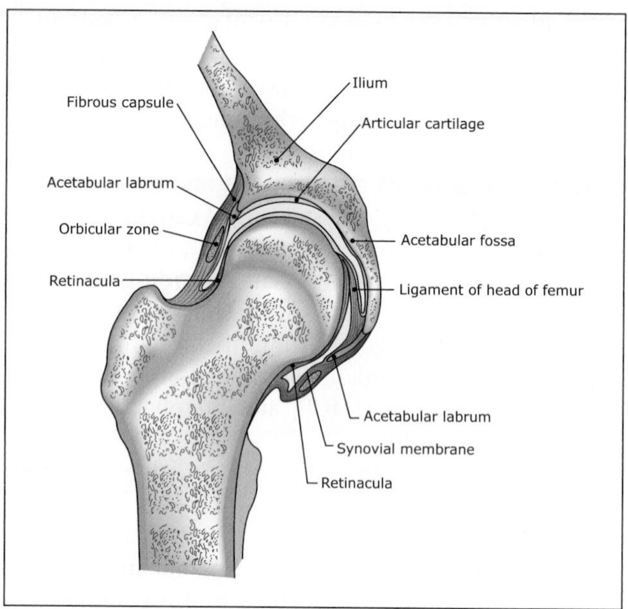

Figure 2-9 **Hip joint osteology: anterior view.**

   b. Acetabulum.
   - Acetabulum faces laterally, inferiorly, and anteriorly.
   - Made of union between ischium, ilium, and pubis bones.
   - Acetabular fossa: center of acetabulum, which is nonarticulating and filled with fat pad for shock absorption.
   - Acetabulum is not completely covered with cartilage. Lined with a horseshoe-shaped articular cartilage with interruption inferiorly forming acetabular notch.

2. Arthrology (coxofemoral).
   a. Synovial joint.
   b. Convex femoral head articulates with concave acetabulum.
   c. Very stable joint due to bony anatomy as well as strength of ligaments and capsule.
   d. Zone of weakness in the femoral neck in where trabeculae are relatively thin and do not cross each other.
3. Muscles (flexors, extensors, adductors, abductors, internal rotators [IRs], and external rotators [ERs]) (see Table 2-5).
4. Noncontractile structures (capsule, labrum, bursae, iliofemoral ligament, ischiofemoral ligament, pubofemoral ligament, and associated nerves and vessels) (see Figure 2-10).
   a. Capsule is strong and dense, and encloses the entire joint.
   b. Labrum.
   - Triangular-shaped, made up of a fibrocartilaginous ring, thickest superiorly.
   - Attaches to bony rim of acetabulum, bridging acetabular notch.

Table 2-5

Pelvic Girdle and Lower Extremity Muscles and Innervation

ACTION TO BE TESTED	MUSCLES	MYOTOMES	REFLEXES	CORD SEGMENT	NERVES
Hip flexion	Iliopsoas	L2		L1–L3	Anterior rami
Hip flexion, abduction, lateral rotation	Sartorius	L2		L2–L3	Femoral
Knee extension	Quadriceps femoris	L3	L4	L2–L4	Femoral
Hip adduction	Pectineus, adductor longus			L2–L3	Obturator
Hip adduction	Adductor brevis			L2–L4	Obturator
Hip adduction	Gracilis			L2–L4	Obturator
Hip abduction, flexion, medial rotation	Gluteus medius, minimus	L5		L4–S1	Superior gluteal
Hip flexion, abduction, medial rotation	Tensor fascia lata			L4–L5	Superior gluteal
Hip lateral rotation	Piriformis			L5–S1	Sacral plexus
Hip extension, lateral rotation	Gluteus maximus			L4–S2	Inferior gluteal
Hip lateral rotation	Obturator internus			L5–S1	Sacral plexus
Hip lateral rotation	Gemelli, quadratus femoris			L5–S1	Sacral plexus
Hip extension, knee flexion, leg lateral rotation	Biceps femoris			L5–S2	Tibial, common fibular
Hip extension, knee flexion	Semitendinosus		L5	L5–S2	Tibial
Leg medial rotation	Semimembranosus			L5–S2	Tibial
Ankle dorsiflexion	Tibialis anterior	L4		L4–L5	Deep fibular
2nd–5th digit MTP extension	Extensor digitorum longus			L4–S1	Deep fibular
Great toe MTP extension	Extensor hallucis longus	L5		L4–S1	Deep fibular
Foot eversion	Fibularis longus/brevis	S1		L5–S2	Superficial fibular
Leg medial rotation	Popliteus			L4–S1	Tibial
Foot inversion	Tibialis posterior	S1		L5–S2	Tibial
Ankle plantar flexion	Gastrocnemius/soleus		S1	L5–S2	Tibial
2nd–5th digit DIP flexion	Flexor digitorum longus			L5–S2	Tibial
Great toe IP flexion	Flexor hallucis longus			L5–S2	Tibial
2nd–5th digit PIP flexion	Flexor digitorum brevis			L5–S1	Medial plantar
Great toe MTP flexion	Flexor hallucis brevis			L5–S2	Medial plantar
Toe adduction/abduction	Dorsal/plantar interossei			S1–S2	Lateral plantar
Pelvic floor control	Perineals and sphincters			S3–4	Sacral plexus

Adapted from Kendall FP, et al: Muscles: Testing and Function, with Posture and Pain, 5th ed. 2005.

- Serves to deepen acetabulum.
- Inner surface is lined with articular cartilage, and outer surface connects to joint capsule.

c. Ligaments.

- Iliofemoral ligament ("Y" or ligament of Bigelow).
    - Two bands, both starting from anterior inferior iliac spine (AIIS). Medial running to distal intertrochanteric line. Lateral running to proximal aspect of intertrochanteric line.
    - Very strong.
    - Both bands taut with extension and ER. Superior band taut with adduction. Inferior band taut with abduction.
- Pubofemoral ligament.
    - Runs from iliopectineal eminence, superior rami of pubis, obturator crest, and obturator membrane, laterally blending with capsule; inserts into same point as medial iliofemoral ligament.
    - Taut with extension, ER, and abduction.
- Ischiofemoral ligament.
    - Runs from ischium and posterior acetabulum, superiorly and laterally, blending with zona articularis, and attaching to greater trochanter.
    - Taut with medial rotation, abduction, and extension.

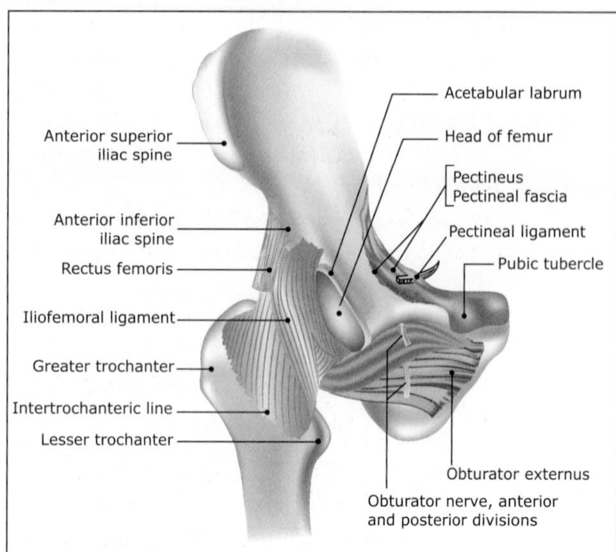

Figure 2-10 Hip joint: ligament and muscular attachments.

- Zona orbicularis.
  - Runs in a circular pattern around femoral neck.
  - Has no bony attachments, but helps to hold head of femur in acetabulum.
- Inguinal ligament.
  - 12–14 cm long, running from anterior superior iliac spine (ASIS) medially and inferiorly, attaching to pubic tubercle.
  - Forms tunnel for muscles, arteries, veins, and nerves.

d. Bursae.
- Subtendinous iliac, located between hip and os pubis.
- Iliopectineal between tendons of psoas major, iliacus, and capsule. Lies close to femoral nerve.
- Ischiofemoral between ischial tuberosity and gluteus maximus. May cause pain in sciatic distribution.
- Deep trochanteric between gluteus maximus and posterior lateral greater trochanter. May cause pain with hip flexion and internal rotation due to compression of gluteus maximus.
- Superficial trochanteric located over greater trochanter.

e. Innervation of hip joint comes from femoral, obturator, sciatic, and superior gluteal nerves.

f. Blood supply.
- Medial and lateral femoral circumflex supplies proximal femur.
- Femoral head is supplied by a small branch off obturator artery.
- Acetabulum is supplied by branches from superior and inferior gluteal arteries.

g. Hip biomechanics.
- Coxofemoral joint arthrokinematics/osteokinematics occur in opposite directions due to relationship of convex femoral head moving within concave acetabulum.
- Normal gait on level ground requires at least the following hip joint ranges of motion: 30° flexion, 10° extension, 5° abduction/adduction, and 5° internal/external rotation.
- Walking on uneven terrain or stairs and activities such as sitting in a chair or sitting cross-legged increase joint range of motion requirements.
- Many movements, such as forward bending, involve combined movements of the femur, pelvis, and lumbar spine, with many factors contributing to the relative contributions.

Knee Region

1. Osteology (femur, tibia, fibula, and patella) (see Figures 2-11 and 2-12).
   a. Femur.
   - Femoral condyles are convex in anterior/posterior and medial/lateral planes.
   - Both femoral condyles are spiral, but lateral one has a longer surface area and medial one descends further inferiorly.

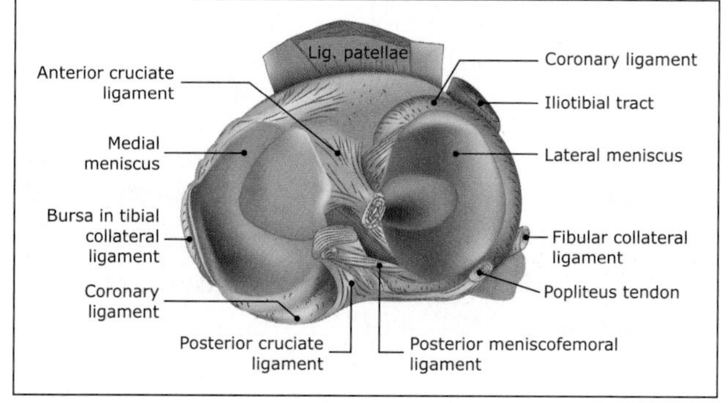

Figure 2-11 Knee: coronal view.

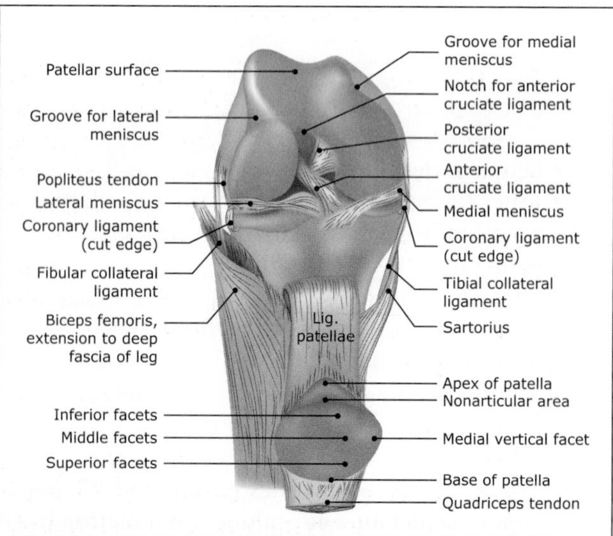

Figure 2-12 Knee: anterior view, cutaway.

b. Tibia.
- Medial tibial condyle is biconcave, has a larger surface area and is more stable, and therefore less mobile.
- Lateral tibial condyle is convex anterior/posterior and concave medial/lateral. Smaller surface area, more circular, and less stable, therefore more mobile.
- Both tibial surfaces are raised where they border intercondylar area.

c. Patella.
- A vertical ridge divides patella into a larger and smaller medial part.
- Patella can further be divided by two faint horizontal ridges that divide it into its facets.

2. Arthrology (tibiofemoral, patellofemoral, and proximal tibiofibular).

a. Proximal tibiofibular joint.
- Oval tibial facet is flat or slightly convex.
- Fibular head has an oval, slightly concave to flat surface.

b. Tibiofemoral joint.
- Synovial hinge joint with two degrees of freedom.
- Minimal bony stability thus relies on capsule, ligaments, and muscles.

c. Patellofemoral joint.
- Patella articular surface is adapted to patellar surface of femur.
- An oblique groove running inferiorly and laterally is the guiding mechanism on femur for patellar tracking. Patellar surface of femur is concave transversely and convex sagittally, creating its saddle (sellar) shape.

3. Muscles (flexors, tibial rotators, and extensors) (see Table 2-5).

4. Noncontractile structures (medial collateral ligament, lateral collateral ligament, anterior cruciate ligament, posterior cruciate ligament, menisci, capsule, bursae and associated nerves and vessels).

a. Capsule.
- Tibiofemoral capsule is a fibrous sleeve attached to distal femur and proximal tibia. Inner wall is covered by a synovium. Shaped as a cylinder with a posterior invagination, which posteriorly divides cavity into medial and lateral halves. Anterior surface has a window cut out for patella.
- Proximal tibiofibular joint has a fibrous capsule, which is continuous with knee joint capsule 10% of time.

b. Ligaments (see Figure 2-12).
- Tibiofemoral and patellofemoral joints (knee joint proper).
  - Medial collateral ligament (MCL): runs from medial aspect of medial femoral condyle to upper end of tibia. Posterior fibers blend with capsule. Runs oblique anteriorly and inferiorly. Taut in extension and slackened in flexion. Prevents ER and provides stability against valgus forces. Runs in same direction as anterior cruciate ligament.
  - Lateral collateral ligament (LCL): runs from lateral femoral condyle to head of fibula. Free of any capsular attachment. Runs oblique inferiorly and posteriorly in same direction as posterior cruciate ligament. Taut in extension and slackened in flexion. Prevents ER and provides stability against varus forces.
  - Anterior cruciate ligament (ACL): attaches to anterior intercondylar fossa of tibia and to femur at medial aspect of lateral condyle. Runs oblique superiorly and laterally. Extracapsular, but more correctly a thickening of the capsule. Limits anterior translation of the tibia on the femur and provides rotational stability.
  - Posterior cruciate ligament (PCL): attaches to posterior intercondylar fossa of tibia and on lateral surface of femoral medial condyle. Runs oblique medially and anteriorly-superiorly. Checks posterior displacement of tibia on femur.
  - Meniscofemoral ligament runs with PCL: attaches below posterior horn of lateral meniscus. Has common insertion into lateral aspect of medial condyle. Occasionally a similar ligament exists medially.
  - Oblique popliteal ligament: inserts into expansion from tendon of semimembranosus. It partially blends with capsule. Forms floor of popliteal fossa and is in contact with popliteal anterior artery. Strengthens posteromedial capsule.
  - Arcuate popliteal ligament: Y-shaped and commonly described as having two bands (medial and lateral). Stem attaches to fibular head. Medial band attaches to posterior border of intercondylar area of tibia. Lateral band extends to lateral epicondyle of femur. Strengthens posterolateral capsule.
  - Transverse ligament: connects lateral and medial meniscus anteriorly.
  - Meniscopatellar ligament: runs from inferolateral edges of patella to lateral borders of each meniscus. Pulls menisci forward with extension.
  - Alar fold: runs from lateral borders of patella to medial and lateral aspects of femoral condyles. Keeps patella in contact with femur.
- Infrapatellar fold: formed by attachments of patella fat pad and tendons via a fibroadipose band lying in intercondylar notch. Acts as stop gap as it is compressed by patella tendon in full flexion.
- Proximal tibiofibular joint ligaments.
  - Anterior tibiofibular ligament: located on anterior aspect of joint. Reinforces capsule anteriorly.
  - Posterior tibiofibular ligament: located on posterior aspect of joint. Reinforces capsule posteriorly.

c. Menisci.
- Medial meniscus.
  - Medial meniscus is large, C-shaped, and fairly stable. Laterally, it is firmly attached to MCL and fibrous capsule. Other structures that attach to the medial meniscus are semimembranosus muscle and medial meniscopatellar ligament.
- Lateral meniscus.
  - Smaller than medial meniscus and more circular. Structures that attach to lateral meniscus include popliteus muscle, lateral meniscopatellar ligament, and meniscofemoral ligament. Lateral meniscus is separated from LCL and lateral capsule by popliteus muscle tendon.
- Function of menisci.
  - Deepens fossa of tibia.
  - Increases congruency of tibia and femur.
  - Provides stability to tibiofemoral joint.
  - Provides shock absorption and lubrication to knee.
  - Reduces friction during movement.
  - Improves weight distribution.
- Movement of menisci.
  - Menisci follow tibia with flexion/extension and femoral condyles with internal/external rotation.
  - Medial meniscus moves a total of 6 mm while lateral moves 12 mm. With isolated tibial rotation, the menisci move opposite; e.g., with tibial IR, the medial meniscus moves anteriorly and the lateral meniscus moves posteriorly.
  - Meniscal motion is also influenced by soft tissue structures. Medial meniscus is pulled posteriorly (flexion) by semimembranosus muscle and ACL. Pulled anteriorly (extension) by medial meniscopatellar ligament. Held firm by attachment to MCL and fibrous capsule.
  - Lateral meniscus pulled posteriorly (flexion) by popliteus muscle and anteriorly (extension) by lateral meniscopatellar ligament and meniscofemoral ligament.

d. Bursae.
- Prepatellar, between skin and anterior distal patella.
- Superficial infrapatellar, anterior to ligamentum patella.
- Deep infrapatellar, between posterior ligamentum patella and anterior tibial tuberosity.
- Suprapatellar, between patella and tibia femoral joint.
- Popliteal, posterior knee often connected to synovial cavity.
- Semimembranosus, between muscle and femoral condyle.
- Gastrocnemius, one for each head. Medial bursa usually communicates with semimembranosus bursa.
- Pes anserine bursa, between pes anserine and MCL.

e. Blood supply comes from descending branch from lateral circumflex femoral branch of the deep femoral artery. Genicular branches of popliteal artery and recurrent branches of anterior tibial artery.

f. Articular innervation is provided by obturator, femoral, tibial, and common fibular nerves.

5. Biomechanics knee joint proper.

a. Arthrokinematics/osteokinematics.
- Movements of femoral condyles during flexion and extension.
  - Condyles roll and glide simultaneously (only way that posterior dislocation of femoral condyle can be avoided). Initially, movement is pure rolling and ends in pure gliding. For medial condyle, pure rolling occurs during first 10°–15° of flexion. For lateral condyle, 20° of flexion.
  - During flexion, femoral condyles roll posteriorly; ACL becomes taut, causing condyles to glide anteriorly.
  - During extension, femoral condyles roll anteriorly; PCL becomes taut, causing condyles to glide posteriorly.
- During walking, normal range of knee flexion is approximately 15°. We are essentially using pure rolling of femur on tibia.

b. Conjunct rotations.
- During flexion at 10°–15°, ACL tightens, causing femur to glide anteriorly, then 5° further, rolling occurs on lateral condyle, causing a conjunct medial rotation of tibia.
- During extension, PCL causes femur to glide posteriorly, while condyles roll anteriorly 10°–15°. Then a further 5° of rolling occurs anteriorly on lateral side, causing a medial femoral rotation or a lateral rotation of tibia as a conjunct rotation with extension.
- "Screw home" mechanism describes the 5° of tibial ER, which occurs during terminal knee extension.
  - Occurs as closed-chain internal femoral rotation during weight-bearing to provide increased stability of knee joint during weight-bearing activities. Can also occur as open-chain external tibial rotation.
  - Lateral or ER of tibia occurs as knee moves toward terminal extension, due to anatomical relationship of surfaces of tibia and femur.
  - Unlocking occurs through action of popliteus. Open-chain unlocking occurs primarily with popliteal action.
- Causes for screw home mechanism.
  - Lateral femoral condyle glides more freely on lateral convex (anterior-posterior) facet of tibia. Causes greater tibial motion in posterior direction on lateral side.
  - Medial femoral condyle has a longer articular surface than lateral condyle. During femoral rolling,

more motion occurs on lateral side (20°) than on medial side (10°–15°).
 - Medial meniscus is attached to MCL, which tightens during extension. Medial meniscus stops gliding, while lateral meniscus continues to glide forward. Creates internal rotation of femur, which is same as ER of tibia.
 - Twisted cruciate ligaments create ER force on tibia, while preventing an internal rotation.
 - Lateral angle of pull of quadriceps muscle creates ER of tibia.

6. Biomechanics proximal tibiofibular joint.
   a. Dorsiflexion of talocrural joint.
      - Fibular head glides superiorly and posteriorly. Fibular shaft rotates externally.
   b. Plantar flexion of talocrural joint.
      - Fibular head glides inferiorly and anteriorly. Fibular shaft rotates internally.

Foot and Ankle Region

1. Osteology and arthrology (talocrural, subtalar, talocalcaneonavicular, calcaneocuboid, transverse tarsal, tarsometatarsal, metatarsophalangeal, and interphalangeal) (see Figures 2-13 and 2-14).
   a. Talocrural joint.
      - Ankle mortise formed by three components: distal end of tibia and its medial malleolus, lateral malleolus of fibula and inferior transverse tibiofibular ligament, and trochlear surface of talus.
      - Three articulations involved in the talocrural joint: tibiofibular, tibiotalar, and fibulotalar.
      - Transversely (medial/lateral), trochlear surface is gently concave. Trochlear surface is wedge-shaped, wider anteriorly than posteriorly.
      - Laterally, talus is triangular-shaped and concave in superior/inferior direction, and convex in anterior/posterior direction. Articulates with reciprocally curved fibula. Medial part of trochlear surface is comparatively flat and articulates with distal end of tibia, which is also flat.
   b. Subtalar joint.
      - Two separate articulations: anterior and posterior talocalcaneal.
        - Posterior talocalcaneal articulation (subtalar joint proper): posterior superior articulation is convex in anterior/posterior direction, and concave in medial/lateral direction. This articulates with reciprocally curved posterior part of inferior surface of talus.
        - Anterior talocalcaneal articulation consists of obliquely oriented surfaces of biconvex inferior surface of neck and head of talus, resting on the biconcave anterior surface of calcaneus. Anterior talocalcaneal articulation, when described functionally, also includes posterior surface of navicular bone, which articulates with head of talus. Joint is properly referred to as talocalcaneonavicular joint.
   c. Talonavicular joint.
      - Biconvex head of talus articulates with biconcavity, formed by posterior navicular surfaces

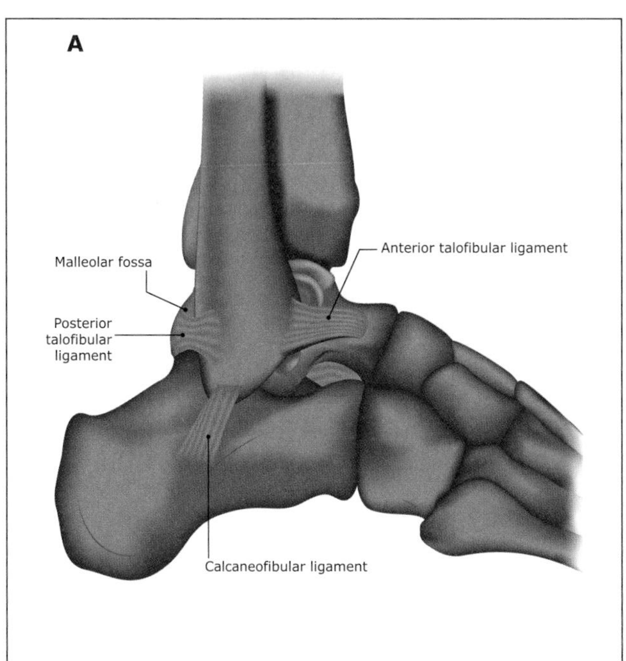

Figure 2-13a Ankle: lateral view.

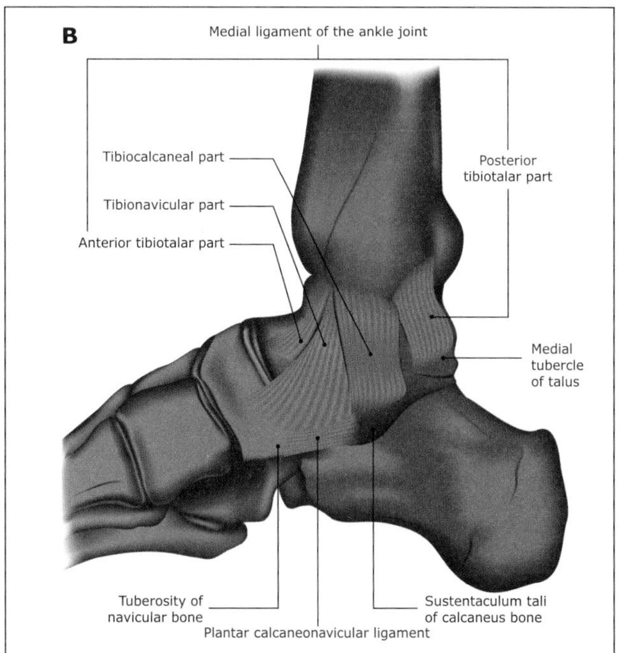

Figure 2-13b Ankle: medial view.

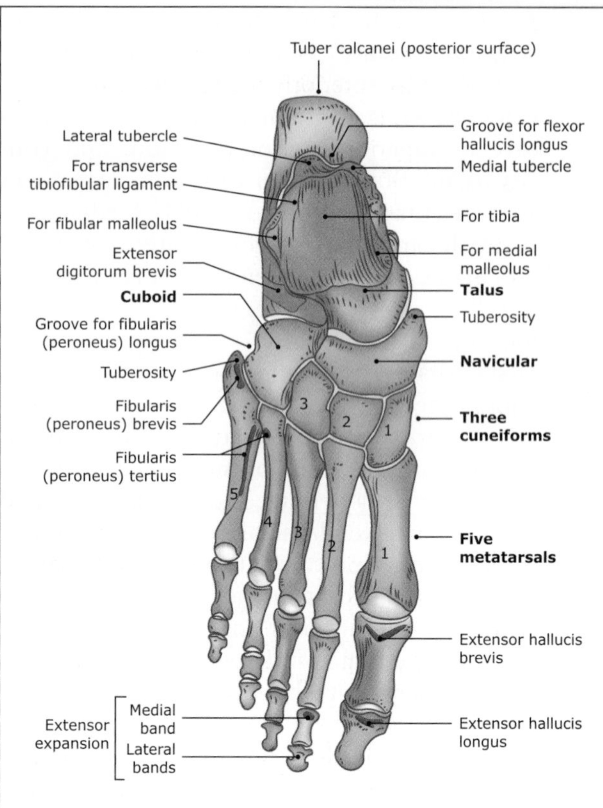

Figure 2-14 **Foot: dorsal view.**

and upper edge of plantar calcaneonavicular ligament.

d. Calcaneocuboid joint.
- Anterior calcaneus is concave medial/lateral and convex superior/inferior. Posterior cuboid is concave superior/inferior and convex medial/lateral.
- Bony prominence on inferior/medial surface of cuboid articulates with inferior surface of calcaneus, making saddle shape deeper. Cuboid is key to lateral arch.

e. Tarsometatarsal joints.
- Proximally, three cuneiforms medially and cuboid laterally. Distally bases of five metatarsals.
- First metatarsal (MT) is largest and strongest, second MT is longest. Third MT articulates primarily with the third cuneiform. Fourth and fifth MT articulate with cuboid.

f. Cuneonavicular joint.
- Biconvex anterior surface of navicular has three facets to articulate with concave posterior surfaces of three cuneiform bones.

g. Metatarsalphalangeal joint.
- Metatarsal heads are convex and proximal phalanges are concave.

h. Interphalangeal joints.
- Same as fingers of hand.

2. Muscles (ankle plantarflexors, ankle dorsiflexors, evertors, invertors, and intrinsics) (see Table 2-5).
3. Noncontractile structures (deltoid ligament, anterior talofibular, posterior talofibular, calcaneofibular, calcaneonavicular [spring ligament], interosseous, bifurcate ligament, plantaraponeurosis, long plantar ligament, and short plantar ligament, capsule, bursae, fascia, nerves, and vessels).

a. Capsule.
- Talocrural joint. Fibrous capsule lined with synovial membrane strengthened by collateral, anterior, and posterior ligaments. Thin anteriorly and posteriorly and thickened laterally.
- Subtalar joint. Posterior articulation has an independent capsule with synovial membrane. Anterior articulation has capsule with synovial membrane that includes talonavicular joint.
- Talonavicular joint. Fibrous capsule with synovial lining is shared with anterior subtalar joint.
- Calcaneocuboid. Independent fibrous capsule with synovial membrane independent from other tarsal articulations.
- Tarsometatarsal (three capsular cavities):
  - First MT with medial cuneiform.
  - Second and third cuneiform capsule is continuous with intercuneiform and cuneonavicular joint cavity.
  - Third cuneiform with base of fourth MT capsule encloses fourth MT with cuboid and third cuneiform.
- Cuneonavicular. Continuous with those of intercuneiform and cuneocuboid joints, as is its synovial cavity. Capsule is connected to second and third cuneometatarsal joints between second and fourth metatarsal bones.
- Metatarsalphalangeal joint. Fibrous capsule present for each articulation.
- Interphalangeal joints. Fibrous capsule present for each articulation.

b. Ligaments.
- Talocrural joint.
  - Medial collateral ligament (deep fibers): anterior talotibial ligament and posterior talotibial ligament.
  - Medial collateral ligament (superficial fibers): deltoid ligament.
  - Lateral collateral ligament: anterior talofibular ligament, calcaneofibular ligament, posterior talofibular ligament.
- Subtalar joint.
  - Interosseous talocalcaneal ligament: two fibrous bands taut with eversion.
  - Lateral talocalcaneal ligament.
  - Posterior talocalcaneal ligament.
  - Medial talocalcaneal ligament.

- Talonavicular joint.
    - Plantar calcaneonavicular ligament (spring ligament).
    - Dorsal talonavicular ligament.
- Calcaneocuboid joint.
    - Medial band of the bifurcate ligament (lateral calcaneonavicular ligament).
    - Medial calcaneocuboid (lateral band of the bifurcated ligament).
    - Long plantar ligament (superficial plantar calcaneocuboid).
    - Plantar calcaneocuboid (short plantar).
- Tarsometatarsal joint.
    - Medially, dorsal ligament runs from medial cuneiform to base of second MT.
    - Laterally, dorsal ligaments with straight fibers from middle cuneiform to second MT, lateral cuneiform to third MT, cruciate fibers from lateral cuneiform to second MT, and middle cuneiform to third MT.
- Cuneonavicular joint.
    - Three dorsal cuneonavicular ligaments, one attached to each cuneiform.
    - Plantar ligaments have similar attachments and receive slips from tendons of posterior tibialis muscle.
- Metatarsalphalangeal (MTP) joint. Plantar ligaments and collateral ligaments present.
- Interphalangeal joints. Plantar ligaments and collateral ligaments present.

c. Plantar fascia.
- Also known as plantar aponeurosis.
- A broad, dense band of longitudinally arranged collagen fibers that can be divided into three components, running from medial calcaneus to phalanges.
- Fascia tightens with dorsiflexion of MTP joints as occurs during push off. Known as "windlass effect." Tightening of this fascia causes supination of calcaneus and inversion of subtalar joint, creating a rigid lever for push off.

d. Bursa.
- Posterior calcaneal bursa.
- Retrocalcaneal bursa.

e. Blood supply comes from malleolar rami of anterior tibial and fibular arteries.

f. Articular innervation comes from deep fibular and tibial nerves.

4. Ankle and foot biomechanics.

a. Talocrural joint.
- Conjunct rotations.
    - Talus rotates medially 30° from dorsiflexion to plantar flexion. Also slight side-to-side gliding, rotation, and abduction/adduction are permitted when foot is plantar flexed.
- Arthrokinematics/osteokinematics.
    - Open chain: During plantar flexion talus describes anterior glide on mortise with slight medial rotation or adduction. Dorsiflexion occurs as reciprocally opposite motion.
    - Closed chain: During plantar flexion tibia glides posteriorly on talus with slight lateral rotation. Dorsiflexion occurs as a reciprocally opposite motion.

b. Subtalar joint.
- Joint axes.
    - Oblique axis extends from posterior, plantar, and lateral to anterior, dorsal, and medial. Joint is oriented obliquely, with the average at 42° from the horizontal and 16° from midline of foot.
    - Variances in joint axis are fairly common.
    - With a high inclination of axis, movement at subtalar joint is increased in transverse plane and decreased in frontal plane.
    - With a low inclination of axis, joint will be more frontal plane dominant, leading to greater calcaneal pronation/supination.
- Conjunct rotation.
    - Calcaneus can move in many directions, due to its multiple articulations. Like a ship in the waves—rotation around a vertical axis, tilts medially and laterally, glides anteriorly and posteriorly.
- Arthrokinematics/osteokinematics.
    - Occurs in same direction when mobilizing calcaneus on a fixed talus. Subtalar joint represents the purest triplanar movement.
    - Open chain: During inversion, calcaneus moves into adduction, supination, and plantar flexion on fixed talus. Eversion occurs as a reciprocally opposite motion.
    - Closed chain: During inversion, supination of calcaneus (talus guides laterally) with abduction and dorsiflexion of talus. Produces ER of tibia. Eversion occurs as a reciprocally opposite motion. Produces internal rotation of tibia.

c. Talonavicular joint.
- Arthrokinematics/osteokinematics.
    - Arthokinematics and osteokinematics occur in same direction when mobilizing navicular on a fixed talus. Rotational movements of midtarsal joint allow forefoot to twist on rearfoot. Talus and navicular rotate in opposite directions.
    - Open chain: During inversion, navicular plantar flexes, adducts, and externally rotates on talus. Eversion occurs as a reciprocally opposite motion.
    - Closed chain: During inversion, navicular plantar flexes (talus glides dorsally on navicular), adducts (talus abducts), and internally rotates. Eversion occurs as a reciprocally opposite motion.

d. MTPs and PIPs same as fingers.

Spine

1. General function of the vertebral column.
   a. Support for head and internal organs.
   b. Stable attachment for all soft tissues, extremities, rib cage, and pelvis.
   c. Protection of internal organs and spinal cord.
   d. Attenuates forces from above and below.
2. Components of the vertebral column.
   a. Consists of 24 freely movable and 9 fused bones.
   b. Divided into five distinct regions (cervical, thoracic, lumbar, sacral, and coccygeal).
3. Osteology.
   a. Typical vertebra (vertebral body, pedicles, lamina which includes superior and inferior articular processes or facets, transverse processes, and the spinous process).
   b. Regional variations.
      - Cervical: two atypical (atlas and axis) which allow for increase active range of motion (AROM) in rotation without compressing the spinal cord, uncinate processes, and transverse foramen.
         - Vertebral body is rectangular-shaped.
         - Uncinate joints (joints of von Luschka) found at C3–C7 limit lateral cervical movement.
      - Costotransverse and costovertebral: articulations between rib and transverse process and vertebral body, respectively.
      - Thoracic: demifacets for articulation with the ribs. Vertebral body is heart-shaped. Prominent spinous processes are angled following "Rules of 3."
         - Rules of 3: spinous process of T1–T3 even with transverse process of same level vertebra; T4–T6 spinous processes are found one-half level below transverse processes of same level; T7–T9 spinous processes are one full level below transverse process of same level; T10 is full level below; T11 is one-half level below; and T12 is level.
      - Lumbar: vertebra larger than other regions and body is kidney-shaped. Very prominent spinous processes (see Figures 2-15 and 2-16).
      - Sacrum is wedge-shaped, both anteriorly/posteriorly and inferiorly/superiorly. Made of five fused vertebrae.
      - Ilium is made up of three fused bones (ischium, ilium, and pubis). Shape varies widely among people, with significant difference in shape between men and women.
4. Arthrology.
   a. Atypical joints.
      - Atlanto-occipital joint: synovial articulation between occiput and C1. Also known as "yes" joint, since much of head nodding motion comes from this articulation.

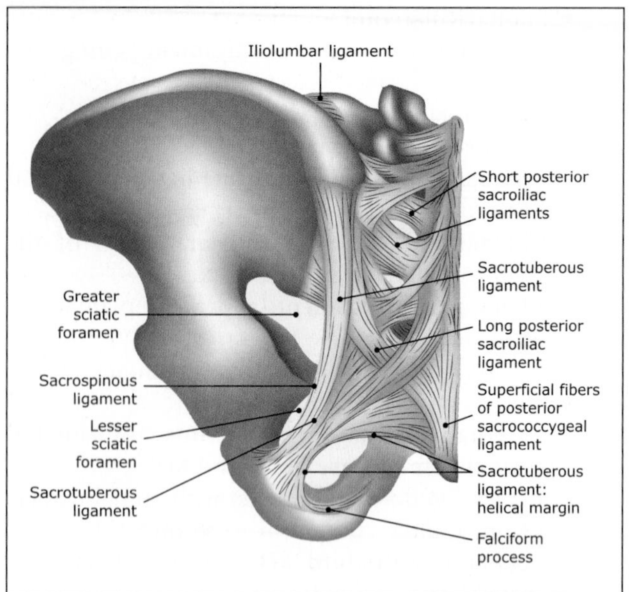

Figure 2-15 Half of pelvis and 5th lumbar vertebra.

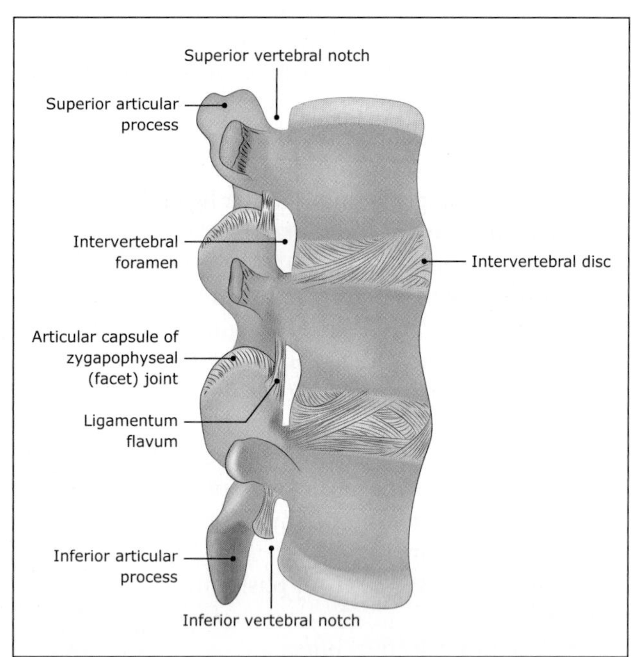

Figure 2-16 Lumbar vertebra.

      - Atlanto-axial joint: nonsynovial articulation between dens of C2 and anterior arch of C1. Known as "no" joint, since much of head rotation comes from this articulation.
   b. Apophyseal or facet joints which guide movement of spine. Synovial/diarthrodial joints with capsule and synovial membrane. Composed of superior and inferior articulatory processes of adjacent vertebrae. In lumbar region, facet surfaces may be flat

or curved. In cervical and thoracic regions, surfaces are generally flat.

c. Intervertebral joints between intervertebral disc and adjacent superior and inferior vertebral bodies. Allow movement between vertebral bodies and transmit loads from one vertebral segment to another.

d. Sacroiliac joint (SIJ): composed of auricular-shaped joint surfaces of sacrum and ilium. Diarthrosis/synarthrosis (syndesmosis) combination. Ilial articulation is primarily convex and covered with a thin layer of fibrocartilage. Sacral articulation is primarily concave and covered with hyaline cartilage. SI joints attenuate forces from trunk and lower extremities.

5. Fibroadipose meniscoid.
   a. Structure composed of dense connective tissue and adipose tissue.
   b. Found at superior and inferior aspects of facet joints.
   c. Protects cartilage of facet surface during extremes in motion.
6. Muscles (see Table 2-6).
7. Intervertebral disc/endplate.
   a. Annulus fibrosis/fibrosus.
      - Concentric layers or lamellae composed of collagen (type I predominates in outer layers to withstand shear; type II in inner portions for weight-bearing) and fibrocartilage. 65% water.
      - Outer one-third of annulus is innervated by branches from sinovertebral nerve.
      - Functions to sustain compressive, torsional, shearing, and distraction loads.
   b. Nucleus pulposis/pulposus.
      - Gel with imbibing capabilities composed of water and proteoglycans with a minimal amount of collagen (type II). 70%–90% water.
      - Avascular and aneural structure.
      - Makes up 20%–33% height of vertebral column.
      - Functions to sustain compressive, torsional, shearing, and distraction loads.
   c. Vertebral endplate.
      - Structure continuous with annulus and nucleus. Sits inside ring apophysis of vertebral body.
      - Composed of proteoglycans, collagen, and water as well as both fibrocartilage (on side closest to disc) and hyaline cartilage (on side closest to vertebral body).
      - Functions to provide passive diffusion of nutrients.
8. Other noncontractile soft tissues.
   a. Ligaments.
      - Alar ligament. Attach dens to occipital condyles. Function to limit flexion, contralateral side-bending, and contralateral rotation.
      - Anterior longitudinal ligament. Courses the anterior and lateral surfaces of the vertebral bodies from the sacrum to the second cervical vertebra. Reinforce the anterolateral portion of the intervertebral discs.
      - Posterior longitudinal ligament. Courses the posterior aspect of the vertebral bodies from C2 to the sacrum. Limits flexion and reinforces the posterior aspect of the intervertebral discs.
      - Tectorial membrane. Superior extension of the posterior longitudinal ligament from C2 to the occiput. Limits flexion.

Table 2-6

Trunk and Rib Cage Muscles and Innervation

ACTION TO BE TESTED	MUSCLES	CORD SEGMENT	NERVES
Inspiration	Diaphragm Levator costarum, external intercostals, anterior internal intercostals	C3–C5 T1–T12	Phrenic Intercostal
Forced expiration	Internal obliques, transverse abdominis, external obliques, posterior internal intercostals, rectus abdominis	T7–L1 T7–T12 T1–T12 T7–T12	Intercostal Intercostal Intercostal Intercostal
Spine extension	Erector spinae, transversospinalis, interspinales, rotatores intertransversarii	Segmental innervation	Posterior rami
Spine flexion	Rectus abdominis/external obliques, internal obliques, psoas minor	T7–T12 T7–L1 L1	Intercostal Intercostal Lumbar plexus
Spine lateral flexion (hip hiking in reverse)	Quadratus lumborum	T12–L3	Lumbar plexus
Spine rotation	Rotators, internal/external obliques, intertransversarii, transversospinalis	Segmental innervation	Posterior rami

Adapted from Chusid JG: Correlative Neuroanatomy and Functional Neurology. Lange Medical Publications, 1970; Kendall FP, McCreary EK, Provance PG: Muscles Testing and Function, 4th ed. Williams & Wilkins, 1993.

- Ligamentum flavum. Courses C2 to the sacrum, connecting lamina of one vertebra to the lamina above it. Limits flexion, particularly in the lumbar region.
- Interspinous ligament. Courses between spinous processes and limits flexion and rotation.
- Supraspinous ligaments. Found in thoracic and lumbar region. Limit flexion.
- Costotransverse ligament (superior, posterior, and lateral). Support costotransverse joint capsule, ribs 1–10.
- Iliolumbar ligaments. Extends from posterior aspect of the ilium to the transverse process of the L5 vertebra. Very strong and functions to limit motion between L5 and S1.
- Posterior sacroiliac ligaments (short, transverse, and long).
- Anterior sacroiliac ligament. Courses the anterior aspect of the ilium to the anterior sacrum. Thickening of the joint capsule.
- Sacrotuberous ligament. Limits sacral anterior rotation and superior translation of the sacrum.
- Posterior interosseous ligament. Courses the posterior superior iliac spine to the 3rd and 4th sacral segments. Limits sacral motion in all directions.

b. Capsules.
- Facet joint: assist ligaments in providing limitation of motion and stability of spine. Strongest in the thoracolumbar and cervicothoracic regions.
- Sacroiliac joints: synovial capsule present in surrounding joint, which is very prominent anteriorly; posteriorly, it is lost within posterior interosseous ligament.

c. Thoracolumbar fascia.
- Provides stability of vertebral column when a force is applied.
- Acts as a corset when tension is created by contraction of abdominals, gluteals, and lumbar muscles.

9. Nerves.

a. Dorsal roots transmit sensory fibers to spinal cord and ventral roots; mainly transmit motor fibers from spinal cord to spinal nerve.

b. Spinal nerves are connected centrally to spinal cord by a dorsal and ventral root, which join to become the spinal nerve in the intervertebral foramen. Spinal nerve divides into dorsal and ventral rami.
- Dorsal rami innervate structures on posterior trunk.
- Ventral rami.
  - Cervical ventral rami form cervical and brachial plexuses (see Figures 2-17 and 2-18).
  - Thoracic ventral rami innervate anterior structures of trunk within thoracic region.
  - Lumbar ventral rami form lumbar and lumbosacral plexuses (see Figures 2-19 and 2-20).

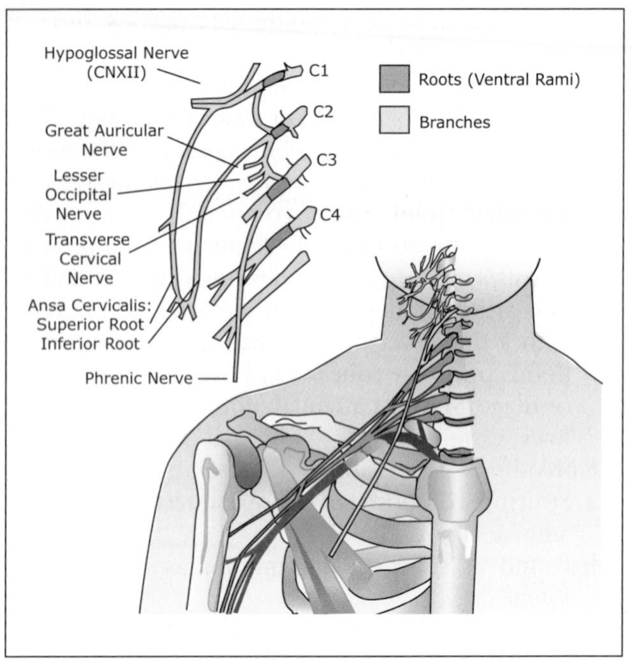

Figure 2-17 Cervical plexus.

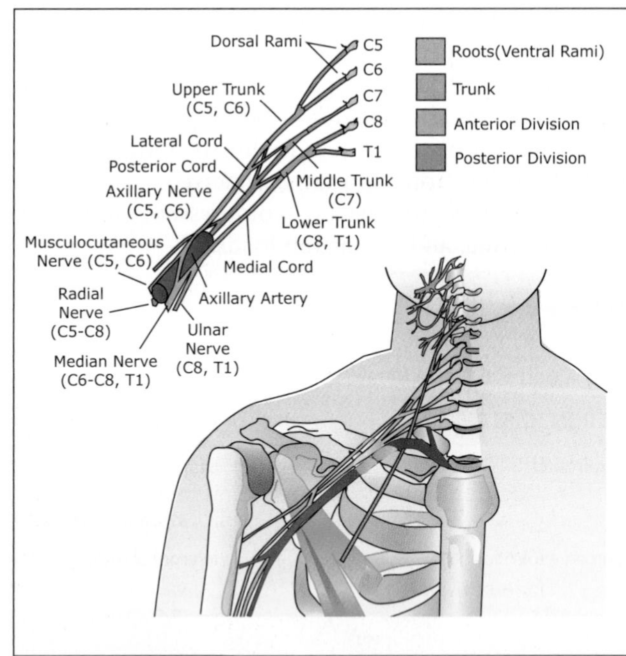

Figure 2-18 Brachial plexus.

c. Spinal nerves in various sections of spine.
- Cervical: spinal nerves come out at the level above its associated vertebra.
- Thoracic/lumbar: spinal nerves come out at level below its associated vertebra.

d. Spinal cord terminates approximately at level of L1–L2 disc (conus medullaris).

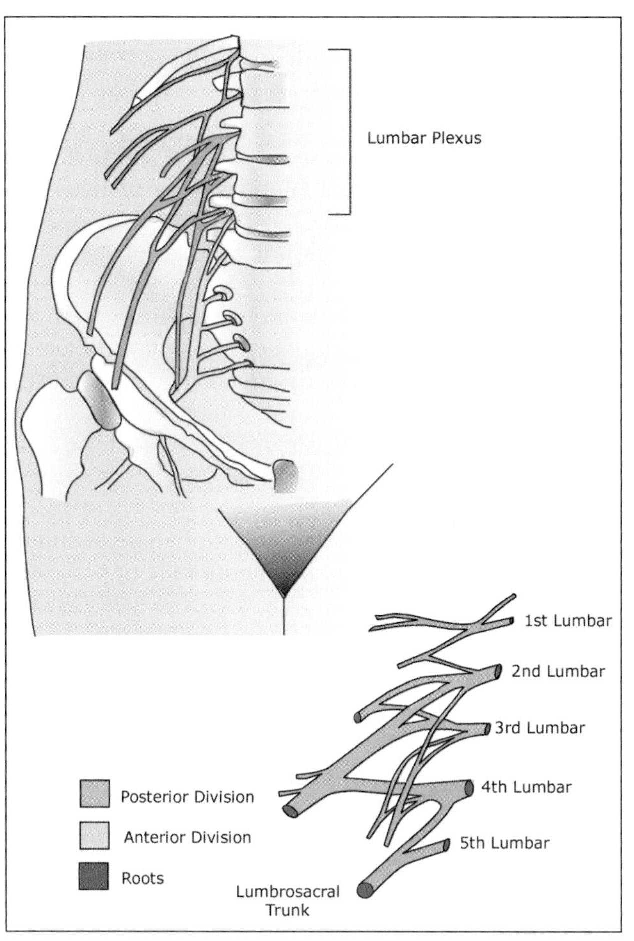

Figure 2-19 **Lumbar plexus.**

Figure 2-20 **Sacral plexus.**

10. Spinal biomechanics.
   a. Arthrokinematics.
      - Flexion: upper facets glide anteroproximally and tilt forward.
      - Extension: upper facets move downward, slightly posterior, and tilt backward.
      - Side-bending: when side-bending right, upper facet moves down and slightly anterior. Left facet moves upward and slightly posterior. Both facets move to the left.
      - Cervical rotation: right rotation causes facets on right to glide down and back, causing approximation of facet joints on right.
      - Lumbar rotation: very little, but clinically important because this motion causes separation and approximation of the facet joints; e.g., if L3 rotates right, there is separation at right L3–L4 joint and approximation at left L3–L4 joint.
   b. Coupled motions.
      - Cervical.
         - Side-bending and rotation occur in same direction from C2–C7, regardless of whether spine is in neutral/extension or flexion. When occiput side bends, C1 rotates in opposite direction.
      - Lumbar/thoracic.
         - Neutral/extension: lumbar segments will side bend and rotate in opposite directions; e.g., side bend right results in segment rotating left.
         - Flexion: lumbar segments will side bend and rotate in the same direction.
         - This coupling described above is a very basic interpretation. In reality, there are significant variations in coupling motions between individuals. Coupling motion may depend on whether a side bend or rotation is done first. Direction of spinal segmental coupling should always be checked with each patient prior to performing a manual technique.
   c. Lumbopelvic rhythm.
      - During flexion, spine (primarily lumbar spine) goes through 60°–70° of motion and then pelvis will rotate anteriorly to allow more movement, eventually followed by flexion of hips.

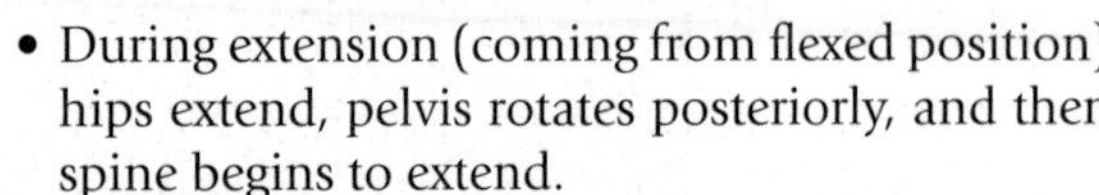

- During extension (coming from flexed position) hips extend, pelvis rotates posteriorly, and then spine begins to extend.

d. Sacroiliac joint osteokinematics.
- Motion limited, but during gait movements takes place in multiple planes.
- Nutation and counternutation: coupling movement that occurs between sacrum and ilium during gait.
  - Nutation: describes a movement that involves flexion of sacrum and posterior rotation of ilium.
  - Counternutation: describes a movement that involves extension of sacrum and anterior rotation of ilium.

Temporomandibular Joint (TMJ)

1. Functional anatomy. A bilateral articulation between mandible and cranium (craniomandibular joint).
2. Arthrology.
   a. Synovial joint with articular surfaces covered by dense fibrous connective tissue rather than hyaline cartilage.
   b. Articular disc composed of dense fibrous connective tissue without blood vessels or nerves in pressure-bearing areas.
   c. Discal ligaments function to restrict movement in sagittal plane.
   d. Superior retrodiscal lamina (superior stratum) composed of elastic connective tissue; counteracts forward pull of superior lateral pterygoid muscle on articular disc.
   e. Retrodiscal pad consists of loose neurovascular connective tissue.
3. Joint movement.
   a. Combination of hinge axis rotation in disc condyle complex and sliding movement of the upper joint.
   b. Functional range of opening is 40 mm, with 25 mm of rotation and 15 mm of translatory glide.

Physical Therapy Examination

Patient/Client History (or Interview), Systems Review, and Tests and Measures

Patient/Client History

1. Gather information to develop a hypothetical diagnosis, which dictates flow of examination. Delineate any precautions and/or contraindications when performing components of examination (see Table 2-7).
2. Components of history.
   a. Demographics: age, gender, diagnosis and referral (if appropriate), hand dominance, etc.
   b. Social and family history.
   c. Current condition(s)/chief complaint.
   d. General health status.
   e. Social health.
   f. Employment/work.
   g. Growth and development.
   h. Living environment.
   i. Functional status and activity level.
   j. Medical/surgical history, including previous treatment and review of systems.

Systems Review

1. Components of system review (see Table 2-8).
   a. Musculoskeletal.
   b. Neuromuscular.
   c. Cardiopulmonary.
   d. Integumentary.
   e. Gastrointestinal/Genitourinary systems.
2. Determine whether identified condition(s) are comorbidity(ies) and/or complicating factor(s).
3. Determine whether a referral to an additional health care provider is appropriate, and if so, make the referral.

Tests and Measures

1. Gather specific data regarding patient/client. Choosing specific components as well as order of exam will be dictated by history.
2. Components that may be a part of tests and measures include:
   a. Anthropometric characteristics.
   b. Postural alignment and position (see Table 2-9, Figure 2-21).
      - Dynamic.
      - Static.
   c. Range of motion (see Tables 2-10 and 2-11).
      - AROM.
      - Passive range of motion (PROM).
      - Flexibility testing.
   d. Muscle performance: resisted tests, manual muscle testing, muscle tension (see Table 2-12).
   e. Motor function.
   f. Cranial and peripheral nerve integrity.

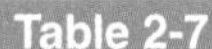

Table 2-7

Questions Related to Specific Areas of Dysfunction

AREA OF DYSFUNCTION	RELATED QUESTIONS
Shoulder	Do you have pain raising your arm up, and if so, at what part of the range does that occur? Have you ever dislocated your shoulder? Do you have pain sleeping on your shoulder at night?
Elbow	Have you recently changed your activities? Have you recently changed the type of tools you use at work or the instruments you use for recreational activities?
Hand	Have you been doing more or different work with your hands than the usual, such as typing, sewing, gardening, etc.?
Cervical	Do you have dizziness when looking overhead? Have you had any previous motor vehicle accidents with resulting neck injury? How many pillows do you use at night?
TMJ	Do you have any popping or clicking in the TMJ? Do you have pain trying to eat specific foods? Does your jaw ever get stuck open or closed?
Thoracic	Do you have pain with breathing? Have you had a recent upper respiratory infection?
Lumbar	Have you had any changes in your ability to urinate or have a bowel movement? Do you have any symptoms such as pain, tingling, burning, etc. in either of your legs?
Sacroiliac	Did you fall onto your buttocks? Did you step off a curb and experience pain? Do you have pain with walking and/or sustained postures?
Hip	Do you have pain in your groin? Do you have stiffness in the morning that feels better with movement?
Knee	Does your knee "pop"? Does your knee ever give way and/or lock? Did your knee swell as soon as you were injured or did the swelling come later?
Ankle/Foot	Have you ever sprained your ankle, and if so, how many times? Do you have pain in your foot when you first try to step out of bed in the morning?

g. Reflex integrity.
h. Sensory integrity.
i. Joint integrity and mobility.
j. Pain.
k. Assistive and adaptive devices.
l. Orthotic, protective, and supportive devices.
m. Ergonomics and body mechanics.
n. Self-care and home management.
o. Gait, locomotion, and balance.
p. Work, community, and leisure integration or reintegration.
q. Special tests (see specifics for each joint/region).

Diagnostic Testing

1. Diagnostic tests are utilized for correlation with history and tests and measures to determine patient's primary physical therapy diagnosis as well as identify any medical conditions that may be contributing factors or comorbidities.
2. If further diagnostic tests are warranted and/or beneficial, make appropriate referral or recommendation.
3. Most common types of diagnostic testing for musculoskeletal dysfunctions include imaging, laboratory tests, and electrodiagnostic testing.
4. Imaging (see Appendix 2B).
   a. Plain film radiograph (x-rays).
      - X-rays are used to demonstrate bony tissues. Beams pass through the tissues resulting in varying shades of gray on film depending on density of tissue it passed through. The more dense the structure (bone), the whiter the structure will appear on the film.
      - Readily available, relatively inexpensive, and shows bony anatomy very well.
      - Negative is patient exposure to radiation.
      - Requires two different projections, since structures may be superimposed on each other, making it difficult to identify pathology with one view. Typical views are anterior-posterior and lateral, although other views may be used.
      - Used for viewing dysfunction and/or disease of bones. Does not demonstrate soft tissues well or at all.

   b. Computed tomography (CT) scan.
      - Uses plain film x-ray slices that are enhanced by a computer to improve resolution. It is multiplanar so can image in any plane; therefore, tissue can be viewed from multiple directions.

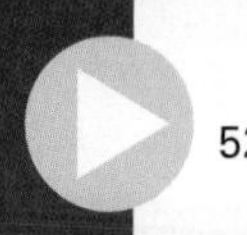

Table 2-8

Summary of Symptoms Observed in Common and Uncommon Dysfunctions

DYSFUNCTION	SYMPTOMS OBSERVED
Degenerative joint disease/osteoarthritis	Pain and stiffness upon rising Pain eases through the morning (4–5 hours) Pain increases with repetitive bending activities Constant awareness of discomfort with episodes of exacerbation Describes pain as more soreness and nagging
Facet joint dysfunction	Stiff upon rising; pain eases within an hour Loss of motion accompanied by pain Patient will describe pain as sharp with certain movements Movement in pain-free range usually reduces symptoms Stationary positions increase symptoms
Discal, with nerve root compromise	No pain in reclined or semireclined position Pain increases with increasing weight-bearing activities Describes pain as shooting, burning, or stabbing Patient may describe altered strength or ability to perform ADLs
Spinal stenosis	Pain is related to position Flexed positions decrease pain, and extended positions increase pain Describes symptoms as a numbness, tightness, or cramping Walking for any distance brings on symptoms Pain may persist for hours after assuming a resting position
Vascular claudication	Pain is consistent in all spinal positions Pain is brought on by physical exertion Pain is relieved promptly with rest (1–5 minutes) Pain is described as a numbness Patient usually has decreased or absent pulses
Neoplastic disease	Patient describes pain as gnawing, intense, or penetrating Pain is not resolved by changes in position, time of day, or activity level Pain will wake the patient

Table 2-9

Effects of Forward Head Posture on the Spine, TMJ, and Associated Soft Tissue Structures

STRUCTURE	POSTURE CHANGES
Cranium	Extended on upper cervical spine
Mandible	Elevated and retruded
TMJ	Posterior close-packed position
Maxillomandibular relationship	Increased freeway space with significant posterior intercuspation
Hyoid	Elevated (suprahyoids shorten, infrahyoids lengthen)
Tongue	Drops to the floor of mouth
Upper cervical spine	Extended (can compress neurovascular structures)
Middle and lower cervical spine	Lordosis decreased (flexed positioning)
First and second ribs	Elevated
Scalenes, suboccipital, sternocleidomastoids, longus colli, upper trapezius, levator scapulae	Shorten
Pectoralis major and minor	Shorten, creating rounded shoulder position
Scapular stabilizers, rectus capitis anterior	Stretched
Longus capitis	Stretched suboccipital region, shorten C2–C6

Adapted from Darnell MA: Proposed chronology of events for forward head posture. *Journal of Craniomandibular Practice,* 1983; 1(4): 50–54.

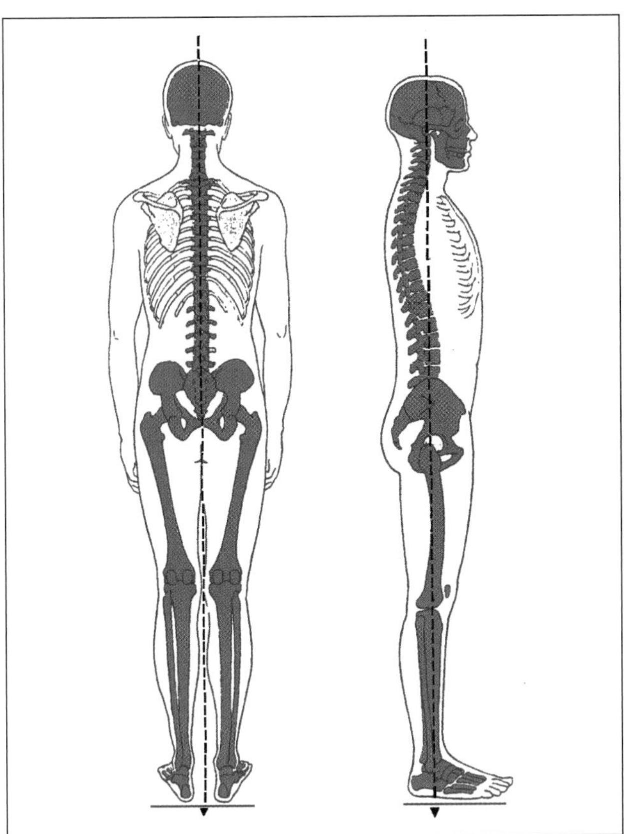

Figure 2-21 **Vertical line of gravity.**

- Typically used to assess complex fractures as well as facet dysfunction, disc disease, or stenosis of the spinal canal or intervertebral foramen. CT demonstrates better quality and better visualization of bony structures than plain films. CT also demonstrates soft tissue structures, although not as well as MRI.
- Fairly expensive, and patient is exposed to radiation.

c. Discography.

- Radiopaque dye is injected into the disc to identify abnormalities within the disc (annulus or nucleus). The needle is inserted into the disc with the assistance of radiography (fluoroscopy).
- Not commonly used. Requires a high level of skill and proper equipment to perform. Fairly specific technique to identify internal disc disruptions of the nucleus and/or annulus.
- Expensive, may be painful, and since it is invasive, there is a risk of infection.

d. Magnetic resonance imaging (MRI).

- Uses magnetic fields rather than radiation.
- Offers excellent visualization of tissue anatomy. Utilizes two types of images: T1 demonstrates fat within the tissues and is typically used to assess bony anatomy, while T2 suppresses fat and demonstrates tissues with high water content. T2 is used to assess soft tissue structures.

Table 2-10

Extremity Range of Motion

JOINT	FLEXION/ EXTENSION	ABDUCTION/ ADDUCTION	EXTERNAL/ INTERNAL ROTATION	HORIZONTAL ADDUCTION	SUPINATION/ PRONATION	RADIAL/ ULNAR DEVIATION	PLANTAR-FLEXION/ DORSIFLEXION
Shoulder	160–180/50–60	170–180/50–75	80–90/60–100	130/45			
Elbow	140–150/0–10				90/80–90		
Wrist	80–90/70–90					15/30–45	
MCP	85–90/30–45						
PIP	100–115/0						
DIP	80–90/20						
1st CMC	45–50	60–70/30					
1st MCP	50–55/0						
1st IP	85–90/0–5						
Hip	110–120/10–15	30–50/30	40–60/30–40				
Knee	135/0–15		30–40/20–30				
Ankle					45–60/15–30		50/20
2nd–5th MTP	40/40						
1st MTP	45/70						
1st IP	90/0						
2nd–5th PIP	35/0						
2nd–5th DIP	60/30						

Table 2-11

Spine Range of Motion

REGION	FLEXION/EXTENSION	SIDE-BENDING	ROTATION	OPENING	PROTRUSION/ RETRUSION	LATERAL DEVIATION
Cervical	80–90/70	20–45	70–90			
Thoracic	20–45/25–45	20–40	35–50			
Lumbar	40–60/20–35	15–20	3–18			
TMJ				35–50 mm	3–6 mm/3–4 mm	10–15 mm

Table 2-12

Muscle Grading

Normal	N	5/5	Lift or hold against gravity with maximal resistance.
Good +	G+	4+/5	Good grades include lifting or holding against gravity with moderate to minimal resistance.
Good	G	4/5	
Good –	G–	4–/5	
Fair +	F+	3+/5	Fair grades include lifting or holding against gravity without resistance.
Fair	F	3/5	
Fair –	F–	3–/5	Some assistance may be required to complete the motion in the minus category.
Poor +	P+	2+/5	Poor grades include movement with gravity eliminated.
Poor	P	2/5	
Poor –	P–	2–/5	Some assistance may be required to complete the motion in the minus category.
Trace	T	1/5	Muscle contraction can be seen or felt. No movement is produced.
Zero	0	0/5	No contraction is seen or felt.

Adapted from Kendall FP, et al: Muscles: Testing and Function, with Posture and Pain, 5th ed. 2005.

- Fairly expensive, and patients with claustrophobia do not tolerate this test well. Quality of open MRI is inferior to closed. May not be able to use with patients who have metallic implants.

e. Arthrography.
- Invasive technique that injects water-soluble dye into area and is observed with a radiograph. Dye is observed as it surrounds tissues, demonstrating the anatomy where fluid moves within joint.
- Typically used to identify abnormalities within joints such as tendon ruptures.
- Expensive and carries risks since it is invasive.

f. Bone scans (osteoscintigraphy).
- Chemicals laced with radioactive tracers are injected.
- Isotope settles in areas where there is a high metabolic activity of bone.
- Radiograph is taken to demonstrate any "hot spots" of increased metabolic activity.
- Patients with dysfunctions, such as rheumatoid arthritis, possible stress fractures, bone cancer, infection within bone, often receive a bone scan, since these dysfunctions increase metabolic activity of bone in the affected regions.

g. Diagnostic ultrasound.
- Utilizes transmission of high-frequency sound waves, similar to therapeutic ultrasound.
- Limited by contrast resolution, small viewing field, how deep it penetrates, and poor penetration of bone. Interpretation of data is subjective, so results depend on skill of operator.
- Provides real-time dynamic images and can assess soft tissue dysfunctions.
- No known harmful effects at this time.

h. Myelography.
- Invasive technique using water-soluble dye. Dye is visualized as it passes through vertebral canal to observe anatomy within region.
- Seldom used due to side effects versus MRI or CT scan, which provide as good, if not better, information. Very expensive, since it often involves a hospital stay overnight.

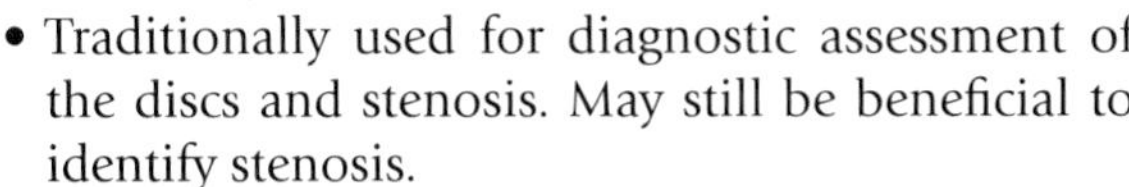

- Traditionally used for diagnostic assessment of the discs and stenosis. May still be beneficial to identify stenosis.

5. Laboratory tests.
   a. Laboratory tests are typically used to screen patients, assist with making a diagnosis, or for monitoring.
   b. Since many patients with musculoskeletal dysfunction present with other medical pathology, it is important to monitor clinical laboratory findings.
   c. Multiple tests available that fall into the following categories.
      - Blood tests.
      - Serum chemistries.
      - Immunological tests.
      - Pulmonary function tests.
      - Arterial blood gases.
      - Fluid analysis.
6. Electrodiagnostic testing (also refer to Chapter 3: Neuromuscular Physical Therapy).
   a. Electroneuromyography (ENMG) and nerve conduction velocity (NCV) tests are commonly used to assess and/or monitor musculoskeletal conditions.

Special Tests of the Upper Extremity

Shoulder Special Tests (See Table 2-13)

1. Glenohumeral joint anterior instability.
   a. Apprehension test.
      - Patient is supine, with shoulder in 90° abduction; slowly take shoulder into full ER.
      - Positive if the patient looks or feels apprehensive/alarmed and resists further motion (apprehension > pain).
   b. Relocation test.
      - With a positive apprehension test, a posterior translation stress is applied to the humeral head.
      - Positive if the patient loses apprehension or pain decreases.
      - Relocation test does not typically change pain with primary impingement.
2. Glenohumeral joint posterior and inferior instability.
   a. Jerk test (posterior).
      - Patient seated; shoulder flexed to 90° and internally rotated.
      - Axially load humerus and horizontally adduct arm.
      - Positive test is production of a sudden jerk or clunk as humeral head subluxes off the back of the glenoid.
   b. Sulcus sign.
      - Patient stands relaxed with arm at side; arm is pulled distally.
      - Positive test is the presence of a sulcus inferior to the acromion combined with reproduction of symptoms.
3. Subacromial impingement.
   a. Hawkins-Kennedy test.
      - Patient is seated or standing; shoulder is passively flexed to 90° and then internally rotated maximally.
      - May be performed in various degrees of forward flexion and horizontal adduction.
      - Positive if reproduces pain within shoulder region.
   b. Neer test (see Figure 2-22).
      - Patient is seated; shoulder is passively internally rotated, then fully abducted.
      - Positive if reproduces pain within shoulder region.
   c. Painful arc.
      - Patient actively abducts the shoulder and reports the start/stop range of any pain.
      - Positive if pain is reported between 60° and 120° of abduction.
   d. Empty can test (see Figure 2-23).
      - Patient seated with shoulder at 90° of abduction and no rotation; resist shoulder abduction.
      - Shoulder placed in "empty can" position (internal rotation and 30° forward (horizontal adduction); resist shoulder abduction.
      - Positive if reproduces pain in supraspinatus tendon and/or weakness while in "empty can" position.
4. Rotator cuff pathology.
   a. Drop arm test.
      - Patient seated with shoulder passively abducted to 120°.
      - Patient instructed slowly to bring arm down to side; guard patient's arm from falling in case it gives way.
      - Positive if patient is unable to lower arm back down to side.
   b. External rotation lag sign.
      - Patient seated or standing; passively abduct shoulder to 90° and externally rotate shoulder to end-range.
      - Positive if unable to maintain externally rotated position.
   c. Infraspinatus muscle test.
      - Patient is seated or standing; resist external rotation with arm neutrally rotated and adducted to the trunk.
      - Positive if patient gives way.
   d. Hornblower sign.
      - Patient is standing; passively elevate the arm to 90° in scapular plane and flex elbow to 90°.
      - Patient externally rotates shoulder against resistance.
      - Positive if unable to laterally rotate the arm.

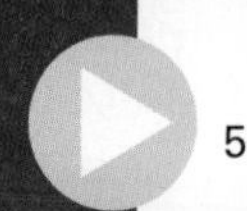

Table 2-13

Diagnostic Accuracy of Shoulder Special Tests

TEST	SN	SP	+LR	–LR
Anterior instability				
- Apprehension test (apprehension)	0.72–1.0	0.86–0.96	7.1–20.2	0.0–0.29
- Apprehension (pain)	0.40–0.50	0.56–0.86	1.1–3.1	0.69–0.90
- Relocation test	0.57–0.81	0.92–1.0	10.4	0.20–0.43
Posterior instability				
- Jerk test	0.98	0.73	36.5	0.27
Subacromial impingement				
- Hawkins-Kennedy test	0.74–0.80	0.56–0.57	1.7–1.8	0.35–0.46
- Neer test	0.72–0.78	0.58–0.60	1.8–1.9	0.38–0.47
- Painful arc	0.53	0.75	2.3	0.62
- Empty can test	0.69	0.62	1.8	0.50
Rotator cuff tears (full-thickness)				
- Drop-arm test	0.35	0.88	2.9	0.74
- External rotation lag sign	0.46	0.94	7.2	0.60
- Infraspinatus muscle test	0.51	0.84	3.2	0.58
- Hornblower sign	1.0	0.93	14.29	0.00
- Internal rotation lag sign	1.0	0.84	6.2	0.00
Acromioclavicular joint				
- Horizontal adduction	0.79	0.77	3.4	0.27
- Paxinos test	0.79	0.50	1.6	0.42
SLAP lesions				
- Active compression (O'Brien) test	0.67	0.37	1.1	0.89
- Biceps load II test	0.30–0.90	0.78–0.90	1.4–30.0	0.10–0.90
- Anterior slide test	0.17	0.86	1.2	0.97
- Compression-rotation	0.61	0.54	1.3	0.72
Combination of tests for instability				
- Apprehension + relocation tests (glenoid labrum tear)	0.38	0.93	5.4	0.67
- Apprehension + relocation tests (anterior instability)	0.82	0.98	39.7	0.19
Combination of tests for SLAP lesion				
- High SN (choose 2) 1. Compression-Rotation test 2. Apprehension test 3. Active compression test	0.75	0.90	7.5	0.28
- High SP (choose 1) 1. Yergason test 2. Biceps load II test 3. Speed test				
Combination of tests for impingement and rotator cuff tear (RCT) 1. Hawkins-Kennedy test 2. Painful arc test 3. Infraspinatus muscle test				
- Impingement: at least 2 positive	0.26	0.98	10.6	0.75
- RCT: all 3 positive	0.33	0.98	15.9	0.69

Adapted from Magee DJ: Orthopedic Physical Assessment, 6th ed. 2014; Cleland AC, Koppenhaver S, Su J: Netter's Orthopaedic Clinical Examination, 3rd ed. 2016.

e. Internal rotation lag sign.
  - Patient seated; hold patient's hand behind the back in the lumbar region in full internal rotation.
  - Positive if patient is unable to maintain position when arm/hand is released.

5. Acromioclavicular (AC) joint.
  a. Horizontal adduction test.
    - Patient standing; shoulder flexed to 90°.
    - Arm is actively or passively fully adducted across the body.
    - Positive test is localized pain over the AC joint.
  b. Paxinos sign.
    - Patient seated; arm relaxed at side.
    - Examiner places thumb under the posterolateral aspect of the acromion and the index/long fingers of the same hand over the middle part of the clavicle.
    - Pressure applied with both the thumb (anterosuperior) and fingers (inferior).
    - Positive test is localized pain in the AC joint.
6. SLAP (superior labrum anterior to posterior) lesions.
  a. Active compression (O'Brien) test.
    - Patient standing; arm flexed to 90° and elbow fully extended.
    - Arm horizontally adducted 10–15°, fully internally rotated, and a downward force applied to the arm.
    - Arm returned to the starting position, now fully externally rotated, and a downward force applied.
    - Positive test is joint pain or painful clicking produced in the first part of the test and eliminated in the second part of the test.
    - Must differentiate between reproduction of glenohumeral vs. acromioclavicular joint symptoms.
  b. Biceps load II test.
    - Patient supine; shoulder abducted 120°, elbow flexed to 90°, forearm supinated.
    - Shoulder is fully externally rotated; if apprehension appears the patient is asked to flex the elbow against resistance.
    - Test is positive if apprehension remains the same or shoulder becomes more painful.
  c. Anterior slide test.
    - Patient seated with hands on waist, thumbs posterior.
    - With scapula stabilized, an anterior-superior force is applied at the elbow.
    - Positive test is pain or click reproduced deep in the shoulder.
  d. Compression-rotation test.
    - Patient supine; shoulder passively abducted to 20° to 90°.
    - Axial compression applied while passively circumducting the glenohumeral joint.
    - Positive test is pain, clicking or catching sensation produced.
  e. Yergason test.
    - Utilized to test for integrity of transverse ligament, bicipital tendinosis/tendinopathy, and SLAP lesions.
    - Patient sitting with shoulder in neutral stabilized against trunk, elbow at 90°, and forearm pronated; resist supination of forearm and ER of shoulder.
    - Tendon of biceps long head will "pop out" of groove. May also reproduce pain in long head of biceps tendon.
  f. Speed's test (biceps straight arm).
    - Utilized to test for bicipital tendinosis/tendinopathy and SLAP lesions.
    - Patient sitting or standing with upper limb in full extension and forearm supinated; resist shoulder flexion.
    - May also place shoulder in 90° flexion and push upper limb into extension, causing an eccentric contraction of the biceps.
    - Positive test is pain in the anterior shoulder.
7. Neurological dysfunction: Upper limb tension tests (see Table 2-14).
  a. Identifies peripheral nerve dysfunction by stressing neurological tissue.
  b. Positive result is reproduction of the patient's symptoms.
8. Thoracic outlet syndrome.
  a. Adson's test (see Figure 2-24).
    - Identifies pathology of structures that pass through thoracic inlet.
    - Patient sitting. Find radial pulse of extremity being tested. Rotate head toward extremity being tested, and then extend and externally rotate the shoulder while extending the head.
    - Neurological and/or vascular symptoms (disappearance of pulse) will be reproduced in upper extremity.
    - SN and SP not available.
  b. Roos elevated arm test.
    - Identifies pathology of structures that pass through thoracic inlet.
    - Patient standing, with shoulders fully externally rotated, 90° abducted, and slightly horizontally abducted. Elbows flexed to 90° and patient opens/closes hands for 3 minutes slowly.
    - Neurological and/or vascular symptoms (disappearance of pulse) will be reproduced in upper extremity.
    - SN and SP not available.

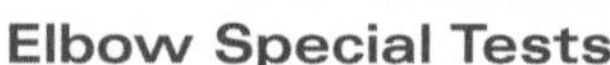

Elbow Special Tests

1. Elbow extension test to rule out fracture or joint injury (see Table 2-15): positive if patient is unable to fully extend the elbow.
2. Ligamentous instability.
   a. Varus/valgus stress test.
      - Patient sitting or supine; entire upper limb is supported and stabilized and elbow placed in 20° to 0° of flexion.
      - Valgus force placed through elbow tests ulnar collateral ligament; varus force placed through elbow tests radial collateral ligament.
      - Primary finding is laxity, but pain may be noted as well.
      - SN and SP not available.

   b. Moving valgus stress test (see Table 2-15).
      - Patient standing or supine; arm abducted, elbow fully flexed.
      - Maintain valgus stress and quickly extend patient's elbow.
      - Reproduction of pain from 120° to 70° elbow flexion indicates partial tear of the ulnar collateral ligament.
3. Biceps rupture: "Popeye" sign.
   a. Distal bunching of the muscle with complete loss of function.
   b. Indicates rupture of the proximal long head of the biceps.
4. Neurological dysfunction.
   a. Elbow flexion test (see Table 2-15).
      - Identifies the presence of cubital tunnel syndrome.
      - Patient supine; performed bilaterally with the shoulder in full ER and the elbow actively held in maximal flexion with wrist extension for one minute.

Table 2-14

Neurodynamic Tension Tests: Upper Limb Tension Test (ULTT)

	ULTT1 (*MEDIAN AND ANTERIOR INTEROSSEOUS NERVE BIAS*)	ULTT2 (*MEDIAN, AXILLARY, AND MUSCULOCUTANEOUS NERVE BIAS*)	ULTT3 (*RADIAL NERVE BIAS*)	ULTT4 (*ULNAR NERVE BIAS*)
Shoulder	Depression and abduction (110°)	Depression and abduction (10°)	Depression and abduction (10°)	Depression and abduction (10° to 90°) with hand to ear (waiter's position)
Elbow	Extension	Extension	Extension	Flexion
Forearm	Supination	Supination	Pronation	Pronation
Wrist	Extension	Extension	Flexion and ulnar deviation	Extension and radial deviation
Fingers and thumb	Extension	Extension	Flexion	Extension
Shoulder		Lateral rotation	Medial rotation	Lateral rotation
Cervical Spine	Contralateral side flexion	Contralateral side flexion	Contralateral side flexion	Contralateral side flexion

Adapted from Magee DJ: Orthopedic Physical Assessment, 6th ed. 2014.

Table 2-15

Diagnostic Accuracy of Elbow Special Tests

TEST	SN	SP	+LR	–LR
Elbow fracture - Elbow extension test	0.91–0.97	0.49–0.69	1.9–3.0	0.04–0.13
Elbow instability - Moving valgus stress test	0.75	1.00	4.0	0.40
Elbow neurologic dysfunction - Elbow flexion test	0.75	0.99	75	0.25

Adapted from Magee, Orthopedic Physical Assessment, 6th Edition; Cleland, Orthopaedic Clinical Examination, 3rd Edition.

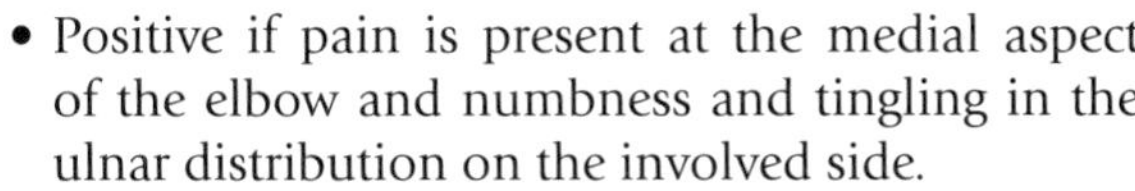

- Positive if pain is present at the medial aspect of the elbow and numbness and tingling in the ulnar distribution on the involved side.

b. Pinch grip test.
- Identifies entrapment of the anterior interosseous nerve.
- Patient asked to pinch tips of index finger and thumb.
- Positive if patient is unable to pinch tip-to-tip; compensatory pulp-to-pulp pinch is present.

Wrist and Hand Special Tests

1. Ligament, capsule, and joint instability.

a. Ulnomeniscotriquetral dorsal glide test (see Table 2-16).
- Patient seated with arm pronated.
- Posteriorly directed force applied with examiner's thumb over ulna dorsally and index finger over the pisotriquetral complex anteriorly.
- Excessive pain or laxity indicates triangular fibrocartilage complex (TFCC) pathology.

b. Watson (scaphoid shift) test (see Table 2-16).
- Patient seated; elbow resting on table, forearm pronated, wrist placed in full ulnar deviation with slight extension while stabilizing metacarpals.
- Place pressure on distal pole of the scaphoid while radially deviating and slightly flexing the patient's hand.
- A painful "shift" of the scaphoid with a "clunk" when pressure is removed indicates carpal instability.

c. Interphalangeal joint varus/valgus stress tests.
- Fingers are supported and stabilized; valgus/varus forces applied to PIP and DIP joints of all digits.
- Primary finding is laxity, but pain may be noted as well.
- SN and SP not available.

2. Tendons and muscles:

a. Eichhoff's test (see Figure 2-26 and Table 2-16).
- Identifies de Quervain's tenosynovitis (tendonitis of the abductor pollicis longus and/or extensor pollicis brevis).
- Patient makes fist with thumb flexed within confines of fingers; examiner passively moves wrist into ulnar deviation.
- Positive test reproduces pain in wrist; often painful with no pathology, so compare to uninvolved side.

b. Finkelstein's test (see Table 2-16).
- Identifies de Quervain's tenosynovitis (tendonitis of the abductor pollicis longus and/or extensor pollicis brevis).
- Examiner passively pulls the wrist and thumb into ulnar deviation and applies longitudinal traction.
- Positive test reproduces pain in wrist; often painful with no pathology, so compare to uninvolved side.

c. Wrist hyperabduction and abduction of the thumb test (WHAT) (see Table 2-16).
- Identifies de Quervain's tenosynovitis (tendonitis of the abductor pollicis longus and/or extensor pollicis brevis).
- Patient's wrist is hyperflexed with the thumb abducted in full MCP and IP extension.
- Resistance is applied against the examiner's index finger.
- Positive test reproduces pain in the wrist.

3. Neurological dysfunction.

a. Phalen's (wrist flexion) test (see Figure 2-28 and Table 2-16).
- Identifies carpal tunnel compression of median nerve.
- Patient maximally flexes both wrists holding them against each other for 1 minute.
- Positive if reproduces tingling and/or paresthesia into hand following median nerve distribution.

Table 2-16

Diagnostic Accuracy of Wrist and Hand Special Tests

TEST	SN	SP	+LR	–LR
Instability				
- Ulnomeniscotriquetral dorsal glide test	0.64	0.66	1.7	0.56
- Watson (scaphoid shift) test	0.66	0.69	2.0	0.47
Muscle and tendon dysfunction				
- Eichhoff's test	0.89	0.14	1.0	0.79
- Finkelstein's test	0.81	0.50	1.6	0.38
- Wrist hyperflexion and abduction test (WHAT)	0.99	0.29	1.39	0.04
Wrist and hand neurologic dysfunction				
- Phalen's (wrist flexion) test	0.34–0.85	0.17–0.92	0.6–9.9	0.19–3.1
Vascular compromise				
- Modified Allen test	0.29–1.00	0.97	0.2–43.5	0.0–0.74

Adapted from Magee, Orthopedic Physical Assessment, 6th Edition; Cleland, Orthopaedic Clinical Examination, 3rd Edition.

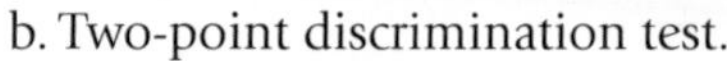

b. Two-point discrimination test.
- Identifies level of sensory innervation within hand that correlates with functional ability to perform certain tasks involving grasp.
- Using a caliper, two-point discriminator, or paper clip, apply device to palmar aspect of fingers to assess patient's ability to distinguish between two points of testing device; record smallest difference that patient can sense two separate points.
- Normal amount that can be discriminated is generally less than 6 mm.

c. Tinel's sign.
- Identifies carpal tunnel compression of median nerve.
- Tap region where median nerve passes through carpal tunnel.
- Reproduces tingling and/or paresthesia into hand following median nerve distribution.
- SN and SP not available.

4. Vascular compromise: modified Allen test (see Figure 2-29 and Table 2-16).
   a. Identify radial and ulnar arteries at wrist; have patient open/close fingers quickly several times and then make a closed fist.
   b. Compress the ulnar artery and have patient open hand; observe palm of hand and then release the compression on artery and observe for vascular filling; perform same procedure with radial artery.
   c. Positive finding will present by abnormal filling of blood within hand during test; under normal circumstances, there is a change in color from white to normal appearance on palm of hand.
5. Finger mobility tests.
   a. Bunnel-Littler test.
   - Identifies joints or intrinsic tightness at the PIP joints.
   - MCP joint is stabilized in slight extension while PIP joint is flexed. Then MCP joint is flexed and PIP joint is flexed.
   - Differentiates between a tight capsule and tight intrinsic muscles. If flexion is limited in both cases, capsule is tight. If more PIP flexion with MCP flexion, then intrinsic muscles are tight.
   - SN and SP not available.

   b. Tight retinacular test (see Figure 2-27).
   - Identifies tightness around proximal interphalangeal joint.
   - PIP is stabilized in neutral while DIP is flexed. Then PIP is flexed and DIP is flexed.
   - Differentiates between a tight capsule and tight retinacular ligaments. If flexion is limited in both cases, capsule is tight. If more DIP flexion with PIP flexion, then retinacular ligaments are tight.
   - SN and SP not available.

Special Tests of the Lower Extremity

Hip Special Tests

1. Hip pathology.
   a. Hip scour test (see Figure 2-31 and Table 2-17).
   - Identifies general hip joint pathology and degenerative joint disease (DJD).
   - Patient supine with hip flexed and adducted to the limit of movement.
   - Hip is taken into abduction while maintaining flexion.
   - May also add compressive load.
   - Positive test is reproduction of familiar pain or apprehension.

   b. Patrick (FABER) test (see Figure 2-30 and Table 2-17).
   - Identifies dysfunction of hip, such as mobility restriction.
   - Patient supine; passively flex, abduct, and externally rotate test leg so that foot is resting just above knee on opposite leg.
   - Slowly lower testing leg down toward table surface.
   - Positive test when involved knee is unable to assume relaxed position and/or reproduction of painful symptoms.
2. Labral lesions: FADDIR/FADIR test (see Figure 2-37 and Table 2-17).
   a. Identifies anterior-superior impingement, iliopsoas tendinopathy, and anterior labral tears.
   b. Patient supine; involved lower extremity is taken from full passive hip flexion, abduction, and ER into a flexed, adducted, and internally rotated position.
   c. Positive test is reproduction of pain with or without click.
3. Muscle length/strength.
   a. Thomas test (see Figure 2-33).
   - Identifies tightness of hip flexors.
   - Patient supine; one hip and knee maximally flexed to chest and held there; opposite limb is kept straight on table.
   - Observe whether hip flexion occurs on straight leg as opposite limb is flexed.
   - Weakness of test is that it does not differentiate between tightness in iliacus versus psoas major.
   - Positive if straight limb's hip flexes and/or patient is unable to remain flat on table when opposite limb is flexed.
   - SN and SP not available.

   b. Ober's test (see Figures 2-34 and 2-35).
   - Identifies tightness of the tensor fascia lata and/or iliotibial band.
   - Patient side lying; lower limb flexed at the hip and the knee.

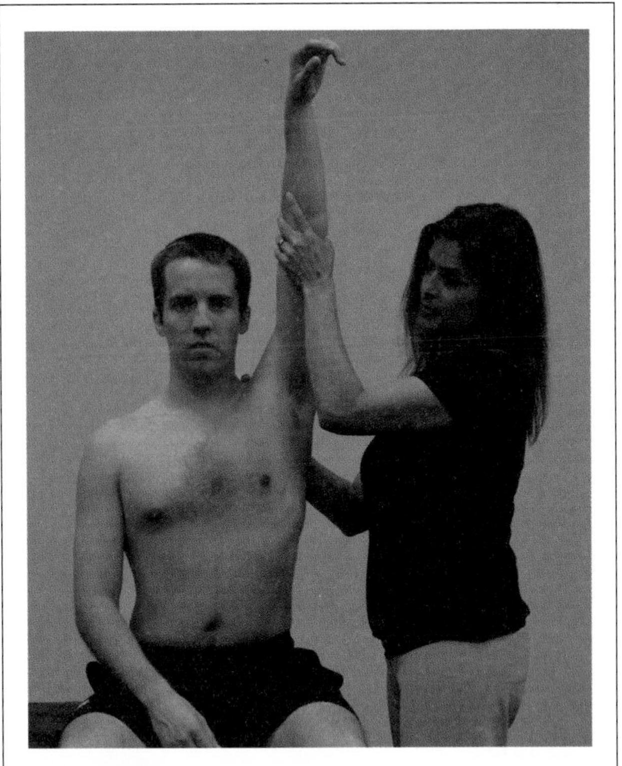

Figure 2-22 Neer's test.

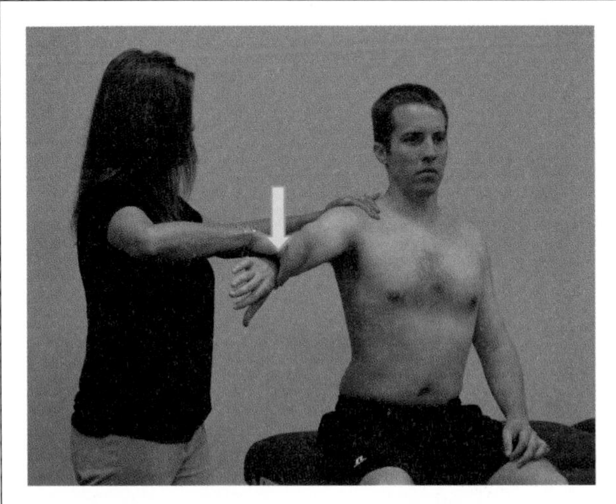

Figure 2-23 Supraspinatus (empty can) test.

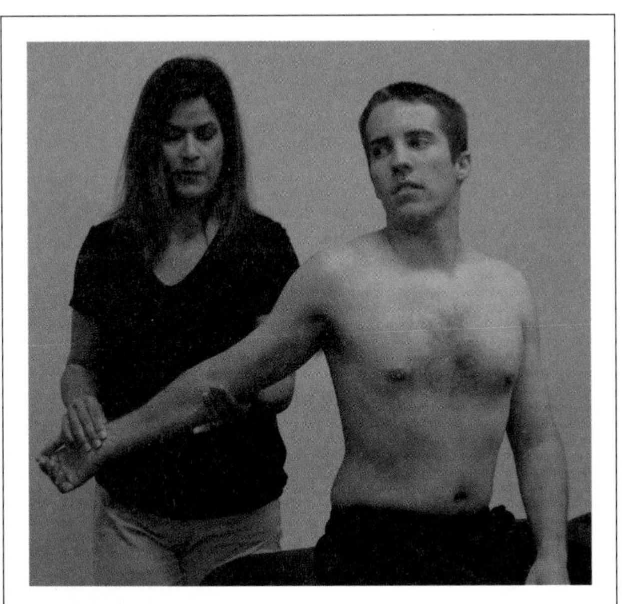

Figure 2-24 Adson's test.

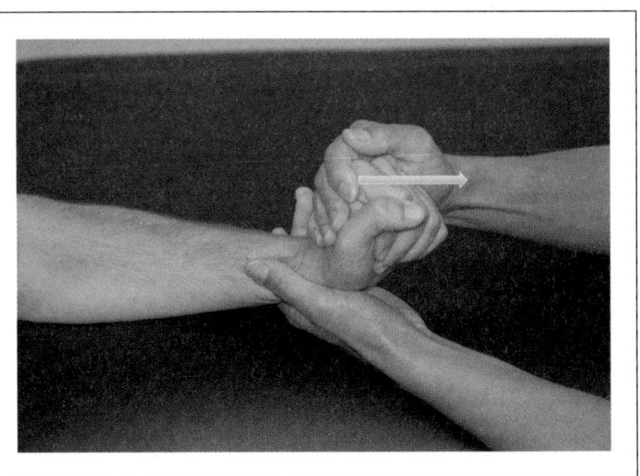

Figure 2-25 Lateral epicondylitis and epicondylopathy ("tennis elbow") test.

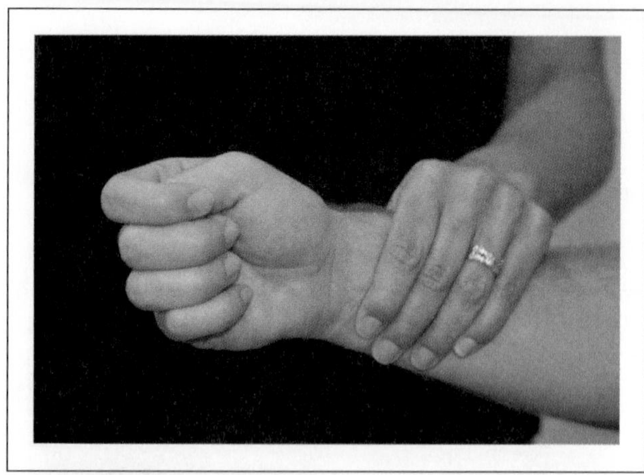

Figure 2-26a Eichhoff's test; start position.

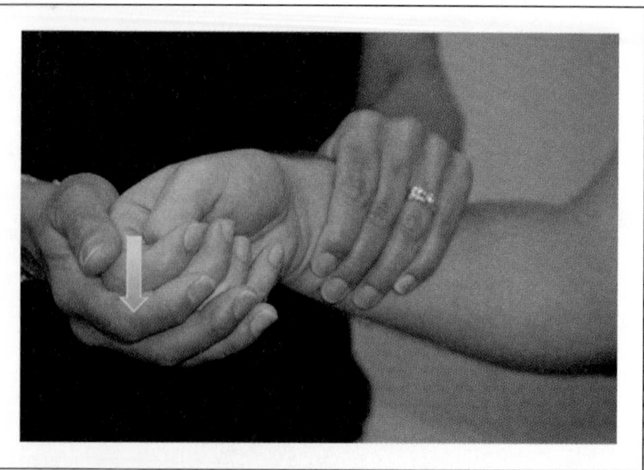

Figure 2-26b Eichhoff's test; passive movement into ulnar deviation.

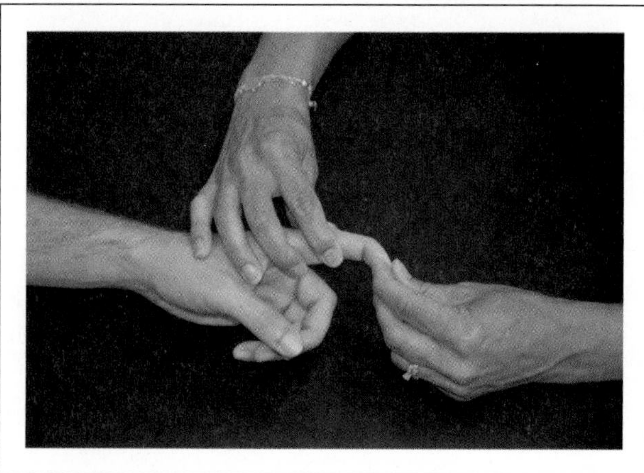

Figure 2-27a Tight retinacular test.

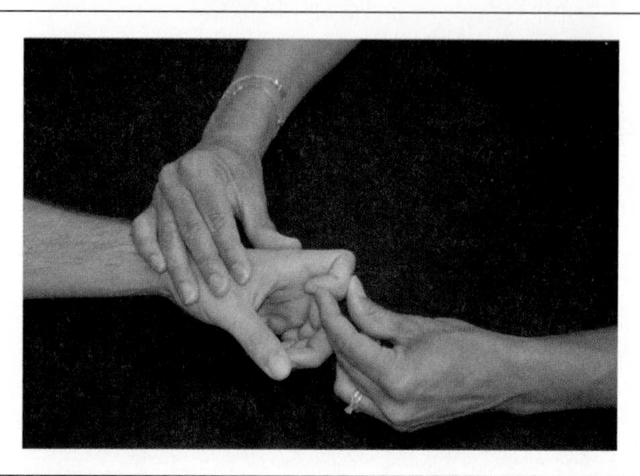

Figure 2-27b Tight retinacular test.

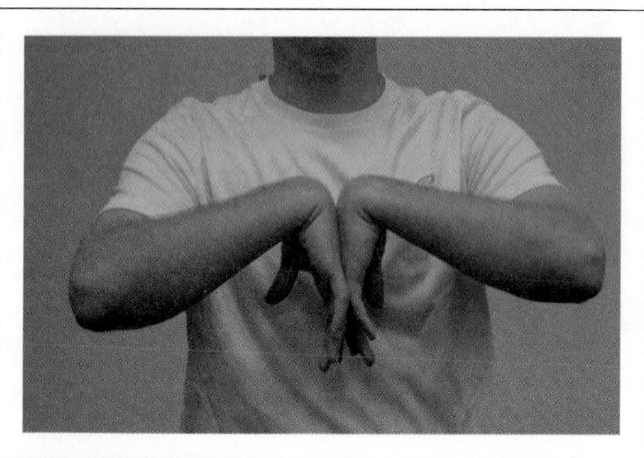

Figure 2-28 Phalen's test.

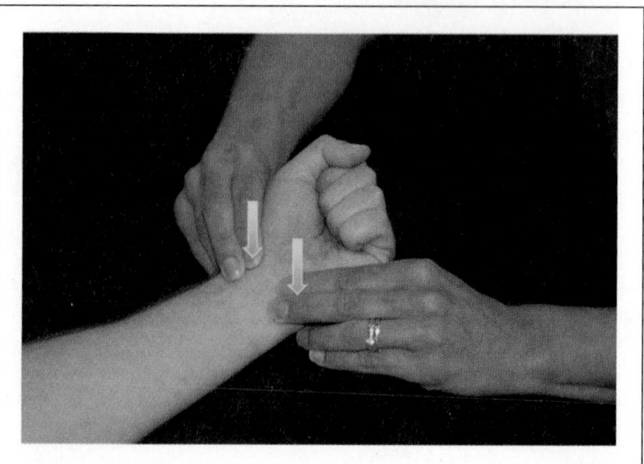

Figure 2-29a Allen test; compress ulnar and radial arteries.

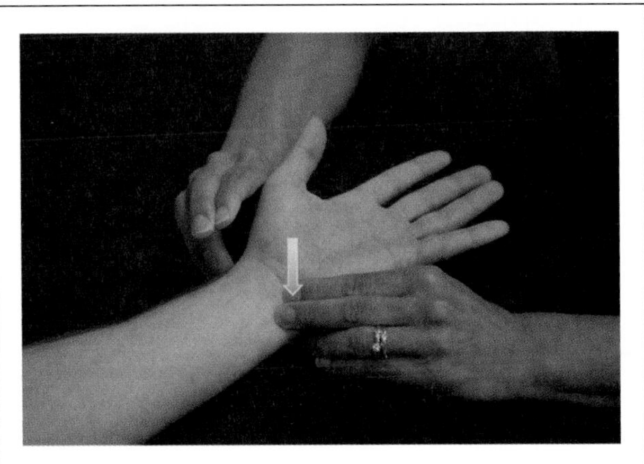

Figure 2-29b Allen test; compress ulnar artery.

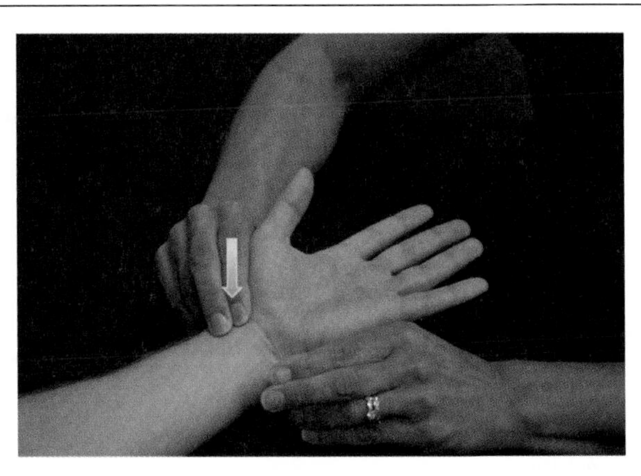

Figure 2-29c Allen test; compress radial artery.

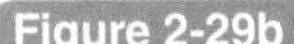

Table 2-17

Diagnostic Accuracy of Hip Special Tests

TEST	SN	SP	+LR	−LR
General hip joint pathology				
- Scour test	0.62	0.75	2.5	0.51
- FABER (flex/abd/ER) test	0.60	0.18	0.73	2.2
Labral lesions				
- FADIR (flex/add/IR) test	0.78	0.10	0.86	2.3
Hip weakness				
- Trendelenburg sign	0.23–0.73	0.77–0.94	3.2–3.6	0.35–0.82
Combination of tests for hip OA: Symptoms increase with squatting Lateral pain with active hip flexion (+) Scour test Pain with active hip extension Passive IR <25 deg				
- 5 of 5 above tests positive	0.14	0.98	7.3	0.87
- 4 of 5	0.48	0.98	24.3	0.53
- 3 of 5	0.71	0.86	5.2	0.33
- 2 of 5	0.81	0.61	2.1	0.31
- 1 of 5	0.95	0.18	1.2	0.27
Hip fracture				
- Patellar-pubic percussion test	0.94–0.96	0.86–0.96	6.7–21.6	0.07–0.14

Adapted from Magee, Orthopedic Physical Assessment, 6th Edition; Cleland, Orthopaedic Clinical Examination, 3rd Edition.

- Passively extend and abduct tested hip with knee flexed to 90° and slowly lower the limb toward the table; modified test starts with knee extended.
- Positive if the uppermost limb remains above horizontal.
- SN and SP not available.

c. Ely's test (see Figure 2-36).
- Identifies tightness of the rectus femoris.
- Patient prone; flex knee of tested limb.
- Positive if hip of tested limb flexes.
- SN and SP not available.

d. 90–90 hamstring test.
- Identifies tightness of the hamstrings.
- Patient supine; hip and knee supported in 90° flexion.
- Passively extend knee until barrier is encountered.
- Positive if knee lacks 10° or greater of knee extension.

e. Piriformis test.
- Identifies piriformis tightness and piriformis syndrome.
- Patient supine; foot of tested limb passively placed lateral to opposite limb's knee with tested hip adducted.
- Observe position of tested knee relative to opposite knee; positive if tested knee is unable to pass over resting knee and/or reproduction of pain/paresthesia in buttock and/or along sciatic nerve distribution.
- SN and SP not available.

f. Trendelenburg sign (see Figure 2-32 and Table 2-17).
- Identifies weakness of the gluteus medius or unstable hip.
- Patient standing and asked to stand on one leg (flex opposite knee).
- Observe pelvis of stance leg; positive when ipsilateral hip drops when lower limb support is removed while standing.

4. Leg length.
   a. Patient supine, with pelvis balanced/aligned with lower limbs and trunk.
   b. Measure distance from ASIS to lateral malleolus or medial malleolus on each limb several times for consistency and compare results.
   c. Unequal girth of the thigh musculature (left versus right) can skew results if using medial malleolus landmark.
   d. A difference in lengths between two limbs identifies a true leg length discrepancy.
   e. True vs. functional leg length discrepancy.
      - True discrepancy is caused by an anatomical difference in bone lengths (either tibia or femur).
      - Functional discrepancies are not anatomical in origin and are the result of compensation due to abnormal position or posture, such as pronation of a foot or pelvic obliquity.
   f. SN and SP not available.
5. Hip fractures: Patellar-Pubic Percussion Test (see Table 2-17).
   a. With patient supine, examiner percusses (taps) each patella separately while auscultating the pubic symphysis with a stethoscope.
   b. A positive test is decreased percussion note on the affected side.

RED FLAG: Timely diagnosis and intervention for a suspected femoral neck fracture, including high-grade femoral neck stress injuries, is critical. Disruption of the circumflex arterial supply potentially leaves the femoral head susceptible to avascular necrosis. Hip fractures carry a substantial health care cost whether managed with conservative or operative treatment.

Knee Special Tests (See Table 2-18)

1. 1-plane anterior instability.
   a. Lachman test (see Figure 2-38).
      - Tests integrity of the anterior cruciate ligament.
      - Patient supine; tested knee flexed 20° to 30°.
      - Stabilize femur and passively translate tibia anteriorly.
      - Positive test is excessive anterior translation of the tibia compared to the uninvolved limb and lack of firm end-feel.
   b. Anterior drawer test.
      - Tests integrity of the anterior cruciate ligament.
      - Patient supine; hip flexed to 45° and knee flexed to 90°.
      - Passively translate tibia anteriorly.
      - Positive test is excessive anterior translation of the tibia compared to the uninvolved limb.
2. 1-plane posterior instability.
   a. Posterior drawer test.
      - Tests integrity of the posterior cruciate ligament.
      - Patient supine; hip flexed to 45° and knee flexed to 90°.
      - Passively translate tibia posteriorly.
      - Positive test is excessive posterior translation of the tibia compared to the uninvolved limb.
   b. Posterior sag sign.
      - Tests integrity of the posterior cruciate ligament.
      - Patient supine; hip flexed to 45° and knee flexed to 90°.
      - Observe to see whether the tibia "sags" posteriorly.
      - Normally, medial tibial plateau extends 1 cm anteriorly beyond the femoral condyle; positive finding is loss of "step."
3. 1-plane medial-lateral instability.
   a. Valgus stress test.
      - Tests integrity of the medial collateral ligament.
      - Patient supine; knee resting on the edge of the exam table.
      - Valgus (medial) stress applied at the knee (both at 0° and 30° of knee flexion).
      - Positive with laxity and/or pain.
      - Positive finding at 0° extension indicates major disruption of the knee with one or more rotary tests also positive.
   b. Varus stress test.
      - Tests integrity of the lateral collateral ligament.
      - Patient supine; knee resting on the edge of the exam table.
      - Varus (lateral) stress applied at the knee (both at 0 and 30° of knee flexion).
      - Positive with laxity and/or pain.
      - Positive finding at 0° extension indicates major disruption of the knee with one or more rotary tests also positive.

Table 2-18

Diagnostic Accuracy of Knee Special Tests

TEST	SN	SP	+LR	–LR
1-plane anterior instability				
- Lachman test	0.81	0.81	4.3	0.24
- Anterior drawer test	0.38	0.81	2.0	0.77
1-plane posterior instability				
- Posterior drawer test	0.56–0.90	0.99	56.0–90.0	0.10–0.44
- Posterior sag sign	0.79	1.0	>100	0.21
Medial instability				
- Pain with valgus stress at 30° of knee flexion	0.78	0.67	2.3	0.30
- Laxity with valgus stress at 30° of knee flexion	0.91	0.49	1.8	0.20
Anterolateral rotary instability				
- Pivot shift test (w/o anesthesia)	0.28	0.81	1.5	0.89
- Pivot shift test (w/anesthesia)	0.73	0.98	36.5	0.28
Meniscus				
- McMurray test	0.51	0.78	2.3	0.63
- Thessaly test	0.31–0.92	0.67–0.95	1.8–39.3	0.09–0.73
Patellofemoral instability				
- Patellar apprehension test	0.32	0.86	2.3	0.79
Ottawa Knee Rules				
- Adults	0.99	0.49	1.9	0.05
- Children	0.99	0.46	1.9	0.07
Combination of tests for meniscus tears				
- Combined history and physical examination (joint effusion, joint line tenderness, McMurray test, hyperflexion text, squat test)	0.86	0.83	5.1	0.17
- Joint line tenderness plus (+) McMurray test	0.75–0.91	0.91–0.99	10.1–75.0	0.10–0.25
- Joint line tenderness plus (+) Thessaly test	0.78–0.93	0.92–0.99	11.6–78.0	0.08–0.22

Adapted from: Magee DJ: Orthopedic Physical Assessment, 6th ed. 2014.; Cleland JA, Koppenhaver S, Su J: Netter's Orthopaedic Clinical Examination, 3rd ed. 2016.

4. Anterolateral instability: pivot-shift test.
   a. Tests integrity of the anterior cruciate ligament.
   b. Patient supine; knee in extension, hip flexed/abducted to 30° with slight internal rotation.
   c. Hold knee with one hand and foot with other hand; place valgus force through knee and flex knee.
   d. Positive test is indicated by tibia relocating during the test; as the knee is flexed, the tibia clunks backward at approximately 30° to 40°.
   e. Tibia was subluxed at the beginning of the test; reduced by pull of the iliotibial band as the knee was flexed.
5. Meniscus tear.
   a. McMurray test (see Figure 2-39).
      - Patient supine; tested knee in maximal flexion.
      - Passively, internally rotate and extend the knee (tests lateral meniscus).
      - Passively, externally rotate and extend the knee (tests medial meniscus).
      - Positive finding is reproduction of click and/or pain in knee joint.
   b. Thessaly test.
      - Patient standing on the symptomatic leg, holding the examiner's hands.
      - Patient rotates the body and leg internally and externally with the knee flexed 5° and then 20°.
      - Positive finding is reproduction of click and/or pain in knee joint.
6. Patellofemoral instability: patellar apprehension test.
   a. Patient supine; knee flexed to 30°, quadriceps relaxed.
   b. Passively translate the patella laterally.
   c. Positive if the patient expresses apprehension or contracts the quadriceps to prevent patella from dislocating.
7. Patellar tilt test.
   a. Patient is supine with the knee extended.
   b. Lift the lateral edge of the patella from the lateral femoral condyle.
   c. Positive test if the patella is not able to be lifted to at least a neutral angle with respect to the horizontal plane.
   d. Sn and Sp not available.

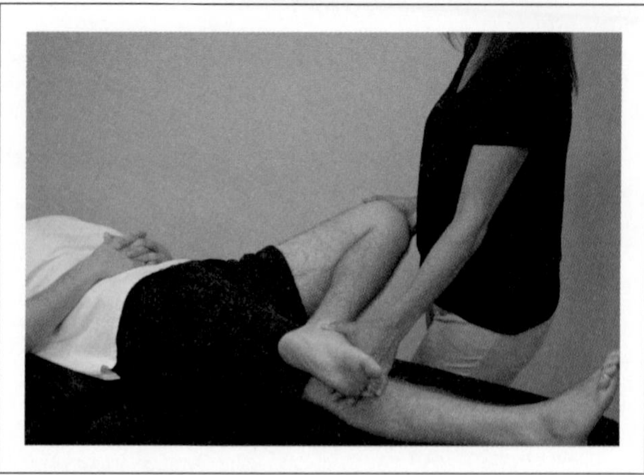

Figure 2-30 Patrick's (FABER) test.

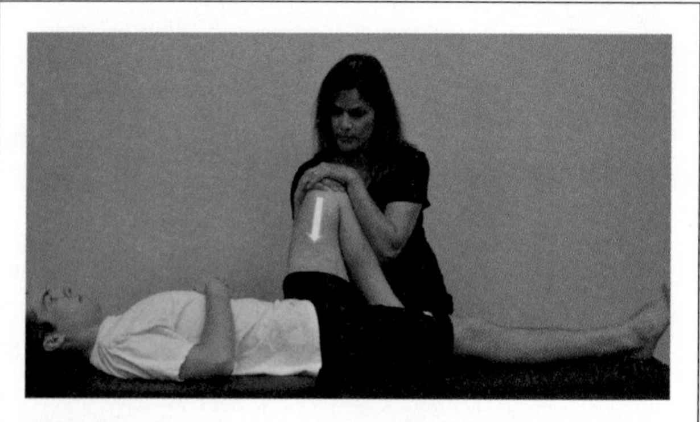

Figure 2-31 Grind (Scouring) test.

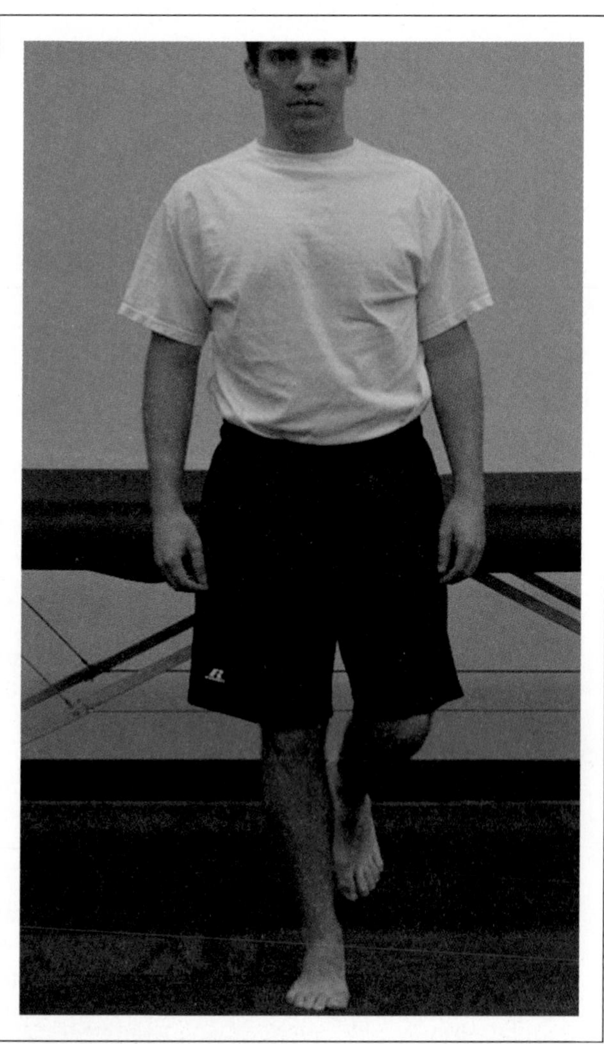

Figure 2-32a Trendelenburg sign; negative test.

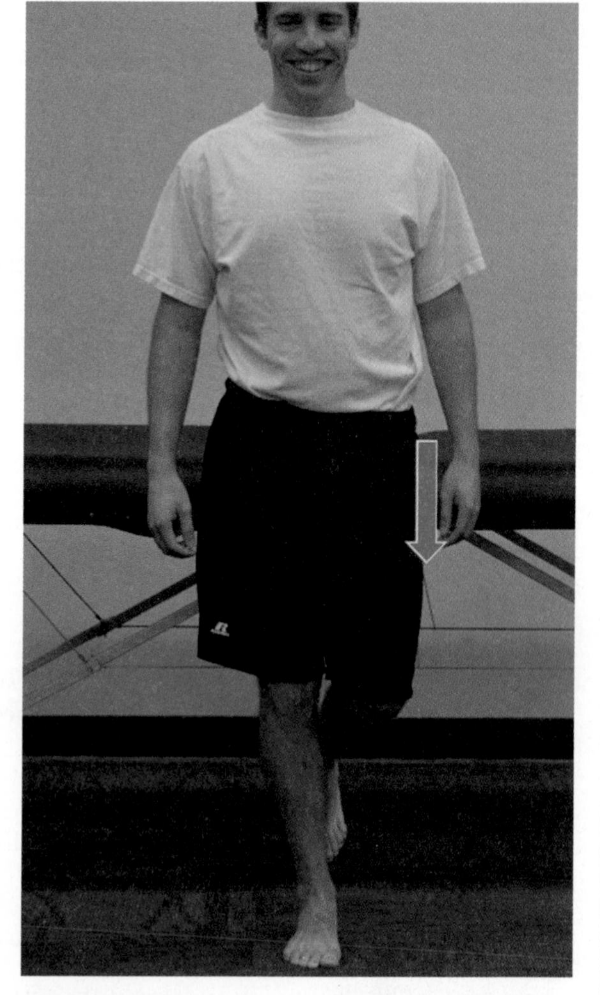

Figure 2-32b Trendelenburg sign; positive test; dropped pelvis.

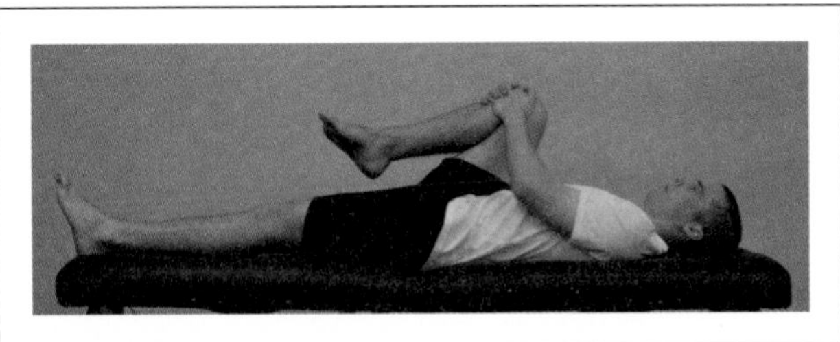

Figure 2-33a Thomas test; negative.

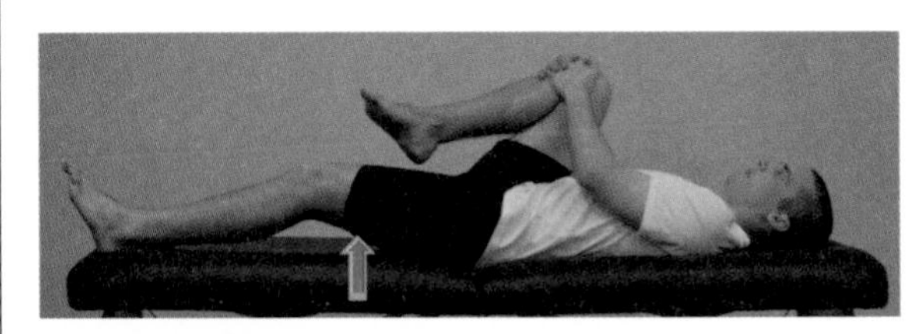

Figure 2-33b Thomas test; positive.

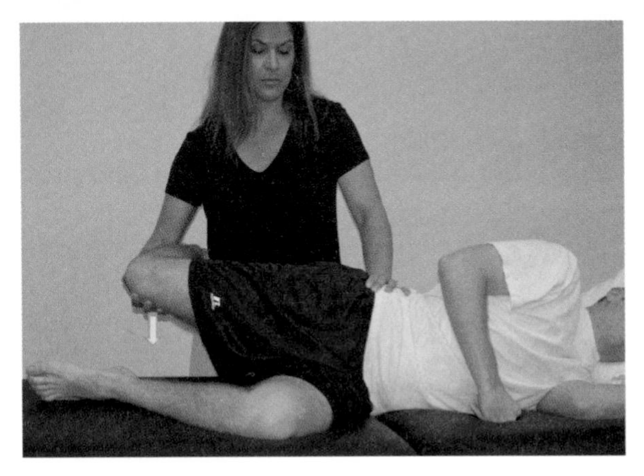

Figure 2-34 Ober test.

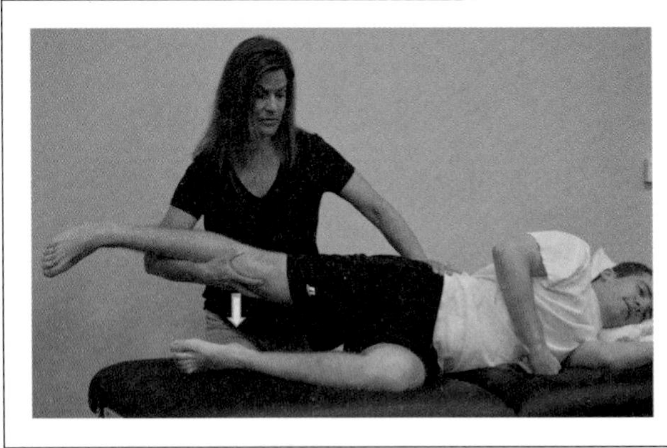

Figure 2-35 Modified Ober test.

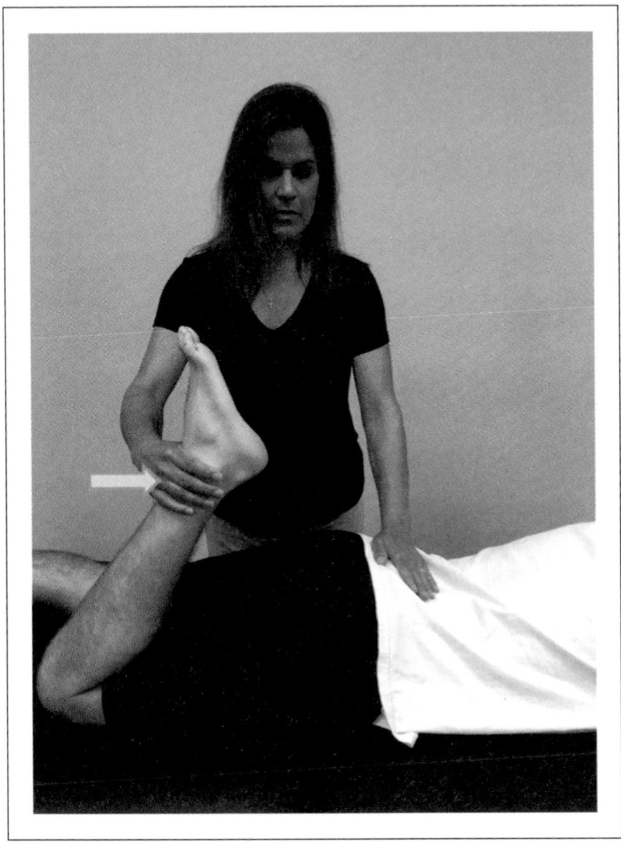

Figure 2-36a Ely's test; negative.

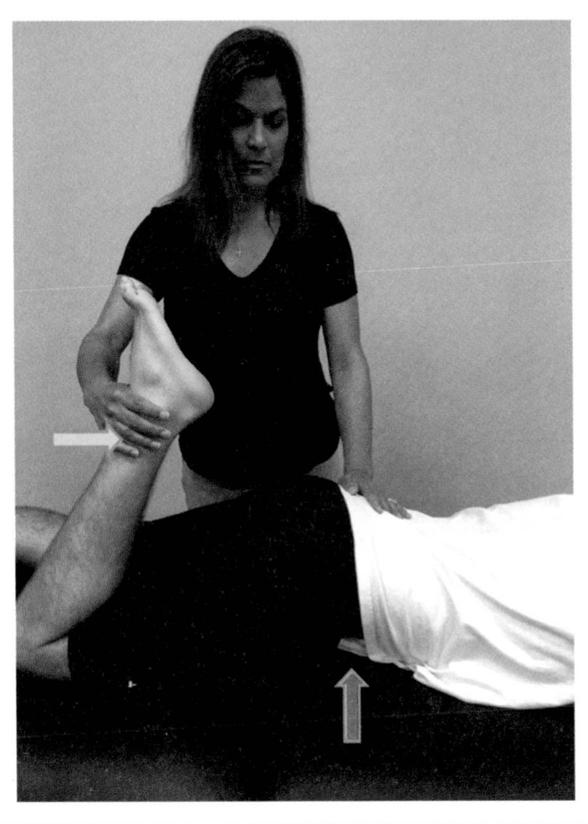

Figure 2-36b Ely's test; positive.

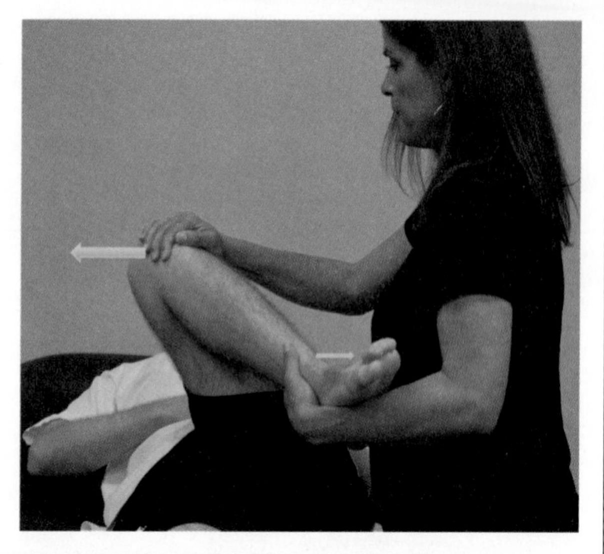

Figure 2-37 FADDIR/FADIR test.

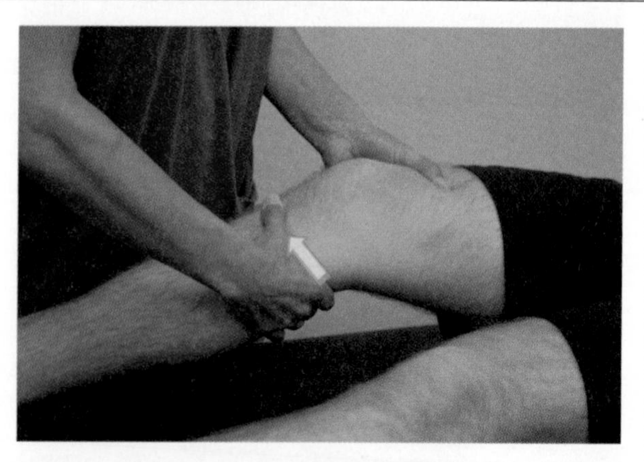

Figure 2-38 Lachman stress test.

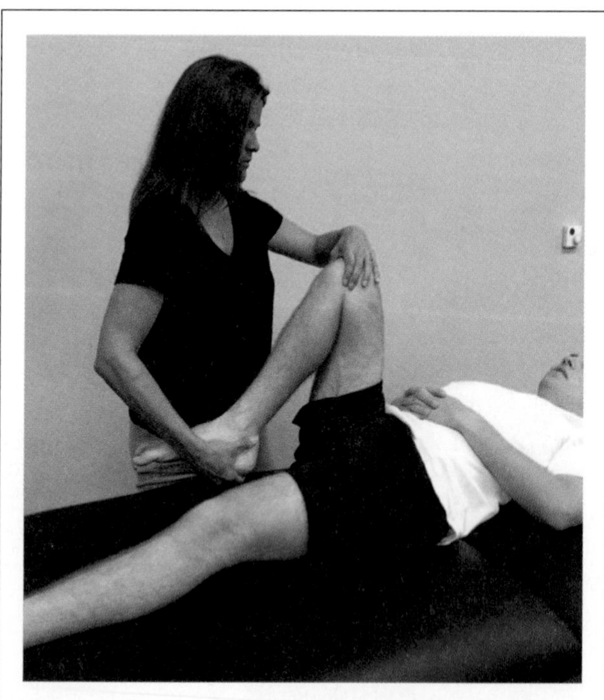

Figure 2-39a McMurray's test; knee flexion.

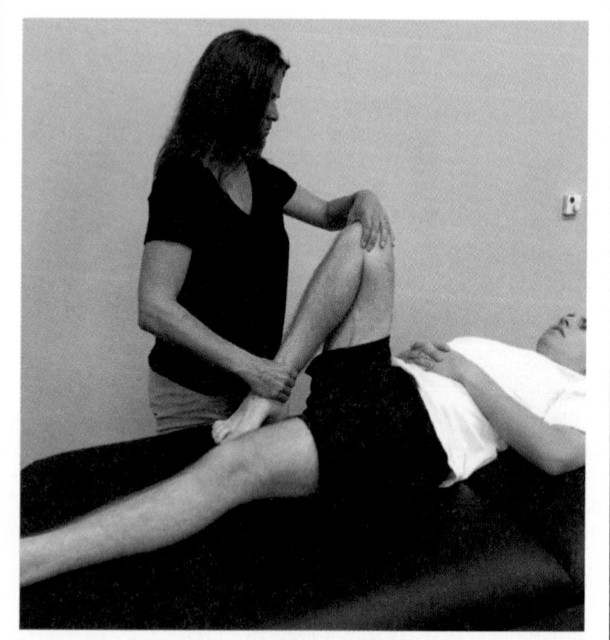

Figure 2-39b McMurray's test; tibial internal rotation.

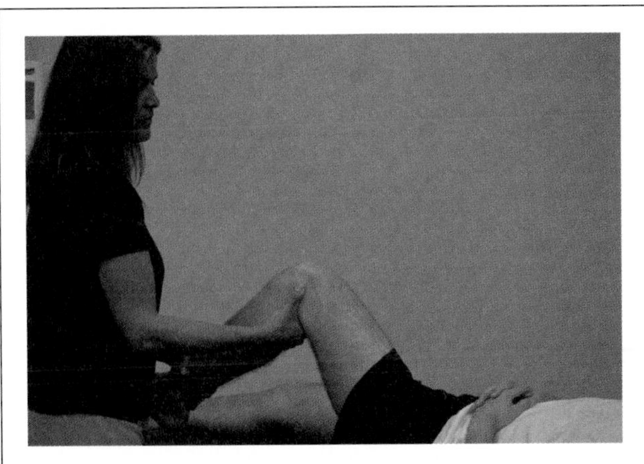

Figure 2-40a Noble compression test; hip and knee flexion.

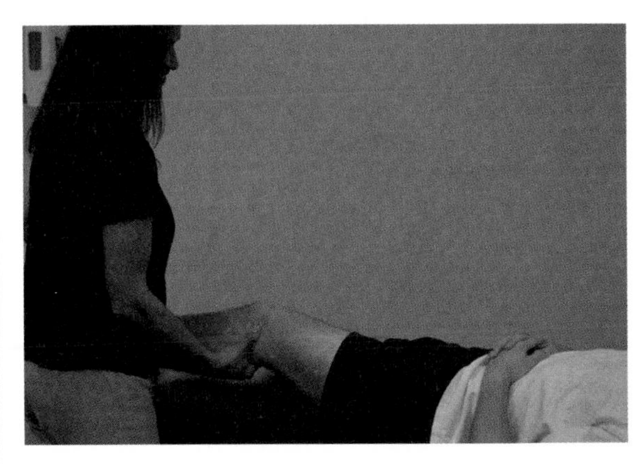

Figure 2-40b Noble compression test; knee extension and pressure.

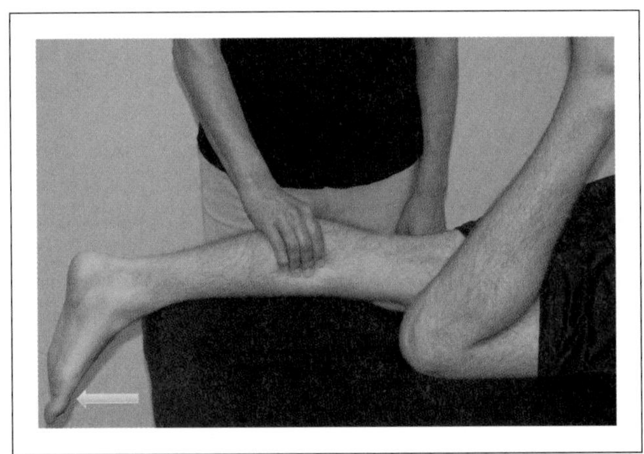

Figure 2-41 Thompson's test.

8. Iliotibial band friction syndrome: noble compression test (see Figure 2-40).
   a. Patient supine; knee flexed to 90° with hip flexion.
   b. Pressure applied 1 to 2 cm proximal to lateral femoral epicondyle; with pressure maintained, patient's knee is passively extended.
   c. Positive if patient experiences pain over the lateral femoral condyle.
9. Swelling: brush (stroke) test.
   a. Patient is supine, knee in full extension.
   b. Starting at the medial tibiofemoral joint, stroke upward two to three times toward the suprapatellar pouch.
   c. Then stroke downward on the distal lateral thigh, just superior to the suprapatellar pouch, toward the lateral joint line.
   d. Positive if fluid is observed on the medial knee.
   e. Quantified with a 5-point scale: 0 = no wave produced on down stroke; trace = small wave; 1+ = larger bulge; 2+ = spontaneous return after upstroke; 3+ = unable to move effusion out of medial knee.
   f. Substantial reliability (Kappa = 0.61).
10. Fractures: Ottawa Knee Rules (see Box 2-10).
    a. SN 0.99; SP 0.49; +LR 1.9; –LR 0.05

> **RED FLAG:** Fractures of the tibia, fibula, or patella may occur with traumatic injuries of the knee. Physical therapists must be able to recognize the signs and symptoms of a possible undiagnosed fracture in their patient. The Ottawa Knee Rules (Box 2-10) provide the therapist with guidelines to determine if a referral for an x-ray is indicated.

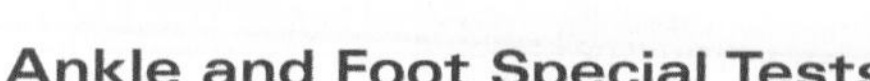

Ankle and Foot Special Tests

1. Ligamentous instability.
   a. Anterior drawer test (see Table 2-19).
      - Primarily tests integrity of the anterior talofibular ligament.
      - Patient supine; foot off edge of table, ankle in 20° plantarflexion.
      - Translate talus anteriorly while stabilizing the lower leg.
      - Positive finding is excessive anterior talar translation and/or pain.

   b. Talar tilt (see Table 2-19).
      - Primarily tests integrity of the calcaneofibular ligament.
      - Patient side lying; knee slightly flexed, ankle in neutral.
      - Move foot into maximal adduction (stresses calcaneofibular ligament) and abduction (stresses deltoid ligament).
      - Positive finding is laxity and/or pain.

   c. Medial subtalar glide test (see Table 2-19).
      - Hold talus in subtalar neutral position with one hand and translate the calcaneus medially on the fixed talus with the other hand.
2. Syndesmosis instability/pain.
   a. External rotation stress (Kleiger) test (see Table 2-19).
      - Tests integrity of the distal tibiofibular syndesmosis.
      - Patient seated; knee flexed to 90°, ankle in neutral.
      - Apply external rotation force to foot while holding tibia in neutral position.
      - Positive with visible joint gapping or reproduction of pain.

   b. Dorsiflexion-external rotation stress test (see Table 2-19).
      - Tests integrity of the distal tibiofibular syndesmosis.
      - Patient seated; knee flexed to 90°, ankle maximally dorsiflexed.
      - Apply external rotation force to foot while holding tibia in neutral position.
      - Positive with visible joint gapping or reproduction of pain.

   c. Squeeze test (see Table 2-19).
      - Tests integrity of the distal tibiofibular syndesmosis.
      - Patient seated; knee flexed to 90°.
      - Apply compression between the middle and distal third of the patient's leg.
      - Positive with pain reproduced at the syndesmosis.
3. Achilles tendon rupture: Thompson's test (see Figure 2-41 and Table 2-19).
   a. Patient prone, with foot off edge of table.
   b. Squeeze calf muscles; ankle should plantarflex under normal circumstances.
   c. Positive test is no movement of foot while squeezing calf.

RED FLAG: A positive Thompson's test indicates an Achilles' tendon rupture. Immediate referral to an orthopedic surgeon for immobilization or surgical repair is recommended. Delayed diagnosis typically results in a less favorable prognosis.

4. Plantar fasciitis: Windlass test (see Table 2-19).
   a. Identifies windlass effect of plantar fascia.

Table 2-19

Diagnostic Accuracy of Ankle and Foot Special Tests

TEST	SN	SP	+LR	–LR
Ligamentous instability				
- Anterior drawer test	0.33–0.58	0.73–1.0	1.27–∞	0.42–0.90
- Talar tilt	0.50	0.88	4.0	0.57
- Medial subtalar glide test	0.58	0.88	4.7	0.48
Syndesmosis instability/pain				
- External rotation stress (Kleiger) test	0.20	0.85	1.31	0.94
- Dorsiflexion-external rotation test	0.71	0.63	1.93	0.46
- Squeeze test	0.26–0.30	0.88–0.93	2.2–4.6	0.75–0.84
Achilles tendon rupture				
- Thompson's test	0.96	0.93	13.5	0.04
Plantar fasciitis				
- Windlass test	0.98	0.20	1.2	0.10
Ottawa Ankle and Foot Rules	0.98	0.20	1.23	0.10

Adapted from: Magee, Orthopedic Physical Assessment, 6th Edition; Cleland, Orthopaedic Clinical Examination, 3rd Edition.

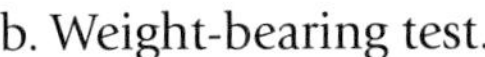

b. Weight-bearing test.
  - Patient standing on step with toes positioned over the edge of the step and equal weight-bearing.
  - Passively extend the patient's first MTP joint.

c. Non–weight-bearing test.
  - The patient seated in non–weight-bearing position with the knee flexed to 90°.
  - Stabilize the ankle and passively extend the patient's first MTP joint.

d. A positive test is the reproduction of plantar surface symptoms. (In a non–weight-bearing test, the symptoms occur at the end of range of motion.)

5. Fracture: Ottawa Ankle and Foot Rules (see Box 2-12).
   a. SN 0.98; SP 0.20; +LR 1.2; –LR 0.10.

> **RED FLAG:** Fractures of the medial and lateral malleolus and foot bones may occur with traumatic injuries of the ankle and foot. Physical therapists must be able to recognize the signs and symptoms of a possible undiagnosed fracture in their patient. The Ottawa Ankle and Foot Rules (Box 2-12) provide the therapist with guidelines to determine if a referral for an x-ray is indicated.

Special Tests of the Spine, Pelvis, and Temporomandibular Joint

Cervical Spine Special Tests

1. Vertebral artery test (see Table 2-20).
   a. Assesses the integrity of the vertebrobasilar vascular system.
   b. Patient supine, with head supported over end of table, eyes open.
      - Passively extend head and neck, hold for 30 seconds. If no symptoms, progress to passive rotation and side-bending with extension in both directions. Hold each position for 30 seconds.
      - Causes reduction of the lumen of the vertebral artery (VA), resulting in decreased blood flow of the intracranial VA of the contralateral side.
      - Symptoms include drop attacks, dizziness, dysphasia, dysarthria, diplopia, ataxic gait, numbness, nausea, or nystagmus.
   c. Patient should be continuously monitored for any change in symptoms during entire test. Test is not progressed beyond that point if symptoms appear.

Table 2-20

Diagnostic Accuracy of Cervical Spine Special Tests

SUSPECTED PATHOLOGY TESTS	SN	SP	+LR	–LR
Cervical Instability				
- Sharp-Purser	0.69	0.96	17.25	0.32
Neurological				
- Distraction Test	0.26–0.43	1.00	—	—
- Foraminal compression (Spurling's)	0.28–0.95	0.74–1.00	1.9–18.6	0.05–0.75
- Shoulder Abduction Test	0.31–0.43	0.80–1.00	1.96–36	0.64–0.77
- Upper Limb Tension A	0.97	0.22	1.3	0.12
- Upper Limb Tension B	0.72	0.33	1.1	0.85
Cervical myelopathy				
- Hoffmann sign	0.44	0.75	1.8	0.70
- Reflex Testing	0.44	0.71	1.5	0.80
- Inverted Supinator sign	0.61	0.78	2.8	0.50
- Babinski sign	0.33	0.92	4.0	0.70
- Clonus	0.11	0.96	2.7	0.90
Vertebral artery test				
- Hold planned mobilization position for at least 30 seconds watching for vertebral-basilar signs and symptoms	N/A			
First rib mobility	Intraexaminer κ = 0.35			
Cervical Muscle Strength (Deep Neck Flexors)				
- Craniocervical flexion test	Intraexaminer κ = 0.72			
Cervical Spine Mobility				
- Cervical flexion rotation test	Intraexaminer κ = 0.50			

Adapted from Magee, Orthopedic Physical Assessment, 6th Edition; Cleland, Orthopaedic Clinical Examination, 3rd Edition.

d. Performing mobilization/manipulation within cervical region without performing this test beforehand would be considered, by most, to be a breach in standard of care even if current evidence demonstrates statistical limitations of this test.

RED FLAG: Life-threatening consequences have been associated with vertebral-basilar artery and cervical arterial dysfunction. Factors associated may include hypermobility, ligamentous instability, or predisposing factors such as anterosclerosis or spondylosis. It is critical to monitor for hallmark signs or symptoms secondary to injury or damage to the vertebral-basilar artery.

Vertebral-basilar artery dysfunction signs and symptoms (adapted from Magee, Orthopedic Physical Assessment, 6th Edition):

- Dizziness/vertigo
- Dysphagia (difficulty swallowing)
- Dysarthria (difficulty with speech)
- Diplopia (double vision)
- Drop attacks
- Ataxia (incoordination)
- Numbness (sensory changes in face or body)
- Nausea
- Nystagmus
- Severe headaches
- Unconsciousness, disorientation, lightheadedness
- Hearing difficulties
- Facial paralysis

2. Flexion rotation test.
   a. Provocative test for atlantoaxial dysfunction and/or cervicogenic headache.
   b. Patient supine, passively perform maximal flexion of the cervical spine then fully rotate the head in each direction.
   c. Positive finding is reproduction of headache symptoms or a loss of 10° range of motion from one side compared to other.
   d. SN 86%; SP 20%.
3. Foraminal compression/Spurling's test (see Table 2-20).
   a. Identifies dysfunction (typically compression) of cervical nerve root.
   b. Patient sitting, with head side bent toward involved side. Apply pressure through head straight down.
   c. Positive finding is pain and/or paresthesia in dermatomal pattern for involved nerve root.
   d. SN 50%; SP 86%.
4. Maximum cervical compression test.
   a. Identifies compression of neural structures at intervertebral foramen and/or facet dysfunction.
   b. Patient sitting. Passively move head into side-bending and rotation toward nonpainful side, followed by extension. Repeat this toward painful side.
   c. Be careful since this is very similar to vertebral artery test.
   d. Positive finding is pain and/or paresthesia in dermatomal pattern for involved nerve root, or localized pain in neck if facet dysfunction.
   e. SN and SP not available.
5. Distraction test (see Table 2-20).
   a. Indicates compression of neural structures at the intervertebral foramen or facet joint dysfunction.
   b. Patient sitting with head passively distracted.
   c. Positive finding is a decrease in symptoms in neck (facet condition) or a decrease in upper limb pain (neurological condition).
6. Shoulder abduction test (see Table 2-20).
   a. Indicates compression of neural structures within intervertebral foramen.
   b. Patient sitting and asked to place one hand on top of their head. Repeat with opposite hand.
   c. Positive finding is a decrease in symptoms into upper limb.
7. Lhermitte's sign (see Figure 2-42).
   a. Identifies dysfunction of spinal cord and/or an upper motor neuron lesion.
   b. Patient long sitting on table. Passively flex patient's head and one hip, while keeping knee in extension. Repeat with other hip.
   c. Positive finding is "electrical" pain down the spine and into the upper or lower limbs.
   d. SN 3%; SP 80%.
8. Alar ligament test.
   a. Determines integrity of the alar ligament.
   b. Patient seated, passively, slightly flex the upper cervical spine and apply a firm pincer grip to the C2 spinous process. Palpate movement at C2 during passive upper cervical side-bending and/or rotation.
   c. Positive finding is an inability to palpate C2 moving in conjunction with C1.
   d. SN and SP not available.
9. Modified Sharp-Purser (see Table 2-20).
   a. Determines integrity of the transverse ligament/atlantoaxial stability.
   b. Patient seated, passively, slightly flex the upper cervical spine and apply a firm pincer grip to the C2 spinous process. Apply a posterior translation and extension force through the forehead while assessing for excessive linear translation or reproduction of myelopathic symptoms.
   c. Positive findings include myelopathic symptoms with upper cervical flexion or a decrease in symptoms or excessive translation during the posterior translation.
10. TOS tests (see shoulder special tests).
11. Upper limb tension tests (see Table 2-14).

RED FLAG: Clinical instability of the cervical spine may exist when physiological loads overcome stabilizing tissues. Patients with neck pain, headache, torticollis, or neurological signs should be screened carefully for upper cervical spine instability, prior to conducting interventions. Ligamentous testing is useful after trauma or in special populations (e.g., rheumatoid arthritis) where degradation of ligamentous tissues may exist. It is critical for the clinician to monitor for hallmark signs and symptoms through a careful subjective history and physical examination.

Cervical instability signs and symptoms:
- Severe muscle spasm
- Patient does not want to move head (especially into flexion)
- Lump in throat
- Lip or facial paresthesia
- Severe headache
- Dizziness
- Nausea
- Vomiting
- Soft-end feel
- Nystagmus
- Pupil changes

Thoracic Spine Special Tests

1. Rib springing.
   a. Evaluates rib mobility.
   b. Patient prone. Begin at upper ribs applying a posterior/anterior force through each rib progressively working through entire rib cage. Following prone test, position patient side-lying and repeat. Be careful with springing the eleventh and twelfth ribs, since they have no anterior attachments and therefore are less stable.
   c. Positive finding is pain, excessive motion of rib, or restriction of rib.
   d. SN and SP not available.
2. Thoracic springing.
   a. Evaluates intervertebral joint mobility in thoracic spine.
   b. Patient prone. Apply posterior/anterior glides/springs to transverse processes of thoracic vertebra. Remember that the spinous process and transverse process of the same vertebra may not be at the same level in the thoracic region.
   c. Positive finding is pain, excessive movement, and/or restricted movement.
   d. SN and SP not available.

Lumbar Spine Special Tests

1. Slump test (see Figure 2-44 and Table 2-21).
   a. Identifies dysfunction of neurological structures supplying the lower limb.
   b. Patient sitting on edge of table with knees flexed. Patient slump-sits, while maintaining neutral position of head and neck. The following progression is then followed.
      - Passively flex patient's head and neck. If no reproduction of symptoms, move on to next step.
      - Passively extend one of patient's knees. If no reproduction of symptoms, move on to next step.
      - Passively dorsiflex ankle of limb with extended knee.
      - Repeat flow with opposite leg.
   c. Positive finding is reproduction of pathological neurological symptoms.
2. Straight leg raise (Lasegue's test) (see Tables 2-21 and 2-22).
   a. Identifies dysfunction of neurological structures that supply lower limb.
   b. Patient supine, with legs resting on table. Passively flex hip of one leg with knee extended until patient complains of symptoms into lower limb. Slowly lower limb until symptoms subside, then passively dorsiflex foot.
   c. Positive finding is reproduction of pathological neurological symptoms when foot is dorsiflexed.
3. Femoral nerve traction test (see Table 2-21).
   a. Identifies compression of femoral nerve anywhere along its course.
   b. Patient lies on nonpainful side with trunk in neutral, head flexed slightly, and lower limb's hip and knee flexed. Passively extend hip while knee of painful limb is in extension. If no reproduction of symptoms, flex knee of painful leg.
   c. Positive finding is neurological pain in anterior thigh.
4. Valsalva's maneuver.
   a. Patient sitting. Instruct patient to take a deep breath and hold while they "bear down" as if having a bowel movement.
   b. Increases pressure in middle ear and in the chest. Used when bracing to lift heavy objects.
   c. Can be used to identify a space-occupying lesion. Positive finding is increased low back pain or neurological symptoms into lower extremity.
   d. SN 22%; SP 94%.
5. Prone instability test (see Table 2-21).
   a. Tests instability of the lumbar spine.
   b. Patient prone with torso resting on the plinth and legs off the edge with feet supported on the ground. Apply PA springing throughout the lumbar spine until a painful segment(s) is identified.
   c. Instruct the patient to lift their legs a few inches off the ground then perform spring testing again on the painful segment(s).
   d. Positive finding is decreased pain during PA springing with the legs raised compared to when the feet were supported on the ground.

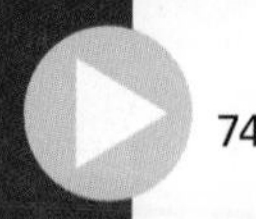

Table 2-21

Diagnostic Accuracy of Lumbar Spine and Pelvis Special Tests

SUSPECTED PATHOLOGY TESTS	SN	SP	+LR	–LR
Neurological				
- Slump test	0.84	0.83	4.94	0.19
- Straight leg raise	0.92	0.28	1.3	0.29
- Cross straight leg raise	0.28	0.90	2.8	0.80
- Femoral nerve traction test	0.84	—	—	—
- Centralization/peripheralization	0.40	0.94	6.9	0.63
		Intraexaminer κ = 0.70		
Lumbar Instability				
- Passive lumbar extension	0.29	0.98	12.8	0.72
- Prone instability test (PIT)	0.72	0.58	1.7	0.48
- Aberrant movement pattern (painful arc in flexion, painful arc in return from flexion, instability catch, Gower sign, lumbopelvic reversal)	0.78	0.50	Intraexaminer κ = 0.60	
Pelvis/sacroiliac joint				
- Patrick's test (FABER)	0.54–0.66	0.51–0.62	1.37–1.43	0.64–0.73
- Thigh thrust	0.88	0.71	2.8	0.66
- Gaenslen's test	0.50–0.53	0.71–0.77	1.84–2.21	0.65–0.66
- Compression test	0.60	0.69	2.2	0.46
- Distraction (Gapping) test	0.23–0.60	0.81	1.24–3.20	0.49–0.94
- Sacral thrust	0.63	0.75	0.49	1.35
- Combined tests (thigh thrust, Gaenslen, compression, distraction, sacral thrust)	0.85	0.76	3.54	0.20

Adapted from Magee, Orthopedic Physical Assessment, 6th Edition; Cleland, Orthopaedic Clinical Examination, 3rd Edition. Hicks GE, Fritz JM, Delitto A, McGill SM. Preliminary development of a clinical prediction rule for determining which patients with low back pain will respond to a stabilization exercise program. *Arch Phys Med Rehab* 2005; 86: 1753–76.

Table 2-22

Lower Extremity Neurotension Tests

VERSION OF SLR	POSITION OF HIP	POSITION OF KNEE	POSITION OF ANKLE	POSITION OF FOOT	POSITION OF TOES	NERVE BIAS
SLR	Flexion and abduction	Extension	Dorsiflexion	N/A	N/A	Sciatic and tibial nerves
SLR2	Flexion	Extension	Dorsiflexion	Eversion	Extension	Tibial nerve
SLR3	Flexion	Extension	Dorsiflexion	Inversion	N/A	Sural nerve
SLR4	Flexion and internal rotation	Extension	Plantarflexion	Inversion	N/A	Common fibular nerve
SLR5 (Well Leg)	Flexion	Extension	Dorsiflexion	N/A	N/A	Spinal nerve root

Adapted from Magee D: Orthopedic Physical Assessment, 6th ed.

6. Quadrant test.
   a. Identifies compression of neural structures at the intervertebral foramen and facet dysfunction.
   b. Patient standing.
      - Intervertebral foramen: cue patient into side-bending left, rotation left, and extension to maximally close intervertebral foramen on the left. Repeat on other side.
      - Facet dysfunction: cue patient into side-bending left, rotation right, and extension to maximally compress facet joint on left. Repeat on other side.
   c. Positive finding is pain and/or paresthesia in the dermatomal pattern for the involved nerve root, or localized pain if facet dysfunction.
   d. SN 70%; SP not available.

7. Aberrant movement testing (see Table 2-21).
   a. If the patient displays any of the five possible movement patterns they are considered positive for aberrant movement.
   b. Instability catch, painful arc in flexion, painful arc in return from flexion, Gower's sign (thigh climbing), reversal of lumbopelvic rhythm.
8. Bicycle (van Gelderen's test).
   a. Differentiates between intermittent claudication and spinal stenosis.
   b. Patient seated on stationary bicycle. Patient rides bike while sitting erect. Time how long the patient can ride at a set pace/speed. After a sufficient rest period, have patient ride bike at same speed while in a slumped position.
   c. Determination is based on length of time patient can ride bike in sitting upright versus sitting slumped. If pain is related to spinal stenosis, patient should be able to ride bike longer while slumped.
   d. SN and SP not available.
9. Crossed straight leg raise (see Table 2-21).
   a. Identifies herniated nucleus pulposis or neural tension/radiculopathy.
   b. Patient supine with head, neck, and torso in neutral, maintain knee extension and neutral dorsiflexion and lift the leg to the point of symptom provocation.
   c. Perform on the contralateral, non-involved lower extremity.
   d. Positive finding is reproduction of low back pain during the straight leg raise of the non-involved lower extremity.
10. Schober test.
   a. Measures the mobility of the lumbar spine.
   b. Patient standing. Examiner marks a point 5 cm below and 10 cm above S2. This distance is measured in the upright position and then in full flexion. The difference between the two measurements is calculated and recorded to the nearest centimeter.
   c. SN 30%; SP 86% in patients with ankylosing spondylitis.

Sacroiliac Joint (SIJ) Special Tests (See Table 2-23)

1. Gillet's test (see Figure 2-44).
   a. Assessing posterior movement of the ilium relative to the sacrum.
   b. Patient standing. Place thumb of the hand under posterior superior iliac spine (PSIS) of limb to be tested and place the other thumb on center of sacrum at same level as thumb under PSIS. Ask patient to flex hip and knee of limb being tested as if bringing the knee to the chest. Assess movement of PSIS via comparison of positions of the thumbs. Make sure eyes are level with thumbs. PSIS should move in an inferior direction.
   c. Positive finding is no identified movement of PSIS as compared to sacrum.
   d. SN 43%; SP 68%.
2. Thigh thrust (see Table 2-21).
   a. Pain provocation test.
   b. Patient supine with hip passively flexed to 90° on the test side. Use one hand to palpate SIJ while thrusting downward through knee and hip.
3. Gaenslen's test (see Table 2-21).
   a. Identifies SIJ dysfunction.
   b. Patient side-lying at edge of table while holding bottom leg in maximal hip and knee flexion (knee to chest). Standing behind patient, passively extend hip of uppermost limb. This places stress on SIJ associated with uppermost limb.
   c. Positive finding is pain in SIJ.

Table 2-23

Positions/Activities That Precipitate SI Dysfunction

TYPE OF DYSFUNCTION	ACTIVITIES THAT PRECIPITATE DYSFUNCTION
Anterior torsion of innominate	Squatting/lifting/lowering Pregnancy Hip at 90° with axial loading Golfing/batting/tennis
Posterior torsion of innominate	Vertical thrust onto extended LE Sprint starting position Fall onto ischial tuberosity Unilateral standing
Sacral dysfunction	Long-term postural abnormalities Fall onto sacrum/coccyx Carrying a load during ambulation Trauma during childbirth Loss of balance during ambulation Sitting combined with rotation and lifting

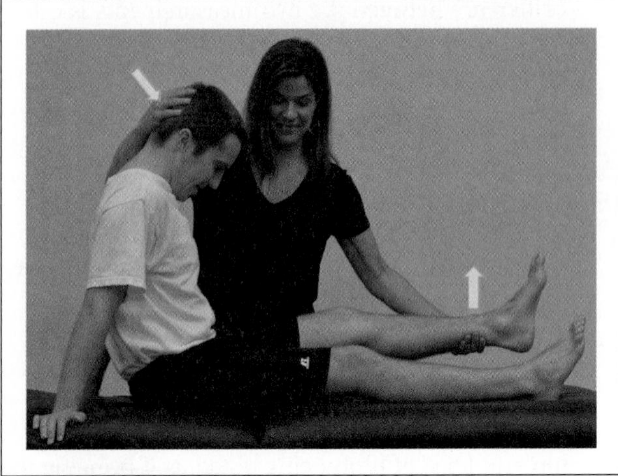

Figure 2-42 **Lhermitte's sign.**

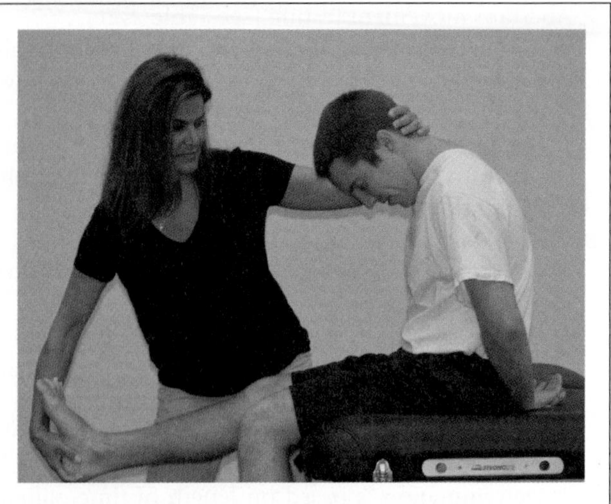

Figure 2-43 **Slump test.**

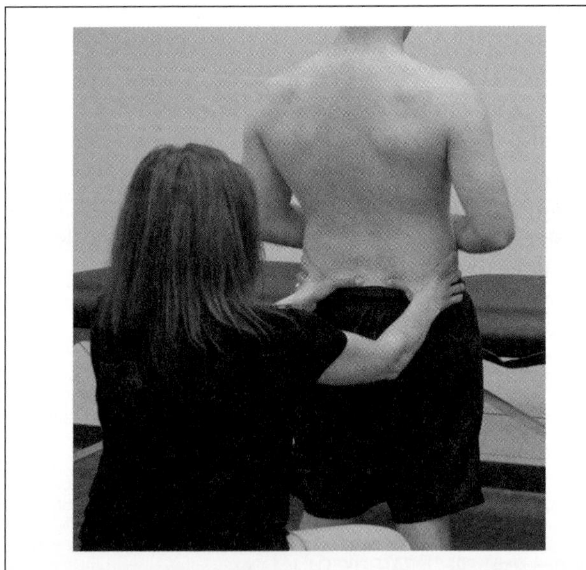

Figure 2-44a **Gillet's test; hand position.**

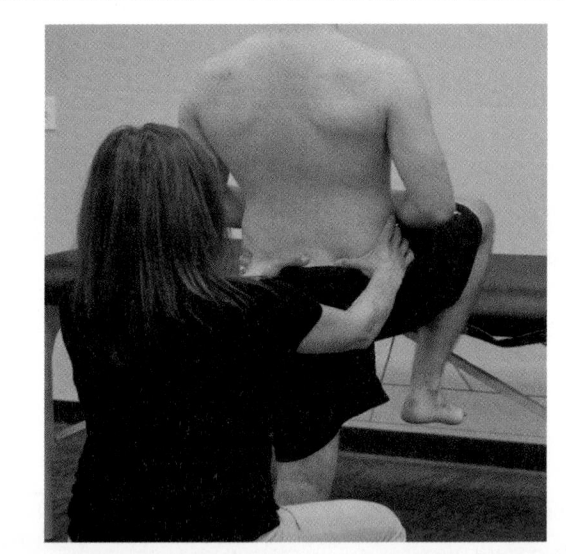

Figure 2-44b **Gillet's test; hip and knee flexion.**

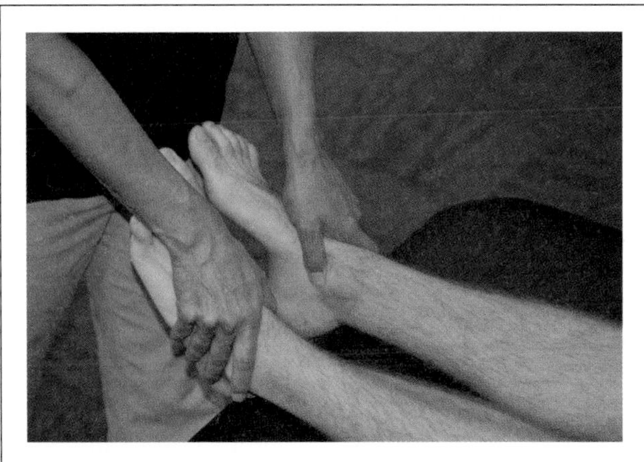

Figure 2-45a Long sitting (supine to sit) test; initial hand position.

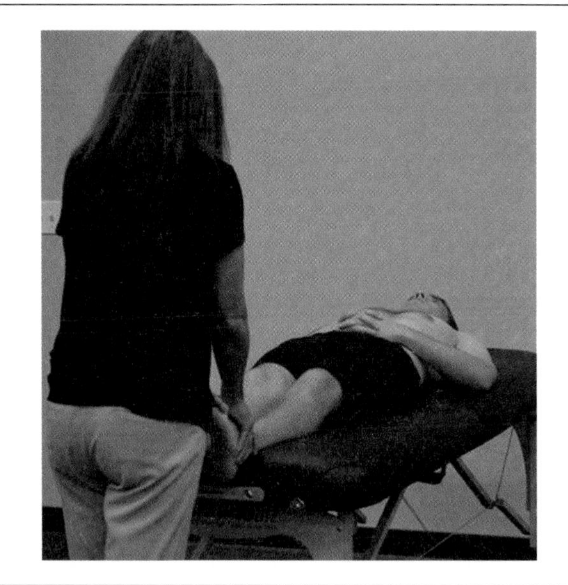

Figure 2-45b Long sitting (supine to sit) test.

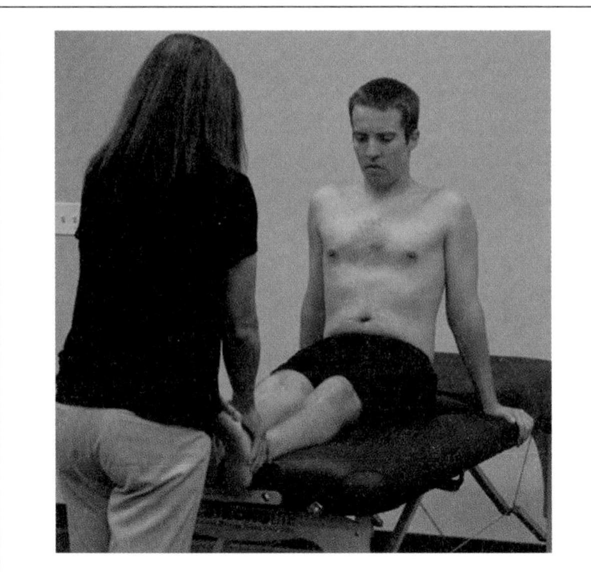

Figure 2-45c Long sitting (supine to sit) test.

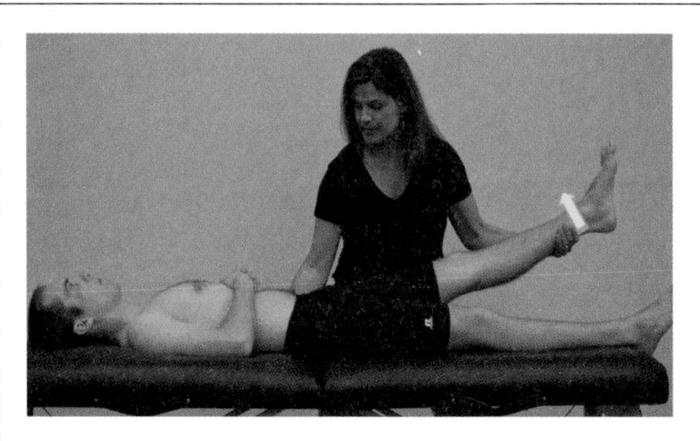

Figure 2-46 Goldthwait's test.

4. Long sitting (supine to sit) test (see Figure 2-45).
   a. Identifies dysfunction of SIJ that may be cause of functional leg length discrepancy.
   b. Patient supine with correct alignment of trunk, pelvis, and lower limbs. Stand at edge of table near patient's feet, palpating the medial malleoli to assess symmetry (one longer than other). Have patient come into long sitting position, and once again assess leg length, making a comparison between supine and long sitting.
   c. Abnormal finding is reversal in limb lengths between supine and long sitting.
   d. SN 44%; SP 64%.
5. Goldthwait's test (see Figure 2-46).
   a. Differentiates between dysfunction in lumbar spine versus SIJ.
   b. Patient supine with examiner's fingers between spinous processes of lumbar spine. With the other hand, passively perform a straight leg raise.
   c. If pain presents prior to palpation of movement in lumbar segments, dysfunction is related to SIJ.
   d. SN and SP not available.
6. Sidelying compression test (see Table 2-21).
   a. Identifies SIJ dysfunction.
   b. Patient lies in side-lying position with painful side up and baseline symptoms are gathered. Examiner places hands on the iliac crest and applies force through the ilium in the downward direction. The examiner may hold the position for 30 seconds and apply continued force.
   c. A positive test reproduces the patient's chief complaint.
7. Supine iliac distraction/gapping test (see Table 2-21).
   a. Identifies SIJ dysfunction.
   b. Patient lies in supine position and baseline symptoms are gathered. Examiner crosses arms and places each hand on the medial aspect of the patient's ASIS and applies a posterior and lateral force. The examiner may hold the position for 30 seconds and apply continued force.
   c. Positive finding is reproduction of patient's chief complaint.

TMJ Special Tests

1. TMJ compression.
   a. Evaluates for pain with compression of the retrodiscal tissues.
   b. Patient sitting or supine. Support/stabilize patient's head with one hand. With other hand, push mandible superior, causing a compressive load to the TMJ.
   c. Positive finding is pain in TMJ.
   d. SN and SP not available.

Gait

See Chapter 12, Figure 12-1 for Phases of Gait

Typical Coupling Patterns Throughout the Lower Kinematic Chain Are Presented in Table 2-24

Lower Kinematic Chain Compensations Are Presented in Table 2-25

Table 2-24

Typical Coupling Patterns Throughout the Lower Kinematic Chain

Lumbar Spine	Lumbar spine flexion is coupled with ilial posterior rotation. Lumbar spine extension is coupled with ilial anterior rotation.
Pelvis	During unilateral ilial posterior rotation, the ilium simultaneously moves in the direction of an outflare, causing ER of the acetabulum (i.e., the hip joint), leading to hip ER.
Femur	ER of the femur causes ER of the tibia.
Tibia	Tibial ER is coupled with an upward glide of the talus and supination of the foot.
Fibula	Supination of the foot is coupled with cranial and anterior glide of the fibula head.

Table 2-25

Lower Kinematic Chain Compensations*,**

REGION	TRUE LEG LENGTH DISCREPANCY ON THE RIGHT
Lumbar Spine	Side bent right. Rotated left.
Pelvis	Right ilium rotated posteriorly.
Femur	Right femur adducted and in ER at hip joint. Right femur in relative extension at hip joint.
Tibia	ER of right tibia.
Fibula	Fibular head glides cranially and anteriorly.
Ankle/Foot	Supination of right foot. Talus rotated externally and glides upwardly.

*Describes the potential functional compensational movements that may be seen in a patient with a leg length discrepancy.
**Individuals may not demonstrate some or any of the compensations for the related conditions listed above. The functional compensations described above are commonly seen, but must be assessed for each patient to determine if they are truly present.

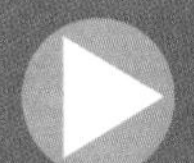

Evaluation, Differential Diagnosis, Prognosis, and Plan of Care of Musculoskeletal Conditions

Evaluation and Clinical Reasoning

1. Process of ongoing cognitive skill used to process information and inform clinical decisions.
2. Synthesize examination findings in relation to the International Classification of Function, Disability and Health (ICF) (see discussion in Chapter 14 and Box 14-1).
   a. Consider all body functions and structures, activities, and participation.
   b. Use evidence-based decision making based on examination findings.
   c. Consider alternative hypotheses based on examination findings.
   d. Document the evidence to support clinical decision making.
3. Integrate relevant evidence to support clinical decision-making process.

Prognosis

1. Anticipated level of optimal functioning and the amount of time required to achieve that level.
2. Barriers to achieving optimal function may include age, medication use, socioeconomic status, co-morbidities, cognitive status, nutrition, social support, and/or environment.

Plan of Care

1. Goal setting.
2. Coordination of care.
3. Progression of care.
4. Discharge.

Arthritic Conditions

Degenerative Joint Disease (DJD); Degenerative Osteoarthritis (OA)/ Osteoarthrosis (See Box 2-1)

1. A degenerative process of varied etiology, which includes mechanical changes, diseases, and/or joint trauma primarily confined to one or more synovial joints and its surrounding soft tissues.
2. Characterized by degeneration of articular cartilage, with hypertrophy of subchondral bone and joint capsule of weight-bearing joints.
3. Most common form of arthritis, affecting men more than women before age 50 and then more women than men after age 50. Differentiated in two ways: primary (idiopathic) and secondary disease (i.e., trauma).
4. Slowly progressive condition with pain initially episodic and triggered activity. Eventually, pain and stiffness become chronic. DJD/OA is a progressive and chronic condition. Knee OA is considered the leading cause of disability in the elderly.
5. Clinical examination assists in confirming diagnosis. Signs and symptoms include pain, swelling, loss of ROM, and bony deformity. Finger DIP and PIP joints and CMC of the thumb are commonly involved. The cervical and lumbar spine, hips, knees, and MTP of the great toe are also often involved.
6. Diagnostic tests utilized: plain film imaging demonstrates characteristic findings of OA (diminished joint space, decreased height of articular cartilage, presence of osteophytes, subchondral cysts) and lab tests help to rule out other disorders such as rheumatoid arthritis (RA).
7. Oral analgesics, NSAIDs, and corticosteroid injections are the primary medications used in medical management. Viscosupplementation (e.g., Synvisc) or intra-articular injections of the knee with a form of hyaluronic acid (HA) can be used.
8. Physical therapy goals, outcomes, and interventions.
   a. Maintain joint and soft tissue mobility.
   b. Physical therapy is most valuable during exacerbation; however, some cases may result in joint surgery including arthrodesis or arthroplasty to help the patient regain function.
   c. Flexibility and general strengthening. Implementation of aerobic capacity/endurance conditioning or reconditioning, such as aquatic programs.

Rheumatoid Conditions

1. Ankylosing spondylitis (Marie-Strümpell disease, Bechterew's disease, rheumatoid spondylitis) (see Table 2-26).
   a. Progressive inflammatory disorder of unknown etiology that initially affects axial skeleton.
   b. Initial onset (usually mid- and low back pain for 3 months or greater) before fourth decade of life.

BOX 2-1 Hip Pain and Mobility Deficits-Hip Osteoarthritis Clinical Practice Guideline

Differential Diagnosis

- Revise diagnosis if impairments are not consistent with the diagnosis/classification or if symptoms are not diminishing with interventions (F-expert opinion, Level V)

Examination

Activity Limitation/Physical Performance Measures (A-strong recommendation, Level I)

- **Throughout the episode of care, should use valid physical performance measures such as 6-minute walk test, timed up-and-go test, single-leg-stance, and others**

Physical Impairment (A-strong recommendation, Level I)

- **Document passive ROM, hip muscle strength, FABER over episode of care with hip pain or osteoarthritis**

Outcome Measures: Activity Limitation (A-strong recommendation, Level I)

- **Use validated outcome measures such as Western Ontario and McMaster Universities Osteoarthritis Index (WOMAC) and others such as a visual analog scale (VAS)**

Diagnosis/Classification (A-strong recommendation, Level I)

- **Hip internal rotation less than 24° or internal rotation/flexion 15° less than nonpainful side**
- **Passive internal rotation increases pain**
- **Morning hip stiffness after awakening**
- **Moderate anterior or lateral hip pain when weight-bearing**

Interventions

Flexibility, Strengthening, and Endurance (A-strong recommendation, Level I)

- **Individualized exercises to address impairments (dosage 1–5 times per week for 6–12 weeks with mild to moderate hip osteoarthritis)**

Manual Therapy (A-strong recommendation, Level I)

- **Manual therapy for mild to moderate hip osteoarthritis that may include soft tissue mobilization, thrust and nonthrust (dosage of 1–3 times per week over 6–12 weeks)**

Patient Education (B-moderate recommendation, Level II)

- Provide patient education consisting of general exercise, weight reduction for the overweight, methods of unloading the painful joint, and activity modification

Functional, Gait, and Balance Training (C-weak recommendation, Level III)

- Impairment-based functional, gait and balance training including use of ambulatory aids, and activity limitations

Modalities (B-moderate recommendation, Level II)

- May use hot packs for pain in short-term and ultrasound

Adapted from Hip Pain and Mobility Deficits—Hip Osteoarthritis, Orthopedic Section, APTA, Summary of Recommendations. *JOSPT;* 6(47): A2, 2017.

Level 1 evidence and Grade A recommendations are highlighted in the table with bold font.

See Table 16-4 in Chapter 16 for Levels of Evidence and Grades of Recommendations.

c. First symptoms include mid- and low back pain, morning stiffness, and sacroiliitis.

d. Results in kyphotic deformity of the cervical and thoracic spine and a decrease in lumbar lordosis.

e. Degeneration of peripheral and costovertebral joints may be observed in advanced stages.

f. Affects men three times more often than women.

g. Medications: NSAIDs, such as aspirin, are used to reduce inflammation and pain. Corticosteroid therapy or medications to suppress immune system may be used to control various symptoms. Cytotoxic drugs (drugs that block cell growth) may be used in people who do not respond well to corticosteroids or who are dependent on high doses of corticosteroids. Tumor necrosis factor (TNF) inhibitors have been shown to improve some symptoms of ankylosing spondylitis.

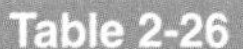

Table 2-26

Differential Diagnosis of Ankylosing Spondylitis and Spinal Stenosis

	ANKYLOSING SPONDYLITIS	SPINAL STENOSIS
History	Morning stiffness Male predominance Sharp pain → ache Bilateral sacroiliac pain may refer to posterior thigh	Intermittent aching pain Pain may refer to both legs with walking (neurogenic intermittent claudication)
Active movements	Restricted	May be normal
Passive movements	Restricted	May be normal
Resisted isometric movements	Normal (in beginning of disorder)	Normal
Posture	Flexed posture of entire spine	Flexed posture of lumbar spine
Special tests	Schober test (mobility less than 4 cm)	Bicycle test of van Gelderen may be positive; Stoop test may be positive
Reflexes	Normal (in beginning of disorder)	May be affected in long-standing cases
Sensory deficit	None (in beginning of disorder)	Usually temporary
Diagnostic imaging	Plain films are diagnostic	Computed tomography scans are diagnostic

Adapted from Magee D: Orthopedic Physical Assessment, 6th ed. 2014. Cleland JA, Koppenhaver S, Su J: Netter's Orthopaedic Clinical Examination, 3rd ed. 2016.

h. Diagnostic tests utilized: HLA-B27 antigen may be helpful, but not diagnostic by itself.
i. Clinical examination will assist in confirming diagnosis.
j. Physical therapy goals, outcomes, and interventions.
  - Implementation of flexibility exercises for trunk to maintain/improve normal joint motion and length of muscles in all directions, especially extension.
  - Implementation of aerobic capacity/endurance conditioning or reconditioning such as aquatic programs.
  - Implementation of relaxation activities to maintain/improve respiratory function.
    - Breathing strategies to maintain/improve vital capacity.

2. Gout.
  a. Genetic disorder of purine metabolism, characterized by elevated serum uric acid (hyperuricemia). Uric acid changes into crystals and deposits into peripheral joints and other tissues (e.g., kidneys).
  b. Most frequently observed at knee and great toe of foot.
  c. Medications: NSAIDS (specifically indomethacin), COX-2 inhibitors (cardiac side effects may limit use), colchicine, corticosteroids, adrenocorticotropic hormone (ACTH), allopurinol, probenecid, and sulfinpyrazone.
  d. Diagnostic tests utilized: lab tests identify monosodium urate crystals in synovial fluid and/or connective tissue samples.
  e. Clinical examination assists in confirming diagnosis.
  f. Physical therapy goals, outcomes, and interventions.
    - Patient/client education for injury prevention and reduction of involved joint(s).
    - Patient/client education on dietary effects on the disease.
    - Early identification of condition, with fast implementation of intervention, is very important.

3. Psoriatic arthritis.
  a. Chronic, erosive inflammatory disorder of unknown etiology, associated with psoriasis.
  b. Erosive degeneration usually occurs in joints of digits as well as axial skeleton.
  c. Both sexes are affected equally.
  d. Medications: acetaminophen for pain, NSAIDs, corticosteroids, disease-modifying antirheumatic drugs (DMARDs) can slow the progression of psoriatic arthritis, and biological response modifiers (BRMs) such as Enbrel (etanercept) are a newly developed class of medicines.
  e. Diagnostic tests utilized: lab tests are not useful except to rule out rheumatoid arthritis.
  f. Clinical examination assists in confirming diagnosis.
  g. Physical therapy goals, outcomes, and interventions.
    - Joint protection strategies.
    - Maintain/improve joint mechanics and connective tissue functions.

- Implementation of aerobic capacity/endurance conditioning or reconditioning, such as aquatic programs.

4. Rheumatoid arthritis (RA).
   a. Chronic systemic autoimmune disorder of unknown etiology thought to have a genetic basis.
   b. Individuals with RA produce antibodies to their own immunoglobulins, such as rheumatoid factor (RF) and anti-citrullinated protein antibody (ACPA). The disease is commonly characterized by periods of exacerbation and remission.
   c. The prevalence of RA among adults in the United States is approximately 1.3 million. Women have two to four times greater incidence than men, with an onset between 40 and 60 years of age.
   d. Onset may be gradual or abrupt. RA is characterized by bilateral and symmetrical synovial joint involvement. Patients often develop limited mobility and present with signs of inflammation (pain, swelling, redness, and increased tissue temperature). The most common joints involved include the hands, feet, and cervical spine.
   e. Systemic features of RA include weight loss, fever, and extreme fatigue.
   f. Juvenile rheumatoid arthritis (JRA) onset prior to age 16, with complete remission in 75% of children.
   g. RA is diagnosed using history, clinical examination of signs and symptoms, and exclusion of other disorders.
   h. Radiographs are essential and may demonstrate symmetrical involvement. Positive laboratory test findings include increased white blood cell count and erythrocyte sedimentation rate. Hemoglobin and hematocrit tests will show anemia, and rheumatoid factor will be elevated.
   i. Pharmacological management varies with disease progression, and may include gold compounds and antirheumatic drugs (DMARDs) (e.g., hydroxychloroquine and methotrexate) early in the course of disease. DMARDs are slow-acting and are known to take several weeks to become effective. NSAIDS (e.g., ibuprofen) and immunosuppressive agents (e.g., cyclosporine, azathioprine, and mycophenolate) may also be prescribed. Corticosteroids are commonly prescribed for acute flare-ups or long-term management.
   j. Physical therapy goals, outcomes, and interventions.
      - Reduce pain and inflammation through modalities and joint protection strategies.
      - Maintain/improve function, joint mechanics, and connective tissue mobility.
      - Implementation of aerobic capacity and endurance conditioning or reconditioning, such as aquatic programs.

Skeletal and Soft Tissue Conditions

Osteoporosis

1. A metabolic disease that depletes bone mineral density/mass, predisposing individual to fracture.
2. Affects women 10 times more frequently than men.
3. Common sites of fracture include thoracic and lumbar spine, femoral neck, proximal humerus, proximal tibia, pelvis, and distal radius.
4. Primary or postmenopausal osteoporosis is directly related to a decrease in estrogen production.
5. Senile osteoporosis occurs due to a decrease in bone cell activity secondary to genetics or acquired abnormalities.
6. Medications: calcium, vitamin D, estrogen, calcitonin, and biophosphonates.
7. Diagnostic tests utilized: CT scan to assess bone density. Single and dual photon absorptiometry are also used, but very expensive.
8. Clinical examination will assist in confirming diagnosis.
9. Physical therapy goals, outcomes, and interventions.
   a. Joint/bone protection strategies.
   b. Maintain/improve joint mechanics and connective tissue functions.
   c. Implementation of aerobic capacity/endurance conditioning or reconditioning, such as aquatic programs.
   d. Patient/client education on dietary changes to improve mineral intake.

Osteomalacia

1. Characterized by decalcification of bones due to vitamin D deficiency.
2. Symptoms include severe pain, fractures, weakness, and deformities.
3. Medications: calcium, vitamin D, and vitamin D injections in the form of calciferol (vitamin D2).
4. Diagnostic tests: plain films, lab tests (urinalysis and blood work), bone scan, and bone biopsy if warranted.
5. Clinical examination assists in confirming diagnosis.
6. Physical therapy goals, outcomes, and interventions.
   a. Joint/bone protection strategies.
   b. Maintain/improve joint mechanics and connective tissue functions.
   c. Implementation of aerobic capacity/endurance conditioning or reconditioning, such as aquatic programs.

Osteomyelitis

1. An inflammatory response within bone caused by an infection.
2. Usually caused by *Staphylococcus aureus*, but could be another organism.

3. More common in children and immunosuppressed adults than healthy adults; more common in males than females.
4. Medical treatment consists of antibiotics. Proper nutrition is important as well. Surgery may be indicated if infection spreads to joints.
5. Diagnostic tests utilized: lab tests for infection and possibly a bone biopsy.
6. Clinical examination will assist in confirming diagnosis.
7. Physical therapy goals, outcomes, and interventions.
   a. Joint/bone protection strategies and cast care.
   b. Maintain/improve joint mechanics and connective tissue functions.

Myofascial Pain Syndrome

1. Characterized by clinical entity known as a "trigger point," which is a focal point of irritability found within a muscle. Trigger point can be identified as a taut, palpable band within the muscle.
2. Trigger points may be active or latent. Active trigger points are tender to palpation and have a characteristic referral pattern of pain when provoked. Latent trigger points are palpable taut bands that are not tender to palpation, but can be converted into an active trigger point.
3. Onset is hypothesized to sudden overload, overstretching, and/or repetitive/sustained muscle activities.
4. Medical intervention may include dry needling (aka intramuscular manual therapy) and/or injection of analgesic, possibly combined with a corticosteroid.
5. Diagnosis is made by clinical assessment, with no diagnostic tests available.
6. Clinical examination will assist in confirming diagnosis.
7. Physical therapy goals, outcomes, and interventions.
   a. Implementation of flexibility exercises to maintain/improve normal joint motion and length of muscles.
   b. Implementation of manual therapy for maintenance of normal joint mechanics.
      - Soft tissue/massage techniques and joint oscillations to reduce pain and/or muscle guarding.
      - Biomechanical faults caused by joint restrictions should be corrected with joint mobilization to the specific restrictions identified during the examination.
      - Use of "spray and stretch" technique.
      - Utilization of dry needling.
      - Cryotherapy, thermotherapy, hydrotherapy, sound agents, and transcutaneous electrical nerve stimulation (TENS) for symptomatic relief of pain.
      - Desensitization of trigger point with manual pressure.
   c. Implementation of strength, power, and endurance exercises.
      - Active assistive, active, and resistive exercises.
      - Task-specific performance training.

Tendonosis/Tendonopathy

1. Common tendon dysfunction caused by an imbalance between tendon loading and recovery, which leads to tendon failure on a microscopic and eventually macroscopic level.
2. Common in many tendons throughout body (supraspinatus, common extensor tendon of elbow, patella, Achilles' tendon, gluteus medius).
3. Histological characteristics include hypercellularity, hypervascularity, no indication of inflammatory infiltrates, and poor organization and loosening of collagen fibrils.
4. Medications: acetaminophen, NSAIDs, and/or steroid injection.
5. Diagnostic tests utilized: possibly MRI.
6. Clinical examination assists in confirming diagnosis. Specific special tests are available to assist with making diagnosis within each region/joint.
7. Physical therapy goals, outcomes, and interventions.
   a. Implementation of flexibility exercises to maintain/improve normal joint motion and length of muscles.
   b. Implementation of manual therapy for maintenance of normal joint mechanics.
      - Soft tissue/massage techniques and joint oscillations to reduce pain and/or muscle guarding.
      - Joint movement restrictions should be addressed by exercises and/or manual therapy tailored to impairments identified during the examination.
   c. Progressive resistance training exercise program with emphasis on eccentric phase of the movement.
   d. Implementation of aerobic capacity/endurance conditioning or reconditioning.
   e. Application of thermal agents for pain reduction.
      - Cryotherapy, thermotherapy, hydrotherapy, and sound agents.
   f. Patient/client education and training/retraining for instrumental activities of daily living (IADLs) as well as activity modification to decrease further tissue damage.
      - Household chores, yard work, shopping, caring for dependents, and home maintenance.

Bursitis

1. Inflammation of bursa secondary to overuse, trauma, gout, or infection.
2. Signs and symptoms of bursitis.
   a. Pain with rest.
   b. PROM and AROM are limited due to pain, but not in a capsular pattern.

3. Medications: acetaminophen, NSAIDs, and/or steroid injection.
4. Clinical examination assists in confirming diagnosis.
5. Physical therapy goals, outcomes, and interventions.
   a. Implementation of flexibility exercises to maintain/improve normal joint motion and length of muscles.
   b. Implementation of manual therapy for maintenance of normal joint mechanics.
      - Soft tissue/massage techniques and joint oscillations to reduce pain and/or muscle guarding.
      - Biomechanical faults caused by joint restrictions should be corrected with joint mobilization to the specific restrictions identified during the examination.
   c. Implementation of aerobic capacity/endurance conditioning or reconditioning.
   d. Application of thermal agents for pain reduction, edema reduction, and muscle performance.
      - Cryotherapy, thermotherapy, hydrotherapy, and sound agents.
   e. Patient/client education and training/retraining for IADLs.
      - Household chores, yard work, shopping, caring for dependents, and home maintenance.

Muscle Strains

1. Inflammatory response within a muscle following a traumatic event that caused microtearing of the musculotendinous fibers.
2. Pain and tenderness within that muscle.
3. Seen within muscles throughout the body.
4. Medications: acetaminophen and/or NSAIDs.
5. Diagnostic tests utilized: MRI if necessary.
6. Clinical examination will assist in confirming the diagnosis.
   a. Muscle strains present with pain on active contraction and passive stretch of the muscle.
   b. Degree of passive motion loss compared with the uninvolved limb can assist with grading the degree of muscle injury.
7. Physical therapy goals, outcomes, and interventions.
   a. Implementation of flexibility exercises to maintain/improve normal joint motion and length of muscles.
   b. Implementation of manual therapy for maintenance of normal joint mechanics.
      - Soft tissue/massage techniques and joint oscillations to reduce pain and/or muscle guarding.
      - Biomechanical faults caused by joint restrictions should be corrected with joint mobilization to the specific restrictions identified during the examination.
   c. Implementation of aerobic capacity/endurance conditioning or reconditioning.
   d. Application of thermal agents for pain reduction, edema reduction, and muscle performance.
      - Cryotherapy, thermotherapy, hydrotherapy, and sound agents.
   e. Patient/client education and training/retraining for IADLs.
      - Household chores, yard work, shopping, caring for dependents, and home maintenance.

Myositis Ossificans

1. Painful condition of abnormal calcification within a muscle belly.
2. Usually precipitated by direct trauma that results in hematoma and calcification of the muscle.
3. Can also be induced by early mobilization and stretching, with aggressive physical therapy following trauma to muscle.
4. Most frequent locations are quadriceps, brachialis, and biceps brachii muscles.
5. Medications: acetaminophen and/or NSAIDs.
6. Surgical care is warranted only in patients with nonhereditary myositis ossificans, and only after maturation of the lesion (6–24 months). Surgery is indicated when lesions mechanically interfere with joint movement or impinge on nerves.
7. Diagnostic tests utilized: imaging (plain films, CT scan, and/or MRI).
8. Clinical examination assists in confirming diagnosis.
9. Physical therapy goals, outcomes, and interventions.
   a. Implementation of flexibility exercises to maintain/improve normal joint motion and length of muscles. Avoid being overly aggressive with muscle flexibility exercises, which may worsen condition.
   b. Implementation of manual therapy for maintenance of normal joint mechanics.
      - Soft tissue/massage techniques and joint oscillations to reduce pain and/or muscle guarding. Avoid aggressive soft tissue/massage techniques, which may worsen condition.
      - Biomechanical faults caused by joint restrictions should be corrected with joint mobilization to the specific restrictions identified during the examination.
   c. Implementation of aerobic capacity/endurance conditioning or reconditioning, such as aquatic programs.

Complex Regional Pain Syndrome (CRPS)

1. Formerly referred to as reflex sympathetic dystrophy (RSD).
2. Etiology largely unknown, but thought to be related to trauma or precipitating event, which can be multifactorial. Can affect upper and lower extremities, trunk, head, and neck.

3. Results in dysfunction of sympathetic nervous system to include pain, circulation, and vasomotor disturbances.
4. Two types of CRPS.
   a. CRPS I is frequently triggered by tissue injury; term describes all patients with the above symptoms, but with no underlying nerve injury.
   b. Patients with CRPS II experience the same symptoms, but their cases are clearly associated with a nerve injury.
5. Medical intervention may include sympathetic nerve block, surgical sympathectomy, spinal cord stimulation, intrathecal drug pumps.
6. Medications: multiple forms including topical analgesic drugs that act locally on painful nerves, skin, and muscles; antiseizure drugs; antidepressants, corticosteroids, and opioids.
7. Long-term changes include muscle wasting, trophic skin changes, decreased bone density, decreased proprioception, loss of muscle strength from disuse, and joint contractures.
8. Diagnostic tests utilized: none.
9. Clinical examination will assist in confirming diagnosis.
10. Physical therapy goals, outcomes, and interventions.
    a. Patient/client education for injury prevention and reduction.
    b. Desensitization activities that focus on return to work/school/home activities.
    c. Implementation of flexibility exercises to maintain/improve normal joint motion and length of muscles.
    d. Electrical stimulation (TENS) for pain relief.

Paget's Disease (Osteitis Deformans)

1. Etiology is largely unknown, but thought to be linked to a type of viral infection along with environmental factors.
2. Considered to be a metabolic bone disease involving abnormal osteoclastic and osteoblastic activity.
3. Results in spinal stenosis, facet arthropathy, and possible spinal fracture.
4. Primary medical intervention is drug therapy, such as acetaminophen for pain control. Drugs such as calcitonin and etidronate disodium may be beneficial, since they limit osteoclast activity.
5. Diagnostic tests utilized: plain film imaging identifies bony changes. Lab tests look for increased levels of serum alkaline phosphatase and urinary hydroxyproline.
6. Clinical examination assists in confirming diagnosis.
7. Physical therapy goals, outcomes, and interventions.
   a. Joint/bone protection strategies should be taught to patient.
   b. Maintain/improve joint mechanics and connective tissue functions.
   c. Implementation of aerobic capacity/endurance conditioning or reconditioning, such as aquatic programs.

Torticollis

1. Spasm and/or tightness of sternocleidomastoid (SCM) muscle, with varied etiology.
2. Dysfunction observed is side-bending toward and rotation away from the affected SCM.
3. Medications: acetaminophen, muscle relaxants, and/or NSAIDs.
4. Diagnostic tests utilized: none.
5. Physical therapy goals, outcomes, and interventions.
   a. Implementation of flexibility exercises to maintain/improve normal joint motion and length of muscles.
   b. Implementation of manual therapy for maintenance of normal joint mechanics.
      - Soft tissue/massage techniques and joint oscillations to reduce pain and/or muscle guarding.
      - Biomechanical faults caused by joint restrictions should be corrected with joint mobilization to the specific restrictions identified during the examination.

Upper Extremity Disorders

Shoulder Conditions (See Tables 2-27 to 2-30)

1. Glenohumeral instability.
   a. Traumatic instability: common in young athletes.
      - Most dislocations occur in the anterior-inferior direction.
      - Anterior-inferior dislocation occurs when abducted upper extremity is forcefully, externally rotated, causing tearing of inferior glenohumeral ligament, anterior capsule, and possibly the glenoid labrum.
      - Posterior dislocations are rare and occur with horizontal adduction and internal rotation of the glenohumeral joint.
      - Diagnosis made by clinical examination; apprehension and relocation tests typically positive for apprehension > pain.
      - Associated injuries.
        - Hill-Sachs lesion: compression fracture of the posterior humeral head.
        - Superior labrum, anterior-to-posterior (SLAP) tear.
        - Bankart lesion: avulsion of the anterior-inferior capsule and glenoid labrum.
        - Axillary nerve injury: exam will demonstrate numbness and tingling in the lateral deltoid and weakness in shoulder abduction.

Table 2-27

Differential Diagnosis of Rotator Cuff Degeneration, Frozen Shoulder, Atraumatic Instability, and Cervical Spondylosis

	ROTATOR CUFF LESIONS	FROZEN SHOULDER	ATRAUMATIC INSTABILITY	CERVICAL SPONDYLOSIS
History	Age 30–50 years Pain and weakness after eccentric load	Age 45+ (insidious type) Insidious onset or after trauma or surgery Functional restriction of lateral rotation, abduction, and medial rotation Normal bone and soft-tissue outlines	Age 10–35 years Pain and instability with activity No history of trauma	Age 50+ years Acute or chronic
Observation	Normal bone and soft-tissue outlines Protective shoulder hike may be seen	Normal bone and soft-tissue outlines	Normal bone and soft-tissue outlines	Minimal or no cervical spine movement Torticollis may be present
Active movement	Weakness of abduction or rotation, or both Crepitus may be present	Restricted ROM Shoulder hiking	Full or excessive ROM	Limited ROM with pain
Passive movement	Pain if impingement occurs	Limited ROM, especially in lateral rotation, abduction, flexion, and medial rotation (capsular pattern)	Normal or excessive ROM	Limited ROM (symptoms may be exacerbated)
Resisted isometric movement	Pain and weakness on abduction and lateral rotation	Normal, when arm by side	Normal	Normal, except if nerve root compressed Myotome may be affected
Special tests	Drop-arm test positive Empty can test positive	None	Load and shift test positive Apprehension test positive Relocation test positive Augmentation tests positive	Spurling's test positive Distraction test positive ULTT positive Shoulder abduction test positive
Sensory function and reflexes	Not affected	Not affected	Anterior or posterior pain	Dermatomes affected Reflexes affected
Palpation	Tender over rotator cuff	Not painful unless capsule is stretched	Negative	Tender over appropriate vertebra or facet
Diagnostic imaging	Radiography: upward displacement of humeral head; acromial spurring MRI diagnostic	Radiography: negative Arthrography: decreased capsular size		Radiography: narrowing osteophytes

Adapted from Magee DJ: Orthopedic Physical Assessment, 6th ed. 2014.
MRI = magnetic resonance imaging; ROM = range of motion; ULTT = upper limb tension test

- Young, active individuals with anterior-inferior labral tears are at greater risk for recurrence of instability without surgical intervention.

b. Atraumatic instability: global hypermobility, throwing athletes.
- Characterized by popping/clicking in the joint.
- Diagnosis made by clinical examination; apprehension and relocation tests typically positive for pain > apprehension.

c. Diagnostic tests utilized: plain film imaging, CT scan, MRI, and/or MRI arthrogram.

d. Physical therapy goals, outcomes, and interventions.
- Physical therapy intervention is varied, depending on specific patient impairments.
- Functional training and resistance training exercises to improve strength, endurance, proprioception, coordination, and flexibility.
- Joint movement restrictions should be addressed by exercises and/or manual therapy tailored to impairments identified during the examination.
- Avoid apprehension position (90/90° abduction/external rotation) for 12 weeks after surgical repairs of the glenoid labrum.

2. Labral tears.

a. Glenoid labrum injuries are classified as either superior (toward the top of the glenoid socket) or inferior (toward the bottom of the glenoid socket). A SLAP lesion is a tear of the rim above the middle

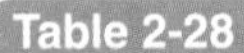

Table 2-28

Differential Diagnosis of Common Shoulder Disorders

SIGNS AND SYMPTOMS	DIFFERENTIAL DIAGNOSIS
Anterolateral shoulder pain with overhead activities and/or painful arc	Subacromial impingement syndrome Rotator cuff tendinopathy Subacromial bursitis
Instability/apprehension (with or without pain) with activity; typically shoulder is abducted and externally rotated	Glenohumeral instability Glenoid labral tear
Decreased range of motion and pain with muscle contraction	Rotator cuff tendinopathy Bicipital tendinopathy
Age >60 with pain, shoulder weakness, and night pain	Rotator cuff tear
Poorly localized shoulder pain and stiffness; typical age over 45	Frozen shoulder
Fall on adducted shoulder	Acromioclavicular joint sprain
Upper extremity paresthesia with prolonged posture or sidelying	Thoracic outlet syndrome Cervical radiculopathy

Adapted from Cleland JA, Koppenhaver S, Su J: Netter's Orthopaedic Clinical Examination, 3rd ed. 2016.

Table 2-29

Signs and Symptoms of Possible Peripheral Nerve Involvement in Shoulder Region

Spinal accessory nerve	Inability to abduct arm beyond 90° Pain in shoulder on abduction
Long thoracic nerve	Pain on flexing fully extended arm Inability to flex fully extended arm Winging starts at 90° forward flexion
Suprascapular nerve	Increased pain on forward shoulder flexion Shoulder weakness (partial loss of humeral control) Pain increases with scapular abduction Pain increases with cervical rotation to opposite side
Axillary (circumflex) nerve	Inability to abduct arm with neutral rotation

of the socket that may also involve the biceps tendon. A tear of the rim below the middle of the glenoid socket is called a Bankart's lesion and also involves the inferior glenohumeral ligament. Tears of the glenoid labrum may often occur with other shoulder injuries, such as a dislocated shoulder.

b. Characterized by the following signs and symptoms.
- Shoulder pain that cannot be localized to a specific point.
- Pain is made worse by overhead activities or when the arm is held behind the back.
- Weakness.
- Instability in the shoulder.
- Pain on resisted flexion of the biceps (bending the elbow against resistance).
- Tenderness over the front of the shoulder.

c. Diagnosis made by clinical examination, through comparing results of AROM, PROM, resistive tests, and palpation. MRI arthrograms are very effective in identifying labral tears. The "gold" standard for identifying a labral tear is through arthroscopic surgery of the shoulder.

d. Medications.
- Acetaminophen for pain.
- NSAIDS for pain and/or inflammation.

e. Physical therapy goals, outcomes, and interventions.
- Physical therapy intervention emphasizes return of function without pain.
- Functional training and resistance training exercises to improve strength, endurance, proprioception, coordination, and flexibility.
- Any underlying causes that contributed to the injury such as shoulder instability should be addressed.
- Joint movement restrictions should be addressed by exercises and/or manual therapy tailored to impairments identified during the examination. Avoid apprehension position (90/90° abduction/external rotation) for 12 weeks after surgical repairs of the glenoid labrum.
- Following surgery, the shoulder is usually kept in a sling for 3–4 weeks. After 6 weeks, more sports-specific training can be done, although full fitness may take 3–4 months.

3. Thoracic outlet syndrome (TOS) (see Table 2-30).

a. Compression of neurovascular bundle (brachial plexus, subclavian artery and vein, vagus and phrenic nerves, and the sympathetic trunk) in thoracic outlet between bony and soft tissue structures.

b. Compression occurs when size or shape of thoracic outlet is altered.

c. Common areas of compression:
- Superior thoracic outlet.
- Scalene triangle.

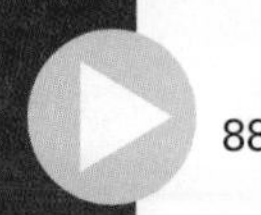

Table 2-30

Differential Diagnosis of Cervical Facet Syndrome, Cervical Spinal Nerve Lesion, and Thoracic Outlet Syndrome

SIGNS AND SYMPTOMS	CERVICAL SPINAL NERVE	CERVICAL FACET SYNDROME	THORACIC OUTLET SYNDROME
Referred pain	Yes	Common	Possible
Pain on hyperextension and rotation of cervical spine	Yes—typically symptoms increase	Yes—typically sharp localized pain at joint (often without increased referral of symptoms)	No
Spine stiffness	Possible	Yes	Possible—typically more muscular as compared to joint stiffness
Paresthesia	Yes	Not likely, but possible	Possible
Reflexes	May be affected	Not affected	May be affected
Muscle guarding	Yes	Yes	Yes
Tension tests	Positive	Typically not positive	May be positive
Pallor and coolness	No	No	Possible—primarily in hands
Muscle weakness	Possible	No	Not early (later smaller muscles)
Muscle fatigue and cramps	No	No	Possible

Adapted from Magee DJ: Orthopedic Physical Assessment, 6th ed. 2014.

- Between clavicle and first rib.
- Between pectoralis minor and thoracic wall.

d. Surgery may be performed to remove a cervical rib or a release of anterior and/or middle scalene muscle.

e. Diagnostic tests utilized: plain film imaging to identify abnormal bony anatomy and MRI to identify abnormal soft tissue anatomy. Electrodiagnostic test to assess nerve dysfunction.

f. Clinical examination including the following special tests will be useful to make diagnosis.
- Adson's test.
- Roos test.
- Wright test.
- Costoclavicular test.

g. Medications.
- Acetaminophen for pain.
- NSAIDs for pain and/or inflammation.

h. Physical therapy goals, outcomes, and interventions.
- Physical therapy intervention varies, depending on the exact cause.
- Includes postural reeducation.
- Functional training and resistance training exercises to improve strength, endurance, proprioception, coordination, and flexibility.
- Joint movement restrictions should be addressed by exercises and/or manual therapy tailored to impairments identified during the examination.
- Manipulations (typically first rib articulation) to diminish pain and soft tissue guarding.

4. Acromioclavicular and sternoclavicular joint disorders.

a. Mechanism of injury is a fall onto shoulder, with upper extremity adducted, or a collision with another individual during a sporting event.

b. Traditionally, degree of injury is graded from first to third degree. Rockwood classification scale uses grades from I to IV, with grades IV–VI as variations of the traditional grade III.

c. Upper extremity is positioned in neutral with use of sling in acute phase. Avoid shoulder elevation during the acute phase of healing.

d. Diagnostic tests utilized: plain film imaging.

e. Clinical examination, including the horizontal adduction test and Paxinos test, will be useful in order to make diagnosis.

f. Surgical repair is rare, due to tendency of acromioclavicular joint degeneration following the repair.

g. Medications.
- Acetaminophen for pain.
- NSAIDs for pain and/or inflammation.

h. Physical therapy goals, outcomes, and interventions.
- Emphasize return of function without pain.
- Functional training and resistance training exercises to improve strength, endurance, proprioception, coordination, and flexibility.
- Manual therapy techniques to AC and SC joints and surrounding connective tissues, such as soft tissue/massage, joint oscillations, and mobilizations to normalize soft tissue and joint biomechanics.

5. Subacromial/subdeltoid bursitis.

a. Subacromial and subdeltoid bursae (which may be continuous) have a close relationship to rotator cuff tendons, making them susceptible to overuse.

b. They can also become impinged beneath the acromial arch.

c. Diagnosis made by clinical examination. Differentiate from contractile condition by comparing results of AROM, PROM, and resistive tests.
d. Medications.
- Acetaminophen for pain.
- NSAIDs for pain and/or inflammation.

e. Physical therapy goals, outcomes, and interventions.
- Refer to intervention for general bursitis/tendonitis/tendonosis.

6. Rotator cuff tendonosis/tendonopathy.
a. Tendons of rotator cuff are susceptible to tendonitis due to relatively poor blood supply near insertion of muscles.
b. May result from mechanical impingement of the distal attachment of the rotator cuff on the anterior acromion and/or coracoacromial ligament with repetitive overhead activities.
c. Diagnostic tests utilized: MRI may be used, but sometimes not sensitive enough for accurate assessment.
d. Clinical examination including the following special tests will be useful to make diagnosis.
- Empty can test.
- Infraspinatus muscle test.

e. Medications.
- Acetaminophen for pain.
- NSAIDs for pain and/or inflammation.

f. Physical therapy goals, outcomes, and interventions.
- Refer to intervention for general bursitis/tendonitis/tendonosis.

7. Impingement syndrome.
a. Characterized by soft tissue inflammation of the shoulder from impingement against the acromion with repetitive overhead AROM.
b. Diagnostic tests utilized: arthrogram or MRI.
c. Clinical examination including the following special tests will be useful to make diagnosis (see Table 2-13).
- Hawkins-Kennedy test.
- Painful arc test.
- Infraspinatus muscle test.

d. Avoid shoulder elevation greater than 90° in early stages following subacromial decompression.
e. Medications.
- Acetaminophen for pain.
- NSAIDs for pain and/or inflammation.

f. Physical therapy goals, outcomes, and interventions.
- Restoration of posture.
- Functional training and resistance training exercises to improve strength, endurance, proprioception, coordination, and flexibility.
- Joint movement restrictions should be addressed by exercises and/or manual therapy tailored to impairments identified during the examination.

8. Internal (posterior) impingement.
a. Characterized by an irritation between the rotator cuff and greater tuberosity or posterior glenoid and labrum.
b. Often seen in athletes performing overhead activities. Pain commonly noted in posterior shoulder.
c. Diagnostic tests utilized: None.
d. Clinical examination, including production of posterior pain with apprehension test and reduction of pain with the relocation test, helps to identify this condition.
e. Medications.
- Acetaminophen for pain.
- NSAIDs for pain and/or inflammation.

f. Physical therapy goals, outcomes, and interventions.
- Functional training and resistance training exercises to improve strength, endurance, proprioception, coordination, and flexibility.
- Joint movement restrictions should be addressed by exercises and/or manual therapy tailored to impairments identified during the examination.

9. Bicipital tendonosis/tendonopathy.
a. Most commonly a tendon degeneration of the long head of the biceps.
b. Results from mechanical impingement of the proximal tendon, between the anterior acromion and the bicipital groove of the humerus.
c. Diagnostic tests utilized: MRI may be used, but sometimes not sensitive enough for accurate assessment.
d. Clinical examination including the following special tests will be useful to make diagnosis.
- Speed's test.

e. Medications.
- Acetaminophen for pain.
- NSAIDs for pain and/or inflammation.

f. Physical therapy goals, outcomes, and interventions.
- Refer to intervention for general bursitis/tendonosis/tendonopathy.

10. Proximal humeral fractures.
a. Humeral neck fractures frequently occur with a fall onto an outstretched upper extremity among older osteoporotic women. Generally does not require immobilization or surgical repair, since it is a fairly stable fracture.
b. Greater tuberosity fractures are more common in middle-aged and elder adults. Usually related to a fall onto the shoulder, and does not require immobilization for healing.
c. Diagnostic tests utilized: plain film imaging.
d. Medications.
- Acetaminophen for pain.
- NSAIDs for pain and/or inflammation.

e. Physical therapy goals, outcomes, and interventions.

- Physical therapy intervention emphasizes return of function without pain.
- Functional training and resistance training exercises to improve strength, endurance, proprioception, coordination, and flexibility.
- Joint movement restrictions should be addressed by exercises and/or manual therapy tailored to impairments identified during the examination.
- Early PROM is important in preventing capsular adhesions.

11. Adhesive capsulitis (frozen shoulder) (see Tables 2-27 and 2-28; Box 2-2).
   a. Characterized by a restriction in shoulder motion as a result of inflammation and fibrosis of the shoulder capsule, usually due to disuse following injury or repetitive microtrauma.
   b. Commonly seen in association with diabetes mellitus and thyroid disease.
   c. Medications.
      - Acetaminophen for pain.
      - NSAIDs for pain and/or inflammation.
   d. Physical therapy goals, outcomes, and interventions.
      - Physical therapy intervention emphasizes return of function without pain.
      - Functional training and resistance training exercises to improve strength, endurance, proprioception, coordination, and flexibility.
      - Joint movement restrictions should be addressed by exercises and/or manual therapy tailored to impairments identified during the examination.

Elbow Conditions

1. Elbow contractures.
   a. Loss of motion in capsular pattern (loss of flexion greater than extension).
   b. Loss of motion in noncapsular pattern as the result of a loose body in the joint, ligamentous sprain, and/or complex regional pain syndrome.
   c. Diagnosis made by clinical examination by comparing results of AROM, PROM, resistive tests, and palpation.
   d. Medications.
      - Acetaminophen for pain.
      - NSAIDs for pain and/or inflammation.
   e. Physical therapy goals, outcomes, and interventions.
      - Joint movement restrictions should be addressed by exercises and/or manual therapy tailored to impairments identified during the examination.
      - Soft tissue/massage techniques, modalities, flexibility exercises, and functional exercises, including strengthening, endurance, and coordination.
      - Splinting may be an effective adjunct to physical therapy management in regaining loss of motion for capsular restrictions.
2. Lateral epicondylalgia/epicondylitis ("tennis elbow").
   a. Most often a chronic degenerative condition of the extensor carpi radialis brevis tendon (ECRB) at its proximal attachment to the lateral epicondyle of the humerus.
   b. Onset is gradual, usually the result of sports activities or occupations that require repetitive wrist extension or strong grip with the wrist extended, resulting in overloading the ECRB.
   c. Must rule out involvement or relationship to cervical spine condition or radial nerve entrapment.
   d. Clinical examination including lateral epicondylitis and epicondylalgia tests helps to identify this condition (see Figure 2-25).
   e. Medications.
      - Acetaminophen for pain.
      - NSAIDs for pain and/or inflammation.
   f. Physical therapy goals, outcomes, and interventions.
      - Resistance training exercises to improve strength and endurance are the cornerstone of treatment.
      - Joint movement restrictions should be addressed by exercises and/or manual therapy tailored to impairments identified during the examination.
      - Education regarding prevention.
      - Patient/client education to avoid gripping or lifting with palm down.
      - Cryotherapy, thermotherapy, hydrotherapy, sound agents, and TENS for symptomatic relief of pain.
      - Counterforce bracing is frequently used to reduce forces along the ECRB.
3. Medial epicondylitis/epicondylalgia ("golfer's elbow").
   a. Usually a degenerative condition of the pronator teres and flexor carpi radialis tendons at their attachment to the medial epicondyle of the humerus.
   b. Occurs with overuse in sports, such as baseball pitching, driving golf swings, swimming, or occupations that require a strong hand grip and excessive pronation of the forearm.
   c. Physical therapy goals, outcomes, and interventions.
      - Intervention is similar to lateral epicondylitis and epicondylalgia.
      - Patient/client education to avoid gripping or lifting with palm down.
4. Distal humeral fractures.
   a. Complications can include loss of motion, myositis ossificans, malalignment, neurovascular compromise, ligamentous injury, and CRPS.

BOX 2-2 Adhesive Capsulitis Clinical Practice Guideline

Differential Diagnosis

- Consider other diagnoses when impairments are not consistent with adhesive capsulitis or when symptoms do not resolve with interventions (F-expert opinion, Level V)

Examination

Risk Factors (C-weak recommendation, Level III)

- Recognize age (40- to 65-years-old); female gender and previous episodes in contralateral arm
- Consider history of diabetes or thyroid disease

Pathoanatomical Features (E-theoretical/foundational, Level V)

- Assess for loss of passive ROM in multiple planes, especially external rotation

Clinical Course (B-moderate recommendation, Level II)

- Recognize a continuum of pathology with a progression of pain and mobility deficits that may persist

Activity Limitation Measures (A-strong recommendation, Level I)

- **Use easily reproducible activity limitations associated with pain and function over the episode of care**

Physical Impairment Measures (E-theoretical/foundational, Level V)

- Measure active and passive ROM, pain
- May assess translational glide loss

Outcome Measures (A-strong recommendation, Level I)

- **Use validated shoulder outcomes measures before and after interventions**

Diagnosis/Classification (F-expert opinion, Level V)

- Recognize a gradual and progressive onset of pain and loss of ROM in elevation and rotation

Interventions

Corticosteroid Injections (A-strong recommendation, Level I)

- **Intra-articular corticosteroid injections combined with shoulder mobility and stretching provide short-term (4–6 weeks) pain relief and improved function as compared to exercises alone**

Patient Education (B-moderate recommendation, Level II)

- Patient education that describes course of the condition, promotes activity modification, and matches stretching to level of irritability

Stretching (B-moderate recommendation, Level II)

- Instruct patients in stretching exercises

Modalities (C-weak recommendation, Level III)

- Ultrasound, shortwave diathermy, or electrical stimulation in conjunction with exercises

Joint Mobilization (C-weak recommendation, Level III)

- Joint mobilization directed at glenohumeral joint to reduce pain and increase function
- Translational manipulation under anesthesia for those not responding to other interventions

Adapted from Adhesive Capsulitis, Orthopedic Section. APTA, Summary of Recommendations. *JOSPT* 5(43): A26, 2013.
Level 1 evidence and Grade A recommendations are highlighted in the table with bold font.
See Table 16-4 in Chapter 16 for Levels of Evidence and Grades of Recommendations.

b. Supracondylar fractures must be examined quickly for neurovascular status due to high number of neurological (typically radial nerve involvement) and vascular structures that pass through this region (may lead to Volkmann's ischemia). In youth, it is important to assess growth plate as well. These fractures have a high incidence of malunion.
c. Lateral epicondyle fractures are fairly common in young people and typically require an open reduction internal fixation (ORIF) to ensure absolute alignment.
d. Diagnostic tests utilized: plain film imaging.
e. Medications.
   - Acetaminophen for pain.
   - NSAIDs for pain and/or inflammation.
f. Physical therapy goals, outcomes, and interventions.
   - Physical therapy intervention includes pain reduction and limiting the inflammatory response following trauma and/or surgery.
   - Improving flexibility of shortened structures, strengthening, and training to restore functional use of UE.

5. Osteochondrosis of humeral capitellum.
   a. Osteochondritis dissecans affects central and/or lateral aspect of capitellum or radial head. An osteochondral bone fragment becomes detached from articular surface, forming a loose body in joint. Caused by repetitive compressive forces between radial head and humeral capitellum. Occurs in adolescents between 12 and 15 years of age.
   b. Panner's disease is a localized avascular necrosis of capitellum leading to loss of subchondral bone, with fissuring and softening of articular surfaces of radiocapitellar joint. Etiology is unknown, but occurs in children age 10 or younger.
   c. Diagnostic tests utilized: plain film imaging.
   d. Medications.
      - Acetaminophen for pain.
      - NSAIDs for pain and/or inflammation.
   e. Physical therapy goals, outcomes, and interventions.
      - Physical therapy intervention includes rest with avoidance of any throwing or upper extremity-loading activities (e.g., gymnastics).
      - When patient is pain-free, initiate flexibility and strengthening/endurance/coordination exercises.
      - During late phases of rehabilitation, a program to slowly increase load on joint is initiated. If symptoms persist, surgical intervention is necessary.
      - After surgery, initial focus of rehabilitation is to minimize pain and swelling using modalities. Flexibility exercises are begun immediately following surgery.
      - Thereafter, a progressive strengthening program is initiated.
      - Joint movement restrictions should be addressed by exercises and/or manual therapy tailored to impairments identified during the examination.

6. Ulnar collateral ligament injuries.
   a. Occurs as result of repetitive valgus stresses to medial elbow with overhead throwing.
   b. Clinical signs include pain along medial elbow at distal insertion of ligament. In some cases, paresthesias are reported in ulnar nerve distribution with positive Tinel's sign.
   c. Diagnostic tests utilized: MRI.
   d. Clinical examination including medial ligament instability test helps to identify this condition.
   e. Medications.
      - Acetaminophen for pain.
      - NSAIDs for pain and/or inflammation.
   f. Physical therapy goals, outcomes, and interventions.
      - Initial intervention includes rest and pain management.
      - After resolution of pain and inflammation, strengthening exercises that focus on elbow flexors are initiated. Taping can also be used for protection during return to activities.

7. Nerve entrapments.
   a. Ulnar nerve entrapment.
      - Various causes including direct trauma at the cubital tunnel, traction due to laxity at medial aspect of elbow, compression due to a thickened retinaculum or hypertrophy of flexor carpi ulnaris muscle, recurrent subluxation or dislocation, and DJD that affects the cubital tunnel.
      - Clinical findings include medial elbow pain, paresthesias in ulnar distribution, and a positive Tinel's sign.
   b. Median nerve entrapment.
      - Occurs within pronator teres muscle and under superficial head of flexor digitorum superficialis with repetitive gripping activities required in occupations (e.g., electricians) and with leisure time activities (e.g., tennis).
      - Clinical signs include an aching pain with weakness of forearm muscles and positive Tinel's sign, with paresthesias in median nerve distribution.
   c. Radial nerve entrapment.
      - Entrapment of distal branches (posterior interosseous nerve) occurs within radial tunnel (radial tunnel syndrome) as result of overhead activities and throwing.
      - Clinical signs include lateral elbow pain that can be confused with lateral epicondylitis and epicondylopathy, pain over supinator muscle, and paresthesias in a radial nerve distribution. Tinel's sign may be positive.
   d. Diagnostic tests utilized: electrodiagnostic tests.

e. Clinical examination helps to identify this condition.
f. Medications.
  - Acetaminophen for pain.
  - NSAIDs for pain and/or inflammation.
  - Neurontin for neuropathic pain.
g. Physical therapy goals, outcomes, and interventions.
  - Early intervention includes rest, avoiding exacerbating activities, use of NSAIDs, modalities, and soft tissue/massage techniques to reduce inflammation and pain.
  - If abnormal neurotension is present, neurodynamic mobilization may be indicated.
  - Protective padding and night splints to maintain slackened position of involved nerves.
  - With reduction in pain and paresthesias, rehabilitation program should focus on strengthening/endurance/coordination exercise of involved muscles to achieve muscle balance between agonists and antagonists, normal flexibility of shortened structures, and normalization of strength/endurance/coordination.
  - Intervention should also include functional training, patient education, and self-management techniques.

8. Elbow dislocations.
a. Posterior dislocations account for most dislocations occurring at elbow.
  - Posterior dislocations are defined by position of olecranon relative to the humerus.
  - Posterolateral dislocations are most common and occur as the result of elbow hyperextension from a fall on the outstretched upper extremity.
  - Posterior dislocations frequently cause avulsion fractures of medial epicondyle secondary to traction pull of medial collateral ligament.
b. Anterior and radial head dislocations account for only 1%–2% of all elbow dislocations.
c. With a complete dislocation, ulnar collateral ligament will rupture, with possible rupture of anterior capsule, lateral collateral ligament, brachialis muscle, and/or wrist flexor and extensor muscles.
d. Clinical signs include rapid swelling, severe pain at the elbow, and a deformity with the olecranon pushed posteriorly.
e. Diagnostic tests utilized: plain film imaging.
f. Medications.
  - Acetaminophen for pain.
  - NSAIDs for pain and/or inflammation.
g. Physical therapy goals, outcomes, and interventions.
  - Initial intervention includes reduction of the dislocation.
  - If elbow is stable, there is an initial phase of immobilization, followed by rehabilitation focusing on regaining flexibility within limits of stability and strengthening.
  - If elbow is not stable, surgery is indicated.

Wrist and Hand Conditions

1. Carpal tunnel syndrome (repetitive stress syndrome). See Box 2-3.
a. Compression of the median nerve at the carpal tunnel of the wrist due to inflammation of the flexor tendons and/or median nerve.
b. Commonly occurs as result of repetitive wrist motions or gripping, with pregnancy, diabetes, and rheumatoid arthritis.
c. Must rule out potential of cervical spine dysfunction, TOS, or peripheral nerve entrapment that mimics this condition.
d. Diagnostic tests utilized: electrodiagnostic testing.
e. Common clinical findings include exacerbation of burning, tingling, pins and needles, and numbness into median nerve distribution at night, and a positive Tinel's sign and/or Phalen's test. Long-term compression causes atrophy and weakness of thenar muscles and lateral two lumbricals.
f. Medications.
  - Acetaminophen for pain.
  - NSAIDs for pain and/or inflammation.
g. Physical therapy goals, outcomes, and interventions.
  - Joint movement restrictions should be addressed by exercises and/or manual therapy tailored to impairments identified during the examination.
  - Soft tissue/massage techniques, modalities, flexibility exercises, and functional exercises including strengthening, endurance, and coordination.

2. de Quervain's tenosynovitis.
a. Inflammation/degeneration of extensor pollicis brevis and abductor pollicis longus tendons at first dorsal compartment.
b. Results from repetitive microtrauma or as a complication of swelling during pregnancy.
c. Diagnostic tests utilized: MRI, but usually not necessary to make diagnosis.
d. Clinical signs include: pain at anatomical snuffbox, swelling, decreased grip and pinch strength, positive Finkelstein's test (which places tendons on a stretch).
e. Medications.
  - Acetaminophen for pain.
  - NSAIDs for pain and/or inflammation.
f. Physical therapy goals, outcomes, and interventions.
  - Joint movement restrictions should be addressed by exercises and/or manual therapy tailored to impairments identified during the examination.

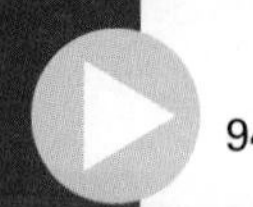

BOX 2-3 Hand Pain and Sensory Deficits: Carpal Tunnel Syndrome (CTS) Clinical Practice Guideline

Examination

Outcome Measures (B-Moderate Recommendation, Level II)

- May use the Boston Carpal Tunnel Questionnaire Symptom Severity Scale (CTQ-SSS) to assess symptoms.
- May use the Boston Carpal Tunnel Questionnaire Functional Scale (CTQ-FS) or Disabilities of the Arm, Shoulder, and Hand (DASH) questionnaire to assess function.

Physical Performance Measures (C-Weak Recommendation, Level III)

- May use Perdue Pegboard (PPB) or Dellon-modified Moberg Pick-Up Test (DMPUT) to quantify dexterity.
- May use DMPUT to assess change following carpal tunnel release (CTR) surgery.

Physical Impairment Measures

- **Should NOT use lateral pinch strength as an outcome (A-strong recommendation, Level I).**
- Should NOT use grip strength as an outcome following CTR surgery (B-moderate recommendation, Level II).
- May use grip strength and 3-point (tip) pinch strength in individuals with signs/symptoms of CTS (C-weak recommendation, Level III).
- Conflicting evidence on 3-point (tip) and abductor pollicis brevis muscle strength testing following CTR surgery (D-contradictory evidence, Level IV).

Sensory and Provocative Measures

- Should not use threshold or vibration testing in individuals undergoing nonsurgical treatment (C-weak recommendation, Level III).
- Conflicting evidence on using sensory measures following CTR surgery (D-contradictory evidence, Level IV).

Diagnosis/Classification

- **Should use Semmes-Weinstein monofilament testing (A-strong recommendation, Level I).**
  - **Assess middle finger with 2.83 or 3.22 monofilament as threshold normal for light-touch sensation and static 2-point discrimination.**
  - **In suspected moderate to severe CTS, assess any radial finger with 3.22 monofilament as threshold for normal.**
- May utilize Katz hand diagram, Phalen test, Tinel sign, and carpal compression test to determine the likelihood of CTS (B-moderate recommendation, Level II).
- A combination of three of the following positive tests is diagnostic for CTS (B-moderate recommendation, Level II).
  - Age >45 years.
  - Shaking hands relieves symptoms.
  - Sensory loss in the thumb.
  - Wrist ratio index >0.67.
  - CTQ-SSS score >1.9.
- Contradictory evidence exists for upper-limb neurodynamic tests, scratch-collapse test, and tests of vibration sense (D-contradictory evidence, Level IV).

Interventions—Assistive Technology

- May educate patients on the effects of mouse use (C-weak recommendation, Level III).
- May recommend keyboards with reduced strike force (C-weak recommendation, Level III).

Interventions—Orthoses

- Should recommend a neutral-positioned wrist orthoses worn at night for short-term symptom relief and functional improvement (B-moderate recommendation, Level II).
- May suggest day-time, symptomatic, or full-time use when night-only use is ineffective (C-weak recommendation, Level III).
- May recommend an orthosis for women during pregnancy (C-weak recommendation, Level III).

(Continued)

BOX 2-3 Hand Pain and Sensory Deficits: Carpal Tunnel Syndrome (CTS) Clinical Practice Guideline (Continued)

Interventions—Biophysical Agents

- May recommend trial of superficial heat, microwave/shortwave diathermy, or interferential current for short-term symptom relief (C-weak recommendation, Level III).
- May perform phonophoresis in nonsurgical treatment of mild to moderate CTS (C-weak recommendation, Level III).
- Should NOT use low-level laser therapy or iontophoresis or use/recommend magnets (B-moderate recommendation, Level II).
- Should NOT use thermal ultrasound (C-weak recommendation, Level III).
- Conflicting evidence on the use of nonthermal ultrasound (D-contradictory evidence, Level IV).

Interventions—Manual Therapy Techniques

- May consider manual therapy at the cervical spine and upper extremity (C-weak recommendation, Level III).
- Contradictory evidence exists on use neurodynamic mobilization (D-contradictory evidence, Level IV).

Interventions—Orthotic/Stretching Program

- May use a combined orthotic/stretching program in individuals with mild-moderate CTS without thenar atrophy and normal two-point discrimination (C-weak evidence, Level III).

Adapted from Hand Pain and Sensory Deficits: Carpal Tunnel Syndrome, Clinical Practice Guidelines, Orthopedic Section, APTA, Summary of Recommendations. *JOSPT* 49(5): 359–360, 2019.

Level 1 evidence and Grade A recommendations are highlighted in the table with bold font.

See Table 16-4 for Levels of Evidence and Grades of Recommendations.

- Soft tissue/massage techniques, modalities, flexibility exercises, and functional exercises including strengthening, endurance, and coordination.

3. Colles' fracture.
   a. Most common wrist fracture, resulting from a fall onto an outstretched upper extremity (UE). These fractures are immobilized for 5–8 weeks. Complication of median nerve compression can occur with excessive edema.
   b. Characteristic "dinner fork" deformity of wrist and hand results from dorsal or posterior displacement of distal fragment of radius, with a radial shift of wrist and hand.
   c. Diagnostic tests utilized: plain film imaging.
   d. Complications may include loss of motion, decreased grip strength, CRPS, and carpal tunnel syndrome.
   e. Medications.
      - Acetaminophen for pain.
      - NSAIDs for pain and/or inflammation.
   f. Physical therapy goals, outcomes, and interventions.
      - Early physical therapy intervention that focuses on normalizing flexibility is paramount to functional recovery of wrist and hand.
      - Joint movement restrictions should be addressed by exercises and/or manual therapy tailored to impairments identified during the examination.
      - Soft tissue/massage techniques, modalities, flexibility exercises, and functional exercises including strengthening, endurance, and coordination.
4. Smith's fracture.
   a. Similar to Colles' fracture, except distal fragment of radius dislocates in a volar direction, causing a characteristic "garden spade" deformity.
   b. Diagnostic tests utilized: plain film imaging.
   c. Medications.
      - Acetaminophen for pain.
      - NSAIDs for pain and/or inflammation.
   d. Physical therapy goals, outcomes, and interventions.
      - Intervention is similar to Colles' fracture.
5. Scaphoid fracture.
   a. Results from a fall onto outstretched UE in a younger person. Most commonly fractured carpal.
   b. Diagnostic tests utilized: plain film imaging, MRI.
   c. Complications include a high incidence of avascular necrosis of the proximal fragment of the scaphoid secondary to poor vascular supply. Carpals are immobilized for 4–8 weeks.
   d. Medications.
      - Acetaminophen for pain.
      - NSAIDs for pain and/or inflammation.
   e. Physical therapy goals, outcomes, and interventions.
      - Early intervention includes maintenance of flexibility of distal and proximal joints while UE is

casted. Later intervention emphasizes strengthening, stretching, and joint and soft tissue mobilizations to regain full functional use of wrist and hand.

RED FLAG: Timely diagnosis and intervention for a suspected scaphoid fracture is critical. The patient should be immobilized and referred to the primary care provider or emergency room with the recommendation to order radiographs. Failure to properly manage a fractured scaphoid may result in avascular necrosis of the bone due to its poor vascular supply.

6. Dupuytren's contracture.
   a. Observed as banding on palm and digit flexion contractures, resulting from contracture of palmar fascia that adheres to skin.
   b. Affects men more often than women.
   c. Contracture usually affects the metacarpophalangeal (MCP) and proximal interphalangeal (PIP) joints of fourth and fifth digits in nondiabetic individuals and affects third and fourth digits most often in individuals with diabetes.
   d. Medications.
      - Acetaminophen for pain.
      - NSAIDs for pain and/or inflammation.
   e. Physical therapy goals, outcomes, and interventions.
      - Physical therapy intervention includes flexibility exercise to prevent further contracture and splint fabrication/application.
      - Once contracture is under control, promote restoration of normal hand function through functional exercises.
      - Physical therapy intervention following surgery includes wound management, edema control, and progression of functional exercise.
7. Boutonnière deformity.
   a. Results from rupture of central tendinous slip of extensor hood.
   b. Observed deformity is extension of MCP and distal interphalangeal (DIP) with flexion of PIP.
   c. Commonly occurs following trauma, or in rheumatoid arthritis with degeneration of the central extensor tendon.
   d. Medications.
      - Acetaminophen for pain.
      - NSAIDs for pain and/or inflammation.
   e. Physical therapy goals, outcomes, and interventions.
      - Physical therapy intervention includes edema management, flexibility exercises of involved and uninvolved joints, splinting or taping, and functional strengthening/endurance/coordination exercises.
8. Swan neck deformity.
   a. Results from contracture of intrinsic muscles with dorsal subluxation of lateral extensor tendons.
   b. Observed deformity is flexion of MCP and DIP with extension of PIP.
   c. Commonly occurs following trauma, or with rheumatoid arthritis following degeneration of lateral extensor tendons.
   d. Diagnostic tests utilized: plain film imaging, but may not be necessary.
   e. Medications.
      - Acetaminophen for pain.
      - NSAIDs for pain and/or inflammation.
   f. Physical therapy goals, outcomes, and interventions.
      - Physical therapy intervention includes edema management, flexibility exercises of involved and uninvolved joints, splinting or taping, and functional strengthening/endurance/coordination exercises.
9. Ape hand deformity.
   a. Observed as thenar muscle wasting, with first digit moving dorsally until it is in line with second digit.
   b. Results from median nerve dysfunction.
   c. Diagnostic tests utilized: electrodiagnostic testing.
   d. Medications.
      - Acetaminophen for pain.
      - NSAIDs for pain and/or inflammation.
   e. Physical therapy goals, outcomes, and interventions.
      - Physical therapy intervention includes edema management, flexibility exercises of involved and uninvolved joints, splinting or taping, and functional strengthening/endurance/coordination exercises.
10. Mallet finger.
    a. Rupture or avulsion of extensor tendon at its insertion into distal phalanx of digit.
    b. Observed deformity is flexion of DIP joint.
    c. Usually occurs from trauma, forcing distal phalanx into a flexed position.
    d. Diagnostic tests utilized: possibly MRI.
    e. Medications.
       - Acetaminophen for pain.
       - NSAIDs for pain and/or inflammation.
    f. Physical therapy goals, outcomes, and interventions.
       - Physical therapy intervention includes edema management, flexibility exercises of involved and uninvolved joints, splinting or taping, and functional strengthening/endurance/coordination exercises.
11. Flexor digitorum profundus tendon rupture/avulsion (Jersey Finger).
    a. Mechanism of injury forced hyperextension of DIP joint with maximal finger flexion contraction.
    b. Ring finger involved in 75% of cases (5 mm more prominent during grip).
    c. May rupture directly from insertion, avulse from bone, or rupture at musculotendinous junction.

d. Key exam finding of Inability to produce isolated flexion of the DIP.
e. Diagnostic tests utilized: finger radiographs.
f. Immediate referral to hand surgeon to avoid loss of finger function.

12. Gamekeeper's thumb.
a. A sprain/rupture of ulnar collateral ligament of MCP joint of first digit.
b. Results in medial instability of thumb.
c. Frequently occurs during a fall while skiing, when increasing forces are placed on thumb through ski pole. Immobilized for 6 weeks.
d. Diagnostic tests utilized: possibly MRI.
e. Medications.
- Acetaminophen for pain.
- NSAIDs for pain and/or inflammation.

f. Physical therapy goals, outcomes, and interventions.
- Physical therapy intervention includes edema management, flexibility exercises of involved and uninvolved joints, splinting or taping, and functional strengthening/endurance/coordination exercises.

13. Boxer's fracture.
a. Fracture of neck of fifth metacarpal.
b. Frequently sustained during a fight, or from punching a wall in anger or frustration.
c. Casted for 2–4 weeks.
d. Diagnostic tests utilized: plain film imaging.
e. Medications.
- Acetaminophen for pain.
- NSAIDs for pain and/or inflammation.

f. Physical therapy goals, outcomes, and interventions.
- Physical therapy intervention includes edema management, flexibility exercise initially at uninvolved joints, followed by involved joints after sufficient healing has occurred.
- Initiation of functional strengthening/endurance/coordination occurs when flexibility is restored.

Lower Extremity Conditions

Hip Conditions (See Boxes 2-1, 2-4 and 2-5)

1. Avascular necrosis (AVN) of the hip (osteonecrosis).
a. Multiple etiologies resulting in an impaired blood supply to the femoral head.
b. Hip ROM is decreased in flexion, internal rotation, and abduction.
c. Diagnostic tests utilized: plain film imaging, bone scans, CT, and/or MRI may be utilized.
d. Symptoms include pain in the groin and/or thigh, and tenderness with palpation at the hip joint.
e. Coxalgic gait.
f. Medications.
- Acetaminophen for pain.
- NSAIDs for pain and/or inflammation.
- Corticosteroids contraindicated since they may be causative factor. Patient taking steroids for some other condition should have dose decreased.

g. Physical therapy goals, outcomes, and interventions.
- Joint/bone protection strategies.
- Maintain/improve joint mechanics and connective tissue functions.
- Implementation of aerobic capacity/endurance conditioning or reconditioning such as aquatic programs.
- Postsurgical intervention includes regaining functional flexibility, improving strength/endurance/coordination, and gait training.

2. Coxa vara and coxa valga.
a. Angle of femoral neck with shaft of femur is <115°; coxa vara results.
b. Angle of femoral neck with shaft of femur is >125°; coxa valga results.
c. Coxa vara usually results from a defect in ossification of head of femur. Coxa vara and coxa valga may result from necrosis of femoral head occurring with septic arthritis.
d. Diagnostic tests utilized: plain film imaging.
e. Physical therapy goals, outcomes, and interventions.
- Maintain/improve joint mechanics and connective tissue functions.

3. Trochanteric bursitis.
a. An inflammation of deep trochanteric bursa from a direct blow, irritation by iliotibial band (ITB), and biomechanical/gait abnormalities causing repetitive microtrauma.
b. This condition is common in patients with rheumatoid arthritis.
c. Diagnostic tests utilized: none.
d. Diagnosis made by clinical examination. Differentiate from contractile condition by comparing results of AROM, PROM, and resistive tests.
e. Medications.
- Acetaminophen for pain.
- NSAIDs for pain and/or inflammation.

f. Physical therapy goals, outcomes, and interventions.
- Refer to intervention for general bursitis/tendonitis/tendonosis.

4. Iliotibial band tightness/friction disorder.
a. Etiology: tight ITB, abnormal gait patterns.
b. Results in inflammation of trochanteric bursa.
c. Noble compression test and/or Ober's test may be positive.
d. Medications.
- Acetaminophen for pain.
- NSAIDs for pain and/or inflammation.

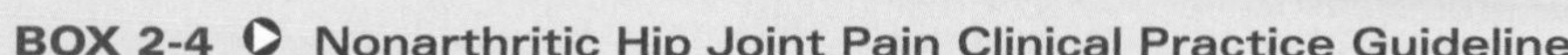

BOX 2-4 Nonarthritic Hip Joint Pain Clinical Practice Guideline

Differential Diagnosis

- Should consider other diagnostic categories if history, activity limitations are not consistent with Diagnosis/Classification, and patient symptoms are not diminishing with interventions (F-expert opinion, Level V)

Examination

Risk Factors (F-expert opinion, Level V)

- Osseous abnormalities, ligamentous laxity, connective tissue disorders, activity level

Physical Impairment Measures (B-moderate recommendation, Level II)

- Assess objective measures of pain, mobility, muscle power, and movement coordination

Outcome Measures (A-strong recommendation, Level I)

- **Use validated hip outcome measures**

Diagnosis/Classification

- Diagnosis of Femoroacetabular Impingement Syndrome can be suspected with the following clinical and radiographic findings: anterior groin or hip pain reproduced by FADIR or FABER; hip internal rotation less than 20° with the hip at 90° of flexion; mechanical symptoms, such as popping or snapping; imaging findings of CAM or pincer impingement (C-weak recommendation, Level III)

Interventions

Patient Education (F-expert opinion, Level V)

- Patient education to manage pain and modify aggravating factors

Manual Therapy (F-expert opinion, Level V)

- Joint mobilization with capsular restrictions
- Soft tissue mobilization if muscles or fascia impair hip mobility

Therapeutic Exercises (F-expert opinion, Level V)

- Therapeutic exercise to address flexibility, strength, deconditioning, and metabolic disorders previously identified

Neuromuscular Reeducation (F-expert opinion, Level V)

- May use neuromuscular reeducation to diminish movement coordination impairments

Adapted from Nonarthritic Hip Joint Pain, Orthopedic Section, APTA, Summary of Recommendations. *JOSPT* 44(6): A2–3, 2014.
Level 1 evidence and Grade A recommendations are highlighted in the table with bold font.
See Table 16-4 in Chapter 16 for Levels of Evidence and Grades of Recommendations.

e. Physical therapy goals, outcomes, and interventions.
   - Reduction of pain and inflammation utilizing modalities, soft tissue techniques, and manual therapy techniques such as soft tissue/massage and joint oscillations.
   - Functional training and resistance training exercises to improve strength, endurance, proprioception, coordination, and flexibility.
   - Joint movement restrictions should be addressed by exercises and/or manual therapy tailored to impairments identified during the examination.
   - Gait training and patient education regarding the selection of running shoes and running surfaces. Orthoses may be fabricated.

5. Piriformis syndrome.
   a. Piriformis muscle is an external rotator of hip at less than 60° of hip flexion and can become overworked with excessive pronation of foot, causing abnormal femoral internal rotation. At 90° of hip flexion, the piriformis becomes an internal rotator and abductor of the hip. Considered a tonic muscle that is active with motion of sacroiliac joint, particularly sacrum.
   b. Tightness or spasm of piriformis muscle can result in compression of sciatic nerve and/or sacroiliac dysfunction.
   c. Diagnostic tests utilized: possibly electrodiagnostic tests for sciatic nerve.
   d. Signs and symptoms include:
      - Restriction in internal rotation.
      - Pain with palpation of piriformis muscle.
      - Referral of pain to posterior thigh.
      - Weakness in ER, positive piriformis test.

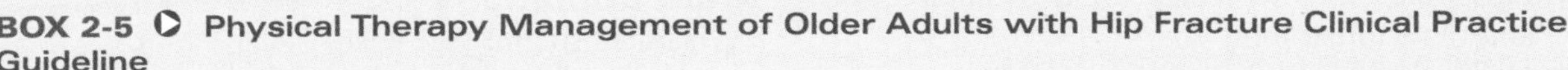

BOX 2-5 Physical Therapy Management of Older Adults with Hip Fracture Clinical Practice Guideline

NOTE: The scope of this CPG is focused on low-energy fractures of the proximal femur in older adults, which are most likely the result of falls and osteoporosis.

Examination

Physical Impairment and Performance Measures – Across the Entire Episode of Care (A-strong recommendation, Level I).

- **Must document knee extension strength.**
- **Must administer/document verbal rating scale for pain.**
- **Should use the gait speed test, documenting comfortable or maximum speed, walking aid, and type of start (rolling vs. static).**
- **Should use the Cumulated Ambulation Score to measure basic mobility.**
- **Should use the timed up-and-go test to measure mobility and risk for falls, documenting comfortable or maximum speed and walking aid use.**

Physical Performance Measures – Across the Entire Episode of Care (B-moderate recommendation, Level II).

- Should use the New Mobility Score to assess status and recovery.
- Should use Falls Efficacy Scale-International to measure concern for falling.

Physical Impairment and Performance Measures – Skilled Nursing and Community Settings (B-moderate recommendation, Level II).

- Should test and document hip extensor and abductor muscle strength.
- Should use the 5-times sit-to-stand or 30-second sit-to-stand test to measure mobility and fall risk.
- Should use the 6-minute walk test.

Interventions

Across the Entire Episode of Care: Must provide structured exercise, to include progressive high-intensity resistance exercises (weight-bearing and non-weight-bearing), balance training exercises, and functional mobility training (A-strong recommendation, Level I)

Early Postoperative Period – Inpatient Setting.

- **Should prescribe a multidisciplinary orthogeriatric program that includes physical therapy and early mobilization (A-strong recommendation, Level I).**
- **Must assist patient out of bed and with ambulation as soon as possible (daily subsequently) after hip fracture surgery (A-strong recommendation, Level I).**
- Should be offered high-frequency (daily) in-hospital physical therapy following surgery (B-moderate recommendation, Level II).

Post-acute Period – Home Care and Community Settings (A-strong recommendation, Level I).

- **Must provide additional physical therapy (strength, balance, functional/gait training) if deficits persist beyond 8–16 weeks after fracture.**
- **Must provide patient education to maximize safe physical activity.**

Interprofessional Management

Prevention and identification of delirium: Should participate in multicomponent nonpharmacological intervention programs delivered by an interdisciplinary team for the entire hospitalization of at-risk patients undergoing surgery (A-strong recommendation, Level I).

Prevention of falls: Must assess and document risk factors for falls and contribute to interdisciplinary management (A-strong recommendation, Level I).

Adapted from Physical Therapy Management of Older Adults With Hip Fracture, Clinical Practice Guidelines, Academy of Orthopaedic Physical Therapy and the Academy of Geriatric Physical Therapy, APTA, Summary of Recommendations.

JOSPT; 2(51): CPG1-CPG47, 2021

Level 1 evidence and Grade A recommendations are highlighted in the table with bold font.

See Table 16-4 in Chapter 16 for Levels of Evidence and Grades of Recommendations

e. Must rule out involvement of the lumbar spine and/or sacroiliac joint.
f. Medications.
- Acetaminophen for pain.
- NSAIDs for pain and/or inflammation.
- Neurontin for neuropathic pain.

g. Physical therapy goals, outcomes, and interventions.
- Reduction of pain utilizing modalities and manual therapy techniques, such as soft tissue/massage to piriformis muscle.
- Functional training and resistance training exercises to improve strength, endurance, proprioception, coordination, and flexibility.
- Joint movement restrictions should be addressed by exercises and/or manual therapy tailored to impairments identified during the examination.
- Restore muscle balance and patient education regarding protection of the sacroiliac joint (e.g., instruction not to step off a curb onto the dysfunctional lower extremity).
- Correction of biomechanical faults may include orthoses or orthotic devices for feet.

6. Femoroacetabular impingement (FAI) (see Box 2-4).
a. Types.
- CAM type: impingement of a large aspherical femoral head in a constrained acetabulum.
- Pincer type: over-coverage of the femoral head by a prominent acetabular rim.

b. Frequently associated with acetabular labral tears.

7. Groin pain in athletes (sports hernia).
a. Common in sports requiring kicking, rapid acceleration/deceleration, and sudden change of direction (hockey, soccer, etc.).
b. May be related to pathology in one or more of the following areas.
- Adductor.
- Iliopsoas.
- Inguinal.
- Pubic.

c. Signs and symptoms.
- Acute or gradual onset.
- Symptoms and painful weakness localized to structures involved.

d. Rule out hip joint involvement.
e. Medications.
- Acetaminophen for pain.
- NSAIDs for pain and/or inflammation.

f. Physical therapy goals, outcomes, and interventions.
- Total length of rehabilitation period 8–12 weeks.
- Reduction of pain utilizing modalities and manual therapy techniques such as soft tissue mobilization to the adductors.
- Functional training and resistance training exercises to improve strength, endurance, proprioception, coordination, and flexibility.

Knee Conditions

1. Ligament sprains (see Boxes 2-6 and 2-7).
a. Four major ligaments may be involved (anterior cruciate [ACL], posterior cruciate [PCL], medial collateral [MCL], and lateral collateral [LCL]).
b. Injury to the ligaments may result in a single plane or rotary instability.
- ACL laxity may result in single plane anterior instability.
- PCL laxity may result in single plane posterior instability.
- ACL and MCL laxity may result in anteromedial rotary instability.
- ACL and LCL laxity may result in anterolateral rotary instability.
- PCL and MCL laxity may result in posteromedial rotary instability.
- PCL and LCL laxity may result in posterolateral rotary instability.

c. Classification of injury.
- First degree, resulting in little or no instability.
- Second degree, resulting in minimal to moderate instability.
- Third degree, resulting in extreme instability.

d. "Unhappy triad" includes injury to the MCL, ACL, and the medial meniscus, resulting from a combination of valgum, flexion, and ER forces applied to knee when the foot is planted.
e. Diagnostic tests utilized: plain film radiographs, MRI.
f. Refer to knee special tests that help to identify ligamentous instabilities of knee joint.
g. Medications.
- Acetaminophen for pain.
- NSAIDs for pain and/or inflammation.

h. Physical therapy goals, outcomes, and interventions.
- Physical therapy intervention is varied depending on whether the patient undergoes a surgical procedure, as well as type of surgery performed.
- Reduction of pain and inflammation utilizing modalities, soft tissue techniques, and manual therapy techniques such as oscillations.
- Functional training and resistance training exercises to improve strength, endurance, proprioception, coordination, and flexibility.
- Joint movement restrictions should be addressed by exercises and/or manual therapy tailored to impairments identified during the examination.
- Progression to functional training based on patient's occupation and/or recreational goals.

i. Prevention of ACL injuries (see Box 2-7).

2. Meniscal and articular cartilage injuries (see Box 2-8).
a. Result from a combination of forces to include tibiofemoral joint flexion, compression, and rotation, which places abnormal shear stresses on the meniscus.

BOX 2-6 Knee Ligament Sprain Clinical Practice Guideline

Differential Diagnosis

- Suspect serious pathological conditions and other ICD classifications when symptoms, impairments, and function are not resolving with intervention (B-moderate recommendation, Level II)

Examination

Physical Performance Measures (B-moderate recommendation, Level II)

- Administer appropriate clinical or field tests (a variety of single-legged hop tests) to establish baseline status relative to function, pain, asymmetries side-to-side, and readiness to return to activities throughout the course of treatment

Physical Impairment Measures (B-moderate recommendation, Level II)

- Use assessments of impairments throughout the episode of care including measures of knee laxity/stability, movement coordination, quadriceps strength, effusion, and ROM

Outcome Measures (B-moderate recommendation, Level II)

- Use validated patient-reported outcome measures to assess knee symptoms and function as well as activity rating scales before and after interventions

Diagnosis/Classification

- **Diagnosis of a knee ligament sprain is made with a reasonable level of certainty when the patient presents with the following clinical findings: symptom onset linked to precipitating trauma; deceleration, cutting, or valgus motion associated with injury; "pop" heard or felt at time of injury; hemarthrosis within 0 to 12 hours following injury; knee effusion; subjective knee instability reported; excessive tibiofemoral laxity with ligament integrity tests (Lachman, Anterior/Posterior Drawer, Varus/Valgus); pain/symptoms with ligament integrity tests; lower-limb strength and coordination deficits; impaired single-leg proprioception/balance; abnormal compensatory strategies observed during deceleration or cutting movements (A-strong recommendation, Level I)**

Interventions

Therapeutic Exercise and Neuromuscular Electrical Stimulation (A-strong recommendation, Level I)

- **Concentric and eccentric exercises in non–weight-bearing and weight-bearing status to increase quad strength and functional performance following ACL reconstruction. Starting within 4–6 weeks and continuing up to 10 months**
- **Neuromuscular electrical stimulation (NMES) following ACL reconstruction (up to 6–8 weeks) to increase quad strength and short-term function**

Neuromuscular reeducation (A-strong recommendation, Level I)

- **Neuromuscular reeducation along with strengthening in patients with knee stability and movement coordination impairments**

Immediate versus Delayed Mobilization (B-moderate recommendation, Level II)

- Use immediate mobilization (within 1 week) following ACL reconstruction to decrease pain, increase ROM, and avoid adverse soft tissue responses

Cryotherapy (B-moderate recommendation, Level II)

- Use cryotherapy immediately after ACL reconstruction

Supervised Rehabilitation (B-moderate recommendation, Level II)

- Exercises and education following ACL reconstruction for supervised in-clinic period and home program

Continuous Passive Motion and Early Weight-Bearing (C-weak recommendation, Level III)

- Use continuous passive motion immediately after ACL reconstruction to decrease pain
- Implement early weight-bearing as tolerated within 1 week after ACL reconstruction Knee Bracing
- Use functional knee bracing with ACL deficiency (C-weak recommendation, Level III)
- Elicit patient preferences regarding bracing following ACL reconstruction (D-conflicting evidence, Level IV)
- May use bracing for PCL and severe MCL injuries (F-expert opinion, Level V)

Adapted from Knee Ligament Sprains Revised 2017, Clinical Practice Guidelines, Orthopedic Section, APTA, Summary of Recommendations. *JOSPT;* 11(47): A2–A3, 2017.

Level 1 evidence and Grade A recommendations are highlighted in the table with bold font.

See Table 16-4 in Chapter 16 for Levels of Evidence and Grades of Recommendations.

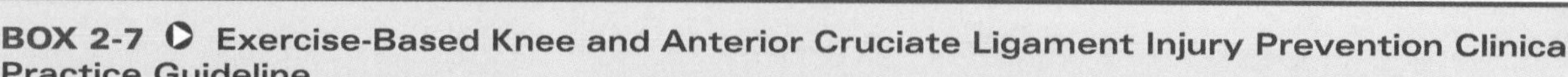

BOX 2-7 Exercise-Based Knee and Anterior Cruciate Ligament Injury Prevention Clinical Practice Guideline

Review Evidence for Prevention Programs

- **Clinicians should recommend use of exercise-based knee injury prevention programs in athletes for prevention knee and anterior cruciate ligament (ACL) injuries (A-strong recommendation, Level I).**

Prevention Program Effectiveness in Subgroups of Athletes

- **To reduce the risk of ACL injuries, female athletes, particularly <18 years of age, should implement knee injury prevention programs prior to training/practice (A-strong recommendation, Level I).**
- **To reduce the risk of severe knee and ACL injuries, soccer players, especially women, should implement knee injury prevention programs (A-strong recommendation, Level I).**
- To reduce the risk of knee injuries, team handball (male and female) players should implement knee injury prevention programs (B-moderate recommendation, Level II).

Evidence for Program Components, Dosage, and Delivery

- **Incorporate multiple components, proximal control exercises, and a combination of strength/plyometric exercises (A-strong recommendation, Level I).**
- **Train multiple times per week, >20 minutes per session, >30 minutes per week (A-strong recommendation, Level I).**
- **Start programs in preseason and continue through the regular season (A-strong recommendation, Level I).**
- **Clinicians, coaches, parents, and athletes ensure high compliance (A-strong recommendation, Level I).**
- May not need balance exercises, and balance should not be the sole component of the program (B-moderate recommendation, Level II).

Provide Suggestions for Program Implementation

- **Implement knee injury prevention programs in all young athletes, not just those identified at risk for ACL injury (A-strong recommendation, Level I).**
- **To reduce future medical costs, implement evidence-based ACL injury prevention programs in athletes 12 to 25 years of age and involved in high-risk sports (A-strong recommendation, Level I).**
- Programs led by either coaches or a group of coaches and medical professionals (B-moderate recommendation, Level II).

Adapted from Exercise-Based Knee and Anterior Cruciate Ligament Injury Prevention, Clinical Practice Guidelines, Orthopedic Section, APTA, Summary of Recommendations. *JOSPT;* 48(9): A1–42, 2018.

Level 1 evidence and Grade A recommendations are highlighted in the table with bold font.

See Table 16-4 for Levels of Evidence and Grades of Recommendations.

b. Symptoms include lateral and/or medial joint pain, effusion, joint popping, knee giving way, limitations in movement, and joint locking.

c. Diagnostic tests utilized: typically MRI (not more sensitive than the clinical exam for diagnosis).

d. Clinical examination for meniscal injuries (see Table 2-18).
   - McMurray's test.
   - Apley's test.

e. Medications.
   - Acetaminophen for pain.
   - NSAIDs for pain and/or inflammation.

f. Physical therapy goals, outcomes, and interventions.
   - Reduction of pain and inflammation utilizing modalities, soft tissue/massage techniques to surrounding muscles, and manual therapy techniques, such as joint oscillations to inhibit pain.
   - Correction of muscle imbalances and biomechanical faults using strengthening, endurance, coordination, and flexibility exercises to gain restoration of normal function.
   - Biomechanical faults caused by joint restrictions should be corrected with joint mobilization to the specific restrictions identified during the examination.
   - Progression to functional training based on patient's occupation and/or recreational goals.

3. Patellofemoral conditions.

   a. Abnormal patella positions.
   - Patella alta.
     - Malalignment in which patella tracks superiorly in femoral intercondylar notch.
     - May result in chronic patellar subluxation; may also be the result of patellar tendon rupture.

BOX 2-8 Meniscal and Articular Cartilage Lesions Clinical Practice Guideline

Differential Diagnosis

- Should consider other diagnoses if impairments are not consistent with Diagnosis/Classification or when the patient's symptoms are not resolving with interventions aimed at normalization of the patient's impairments of body function (C-weak recommendation, Level V)

Examination

Risk Factors

- Cutting and pivoting sports are risk factors for meniscus tears (B-moderate recommendation, Level II)
- Older age and delayed ACL reconstruction are risk factors for future meniscus tear (C-weak recommendation, Level III)

Physical Performance Measures

- Administer appropriate clinical tests such as a single-legged hop to assess pain and function, detect side-to-side asymmetries, determine readiness to return to activities (C-weak recommendation, Level III)

Physical Impairment Measures

- Administer appropriate physical impairment measures to establish baseline and at discharge and other points for all patients with meniscus tears, including the modified stroke test for effusion; active knee ROM; maximum isometric or isokinetic quadriceps strength; McMurray's test and palpation of joint-line tenderness (B-moderate recommendation, Level II)
- Administer appropriate physical impairment measures to establish baseline and at discharge and other points for all patients with articular cartilage lesion, including the modified stroke test for effusion; active knee ROM; maximum isometric or isokinetic quadriceps strength; palpation of joint-line tenderness (D-conflicting evidence, Level-higher quality studies disagree on conclusions)

Outcome Measures; Activity Limitations

- Outcome measures include a general health questionnaire and a validated activity scale for patients with knee pain and mobility impairments before and after interventions. These may include the SF-36 and Knee Quality of Life Questionnaire (C-weak recommendation; Level III)
- Knee-specific outcomes use Knee Injury and Osteoarthritis Outcome Score (KOOS) among others (B-moderate recommendation, Level II)

Diagnosis/Classification

- Diagnosis of a meniscal tear is made with a fair level of certainty when the patient presents with the following findings: twisting injury; tearing sensation at the time of injury; delayed effusion (6–24 hours postinjury); history of "catching" or "locking"; pain with forced hyperextension; pain with maximum flexion; pain or audible click with McMurray's maneuver; joint line tenderness; discomfort or sense of locking or catching in the knee over either the medial or lateral joint line during the Thessaly Test when performed at 5 or 20° of knee flexion (C-weak recommendation, Level II)
- Diagnosis of articular cartilage defect is made with a low level of certainty when the patient presents with the following clinical findings: acute trauma with hemarthrosis (0–2 hours) (associated with osteochondral fracture); insidious onset aggravated by repetitive impact; intermittent pain and swelling; history of "catching" or "locking"; joint line tenderness (C-weak recommendation, Level V)

Interventions

Progressive Knee Motion (B-moderate recommendation, Level II)

- Early, progressive active knee motion following meniscal or cartilage surgery

Supervised Rehabilitation (B-moderate recommendation, Level II)

- Supervised clinic and home-based exercise programs following arthroscopic meniscectomy

Therapeutic Exercises (B-moderate recommendation, Level II)

- Supervised, progressive ROM exercises; strength training for knee and hip muscles and neuromuscular training for meniscal and articular cartilage lesions or following surgery

Neuromuscular Electrical Stimulation (NMES) (B-moderate recommendation, Level II)

- NMES can be used to increase quadriceps strength, functional performance, and knee function following meniscal procedures

(Continued)

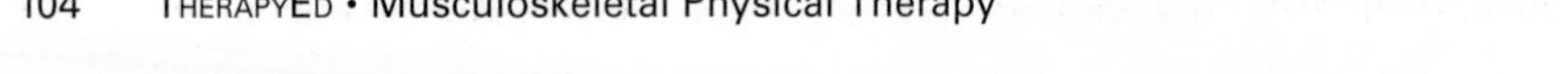

BOX 2-8 Meniscal and Articular Cartilage Lesions Clinical Practice Guideline (Continued)

Progressive Weight-Bearing

- Early progressive weight-bearing following meniscal repairs (C-weak recommendation, Level III)
- Stepwise progression of weight-bearing following articular cartilage surgery to reach full weight-bearing at 6 to 8 weeks (B-moderate recommendation, Level II)

Progressive Return to Activity

- Early, progressive return to activity following meniscal repair surgery (C-weak recommendation, Level III)
- Delayed return to activity following articular cartilage surgery (E-theoretical/foundational, Level V)

Note that these guidelines are aimed primarily at postsurgical care.

Adapted from Knee Pain and Mobility Impairments: Meniscal and Articular Cartilage Lesions Revised, Orthopedic Section, APTA, Summary of Recommendations. *JOSPT;* 48: A2, 2018.

Level 1 evidence and Grade A recommendations are highlighted in the table with bold font.

See Table 16-4 in Chapter 16 for Levels of Evidence and Grades of Recommendations

Chapter 2 MS

  - Positive camel back sign (two bumps over anterior knee region instead of typical one). Two bumps, since patella rides high within femoral condyles, creating a superior bump with tibial tuberosity forming second bump inferiorly.
- Patella baja.
  - Malalignment in which patella tracks inferiorly in femoral intercondylar notch.
  - Results in restricted knee extension with abnormal cartilaginous wear, resulting in DJD; may also be the result of quadriceps tendon rupture.
- Diagnostic tests utilized: plain film imaging including "sunrise" view.
- Physical therapy goals, outcomes, and interventions.
  - Regaining functional strength of the lower extremity, including quadriceps and gluteal musculature; regain normal flexibility of the quadriceps, hamstrings, and gluteal muscles; orthoses (if appropriate); and patellar taping/bracing.

b. Patellofemoral pain syndrome (PFPS; see Box 2-9).
- Common dysfunction that is the result of elevated patellofemoral joint loading caused by trauma, biomechanical factors, and/or muscle tightness and weakness.
- May be associated with patellar tendinopathy and/or chondromalacia patellae. Differentiate from infrapatellar bursitis and/or fat pad syndrome (Hoffa's syndrome).
- Medications.
  - Acetaminophen for pain.
  - NSAIDs for pain and/or inflammation.
- Physical therapy goals, outcomes, and interventions (see Box 2-9).

c. Patellar tendonosis/tendonopathy ("jumper's knee").
- This is a degenerative condition of the patellar tendon, typically of the deep aspect of the tendon.
- May be related to overload and/or jumping-related activities/sports.
- May also be interrelated to patellofemoral dysfunction.
- Diagnosis made by clinical examination.
- Medications.
  - Acetaminophen for pain.
  - NSAIDs for pain and/or inflammation.
  - Corticosteroid injection or by mouth.
- Physical therapy goals, outcomes, and interventions.
  - Refer to intervention for general tendonosis/tendonopathy.

4. Pes anserine bursitis.
   a. Typically caused by overuse or a contusion.
   b. Must be differentiated from tendonitis.
   c. Diagnosis made by clinical examination. Differentiate from contractile condition by comparing results of AROM, PROM, and resistive tests.
   d. Medications.
   - Acetaminophen for pain.
   - NSAIDs for pain and/or inflammation.
   - Corticosteroid injection or by mouth.
   e. Physical therapy goals, outcomes, and interventions.
5. Fractures involving knee joint.
   a. Femoral condyle.
   - Medial femoral most often involved due to its anatomical design.
   - Numerous etiological factors include trauma, shearing, impacting, and avulsion forces.
   - Common mechanism of injury is a fall, with knee subjected to a shearing force.

BOX 2-9 Patellofemoral Pain Clinical Practice Guidelines

Diagnosis

Should use reproduction of retropatellar or peripatellar pain with squatting and other functional activities that load the patellofemoral joint (PFJ) in flexed positions as diagnostic tests (A-strong recommendation, Level I).

Should diagnose PFP with the following criteria (B-moderate recommendation, Level II):

- Presence of retropatellar or peripatellar pain
- Reproduction of pain with squatting, stair climbing, prolonged sitting, or other functional activities that load the PFJ in a flexed position
- Exclusion of all other conditions that may cause anterior knee pain

May use the patellar tilt test to support diagnosis of PFP (C-weak recommendation, Level III).

Classification

Four subcategories based on predominant impairments present (F-expert opinion, Level V).

- Overuse/overload without other impairment: increase in frequency/intensity/duration of loading that surpasses ability to recover
- Muscle performance deficits: impaired hip or knee muscle performance
- Movement coordination deficits: excessive or poorly controlled knee valgus during dynamic tasks
- Mobility impairments: foot hypermobility and/or flexibility deficits in the hamstrings, quadriceps, gastrocnemius, soleus, lateral retinaculum, or iliotibial band

Examination

Outcome measures (A-strong recommendation, Level I).

- **Should use Anterior Knee Pain Scale (AKPS), patellofemoral pain and osteoarthritis subscale of the Knee Injury and Osteoarthritis Outcome Score (KOOS-PF), or the visual analog scale (VAS) for activity to measure pain and function. Should use VAS for worst pain, VAS for usual pain, or Numeric Pain-Rating Scale (NPRS) to measure pain.**

Activity limitations/physical performance measures: should administer clinical or field tests that reproduce pain and assess lower extremity movement coordination, such as squatting, step-downs, and single leg squats (B-moderate recommendation, Level II).

Activity limitations/physical impairment measures: may assess patellar provocation, patellar mobility, foot position, hip and thigh muscle strength, and muscle length (C-weak recommendation, Level III).

Interventions

Combined interventions (A-strong recommendation, Level I).

- **Should combine PT interventions with exercise as the critical component**
- **Should consider addition of foot orthoses, patellar taping, patellar mobilizations, and lower extremity stretching**

Specific modes of exercise therapy (A-strong recommendation, Level I).

- **Should include both hip and knee exercises.**
- **Hip exercises should target posterolateral hip muscles.**
- **Knee exercises may include weight-bearing or non-weight-bearing exercises.**

Patellar taping: may use tailored patellar taping in combination with exercise therapy (B-moderate recommendation, Level II).

Patellofemoral knee orthoses (bracing): should not prescribe patellofemoral knee orthoses (B-moderate recommendation, Level II).

Foot orthoses: should prescribe prefabricated foot orthoses for patients with greater than normal pronation, only for the short-term (up to 6 weeks) (A-strong recommendation, Level I).

Should not use visual biofeedback on lower extremity (B-moderate recommendation, Level II).

Running gait retraining (B-moderate recommendation, Level II).

- May use gait retraining consisting of multiple sessions of cuing to adopt a forefoot-strike pattern (for rearfoot strike runners)

(Continued)

BOX 2-9 Patellofemoral Pain Clinical Practice Guidelines (Continued)

- May use cuing to increase running cadence
- May use cuing to reduce peak hip adduction while running

Blood flow restriction training plus high-repetition knee-targeted exercises: may use blood flow restriction plus high-repetition knee exercises for those with limiting painful resisted knee extension (F-expert opinion, Level V).

Needling Therapies

- **Should not use dry needling (A-strong recommendation, Level I)**
- May use acupuncture to reduce pain (C-weak recommendation, Level III)

Manual therapy as a stand-alone treatment: should not use manual therapy, including lumbar, knee, or patellofemoral manipulation/mobilization (A-strong recommendation, Level I).

Should not use biophysical agents, including ultrasound, cryotherapy, iontophoresis, electrical stimulation, and therapeutic laser (B-moderate recommendation, Level II).

May include specific patient education on load management, body-weight management, when appropriate, and the importance of adherence to active treatments (F-expert opinion, Level V).

Adapted from Patellofemoral Pain, Clinical Practice Guidelines, Orthopedic Section, APTA, Summary of Recommendations. *JOSPT;* 9(49): CPG1-CPG95, 2019.

Level 1 evidence and Grade A recommendations are highlighted in the table with bold font.

See Table 16-4 in Chapter 16 for levels of evidence and grades of recommendation.

b. Tibial plateau.
- Common mechanism of injury is a combination of valgum and compression forces to knee when knee is in a flexed position.
- Often occurs in conjunction with a medial collateral ligamentous injury.

c. Epiphyseal plate.
- Mechanism of injury is frequently a weight-bearing torsional stress.
- Presents more frequently in adolescents where an ACL injury would occur in an adult.

d. Patella.
- Most common mechanism of injury is a direct blow to patella due to a fall.

e. Plain film imaging most likely unless complex fracture, which requires CT (see Box 2-10).

f. Medications.
- Acetaminophen for pain.
- NSAIDs for pain and/or inflammation.

g. Physical therapy goals, outcomes, and interventions.
- Physical therapy intervention emphasizes return of function without pain.

Conditions of the Lower Leg

1. Acute compartment syndrome.
   a. Elevated compartment (anterior, lateral, posterior) pressure that results in local ischemic condition.
   b. Usually the result of direct trauma and/or fracture.
   c. Six "P's" of compartment syndromes.
   - Pain.
   - Palpable tenderness.
   - Paresthesia.
   - Paresis.
   - Pallor.
   - Pulselessness.

   d. Diagnosis made by clinical examination; compartment pressure testing after exercise may confirm the diagnosis.

RED FLAG: Acute compartment syndromes are medical emergencies that may require immediate surgical intervention (fasciotomy) to relieve the pressure on the muscles and neurovascular contents of the compartment.

2. Chronic exertional compartment syndrome.
   a. Result of elevated compartment (anterior, lateral, posterior) pressure that restricts blood flow to muscles.
   b. Symptoms depend on the compartment involved; anterior is most common with resulting pain in the anterolateral leg region but may also present with paresthesia.
   c. Diagnosis made by clinical examination; compartment pressure testing after exercise may confirm the diagnosis.
   d. Physical therapy goals, outcomes, and interventions.
   - Reduction in loading with a gradual return to activity; may require orthoses, change in footwear, or change in training surface.
   - Run retraining to a nonrearfoot strike may decrease forces in the anterior compartment.
   - Functional training and resistance training exercises to improve strength, endurance, proprioception, coordination, and flexibility.

BOX 2-10 Ottawa Knee Rules

A knee x-ray series is only required for patients with knee injury and who have any of the following:

- Age 55 years or older, *or*
- Isolated patellar tenderness without other bone tenderness, *or*
- Tenderness of the fibular head, *or*
- Inability to flex knee to 90°, *or*
- Inability to bear weight immediately after injury and in the emergency department.

To apply the Ottawa Knee Rules accurately:

- Test is designed to rule out fractures after acute knee injury.
- Advised to order radiography with one or more positive answers.
- Negative rest results are considered highly diagnostic of the absence of fracture.

Adapted from: Bachmann LM, Haberzeth S, Steurer J, ter Riet G. The accuracy of the Ottawa Knee Rules to rule out knee fractures: a systematic review. *Ann Intern Med.* 2004; 140: 121–124.

3. Medial tibial stress syndrome.
   a. Overuse injury of the posterior tibialis and/or the medial soleus, resulting in periosteal inflammation at the muscular attachments.
   b. Etiology is thought to be excessive pronation.
   c. Pain elicited with palpation of the distal posteromedial border of the tibia.
   d. Diagnosis made by clinical examination.
   e. Medications.
      - Acetaminophen for pain.
      - NSAIDs for pain and/or inflammation.
   f. Physical therapy goals, outcomes, and interventions.
      - Correction of muscle imbalances and biomechanical faults using strengthening, endurance, and coordination exercises.
      - Flexibility exercises for anterior compartment muscles as well as the triceps surae to gain restoration of normal function.
4. Stress fractures.
   a. Overuse injury resulting most often in microfracture of the tibia or fibula.
   b. 49% of all stress fractures involve the tibia, and 10% involve the fibula.
   c. Three common etiologies: abnormal biomechanical alignment, poor conditioning, and improper training methods.
   d. Diagnostic tests utilized: plain film imaging, bone scan, MRI.
   e. Medications.
      - Acetaminophen for pain.
      - NSAIDs for pain and/or inflammation.
   f. Physical therapy goals, outcomes, and interventions.
      - Correction of muscle imbalances and biomechanical faults using strengthening, endurance, and coordination exercises.
      - Flexibility exercises for anterior compartment muscles as well as the triceps surae to gain restoration of normal function.

Foot and Ankle Conditions

1. Ligament sprains (see Box 2-11).
   a. 95% of all ankle sprains involve lateral ligaments.
   b. The most common grading system is as follows:
      - Grade I: no loss of function, with minimal tearing of the anterior talofibular ligament.
      - Grade II: some loss of function, with partial disruption of the anterior talofibular and calcaneofibular ligaments.
      - Grade III: complete loss of function, with complete tearing of the anterior talofibular and calcaneofibular ligaments, with partial tear of the posterior talofibular ligament.
   c. Diagnostic tests utilized: plain film imaging (see Box 2-12).
   d. Instability is evaluated using anterior drawer and talar tilt special tests.
   e. Medications.
      - Acetaminophen for pain.
      - NSAIDs for pain and/or inflammation.
   f. Physical therapy goals, outcomes, and interventions.
      - Physical therapy intervention is varied, depending on whether the patient undergoes a surgical procedure as well as type of surgery that is performed.
      - Reduction of pain and inflammation utilizing modalities, soft tissue techniques, and manual therapy techniques, such as oscillations.
      - Correction of muscle imbalances and biomechanical faults using strengthening, endurance, coordination, and flexibility exercises to gain restoration of normal function.

BOX 2-11 Ankle Ligament Sprains Clinical Practice Guideline

Diagnosis/Classification

Acute lateral ankle sprain (LAS) (B-moderate recommendation, Level II)

- Evaluation should include: age, BMI, pain coping strategies, report of instability, history of previous sprain, ability to bear weight, pain with weight-bearing, ankle dorsiflexion range of motion, medial joint line tenderness, balance, and jumping ability.
- Use special tests, such as reverse anterolateral drawer test, anterolateral talar palpation, and traditional anterior drawer test, with a thorough history and physical examination to aid in diagnosis.

Chronic ankle instability (CAI) (B-moderate recommendation, Level II)

- Evaluation may include: previous treatment, number of sprains, pain level, self-report function, sensorimotor movement system assessment.
- To assist with diagnosis, use valid/reliable discriminative instruments (Cumberland Ankle Instability Tool or Identification of Functional Ankle Instability) and a battery of functional performance tests.

Examination

Patient-reported Outcome Measures (A-strong recommendation, Level I)

- **Use valid/reliable measures: PROMIS physical function and pain interference, Foot and Ankle Ability Measure (FAAM), and Lower Extremity Functional Scale (LEFS).**
- **Utilize at baseline and at least 1 follow-up.**

Physical Impairment Measures (A-strong recommendation, Level I)

- **Include objective measures of ankle swelling; ROM; talar translation and inversion, and single-leg balance.**
- **Specifically include: weight-bearing lunge test, static single leg balance on firm surface with eyes closed, dynamic balance the Star Excursion Balance Test.**

Physical Performance Measures (B-moderate recommendation, Level II)

- Use valid/reliable measures at baseline and 2 or more follow-up periods.
- Specifically include: single leg hopping under timed conditions.

Interventions

Acute Lateral Ankle Sprain (A-strong recommendation, Level I)

- **For primary prevention, should prescribe prophylactic bracing, particularly with risk factors.**
- **For secondary prevention, should prescribe prophylactic bracing and use proprioception/balance training.**
- **Should advise patients on external support (brace/tape) and progressive weight-bearing.**
- **For severe injuries, may immobilize for up to 10 days postinjury.**
- **Should implement structured therapeutic exercise program that includes protected active ROM, stretching, neuromuscular training, postural reeducation and balance training, both in the clinic and at home.**
- **Should use manual therapy (lymphatic drainage, soft tissue mobilization, and joint mobilization) in conjunction with exercise to reduce swelling, improve mobility, and normalize gait.**
- **Should NOT use ultrasound.**

Chronic Ankle Instability (A-strong recommendation, Level I)

- **Should prescribe proprioceptive and neuromuscular therapeutic exercise to improve dynamic postural stability and patient perceived stability.**
- **Should use manual therapy (grade joint mobilizations, manipulations, and mobilizations with movement) to improve weight-bearing dorsiflexion and dynamic balance in the short-term.**

Grade=recommendation strength; Level=Level of Evidence

Level 1 evidence and Grade A recommendations are highlighted in the table with bold font.

See Table 16-4 in Chapter 16 for Levels of Evidence and Grades of Recommendations

Adapted from Ankle Stability and Movement Coordination Impairments: Ankle Ligament Sprains Revision 2021, Orthopedic Section, APTA, Summary of Recommendations.

JOSPT; (4)51: CPG1-54., 2021.

BOX 2-12 Ottawa Ankle and Foot Rules

An ankle x-ray series is only required if there is any pain in the malleolar zone and any of these findings:
1. Bone tenderness from the posterior edge or tip of the lateral malleolus extending 6 cm proximally, *or*
2. Bone tenderness from the posterior edge or tip of the medial malleolus extending 6 cm proximally, *or*
3. Inability to take 4 complete steps both immediately and in the emergency department.

A foot x-ray series is only required if there is any pain in the midfoot zone and any of these findings:
1. Bone tenderness at the base of the fifth metatarsal, *or*
2. Bone tenderness of the navicular, *or*
3. Inability to take four complete steps both immediately and in the emergency department.

To apply the Ottawa Ankle Rules accurately:
- Palpate the entire distal 6 cm of the fibula and tibia.
- Do not neglect the importance of medial malleolar tenderness.
- Do not use for patients under 18 years of age.

Adapted from Stiell IG, McKnight RD, Greenberg GH, et al. Implementation of the Ottawa Ankle Rules. *JAMA.* 1994; 271: 827–832.

- Biomechanical faults caused by joint restrictions should be corrected with joint mobilization to the specific restrictions identified during the examination.
- Progression to functional training based on patient's occupation and/or recreational goals.

2. Achilles tendinosis/tendinopathy (see Box 2-13).
   a. This is a degenerative condition of the Achilles' tendon.
   b. Clinical examination including Thompson's test helps to identify this condition.
   c. Medications.
      - Acetaminophen for pain.
      - NSAIDs for pain and/or inflammation.
      - Corticosteroid injection or by mouth.
   d. Physical therapy goals, outcomes, and interventions.
      - Refer to intervention for general bursitis/tendonitis/tendonosis.
3. Fractures of the foot and ankle (see Box 2-12).
   a. Unimalleolar involves the medial or lateral malleolus.
   b. Bimalleolar involves the medial and lateral malleoli.
   c. Trimalleolar involves the medial and lateral malleoli, and the posterior tubercle of the distal tibia.
   d. Diagnostic tests utilized: plain film imaging.
      - Growth plate fractures are a concern, since bone growth can be affected. Types III and IV fractures, according to the Salter Harris classification, are of most concern and can have a high complication rate (see Table 2-31).
   e. Medications.
      - Acetaminophen for pain.
      - NSAIDs for pain and/or inflammation.
   f. Physical therapy goals, outcomes, and interventions.
      - Physical therapy intervention emphasizes return of function without pain.
      - Functional training and restoration of muscle imbalances using exercise to normalize strength, endurance, coordination, and flexibility.
      - Early PROM is important in preventing capsular adhesions.
4. Tarsal tunnel syndrome.
   a. Entrapment of the posterior tibial nerve or one of its branches within the tarsal tunnel.
   b. Over/excessive pronation, overuse problems resulting in tendonitis of the long flexor and posterior tibialis tendon, and trauma may compromise space in the tarsal tunnel.
   c. Symptoms include pain, numbness, and paresthesias along the medial ankle to the plantar surface of the foot.
   d. Diagnostic tests utilized: electrodiagnostic tests.
   e. Positive Tinel's sign at the tarsal tunnel.
   f. Medications.
      - Acetaminophen for pain.
      - NSAIDs for pain and/or inflammation.
      - Neurontin for neuropathic pain.
   g. Physical therapy goals, outcomes, and interventions.
      - Intervention includes the use of orthoses to maintain neutral alignment of the foot.
      - If abnormal neurotension is present, neurodynamic mobilization may be indicated.
5. Flexor hallucis tendonopathy.
   a. Identified as a tendonitis in the acute stage, or can present as a chronic tendonosis. Commonly seen in ballet performers.

BOX 2-13 Achilles' Tendinopathy Clinical Practice Guideline

Differential Diagnosis

- Consider other diagnoses when activity limitations or function are not consistent with Diagnosis/Classification or symptoms do not resolve with interventions (F-expert opinion, Level V)

Examination

Risk Factors (B-moderate recommendation, Level II)

- Abnormal ankle dorsiflexion and subtalar ROM, decreased plantar flexion strength, increased foot pronation
- Obesity, hypertension, hyperlipidemia, and diabetes
- Faulty equipment, training errors, and environmental factors

Activity Limitation Measures (B-moderate recommendation, Level II)

- Include objective and reproducible assessment of ability to walk, descend stairs, perform unilateral heel raises, and single limb hop

Physical Impairment Measures (B-moderate recommendation, Level II)

- Include measuring dorsiflexion and subtalar ROM, plantar flexion strength, static arch height, forefoot alignment, endurance, and pain on palpation over the episode of care

Outcome and Physical Performance Measures

- **Use the Victorian Institute of Sport Assessment-Achilles (VISA-A) to assess pain and stiffness (A-strong recommendation, Level I)**
- **Use the Foot and Ankle Ability Measure (FAAM) or the Lower Extremity Functional Scale (LEFS) to assess activity and participation (A-strong recommendation, Level I)**
- Include hop tests and heel raise endurance tests, as appropriate (B-moderate recommendation, Level II)

Diagnosis/Classification

- Pain located 2–6 cm proximal to Achilles tendon insertion that began gradually (C-weak recommendation, Level III)
- Positive arc sign and Royal London Hospital test (C-weak recommendation, Level III)

Interventions

- **Use mechanical loading (eccentric or heavy-load, slow velocity) exercise to decrease pain and increase function (A-strong recommendation, Level I)**
- Educate patient that complete rest is not indicated; continue with activity within pain tolerance while participating in rehabilitation (B-moderate recommendation, Level II)
- Dexamethasone iontophoresis to decrease pain and improve function (B-moderate recommendation, Level II)
- Stretching to reduce pain and improve function with those that have limited dorsiflexion ROM (C-weak recommendation, Level III)
- Soft tissue and joint mobilization may reduce pain and increase mobility (F-expert opinion, Level V)
- May use rigid tape to decrease stress on Achilles' tendon; should not use therapeutic elastic tape (F-expert opinion, Level V)
- Contradictory evidence exists on use of heel lifts and low-level laser to decrease pain and stiffness (D-contradictory evidence, Level IV)
- Contradictory evidence exists for the use of foot orthosis (D-contradictory evidence, Level IV)
- Night splints are not beneficial in reducing pain when compared with eccentric exercise (C-weak evidence, Level III)

Adapted from Achilles' Tendinopathy, Clinical Practice Guidelines, Orthopedic Section, APTA, Summary of Recommendations. *JOSPT;* 48(5): A1–38, 2018.

Level 1 evidence and Grade A recommendations are highlighted in the table with bold font.

See Table 16-4 in Chapter 16 for Levels of Evidence and Grades of Recommendations.

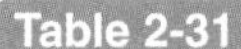

Table 2-31

Salter-Harris Fracture Classification

TYPE	ANATOMICAL DEFORMITY	COMMON CAUSE	GENERAL PROGNOSIS	MEDICAL MANAGEMENT
I	Entire epiphysis	Caused by shearing, torsion, or avulsion forces.	Good, with very few complications to growth of the bone.	Relocated if necessary, and immobilized with cast.
II	Entire epiphysis and portion of the metaphysis	Usually caused by a shear or avulsion with angular force. Most common type.	May cause decreased bone growth, but typically minimal, so limited negative impact on long-term function.	Relocated and immobilized with cast.
III	Portion of the epiphysis	Typically occurs when the growth plate is partially fused. Rare, but most commonly occurs to the distal tibia in adolescents.	This type of fracture may lead to long-term problems secondary to the fracture, crossing the physis and extending into the articular surface of the bone. Even with this potential, the prognosis is typically favorable, since these fractures rarely result in significant deformity.	Relocated and immobilized. Occasionally requires surgical intervention (e.g., ORIF). A specific fracture known as the Tillaux fracture (a Type III fracture of the distal tibia) has a particularly poor prognosis.
IV	Portion of the epiphysis and portion of the metaphysis	Similar to Type III. Most commonly seen in the distal humerus.	Since this fracture interferes with the cartilage growth, it may lead to premature focal fusion of the involved bone causing deformity of the joint.	Generally, surgery (e.g., ORIF) is necessary to restore alignment. Prognosis is correlated to quality of alignment achieved.
V	Nothing "broken off"; compression injury of the epiphyseal plate	This is caused by a compression or crush injury of the epiphyseal plate, with no associated epiphyseal or metaphyseal fracture.	Type V fractures are associated with growth disturbances at the physis, and generally will have a poor functional prognosis.	These are usually found "after the fact," so no immediate intervention is provided. If it is identified acutely, patient is placed on non-weight-bearing protocols.

b. Medications.
   - Acetaminophen for pain.
   - NSAIDs for pain and/or inflammation.
   - Corticosteroid injection or by mouth.

c. Physical therapy goals, outcomes, and interventions.
   - Refer to intervention for general bursitis/tendonitis/tendonosis.

6. Pes cavus (hollow foot).
   a. Numerous etiologies to include genetic predisposition, neurological disorders resulting in muscle imbalances, and contracture of soft tissues.
   b. Deformity observed includes an increased height of longitudinal arches, dropping of anterior arch, metatarsal heads lower than hindfoot, plantar flexion and splaying of forefoot, and claw toes.
   c. Function is limited due to altered arthrokinematics, reducing ability to absorb forces through foot.
   d. Diagnosis made by clinical examination including thorough biomechanical lower quarter exam.
   e. Physical therapy goals, outcomes, and interventions.
      - Intervention includes patient education emphasizing limitation of high-impact sports (e.g., long-distance running and ballet), use of proper footwear, and fitting for orthoses.
7. Equinus.
   a. Etiology can include congenital bone deformity, neurological disorders such as cerebral palsy, contracture of gastrocnemius and/or soleus muscles, trauma, or inflammatory disease.
   b. Deformity observed: plantar flexed foot.
   c. Compensation secondary to limited dorsiflexion includes subtalar or midtarsal pronation.
   d. Diagnosis made by clinical examination, including thorough biomechanical lower quarter exam.
   e. Physical therapy goals, outcomes, and interventions.
      - Physical therapy intervention includes flexibility exercises of shortened structures within foot, joint mobilization to joint restrictions identified in examination, strengthening to intrinsic and extrinsic foot muscles, and orthotic management.
8. Hallux valgus.
   a. Etiology is varied to include biomechanical malalignment (excessive pronation), ligamentous laxity, heredity, weak muscles, and footwear that is too tight.
   b. Deformity observed: a medial deviation of head of first metatarsal from midline of body; metatarsal

and base of proximal first phalanx move medially, while distal phalanx then moves laterally.

c. Normal metatarsophalangeal angle is 8°–20°.

d. Diagnosis made by clinical examination, including thorough biomechanical lower quarter exam.

e. Physical therapy goals, outcomes, and interventions.
   - Early orthotic fitting and patient education.
   - Later management requires surgery, followed by flexibility exercises to restore normal function, strengthening exercises, and possible joint mobilization to identified restrictions.

9. Metatarsalgia.
   a. Etiologies.
      - Mechanical: tight triceps surae group and/or Achilles' tendon, collapse of transverse arch, short first ray, pronation of forefoot.
      - Structural changes in transverse arch, possibly leading to vascular and/or neural compromise in tissues of forefoot.
      - Changes in footwear.
   b. Complaint frequently heard is pain at first and second metatarsal heads after long periods of weight-bearing.
   c. Diagnosis made by clinical examination including thorough biomechanical lower quarter exam.
   d. Medications.
      - Acetaminophen for pain.
      - NSAIDs for pain and/or inflammation.
      - Neurontin for neuropathic pain.
   e. Physical therapy goals, outcomes, and interventions.
      - Intervention includes correction of biomechanical abnormality (improving flexibility of triceps surae), modalities to decrease pain.
      - Prescription and/or creation of orthoses.
      - Patient education regarding selection of footwear.

10. Charcot-Marie-Tooth disease.
   a. Peroneal muscular atrophy that affects motor and sensory nerves.
   b. May begin in childhood or adulthood.
   c. Initially affects muscles in lower leg and foot, but eventually progresses to muscles of hands and forearm.
   d. Slowly progressive disorder with varying degrees of involvement, depending on degree of genetic dominance.
   e. Diagnostic tests utilized: electrodiagnostic tests.
   f. Diagnosis made by clinical examination including thorough biomechanical lower quarter exam.
   g. Medications.
      - Acetaminophen for pain.
      - NSAIDs for pain and/or inflammation.
      - Neurontin for neuropathic pain.
   h. Physical therapy goals, outcomes, and interventions.
      - No specific treatment to prevent, since it is an inherited disorder.
      - Physical therapy intervention centers on preventing contractures/skin breakdown and maximizing patient's functional capacity to perform activities.
      - Patient education and training regarding braces and ambulatory assistive devices.

11. Plantar fasciitis (see Box 2-14).

12. Forefoot/rearfoot deformities.
   a. Rearfoot varus (subtalar varus, calcaneal varus).
      - Etiology: abnormal mechanical alignment of tibia, shortened rearfoot soft tissues, or malunion of calcaneus.
      - Deformity observed: rigid inversion of calcaneus when subtalar joint is in neutral position.
      - Diagnosis made by clinical examination including thorough biomechanical lower quarter exam.

BOX 2-14 Heel Pain-Plantar Fasciitis Clinical Practice Guideline

Examination

Risk Factors (B-moderate recommendation, level II)

- Limited ankle dorsiflexion range of motion, high body mass index in nonathletic individuals, running, and work-related weight-bearing activities (particularly under conditions with poor shock absorption)

Activity Limitation Measures (Expert opinion, Level V)

- Utilize easily reproducible performance-based measures of activity limitation

Outcome Measures (A-strong recommendation, level I)

- **Use outcome measures such as Foot and Ankle Ability Measure (FAAM), Foot Function Index (FFI), and others**

Diagnosis/Classification

- Diagnose plantar fasciitis based on the following clinical findings: plantar medial heel pain after initial steps, pain with palpation of proximal insertion of plantar fascia, positive windlass test, negative tarsal tunnel tests such as Tinel's sign, limited ankle dorsiflexion, high body mass index, work-related weight-bearing with poor shock absorption (B-moderate recommendation, level II)

(Continued)

BOX 2-14 Heel Pain-Plantar Fasciitis Clinical Practice Guideline (Continued)

Interventions

Manual Therapy (A-strong recommendation, level I)

- **Joint and soft tissue mobilization**

Stretching (A-strong recommendation, level I)

- **Should use fascia-specific and gastrocnemius-soleus stretching (1–4 months)**

Taping, Orthoses, and Night Splints (A-strong recommendation, level I)

- **Should use taping (1–3 weeks)**
- **Should use foot orthoses to support medial longitudinal arch and cushion the heel (2 weeks to 1 year)**
- **Should prescribe night splints (1–3 months)**

Physical Agents

- Other therapeutic modalities are not particularly recommended. May use low-level laser (C-weak recommendation, levels II, III, and IV) and phonophoresis (C-weak recommendation, levels II, III, and IV) to reduce pain. Ultrasound and dry needling cannot be recommended

Adapted from Heel Pain, Plantar Fasciitis, Orthopedic Section, APTA, Summary of Recommendations. *JOSPT;* 4(38): A2–A3, 2014.
Level 1 evidence and Grade A recommendations are highlighted in the table with bold font.
See Table 16-4 in Chapter 16 for Levels of Evidence and Grades of Recommendations.

- Physical therapy goals, outcomes, and interventions.
  - Regaining proper mechanical alignment.
  - Improving flexibility of shortened soft tissues.
  - Orthotic fitting and patient education regarding selection of footwear.

b. Rearfoot valgus.
- Etiology: abnormal mechanical alignment of the knee (genu valgum), or tibial valgus.
- Deformity observed: eversion of calcaneus with a neutral subtalar joint.
- Due to increased mobility of hindfoot, fewer musculoskeletal problems develop from this deformity than with rearfoot varus.
- Diagnosis made by clinical examination, including thorough biomechanical lower quarter exam.
- Physical therapy goals, outcomes, and interventions.
  - Regaining proper mechanical alignment.
  - Improving flexibility of shortened soft tissues.
  - Orthotic fitting and patient education regarding selection of footwear.

c. Forefoot varus.
- Etiology: congenital abnormal deviation of head and neck of talus.
- Deformity observed: inversion of forefoot when subtalar joint is in neutral.
- Diagnosis made by clinical examination, including thorough biomechanical lower quarter exam.
- Physical therapy goals, outcomes, and interventions.
  - Regaining proper mechanical alignment.
  - Improving flexibility of shortened soft tissues.
  - Orthotic fitting and patient education regarding selection of footwear.

d. Forefoot valgus.
- Etiology: congenital abnormal development of head and neck of talus.
- Deformity observed: eversion of forefoot when the subtalar joint is in neutral.
- Diagnosis made by clinical examination, including thorough biomechanical lower quarter exam.
- Physical therapy goals, outcomes, and interventions.
  - Regaining proper mechanical alignment.
  - Improving flexibility of shortened soft tissues.
  - Orthotic fitting and patient education regarding selection of footwear.

Spinal Conditions (See Boxes 2-15 and 2-16)

Muscle Strain

1. May be related to sudden trauma, chronic or sustained overload, or abnormal muscle biomechanics secondary to faulty function (abnormal joint or muscle biomechanics).
2. Commonly will resolve without intervention, but if trauma is too great or if related to chronic etiology, patient will benefit from intervention.
3. Diagnosis made by clinical examination through comparing results of flexibility (AROM/PROM), resistive tests, and palpation.
4. Physical therapy goals, outcomes, and interventions.
   a. Biomechanical faults caused by joint restrictions should be corrected with joint mobilization.

BOX 2-15 Neck Pain Clinical Practice Guideline

Differential Diagnosis (A-strong recommendation, Level I)

- **Determine appropriateness of physical therapy and need for referral by performing assessments and utilizing existing imaging studies to determine presence of serious pathology (fracture, unexplained cranial nerve dysfunction, cancer, ligamentous instability, arterial insufficiency, infection)**

Examination

- **Risk factors: female gender and prior history of neck pain are the strongest and most consistent risk factors. Older age, high job demands, smoking history, low social/work support, and prior history of low back pain may also be risk factors (A-strong recommendation, Level I)**
- **Use validated outcome measures (e.g., Neck Disability Index, Patient Specific Functional Scale) for neck pain relative to pain, function and psychosocial matters to establish baseline (A-strong recommendation, Level I)**
- Assess physical impairments to establish baselines, monitor changes over time and guide clinical decision making. For neck pain with mobility deficits include cervical active ROM, cervical flexion-rotation test, and thoracic segment mobility. For neck pain with headache add or include upper cervical mobility testing. For neck pain with radiating pain add or include neurodynamic testing, Spurling's test, distraction test, and Valsalva test. For neck pain with movement coordination impairment add or include neck flexor muscle endurance tests (B-moderate recommendation, Level II)

Diagnostic Classification

- Determine if acute, subacute, or chronic and consider other factors, such as biopsychosocial elements and tissue irritability, in deciding treatment types and dosage
- Use motion limitations, headache, trauma history, and referred or radiating pain to classify the neck pain into categories (C-weak recommendation, Level III)
  - Neck pain with mobility deficits
  - Neck pain with movement coordination impairments (including whiplash associated disorder (WAD)
  - Neck pain with headache of cervicogenic origin
  - Neck pain with radiating pain

Interventions: Neck Pain with Mobility Deficits

- Acute: thoracic manipulation, neck ROM, home ROM exercise, scapulothoracic and upper extremity stretching and strengthening (B-moderate recommendation, Level II)
- Acute: cervical mobilization/manipulation (C-weak recommendation, Level III)
- Subacute: neck and shoulder girdle endurance (B-moderate recommendation, Level II)
- Subacute: thoracic manipulation, cervical mobilization/manipulation (C-weak recommendation, Level III)
- Chronic: thoracic manipulation and cervical mobilization/manipulation, neuromuscular types of exercises (coordination, proprioception, etc.); stretching, strengthening, endurance, aerobic conditioning, cognitive; dry needling, intermittent traction (B-moderate recommendation, Level II)
- Chronic: advice to remain active, endurance exercises for trunk, shoulder, and neck that promote active lifestyle and address any cognitive or affective disorders (C-weak recommendation, Level III)

Interventions: Neck Pain with Movement Coordination Impairments (Including WAD)

- Acute: advice to remain active, education to return to preaccident activities as soon as possible; minimize use of a cervical collar; perform postural and mobility exercises to decrease pain and increase ROM; reassurances that recovery will occur within first 2 to 3 months, multimodal interventions including mobilization; strengthening; endurance; flexibility; postural; aerobic for those patients predicted to have a moderate to slow recovery (B-moderate recommendation, Level II)
- Acute: transcutaneous electrical nerve stimulation (C weak recommendation, Level III)
- Chronic: patient education; mobilization; submaximal exercise program including strengthening, flexibility, endurance, and coordination using principles of cognitive behavioral therapy, transcutaneous electrical nerve stimulation (C-weak recommendation, Level III)

Interventions: Neck Pain with Headache

- Acute: supervised active mobility exercises (B-moderate recommendation, Level II)
- Acute: C1–2 self-sustained natural apophyseal glide (self-SNAG) (C-weak recommendation, Level III)

(Continued)

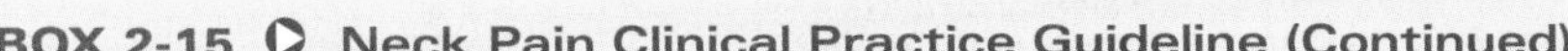

BOX 2-15 Neck Pain Clinical Practice Guideline (Continued)

- Subacute: cervical mobilization/manipulation (B-moderate recommendation, Level II)
- Subacute: C1–2 self-SNAG (C-weak recommendation, Level III)
- Chronic: cervical or thoracic mobilization/manipulation, shoulder girdle and neck stretching, endurance and strengthening (B-moderate recommendation, Level II)

Interventions: Neck Pain with Radiating Pain

- Acute: mobilizing and stabilizing exercises; low-level laser, possible short-term use of a cervical collar (C-weak recommendation, Level III)
- Chronic: stretching, strengthening, cervical/thoracic mobilization/manipulation, education and counseling to participate in activities and movement, mechanical intermittent cervical traction (B-moderate recommendation, Level II)

Adapted from Neck Pain: Revision 2017, Orthopedic Section, APTA, Summary of Recommendations. *JOSPT*; 7(47): A2–A3, 2017.
Level 1 evidence and Grade A recommendations are highlighted in the table with bold font.
See Table 16-4 in Chapter 16 for Levels of Evidence and Grades of Recommendations.

BOX 2-16 Low Back Pain Clinical Practice Guideline

Differential Diagnosis

- **Consider serious medical conditions or psychosocial factors and refer to an appropriate medical practitioner, if activity limitations or body structure are not consistent with low back pain diagnosis/classifications, or if symptoms are not resolving with interventions (A-strong recommendation, Level I)**

Examination

Risk Factors

- Multifactorial, population specific, and only weakly associated with the development of low back pain; two categories of suspected risk factors for low back pain are individual and activity-related (work and leisure) factors (B-moderate recommendation, Level II)

Outcome Measures

- **Should use validated self-report questionnaires (e.g., Oswestry Disability Index) to establish baseline and on-going status relative to pain, function, and disability (A-strong recommendation, Level I)**

Activity Limitation Measures

- Should routinely assess activity limitation using validated performance-based measures throughout the episode of care (F-expert opinion, Level V)

Diagnostic Classification

- Determine clinical course of low back pain as acute, subacute, recurrent, or chronic
- If no signs/symptoms of serious medical or psychological conditions, should classify based on associated findings (B-moderate recommendation, Level II):
  - Mobility impairments in thoracic, lumbar, or sacroiliac regions
  - Referred or radiating pain to a lower extremity
  - Generalized low back pain

Interventions

Clinical Course (E-theoretical/foundational, Level V)

- Should place emphasis on interventions that prevent recurrences or transition from acute and subacute to chronic low back pain

Manual Therapy (A-strong recommendation, Level I)

- **Thrust manipulation to reduce pain with acute low back and back-related buttock or thigh pain**

(*Continued*)

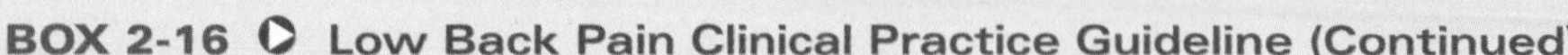

BOX 2-16 Low Back Pain Clinical Practice Guideline (Continued)

- **Thrust and nonthrust mobilization to reduce pain and improve spine and hip mobility with subacute and chronic low back involvement**

Trunk Coordination, Endurance, and Strengthening Exercises (A-strong recommendation, Level I)

- **Trunk coordination, endurance and strengthening exercises with subacute and chronic low back pain and post-lumbar micro-discectomy**

Centralization Procedures (A-strong recommendation, Level I)

- **Repeated movements, exercises or procedures to promote reductions of symptoms with acute low back pain with related lower extremity pain**
- **Repeated exercises in a specific direction (determined by response) to improve mobility and reduce symptoms with acute, subacute, or chronic low back pain**

Flexion Exercises (C-weak recommendation, Level III)

- Flexion exercises in older patients with chronic low back pain with radiation combined with manual therapy, strengthening, nerve mobilization, and progressive walking

Lower-Quarter Nerve Mobilization (C-weak recommendation, Level III)

- Lower-quarter nerve mobilization with subacute and chronic low back pain with accompanying radiating pain

Traction (D-conflicting evidence, Level IV)

- There is conflicting evidence for use of intermittent lumbar traction
- A subgroup of patients may benefit from prone traction if there are signs of nerve root compression or a positive crossed straight leg raise
- Should NOT use traction with acute or subacute nonradicular pain or at any time with chronic low back pain

Patient Education and Counseling (B-moderate recommendation, Level II)

- Emphasize neuroscience that explains pain perception, anatomy of the spine and musculature, overall favorable prognosis of low back pain, use of active pain coping strategies, and early resumption of activities or work even if experiencing some pain
- Should NOT promote extended bed rest or in-depth pathoanatomical explanations of low back pain

Progressive Endurance and Fitness (A-strong recommendation, Level I)

- **Moderate- to high-intensity exercise for chronic low back pain without generalized pain**
- **Progressive, low-intensity, submaximal fitness, and endurance activities with chronic low back pain with generalized pain**

Adapted from Low Back Pain, Orthopedic Section, APTA, Summary of Recommendations. *JOSPT;* 4(42): A44–A46, 2012.

Level 1 evidence and Grade A recommendations are highlighted in the table with bold font.

See Table 16-4 in Chapter 16 for Levels of Evidence and Grades of Recommendations.

b. Patient education regarding the elimination of harmful positions and postural reeducation.
c. Spinal manipulation for pain inhibition is generally indicated for this condition.

Spinal or Intervertebral Stenosis (See Table 2-26)

1. Etiology: congenital narrow spinal canal or intervertebral foramen, coupled with hypertrophy of the spinal lamina and ligamentum flavum or facets, as the result of age-related degenerative processes or disease.
2. Results in vascular and/or neural compromise.
3. Signs and symptoms (see Table 2-8).
   a. Bilateral pain and paresthesia in back, buttocks, thighs, calves, and feet.
   b. Pain decreases in spinal flexion, increases in extension.
   c. Pain increases with walking.
   d. Pain relieved with prolonged rest or activity modification, such as leaning on a shopping cart.
4. Diagnostic tests utilized: imaging including plain films, MRI, and/or CT scan. Occasionally, myelography is helpful.
5. Clinical examination, including bicycle (van Gelderen's test), helps identify this condition and differentiate it from intermittent claudication. The two-stage treadmill test may also be performed.
6. Medications.
   a. Acetaminophen for pain.
   b. NSAIDs for pain and/or inflammation.
   c. Corticosteroid injection or by mouth.
   d. Muscle relaxants.
   e. Trigger point injections.
7. Physical therapy goals, outcomes, and interventions.
   a. Biomechanical faults caused by joint restrictions should be corrected with joint mobilization to the specific restrictions identified during the examination.

b. Perform flexion-based exercise and exercises that promote dynamic stability throughout the trunk and pelvis.
c. Avoid extension and/or other positions that narrow the spinal canal or intervertebral foramen (i.e., extension, ipsilateral side-bending, and ipsilateral rotation).
d. Manual and/or mechanical traction.
   - Traction.
     - Cervical spine positioned at 15° of flexion to provide the optimum intervertebral foraminal opening.
     - Contraindications include joint hypermobility, pregnancy, rheumatoid arthritis, Down syndrome, or any other systemic disease that affects ligamentous integrity.

Disc Conditions

1. Internal disc disruption (see Table 2-8).
   a. Internal structure of disc annulus is disrupted; however, external structures remain normal. Most common in lumbar region.
   b. Symptoms include constant deep, achy pain, and increased pain with movement. No objective neurological findings, although patient may have referred pain in lower extremity.
   c. Regular CT or myelogram will not demonstrate any abnormal findings. Can be diagnosed by CT discogram or an MRI.
   d. Clinical examination helps to identify this condition.
   e. Medications.
      - Acetaminophen for pain.
      - NSAIDs for pain and/or inflammation.
      - Muscle relaxants.
      - Trigger point injections.
      - Corticosteroid injection or by mouth.
   f. Physical therapy goals, outcomes, and interventions.
      - Biomechanical faults caused by joint restrictions should be corrected with joint mobilization to the specific restrictions identified during the examination.
      - Spinal manipulation may be contraindicated for this condition.
      - Patient education regarding proper body mechanics, positions to avoid, limiting repetitive bending and twisting movements, limiting upper extremity overhead and sitting activities, and carrying heavy loads.
2. Posterolateral bulge/herniation.
   a. Most commonly observed disc disorder of lumbar spine due to three structural deficiencies:
      - Posterior disc is narrower in height than anterior disc.
      - Posterior longitudinal ligament is not as strong and only centrally located in lumbar spine.
      - Posterior lamellae of annulus are thinner.
   b. Etiology: overstretching and/or tearing of annular rings, vertebral endplate and/or ligamentous structures, from high compressive forces or repetitive microtrauma.
   c. Results in loss of strength, radicular pain, paresthesia and inability to perform activities of daily living.
   d. Diagnostic tests utilized: MRI.
   e. Clinical examination helps to identify this condition.
   f. Medications.
      - Acetaminophen for pain.
      - NSAIDs for pain and/or inflammation.
      - Muscle relaxants.
      - Trigger point injections.
      - Corticosteroid injection or by mouth.
   g. Physical therapy goals, outcomes, and interventions.
      - Exercise program to promote dynamic stability throughout trunk and pelvis and to provide optimal stimulus for regeneration of disc.
      - Positional gapping for 10 minutes to increase space within region of space occupying lesion. If left posterolateral lumbar is herniation present:
        - Have patient side-lying on right side, with pillow under right trunk (accentuating trunk side-bending right).
        - Flex both hips and knees.
        - Rotate trunk to left (or pelvis to right).
        - Patient can be taught to perform this at home.
      - Spinal manipulation may be contraindicated for this condition, particularly at the level of the herniation.
      - Patient education regarding proper body mechanics, positions to avoid, limiting repetitive bending and twisting movements, limiting upper extremity overhead and sitting activities, and carrying heavy loads.
      - Manual and/or mechanical traction.
        - Traction: cervical spine positioned at 15° of flexion to provide the optimum intervertebral foraminal opening.
        - Contraindications include joint hypermobility, pregnancy, rheumatoid arthritis, Down syndrome, or any other systemic disease that affects ligamentous integrity.
        - Efficacy of traction for intervention of disc conditions is currently under scrutiny.
3. Central posterior bulge/herniation.
   a. More commonly observed in the cervical spine but can also be seen in the lumbar spine.
   b. Etiology: overstretching and/or tearing of annular rings, vertebral endplate, and/or ligamentous structures (posterior longitudinal ligament) from high compressive forces and/or long-term postural malalignment.

c. Results in loss of strength, radicular pain, paresthesia, inability to perform activities of daily living, and possible compression of the spinal cord. Patient exhibits central nervous system symptoms, e.g., hyperreflexia and a positive Babinski reflex.
d. Diagnostic tests utilized: MRI.
e. Clinical examination helps to identify this condition.
f. Medications.
- Acetaminophen for pain.
- NSAIDs for pain and/or inflammation.
- Muscle relaxants.
- Trigger point injections.
- Corticosteroid injection or by mouth.

g. Physical therapy goals, outcomes, and interventions.
- Refer to posterolateral intervention above.

4. Anterior bulge/herniation is very rare due to structural integrity of anterior intervertebral disc.

Facet Joint Conditions

1. Degenerative joint disease (DJD) Tables 2-8 and 2-27.
   a. Etiology: Part of normal aging process due to weight-bearing properties of facets and intervertebral joints (see Table 2-8).
   b. Results in bone hypertrophy, capsular fibrosis, hypermobility or hypomobility of joint, and proliferation of synovium.
   c. Symptoms include reduction in mobility of the spine, pain, and possible impingement of associated nerve root, resulting in loss of strength and paresthesias.
   d. Diagnostic tests utilized: plain film imaging.
   e. Clinical examination including lumbar quadrant test helps to identify this condition.
   f. Medications.
   - Acetaminophen for pain.
   - NSAIDs for pain and/or inflammation.
   - Muscle relaxants.
   - Trigger point injections.
   - Corticosteroid injection or by mouth.

   g. Physical therapy goals, outcomes, and interventions.
   - Exercise program to promote dynamic stability throughout trunk and pelvis and to provide optimal stimulus for regeneration of facet cartilage and/or capsule.
   - Biomechanical faults caused by joint restrictions should be corrected with joint mobilization to the specific restrictions identified during the examination.
   - Spinal manipulation may be useful.
2. Facet entrapment (acute locked back).
   a. Caused by abnormal movement of fibroadipose meniscoid in facet during extension (from flexion). Meniscoid does not properly reenter joint cavity and bunches up, becoming a space-occupying lesion, which distends capsule and causes pain.
   b. Flexion is most comfortable for patient, and extension increases pain.
   c. Clinical examination, including lumbar quadrant test, helps to identify this condition.
   d. Medications.
   - Acetaminophen for pain.
   - NSAIDs for pain and/or inflammation.
   - Muscle relaxants.
   - Trigger point injections.
   - Corticosteroid injection or by mouth.

   e. Physical therapy goals, outcomes, and interventions.
   - Positional facet joint gapping and/or manipulation are appropriate treatments.

Acceleration/Deceleration Injuries of Cervical Spine

1. Also known as Whiplash Associated Disorder or WAD (see Box 2-15).
2. Occurs when excess shear and tensile forces are exerted on cervical structures.
3. Structures injured may include facets/articular processes, facet joint capsules, ligaments, disc, anterior/posterior muscles, fracture to odontoid process and spinous processes, TMJ, sympathetic chain ganglia, spinal and cranial nerves.
4. Signs and symptoms.
   a. Early signs and symptoms include headaches, neck pain, limited flexibility, reversal of lower cervical lordosis and decrease in upper cervical kyphosis, vertigo, change in vision and hearing, irritability to noise and light, dysesthesias of face and bilateral upper extremities, nausea, difficulty swallowing, and emotional lability.
   b. Late include chronic head and neck pain, limitation in flexibility, TMJ dysfunction, limited tolerance to ADLs, disequilibrium, anxiety, and depression.
5. Common clinical findings include postural changes, excessive muscle guarding with soft tissue fibrosis, segmental hypermobility, and gradual development of restricted segmental motion, cranial and caudal to the injury (segmental hypomobility).
6. Diagnostic tests utilized: plain film imaging, CT, and/or MRI (see Box 2-17).

RED FLAG: Physical therapists must be able to recognize the signs and symptoms of possible undiagnosed spine injuries in their patient. Fractures and/or instability may occur following traumatic injuries of the cervical spine. The Canadian C-Spine Rules (SN 0.99; SP 0.45; +LR 1.8; –LR 0.02) provide the therapist with guidelines to determine if a referral for an x-ray or other imaging study is indicated.

7. Clinical examination helps to identify this condition.
8. Medications.
   a. Acetaminophen for pain.
   b. NSAIDs for pain and/or inflammation.

BOX 2-17 Canadian C-Spine Rules

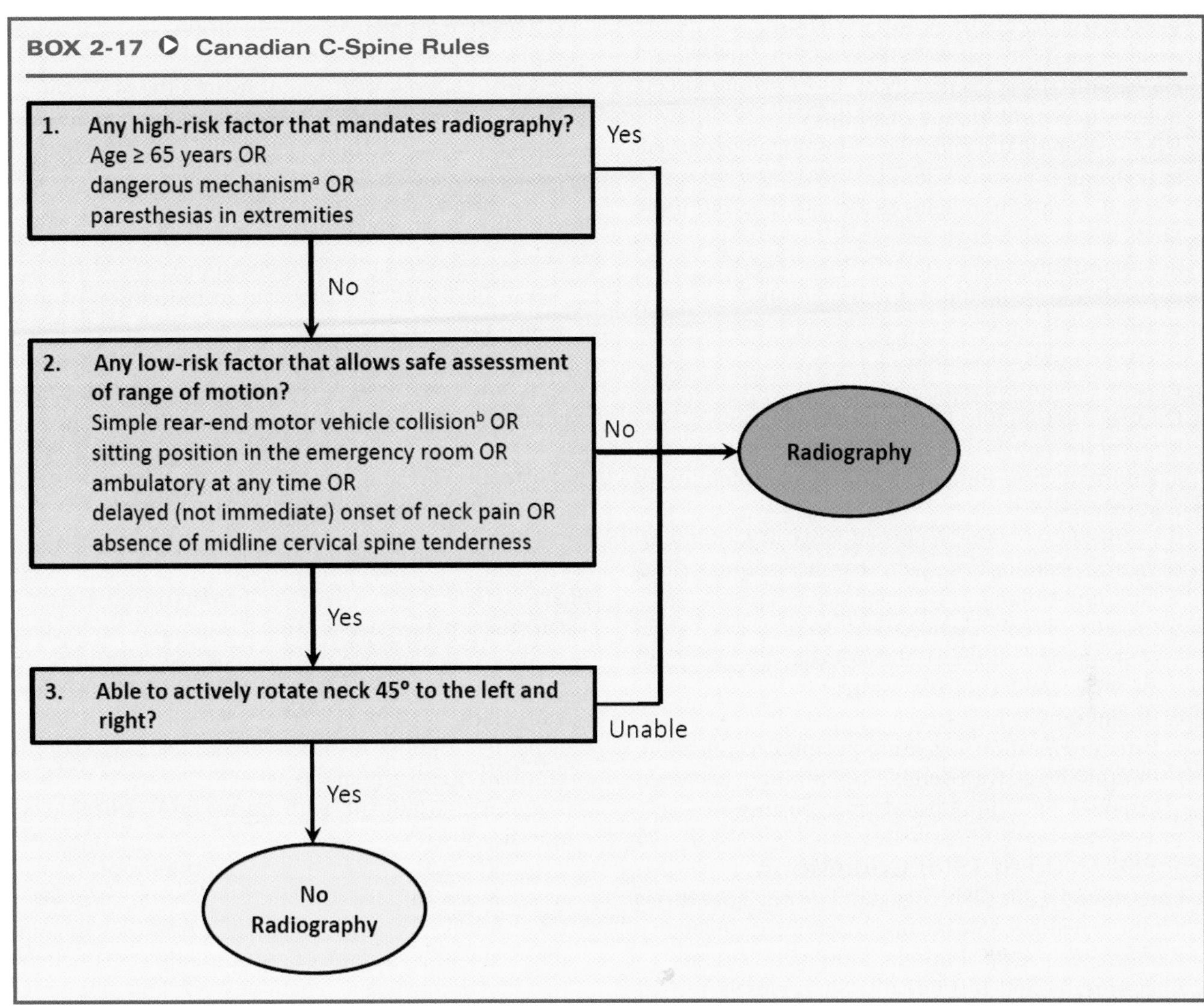

[a]A dangerous mechanism is considered to be a fall from an elevation of 3 feet or greater or three to five stairs; an axial load to the head (e.g., diving); a motor vehicle collision at high speed (>100 km/hr) or with rollover or ejection.

[b]A simple rear-end motor vehicle collision excludes being pushed into oncoming traffic, being hit by a bus or a large truck, a roll-over, or being hit by a high-speed vehicle.

Adapted from: Stiell IG, et al. The Canadian C-Spine Rule versus the NEXUS Low-Risk Criteria in Patients with Trauma. *N Eng J Med.* 2003; 349: 2510–2518.

c. Muscle relaxants.
d. Trigger point injections.
e. Corticosteroid injection or by mouth.

9. Physical therapy goals, outcomes, and interventions.
   a. Spinal manipulation is generally indicated.
   b. Correction of muscle imbalances and biomechanical faults using strengthening, endurance, coordination, and flexibility exercises to gain restoration of normal function.
   c. Biomechanical faults caused by joint restrictions should be corrected with joint mobilization to the specific restrictions identified during the examination.
   d. Progression to functional training based on patient's occupation and/or recreational goals.
   e. Patient education regarding the elimination of harmful positions and postural reeducation.
   f. Manual and/or mechanical traction.
      - Traction.
        - Cervical spine positioned at 15° of flexion to provide the optimum intervertebral foraminal opening.
        - Contraindications include joint hypermobility, pregnancy, rheumatoid arthritis, Down syndrome, or any other systemic disease that affects ligamentous integrity.

Hypermobile Spinal Segments

1. An abnormal increase in ROM at a joint due to insufficient soft tissue control (i.e., ligamentous, discal, muscle, or a combination of all three).
2. Diagnostic tests utilized: plain film imaging, particularly dynamic flexion/extension views.
3. Clinical examination helps to identify this condition.
4. Medications.
   a. Acetaminophen for pain.
   b. NSAIDs for pain and/or inflammation.
   c. Muscle relaxants.
   d. Trigger point injections.
   e. Sclerosing injections.
   f. Corticosteroid injection or by mouth.
5. Physical therapy goals, outcomes, and interventions.
   a. Pain reduction modalities to reduce irritability of structures.
   b. Passive ROM within a normal range of movement.
   c. Passive stabilization with corsets, splints, casts, tape, and collars.
   d. Increase strength/endurance/coordination, especially in the multifidus, abdominals, extensors, and gluteals, which control posture.
   e. Regain muscle balance.
   f. Patient education regarding postural reeducation, limiting excessive overloading, limiting sustained activities, and limiting end range postures.

Sacroiliac Joint (SIJ) Conditions

1. Cause and specific pathology is unknown. Since this is a joint, it may become inflamed, develop degenerative changes, or develop abnormal movement patterns.
2. Anatomically and functionally, SIJ is closely related to lumbar spine, so a thorough examination of both regions is indicated if a patient presents with pain in either.
3. Diagnostic tests utilized: plain film imaging and possibly MRI. Occasionally, double-blind injections may be used to assist in making the diagnosis (first injection is provocative in nature, and second injection is analgesic). If increased "same" pain with first injection and decreased pain following second injection, joint is determined to be pathological.
4. Clinical examination, including the following special tests, will be useful to make diagnosis. In SIJ two of the following four tests should be positive to indicate SIJ, or three out of five when Gaenslen's test is included:
   a. SI gapping.
   b. SI compression test.
   c. Gaenslen's test.
   d. Sacral thrust.
   e. Thigh thrust.
5. Medications.
   a. Acetaminophen for pain.
   b. NSAIDs for pain and/or inflammation.
   c. Muscle relaxants.
   d. Trigger point injections.
   e. Corticosteroid injection or by mouth.
6. Physical therapy goals, outcomes, and interventions.
   a. Spinal manipulation such as SIJ gapping is generally indicated to inhibit pain, reduce muscle guarding, and restore normal joint motion.
   b. Correction of muscle imbalances throughout pelvis using strengthening, endurance, coordination, and flexibility exercises to gain restoration of normal function.
   c. Biomechanical faults caused by joint restrictions should be corrected with joint mobilization to the specific restrictions identified during the examination.
   d. Patient education regarding the elimination of harmful positions and postural reeducation.
   e. Sacroiliac belts may be useful in some patients.

Repetitive/Cumulative Trauma to Back

1. Disorders of the nerves, soft tissues, and bones precipitated or aggravated by repeated exertions or movements of the back, occurring most often in the workplace.
2. Repetitive trauma disorders account for 48% of all reported occupational diseases.
3. Diagnosis is difficult, with up to 85% of back pain nondiagnosed.
4. Typically causes one of the conditions previously listed above: muscle, disc, and/or joint impairment.
5. Vocational factors that contribute to back pain include physically heavy static work postures, lifting, frequent bending and twisting, repetitive work, and vibration.
6. Chronic disability may be reduced by enrollment in a work-conditioning program, including patient education, aerobic exercises, general strengthening, and functional stability exercises that promote endurance for work-related activities.
7. Clinical examination helps to identify this condition.
8. Intervention should focus on prevention, consisting of education. If this phenomenon leads to a condition listed above, follow the specific intervention associated with that condition.

Masqueraders of Musculoskeletal Pain

1. Bone tumors.
   a. May be primary or metastatic.
      - Primary tumors include multiple myeloma (the most common primary bone tumor), Ewing's sarcoma, malignant lymphoma, chondrosarcoma, osteosarcoma, and chondromas.
      - Metastatic bone cancer has primary sites in lung, prostate, breast, kidney, and thyroid.
      - Patient history should always include questions about a prior episode of cancer.

- Signs and symptoms include pain that is unvarying and progressive, is not relieved with rest or analgesics, and is more pronounced at night.
- Diagnostic tests utilized: plain film imaging, CT, and/or MRI as well as laboratory tests.

2. Visceral tumors.
   a. Esophageal cancer symptomatology may include pain radiating to the back, pain with swallowing, dysphagia, and weight loss.
   b. Pancreatic cancer symptomatology includes a deep, gnawing pain that may radiate from the chest to the back.
   c. Diagnostic tests utilized: plain film imaging, CT, and/or MRI as well as laboratory tests.
3. Gastrointestinal conditions (See Chapter 8).
   a. Acute pancreatitis may manifest itself as mid-epigastric pain radiating through to the back.
   b. Cholecystitis may present with abrupt, severe abdominal pain and right upper quadrant tenderness, nausea, vomiting, and fever.
   c. Diagnostic tests utilized: plain film imaging, CT, and/or MRI as well as laboratory tests.
   d. May be identified as pain during palpation of abdominal region.
4. Cardiovascular and pulmonary conditions.
   a. Heart and lung disorders can refer pain to chest, back, neck, jaw, and upper extremity.
   b. Abdominal aortic aneurysm (AAA) usually appears as nonspecific lumbar pain.
   c. AAA may be identified as pulsatile mass during examination of abdominal region.
   d. Diagnostic tests utilized: US, plain film imaging, CT, and/or MRI as well as laboratory tests.
5. Urological and gynecological conditions.
   a. Kidney, bladder, ovary, and uterus disorders can refer pain to the trunk, pelvis, and thighs.
   b. Diagnostic tests utilized: plan film imaging, CT, and/or MRI as well as other laboratory tests.
6. See Figure 2-47 for pain referral patterns from viscera.

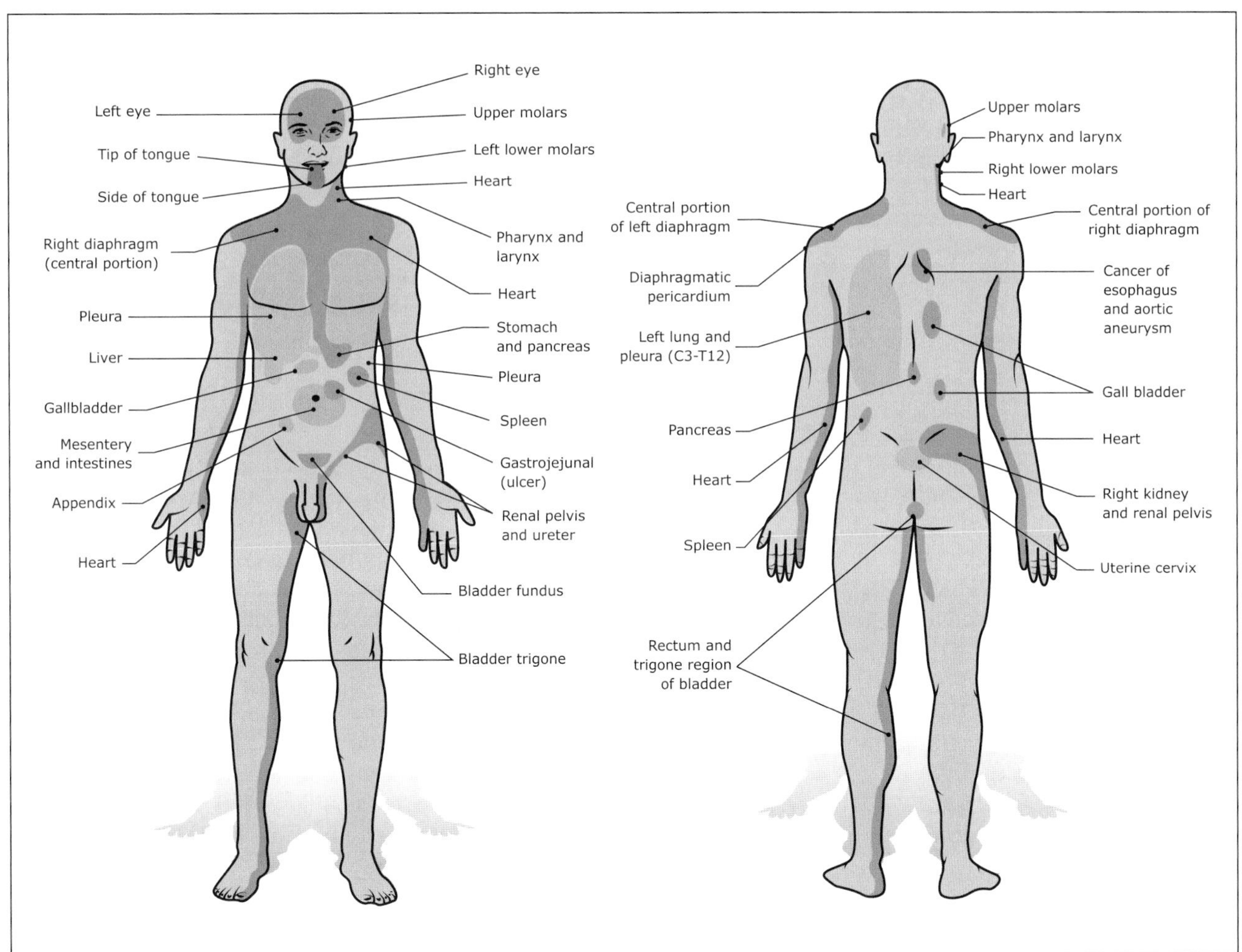

Figure 2-47 Pain referred from viscera.

From Roy S, Wolf S, Scalzitti D (2012) Rehabilitation Specialist's Handbook, 4th ed., Philadelphia, FA Davis, pp. 190–191, with permission.

Chapter 2 MS

Temporomandibular Joint Conditions

1. Common signs and symptoms include joint noise (i.e., clicking, popping, and/or crepitation), joint locking, limited flexibility of jaw, lateral deviation of mandible during depression or elevation of mandible, decreased strength/endurance of muscles of mastication, tinnitus, headaches, forward head posture, and pain with movement of mandible.
2. Cervical spine must be thoroughly examined due to close biomechanical and functional relationships between TMJ and the cervical region. Many patients with a TMJ condition have a component of cervical dysfunction.
3. Dysfunctions fall into three diagnostic categories.
   a. DJD, such as OA or RA in TMJ (refer to OA and RA for causes, characteristic findings, diagnostic methods, medical and physical therapy intervention).
   b. Myofascial pain is most common form of temporomandibular dysfunction (TMD), which is discomfort or pain in muscles controlling jaw function, as well as neck and shoulder muscles (refer to myofascial pain syndrome for causes, characteristic findings, diagnostic methods, medical and physical therapy intervention).
   c. Internal derangement of joint, meaning a dislocated jaw, displaced articular disc, or injury to condyle.
      - Loss of functional mobility may result from increased activity in muscles of mastication due to stress and anxiety.
      - Causes.
         - Trauma: leading to joint edema, capsulitis, hypomobility/hypermobility, or abnormal function of ligaments, capsule, and/or muscles.
         - Congenital anatomical anomalies: change in shape of palate.
         - Abnormal function, such as repeatedly chewing ice or hard candy, paranormal breathing (mouth breather), forward head posture.
      - Diagnostic tests utilized: plain film imaging and/or MRI if necessary.
      - Clinical examination helps to identify this condition.
      - Medications.
         - Acetaminophen for pain.
         - NSAIDs for pain and/or inflammation.
         - Muscle relaxants.
         - Trigger point injections.
         - Corticosteroid injection or by mouth.
      - Physical therapy goals, outcomes, and interventions.
         - Postural reeducation regarding regaining the normal anterior-posterior curves and left-right symmetry of the spine.
         - Modalities for reduction of pain and inflammation.
         - Biofeedback to minimize effects of stress and/or anxiety.
         - Joint mobilization if restriction in TMJ is present. Primary glide is inferior, which gaps joint, stretches the capsule, and allows relocation of anteriorly displaced disc.
         - Flexibility and muscle-strengthening exercises (e.g., Rocabado's jaw opening while maintaining the tongue in contact with the palate and isometric mandibular exercises).
         - Patient education (e.g., foods to avoid, maintaining proper postural alignment).
         - Night splints may be prescribed by the dentist to maintain resting jaw position.
         - Educate patient regarding resting position of tongue on hard palate.
         - It is critical to normalize the cervical spine posture before the patient receives any permanent dental procedures and/or appliances.

Pediatric Orthopedic Conditions

Torsional Conditions

1. Toeing in/out.
   a. Foot progression angle (gait angle) is the angle made by the foot with respect to a straight line plotted in the direction the child is walking.
   b. It can be normal in children with combined torsional deformity.
      - + sign denotes out-toeing angle.
      - – sign denote in-toeing angle.
   c. Thigh–foot angle is the angle between axis of the foot and axis of thigh measured with child prone and knees at 90°.
      - The angle describes the degrees of tibial torsion.
   d. Toeing in (pigeon-toed) is common in W sitting (hips and knees bent in front of the body) and is caused by three types of deformity depending on the age of the child including metatarsus adductus, internal tibial torsion, and increased femoral anteversion.
   e. Metatarsus adductus is the most common congenital foot deformity; greater occurrence in females and more common on left side.
      - The most common cause is intrauterine packing.
      - There are two types, including rigid and flexible.
      - Rigid form results in a medial subluxation of tarsometatarsal joints.
      - Hindfoot slightly in valgus with navicular lateral to head of talus.
      - Flexible form is observed as adduction of all five metatarsals at the tarsometatarsal joints.
         - Diagnosis through clinical exam.
         - Treatment includes stretching exercises and casting if needed.

- Surgical option is release of abductor hallucis tendon.
- Strengthening and regaining proper alignment of the foot (use of orthoses).
- 85%–90% of cases identified at birth resolve without treatment by 1 year.

f. Internal tibial torsion is the most common cause of in-toeing.
- There is a high complication rate with osteotomy of tibia and is associated with W sitting.

g. Increased femoral anteversion.
- The femoral neck angles anteriorly 10°–25° from the frontal plane to form anterior antetorsion angle.
- It is considered excessive if angle is >25°–30° and is associated with W sitting.

h. Toeing-out is less common and can be caused by: femoral retroversion, external tibial torsion, and flat feet.
- The femoral neck angles anteriorly 10°–25° from the frontal plane to form anterior antetorsion angle.
  - It is considered excessive if anterior antetorsion angle <10°.
- External tibial torsion correction has a high complication rate with surgery.

Talipes Equinovarus (Clubfoot)

1. Etiology: postural or talipes equinovarus.
   a. Postural from intrauterine malposition.
   - Abnormal development of the head and neck of talus, due to hereditary or neuromuscular disorders.
   - Observation: plantar flexed, adducted and inverted foot (postural).
2. Talipes equinovarus: plantar flexion at talocrural joint.
   a. Inversion at subtalar, talocalcaneal, talonavicular, and calcaneocuboid joints.
   b. Supination at midtarsal joints.
3. Diagnosis: at birth and can be detected with prenatal ultrasound.
   a. Thorough biomechanical lower quarter exam.
   b. Affected foot is a half size smaller and less mobile. The calf muscles will be smaller.
   c. 50% can be affected bilaterally.
4. Physical therapy goals, outcomes, and interventions.
   a. Postural condition: manipulation followed by casting or splinting (Ponseti method).
   b. Following casting, stretching is important. Orthoses (Denis-Browne splints) throughout the day for up to 3 months and then at night for up to 3 years.
   c. Talipes equinovarus (non-postural) requires surgical intervention to correct deformity followed by casting or splinting.
   - Achilles' tenotomy may be necessary.

Angular Conditions

1. Genu valgum: excessive lateral tibial torsion, referred to as knock-knees; excessive lateral patellar positioning.
2. Genu varum: excessive medial tibial torsion, referred to as bowlegs.
3. Excessive medial patellar positioning; pigeon-toed orientation of the feet.
4. Age norms.
   a. Genu varum is normal in newborn and infants.
   b. Maximal varum present at 6–12 months of age.
   c. Lower limbs gradually straighten with a zero tibiofemoral angle by 18–24 months.
   d. Knees gradually drift into valgus and is maximal around 3–4 years with an average medial tibiofemoral angle of 12°.
   e. Genu valgum spontaneously corrects by age 7 to the adult alignment of lower limbs.
   f. 8° of valgum in females and 7° in the male.
5. Diagnosis: plain film imaging consisting of standing long films (AP and lateral).
   a. Clinical examination.
6. Physical therapy goals, outcomes, and interventions: decreased loading of knee while maintaining strength and endurance.

Hip Dysplasia

1. Etiology: abnormality in the size, shape, orientation, or organization of the femoral head, acetabulum, or both.
   a. Can result in subluxations or dislocation.
2. Risk factors: females > males, breech position, family history of hip dysplasia, low levels of amniotic fluid, swaddling an infant too tightly.
3. Diagnosis: US screening after 4 weeks.
   a. Radiographs for infants 4–6 months can be used to assess the hips, monitor development after treatment, and assess long term outcomes.
   b. Clinical/physical exam: Barlow test, Ortolani test, Limited hip abduction, Galeazzi sign, Klisic sign.
4. Treatment: Pavlik harness current gold standard treatment.
   a. Maintain the hip in flexion and abduction position to maintain femoral head in acetabulum; recommendation for time frame varies. 85%–95% success rate with use in newborns to 6 months.
   b. Closed reduction under anesthesia followed by spica cast for 12 weeks for children 6 months to 2 years.
   c. Open reduction under anesthesia followed by spica cast for 6–12 weeks for children older than 2 years.
5. Physical therapy goals, outcomes, and interventions.
   a. Moderate resistance exercise program, delay deformities, and maximize function and patient education.

Transient Synovitis in Children

1. Etiology: acute onset of sudden hip pain in children ages 3–10.
   a. Transient inflammation of the synovium of the hip.
2. Diagnosis: clinical exam shows decreased hip abduction and internal rotation.
   a. Biopsy, ultrasonography shows effusion that causes bulging of the anterior joint capsule.
3. Signs and symptoms.
   a. Unilateral hip or groin pain.
   b. Less common medial thigh or knee pain.
   c. Crying at night.
   d. Antalgic limp.
   e. Pain not common.
   f. Recent history of upper respiratory tract infection.
4. Treatment: NSAIDs, rest while healing; lasts about 7–10 days.

Legg-Calvé-Perthes Disease

1. Etiology: blood supply interrupted to the femoral head.
   a. Age of onset between 2–13 years.
   b. Four times greater incidence in males than females.
2. Diagnosis: MRI showing positive bony crescent sign.
3. Clinical exam.
   a. Characteristic psoatic limp due to weakness of psoas major; moves in ER, flexion, and adduction.
   b. Gradual onset of aching pain at hip, thigh, and knee.
   c. AROM limited in abduction and extension (collapse of subchondral bone at femoral neck/head).
4. Treatment: medications include acetaminophen for pain, NSAIDs for pain and/or inflammation.
   a. Cast for 4–6 weeks, surgery if necessary.
5. Physical therapy goals, outcomes, and interventions.
   a. Joint/bone protection strategies.
   b. Maintain/improve joint mechanics and connective tissue functions.
   c. Implementation of aerobic capacity/endurance conditioning activities or reconditioning such as aquatic programs.
   d. Postsurgical interventions: regaining functional flexibility; improving strength, endurance, coordination, and gait training.

Slipped Capital Femoral Epiphysis

1. Etiology: most common hip disorder observed in adolescents of unknown etiology.
   a. Femoral head is displaced posteriorly and inferiorly in relation to the femoral neck and within the confines of the acetabulum.
   b. Onset in males 10–17 years, with average onset at 13 years.
   c. Onset in females 8–15 years, with average onset at 11 years.
   d. Two times greater incidence in males than females.
2. Diagnosis based on clinical examination.
   a. AROM restricted in abduction, flexion, and internal rotation.
   b. Patient describes pain as vague at knee, thigh, and hip.
   c. In chronic conditions, may demonstrate a Trendelenburg gait.
   d. Plain film imaging shows positive displacement of upper femoral epiphysis.
3. Treatment: operative internal fixation—prevention of complications such as avascular necrosis.
   a. Medications: acetaminophen for pain, NSAIDs for pain and inflammation.
4. Physical therapy goals, outcomes, and interventions.
   a. Joint/bone protection strategies.
   b. Maintain/improve joint mechanics and connective tissue functions.
   c. Implementation of aerobic capacity/endurance conditioning or reconditioning.
   d. Postsurgical intervention includes regaining functional flexibility; improving strength, endurance, coordination, and gait training.

Tendon Lengthening Conditions

1. Osgood-Schlatter disease.
   a. Etiology: mechanical dysfunction resulting in traction apophysitis of the tibial tubercle at the patellar tendon insertion.
   b. Diagnosis: plain film findings demonstrate irregularities of the epiphyseal line and/or clinical examination.
   c. Treatment.
      - Medications: acetaminophen for pain, NSAIDs for pain and inflammation.
      - Occasionally surgery is indicated.
   d. Physical therapy goals, outcomes, and interventions.
      - Modify activities to prevent excessive stress to irritated site.
      - Flexibility is important especially for prevention.
2. Sever's disease (calcaneal apophysitis).
   a. Etiology: most common cause of heel pain in growing children, occurs before or during peak growth spurt.
      - Caused by repetitive microtrauma due to increased traction by the Achilles tendon on its insertion site.
      - Bilateral involvement in 60% of cases.
   b. Diagnosis based on plain film imaging.
   c. Treatment: NSAIDs; temporary cessation of running, jumping activities, heel lifts/heel cups.
   d. Physical therapy goals, outcomes, and interventions.
      - Stretching and strengthening exercises.
3. Sinding-Larsen Johannson's disease.
   a. Etiology: traction apophysitis at the patella-patellar tendon junction, overuse injury due to repeated

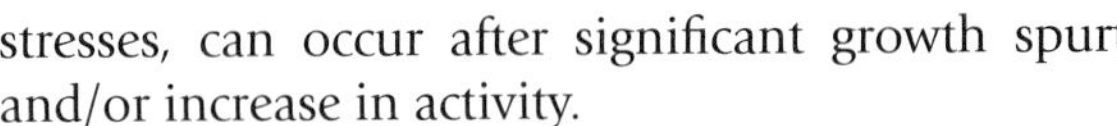

stresses, can occur after significant growth spurt and/or increase in activity.
   b. Diagnosis based on plain film imaging and/or clinical examination.
   c. Treatment includes NSAIDs, temporary cessation of activity.
   d. Physical therapy goals, outcomes, and interventions.
      - Stretching and strengthening exercise.
      - Activity modification.

Growing Pains (Benign Nocturnal Pains of Childhood)

1. Etiology is unknown but could be due to muscular fatigue, poor posture, stress, etc.
   a. No evidence linking growing pains and growing.
   b. Can affect 20% of children most likely between ages 3–5 and 8–11.
2. Diagnosis based on clinical exam.
   a. Increased pain at night, typically bilateral leg pain.
   b. Not associated with redness, temperature, swelling, and tenderness.
3. Treatment primarily related to managing the pain.

Osteochondritis Dissecans

1. Etiology: occurs in adolescents between ages of 12–15 years.
   a. Most common is a separation of articular cartilage from underlying bone (osteochondral fracture), usually involving medial femoral condyle near intercondylar notch.
   b. Can also be observed less frequently at femoral head and talar dome.
   c. Osteochondritis of humeral capitellum affects central and/or lateral aspect of capitellum or radial head. Osteochondral bone fragment becomes detached from articular surface, forming a loose body in the joint. Caused by repetitive compressive forces.
2. Diagnosis based on plain film imaging or CT scan to identify defect and/or clinical examination.
3. Treatment: if fracture is displaced, surgical intervention required.
   a. Medications: acetaminophen and/or NSAIDs.
4. Physical therapy goals, outcomes, and interventions.
   a. Rest and avoidance of aggravating factors.
   b. Joint/bone protection strategies.
   c. Correct biomechanical faults.
   d. Implementation of flexibility, strengthening, endurance, and coordination exercises to maintain/improve normal joint motion and length of muscles.
   e. Implementation of aerobic capacity/endurance conditioning or reconditioning.
   f. Implementation of strength, power, and endurance exercises to increase load on joints in late phases of rehabilitation.

Panner's Disease

1. Etiology: Localized avascular necrosis of capitellum leading to loss of subchondral bone, with fissuring and softening of articular surfaces of radiocapitellar joint.
   a. Unknown etiology but occurs in children age 10 or younger.
2. Diagnosis based on plain film imaging or CT scan to identify defect and/or clinical examination.

Leg Length Discrepancies

1. Etiology: congenital disorders of bones, muscles, or joints.
   a. Disuses or overuse of the bones, muscles, or joints caused by illness or disease.
   b. Disease such as bone cancer.
   c. Traumatic injuries, such as severe fractures that damage growth plates.
2. Diagnosis based on clinical exam.
   a. Leg length test: patient supine with pelvis balanced/aligned with lower limbs and trunk. Measure distance from ASIS to lateral malleolus or medial malleolus on each limb three times. Will determine true or functional limb discrepancy.
3. Treatment: noninvasive therapy and/or shoe inserts.
   a. Invasive: surgical.
4. Physical therapy goals, outcomes and interventions.
   a. Biomechanical corrections.

Scoliosis

1. Etiology: structural and nonstructural, both of unknown etiology.
   a. Structural is an irreversible lateral curvature of the spine with a rotational component.
   b. Nonstructural is a reversible lateral curvature of spine without a rotational component which straightens as individual flexes the spine.
2. Diagnosis: plain film imaging—full length Cobb's method.
   a. CT and/or MRI to rule out other associated conditions.
   b. Clinical examination.
3. Treatment.
   a. Conservative.
      - Degree of curvature less than 25°.
   b. Bracing.
      - Degree curvature 25°–45°.
   c. Surgery with placement of Harrington rod instrumentation.
      - Curvature greater than 45°.
4. Physical therapy goals, outcomes, and interventions.
   a. Flexibility exercises to maintain/improve normal joint motion and length of muscles throughout trunk and pelvis.
   b. Implementation of strength, power, and endurance exercises.
   c. Patient education.

Pes Planus (Flat Foot)

1. Etiology: can include genetic predisposition, muscle weakness, ligamentous laxity, paralysis, excessive pronation, trauma, or disease.
   a. Normal in infant and toddler feet and develop normal arches around 2–3 years.
2. Diagnosis based on clinical examination.
   a. Biomechanical lower quarter exam.
      - Reduction in height of medial longitudinal arch.
      - Decreased ability of foot to provide a rigid lever for push off during gait due to altered arthrokinematics.
3. Physical therapy goals, outcomes, and interventions.
   a. Patient education.
   b. Postural corrections.
   c. Use of proper footwear and orthotic fitting.

Congenital Muscular Torticollis

1. Spasm and/or tightness of SCM muscle.
2. Etiology: Fibrosis related to birth trauma; breech births, forceps birth, vacuum extraction, or C-section; restrictive intrauterine environment; genetic predisposition; cervical-vertebral abnormalities.
3. Observation: side-bending toward and rotation away from the affected SCM.
4. Diagnosis based on clinical exam and plain film imaging to rule out cervical spine abnormality or tumor.
5. Treatment.
   a. Medications: acetaminophen, muscle relaxants and/or NSAIDs.
   b. Physical therapy and positioning techniques.
   c. Splinting in older children (>4 months) with continued head tilt.
6. Physical therapy goals, outcomes, and interventions.
   a. Flexibility exercises to maintain/improve normal joint motion and length of muscles.
   b. Manual therapy including soft tissue/massage techniques and/or joint oscillations for maintenance and to reduce pain and/or muscle guarding.
   c. Therapeutic exercises.
   d. Education to parents on positioning.
   e. Good prognosis; poor if left untreated.

Spasmodic Torticollis

1. Movement disorder with CNS pathology.

Plagiocephaly (Flat Head Syndrome)

1. Etiology: development of a flat spot on the back or side of the head as the skull is soft and malleable and can be misshapen easily.
2. Diagnosis: clinical examination.
3. Treatment: repositioning techniques, parent education, use of helmet. (See additional information in Chapter 9 Pediatric Physical Therapy).

Arthrogryposis Multiplex Congenita

1. Etiology: congenital deformity of skeleton and soft tissues, characterized by limitation in joint motion and a "sausage-like" appearance of limbs.
   a. Nonprogressive contractures.
   b. Intelligence develops normally.
2. Diagnosis: plain films and/or clinical examination.
3. Treatment.
   a. Ongoing communication with patient and family.
4. Physical therapy goals, outcomes, and interventions.
   a. Joint/bone protection strategies.
   b. Maintain/improve joint mechanics and connective tissue functions.
   c. Implementation of aerobic capacity/endurance conditioning or reconditioning.
   d. Patient education regarding adaptive devices, assistive devices, orthotic devices, and supportive devices.
   e. Implementation of flexibility, coordination, endurance, and strength exercises.

Osteogenesis Imperfecta (OI)

1. Etiology: inherited disorder transmitted by autosomal dominant gene.
   a. Characterized by abnormal collagen synthesis leading to imbalance between bone deposition and reabsorption.
   b. Cortical and cancellous bones become very thin, leading to fractures and deformity of weight-bearing bones.
2. Diagnosis: bone scan and plain films to show old fractures and deformities; serological testing; clinical examination.
3. Treatment.
   a. Medications: calcium, vitamin D, estrogen, calcitonin, and bisphosphonates.
4. Physical therapy goals, outcomes, and interventions.
   a. Joint/bone protection strategies.
   b. Maintain/improve joint mechanics and connective tissue functions.
   c. Implement of aerobic capacity/endurance conditioning or reconditioning.
      - Aquatic therapy.

Spondylolisthesis

1. Etiology: congenitally defective pars interarticularis.
   a. Spondylolysis is a fracture of the pars interarticularis with positive "Scotty dog" on oblique radiographic view of the spine.
   b. Spondylolisthesis is the actual anterior or posterior slippage of one vertebra on another, following bilateral fracture of pars interarticularis.
   c. Can be graded from grade 1 (25% slippage) to 4 (100% slippage).
2. Diagnosis: plain films; oblique views to see fracture, lateral views to see slippage.
   a. Clinical examination: Stork test.

3. Treatment.
   a. Medication.
      - Acetaminophen for pain.
      - NSAIDs for pain and/or inflammation.
      - Corticosteroid injection or by mouth.
      - Muscle relaxants.
4. Physical therapy goals, outcomes, and interventions.
   a. Correct biomechanical faults caused by joint restriction.
   b. Dynamic stabilization exercises for the trunk with emphasis on abdominals.
   c. Avoid extension and/or other positions that cause stress to defect.
   d. Patient education on positioning and postural education.
   e. Orthoses if needed.
   f. Spinal manipulation is contraindicated.

Orthopedic Surgical Procedures

General Guidelines

1. Broadly categorized into soft-tissue and bony procedures; categories are not exclusive.
2. Not all surgical procedures are discussed, new procedures are constantly being developed, and rehabilitation protocols may differ based on surgeon preferences.
3. Physical therapist should focus on principles of rehabilitation.

Soft-Tissue Procedures

1. General guidelines and considerations.
   a. Consider stages of healing and the effect of immobilization on connective tissue.
   b. Consider adjacent tissues affected by the surgery.
   c. Goals in perioperative period are to reduce pain and restore motion, strength, and function.
2. Ligament reconstruction.
   a. Commonly at the knee (ACL, PCL, MCL), ankle (ATFL, CFL), and elbow (UCL).
   b. Generally, utilize auto or allograft tissue to create a new ligament versus repairing the original ligament.
   c. Communicate with surgeon on specifics of the procedure.
      - Important factors include graft material, fixation, quality of tissue, status of joint surfaces, and comorbidities.
      - Associated injuries frequently impact rehabilitation.
   d. ACL reconstruction (see Box 2-6 and Table 2-32).
   e. PCL reconstruction: frequently immobilized in full extension for a period of 6 weeks.
   f. Lateral ankle reconstruction.
      - Immobilized for 4–6 weeks in a combination of cast and/or rigid walking boot.
      - Focus on regaining range of motion after immobilization.
3. Tendon surgery.
   a. Commonly at the hand, rotator cuff, Achilles, and patellar tendons.
   b. Key issues are prevention of mobility impairments without overloading tendon repair and preventing excessive atrophy.
   c. Communicate with the surgeon to ensure an understanding of the quality of the repair to avoid over-loading or under-loading healing tissue.
   d. Tendon repairs of the hand.
      - Flexor tendon repairs.
        - Immobilized 3–4 weeks with wrist and digits flexed.
        - Resisted extension and passive flexion within limits of splint.
        - AROM to tolerance initiated at 4 weeks.
      - Distal repairs.
        - Immobilized with DIP joints in neutral for 6–8 weeks.

Table 2-32

Hamstring versus Patella Tendon Graft for ACL Reconstruction

HAMSTRING GRAFTS	PATELLA TENDON GRAFTS
Pros	
1. Typically fewer symptoms postoperatively.	1. Better at maintaining graft tension postoperatively.
2. Greater return to preinjury level of activity.	2. Typically less expensive.
3. Typically allows earlier rehabilitation.	3. Faster healing time.
Cons	
1. Typically more expensive.	1. Increased potential for anterior knee pain and later patellofemoral osteoarthrosis.
2. Believed to be more technically difficult procedure.	2. Increased potential for knee extension deficit.
3. Rehabilitation can be more difficult (i.e., slower).	3. Potential delay in rehabilitation secondary to more atrophy of quadriceps.

 - AROM initiated at 6 weeks with PIP in neutral.
 - Active extension initiated first, followed by flexion.
- Proximal repairs.
 - Immobilized with wrist and digital joints in extension for 4 weeks.
 - Early AROM/PROM in flexion with MCP joints in extension.
 - Full AROM initiated into flexion/extension at 6 weeks.

e. Rotator cuff repair.
- Typically immobilized for 4–6 weeks.
- No active shoulder motion or weight-bearing through shoulder for 4–6 weeks.
- Isometric exercise initiated at 6 weeks.

4. Soft-tissue stabilization procedures.
 a. Performed for joint instability resulting from capsular laxity (frequently in the shoulder).
 b. Fixation is usually soft-tissue to soft-tissue, without bony stability.
 c. Loading of the repair site is controlled for a lengthy period because of the lack of rigid fixation and length of soft-tissue healing.
 d. Repaired tissue is noncontractile; muscle activation is allowed as long as ROM restrictions are considered.
5. Meniscal and labral repairs and debridement.
 a. Commonly at the knee (meniscus), hip (labrum), and shoulder (labrum).
 b. Debridement requires less early protection than repair.
 c. Must understand loads on the repair in different joint positions.
 d. Avoid provocative positions early when repair is still fragile.
 - Knee meniscus: weight-bearing with flexion.
 - Shoulder anterior-inferior labrum (Bankart): external rotation.
 - Hip labrum: passive unilateral hip extension, excessive hip flexion, abduction, and external rotation.
 e. Communicate with the surgeon on the type, location, extent, and stability of the repair.

Bony Procedures

1. Most procedures involving articular cartilage also involve bone.
2. No optimal treatment for patients with articular cartilage injuries.
3. Lavage/debridement.
 a. Removes loose fragments and other mechanical or chemical irritants.
 b. Does not address underlying pathology; improvements frequently short-lived.
4. Microfracture.
 a. Small holes or "microfractures" stimulate a healing response and local fibrocartilage in-growth; mechanical properties are inferior to hyaline cartilage.
 b. Weight-bearing limited for up to 8 weeks.
 c. Many surgeons advocate continuous passive motion for up to 6 weeks.
5. Procedures to restore and preserve articular cartilage.
 a. Common procedures.
 - Osteochondral autograft transplantation (OAT): transfers articular cartilage from areas of low-loading to areas of high-loading.
 - Autologous chondrocyte implantation (ACI): healthy articular cartilage is harvested from the patient and injected under a periosteal flap closed with additional sutures and fibrin glue.
 b. Early non–weight-bearing followed by gradual progression of weight-bearing.
 c. Higher impacted activities limited until 6+ months, depending on the lesion, patient factors, type of activity, and procedure.
6. Open reduction–internal fixation (ORIF).
 a. Closed reduction is either not possible or fracture healing would be protracted.
 b. Post-op restrictions (weight-bearing, motion) depend on the location and severity of the fracture and the extent of associated soft-tissue injury.
7. Osteotomy.
 a. Surgical cutting of bone to correct bony alignment.
 b. Commonly performed at the knee to correct excessive genu varum or valgum.
 c. Weight-bearing is limited for 6–8 weeks to allow bone healing.

Total Joint Arthroplasty

1. Performed as a result of severe joint degeneration that has failed all other conservative or surgical treatment options.
2. Primary goal of joint arthroplasty is pain relief; increased ROM, strength, or function cannot be expected.
3. In general, postoperative rehabilitation should focus on restoration of motion, strength, and function and consideration of the underlying cause of the surgery.
4. Cemented versus noncemented.
 a. Cemented hips can tolerate full weight-bearing immediately following surgery.
 b. Cement may crack with aging, causing a loosening of prosthesis.
 c. Noncemented technique is more stressful on bones during the surgical procedure.
 d. Noncemented procedures are typically used with younger and/or more active individuals.
 e. Cemented technique may be better for individuals with fragile bones, or for those who will benefit from immediate ability to weight bear (e.g., those with dementia or significant debilitation).
5. Total hip replacement/arthroplasty (THR/THA).
 a. See Table 2-33 for general THR rehabilitation guidelines and precautions.
 b. Bed positioning with a wedge to prevent adduction.

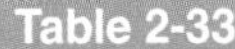

Table 2-33

Total Hip Replacement Guidelines/Precautions

ACTIVITY	CEMENTED	CEMENTLESS	
Internal rotation of hip joint	Do not perform for 3–6 months.	Do not perform for 3–6 months.	
Adduction of hip joint	Do not perform for 3–6 months.	Do not perform for 3–6 months.	
Flexion of hip joint beyond 90°	Do not perform for 3–6 months.	Do not perform for 3–6 months.	
Ambulation	Partial weight-bearing (PWB) for approximately 3 weeks. Begin ambulation with cane at week 4 postop. Begin transition to full weight-bearing at week 5.	Varies from weight-bearing as tolerated (WBAT) to touch-down weight-bearing (TDWB), based on the surgeon's philosophy and the surgical approach.	
		WBAT (WB as Tolerated)	**TDWB (Touch Down)**
		Partial weight-bearing (PWB) for approximately 3 weeks. Begin ambulation with cane at week 4 postop. Begin transition to full weight-bearing at week 6.	Progress to 1/3 weight-bearing at week 6. Progress to 2/3 weight-bearing at week 8. Progress to full weight-bearing at week 10 with walker. Begin transition to cane at week 12. Progress to no assistive device when safe and no Trendelenberg gait.
Isometric exercise	Immediately postop as tolerated by the patient.	Immediately postop as tolerated by the patient.	
Active exercise	Initiation is variable between weeks 1 through 4, depending on the surgeon's guidelines.	Initiation is variable between weeks 1 through 4, depending on surgeon's guidelines.	

RED FLAG: Patients should avoid the positions of hip flexion >90°, adduction past midline, and internal rotation for the first 6 weeks after surgery. These positions place the hip at risk for dislocation and other complications.

6. Total knee replacement/arthroplasty (TKR/TKA).
   a. See Table 2-34 for general TKR rehabilitation guidelines and precautions.
   b. Do not use continuous passive motion machines for postoperative management of patients following uncomplicated total knee replacement (White N, et al. Phys Ther. 2015).
   c. Avoid forceful mobilization and PROM into flexion because of the mechanical restraints of the prosthesis.

Spine Procedures

1. Rehabilitation and precautions vary according to the type of surgery performed.
2. A solid walking program is a foundation for both lumbar and cervical procedures.
3. A muscle strength and stabilization program and early mobilization exercises should be initiated prior to surgery.
4. Harrington rod placement for idiopathic scoliosis.
   a. Focus on early mobilization in bed and effective coughing.
   b. Begin ambulation between the fourth and seventh postoperative days.
   c. The patient should avoid heavy lifting and excessive twisting and bending.
5. Lumbar nonfusion (laminectomy/discectomy, microdiscectomy).
   a. Precautions: avoid end-range rotation and flexion, no joint mobilizations for 3 months.
   b. With microdiscectomies, rehabilitation time is decreased because the fibers of the annulus fibrosus are not damaged.
   c. With laminectomy/discectomy, early movement and activation of spinal musculature (especially multifidus) is necessary.
6. Fusion procedures.
   a. Adjacent joints compensate to restore mobility, possibly creating pain above or below the fusion.
   b. Muscles must be retrained to adapt to a new movement pattern.
      - Lumbar: core stabilization exercises.
      - Cervical deep neck flexor strengthening and stabilization exercises.
   c. Lumbar precautions: avoid end-range rotation and extension, no intensive abdominals, and no impact loading for 3 months.
   d. Cervical precautions: no lifting >5–10 lbs. for 4 weeks.
7. Total disc replacements.
   a. Aims to preserve normal spine motion while relieving pain.
   b. Similar precautions to cervical and lumbar fusion procedures.

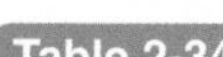

Table 2-34

Total Knee Replacement Guidelines/Precautions

ACTIVITY	CEMENTED	CEMENTLESS	
Range of motion	0°–90° within 2 weeks 0°–120° within 3–4 weeks	0°–90° within 2 weeks 0°–120° within 3–4 weeks	
Ambulation	Weight-bearing as tolerated with walker immediately postop. Ambulation with cane at week 3. Transition to full weight-bearing at week 4.	Varies from weight-bearing as tolerated (WBAT) to touch-down weight-bearing (TDWB) based on surgeon's philosophy and surgical approach.	
		WBAT	**TDWB**
		Weight-bearing as tolerated with walker immediately postop. Ambulation with cane at week 5–6. Transition to full weight-bearing at week 6.	Touch down weight-bearing with walker immediately postop. Weight-bearing as tolerated with walker at week 6. Ambulation with cane at week 8–10. Transition to full weight-bearing at week 10.
Isometric and active exercise	Immediately postop	Immediately postop	
Resisted exercise	Begin at week 2–3	Begin at week 2–3	

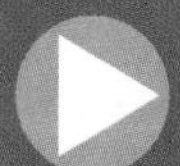

Interventions for Patients/Clients with Musculoskeletal Conditions

Interventions for Patients/Clients with Acute Conditions

Severity of Tissue Injury

1. Grade 1 (first degree). Mild pain and swelling and pain with tissue tension.
2. Grade 2 (second degree). Moderate pain and swelling requiring activity modification. Tissue is focally tender to palpation. Partial ligament tear may result in some increased joint laxity.
3. Grade 3 (third degree). Near-complete or complete tear with severe pain. Minimal or no pain with tissue tension. Palpable defect. Complete ligament tear will result in joint instability.

Stages of Soft Tissue Healing

1. Inflammatory Stage
   a. Physiology. This phase begins immediately and lasts 3–5 days.
      - Vascular changes mobilize and transport cells. Injured cells in the area release chemical substances (e.g., prostaglandins, bradykinin) to initiate the inflammatory response.
      - Platelets form a plug to contain bleeding and provide tissue scaffolding.
      - Vasodilation occurs to increase local blood flow while capillary permeability altered to allow cellular exudation.
      - Damaged tissues and microorganisms are removed.

   b. Treatment Principles: Treatment principles in the early phase include optimal loading and prevention of secondary complications.
      - Set conducive healing environment.
      - Balance of rest and loading.
      - Overload may perpetuate bleeding or the inflammatory response.
2. Proliferative Stage
   a. Physiology: This phase lasts from 48 hours to 6–8 weeks.
      - Fibroblasts actively resorb collagen and synthesize new collagen.
      - New tissue is vulnerable and susceptible to disruption by overload.
      - Decreased macrophages and fibroblasts with corresponding scar formation.

   b. Treatment Principles: Focus on restoration of normal tissue function, optimal loading, and avoiding complications.
      - Complications may result from changes in movement patterns to accommodate pain, weakness, or motion loss.
      - Correct faulty movement patterns that otherwise may create excessive loads on uninjured tissues.
3. Remodeling Stage
   a. Physiology: Tissue will continue to remodel and mature for 1–2 years postinjury.
      - Increased organization of extracellular matrix.
      - Collagen begins to organize into randomly placed fibrils.
      - Tension is required to provide tissue orientation.

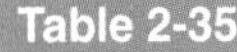

Table 2-35

Stages of Soft-Tissue Healing

INFLAMMATORY STAGE (ACUTE)	PROLIFERATIVE STAGE (SUBACUTE)	REMODELING STAGE (CHRONIC)
0–5 days	48 hours to 8 weeks	Weeks to 1–2 years postinjury
Vascular changes	Removal of noxious stimuli	Maturation of connective tissue
Exudation of cells and chemicals	Growth of capillary beds	Contracture of scar tissue
Clot formation	Collagen formation	Remodeling of scar
Phagocytosis	Granulation tissue	Collagen aligns to stress
Inflammation	Decreasing inflammation	Absence of inflammation
Pain before tissue resistance	Pain synchronous with tissue resistance	Pain after tissue resistance
	TREATMENT CONSIDERATIONS	
ACUTE PHASE	**SUBACUTE PHASE**	**FUNCTIONAL RESTORATION PHASE**
Maximum Protection	Moderate Protection/Controlled-Motion	Minimum Protection/Return to Function
Control effects of inflammation: selective rest, ice, compression, elevation	Develop mobile scar: selective stretching, loading of restrictions	Increase tensile quality of scar: progressive strengthening and endurance exercises
Prevent deleterious effects of rest: well-tolerated movement: passive ROM, massage, and muscle setting with caution	Promote healing: controlled active, resistive, stabilization, muscular endurance, and cardiopulmonary endurance exercises, progressed in intensity and range	Develop functional independence: functional exercises and specificity drills

Adapted from: Kisner C, et al: Therapeutic Exercise, 7th edition, 2018.

b. Treatment Principles: Return to function with optimal loading.
- Goal to enhance mobility and functional movement patterns.
- Use loading patterns and functional activities tailored to the patient.
- Consider healing tissue and graded loading to achieve optimal function.

4. See Table 2-35 for stages of soft-tissue healing characteristics and treatment considerations.
5. Complete healing times for specific musculoskeletal tissues.
   a. Muscle
   - Delayed onset muscles soreness (DOMS): 0–3 days
   - Grade 1 muscle strain: 0–4 weeks
   - Grade 2 muscle strain: 3–12 weeks
   - Grade 3 muscle strain: 4 weeks to 6 months

   b. Tendon: 8 weeks to 6 months
   c. Ligament
   - Grade 1 ligament sprain: 0–4 weeks
   - Grade 2 ligament sprain: 3 weeks to 6 months
   - Grade 3 ligament sprain: 5 weeks to >1 year

   d. Bone injury/fracture: 6–12 weeks
   e. Cartilage (fibrocartilage): 8 weeks to 12 months; healing times vary depending on structure (menisci, labrum, TFCC, articular disc of TMJ), weight-bearing constraints, conservative vs. surgical management, etc.

Interventions for Patients/ Clients with a Chronic Condition

Determine Possible Causative Factors

1. Abnormal remodeling of injured tissues.
2. Chronic low-grade inflammation due to repetitive stresses of tissues.

Reduce Stresses to Tissues

1. Identify/eliminate the magnitude of loading.
2. Identify/eliminate direction of forces.
3. Identify and eliminate any biomechanical barriers that are preventing healing; e.g., leg length discrepancy.
4. Patient education regarding protection of joints and associated soft tissues.

Regain Structural Integrity

1. Improving flexibility.
2. Postural reeducation.
3. Increasing tissue's capacity to tolerate loading.
4. Functional strengthening, endurance, and coordination exercises.

Resume Optimal Patient Function and Prevention of Reoccurrence

1. Patient education regarding causative factors in dysfunction.
2. Work conditioning.

Specific Interventions

Soft Tissue/Myofascial Techniques

1. Aid in reduction of metabolites from muscle, reactivating a muscle that has not been functioning secondary to guarding and ischemia, revascularization of muscle, and also decrease guarding in a muscle.
2. Autonomic: stimulation of skin and superficial fascia to facilitate a decrease in muscle tension.
3. Mechanical: movement of skin, fascia, and muscle causes histological and mechanical changes to occur in soft tissues to produce improved mobility and function (e.g., acupressure and osteopathic mechanical stretching techniques).
4. Goals: decrease pain, edema, and muscle spasm, increase metabolism and cutaneous temperature, stretch tight muscles and other soft tissues, improve circulation, strengthen weak muscles, and mobilize joint restrictions.
5. Indications: patients with soft tissue and joint restriction that results in pain and limits ADLs.
6. Contraindications.
   a. Absolute: soft tissue breakdown, infection, skin disease, cellulitis, osteomyelitis, contagious illness, malignant tumor, and/or aneurysms.
   b. Neuroses, lymphangitis, hemophilia, sensory impairment, deep vein thrombosis, hematoma.
7. Traditional massage techniques, such as effleurage and petrissage.
8. Functional massage.
   a. Three techniques used to assist in reactivation of a debilitated muscle and/or to increase vascularity to a muscle.
      - Soft tissue without motion.
         - Traditional technique; however, hands do not slide over skin; instead, they stay in contact with skin while hands and skin move together over the muscle.
         - Direction of force is parallel to muscle fibers, and total stroke time should be 5–7 seconds.
      - Soft tissue with passive pumping.
         - Place muscle in shortened position and with one hand place tension on muscle parallel to muscle fibers.
         - Other hand passively lengthens muscle and simultaneously gradually releases tension of hand in contact with muscle.
      - Soft tissue with active pumping.
         - Place muscle in lengthened position, and with one hand place tension on muscle perpendicular to muscle fibers.
         - Other hand guides limb as patient actively shortens muscle. As muscle shortens, gradually release tension of hand in contact with muscle.
9. Transverse friction massage.
   a. Used to initiate an acute inflammatory response for a tissue that is in metabolic stasis, such as a tendonosis.
   b. Involved tendon is briskly massaged in a transverse fashion (perpendicular to the direction of the fibers).
   c. Performed for 5–10 minutes and tends to be very uncomfortable for the patient.
10. Instrument-assisted technique.
   a. Cross friction technique used to enhance collagen formation and reorganization.
11. Myofascial release.
   a. Stretching the fascia to release restrictions.
   b. Allows connective tissue fibers to optimally reorganize.
12. Lymphatic drainage.
   a. Assist lymphatic system through slow and gentle stroking.
   b. Move fluid through lymph glands and vessels to decrease swelling (see Chapter 4).
13. Movement approaches require the patient to actively participate in treatment. Examples include:
   a. Feldenkrais.
      - Facilitates development of normal movement patterns.
      - The practitioner uses skillful, supportive, gentle hands to create a sense of safety, maintain supportive contact, while introducing new movement possibilities in small, easily available increments.
   b. Muscle energy techniques.
      - Include voluntary contraction in a precisely controlled direction, at varying levels of intensity, against an applied counterforce from the clinician.
      - Purpose is to gain motion that is limited by restrictions of the neuromuscular system.
      - Modification of proprioceptive neuromuscular facilitation (PNF) technique.
   c. PNF hold-relax-contract technique.
      - Antagonist of the shortened muscle is contracted to achieve reciprocal inhibition and increased range.
      - Refer to Chapter 3: Neuromuscular Physical Therapy for details.

Manual Mobilization/Manipulation

1. Joint mobilization (nonthrust manipulation).
   a. Utilization.
      - Inhibit pain and/or muscle guarding.
      - Lubricate joint surfaces and provide nutrition to joint structures.
      - Stretch/lengthen/deform connective tissue and normalize joint movement.
   b. Four grades of movement, as described by Maitland (see Figure 2-48).

- Grade I oscillations: small amplitude before the beginning of tissue resistance.
- Grade II oscillations: large amplitude before the beginning of tissue resistance.
- Grade III oscillations: large amplitude into tissue resistance.
- Grade IV oscillations: small amplitude into tissue resistance.
- Grade V: high-velocity, low amplitude thrust at the end of joint movement; technically, this is not an oscillation but rather a single movement.
- Indications for different grades.
  - Grades I and II are used to improve joint lubrication/nutrition and decrease pain/guarding.
  - Grades III and IV are used to stretch tight muscles, capsules, and ligaments.
  - Grade V is used to regain normal joint mechanics, as well as decrease pain and guarding.

c. Grades of movement, as described by Kaltenborn.
- Grade I: "loosening" translatoric glide; very small amplitude traction force; used to relieve pain and/or decompress a joint during joint glides, performed within examination or intervention.
- Grade II: "tightening" translatoric glide; movement takes up slack in tissues surrounding joint; used to alleviate pain, assess joint play, and/or reduce muscle guarding.
- Grade III: "stretching" translatoric glide; movement stretches the tissues crossing the joint; used to assess end-feel, or to increase movement.

d. Traction: manual, mechanical, and self- or autotraction.
- Vertebral bodies setting.
- Distraction and gliding of facet joints.
- Tensing of the ligamentous structures of the spinal segment.
- Intervertebral foramen widening.
- Spinal muscle stretching.

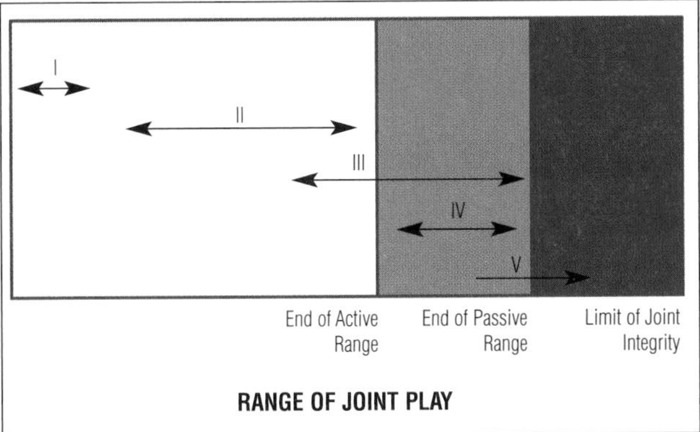

Figure 2-48 Grades of movement.

Adapted from Grieve GP: Mobilization of the Spine: A Primary Handbook of Clinical Method, 5th ed. Churchill Livingstone, 1991.

> RED FLAG: Absolute contraindications for joint mobilization/manipulation/traction include joint ankyloses, malignancy, diseases that affect the integrity of ligaments (RA, Down syndrome), arterial insufficiency, and active inflammatory and/or infectious process. Relative contraindications are arthrosis, metabolic bone disease (osteoporosis, Paget's disease, tuberculosis), hypermobility, total joint replacement, pregnancy, spondylolisthesis, use of steroids, radicular symptoms.

2. Manipulation (thrust).

a. Inhibit pain and/or muscle guarding.

b. Improve translatoric glide in cases of joint dysfunction due to restriction.

c. Health care practitioners who commonly perform manipulative thrusts include physical therapists, osteopaths, chiropractors, and medical doctors.

d. Types of manipulations.
- Generalized.
  - Fairly forceful, long lever techniques intended to include as many vertebral segments as possible.
  - More commonly performed by chiropractic practitioners.
- Specific.
  - Aimed at having an effect on either a specific segment or only a few vertebral segments.
  - Uses minimal force with short lever arms.
  - Often includes "locking" techniques based on biomechanics to ensure that a specific vertebral segment receives the manipulative thrust.
  - More commonly performed by physical therapists.
- Mid-range.
  - Very gentle, short lever arm techniques.
  - Barrier is created in mid-range by specific positioning of patient as well as creating tautness in surrounding soft tissues.
  - More commonly performed by osteopathic practitioners.

e. Contraindications.
- Absolute: joint ankylosis, malignancy involving bone, diseases that affect the integrity of ligaments (RA and Down syndrome), arterial insufficiency, and active inflammatory and/or infective process.
- Relative: arthrosis (DJD), metabolic bone disease (osteoporosis, Paget's disease, and tuberculosis), hypermobility, total joint replacement, pregnancy, spondylolisthesis, use of steroids, and radicular symptoms.

f. Common mistakes in performing a thrust manipulation.
- Not communicating clearly with the patient regarding the technique.

- Taking too long to properly position the patient.
- Not performing the "trial" thrust prior to the actual thrust.
- Not allowing the person to "bottom out" with their breath prior to performing the thrust.
- Taking up the slack while the patient exhales and then letting off with pressure prior to the thrust.
- Velocity too slow.
- Amplitude too great.

g. Suggested algorithm to perform a manipulation.
- Consider indications and contraindications.
- Explain the intentions and implications regarding manipulation to the patient.
- Describe the actual technique to the patient.
- Place patient into position and assess for patient comfort.
- Perform a prethrust force into the range to determine patient tolerance.
- Ask patient to inhale and then exhale. Take up the slack into the range as they exhale.
- When they reach the end of exhalation, perform the thrust.
- Specific thoughts for thrusting the cervical region.
- Perform vertebrobasilar testing when performing manipulations to cervical segments.
- Consider performing thrusts to thoracic region to attain the result that was sought after for the cervical thrust.
- Headaches in the cervical region are a common indication for thrusts, but are also a contraindication. Query female patients regarding birth control combined with smoking since this may be a cause for vascular accidents. Consider that headaches frequently precede a cerebrovascular accident.

Neural Tissue Mobilization

1. Movement of neural structures to regain normal mobility.
2. Tension or gliding techniques to reduce neuropathic symptoms for upper and lower extremities.
   a. Movement of soft tissues that may be restricting neural structures (e.g., cross friction massage for adhesions of the radial nerve to the humerus at a fracture site).
   b. Indications: used for patients who have some type of restriction in neural mobility, anywhere along the course of the nerve.
   c. Postural reeducation: to open up the intervertebral foramen, and decrease tension to tissues.
   d. Contraindications: extreme pain and/or increase in abnormal neurological signs.
3. Perform assessment with neurotension testing.
4. Determine whether managing irritated or nonirritated neurologic tissue.
   a. Irritated tissue.
   - Utilize grade II mobilizations (based on Maitland scale); should be nonpainful.

   b. Nonirritated tissue.
   - Utilize grade III mobilizations (based on Maitland scale) to engage the barrier but remain nonpainful.

Therapeutic Exercise for Musculoskeletal Conditions

1. Therapeutic exercise is indicated to:
   a. Decrease muscle guarding.
   b. Decrease pain.
   c. Increase vascularity of tissue.
   d. Promote regeneration and/or speed up recovery of connective tissues, such as cartilage, tendons, ligaments, capsules, intervertebral discs.
   e. Mobilize restricted tissue to increase flexibility.
   f. Increase endurance of muscle.
   g. Increase coordination of muscle.
   h. Increase strength of muscle.
   i. Sensitize muscles to minimize joints going into excessive range in cases of hypermobility.
   j. Develop dynamic stability and functional movement patterns, allowing for optimal function within the environment.
2. Home exercise program for patients/clients with musculoskeletal conditions.
   a. Patient's home program will consist of exercises to reinforce clinical program.
   b. Necessary to perform enough repetitions for desired physiological effect on appropriate tissues, as well as to develop coordination and endurance in order to promote dynamic stability within functional patterns.
3. See Chapter 6: Therapeutic Exercise.

Dry Needling

1. Also referred to as intramuscular manual therapy (IMT).
2. Utilized to break up trigger points in myofascial pain syndrome.
3. A solid filiform needle is inserted into the trigger point (within the muscle).
4. Dry needling is not part of the NPTE.
5. There are continued discussions about dry needling secondary to variations in state law practice acts and whether this should be considered part of an entry level or advanced practice.

Relevant Pharmacology

Nonsteroidal Anti-Inflammatory Drugs (NSAIDs)

1. Most commonly prescribed medication for pain relief for musculoskeletal dysfunction.
2. Examples include ibuprofen (Motrin), naproxen sodium (Aleve), salsalate (Discalced), and indomethacin (Indocin).

3. Provide analgesic, anti-inflammatory, and antipyretic capabilities.
4. Adverse side effects could include gastrointestinal irritation, fluid retention, renal or liver problems, and prolonged bleeding.
5. COX-2 inhibitors have decreased gastrointestinal irritation, but rofecoxib (Vioxx) was withdrawn from the market secondary to its relationship with heart-related conditions. Other COX-2 inhibitors such as colecoxib (Celebrex) and valdecoxib (Bextra) are being evaluated for their safety and possible association with heart-related conditions.

Muscle Relaxants

1. Commonly prescribed for skeletal muscle spasm.
2. Examples include cyclobenzaprine HCl (Flexeril), methocarbamol (Robaxin), and carisoprodol (Soma).
3. Act on the central nervous system to reduce skeletal muscle tone by depressing the internuncial neurons of the brain stem and spinal cord.
4. Adverse side effects could include drowsiness, lethargy, ataxia, and decreased alertness.

Nonnarcotic Analgesics

1. Prescribed when NSAIDs are contraindicated.
2. Examples include acetaminophen (Tylenol).
3. Act on the central nervous system to alter response to pain, and have antipyretic capabilities.
4. Adverse side effects are negligible when taken in recommended doses. Excessive amounts of acetaminophen may lead to liver disease or acute liver shutdown.

Narcotic Analgesics

1. Prescribed for acute, moderate to severe pain.
2. Examples include codeine, fentanyl, hydrocodone, hydromorphone, and oxycodone.
3. Prevents pain input by binding to CNS opioid receptors.
4. Adverse side effects could include sedation, confusion, vertigo, orthostatic hypotension, constipation, incoordination, physical dependence, tolerance.

RED FLAG: Patients with a wide variety of musculoskeletal disorders may be prescribed narcotics (opioids). There is an increasing number of individuals who suffer from opioid dependency. Physical therapists should recognize the signs and symptoms of the "opioid overdose triad": pinpoint pupils, respiratory depression, and unconsciousness. The therapist should initiate emergency response procedures if a patient exhibits any signs or symptoms consistent with an opioid crisis. (See the APTA white paper on the opioid epidemic dated June 1, 2018.)

Corticosteroids

1. Prescribed for hormonal and anti-inflammatory effect.
2. Examples include prednisone, hydrocortisone, prednisolone, methylprednisolone, dexamethasone.
3. Prevents or slows the immune system responses that trigger inflammation.
4. Short-term use can cause weight gain, puffy face, nausea, mood swings, and trouble sleeping.
5. Long-term use can cause osteoporosis.

Psychosocial Considerations

Malingering (Symptom Magnification Syndrome)

1. Defined as a behavioral response where displays of symptoms control the life of the patient, leading to functional disability.
2. There may be psychological advantages to illness.
   a. The patient may feel protected from the threatening world.
   b. Uncertainty or fear about the future.
   c. Social gain.
   d. Reduces stressors.
3. Therapist needs to recognize symptoms and respond to the patient.
   a. Tests to evaluate malingering back pain may include Hoover test, Burn's test, and Waddell's signs.
      - Hoover test involves the therapist's evaluation of the amount of pressure the patient's heels place on the therapist's hands when the patient is asked to raise one lower extremity while in a supine position.
      - Burn's test requires the patient to kneel and bend over a chair to touch the floor.
      - Waddell's signs evaluate tenderness, simulation tests, distraction tests, regional disturbances, and overreaction. Waddell's scores can be predictive of functional outcome.
   b. Functional capacity evaluations are used to evaluate psychosocial as well as physical components of disability.
   c. Emphasize regaining functional outcomes, not pain reduction.

Secondary Gain

1. Usually some type of financial gain for staying ill.
   a. Workers' compensation.
   b. Larger settlement for injury claims.
2. Frequently seen in clinics that manage industrial injuries.
3. May not want to return to work for various reasons associated with the work environment; e.g., stress, disliking coworkers.

Acknowledgment to Robert Rowe PT, DPT, DMT, MHS, FAAOMPT for his original contribution in formulating this chapter.

APPENDIX 2A

Selected Musculoskeletal Outcome Measures

Table 2A-1

SELF-REPORT OUTCOME MEASURE	DESCRIPTION	RELIABILITY	VALIDITY
General Musculoskeletal			
Numerical Pain Rating Scale (NPRS)[3]	Pain on 11-point scale (0–10). Higher scores = more pain. Often asked as "current pain" and "least," "worst," and "average pain" in the past 24 hours	ICC 0.76	MCID 1.3
Fear Avoidance Beliefs Questionnaire (FABQ)[3]	2 parts 1. 7-item work subscale (FABQW) 2. 4-item physical activity subscale (FABQPA) Each scale scored separately Higher scores = higher levels of fear avoidance	FABQW: ICC = 0.82 FABQPA: ICC = 0.66	N/A
Patient Specific Functional Scale (PSFS)[1,2,4,10]	Rate ability to perform 1–5 functional activities on a 0–10 scale Individual task scores are averaged Lower average scores = more disability	ICC = 0.71	MCID: 1.34 = small change 2.30 = medium change 2.70 = large change
Global Rating of Change[7]	Single-item, recall-based rating of change in well-being since the previous week's treatment on an 11-point scale where 0 equals no change, +5 is completely recovered, and −5 is very much worse	ICC = 0.90	MCID = 2
Cervical Spine			
Neck Disability Index (NDI)[3]	10 tasks rated from 0–5 Scores range from 0–100 Higher scores = greater disability	ICC = 0.64	MCID = 10.2

(*Continued*)

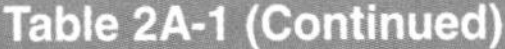
Table 2A-1 (Continued)

SELF-REPORT OUTCOME MEASURE	DESCRIPTION	RELIABILITY	VALIDITY
Lumbar Spine			
Modified Oswestry Disability Index (modified ODI)[3]	10 tasks rated from 0–5 Scores range from 0–100 Higher scores = greater disability	ICC = 0.90	MCID = 6
Subgroups for Targeted Treatment (STarT)[5,6]	9 items: referred leg pain, comorbid pain, disability (2 items), psychosocial (5 items; bothersomeness, catastrophizing, fear, anxiety, and depression) Low risk = 0–3 High risk = 4–5 psychosocial subscale Medium risk = remainder	Kappa = 0.73	N/A
Osteoarthritis			
Western Ontario and McMaster Universities Osteoarthritis Index (WOMAC)[3]	3 subscales: pain (5 items), stiffness (2 items), and physical function (17 items) Item scores range from 0 (no symptoms) to 10 (extreme symptoms), or alternatively on a Likert-type scale from 0–4 Higher scores = more pain, stiffness, and disability	ICC = 0.90	MCID = 6.7% for improvement MCID = 12.9% for worsening
General Lower Extremity			
Lower Extremity Functional Scale (LEFS)[3]	20 functional tasks rated from 0 (extremely difficult or unable to perform activity) to 4 (no difficulty) Scores range from 0–80 Lower scores = more disability	ICC = 0.92	MCID = 9
Knee			
Knee Outcome Survey (KOS) Activity of Daily Living Scale (ADLS)[3]	Sections on symptoms and functional disability Rate symptoms from 5 (never have) to 0 (prevent me from all daily activity) and function from 5 (not difficult at all) to 0 (unable to do) Scores expressed as percentage (sum divided by 80) Higher scores = fewer symptoms and higher function	ICC = 0.93	MCID = 7.1%
Foot and Ankle			
Foot and Ankle Ability Measure (FAAM)[8]	29 items rated 0 (no difficulty) to 4 (unable to do) 21-item ADL subscale 8-item sports subscale The total score for the items is divided by the highest possible score and multiplied by 100 to obtain a percentage Higher scores = higher function	ICC: ADL = 0.89 Sports = 0.87	MCID: ADL = 8 Sports = 9
Foot Function Index (FFI)[3]	23 items: pain, disability, and activity restriction subscales Scores range from 0–100 Higher scores indicate more impairment	ICC = 0.85	Unknown
General Upper Extremity			
Disabilities of the Arm, Shoulder and Hand Outcome Measure (DASH)[3]	30 items (21 physical function, 5 pain, 4 emotional/social) rated on a Likert-type scale Scores range from 0–100 Higher scores = more disability	ICC = 0.90	MCID = 10.2
Shortened Version of Disabilities of the Arm, Shoulder, and Hand Questionnaire (Quick-DASH)[3]	11 items addressing symptoms and physical function Scores range from 0–100 Higher scores = more disability	ICC = 0.90	MCID = 8.0

(Continued)

Table 2A-1 (Continued)

SELF-REPORT OUTCOME MEASURE	DESCRIPTION	RELIABILITY	VALIDITY
Shoulder			
Shoulder Pain and Disability Index (SPADI)[9]	13 items (5 pain, 8 disability) rated on a 0–10 scale Scores range from 0–100 Higher scores = more disability	ICC = 0.89	MCID = 8
Penn Shoulder Score (PSS)[3]	Rate level of pain, satisfaction, and function on three subscales. The pain subscale is a 10-point numeric rating scale with "no pain" and "worst pain possible" as end points. The satisfaction subscale is also based on a 10-point numeric rating scale with "not satisfied" and "very satisfied" as end points. The function subscale is based on a 4-point Likert scale with "can't do at all," "much difficulty," "with some difficulty," and "no difficulty" as response options. Scores range from 0–100 Higher scores = low pain, high satisfaction, and high function	ICC = 0.94	MCID = 11.4
HAND			
Michigan Hand Outcomes Questionnaire (MHQ)[3]	37-items on 6 scales: (1) overall hand function, (2) activities of daily living (ADLs), (3) work performance, (4) pain, (5) aesthetics, and (6) satisfaction with hand function rated on a 5-point Likert-type scale. Scores range from 0–100. Higher scores = better hand function.	ICC = 0.95	MCID: Pain = 23 Function = 13 ADL = 11 Work = 8
TMJ			
Mandibular Function Impairment Questionnaire[3]	17 questions rating perceived level of difficulty on a Likert scale ranging from 0 (no difficulty) to 4 (very great difficulty or impossible without help) Total scores range from 0–68 Higher scores = more disability	Spearman's r = 0.69-0.96	MCID = 14

Abbreviations: ICC, Intraclass Correlation Coefficient; MCID, Minimum Clinically Important Difference; MDC, Minimum Detectable Change

References

1. Abbott JH, Schmitt J. Minimum important differences for the Patient-Specific Functional Scale, 4 Region-Specific Outcome Measures, and the Numeric Pain Rating Scale. *J Orthop Sports Phys Ther*. May 2014. doi:10.2519/jospt.2014.5248.
2. Chatman AB, Hyams SP, Neel JM, et al. The Patient-Specific Functional Scale: measurement properties in patients with knee dysfunction. *Phys Ther*. 1997; 77(8): 820–829.
3. Cleland J, Koppenhaver S, Su J, Netter FH. *Netter's Orthopaedic Clinical Examination: An Evidence-Based Approach*. 3rd ed. Philadelphia, PA: Elsevier; 2016. https://www-clinicalkey-com.stimson.idm.oclc.org/#!/browse/book/3-s2.0-C20140013111. Accessed April 21, 2018.
4. Hefford C, Abbott JH, Arnold R, Baxter GD. The patient-specific functional scale: validity, reliability, and responsiveness in patients with upper extremity musculoskeletal problems. *J Orthop Sports Phys Ther*. 2012; 42(2): 56–65. doi:10.2519/jospt.2012.3953.
5. Hill JC, Dunn KM, Lewis M, et al. A primary care back pain screening tool: identifying patient subgroups for initial treatment. *Arthritis Rheum*. 2008; 59(5): 632–641. doi:10.1002/art.23563.
6. Hill JC, Whitehurst DGT, Lewis M, et al. Comparison of stratified primary care management for low back pain with current best practice (STarT Back): a randomised controlled trial. *Lancet*. 2011; 378(9802): 1560–1571. doi:10.1016/S0140-6736(11)60937-9.
7. Kamper SJ, Maher CG, Mackay G. Global rating of change scales: a review of strengths and weaknesses and considerations for design. *J Man Manip Ther*. 2009; 17(3): 163–170. doi:10.1179/jmt.2009.17.3.163.
8. Martin RL, Irrgang JJ, Burdett RG, Conti SF, Van Swearingen JM. Evidence of validity for the Foot and Ankle Ability Measure (FAAM). *Foot Ankle Int Am Orthop Foot Ankle Soc Swiss Foot Ankle Soc*. 2005; 26(11): 968–983.
9. Roy JS, MacDermid JC, Woodhouse LJ. Measuring shoulder function: a systematic review of four questionnaires. *Arthritis Rheum*. 2009; 61(5): 623–632. doi:10.1002/art.24396.
10. Stratford PW, Gill C, Westaway MD, Binkley JM. Assessing disability and change on individual patients; a report of a patient specific functional measure. *Phys Can*. 1995; 47(4): 258–263.

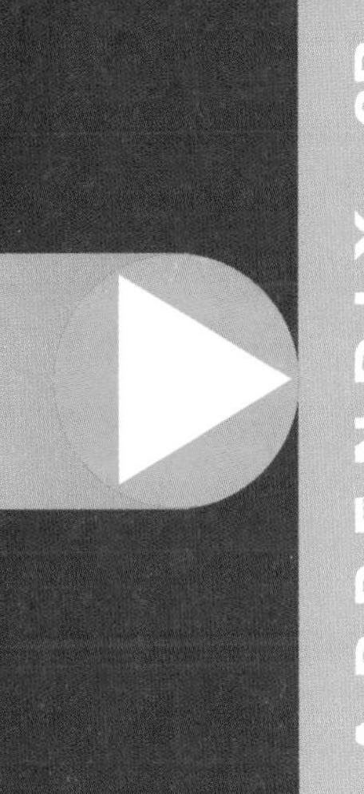

APPENDIX 2B

Musculoskeletal Imaging

THOMAS SUTLIVE
L. VINCENT LEPAK III

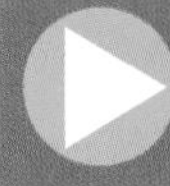

Radiology

Professionals

Radiologists: Physicians That Train and Subspecialize in Different Types of Imaging

Radiographers: The Technicians Trained to Perform Specific Types Ofimaging

Physical Therapists: Receive Basic Training in the Interpretation of These Studies and the Type of Studies Indicated for Their Clients

Diagnostic Exams and Procedures

Radiography (X-Rays)

1. Noninvasive test used to identify and screen for lung or heart disease, fractures, dislocations, bone growth, foreign objects, etc.
2. X-ray photons pass through the body and are captured on plain film or digitally. The radiodensity of the anatomical structure determines whether the object is seen as white, black, gray-black, or gray.
   a. A structure that is radiodense (bone) will absorb more x-rays and leave the film white, while a less radiodense structure (air) will not absorb as much X-radiation, allowing penetration to the film and turning it black.
   b. The radiograph (x-ray) is a 2-D (dimensional) view of a 3-D object, causing structures to be superimposed. At least two views (often three) are required so the diagnostician does not neglect an abnormality that is viewable in another plane (sagittal, frontal, or transverse).
3. Use the ABCs to interpret the musculoskeletal radiograph: Alignment: size, contour, alignment with adjacent bones; Bone density: density and texture; Cartilage spaces: joint space width, presence of subchondral bone, epiphyseal plates.
4. Advantages: quick, easy, portable, and relatively inexpensive.
5. Disadvantages: ionizing radiation, poor at visualizing soft tissues and small fractures.

Magnetic Resonance Imaging (MRI) (See Table 2B-1)

1. Noninvasive test that provides sectional imaging of anatomy that is especially helpful for visualizing soft tissues. These images can be configured into detailed 3-D models.
2. MRI uses radio waves and magnetic fields to provide detailed imaging of the body that is often not visible to other types of imaging. The two basic types of an MRI are T1 and T2.
   a. T1: fat is brighter and is helpful in defining anatomy.
   b. T2: fluid appears brighter, and the fat is suppressed, which is helpful for various joint pathologies.
3. Functional MRIs are used to detect metabolic changes in the brain.
4. Advantages: high-quality imaging of almost any structure of the body (e.g., organs, bone, soft tissues). Does not rely on ionizing radiation. Contrasts can be used to increase details.
5. Disadvantages: expensive, time-consuming, must remain perfectly still to avoid artifacts, may not be able to distinguish between edema and cancer tissue, may cause implanted metal device to malfunction, claustrophobic environment, and relatively nonportable.

Computed Tomography (CT) or CAT Scan

1. Noninvasive test that provides sectional imaging of bone and most soft tissues. Especially useful for the chest and abdomen, with better anatomical resolution than an x-ray. Able to measure bone density (predict fractures) and identify tumors.
2. A special radiography device with advanced computer analysis that configures images from x-rays at various angles to show high-quality cross-sectional and 3-D imaging of body tissues (e.g., bone, lungs, vessels, brain, tendons) and organs.
3. Advantages: fast; provides high-quality imaging of bone, soft tissue, and blood vessels all at the same time. Contrasts can be used to increase details.
4. Disadvantages: large amounts of ionizing radiation; not as good at soft-tissue structures as MRI. Not portable, expensive, may result in a claustrophobic reaction, and has bariatric limits.

Bone Scan or Bone Scintigraphy

1. Helps to diagnose fractures not detected by x-ray and areas of damage to bone caused by cancer, trauma, infection, or other conditions.
2. Uses gamma ray emission to detect newly forming bone. A radionuclide is injected intravenously, and the distribution (uptake) is recorded on radiographic film. Increased areas of uptake equal increased metabolic activity and show up on the film as black. This test has poor specificity and good sensitivity.
3. Advantages: noninvasive, small amounts of radiation, and improved detection of abnormal bone metabolism.
4. Disadvantages: time-consuming (about 1 hour for whole body), ionizing radiation, potential adverse reaction from contrast.

Angiography

1. A common procedure that helps the medical team evaluate and diagnose a client's condition. Also provides valuable information for prognosis and treatment intervention.
2. A catheter and a contrast material are often used in conjunction with x-rays, CT-scan, or MRI. The primary purpose of this procedure is to examine blood vessels throughout the body. Also may be used to guide intervention, e.g., stent placement.

Bone Density Scan or Dual-Energy X-Ray Absorptiometry (DEXA) or Bone Densitometry

1. Measures bone mineral density. Used to delineate osteopenia from osteoporosis.
2. An enhanced x-ray technique; gold standard for measuring bone mineral density.

Table 2B-1

Tissue Appearance According to Imaging Study

	RADIOGRAPH	CT	T1 MRI	T2 MRI
Air	Black	Black	Black	Black
Fat	Poorly visualized or absent	Black	White	Gray
Bone cortex	White	White	Black	Black
Bone marrow	White	Gray	White	Gray

Ultrasound (US)

1. Purpose: With regards to the musculoskeletal system, it helps diagnose partial tendon tears, soft-tissue masses (e.g., tumors, hematomas), pockets of fluid, muscle development or activation.
2. Description: sound waves capture real-time images of various body structures and blood flowing through the vessels. Structures that have more collagen will create a whiter image (hyperechoic) because they reflect the US better than an object that lacks collagen. Muscles appear darker (hypoechoic) relative to tendon. Structures that lack collagen (e.g., blood) will be dark and void of an echo because it allows the US to pass through the object resulting in an anechoic image. Physical therapists are increasingly using this modality to assess the structure, function, and movement of muscles and peripheral nerves in both healthy and unhealthy populations. US is a reliable and valid method to examine muscle thickness and diagnose soft-tissue injury.
3. Advantages: noninvasive, quick, easy, provides real-time imagery, relatively low cost when compared to other diagnostic imaging equipment (e.g., CT and MRI). It has great resolution for soft-tissue lesions when compared to an MRI.
4. Disadvantages: unable to penetrate bone, requires a practitioner that is experienced and well trained at performing US.

Positron Emission Tomography (PET) Scan

1. Used to detect nonperfusing areas of the heart or to evaluate the brain in cases of undetermined dementia, stroke, seizures, memory disorders, or suspected tumors.
2. Captures positrons emitted from radioactive substance.

Region: Head and Neck

Figure 2B-1 Lateral Radiographic View of Cervical Spine:

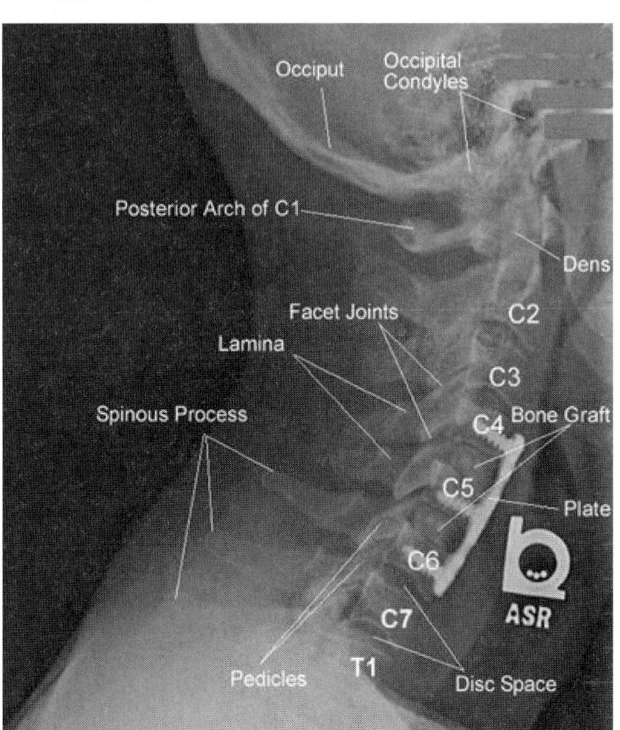

From: http://www.neckpainexplained.com/degenerative-disc-disease.htm

Region: Thorax and Spine

Figure 2B-2 Lateral Radiographic View of Normal Lumbar Spine:

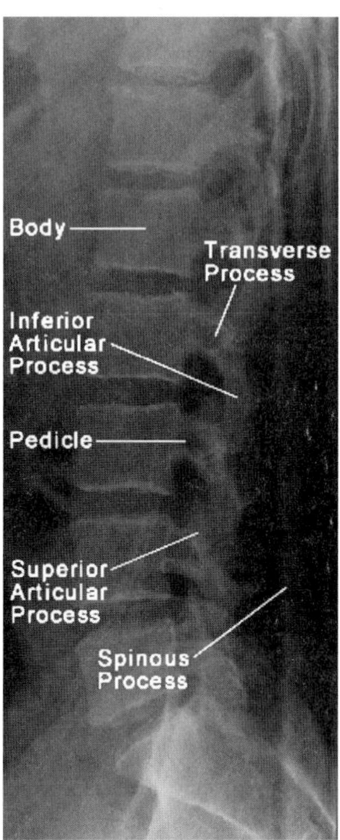

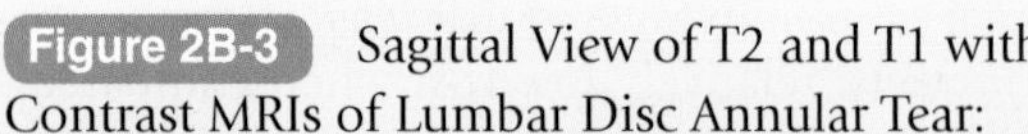

Figure 2B-3 Sagittal View of T2 and T1 with Contrast MRIs of Lumbar Disc Annular Tear:

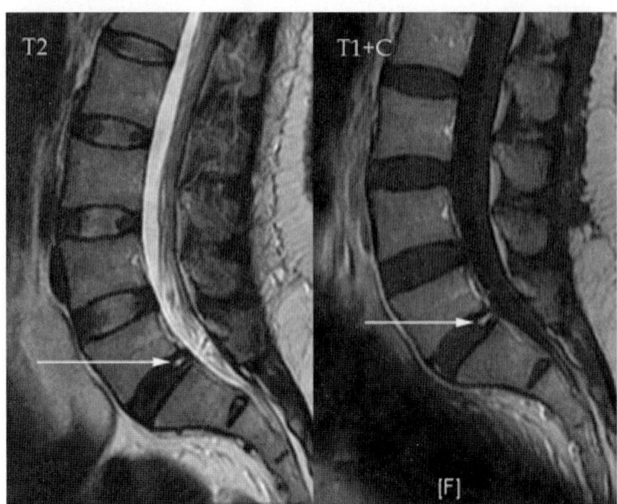

Figure 2B-4 Oblique Radiographic View Demonstrates Fracture Through the Pars Interarticularis (arrows):

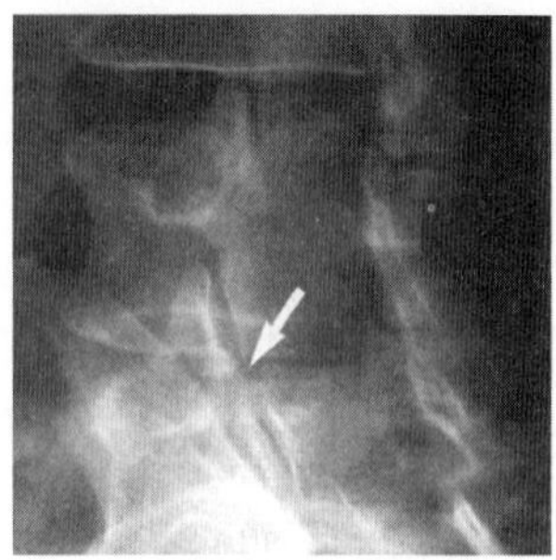

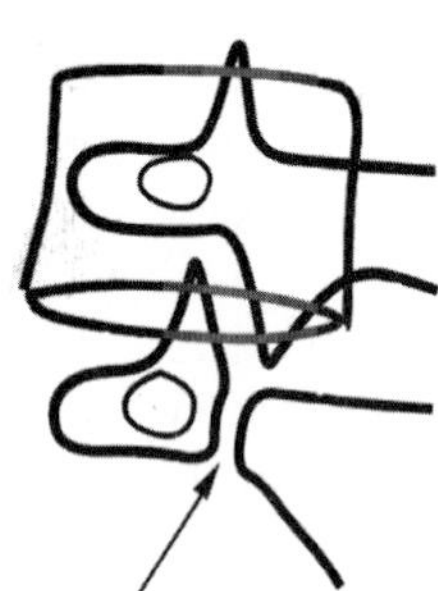

Region: Upper Extremity

Figure 2B-5 Anterior-Posterior (AP) Radiographic View of Right Shoulder in ER:

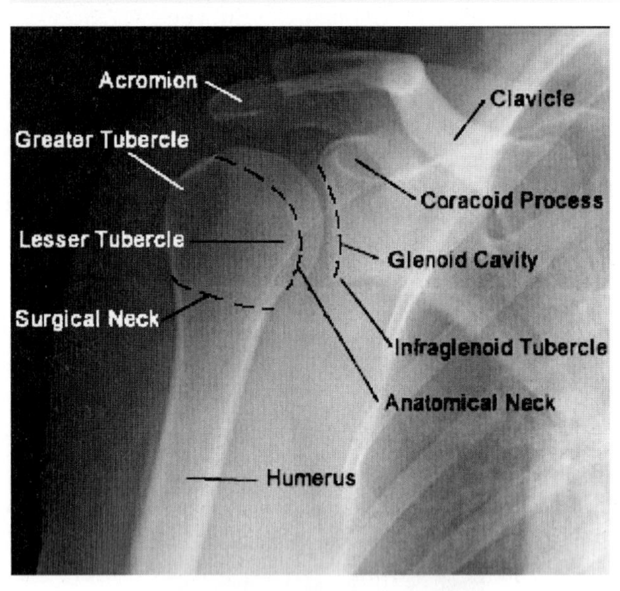

Figure 2B-6 AP Radiographic Stress View of Type II Separation:

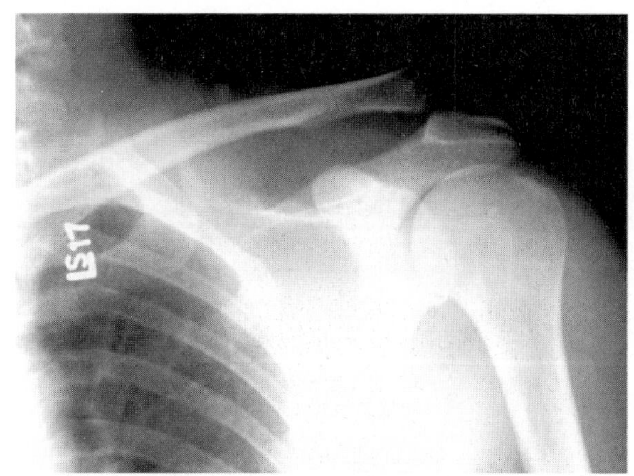

Figure 2B-7 Coronal T1 (left image—normal) and T2 (right image—torn supraspinatus):

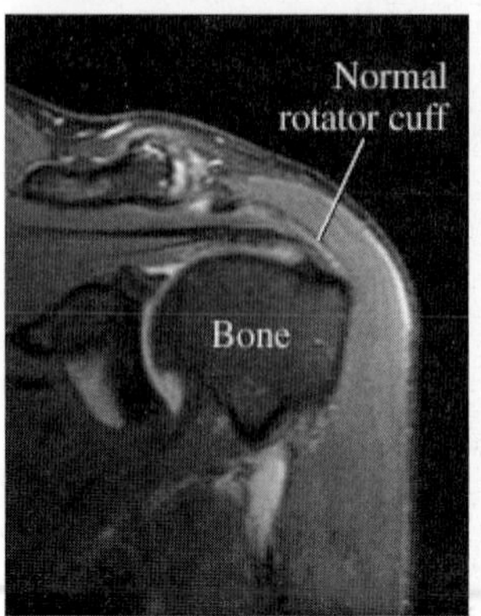

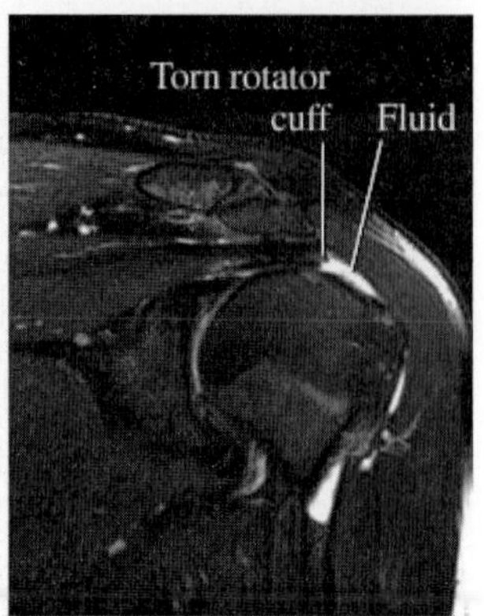

Figure 2B-8 Coronal T1 MRI of right SLAP Lesion (Superior Labrum Anterior to Posterior):

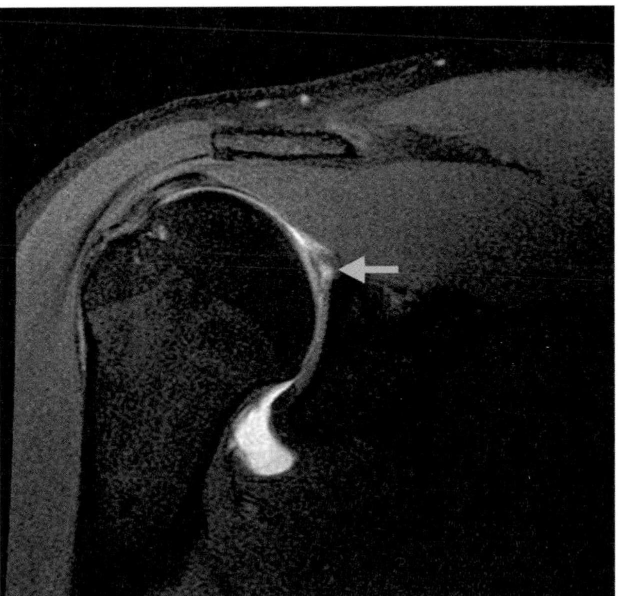

From: *J Orthop Sports Phys Ther 2012; 42(12):1050. doi:10.2519/jospt.2012.0420*

Figure 2B-9 AP Radiographic View of Left Humerus Fracture with Open Reduction/Internal Rotation. Bullet fragments can be seen in the inset picture (arrows):

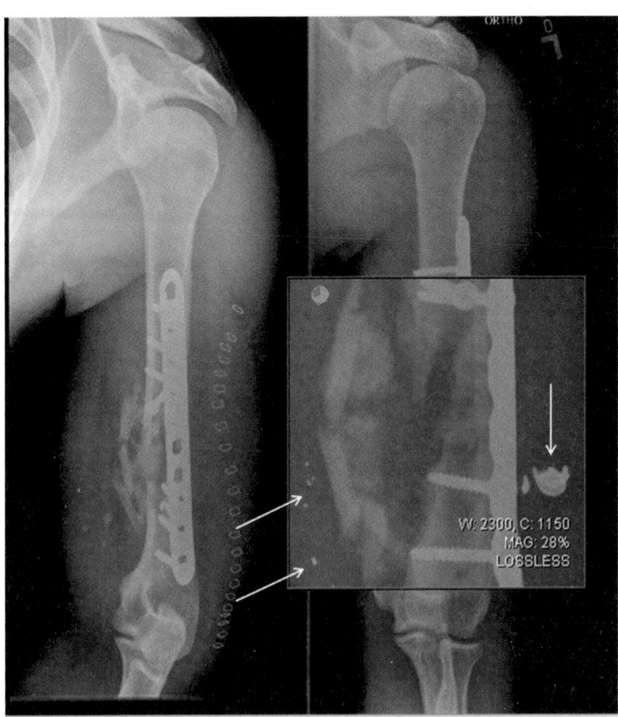

Figure 2B-10 Lateral and AP Radiographic Views of Normal Elbow:

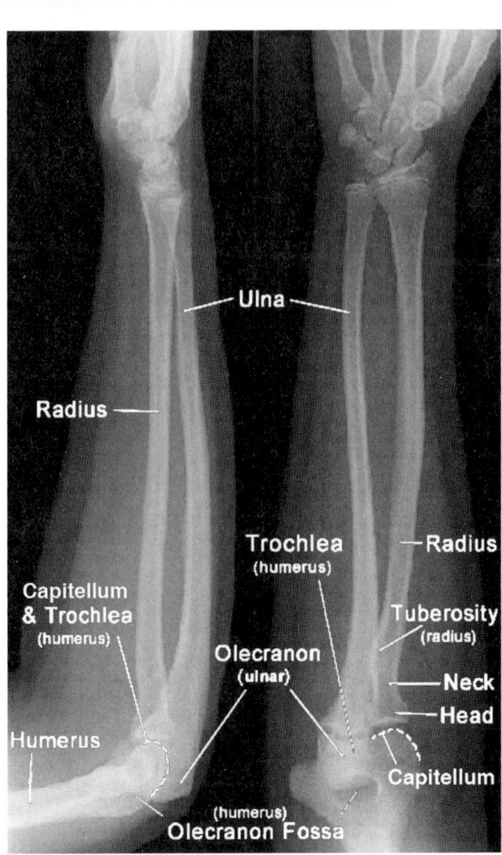

Figure 2B-11 AP Radiographic View of Wrist:

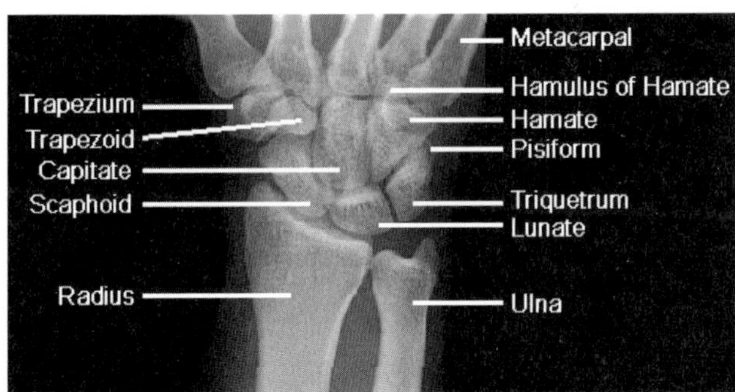

Mnemonic for remembering carpals: Some Lovers Try Positions That They Can't Handle. Scaphoid, Lunate, Triquetrum, Pisiform, Trapezium, Trapezoid, Capitate, Hamate

From: http://www.med-ed.virginia.edu/courses/rad/

Figure 2B-12 Radiographic View of Boxer's Fracture of Fifth Metacarpal (white pointer):

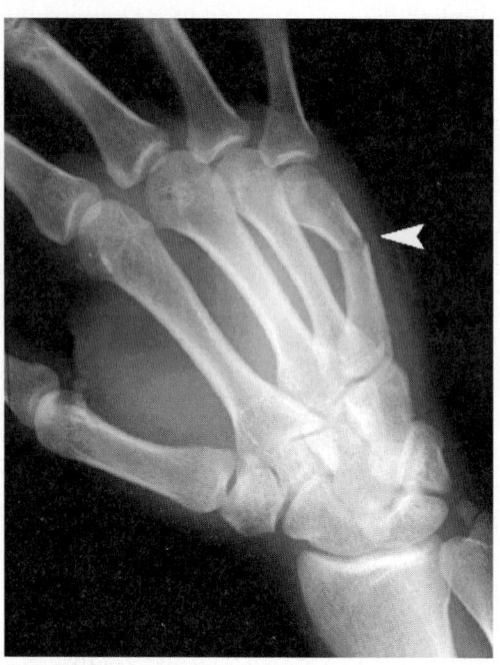

Figure 2B-13 Radiograph Demonstrates Ulnar Deviation of the Metacarpophalangeal Joints Due to Rheumatoid Arthritis:

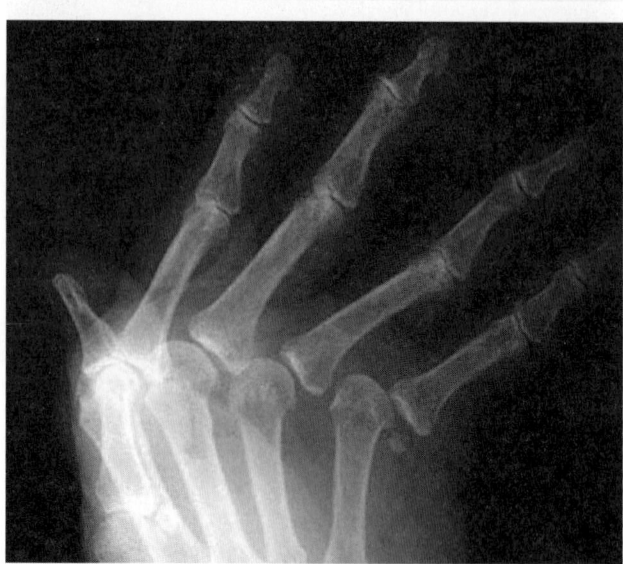

Region: Lower Extremity

Figure 2B-14 AP Radiographic View of Normal Pelvis:

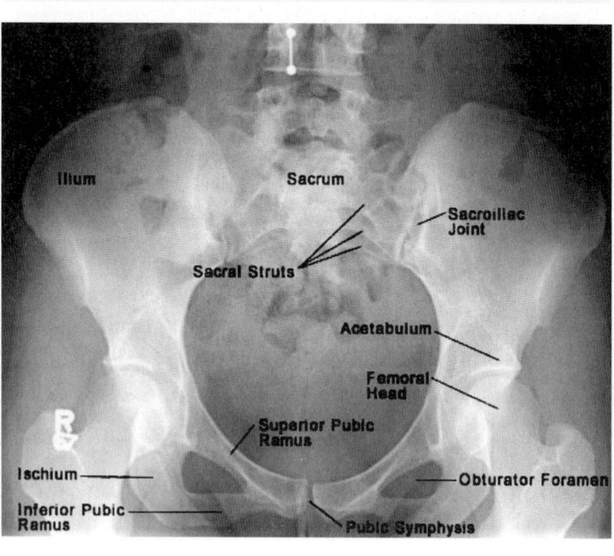

Figure 2B-15 AP Radiographic View of Right Acetabular Fracture (arrow):

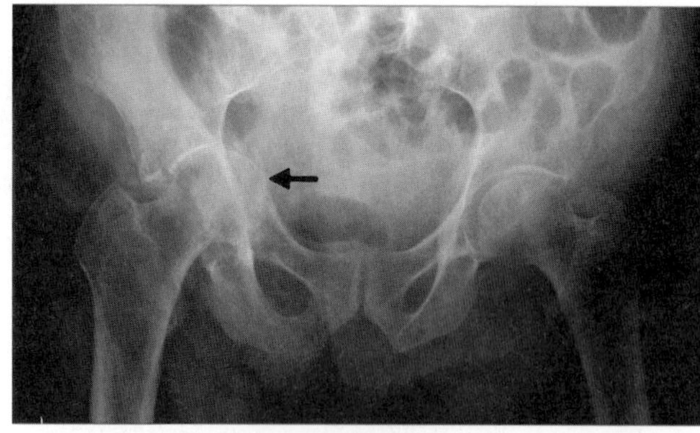

Figure 2B-16 AP Radiographic of Pelvis showing Left Femoral Neck Stress Fracture:

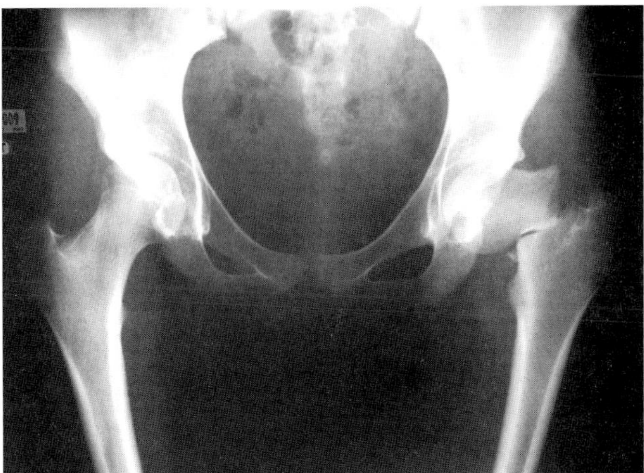

From: http://www.ncbi.nlm.nih.gov/pmc/articles/PMC3435922/

Figure 2B-17 AP Radiographic View of Normal Child's Leg:

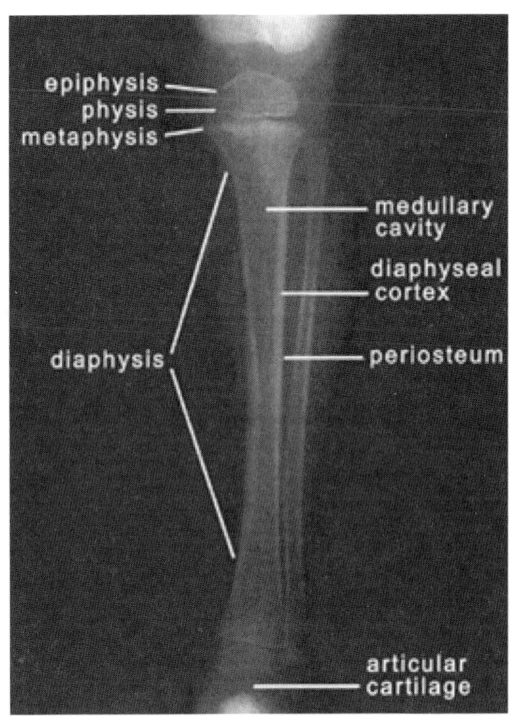

Figure 2B-18 MRI Normal ACL:

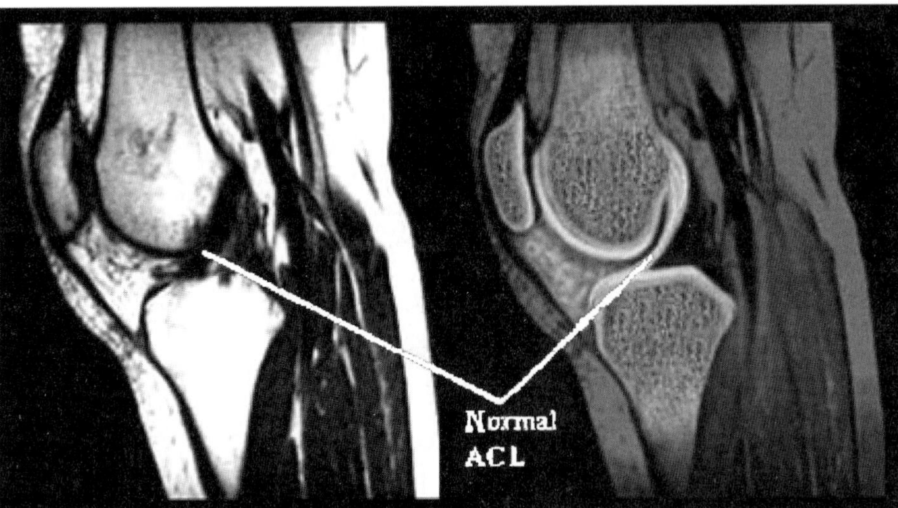

Figure 2B-19 Axial MRI of Longitudinal Tibial Stress Fracture:

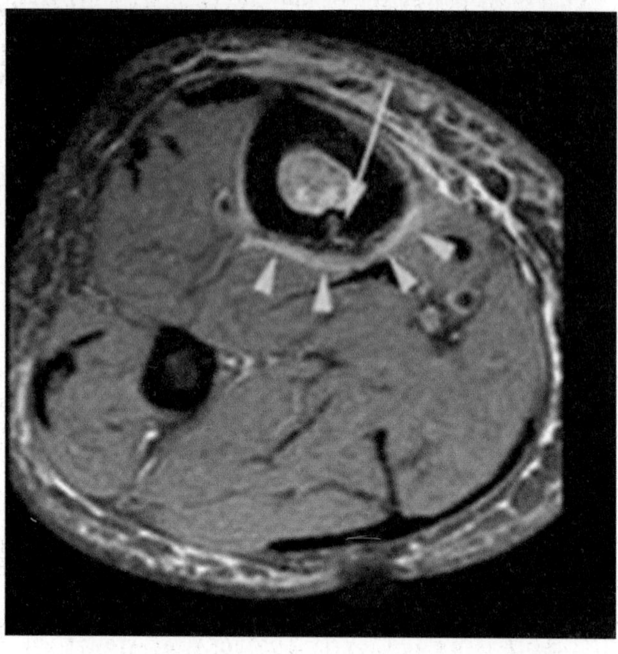

Figure 2B-20 Sagittal T2 Image of Longitudinal Tibial Stress Fracture (arrows):

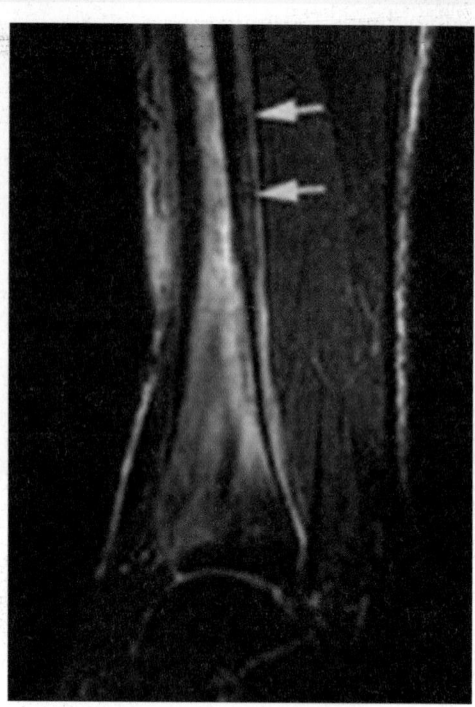

Figure 2B-21 Lateral Radiographic View of Normal Ankle:

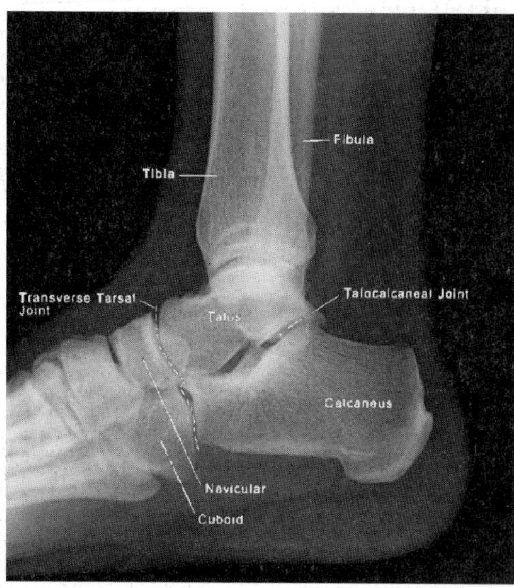

Figure 2B-22 Lateral Radiographic View of Heel Spur:

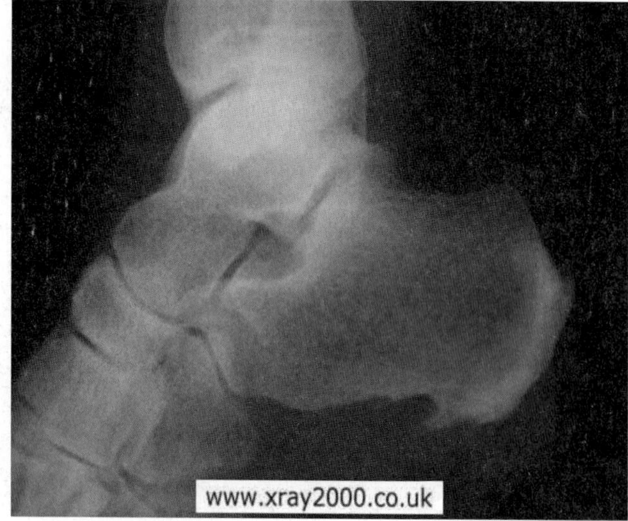

Figure 2B-23 AP Radiographic View of Left Ankle Showing Oblique Fibular Fracture with Deltoid Ligament Tear (Weber C Injury):

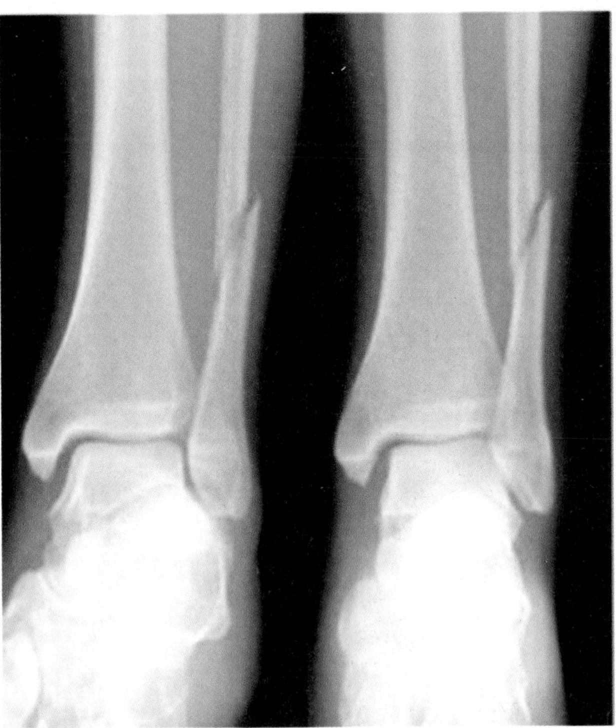

Figure 2B-24 AP Radiographic View of Right Ankle Medial Malleolus Fracture:

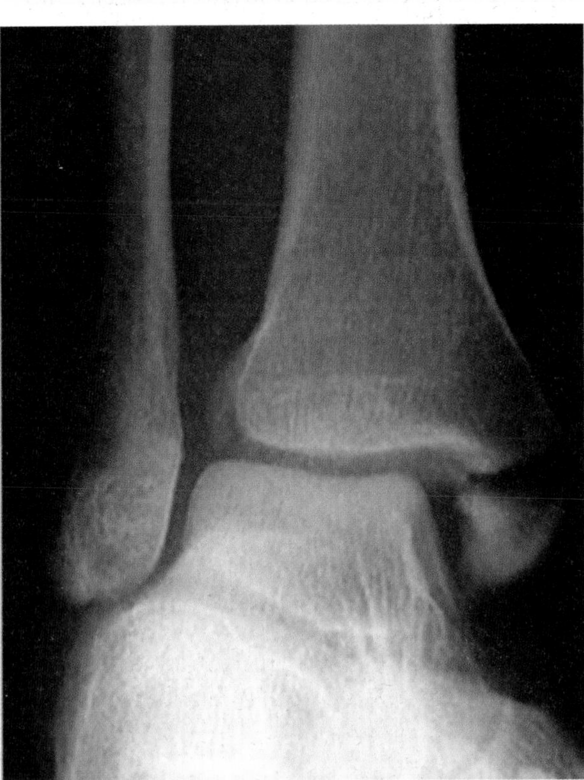

Figure 2B-25 Maisonneuve Fracture. AP Radiographic image showing abduction (eversion) injury to left ankle (image on left). Forces were transmitted through the syndesmosis, exiting through proximal fibula (arrow seen on lateral view at right):

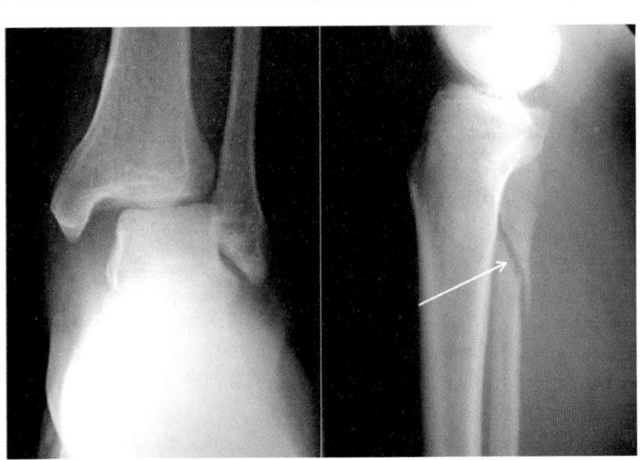

Figure 2B-26 Lateral Radiographic View Showing Shrapnel in Leg, Ankle, and Foot:

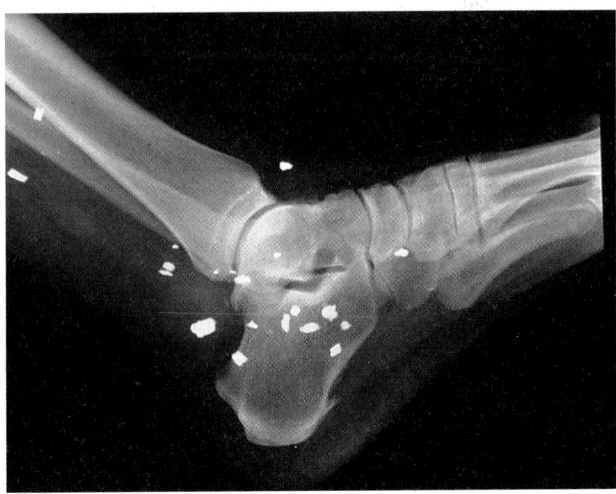

From: https://commons.wikimedia.org/wiki/File:Korean_War_shrapnel_ankle_X-ray.jpg

Figure 2B-27 Lateral Radiographic View of Right Foot Showing Jones' Fracture (base of 5th metatarsal):

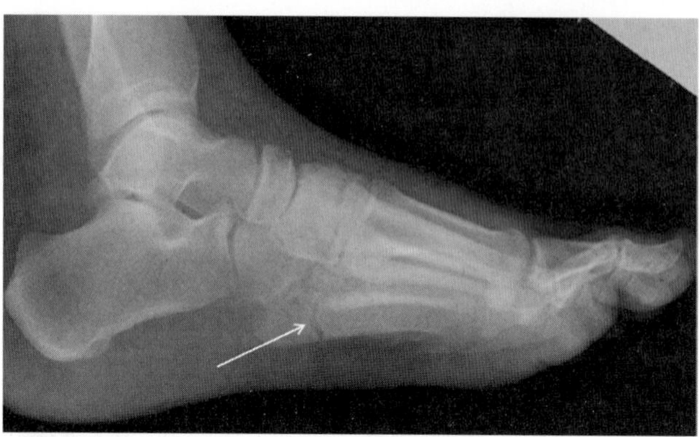

Figure 2B-28 T1 MRI (left image) and T2 MRI (right image) of Torn Achilles Tendon:

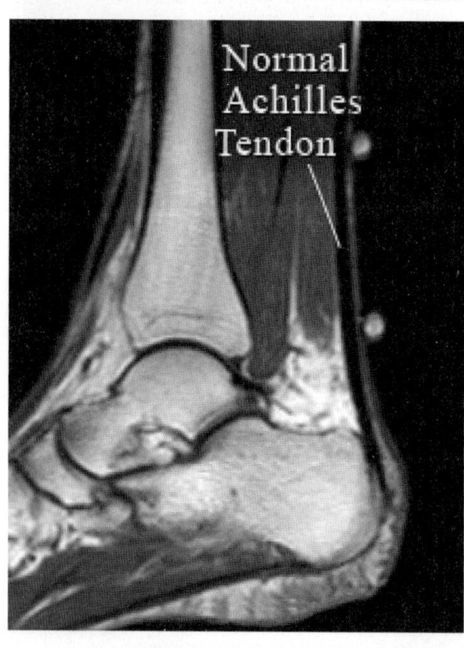

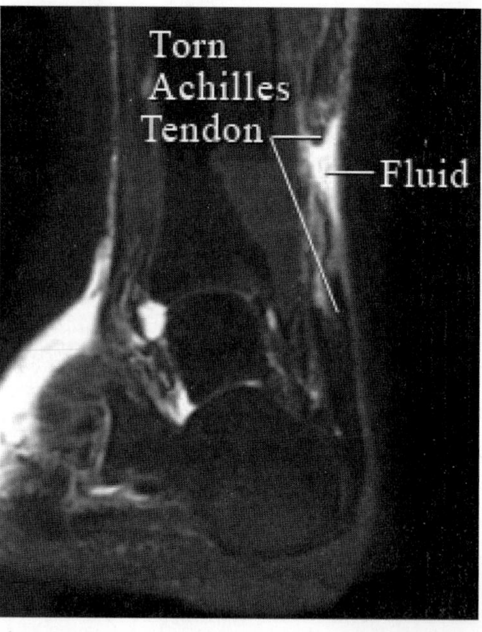

Figure 2B-29 Coronal T1 MRI of Talar Dome Osteochondral Defect:

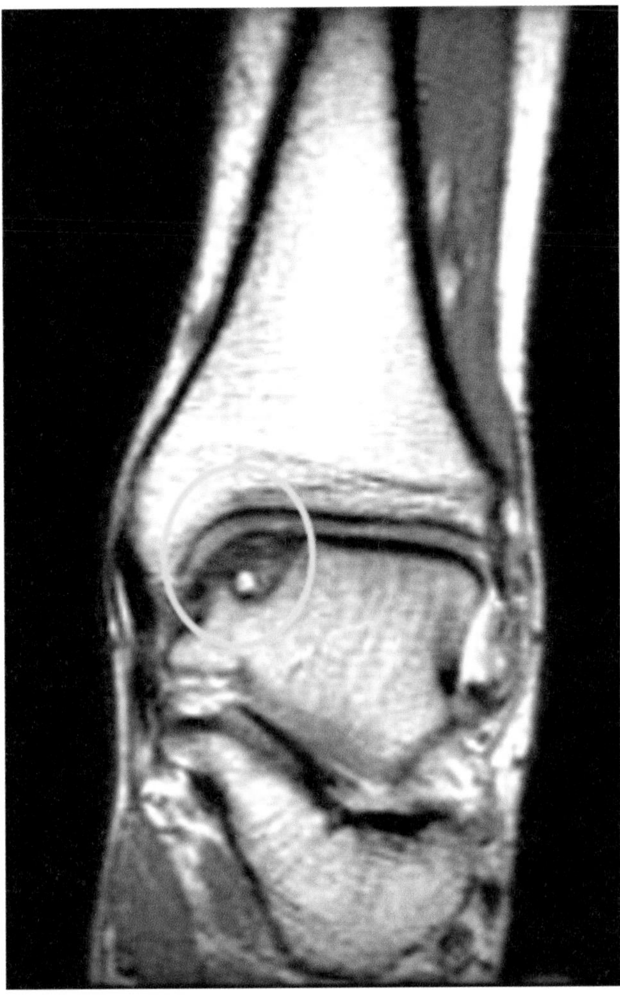

Figure 2B-30 Coronal T1 MRI (left image) and Axial T2 MRI (right image) of Posterior Tibial Tendonitis (arrow):

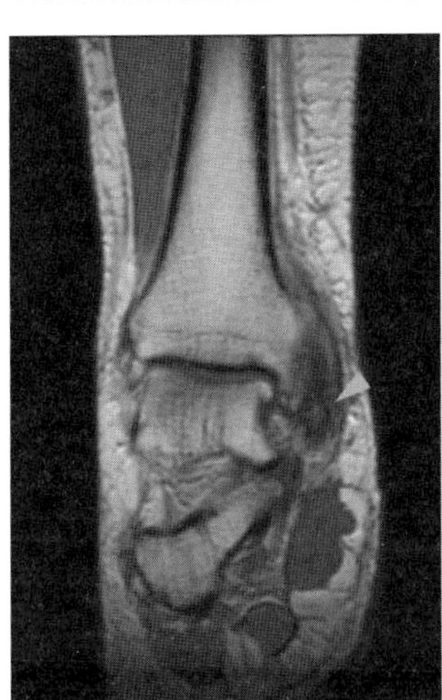

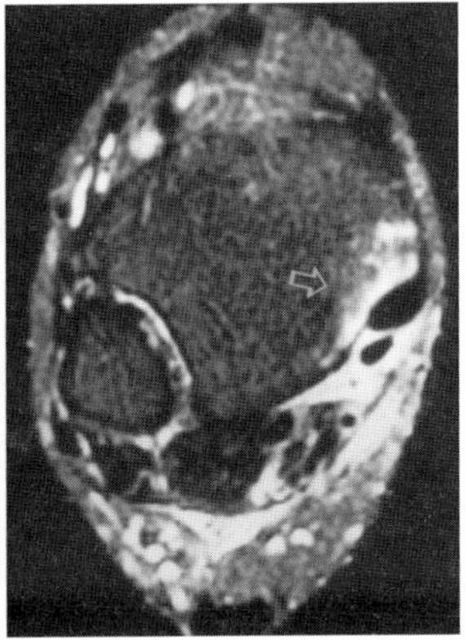

Figure 2B-31 AP Radiographic View of Normal Foot:

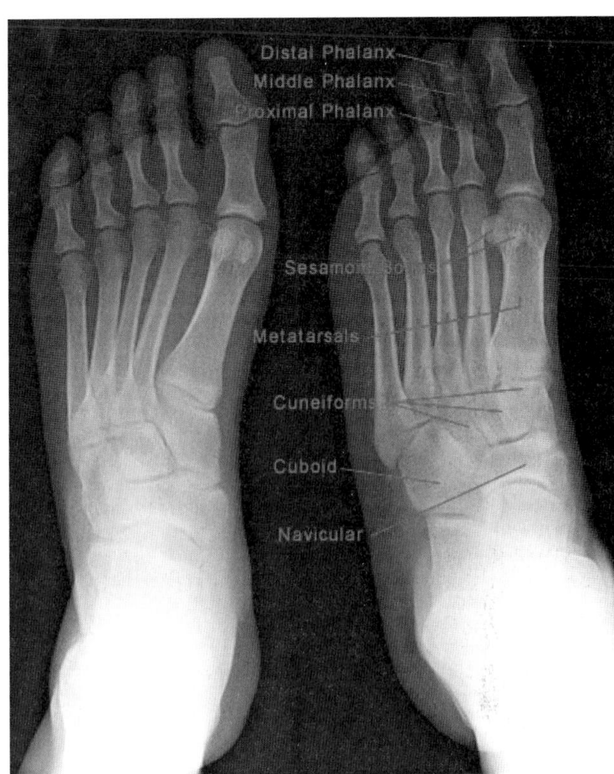

Figure 2B-32 Full Body Bone Scan of Insufficiency Rib Fractures:

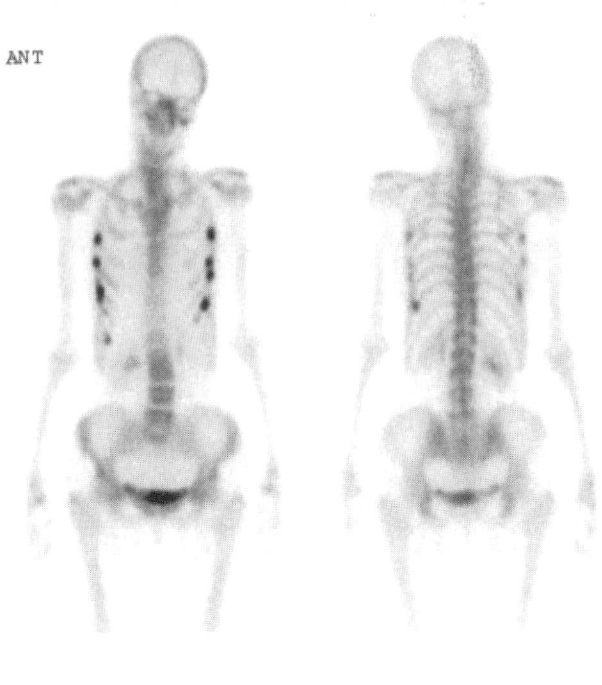

Ultrasound Images

Figure 2B-33 Ultrasound Image of Muscles of the Anterolateral Abdominal Wall:

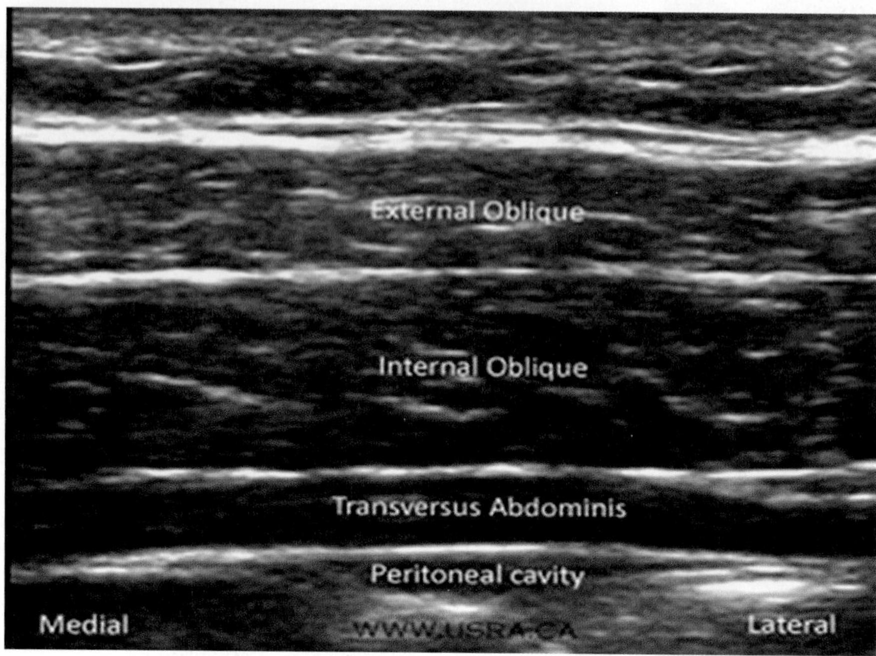

From: http://www.usra.ca/tapscan.php

Figure 2B-34 Lateral Ultrasound Image of Achilles Tendon Rupture:

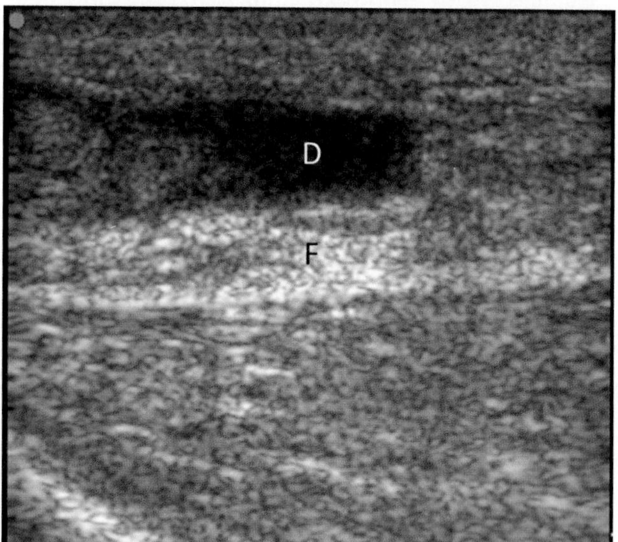

Dark, anechoic area is the palpable defect (D). White, hyperechoic area just below the defect is the fascia/tendon sheath separating the deep compartment muscles/tendons from the superficial muscles (F). Proximal segment is to the right on this image; distal segment is to the left.

Figure 2B-35 AP Ultrasound Image of Partially Denervated Infraspinatus Muscle:

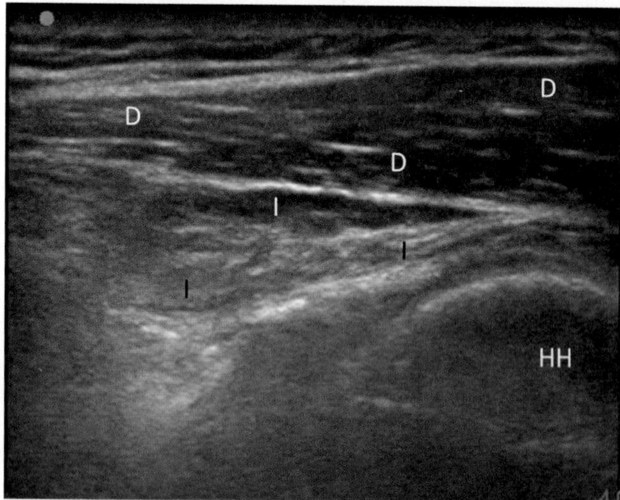

I = the infraspinatus muscle. Since the muscle is mostly denervated as confirmed by EMG, most of the infraspinatus appears hyperechoic (white or light). The darker, hypoechoic area is the posterior deltoid muscle (D).
HH = The posterior aspect of the head of the humerus.

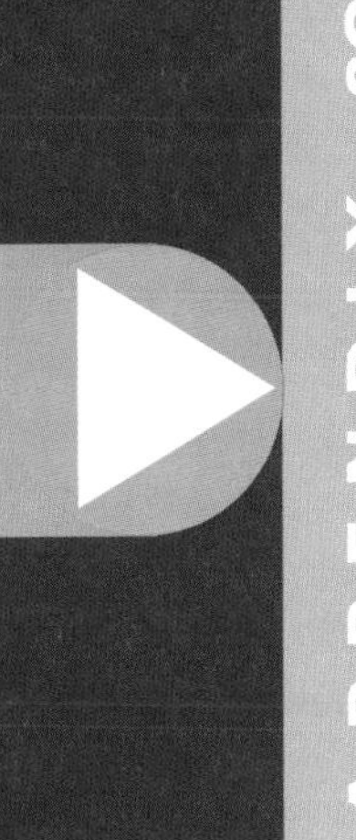

APPENDIX 2C

Review Questions and Case Studies

(Answers to all Review Questions and Case Studies can be found in Chapter 17)

1. Which motion at the glenohumeral joint has the greatest limitation if the diagnosis is adhesive capsulitis?

2. When considering the concave-convex rule, to which joints in the spine does the concave rule apply?

3. Which special test when applied to the ankle/foot is BEST used to identify ligamentous instability of the calcaneofibular ligament?

4. What are the major differences in diagnostic characteristics and pattern of joint dysfunction between osteoarthritis and rheumatoid arthritis?

5. Based on Clinical Practice Guidelines for Knee Ligament Sprain, which intervention has the strongest overall evidence for effectiveness?

6. Following a total hip replacement, in the acute phase, which positions should be avoided in bed positioning and activities involving bed mobility?

7. For an anteriorly displaced articular disc at the TMJ, what is the primary joint mobilization technique?

Case Study #1

Patient Profile

- Gender: Female
- Age: 49

Presenting Problem/Current Condition

- Patient referred to outpatient physical therapy with a chief complaint of right-sided neck pain
- Insidious onset upon waking up 3 days ago
- Pain and numbness extending to right posterior forearm and dorsum of hand, occasionally extending to the 3rd digit
- Arm weakness

Past Medical History

- History of hypertension
- Occasional headaches associated with neck pain

Other Information

- School teacher
- Obese, BMI=34
- Occasional consumption of alcohol

Question #1

What elements from the patient interview make a diagnosis of cervical radiculopathy most likely?

1. Associated referred pain to the right upper extremity.
2. Acute onset of unilateral neck pain.
3. Dermatomal paresthesia or numbness and myotomal muscle weakness.
4. History of headaches associated with neck movements.

Question #2

What are most common findings in the clinical examination for patients with cervical radiculopathy?

1. (+) ULTT, (–) Spurling's test, (–) cervical distraction test, painful ROM.
2. (+) ULTT, (+) Spurling's test, (–) cranial cervical flexion test, painful ROM.
3. (+) ULTT, (+) Spurling's test, (+) cervical distraction test, painful ROM.
4. (+) ULTT, (+) Spurling's test, (+) cranial cervical flexion test, painful ROM.

Question #3

What intervention is the **BEST** choice for reducing pain and improving function in acute cervical radiculopathy?

1. Transcutaneous electrical nerve stimulation (TENS).
2. Cryotherapy.
3. Thoracic manipulation.
4. Cervical mobilizing and stabilizing exercises.

Question #4

During the patient interview, the therapist learns that the patient has rheumatoid arthritis. What special test is most appropriate to determine if the patient has upper cervical spine instability?

1. Spurling's test.
2. Sharp Purser test.
3. Quadrant test.
4. Neck flexor muscle endurance test.

Case Study #2

Patient Profile

- Gender: Female
- Age: 68

Presenting Problem/Current Condition

- Referred to physical therapy with a chief complaint of right posterior thigh/knee pain for the past 6 weeks
- Onset after a long period of sitting during a train ride
- Knee stiffness on waking in the morning that lasts for less than 30 minutes
- Pain worsens with inactivity and improves with staying active

Past Medical History

- History of left knee replacement 2 years ago

Other Information

- DVT ruled out with Doppler ultrasound
- Denies any neurologic symptoms or low back pain

Question #1

What elements from the patient interview make a diagnosis of knee osteoarthritis (OA) more likely?

1. Knee stiffness upon first waking that lasts less than 30 minutes.
2. Knee stiffness upon first waking that lasts greater than 60 minutes.
3. Report of bilateral pain affecting multiple joints.
4. Joint swelling, warmth, and stiffness.

Question #2

What are most common findings in the clinical examination and diagnostic imaging for patients with knee osteoarthritis?

1. Hypomobile, painful joint; increased joint space and osteophytes on radiographs.
2. Hypomobile, painful joint; decreased joint space and osteophytes on radiographs.
3. Hypermobile, painful joint; increased joint space and osteophytes on radiographs.
4. Hypermobile, painful joint; decreased joint space and osteophytes on radiographs.

Question #3

What interventions offer strong evidence for reducing pain and improving function in osteoarthritis?

1. Transcutaneous electrical nerve stimulation (TENS).
2. Cryotherapy.
3. Therapeutic ultrasound.
4. Therapeutic exercise (neuromuscular and functional exercises).

3

Neuromuscular Physical Therapy

SUSAN B. O'SULLIVAN, CARRIE W. HOPPES, AND SCOTT W. SHAFFER

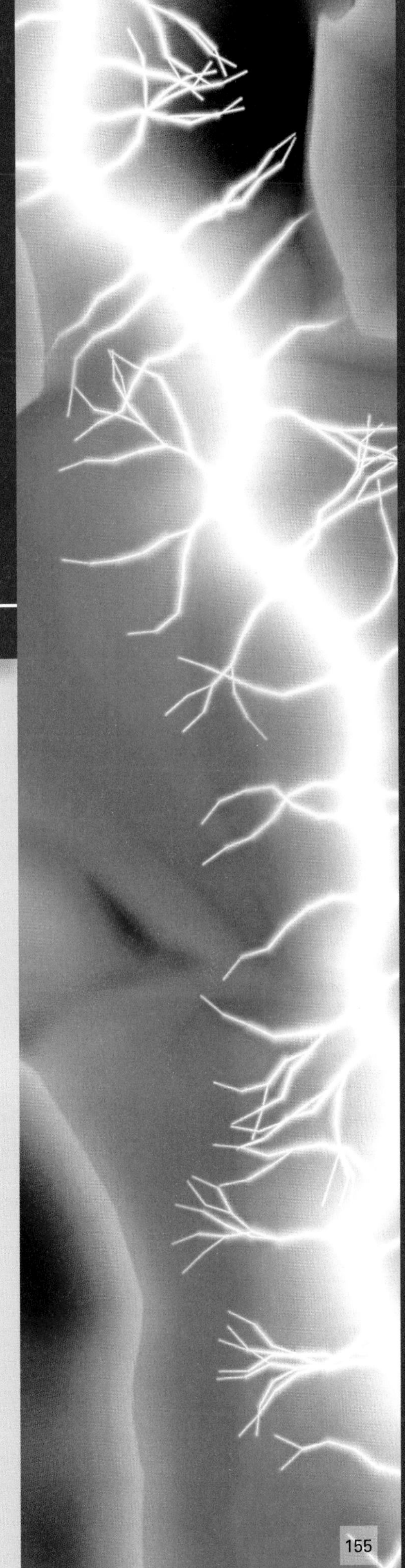

Chapter Outline

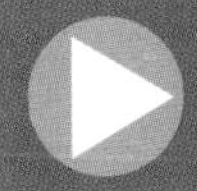

Study Tactics

Questions About the Neuromuscular System Comprise 23.5% of the NPTE, or a Total of 44–50 Questions.

The Number of Questions by Category Are:

- Examination of the Patient/Client: 15–17
- Evaluation, Differential Diagnosis, Prognosis: 14–16
- Interventions: 15–17

Examination of the Patient/Client. Focus on:

- Neuroanatomy. Comprehensive foundational knowledge of central nervous system (CNS) and peripheral nervous system (PNS) anatomy is critical to understanding components of the neuromuscular examination.
- Major neuromuscular health conditions across the lifespan seen by physical therapists. These include Parkinson's disease, multiple sclerosis, Guillain-Barré syndrome, stroke, spinal cord injuries, traumatic brain injuries, amyotrophic lateral sclerosis, cerebral palsy, Down syndrome, myopathies (e.g., muscular dystrophies), peripheral neuropathies, and neuromuscular junction disorders.
- Components of a comprehensive neurological examination and the relevance of the information for differential diagnosis and intervention
- Common tests and measures of cognition, strength, sensation, reflexes, tone assessment, coordination, mobility (sit to stand, stairs, and gait), balance, and fall risk that are used to assess patients with neuromuscular conditions
- Neuromuscular and nervous system outcomes measures and their application to effective patient management and interventions

Evaluation, Differential Diagnosis, and Prognosis. Focus on:

- Foundational knowledge of the CNS, PNS, and autonomic nervous system (ANS). Differential diagnosis questions may test knowledge of blood supply of the brain, specific domains of function in the CNS, somatotopic organization of the cerebral cortex (homunculus), and other areas of the CNS, spinal cord tracts, etc.
- The clinical features (signs and symptoms) and differential diagnosis of prevalent neuromuscular conditions across the lifespan. These include conditions that affect the CNS, PNS, and ANS.
- Development of a plan of care to include prognosis for common neuromuscular disorders
- Medical management and diagnostic studies of the neuromuscular and nervous systems to include imaging, laboratory tests, and surgical procedures
- Actions and side effects of pharmacological management of neuromuscular problems

Interventions. Focus on:

- Physical therapy interventions for neuromuscular conditions and their applications for rehabilitation, health promotion, and performance according to current best evidence
- Interventions for neuromuscular and neurologic disorders are often focused on a task specific approach. Intervention questions may also test knowledge of a specific neurotherapeutic technique (e.g., slow sustained stretching) for a given examination finding/impairment (e.g., hypertonicity or spasticity).
- Management of pediatric conditions. Knowledge of developmental milestones, reflexes, facilitation, and inhibition techniques are important.
- Motor control and motor learning strategies (when to use knowledge of results versus knowledge of performance, when to use different types of feedback) as related to interventions for neuromuscular conditions
- Potential adverse side effects or complications on the neuromuscular and nervous systems from physical therapy interventions (e.g., fatigue or weakness with exercise in patients with multiple sclerosis, Guillain-Barré, myasthenia gravis)

Anatomy and Physiology of the Nervous System

Brain

Cerebral Hemispheres (Telencephalon) (See Figure 3-1)

1. Convolutions of gray matter composed of gyri (crests) and sulci (fissures).
   a. Lateral central fissure (fissure of Sylvius) separates temporal lobe from frontal and parietal lobes.
   b. Longitudinal cerebral fissure separates the two hemispheres.
   c. Central sulcus separates the frontal lobe from the parietal lobe.
2. Paired hemispheres, consisting of six lobes on each side: frontal, parietal, temporal, occipital, insular, limbic.
   a. Frontal lobe.
      - Precentral gyrus: primary motor cortex for voluntary muscle activation.
      - Prefrontal cortex: controls emotions and judgments.
      - Broca's area: controls motor aspects of speech.
   b. Parietal lobe.
      - Postcentral gyrus: primary sensory cortex for integration of sensation.
      - Receives fibers conveying touch, proprioceptive, pain and temperature sensations from opposite side of body.
      - See Figure 3-2 for sensory cortical somatotopic organization.

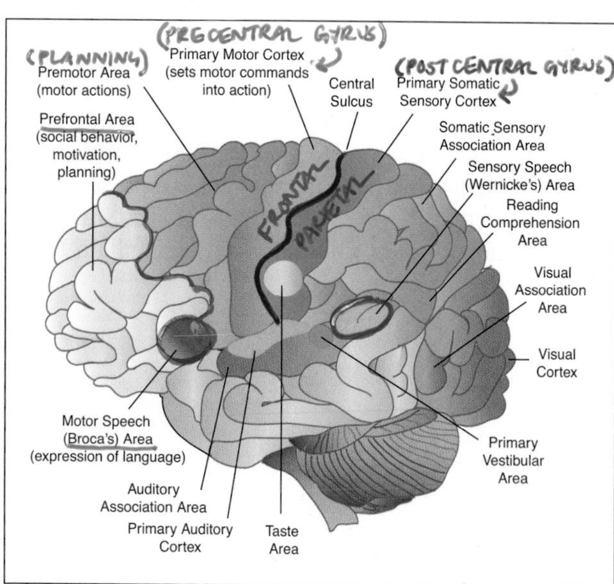

Figure 3-1 **Functional areas of the brain.**

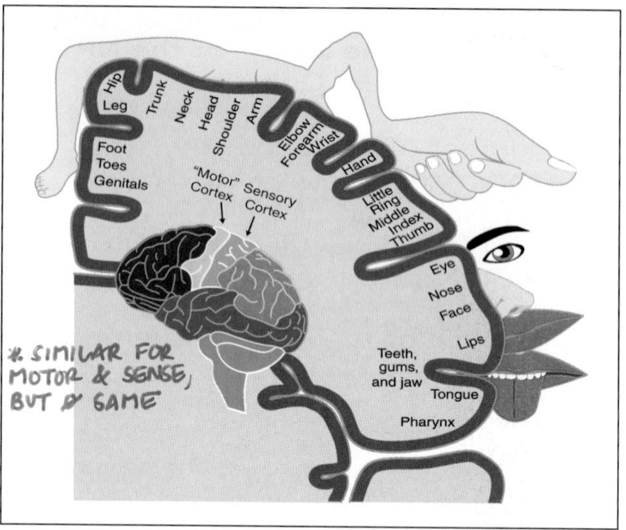

Figure 3-2 **Sensory Homunculus.**

Adapted from Nguyen JD, Duong H. Neurosurgery, Sensory Homunculus. 2020 Jul 31. In: StatPearls [Internet]. Treasure Island (FL): StatPearls Publishing; 2021 Jan (Image S. Bhimji MD). Image is a licensed with Creative Commons Attribution 4.0 International License, http://creativecommons.org/licenses/by/4.0/. Photo color scheme was adapted to a white background and black font.

   c. Temporal lobe.
      - Primary auditory cortex: receives/processes auditory stimuli.
      - Associative auditory cortex: processes auditory stimuli.
      - Wernicke's area: language comprehension.
      - Primary vestibular area: head position and movement, perception of vertical.
   d. Occipital lobe.
      - Primary visual cortex: receives/processes visual stimuli.
      - Visual association cortex: processes visual stimuli.
   e. Insula.
      - Deep within lateral sulcus, associated with visceral functions.
   f. Limbic system.
      - Consists of the limbic lobe (cingulate, parahippocampal and subcallosal gyri), hippocampal formation, amygdaloid nucleus, hypothalamus and anterior nucleus of thalamus.
      - Phylogenetically oldest part of the brain, concerned with instincts and emotions contributing to preservation of the individual.
      - Basic functions include feeding, aggression, emotions, and endocrine aspects of sexual response.

- Critical role in memory (especially emotionally memories), motivation, and learning.

3. White matter: myelinated nerve fibers located centrally.
   a. Transverse (commissural) fibers: interconnect the two hemispheres, including the corpus callosum (the largest), anterior commissure, and hippocampal commissure.
   b. Projection fibers: connect cerebral hemispheres with other portions of the brain and spinal cord.
   c. Association fibers: connect different portions of the cerebral hemispheres, allowing cortex to function as an integrated whole.
4. Basal ganglia (BG).
   a. Masses of gray matter deep within the cerebral hemispheres, including the striatum (caudate nucleus, nucleus accumbens, putamen), globus pallidus (external segment, internal segment), subthalamic nucleus and substantia nigra (compact part, reticular part). The term *lenticular nucleus* refers to the putamen and globus pallidus.
   b. Forms an associated motor system (extra-pyramidal system) with other nuclei in the subthalamus and the midbrain.
   c. Multiple circuits exist in the BG.
      - Oculomotor circuit (caudate loop): originates in frontal and supplementary motor eye fields; projects to caudate; functions with saccadic eye movements.
      - Motor loop (putamen loop): originates in precentral motor and postcentral somatosensory areas; projects to and excites putamen neurons; putamen cells inhibit globus pallidus neurons, which in turn boosts activity in the ventral lateral nucleus and supplemental motor area; functions to scale amplitude and velocity of movements; reinforces selected pattern, suppresses conflicting patterns; preparatory for movement (i.e., motor set, anticipatory movement).
      - Limbic circuit: originates in prefrontal and limbic areas of cortex; to BG; to prefrontal cortex; functions to organize behaviors (executive functions, problem-solving, motivation) and for procedural learning.

Diencephalon

1. Thalamus.
   a. Sensory nuclei: integrate and relay sensory information from body, face, retina, cochlea, and taste receptors to cerebral cortex and subcortical regions; smell (olfaction) is the exception.
   b. Motor nuclei: relay motor information from cerebellum and globus pallidus to precentral motor cortex.
   c. Other nuclei: assist in integration of visceral and somatic functions.
2. Subthalamus: involved in control of several functional pathways for sensory, motor, and reticular function.
3. Hypothalamus.
   a. Integrates and controls the functions of the autonomic nervous system and the neuroendocrine system.
   b. Maintains body homeostasis: regulates body temperature, eating, water balance, anterior pituitary function/sexual behavior, and emotion.
4. Epithalamus.
   a. Habenular nuclei: integrate olfactory, visceral, and somatic afferent pathways.
   b. Pineal gland: secretes hormones that influence the pituitary gland and several other organs; influences circadian rhythm.

Brainstem

1. Midbrain (mesencephalon).
   a. Connects pons to cerebrum; superior peduncle connects midbrain to cerebellum.
   b. Contains cerebral peduncles (two lateral halves), each divided into an anterior part or basis (crus cerebri and substantia nigra) and a posterior part (tegmentum).
   c. Tegmentum contains all ascending tracts and some descending tracts; the red nucleus receives fibers from the cerebellum; is the origin for the rubrospinal tract, important for coordination; contains cranial nerve nuclei: oculomotor III and trochlear. IV
   d. Substantia nigra is a large motor nucleus connecting with the basal ganglia and cortex; it is important in motor control and muscle tone.
   e. Superior colliculus is an important relay station for vision and visual reflexes; the inferior colliculus is an important relay station for hearing and auditory reflexes.
   f. Periaqueductal gray contains endorphin-producing cells and descending tracts that are important for pain and reflex modulation.
2. Pons. resp. rate, HR
   a. Connects the medulla oblongata to the midbrain, allowing passage of important ascending and descending tracts.
   b. Anterior basal part acts as a bridge to cerebellum (middle cerebellar peduncle).
   c. Midline raphe nuclei project widely and are important for modulating pain and controlling arousal.
   d. Tegmentum contains several important cranial nerve nuclei: abducens VI, trigeminal V, facial VII, vestibulocochlear. VIII
3. Medulla oblongata.
   a. Connects spinal cord with pons.
   b. Contains relay nuclei of dorsal columns (gracilis and cuneatus); fibers cross to give rise to medial lemniscus.
   c. Inferior cerebellar peduncle relays dorsal spinocerebellar tract to cerebellum.

d. Corticospinal tracts cross (decussate) in pyramids.
e. Medial longitudinal fasciculus arises from vestibular nuclei and extends throughout brainstem and upper cervical spinal cord; important for control of head movements and gaze stabilization (vestibulo-ocular reflex).
f. Olivary nuclear complex connects cerebellum to brainstem and is important for voluntary movement control.
g. Contains several important cranial nerve nuclei: hypoglossal, dorsal nucleus of vagus and vestibulocochlear.
h. Contains important centers for vital functions: cardiac, respiratory, and vasomotor centers.

4. Reticular Activating System (RAS).
   a. Anterior-most segment of the brainstem (midbrain, pons, and medulla).
   b. Includes four nuclei that produce key neurotransmitters (e.g., serotonin, norepinephrine, acetylcholine) that assist with attention, arousal, and modulation of muscle tone.
   c. Damage to the RAS or circuits to or from the cortex result in dysregulation of sleep-wake cycles, impaired arousal, and ability to focus.

Cerebellum

1. Located behind dorsal pons and medulla in posterior fossa.
2. Structure.
   a. Joined to brainstem by three pairs of peduncles: superior, middle, and inferior.
   b. Comprises two hemispheres and midline vermis; cerebellar cortex, underlying white matter; and four paired deep nuclei.
   c. Archicerebellum (flocculonodular lobe) connects with vestibular system and is concerned with equilibrium and regulation of muscle tone; helps coordinate vestibulo-ocular reflex.
   d. Paleocerebellum (rostral cerebellum, anterior lobe; also known as spinocerebellum) receives input from proprioceptive pathways and is concerned with modifying muscle tone and synergistic actions of muscles; it is important in maintenance of posture and voluntary movement control.
   e. Neocerebellum (lateral cerebellar hemispheres, posterior lobe; also known as pontocerebellum or functionally as cerebrocerebellum); receives input from corticopontocerebellar tracts and olivocerebellar fibers; it is concerned with the smooth coordination of voluntary movements; ensures accurate force, direction, and extent of movement. Important for motor learning, sequencing of movements, and visually triggered movements. May have a role in assisting cognitive function and mental imagery.

Spinal Cord

General Structure (See Figure 3-3)

1. Cylindrical mass of nerve tissue extending from the foramen magnum in the skull continuous with the medulla to the lower border of the first lumbar vertebra in the conus medullaris.
2. Divided into 30 segments—8 cervical, 12 thoracic, 5 lumbar, 5 sacral—and a few coccygeal segments.

Central Gray Matter

1. Two anterior (ventral) and two posterior (dorsal) horns united by gray commissure with central canal (Figure 3-4).
2. Anterior horns contain cell bodies that give rise to efferent (motor) neurons: alpha motor neurons to affect muscles and gamma motor neurons to affect muscle spindles.
3. Posterior horns contain afferent (sensory) neurons with cell bodies located in the dorsal root ganglia.
4. Two enlargements (cervical and lumbosacral) for origins of nerves of upper and lower extremities.
5. Lateral horn is found in thoracic and upper lumbar segments for preganglionic fibers of the autonomic nervous system.

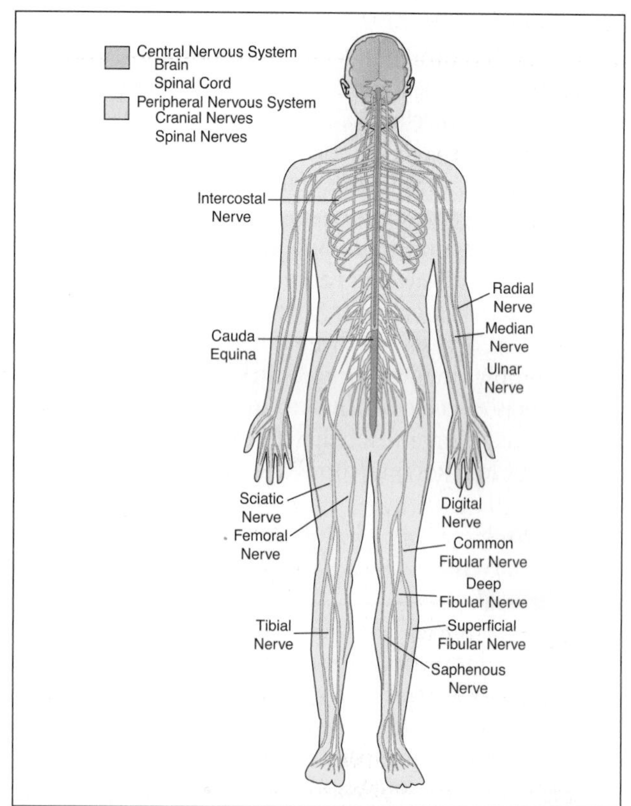

Figure 3-3 Overview of nervous system.

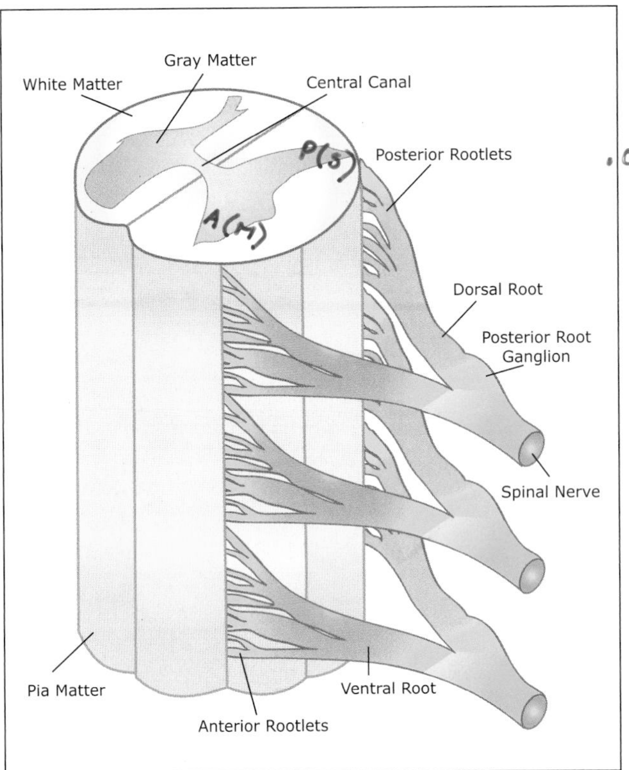

Figure 3-4 **Spinal cord: Anterior cross section.**

White Matter

1. Anterior (ventral), lateral, and posterior (dorsal) myelinated columns or funiculi.
2. Ascending fiber systems (sensory pathways).
   a. Dorsal columns/medial lemniscal system: convey sensations of proprioception, vibration, and tactile discrimination; divided into fasciculus cuneatus (upper extremity tracts, laterally located) and fasciculus gracilis (lower extremity tracts, medially located); neurons ascend to medulla where fibers cross (lemniscal decussation) to form medial lemniscus; ascend to thalamus and then to somatosensory cortex.
   b. Spinothalamic tracts: convey sensations of pain and temperature (lateral spinothalamic tract), and crude touch (anterior spinothalamic tract); tracts ascend one or two ipsilateral spinal cord segments (Lissauer's tract), synapse and cross in spinal cord to opposite side and ascend in ventrolateral spinothalamic system.
   c. Spinocerebellar tracts: convey proprioception information from muscle spindles, Golgi tendon organs, and touch and pressure receptors to cerebellum for control of voluntary movements; dorsal spinocerebellar tract ascends to ipsilateral inferior cerebellar peduncle, and ventrospinocerebellar tract ascends to contralateral and ipsilateral superior cerebellar peduncle.
   d. Spinoreticular tracts: convey deep and chronic pain to reticular formation of brainstem via diffuse, polysynaptic pathways.
3. Descending fiber systems (motor pathways).
   a. Corticospinal tracts: arise from primary motor cortex, descend in brainstem, cross in medulla (pyramidal decussation), via lateral corticospinal tract to ventral gray matter (anterior horn cells); 10% of fibers do not cross and travel in anterior corticospinal tract to cervical and upper thoracic segments; important for voluntary motor control.
   b. Vestibulospinal tracts: arise from vestibular nucleus and descend to spinal cord in lateral (uncrossed) and medial (crossed and uncrossed) vestibulospinal tracts; important for control of muscle tone, antigravity muscles, and postural reflexes.
   c. Rubrospinal tracts: arise in contralateral red nucleus and descend in lateral columns to spinal gray matter; assist in motor function.
   d. Reticulospinal system: arises in the reticular formation of the brainstem and descends (crossed and uncrossed) in ventral and lateral columns, terminates both on dorsal gray (modifies transmission of sensation, especially pain) and on ventral gray (influences gamma motor neurons and spinal reflexes).
   e. Tectospinal tract: arises from superior colliculus (midbrain) and descends to ventral gray; assists in head-turning responses to visual stimuli.
4. Somatotopic organization spinal cord pathways.
   a. Spinal cord pathways maintain somatotopic organization (please see Figure 3-5).
   b. Explains variability in patients with partial spinal cord injuries, chronic compression (e.g., cervical myelopathy), or disease (e.g., multiple sclerosis with demyelinating plaques).
   c. See Table 3-22 for clinical examples of spinal cord injuries.

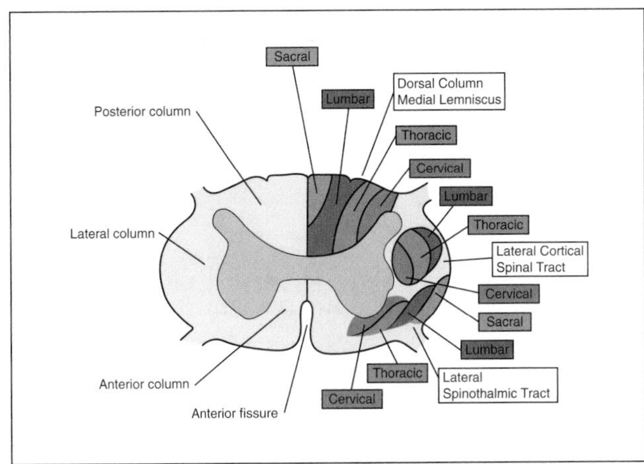

Figure 3-5 **Spinal cord somatotopic organization.**

Autonomic Nervous System (ANS)

1. Concerned with innervations of involuntary structures: smooth muscle, heart, glands; helps maintain homeostasis (constant internal body environment).
2. Two divisions: sympathetic and parasympathetic; both have afferent and efferent nerve fibers; preganglionic and postganglionic fibers.
   a. Sympathetic (thoracolumbar division, T1–L2): prepares body for fight or flight, emergency responses; increases heart rate and blood pressure, constricts peripheral blood vessels (with exception of vasodilation of skeletal muscles), and redistributes blood; inhibits peristalsis (Figure 3-6).
   b. Parasympathetic (craniosacral division, CN III, VII, IX, X; pelvic nerves): conserves and restores homeostasis; slows heart rate and reduces blood pressure; increases peristalsis and glandular activity (Figure 3-7).
3. Autonomic plexuses: cardiac, pulmonary, celiac (solar), hypogastric, pelvic.
4. Modulated by brain centers.
   a. Descending autonomic system: arises from control centers in hypothalamus and lower brainstem (cardiac, respiratory, vasomotor) and projects to preganglionic ANS segments in thoracolumbar (sympathetic) and craniosacral (parasympathetic) segments.

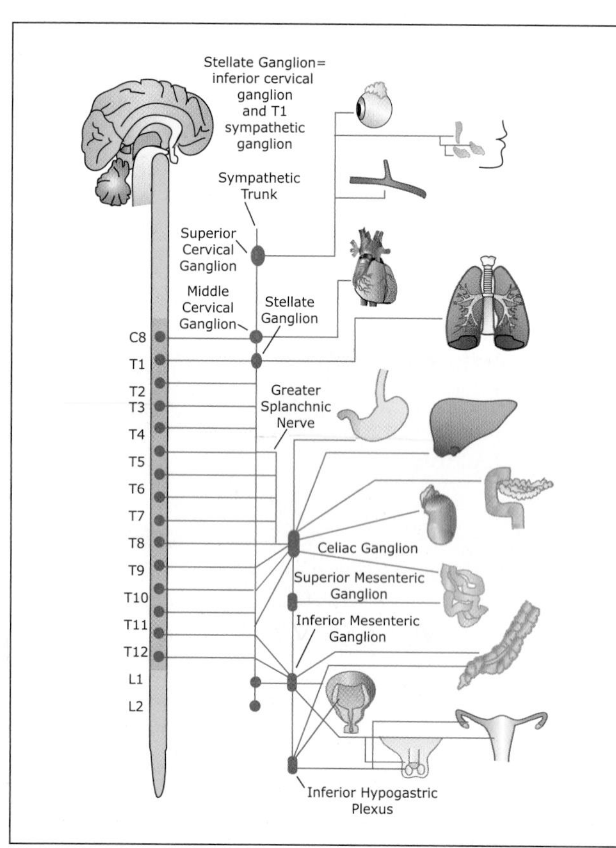

Figure 3-6 ANS-sympathetic division.

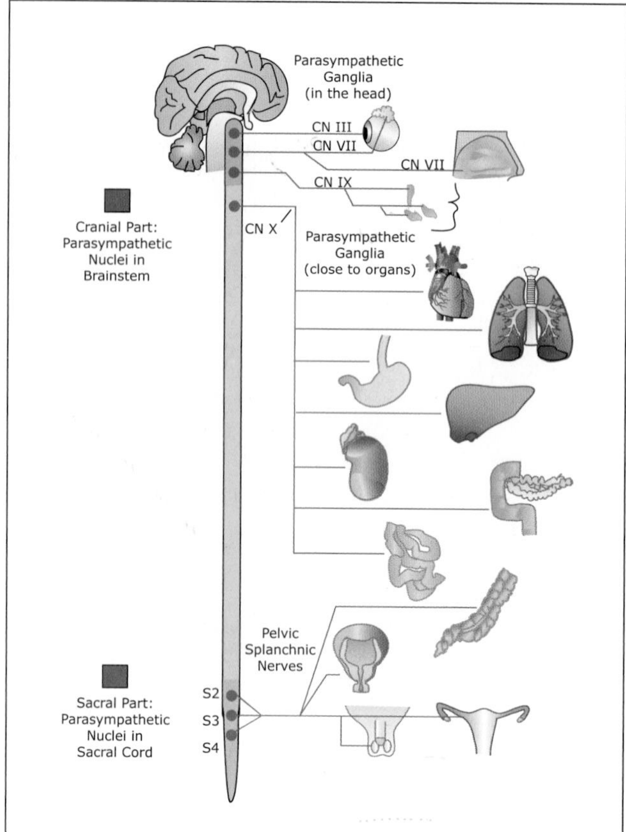

Figure 3-7 ANS-parasympathetic division.

   b. Cranial nerves: visceral afferent sensations via glossopharyngeal and vagus nerves; efferent outflow via oculomotor, facial, glossopharyngeal, and vagus nerves.

CNS Support Structures

Bony Structure

1. Skull (cranium): rigid bony chamber that contains the brain and facial skeleton, with an opening (foramen magnum) at its base.

Meninges

1. Three membranes that envelop the brain.
   a. Dura mater: outer, tough, fibrous membrane attached to inner surface of cranium; forms falx and tentorium.
   b. Arachnoid: delicate, vascular membrane.
   c. Pia mater: thin, vascular membrane that covers the brain surface; forms tela choroidea of ventricles.
2. Subarachnoid space: formed by arachnoid and pia mater, contains cerebrospinal fluid (CSF) and cisterns, major arteries.

Ventricles

1. Four cavities or ventricles that are filled with CSF and communicate with each other and with the spinal cord canal.

2. Lateral ventricles: large, irregularly shaped with anterior (frontal), posterior (occipital), and inferior (temporal) horns; communicates with third ventricle through foramen of Monro.
3. Third ventricle: located posterior and deep between the two thalami; third ventricle communicates with fourth ventricle through cerebral aqueduct.
4. Fourth ventricle: pyramid-shaped cavity located in pons and medulla; foramina (openings) of Luschka and Magendie communicate with fourth ventricle through subarachnoid space.

Cerebrospinal Fluid (CSF)

1. Provides mechanical support (cushions brain), controls brain excitability by regulating ionic composition, aids in exchange of nutrients and waste products.
2. Produced in choroid plexuses in ventricles.

Blood-Brain Barrier

1. Selective restriction of blood-borne substances from entering the CNS.
2. Associated with capillary endothelial cells.

Blood Supply

1. Brain is 2% of body weight with a circulation of 18% of total blood volume.
2. Carotid system: internal carotid arteries arise off common carotids and branch to form anterior and middle cerebral arteries; supplies a large area of brain and many deep structures.
3. Vertebrobasilar system: vertebral arteries arise off subclavian arteries and unite to form the basilar artery; this vessel bifurcates into two posterior cerebral arteries; supplies the brainstem, cerebellum, occipital lobe, and parts of thalamus.
4. Circle of Willis: formed by anterior communicating artery, connecting the two anterior cerebral arteries and the posterior communicating artery, connecting each posterior and middle cerebral artery (Figure 3-8).
5. See Figure 3-9 for associated Cortex Vascular Zones.
6. Venous drainage: includes cerebral veins and dural venous sinuses.
7. See Neurological Dysfunction, Cerebrovascular Accident for a discussion of specific stroke syndromes (characteristic signs and symptoms associated with occlusion of specific cerebral vessels).

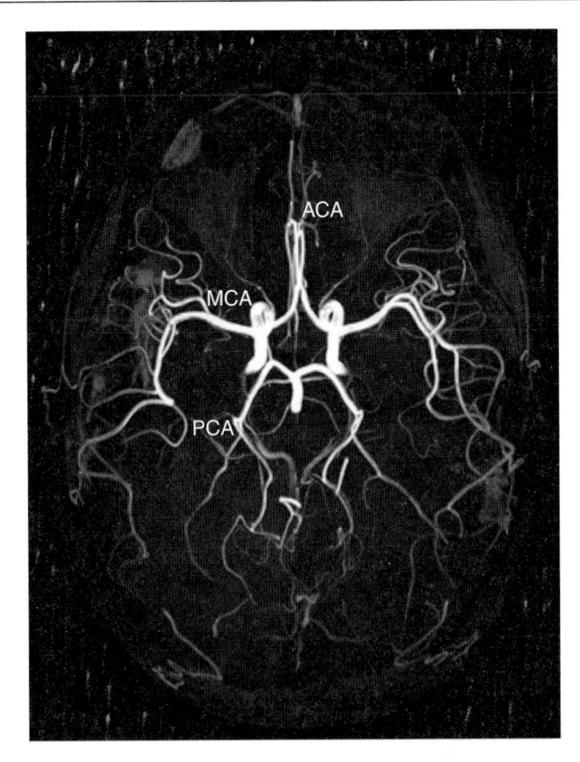

Figure 3-8 **MRI of circle of Willis and other cerebral arteries.**

ACA = anterior cerebral artery, MCA = middle cerebral artery, PCA = posterior cerebral artery.

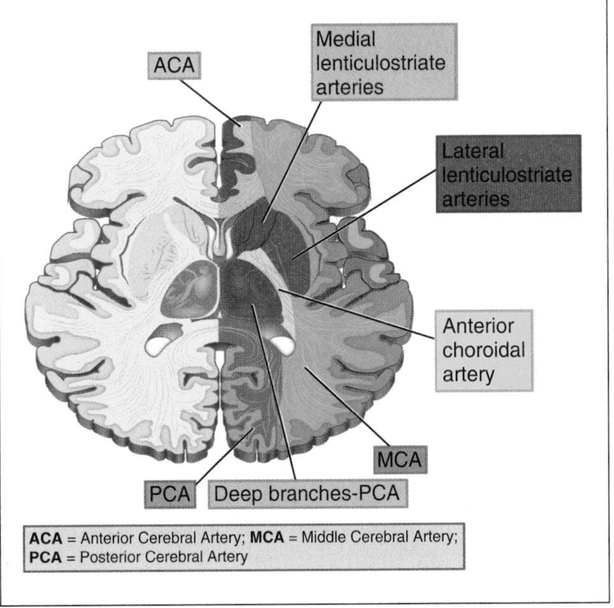

Figure 3-9 **Cortex vascular zones.**

Neurons

Structure

1. Neurons vary in size and complexity.
   a. Cell bodies (genetic center) with dendrites (receptive surface area to receive information via synapses).
   b. Axons conduct impulses away from the cell body (one-way conduction).

c. Synapses allow communication between neurons; chemical neurotransmitters are released (chemical synapses) or electrical signals pass directly from cell to cell (electrical synapses).

2. Neuron groupings and types.
   a. Nuclei are compact groups of nerve cell bodies; in the peripheral nervous system, these groups are called ganglia.
   b. Projection neurons carry impulses to other parts of the CNS.
   c. Interneurons are short relay neurons and assist in the inhibition or excitation of projection neurons and/or alpha motor neurons (e.g., reflexes).
   d. Axon bundles are called tracts or fasciculi; in the spinal cord, collections of tracts are called columns or funiculi.
3. Neuroglia: support cells that do not transmit signals; important for myelin production (oligodendrocytes-central nervous system; Schwann cell peripheral nervous system) and neuronal support, maintenance of K+ levels, form tight junction for blood-brain barrier, and reuptake of neurotransmitters after neural transmission at synapses (Astrocytes).

Function. Neuronal Signaling

1. Resting membrane potential: positive on outside, negative on inside (about –70 mV).
2. Action potential: increased permeability of Na+ and influx into cell with outflow of K+ results in polarity changes (inside to about +35 mV) and depolarization; generation of an action potential is all-or-none.
3. Conduction velocity is proportional to axon diameter and the degree of myelination.
4. Repolarization results from activation of K+ channels.
5. Myelinated axons: axons are covered with myelin with small gaps (nodes of Ranvier) where myelin is absent; the action potential jumps from one node to the next, termed *saltatory conduction*; myelin functions to increase speed of conduction and conserve energy.
6. Nerve fiber types.
   a. A fibers: larger diameter, myelinated, and faster conduction (degree of myelination and fiber size decreases from A-alpha to A-delta).
      - Alpha: proprioception, somatic motor.
      - Beta: touch, pressure.
      - Gamma: motor to muscle spindles.
      - Delta: fast/sharp/localized pain, temperature, and crude touch.
   b. B fibers: small, myelinated, conduct less rapidly; preganglionic autonomic.
   c. C fibers: smallest, unmyelinated, slowest conducting. Polymodal fibers that respond to mechanical, chemical, and thermal stimuli.
      - Dorsal root: pain, temperature, and reflex responses.
      - Sympathetic: postganglionic sympathetics.

Peripheral Nervous System

Peripheral Nerve (Lower Motor Neuron [LMN])

1. Motor (efferent) fibers originate from motor nuclei (cranial nerves) or anterior horn cells (spinal nerves).
2. Sensory (afferent) fibers originate in cells outside of brainstem or spinal cord with sensory ganglia (cranial nerves) or dorsal root ganglia (spinal nerves) (Figure 3-4).
3. Autonomic nervous system fibers: sympathetic fibers (Figure 3-6) at thoracolumbar spinal segments and parasympathetic fibers at craniosacral segments (Figure 3-7).

Cranial Nerves (CN)

1. Twelve pairs of cranial nerves; all nerves are distributed to the head and neck, except CN X, which is distributed to the thorax and abdomen.
2. Cranial nerve (CN) assessment provides information on specific CN function and assists practitioners in localizing brain stem/cortical lesions (Table 3-1).
3. CN I, II, and VIII are pure sensory, carry special senses of smell, vision, hearing, and equilibrium.
4. CN III, IV, and VI are pure motor, controlling eye movements and pupillary constriction.
5. CN XI and XII are pure motor, innervating sternocleidomastoid, trapezius, and tongue.
6. CN V, VII, IX, and X are mixed motor and sensory; involved in chewing (V), facial expression (VII), swallowing (IX, X), vocal sounds (X); sensations from head (V, VII, IX), alimentary tract, heart, vessels, and lungs (IX, X), and taste (VII, IX, X).
7. CN III, VII, IX, and X carry parasympathetic fibers of ANS; involved in control of smooth muscles of inner eye (III); salivatory and lacrimal glands (VII); parotid gland (IX); muscles of heart, lung, and bowel (X).

Spinal Nerves

1. 31 pairs of spinal nerves; spinal nerves are divided into groups (8 cervical, 12 thoracic, 5 lumbar, 5 sacral, and 1 coccygeal) and correspond to vertebral segments; each has a ventral root and a dorsal root.
2. Ventral (anterior) root: efferent (motor) fibers to voluntary muscles (alpha motor neurons, gamma motor neurons), and to viscera, glands, and smooth muscles (preganglionic ANS fibers).
3. Dorsal (posterior) root: afferent (sensory) fibers from sensory receptors from skin, joints, and muscles; each dorsal root possesses a dorsal root ganglion (cell bodies of sensory neurons); there is no dorsal root for C1.
4. The term *dermatome* refers to a specific segmental skin area innervated by spinal sensory axons (Figure 3-10).

Table 3-1

Examination of Cranial Nerve Integrity

NERVE	FUNCTION	TEST	POSSIBLE ABNORMAL FINDINGS
I Olfactory	Smell	Test sense of smell on each side: use common, nonirritating odors; close off other nostril	Anosmia (inability to detect smells), seen with frontal lobe lesions
II Optic	Vision	Test visual acuity Central: Snellen eye chart; test each eye separately by covering other eye; test at distance of 20 feet Visual fields: test peripheral vision by confrontation	Blindness, myopia (impaired far vision); presbyopia (impaired near vision) Visual field defects: (homonymous hemianopsia and bitemporal hemianpsia)
III Oculomotor	Pupillary reflex (tests CN II-afferent response and CN III-efferent response) Accommodation Convergence	Shine light in eye: pupil Eye accommodates to light Pupils move medially when viewing object at close range	Absence of pupillary constriction in both eyes indicates CN II lesion and absent in tested eyes indicates CN III lesion Lateral strabismus (Exotropia) Unequal pupils (Anisocoria)
III, IV, VI Oculomotor, Trochlear, and Abducens	Extraocular movements CN III: turns eye up, down, in; constricts pupil and elevates eyelid CN IV: turns adducted eye down CN VI: turns eye out	Test extraocular movements: ask patient to look up, down, medial, and lateral Ask patient to look in and down Ask patient to look lateral	Lateral strabismus: eyeball turns lateral; can cause diplopia or nystagmus CN III lesions also result in complete ptosis and dilated pupil Inability to look down and in Medial strabismus: eyeball turns inward; can cause diplopia or nystagmus
V Trigeminal	Sensory: face Sensory: cornea Motor: temporal and masseter muscles	Test pain, light touch sensations: forehead, cheeks, jaw (eyes closed) Test corneal reflex: touch lightly with wisp of cotton Palpate muscles; have patient clench teeth, hold against resistance	Loss of facial sensations Loss of corneal reflex ipsilaterally Weakness, wasting of muscles of mastication Deviation of jaw when opened to ipsilateral side abnormal findings: Assymetry of jaw movement Assymetry of jaw strength
VII Facial	Facial expression Sensory Function: taste to anterior two thirds of tongue	Test motor function facial muscles: raise eyebrows, frown, show teeth, smile, close eyes tightly, puff out both cheeks Apply sweet, salty, and sour solutions to outer and lateral portions of anterior tongue using a cotton swab (occlude vision)	Paralysis ipsilateral facial muscles: inability to close eye, droop in corner of mouth, difficulty with speech articulation; PNI: Bell's palsy (CN VII) results in complete ipsilateral facial paralysis; UMN lesion: above the facial nucleus results in paralysis in the contralateral lower part of the face Incorrectly identifies solution Decreased taste
VIII Vestibulocochlear (Acoustic)	Vestibular function Test eye-head coordination: vestibulo-ocular reflex (VOR) Cochlear function	Test balance: vestibulospinal function Test eye–head coordination: vestibulo-ocular reflex (VOR) Test auditory acuity Test for lateralization (Weber's test): place vibrating tuning fork on top of head, mid position; check if sound heard in one ear, or equally in both Compare air and bone conduction (Rinne's test): place vibrating tuning fork on mastoid bone, then close to ear canal; sound heard longer through air than bone	Vertigo, dysequilibrium Gaze instability with head movement, nystagmus (an involuntary, rapid, rhythmic, oscillatory eye movement) Deafness, impaired hearing, tinnitus Unilateral sensorineural loss: sound lateralized to good ear Sensorineural loss: sound heard in good ear Conductive loss: sound heard through bone is equal to or longer than air

(Continued)

Table 3-1

Examination of Cranial Nerve Integrity (Continued)

NERVE	FUNCTION	TEST	POSSIBLE ABNORMAL FINDINGS
IX Glossopharyngeal	Sensory function: posterior one-third of tongue, pharynx, middle ear	Apply sweet, salty, and sour solutions to posterior tongue	Incorrectly identifies solution, loss of taste on posterior tongue
IX/X Glossopharyngeal and Vagus	Phonation	Listen to voice quality	Dysphonia: hoarseness denotes vocal cord paralysis; nasal quality denotes palatal weakness
	Swallowing	Examine for difficulty in swallowing	Dysphagia: difficulty swallowing; loss of swallowing refexes
IX/X Glossopharyngeal and Vagus	Palatal, pharynx control	Have patient say "ah"; observe motion of soft palate (elevates) and position of uvula (remains midline)	Dysarthria: difficulty articulating words clearly, slurs words
	Gag reflex	Stimulate back of throat lightly on each side	Paralysis: palate fails to elevate (lesion of CN X); asymmetrical elevation: unilateral paralysis Absent reflex: lesion of CN IX; possibly CN X
XI Accessory	Muscle function Trapezius muscle	Examine bulk, strength Inability to elevate shoulder girdle or put shoulder to ear	Atrophy, fasciculations, weakness (PNI): Inability to shrug ipsilateral shoulder; shoulder droops; + scapular flip test (scapular winging)
	Sternocleidomastoid (involvement raises concern of brain-stem involvement secondary to proximal innervation)	In supine, ask patient to flex head anterolaterally and rotate head to opposite side; resistance is applied in an obliquely posterior direction	Weakness, inability to flex head laterally and forward, rotate head to contralateral side Contracture produces torticollis (wry neck), a dystonic condition that produces a fixed abnormal head position (tilted, rotated, with flexion or extension)
XII Hypoglossal	Tongue movements	Listen to patient's articulation Examine resting position of tongue Examine tongue movements (move side-to-side, protrude)	Dysarthria (lesions of CN X or CN XII) UMN (supranuclear) lesion: produces mild to moderate contralateral weakness; may be transient. LMN (nuclear or infranuclear) lesion: produces paralysis, atrophy, and fasciculations of the tongue on involved side; deviation on protrusion is to the weak side. Bilateral supranuclear lesions (pseudobulbar palsy) produce moderate to severe loss of tongue function. Check for tongue tremors or involuntary tongue movements

Key: CN = cranial nerve; CNS = central nervous system; PNI = peripheral nerve injury; UMN = upper motor neuron

5. The term *myotome* refers to the skeletal muscles innervated by motor axons in a given spinal root. A motor unit consists of the alpha motor neuron and the muscle fibers it innervates.
6. Nerve roots exit from the vertebral column through the intervertebral foramina.
   a. In the cervical spine, numbered roots exit horizontally above the corresponding vertebral body, with C8 exiting below C7 and above T1.
   b. In the thoracic, lumbar, and sacral spine, the roots exit below the corresponding vertebral body.
   c. Spinal cord ends at the level of L1; in the lumbosacral region, the nerve roots descend almost vertically below the cord to form the cauda equina (horse's tail).
7. After emerging from the intervertebral foramen, each spinal nerve divides into a large anterior ramus (supplying the muscles and skin of the anterolateral body wall and limbs) and a small posterior ramus (supplying the muscles and skin of the back); each ramus contains motor and sensory fibers.
8. The anterior rami join at the root of the limbs to form nerve plexuses. The cervical and brachial plexuses are at the root of the upper limbs; the lumbar and sacral plexuses are at the root of the lower limbs.
   a. The cervical plexus arises from C1 through C4 nerve roots (see Figure 2-17). The brachial plexus arises from C5 through T1 nerve roots that split into three trunks (upper, middle, lower), anterior and posterior divisions, redistributing fibers into

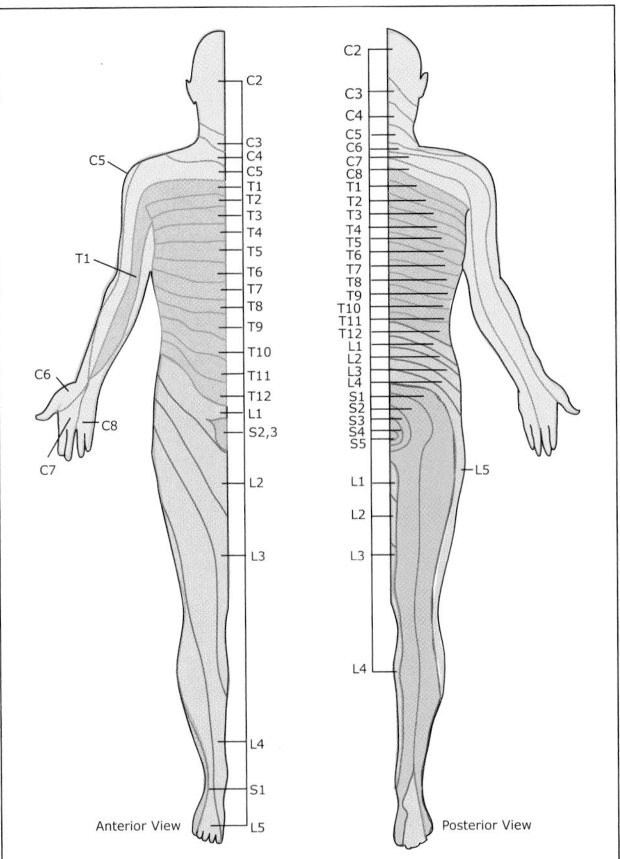

Figure 3-10 Dermatomes.

Note: Studies show variability in dermatomes. Recommend use of specific autonomous zones highlighted on anterior view for C5-T1, T4, T10, and L1-S1.

three cords (lateral, posterior, and medial) and finally into the peripheral nerves that supply the upper extremity (see Figure 2-18).

b. The lumbar plexus arises from T12 through L4 nerve roots (see Figure 2-19). The sacral plexus arises from L4 through S3 nerve roots (see Figure 2-20). Nerve fibers from both are redistributed into the peripheral nerves that supply the lower extremity.

c. Refer to Table 2-4 (Shoulder Girdle and Upper Extremity Muscular and Neurological Screening), Table 2-5 (Pelvic Girdle and Lower Extremity Muscular and Neurological Screening), and Table 2-6 (Trunk and Ribcage Muscular and Neurological Screening).

Spinal Level Reflexes—Basic Functions and Motor Control

1. Involuntary responses to stimuli; basic, specific, and predictable; dependent on intact neural pathway (reflex arc); reflexes result in a behavioral response that may be monosynaptic or polysynaptic (involving interneurons); impact a single level and one side of the spinal cord (e.g., monosynpatic reflex); impact multiple levels and both sides of the spinal cord (e.g., flexor withdrawal reflex, crossed extension reflex); provides basis for unconscious motor function and basic defense mechanisms.
2. Key understanding of reflexes is required and allows practitioners to assess for upper (hyper-reflexia and/or pathologic reflexes) or lower (hyporeflexia with low tone) motor neuron lesions. Physical therapists also use various positioning and treatment techniques to facilitate or inhibit reflexes/tone to improve function.

Stretch (Myotatic) Reflexes

1. Stimulus: muscle stretch.
2. Reflex arc: afferent Ia fiber from muscle spindle to alpha motor neurons projecting back to muscle of origin (monosynaptic).
3. Functions for maintenance of muscle tone, support agonist muscle contraction, and provide feedback about muscle length.
4. Clinically, sensitivity of the stretch reflex and intactness of spinal cord segment are tested by applying tap to the deep tendons, thus resulting in a muscle stretch reflex (also called deep tendon reflexes).
5. Reciprocal inhibition: via an inhibitory interneuron, the same stretch stimulus inhibits the antagonist muscle.
6. Reciprocal innervation: describes the effects of a stretch stimulus on agonist (autogenic facilitation), antagonist (reciprocal inhibition), and synergistic muscles (facilitation).

Inverse Stretch (Myotatic) Reflex

1. Stimulus: muscle contraction.
2. Reflex arc: Multiple sensory receptors and corresponding fiber types activate inhibitory interneuron to muscle of origin (polysynaptic).
3. Functions to provide agonist inhibition, diminution of force of agonist contraction, stretch-protection reflex.

Gamma Reflex Loop

1. Stretch reflex forms part of this loop.
2. Allows muscle tension to come under control of descending pathways (reticulospinal, vestibulospinal, and others).
3. Descending pathways excite gamma motor neurons, causing contraction of muscle spindle, and in turn increased stretch sensitivity and increased rate of firing from spindle afferents; impulses are then conveyed to alpha motor neurons.

Flexor Withdrawal Reflex

1. Stimulus: cutaneous sensory stimuli.
2. Reflex arc: cutaneous receptors via interneurons to largely flexor muscles; multisegmental response involving groups of muscles (polysynaptic).
3. Functions as a protective withdrawal mechanism to remove body part from harmful stimuli.

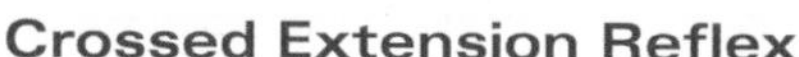

Crossed Extension Reflex

1. Stimulus: noxious stimuli and reciprocal action of antagonists; flexors of one side are excited, causing extensors on same side to be inhibited; opposite responses occur in opposite limb.
2. Reflex arc: cutaneous and muscle receptors diverging to many spinal cord motor neurons on same and opposite side (polysynaptic).
3. Function: coordinates reciprocal limb activities such as gait.

Brain Stem Functions and Motor Control

Brainstem Functions

1. Controls flow of information between cortex and spinal cord/peripheral nervous system.
2. Critical functions such as breathing, swallowing, heart rate, blood pressure, consciousness, and arousal.
3. Houses nuclei for various neurotransmitters that influence both the cortex (e.g., arousal, attention) and spinal cord (e.g., descending pain modulation).
4. Contains cranial nerve nuclei (please see Table 3-1).

Brain Stem and Motor Control

1. Brain stem is critical for maintaining autonomous rhythmic movements (e.g., walking, chewing, swallowing).
2. Critical cranial nerve reflexes to include pupillary light reflex, corneal blink reflex, and gag reflex.
3. Medial descending brain stem pathways (vestibulospinal, reticulospinal, tectospinal) important for head/neck control and postural stability.
4. Assists in unconscious integration of visual, vestibular, and somatosensory information with trunk and proximal muscle activation.
5. Allows integration of visual and vestibular input during rapid head/body movements (vestibulo-ocular reflex).

Cortex Functions and Motor Control

Cortex Functions

1. Higher thought processes such as decision-making and language.
2. Processes information from the five senses.
3. Memory
4. Personality
5. Executive function

Cortex and Motor Control

1. Controls purposeful, goal-orientated, learned voluntary movements.
2. Utilizes feedback and feed forward mechanisms.
3. See Table 3-26 for additional information on Stages of Motor Learning and Training Strategies.

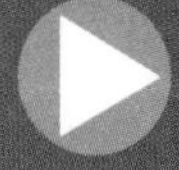

Neurological Examination: History, Systems Review, Tests, and Measures

Patient Interview

Presenting Symptoms

1. Onset, progression, nature of symptoms.
2. Patient's insight into medical condition and functional abilities.

Past Medical History

1. Other diagnoses, surgeries.
2. Health status.

Social History

1. Family/social support.
2. Current living situation.
3. Education level.
4. Employment.
5. Lifestyle.

Examine Level of Consciousness

Determine Orientation to Person, Place, and Time (Oriented ×3)

Determine Response to Stimuli

1. Purposeful, nonpurposeful, no response.
2. Verbal, tactile, simple commands.
3. Painful stimuli: pinch, pinprick.

Determine Level of Consciousness

1. Alertness: alert patient responds appropriately; can open eyes, look at examiner, respond fully and appropriately to stimuli.
2. Lethargy: patient appears drowsy; can open eyes and look at examiner, respond to questions, but falls asleep easily.

3. Obtundation: patient can open eyes, look at examiner, but responds slowly and is confused; demonstrates decreased alertness and interest in environment.
4. Stupor: patient can be aroused from sleep only with painful stimuli; verbal responses are slow or absent; patient returns to unresponsive state when stimuli are removed; demonstrates minimal awareness of self and environment.
5. Coma: a state of unconsciousness from which patient cannot be aroused, eyes remain closed; no response to external stimuli or environment.
6. Unresponsive Wakefulness Syndrome (also referred to as vegetative state): a state characterized by the return of sleep/wake cycles, normalization of vegetative functions (respiration, heart rate, blood pressure, digestion) and lack of cognitive responsiveness (can be aroused but is unaware). Persistent vegetative state: a state lasting >1 year for traumatic brain injury (TBI) and >3 months for anoxic brain injury.
7. Minimally conscious state (MCS): a state characterized by severely altered consciousness with minimal but definite evidence of self or environmental awareness.

Glasgow Coma Scale (GCS) (Teasdale and Jennette, 1974)

1. Relates consciousness to three elements of response: eye opening, motor response, and verbal response.
2. Scoring range from 3 to 15: severe brain injury (scores 1–8); moderate brain injury (scores 9–12); minor brain injury (scores 13–15).
3. Typically used to assess acute concussions/TBIs.

Coma Recovery Scale-Revised (McCulloch KL et al., 2016)

1. Examines multiple domains (auditory, visual, motor, verbal, communication, and arousal) of consciousness and function.
2. Includes brain stem reflexes (pupillary light reflex, corneal reflex, spontaneous eye movements, oculocephalic reflex, and postural responses).
3. Recommended for use in multiple rehabilitation settings (acute care, inpatient/outpatient, long-term acute care/skilled nursing, home health) and patients with various health conditions (moderate to severe TBI, stroke).

Examine Cognitive Function

Memory

1. Immediate recall: name three items previously presented after a brief interval (i.e., 5 minutes).
2. Recent memory (short-term): recall of recent events (i.e., What did you have for breakfast?).
3. Remote memory (long-term): recall of past events (i.e., Where were you born? Where did you grow up?).

Attention

1. Length of attention span: digit span retention test (i.e., ability to recall seven numbers in order presented).
2. Ability to attend to task without redirection (sustained attention); determine time on task, frequency of redirection.
3. Ability to shift attention from one task to another (divided attention); assess ability of dual task control; assess also for perseveration (mental inertia): getting stuck on a task.
4. Ability to stay on task in presence of detractors (focused attention); assess impact of environmental versus internal detractors.
5. Ability to follow commands: one- or two-step, multilevel commands.
6. Documentation: ability to follow specific requests (e.g., able to follow 2/5 verbal requests).

Emotional Responses/Behaviors

1. Safety, judgment: impulsivity and lack of inhibition.
2. Affect, mood: irritability, agitation, depression, and withdrawal.
3. Frustration tolerance.
4. Self-centeredness (egocentricity).
5. Insight into disability.
6. Ability to follow rules of social conduct.
7. Ability to tolerate criticism.

Higher-Level Cognitive Abilities

1. Judgment, problem-solving.
2. Abstract reasoning.
3. Fund of general knowledge: current events, ability to learn new information, generalize learning to new situations.
4. Calculation: serial 7 test (count backward from 100 by 7s).
5. Sequencing: ability to order components of cognitive or functional task; assess if cueing is necessary, frequency of cues.

Mini-Mental State Examination (MMSE) (Folstein, Flostein, and McHugh, 1975)

1. Brief screening test for cognitive dysfunction.
2. Includes screening items for orientation, registration, attention and calculation, recall and language.
3. Maximum score is 30; 21–24 indicates mild cognitive impairment, 16–20 indicates moderate impairment, 15 or less indicates severe impairment.
4. The MMSE has evidence for screening but is not a stand-alone tool for diagnosis of cognitive impairment/dementia.

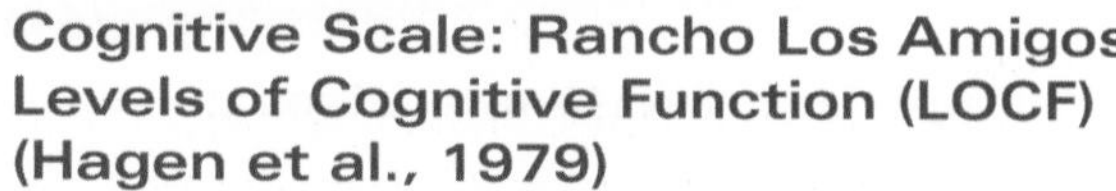

Cognitive Scale: Rancho Los Amigos Levels of Cognitive Function (LOCF) (Hagen et al., 1979)

1. Assesses cognitive recovery from TBI.
2. Includes eight levels of behavior: No response (I), decreased response levels (II and III), confused levels (IV, V, and VI), appropriate (automatic, purposeful) levels (VII and VIII).
3. Delineates emerging behaviors; patients may plateau at any level (see Table 3-17).

Examine Speech and Communication

Expressive Function

1. Examine fluency of speech, speech production.
2. Nonfluent aphasia (Broca's motor aphasia, expressive aphasia).
   a. A central language disorder in which speech is typically awkward, restricted, interrupted, and produced with effort.
   b. The result of a lesion involving the third frontal convolution of the left hemisphere (Broca's area).
3. Verbal apraxia: impairment of volitional articulatory control secondary to a cortical, dominant hemisphere lesion.
4. Dysarthria: impairment of speech production resulting from damage to the central or peripheral nervous system; causes weakness, paralysis, or incoordination of the motor-speech system (respiration, articulation, phonation, and movements of jaw and tongue).

Receptive Function

1. Examine comprehension.
2. Fluent aphasia (Wernicke's aphasia, receptive aphasia).
   a. A central language disorder in which spontaneous speech is preserved and flows smoothly, while auditory comprehension is impaired.
3. The result of a lesion in the posterior first temporal gyrus of the left hemisphere (Wernicke's area).

Global Aphasia

1. Severe aphasia.
2. Examine for marked impairments in comprehension and production of language.

Conduction/Association Aphasia

1. Result of damage to the arcuate fasciculus (association neural fibers) that connect Wernicke's and Broca's areas.
2. Causes word finding issues and problems with repeating phrases.
3. Treatment strategies: Give the patient time to correct and repeat phrases. Also allow patients to write down words or sentences they hear to assist with recall.

Nonverbal Communication

1. Examine ability to read and write.
2. Use of gestures, symbols, and pictographs.

Examine Cranial Nerves

Examination of Cranial Nerve Integrity (Table 3-1)

Examine Vital Signs

Determine Heart Rate (HR), Blood Pressure (BP), and Oxygen Saturation (O_2 Sat)

1. Examine for any irregularities in pulse: bounding, thready (fine, barely perceptible), tachycardia, or bradycardia.
2. Examine for increase or decrease in BP (see Table 4-3). American Heart Association (AHA) Blood Pressure Guidelines.
3. Examine for changes in response to activity: normally, HR increases in direct proportion to intensity of exercise; SBP increases, while DBP remains the same or slightly decreases.
4. O_2 Sat should be >94% in patients with central nervous system damage and ideally between 97%–100% (American Heart & Stroke Associations).

Examine Respiration

1. Examine respiratory rate (RR), depth, rhythm, and characteristics of inspiratory and expiratory phases.
2. Cheyne-Stokes respiration: a period of apnea lasting 10–60 seconds followed by gradually increasing depth and frequency of respirations; accompanies depression of frontal lobe and diencephalic dysfunction.
3. Hyperventilation: increased rate and depth of respirations; accompanies dysfunction of lower midbrain and pons.
4. Apneustic breathing: abnormal respiration marked by prolonged inspiration; accompanies damage to upper pons.

Examine Temperature

1. Elevation may indicate infection, damage to hypothalamus or brainstem.

Examine for Meningeal Irritation/Brain Infection

Signs and Symptoms

1. Impaired neck mobility: stiffness and pain with limitation and guarding into neck flexion.
   a. Kernig's sign.
   b. Brudzinski's sign.
2. Irritability, visual discomfort with bright light.
3. Altered level of consciousness: sleepiness, confusion; can progress to complete loss of consciousness and coma.
4. Severe headache, nausea, vomiting.
5. Altered vital signs, high fever.
6. Generalized weakness.

Examine for Increased Intracranial Pressure/Cerebral Edema and Brain Herniation

Signs and Symptoms

1. Altered level of consciousness: progresses from restlessness and confusion to decreasing level of consciousness, unresponsiveness, and coma.
2. Altered vital signs: examine for increased systolic BP; widening pulse pressure and bradycardia; irregular respirations including bradypnea (<12 breaths/min), periods of apnea, Cheyne-Stokes respirations; elevated temperature.
3. Headache.
4. Vomiting secondary to irritation of vagal nuclei, CN X.
5. Pupillary changes (CN III signs): examine for ipsilateral dilation of pupil (unequal pupils), slowed reaction to light. Progression to fixed, dilated pupils (a poor prognositic sign).
6. Papilledema at entrance to eye.
7. Progressive impairment of motor function. Examine for weakness, hemiplegia, positive Babinski response, decorticate or decerebrate rigidity.
8. Seizure activity.

Examine Autonomic Nervous System Function

See Table 3-2

Examine Sensory Function

Subjective

1. Ask patient to describe (map out areas) where sensation does not feel normal; provide sensory clues.

Testing Considerations

1. Consider the body area and type of impairment (parethesia, hypoethesia, anesthesia, hyperethesia) reported by the patient.

Table 3-2

Autonomic Nervous System Functions

SYMPATHETIC NERVOUS SYSTEM	PARASYMPATHETIC NERVOUS SYSTEM
Activated in stressful situations, producing an arousal reaction (fight or flight)	Results in conservation and restoration of body energy and homeostasis (system balance)
Effects are widespread	Effects are localized and short-acting
Inhibits salivation and tearing	Stimulates salivation and tearing
Dilates pupils (mydriasis)	Constricts pupils
Accelerates heart rate and output	Slows heart rate
Constricts or dilates blood flow in skeletal muscles	Dilates blood vessels in gut
Constricts blood flow to skin and viscera	
Relaxes airways	Constricts airways
Stimulates secretion of epinephrine and norepinephrine from adrenal medulla	
Decreases peristalsis, intestinal motility; inhibits digestion	Stimulates pancreas to release insulin and digestive enzymes Stimulates digestion
Increases sweating	
Stimulates glucose production and release	
Relaxes urinary bladder	Stimulates urinary bladder to contract

2. Does the sensory impairment follow a specific nerve, dermatome, portion of the extremity (e.g., sensory homunculus)?
3. Is the sensory loss unilateral (e.g., mononeuropathy, radiculopathy, cortical stroke), bilateral (e.g., polyneuropathy, lumbar spinal cord injury), involve all extremities (e.g., polyneuropathy, cervical myelopathy, cervical spinal cord injury), or sporadic (e.g., multiple sclerosis)?

Sensory Examination

1. Test superficial and proprioceptive sensations first.
   a. Provides insight into ability to detect pain, discriminate touch, vibration, and proprioception.
   b. Correlates with spinothalamic and dorsal column medial lemniscus pathways.
   c. See Table 3-3.
2. Test combined sensations after determining superficial and proprioceptive touch is intact.
   a. Combined sensation requires communication between various areas of the cortex (somatosensory association and primary cortex).
   b. Allows patients to know what they are touching or holding.
3. Ensure that patient comprehends instructions and can reliably communicate responses.
4. Occlude vision: consider barrier method (use a piece of paper to block vision) versus blindfolding the patient.
5. Apply stimulus in random, unpredictable order; avoid summation.
6. To assess responses, pose a choice (e.g., hot or cold).
7. Examine for objective manifestations: withdrawal, wincing, blinking.
8. Consider skin condition (calluses, scars) for areas of desensitivity.
9. Look for signs of repetitive trauma, skin lesions.
10. Examine for hair loss and skin color changes and consider if vascular/autonomic changes are also present.

Evaluation and Documentation

1. Determine whether the patient can readily distinguish one sensation from another.
2. Determine the sensory threshold, the lightest stimulus perceived.
3. Determine the degree and location of deficits. Document the specific area and type (e.g., light touch, sharp/dull, vibration) of sensory impairment.
4. Document the device (e.g., 5.07/10 gram-monofilament), location (dorsum of great toe), and quantify (e.g., able to detect 1 of 3 trials) the specific sensory loss.
5. Determine functional impact of sensory losses (e.g., if large fiber neuropathy patients will have balance/coordination impairments; small fiber neuropathy = pain; small and large fiber neuropathy = paresthesia, loss of protective sensation and problems with balance/coordination).

Table 3-3

Examination of Sensory Integrity*

Test Superficial Sensations	
Pain	Test sharp/dull stimuli with paper clip.
Temperature	Test response to hot/cold stimuli with test tubes filled with hot or cold water.
Touch	Test touch/nontouch in response to slight touch stimulus (cotton ball) or no touch.
Test Proprioceptive (Deep) Sensations	
Joint position sense:	Test ability to perceive joint position at rest in response to your positioning the patient's limb (up or down, in or out).
Kinesthesia (movement sense)	Test ability to perceive movement in response to your moving the patient's limb; patient can duplicate movement with opposite limb or give a verbal report.
Vibration sense (pallesthesia)	Test proprioceptive pathways by applying vibrating tuning fork or pressure only (sham vibration) on bony areas. Can also test specific time(s) patients can perceive vibration.
Test Combined (Cortical) Sensations (Use a sample of two or three from this group.)	
Stereognosis	Test ability to identify familiar objects placed in the hand by manipulation and touch.
Tactile localization	Test ability to identify location of a touch stimulus on the body by verbal report or pointing.
Two-point discrimination	Test ability to recognize one or two blunt points applied to the skin simultaneously; determine minimal distance on skin where two points can still be distinguished in millimeters using an aesthesiometer (the two tips must be applied simultaneously).
Barognosis	Test ability to identify similar size/shaped objects placed in the hand with different gradations of weight.
Graphesthesia	Test ability to identify numbers, letters, or symbols traced on skin, typically the hand.
Bilateral simultaneous stimulation	Test ability to identify simultaneous touch on the two sides/segments of the body.

*All tests are with vision occluded.

Examine Perceptual Function

Testing Considerations

1. Suspect perceptual dysfunction if patient has difficulty with functional mobility skills or activities of daily living for reasons that cannot be accounted for by specific sensory, motor, or comprehension deficits.
2. Rule out specific sensory and motor loss, language impairment, hearing loss, or visual disturbance as cause of loss of function.
3. Rule out psychological/emotional and cognitive factors.

Test for Visual Field Impairments

1. Slowly bring two fingers from behind head into the patient's visual field while asking the patient to gaze straight ahead; the patient indicates when and where the fingers first appear.
2. Homonymous hemianopsia: Loss of half of visual field in each eye, contralateral to the side of a cerebral hemisphere lesion.
3. Bitemporal hemianopsia: Loss of outer half of both the right and left visual field resulting in a loss of peripheral vision. Occurs with damage at the optic chiasm.

Examine for Body Scheme/Body Image Disorders

1. Body scheme disorder (somatognosia): have patient identify body parts or their relationship to each other.
2. Visual spatial neglect (unilateral neglect): determine whether patient ignores one side of the body and stimuli coming from that side.
3. Right/left discrimination disorder: have patient identify right and left sides of his or her own body and your body.
4. Anosognosia: severe denial, neglect or lack of awareness of severity of condition; determine whether patient shows severe impairments in neglect and body scheme.

Examine for Spatial Relations Syndrome

1. Figure-ground discrimination: have patient pick out an object from an array of objects (e.g., brake from rest of wheelchair).
2. Form constancy: have patient pick out an object from an array of similarly shaped but different-sized objects (e.g., large block from group of blocks).
3. Spatial relations: have patient duplicate a pattern of two or three blocks.
4. Position in space: have patient demonstrate different limb positions (e.g., put your arm overhead; put your foot underneath the chair).
5. Topographical disorientation: determine whether patient can navigate a familiar route on his or her own (e.g., travel from room to physical therapy clinic).
6. Depth and distance imperceptions: determine whether patient can judge depth and distance (e.g., navigate stairs, sit down in chair).
7. Vertical disorientation: determine whether patient can accurately identify when something is upright (e.g., hold a cane, ask patient when it is vertical; ask patient to determine whether own body is vertical).

Examine for Agnosia

1. Inability to recognize familiar objects with one sensory modality while retaining ability to recognize same object with other sensory modalities.
2. Subject doesn't recognize an object (clock) by sight, but can recognize it by sound (ticking).

Examine for Apraxia

1. Inability to perform voluntary, learned movements in the absence of loss of sensation, strength, coordination, attention, or comprehension; represents a breakdown in the conceptual system or motor production system or both.
2. Ideomotor apraxia: patient cannot perform the task on command but can do the task when left on own.
3. Ideational apraxia: patient cannot perform the task at all, either on command or on own.
4. Apraxia correlates with damage to the prelateral frontal cortex and somatosensory association cortex.

Examine Motor Function

Examine Muscle Bulk, Firmness (See Tables 3-4 and 3-5)

1. Determine whether there is atrophy.
   a. Determine whether atrophy is due to denervation, disuse, or primary atrophy.
   b. The presence of persistent fasciculations suggests lower motor neuron (LMN) injury.
   c. Examine by inspection, palpation, and girth measurement.
2. Check muscle firmness, tenderness, and reactivity.

Examine Muscle Tone

1. Use passive range of motion (PROM) to assess muscle stretch reflexes and responsiveness to passive elongation.
2. Flaccidity (absent tone), hypotonia (decreased tone).
   a. Seen in segmental/LMN lesions: nerve roots and peripheral nerve injury.
   b. Seen initially after suprasegmental/upper motor neuron (UMN) lesions (i.e., brief period of spinal shock in spinal cord injuries, cerebral shock in stroke). There is decreased or no resistance to PROM.

Table 3-4

Differential Diagnosis: Comparison of Major Types of Central Nervous System Disorders

DISORDER	STROKE	PARKINSONISM	CEREBELLAR LESION (TUMOR, STROKE)	SPINAL CORD INJURY (COMPLETE/INCOMPLETE)
Location of Lesion	Cerebral Cortex Corticospinal Tracts	Basal Ganglia: Subcortical Gray	Cerebellum	Spinal Cord
Sensation	Impaired or absent, depending on lesion location; contralateral sensory loss	Not affected	Not affected	Impaired or absent below
Tone	Hypertonia/spasticity; clasp-knife phenomena present; spasticity is velocity-dependent; with cerebral shock may see initial flaccidity	Leadpipe rigidity: uniform increased resistance to movement; cogwheel rigidity: rachet-like resistance to movement; rigidity is not velocity-dependent	Normal or may be decreased secondary to decreased ability to produce force when needed	Hypertonia/spasticity below the level of the lesion; initial flaccidity: spinal shock
Reflexes	Increased/hyperreflexia	Normal or may be decreased/hyporeflexia	Normal or decreased/ hyporeflexia	Increased/hyperreflexia
Strength	Contralateral weakness or paralysis: hemiplegia	Slowness of movement	Normal or weak: asthenia	Impaired or absent below the level of the lesion: paraplegia or tetraplegia
Bulk	Normal: acute; disuse atrophy: chronic	Normal or disuse atrophy	Normal	Disuse atrophy
Involuntary Movements	Spasms	Resting tremor	None	Spasms
Voluntary Movements	Dyssynergic: abnormal timing, coactivation, activation, fatigability	Bradykinesia/akinesia slowness, lack of spontaneous and automatic movements	Ataxia: intention tremor dysdiadochokinesia, dysmetria, dyssynergia nystagmus	Intact: above level of lesion
Postural Control/Stability	Impaired or absent, depends on lesion location	Impaired: stooped	Impaired: truncal ataxia, dysequilibrium	Impaired below level of lesion
Gait	Impaired: gait deficits due to abnormal synergies, spasticity, timing deficits	Impaired: shuffling, festinating gait	Impaired: ataxic gait deficits, wide-based, unsteady	Impaired or absent: depends on level of lesion

3. Spasticity (spastic hypertonia).
   a. Seen in suprasegmental/UMN lesions.
   b. There is increased resistance to PROM; determine whether increasing the speed increases the resistance (spasticity is velocity-dependent) (Table 3-6).
   c. Examine for additional signs of spastic hypertonia.
      - Clasp-knife response: marked resistance to PROM suddenly gives way.
      - Clonus: maintained stretch stimulus produces a cyclical, spasmodic contraction; common in plantar flexors, also seen in wrist flexors and jaw.
      - Hyperactive cutaneous reflexes, positive Babinski response: dorsiflexion of great toe with fanning of other toes in response to stroking up the lateral side of the sole of the foot; indicative of corticospinal (pyramidal) tract disruption.
      - Hyperreflexia: increased deep tendon reflexes (DTRs).
      - Some degree of muscle weakness is usually present.
   d. Modified Ashworth Scale: six grades are used for grading spasticity:
      0—No increase in muscle tone.
      1—Slight increase in muscle tone, minimal resistance at end of ROM.
      1+—Slight increase in muscle tone, minimal resistance through less than half of ROM.
      2—More marked increase in muscle tone, through most of ROM, affected part easily moved.
      3—Considerable increase in muscle tone, passive movement difficult.
      4—Affected part rigid in flexion or extension.

Table 3-5

Differential Diagnosis: Comparison of Upper Motor Neuron (UMN) and Lower Motor Neuron (LMN) Syndromes

	UMN LESION	LMN LESION
Location of Lesion	Central nervous system	Peripheral nervous system
Structures Involved	Cortex, brainstem, corticospinal tracts, spinal cord	SC: anterior horn cell, spinal roots, peripheral nerves CN: cranial nuclei and peripheral axons
Disorders	Stroke, traumatic brain injury, spinal cord injury	Polio, Guillain-Barré, PNI, peripheral neuropathy, radiculopathy
Tone	Increased: hypertonia Velocity-dependent	Decreased or absent: hypotonia, flaccidity Not velocity dependent
Reflexes	Increased: hyperreflexia, clonus Exaggerated cutaneous and autonomic reflexes: + Babinski response	Decreased or absent: hyporeflexia Cutaneous reflexes decreased or absent
Involuntary Movements	Muscle spasms: flexor or extensor	With denervation: fasciculations
Strength	Stroke: weakness or paralysis on one side of the body Corticospinal lesions: contralateral if above decussation in medulla, ipsilateral if below Spinal cord lesions: unilateral (partial spinal cord injuries), bilateral (complete thoracic/lumbar cord) and quadrilateral (cervical cord) loss below level of lesion	Mononeuropathy: Muscles impacted from one nerve (e.g., carpal tunnel snydrome) Radiculopathy: muscles from a specific myotome (e.g., L5 nerve root) Polyneuropathy: Initially distal extremity muscles and progresses to proximal muscles
Muscle Bulk	Variable, disuse atrophy	Neurogenic atrophy: rapid, focal, significant muscles wasting consistent with degree of axonal/myelin damage
Voluntary Movements	Impaired or absent: dyssynergic patterns, obligatory synergies	Weak or absent if nerve interrupted

Key: CN = cranial nerve; PNI = peripheral nerve injury; SC = spinal cord

4. Rigidity: increased resistance to PROM that is independent of the velocity of movement.
   a. Rigidity seen in basal ganglia/nigrostriatal disorders: increased resistance to passive movement in agonist and antagonist muscle.
   b. Rigidity can be leadpipe (uniform throughout the range) or cogwheel (interrupted by a series of jerks).
   c. Associated with Parkinson's disease, resting tremor, bradykinesia; strength is affected with immobility and deconditioning.
5. Decerebrate rigidity/posturing.
   a. Seen in comatose patients with brainstem lesions between the superior colliculus and the vestibular nucleus.
   b. Results in increased tone and sustained posturing in rigid extension of all four limbs and trunk/neck.
6. Decorticate rigidity/posturing.
   a. Seen in comatose patients with lesions above the superior colliculus.
   b. Results in increased tone and sustained posturing of upper limbs in flexion and the lower limbs in extension.
7. Opisthotonos.
   a. Prolonged, severe spasm of muscles, causing the head, back, and heels to arch backward; arms and hands are held rigidly flexed.
   b. Seen in severe meningitis, tetanus, epilepsy, and strychnine poisoning.
8. Use active ROM, active movement control to assess tone in automatic postural adjustments.
   a. Check stiffness of limbs and trunk in maintaining posture against gravity.
   b. Examine for abnormal movements: are movements restricted, are they performed with great effort, are there limitations in voluntary movements?
9. Evaluation and documentation.
   a. Determine which body parts and muscles have abnormal tone.
   b. Determine whether asymmetries exist, upper extremities versus lower extremities, axial (trunk) versus appendicular (limbs), distal versus proximal.
   c. Describe the character of the resistance (e.g., velocity-dependent versus uniform, clasp-knife, leadpipe, cogwheel).
   d. Describe the effects of tone on active movements, posture, and functional activities.

Table 3-6

Typical Patterns of Spasticity in Upper Motor Neuron Syndrome

UPPER LIMBS	ACTIONS	MUSCLES AFFECTED
Scapula	Retraction, downward rotation	Rhomboids
Shoulder	Adduction and internal rotation, depression	Pectoralis major, latissimus dorsi, teres major, subscapularis
Elbow	Flexion	Biceps, brachialis, brachioradialis
Forearm	Pronation	Pronator teres, pronator quadratus
Wrist	Flexion, adduction	F. carpi radialis
Hand	Finger flexion, clenched fist Thumb adducted in palm	F. dig. profundus/sublimis, Add. pollicis brevis, F. pollicis brevis
LOWER LIMBS		
Pelvis	Retraction (hip hiking)	Quadratus lumborum
Hip	Adduction (scissoring) Internal rotation Extension	Add. longus/brevis Add. magnus, gracilis Gluteus maximus
Knee	Extension	Quadriceps
Foot and ankle	Plantarflexion Inversion Equinovarus Toes claw (MP ext., PIP flex, DIP ext.) Toes curl (PIP, DIP flex)	Gastrocsoleus Tibialis posterior Long toe flexors Ext. hallucis longus Peroneus longus
Hip and knee (prolonged sitting posture)	Flexion Sacral sitting	Iliopsoas Rectus femoris, pectineus Hamstrings
Trunk	Lateral flexion with concavity rotation	Rotators Internal/external obliques
COG forward (prolonged sitting posture)	Excessive forward flexion Forward head	Rectus abdominis, external obliques Psoas minor

The form and intensity of spasticity may vary greatly, depending upon the CNS lesion site and extent of damage. The degree of spasticity can fluctuate within each individual (i.e., due to body position, level of excitation, sensory stimulation, and voluntary effort). Spasticity predominates in antigravity muscles (i.e., the flexors of the upper extremity and the extensors of the lower extremity). If left untreated, spasticity can result in movement deficiencies, subsequent contractures, degenerative joint changes, and deformity.

Adapted from Mayer NH, Esquenazi A, Childers MK. Common patterns of clinical motor dysfunction. *Muscle and Nerve* 6:S21, 1997.

Examine Reflexes (See Table 3-7)

1. Reflex categories.
   a. Deep tendon reflexes: normally occurring reflexes in response to stretch of muscle.
   b. Superficial cutaneous reflexes: normally occurring reflexes in response to noxious stimulus (light scratch) applied to skin.
   c. Primitive spinal reflexes (Babinski).
   d. Midbrain/cortical reactions (e.g., protective extension, optical righting).
2. Reflex Scoring Scale (Capute) for primitive/spinal and tonic/brainstem reflexes:
   0—absent.
   1+—Tone change; no visible movement of extremities.
   2+—Visible movement of extremities.
   3+—Exaggerated, full movement of extremities.
   4+—Obligatory and sustained movement, lasting for >30 seconds.

Table 3-7

Examination of Reflexes

Muscle Stretch Reflexes/Deep Tendon Reflexes (DTRs)	Tap directly on tendon: stretch stimulus produces contraction of agonist muscle with corresponding quick movement Reflexes commonly tested: jaw reflex, trigeminal CN V; biceps, C5–C6; triceps, C7–C8; brachioradialis, C5–C6; hamstrings, L5–S3; quadriceps (knee jerk, patellar), L2–4; Achilles (ankle jerk), S1–2 Scoring: 0 absent reflex; 1+ low normal, diminished; 2+ normal; 3+ brisker response, may or may not be normal; 4+ hyperreflexive with clonus DTRs: may be abnormal in CNS lesions (hyporeflexia with spinal or cerebral shock-acute phase, hyperreflexia/hypertonia after a few weeks) or PNS lesions (hyporeflexia)
Superficial Cutaneous Reflexes	
Plantar Reflex (S1–2, tibial nerve) or Negative Babinski Response	Stroking of the lateral sole of foot from calcaneus to base of fifth metatarsal and medially across metatarsal heads produces plantar flexion of the toes Occurs in neurologically intact individual
Positive Babinski Response	Stroking of the lateral sole of foot from calcaneus to base of fifth metatarsal and medially across metatarsal heads produces dorsiflexion of the great toe and fanning (abduction) of the four lesser toes Seen in patients with corticospinal lesions
Abdominal Reflexes (T6–L1)	Lateral to medial scratching of skin (toward umbilicus) in each of four quadrants produces deviation of the umbilicus toward the stimulus Occurs in neurologically intact individual Loss of abdominal reflexes is a sign of corticospinal lesions
Cremasteric Reflex (L1–L2)	Stroking of skin of the proximal and medial thigh produces elevation of the testicle (neurologically intact individuals) Absent in spinal cord injury and corticospinal lesions
Primitive/Spinal Reflexes	Present developmentally in normal infants (see Chapter 9) and in some patients with brain injury
Flexor Withdrawal	Noxious stimulus (pinprick) to sole of foot produces toe extension, dorsiflexion of the foot, and flexion of entire LE
Crossed Extension Reflex	Noxious stimulus to sole of foot produces flexion of stimulated leg, then extension with adduction of opposite leg
Traction	Stretch stimulus from grasping the forearm and pulling produces total flexion response of the UE
Grasp	Maintained pressure to palm of hand (palmar grasp) or ball of foot (plantar grasp) produces maintained flexion of fingers or toes
Tonic/Brainstem Reflexes	Present developmentally in normal infants (see Chapter 9) and in some patients with brain injury
Asymmetrical Tonic Neck (ATNR)	Rotation of the head to one side produces flexion of the skull side limb and extension of the jaw side limb
Symmetrical Tonic Neck (STNR)	Flexion of the head produces flexion of the UEs with extension of the LEs Extension of the head produces extension of the UEs and flexion of the LEs
Positive Supporting	Contact to the ball of the foot in the standing position produces rigid extension (co-contraction) of the LEs
Associated Reactions	Strong voluntary movement in one body segment produçes involuntary movement in another resting extremity

LE = lower extremity; UE = upper extremity

Examine Voluntary Movement and Range of Motion

1. Determine/document.
   a. Quality (synergistic organization) of muscle activation patterns.
   b. Are movements fractionated, appropriate and timely in response to stimulus or command?
   c. Able to easily vary the type of contraction pattern (i.e., isometric, concentric, eccentric)?
   d. Are movements symmetrical?
   e. Adequate control of multiple body segments, postural stabilization?
   f. Assess for presence of abnormal synergy patterns: muscle synergistic patterns that are highly stereotyped and obligatory; commonly seen in UMN dysfunction (e.g., cerebrovascular accident, TBI) (Table 3-8).

Examine for Presence of Involuntary Movements

1. Extrapyramidal disorders, basal ganglia dysfunction.
   a. Tics: spasmodic contractions of specific muscles, commonly involving face, head, neck, or shoulder muscles.
   b. Chorea: relatively quick twitches or "dancing" movements.
   c. Athetosis: slow, irregular, twisting, sinuous movements, occurring especially in upper extremities.
   d. Tremor: continuous quivering movements; rhythmic, oscillatory movement observed at rest (resting tremor).
   e. Myoclonus: single, quick jerk.
2. Cerebellar disorders: intention tremor occurring when voluntary movement is attempted.

Table 3-8

Abnormal Synergy Patterns of the Extremities Seen in Patients Following Stroke
UPPER EXTREMITY
Flexion synergy components: scapular retraction/elevation, shoulder abduction, external rotation, elbow flexion,* forearm supination, wrist and finger flexion*
Extension synergy components: scapular protraction, shoulder adduction,* internal rotation, elbow extension, forearm pronation, wrist and finger flexion
LOWER EXTREMITY
Flexion synergy components: hip flexion, abduction, external rotation, knee flexion, ankle dorsiflexion/inversion
Extension synergy components: hip extension, adduction,* internal rotation, knee extension,* ankle plantarflexion*/inversion

The form and intensity of abnormal synergy patterns may vary greatly, depending upon the CNS lesion site, age when the lesion occurs (e.g., cerebral palsy vs. older adult with stroke), extent of damage, and stage of recovery. Synergies can fluctuate due to body position (presence of reflexes), degree of spasticity, level of excitation, sensory stimulation, and voluntary effort.

*Generally the strongest components are starred.

3. Cortical disorders: epileptic seizures, tonic/clonic convulsive movements.
4. Determine/document.
   a. Are movements extraneous and spontaneous, apparently unintended?
   b. Part of body involved, orientation in space.
   c. Frequency, amplitude, pattern.
   d. Effect of triggering stimuli or changes in environment.
   e. Methods: patient's self-report, observation/functional assessment, videotaped analysis.

Examine Muscle Performance. Strength, Power, and Endurance

1. Determine/document: relative strength/peak power, ability to initiate/accelerate contraction, control torque output at varying speeds.
2. Methods: patient's self-report, manual muscle test (MMT), dynamometry, muscle performance tests, physical capacity tests, technology-assisted analyses, timed activity tests.
3. Observe muscle strength, power, and endurance during functional activities (e.g., basic and instrumental activities of daily living, functional mobility skills).
4. Decreased strength: paresis (weakness) or paralysis (loss of voluntary motion).
   a. Cerebrovascular accident: hemiparesis or hemiplegia.
   b. Spinal cord injury: paraplegia or tetraplegia (quadriplegia).
   c. Traumatic brain injury: any level or degree possible.
5. Clinical issues with strength testing (standard MMT): patients with CNS, UMN lesions.
   a. Passive restraint: soft tissue changes restrict ability to move (e.g., contractures).
   b. Active restraint: spastic muscles restrict ability to move.
   c. Abnormal synergistic activity, inappropriate coactivation of muscles.
   d. Recruitment problems: abnormal type II fiber recruitment.
   e. Abnormal reflex activity: restricts ability to move.
   f. Isokinetic dynamometry: patients with UMN syndrome (i.e., stroke) typically demonstrate decreased torque development with increased problems at higher speeds, decreased limb excursion, extended time to peak torque development, extended time peak torque held, increased time intervals between reciprocal contractions, and changes on "supposedly normal" extremities.
6. Clinical issues with strength testing: patients with PNS, LMN lesions.
   a. With myopathies: typically see proximal weakness of extremities.
   b. With neuropathies: typically see distal weakness of extremities.
   c. Some conditions produce decremental strength losses (e.g., myasthenia gravis) that are more pronounced with repetitive testing.

Examine for Fatigue

1. Fatigue is the failure to generate the required or expected force during sustained or repeated contractions.
   a. Fatigue is protective: guards against overwork and injury.
   b. Fatigue is task-dependent.
   c. Sources of fatigue.
      - CNS/central fatigue: seen in multiple sclerosis, amyotrophic lateral sclerosis, chronic fatigue syndrome.
      - Neural/myoneural junction: seen in multiple sclerosis, postpolio syndrome, Guillain-Barré syndrome, myasthenia gravis.

- Muscle contractile failure: metabolic changes at the level of the muscle (e.g., depleted Ca^{2+} stores) seen in muscular dystrophy.

2. Determine/document.
   a. Source of fatigue.
   b. Frequency and severity of fatigue episodes.
   c. Threshold for fatigue: level of exercise that cannot be sustained indefinitely.
      - Onset is typically gradual, not abrupt.
      - Dependent on the intensity and duration of activity attempted.
   d. Factors that influence fatigue: health status, environmental temperature, stress.
   e. Level of functional performance: independence, modified dependence, dependence, level of assistance, assistive devices.
   f. Episodes of exhaustion: limit of endurance beyond which no further performance is possible.
   g. Overwork weakness or injury: prolonged decrease in absolute strength and endurance due to excessive activity of partially denervated muscle. Common in postpolio syndrome, Duchenne's muscular dystrophy.
   h. Test and measures.
      - Modified Fatigue Impact Scale (MFIS): subjective scale that includes three subscales assessing the impact of fatigue on physical, cognitive, and psychosocial function.
      - Isokinetic dynamometry, electromyography (EMG): can observe decrements in force production.
      - Repetitive muscle or functional testing: Patients with neuromuscular conditions (e.g., neuromuscular junction disease) may have normal muscle testing with one repetition but may show signs of fatigue/weakness with repetitive testing (e.g., five repetitions of sit to stand).

Examine Coordination

1. Gross motor coordination: body posture, balance, and extremity movements involving large muscle groups.
   a. Upper extremity tests: unilateral (finger to nose); rapid alternating movements (RAM), supination/pronation; bilateral symmetrical movements (clapping, RAM), bilateral asymmetrical movements (alternate touch knee/shoulder), bilateral unrelated movements (knee pat/elbow extension).
   b. Lower extremity tests: unilateral (heel to shin, foot tapping); bilateral symmetrical (foot tapping, alternate knee flexion/extension); bilateral asymmetrical (alternate knee flexion/extension); bilateral unrelated movements (knee flexion/extension and hip abduction/adduction).
   c. Postural/trunk tests: whole body movements.
2. Fine motor coordination: extremity movements concerned with use of small muscle groups.
   a. Thumb to finger opposition (unilateral, bilateral).
   b. Manual/finger dexterity: grasp and release.
   c. Standardized tests and measures: Jebsen-Taylor Hand Function Test, Minnesota Rate of Manipulation Test, Purdue Pegboard.
3. Evaluation and documentation.
   a. Speed/rate control: Does increasing the speed of performance affect quality of motor performance?
   b. Control: Are movements precise? Are continuous and appropriate motor adjustments made if speed and direction are changed? Can movement and distance be judged following a moving target? Does occluding vision alter performance?
   c. Steadiness: Is there consistency over time? Can a position be maintained without swaying, tremors, or extra movements? Does patient fatigue rapidly?
   d. Response orientation: Does correct movement occur in response to a specific stimulus?
   e. Reaction time: Does movement occur in a reasonable amount of time?
   f. Descriptive comments/terms.
      - Dyssynergia: impaired ability to associate muscles together for complex movement.
      - Dysmetria: impaired ability to judge the distance or range of movement.
      - Dysdiadochokinesia: impaired ability to perform rapid alternating movements.
   g. Scoring: 0 (unable), 1 (severe impairment), 2 (moderate impairment), 3 (minimal impairment), 4 (normal performance).
   h. Methods.
      - Patient's self-report.
      - Observation/functional assessment.
      - Timed tests.
      - Videotaped analysis.

Examine Balance/Postural Stability

1. Balance refers to an individual's ability to maintain their center of gravity within their base of support (BOS).
2. Components of Balance (see Table 3-9).
3. Sensory integration.
   a. Visual system: examine visual acuity, depth perception, visual field deficits.
   b. Somatosensory: examine proprioception, cutaneous sensation (touch, pressure), lower extremities and trunk, especially feet and ankles.
   c. Vestibular: examine Head Impulse test, observe balance with changes in head position or head movement.
   d. Sensory Organization Test (SOT)
      - Equipment: computerized moving platform (e.g., NeuroComBasic and Balance Master Systems, Bertec Computerized Dynamic Posturography/Immersive Virtual Reality); stopwatch.

Table 3-9

Components of Postural Stability/Balance

COMPONENTS OF BALANCE	OPERATIONAL DEFINITION	EXAMPLE OF EXAMINATION ITEM(S)
Sensory Integration	Ability to integrate varying degrees of sensory information (vision, vestibular, somatosensory)	modified Clinical Test of Sensory Interaction in Balance (mCTSIB)
Motor Systems	Tone, strength, and coordination to maintain postures	Ashworth Scale, Strength/Coordination Assessment
Verticality and Orientation in Space	Ability to align body appropriately in standing/sitting	Ability to stand/sit upright Balance Evaluation Systems Test (BEST): Standing Incline Eyes Closed
Static Stability	Ability to maintain center of mass (COM) in varied stance when base of support (BOS) does not change	Narrow stance, semi-tandem stance, tandem stance, single legged stance
Functional Stability Limits	Ability to move COM as far as possible in mediolateral/anteroposterior direction within BOS	Functional Reach Test, Multidirectional Reach Test
Dynamic Stability	Ability to exert control of COM when BOS is changing (e.g., during gait and postural movements)	Functional Gait Index, Four Square Step Test, Sit to Stand
Anticipatory Postural Control	Ability to shift COM before a specific voluntary movement	Functional Gait Assessment, BEST, Functional Gait Index, Star Excursion Balance Test
Reactive Postural Control	Ability to recover balance after an external perturbation and bring COM within BOS by corrective strategies (ankle, hip, stepping, suspensory)	BEST, Mini-BEST, Performance Orientated Mobility Assessment (POMA)
Cognition: Multi-Tasking	Ability to maintain stability while reacting to commands/stimuli of a different task	Fullerton Advanced Balance Scale, BEST, Mini-BEST, Timed Up and Go while counting by 7's

Adapted from Sibley KM, Beauchamp MK, Van Ooteghem K, Straus SE, Jaglal SB. Using the systems framework for postural control to analyze the components of balance evaluated in standardized balance measures: a scoping review. *Arch Phys Med Rehabil.* 2015 Jan; 96 (1): 122–132.

- Examines six different sensory conditions, progressing in difficulty.
  Condition 1: eyes open, stable surface (EOSS).
  Condition 2: eyes closed, stable surface (ECSS).
  Condition 3: visual conflict (sway-referenced vision using a moving surround screen or virtual reality surround screen), stable surface.
  Condition 4: eyes open, moving surface (EOMS).
  Condition 5: eyes closed, moving surface (ECMS).
  Condition 6: visual conflict, moving surface.
- Non-instrumented evaluation and documentation.
  - Record time that standing posture is maintained (30 seconds); record changes in the amount and direction of postural sway, on a scale of 1 (minimal sway) to 4 (fall).
  - Patients dependent on vision become unstable in conditions 2, 3, 5, and 6.
  - Patients dependent on surface/somatosensory inputs become unstable in conditions 4, 5, and 6.
  - Patients with vestibular deficits become unstable in conditions 5 and 6.
  - Patients with sensory selection problems become unstable in conditions 3, 4, 5, and 6.

e. Clinical Test for Sensory Interaction in Balance (CTSIB) (Shumway-Cook and Horak, 1986): uses medium-density foam to substitute for a moving platform and a modified visual dome to substitute for a moving visual surround. Tests six conditions, similar to SOT.

f. Modified Clinical Test of Sensory Interaction on Balance (mCTSIB)
  - A simpler test that uses four different sensory conditions: eyes open and eyes closed on stable surface and on foam (EOSS, ECSS, EOFS, ECFS).
  - Three 30-second trials are used.
  - Time in balance and changes in sway are recorded. Test is stopped if patient alters position of feet (takes a step), opens eyes, or loses balance.
  - Patient subjective complaints are also recorded (e.g., nausea, dizziness).

4. Musculoskeletal systems.
   a. Examine musculoskeletal strength, coordination, and range of motion (ROM) of the lower extremities and trunk.
5. Verticality and body orientation in space: Determine patient's ability to orient body in appropriate vertical position
   a. Test sit to stand.
   b. Patients may exhibit Pusher's syndrome (push to weak side).
6. Examine static balance: ability to maintain a sitting or standing position with varying BOS (document time, postural sway, and postural synergies/strategies).
   a. Sitting: maintaining a vertical posture with and without arm support.

b. Standing, double limb support progression: feet apart (eyes open), feet apart (eyes closed), feet together (eyes open), feet together (eyes closed).
c. Standing, semi-tandem stance: lunge position (feet apart eyes open); lunge position (feet apart eyes closed).
d. Standing, tandem stance: heel to toe position (eyes open progress to eyes closed).
e. Standing, single limb leg support: eyes open progress to eyes closed.
f. Determine postural synergies/strategies to maintain balance.
 - Ankle strategy: ankle muscles and leg/foot proprioception utilized to maintain balance.
 - Hip strategy: hip and lower trunk muscles maintain balance by shifting center of mass (COM) using hip motions (flexion or extension).
 - Stepping strategy: rapid step(s) taken to realign COM within BOS.
 - Suspensory strategy: bending the knees to lower the center of gravity.

7. Functional stability limits.
 a. Ability to move COM in anterior/posterior or mediolateral directions.
 b. Important for reaching task (e.g., Functional Reach Test).
8. Dynamic stability.
 a. Additional complexity required to maintain control of COM when BOS is changing (e.g., sit to stand and gait).
9. Anticipatory postural control.
 a. Ability to shift COM before a specific voluntary movement (e.g., stepping, head turn, arm raise).
10. Reactive postural control (document postural strategies required to maintain balance).
 a. Response to external perturbations and ability to bring COM back within BOS by use of postural strategies (ankle, hip, stepping, or suspensory).
 b. Perturbations: can include force against the COM (push or pull) or displacement of the BOS (using a moveable surface such as platform, ball, or equilibrium board).
 c. Used for patients who have exhibited static/dynamic stability and anticipatory postural control.
 d. Important to make sure patients are safe (use of harness or positional support).
11. Cognition: multi-tasking.
 a. Ability to maintain balance while challenged with verbal requests or cognitive (counting backwards)/physical (carrying a cup while walking) tasks.
12. See Table 3-10 for functional balance grades.
13. See Box 3-1 and Table 3-11 for recommended and selected functional balance and mobility tests.
14. Selected neuromuscular outcomes measures and references are presented in Appendix 3A.

Examine Gait and Mobility (See also Chapter 12)

1. Gait is the manner in which a person walks, characterized by rhythm, cadence, step, stride, and speed (Guide to Physical Therapist Practice).
 a. Kinematic gait analysis: analyzes gait characteristics and deviations.
 b. Consider how various neuromuscular conditions impact gait characteristics (e.g., Parkinson's disease results in decreased stride length but has increased cadence and step count).
 c. Determine the impact visual (looking up or down), vestibular (head and body turns), and cognitive (walk and talk) cues have on gait characteristics for higher functioning patients.
2. Common neuromuscular gait deviations:
 a. Ataxia: wide-based gait with uncoordinated movements. Multiple causes:
 - Polyneuropathy: ataxic gait that is typically improved with looking down.
 - Cerebellar disorder: ataxic gait that is also associated with postural and limb intention tremor. Not typically improved with looking down.

Table 3-10

Functional Balance Grades	
Normal	Patient is able to maintain steady balance without hand-hold support (static). Patient accepts maximal challenge and can shift weight easily at full range in all directions (dynamic).
Good	Patient is able to maintain balance without hand-hold support, limited postural sway (static). Patient accepts moderate challenge; able to maintain balance while picking object off floor (dynamic).
Fair	Patient is able to maintain balance with hand-hold support; may require occasional minimal assistance (static). Patient accepts minimal challenge; able to maintain balance while turning head/trunk (dynamic).
Poor	Patient requires hand-hold support and moderate to maximal assistance to maintain position (static). Patient unable to accept challenge or move without loss of balance (dynamic).
0 Absent	Patient unable to maintain balance.

From: O'Sullivan S, Schmitz, Fulk G, ed 7. Philadelphia, FA Davis, 2019, pg 212, with permission.

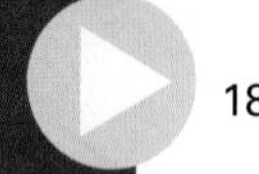

BOX 3-1 Core Outcome Measures for Adult Neurologic Rehabilitation

Examination

APTA Neurology Section recommends the following outcome measures for patients with various neurologic conditions:

Outcome Measures

- **The Berg Balance Scale (BBS) assesses sitting/standing balance and is applicable for patients with acute, chronic, and chronic progressive conditions (A-strong recommendation, Level I).**
- **The Activities-specific Balance Confidence (ABC) Scale is appropriate for patients with acute, chronic, and chronic progressive neurologic conditions (A-strong recommendation, Level I).**
- **Functional Gait Assessment (FGA) examines balance while walking and strong evidence for patients with acute and chronic neurologic conditions (A-strong recommendation, Level I) and moderate evidence (B-moderate recommendation, Level 1) for chronic progressive conditions.**
- **The 10-meter Walk Test (10mWT) and 6-Minute Walk Test (6MWT) have strong evidence for patients with chronic and chronic progressive neurologic conditions (A-strong recommendation, Level I).**
- The 10mWT and the 6MWT are recommended as best practice for patients with acute neurologic conditions but require additional research (P-Best practice/expert opinion recommendation, Level V).
- The 5-times Sit to Stand test (5TSTS) measures transfer capability and is recommended for use at admission and discharge for adult patients with neurologic conditions (P-Best practice/expert opinion recommendation, Level V).

The APTA Neurologic Section Clinical Practice Guideline recommends that the core set of outcome measures (BBS, ABC scale, FGA, 10mWT, 6MWT, and 5TST) should be administered to patients during the initial evaluation and discharge (B-moderate recommendation, Level 2).

Adapted from Moore JL et al. A core set of measures for adults with nuerologic conditions undergoing rehabilitation: A clinical practice guideline. *J Neurol Phys Ther.* 2018; 42(3): 174–220.

Additional information regarding this clinical practice guideline is located at https://www.neuropt.org/practice-resources/anpt-clinical-practice-guidelines/core-outcome-measures-cpg.

Table 3-11

Selected Functional Balance and Mobility Tests

TEST	DESCRIPTION	SCORING
Berg Balance Scale	Examines functional balance (14 items) including sitting unsupported, sit-to-stand, stand-to-sit, transfers; in standing: EO to EC, feet together, forward reach, pick object off floor, head turns, turning 360°, stepping up, tandem stand, stand on one leg	Uses ordinal scale with specific scoring criteria for each activity. Some items are timed. Maximum score is 56; patients who score <45 are at high risk for falls; with scores 54–46, a 1-point drop is associated with a 6%–8% increase in fall risk
Activities-Specific Balance Confidence (ABC) Scale	Examines level of confidence using percentage points; activities rated include 16 daily activities, e.g., reaching, walking (in house, outside, ramps, stairs), stepping on escalator	0%–100% scoring scale with 0 being no confidence and 100% being full confidence
10 Meter Comfortable/Fast Gait Speed	Test examines comfortable ("walk at your own comfortable walking speed") and fast ("walk as fast as you can safely walk") gait speed for 10 meters. Time to complete central 6 meters is specifically timed. Level of assistance and assistive device (if required) should also be recorded	Reported as meters/seconds. Various normative values based on age and health conditions
Functional Gait Assessment (FGA)	A 10-item gait assessment is based on the Dynamic Gait Index. It includes additional items on walking (ambulating backward, with narrow base of support, with eyes closed)	Items are scaled using an ordinal scale; total possible score is 30
Five Times Sit to Stand Test	Examines sit-to-stand-to-sit transitions five times with arms crossed on chest	Test is timed using a stopwatch

(*Continued*)

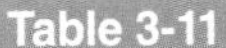

Selected Functional Balance and Mobility Tests (Continued)

TEST	DESCRIPTION	SCORING
6-Minute Walk Test	Examines endurance and distance walked over 6 minutes. Requires level hallway or open area at least 12 meters and at least 49 inches (124 cm) wide for turns. Vital signs should also be recorded before and after testing.	Reported as distance walked in meters. Various normative values based on age, health conditions, or setting (hallway versus open community setting).
Timed Up and Go (TUG), TUG cognitive/manual	Examines functional balance during rise from a chair, walk 3 m, turn, and return to chair. Performance on the TUG is timed. May also include cognitive (count backward by 3s) or manual (hold a cup of water) task	Normal intact adults can perform the TUG in ≤10 seconds; 11–20 seconds is considered normal for frail elderly or disabled patients; patients who take >20 seconds are at increased risk for falls; patients who take >30 seconds are at high risk
Functional Reach (FR)	Examines maximal distance a person can reach forward beyond arm's length while maintaining a fixed position in standing (single item test)	Forward reach norms: age — Men (inches) — Women (inches) 20–40 — 16.7 ± 1.9 — 14.6 ± 2.2 41–69 — 14.9 ± 2.2 — 13.8 ± 2.2 70–87 — 13.2 ± 1.6 — 10.5 ± 3.5 A score of 6 or less indicates a significant risk for falls; scores between 6–10 indicate a moderate risk for falls.
Multidirectional Reach Test (MDRT)	Examines maximal distance a person can reach forward, backward, and lateral to right and left	Backward: above average >7.6 inches, below average <1.6 inches; lateral: above average >9.4 inches, below average <3.8 inches
The Balance Evaluation Systems Test (BESTest)	A comprehensive instrument with six sections. Examines biomechanical constraints, stability limits/verticality, transitions/anticipatory, reactive, sensory integration; includes assessment of posture, gait, transfers, and balance/falls	Specific scoring criteria for each section. Uses ordinal scale, timed items, and observation
The Mini-BESTest Items are scored . . .	A shorter version of the test with 14 items	Items are scored from 0–2 with a maximum score of 28
Performance-Oriented Mobility Assessment (POMA,Tinetti)	Exams balance (sitting, sit to stand, stand to sit, standing feet together, 360° turn, and sternal nudge) and gait subsets (gait initiation, turning, step-over obstacle).	Maximum score is 28; patients who score <19 are at high risk for falls; patients who score 19–24 are at moderate risk
High-Level Mobility Assessment Tool (Hi-MAT)	Examines high-level balance and mobility problems. Minimal requirement for testing is independent walking for 20 m without gait aids. Includes walking tasks, running, skipping, hopping, bounding, and stairs	Items are scored using time or distance on a 0–5 scale. Total Hi-MAT score is 54
Short Physical Performance Battery (SPPB)	Includes repeated chair stands (sit-to-stand rises), semitandem, tandem, and side-by-side stands as well as a timed 8-ft (2.44 meter) walk	Tests are scored in terms of time to complete: Five sit-to-stands, 10 sec in each of the standing conditions and 8-ft walk An ordinal score is given for each section. Summary ordinal score: 0 (worst performance) to 12 (best performance).
Balance Efficacy Scale (BES)	Examines level of self-confidence when performing functional tasks encountered in daily life; 18 questions are scored from 0%–100% confidence; activities include getting out of chair, walking up and down flight of 10 stairs, getting out of bed, getting into and out of tub or shower, removing items from cupboard, walking on uneven ground, standing on one leg	Total score is divided by 18 to yield mean BES score; scores <50 indicate low confidence
Dynamic Gait Index (DGI)	Examines dynamic gait (eight items) including changes in gait speed, head turns, pivot turns, obstacles, and stairs	Uses a 4-point ordinal scale; total score is 24. Scores of 22/24 indicate safe ambulation while scores <19/24 are predictive of falls in the elderly.

For additional information on outcome measures please see Shirley Ryan Agility Lab. Rehabilitation Measures Database, https://www.sralab.org/rehabilitation measures and the APTA Neurology Section Outcome Measure Recommendations, https://www.neuropt.org/practice-resources/neurology-section-outcome-measures-recommendations

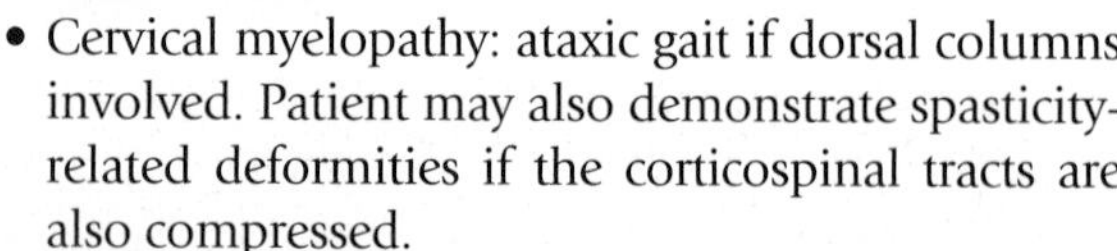

- Cervical myelopathy: ataxic gait if dorsal columns involved. Patient may also demonstrate spasticity-related deformities if the corticospinal tracts are also compressed.

b. Hemiplegic gait: gait is altered following stroke owing to a number of factors, including obligatory synergies, weakness, spasticity, sensory loss, and impaired balance. Gait is typically slow and asymmetrical, with decreased stance time and push off on the stroke-affected side. The stroke-affected UE and LE move as a unit rather than with a dissociating arm swing from the LE on forward progression.

c. Festinating/Parkinson gait: characterized by freezing with initiation/termination and short, rapid steps once gait starts.

d. Myopathic gait: pelvic girdle and proximal muscle weakness results in hyperlordosis and compensated Tredenlenburg on weight-bearing limb.

e. Please see Chapter 12 for gait deviations secondary to weakness at the hip, knee, and ankle.

3. Common gait/mobility outcome measures (see Box 3-1 and Table 3-11).

Imaging, Electrophysiologic, and Laboratory Procedures

Imaging

1. X-rays: delineates skull or spine trauma (fracture) and alignment.
2. Computed tomography (CT): neuroimaging technique in which narrow x-ray beams are transmitted through tissues of varying densities and precisely measured.
   a. CT provides cross sections (slices) of the brain and spinal cord for three-dimensional analysis.
   b. Contrast agents (intravenous iodinated agents) can be used to increase diagnostic sensitivity, to detect brain abnormalities (e.g., tumor, calcifications). Useful for showing presence of abnormal changes in tissue density: areas of acute bleeding (hemorrhage in developing stroke), cerebral edema (within 3 days poststroke), and cerebral infarction (within 3–5 days' poststroke).
   c. Diagnostic in acute stroke: allows administration of TPA (clot busting drug) in absence of evidence of hemorrhage within 3 to 4 1/2 hours of thromboembolic stroke. CT myelography: uses contrast dye and allows for visualization of spinal cord, nerve roots, and spinal lining (meninges).
      - Often used in patients with metal or suspected scar tissue in the area of imaging (e.g., history of spinal fusion).
      - Complications: dye may result in allergic reaction or meningeal irritation.
   d. See images of CT scans in Figures 3-11 and 3-12.
3. Advantages: CT scans take minimal time (a few minutes), helpful following trauma or hemorrhagic stroke, and good visualization of osseous tissue (e.g., skull fracture) and larger cortical lesions.
4. Disadvantages: Limited visualization of small/ischemic lesions, and patient has exposure to radiation.
5. Please see Appendix 2B for additional details.

Magnetic Resonance Imaging (MRI)

1. Neuroimaging technique in which nuclear particles (protons and neutrons) are depicted in a strong external magnetic field; no radiation is used.
2. Useful for superior imaging of brain, providing greater resolution of tissues and flow of blood within medium and larger arteries and veins.
3. Allows three-dimensional localization with high spatial resolution.
4. More sensitive in diagnosis of acute stroke: allows detection of cerebral edema within 30 minutes after vascular occlusion and infarction within 2 to 6 hours.
5. Primary method of examination of tumors, demyelination, and vascular abnormalities.

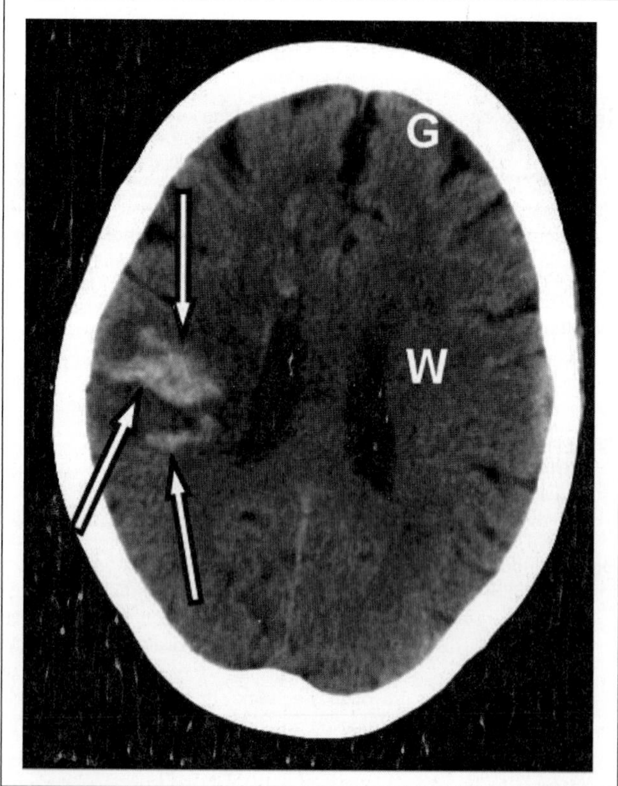

Figure 3-11 Axial CT of hemorrhagic stroke. The blood is white, with slightly darker than normal areas surrounding this, due to local brain swelling (edema). G = normal brain gray matter; W = normal brain white matter (darker on CT scans than gray matter).
From: www.radiologyinfo.org

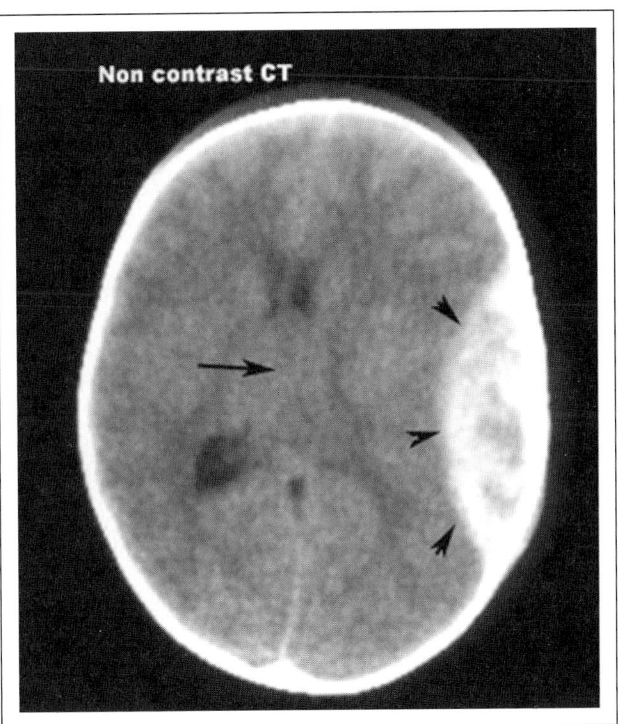

Figure 3-12 **Axial CT of epidural hematoma.**
Arrowheads point to the collection of blood between the skull and dura. The arrow demonstrates a shift of midline to the right.
From: www.meddean.luc.edu

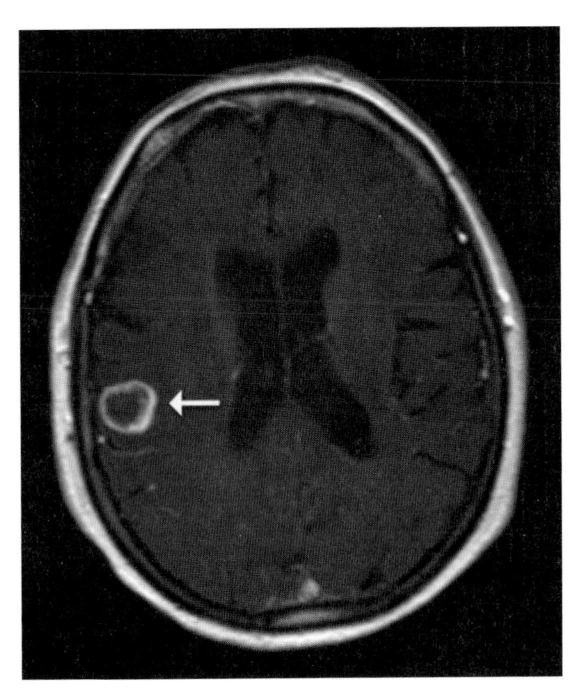

Figure 3-13 **MRI-brain metastasis.**
A cross section through a patient's brain after administration of intravenous contrast shows the contrast accumulating in the periphery of a cancerous deposit that has traveled to the brain, giving a characteristic ring-enhancing appearance.

6. Magnetic resonance angiography (MRA) uses special software to create an image of the arteries in the brain; identifies vascular abnormalities similar to angiography (x-ray of the brain) with increased sensitivity and lowered risks.
7. Contraindications: metal implants, pacemakers.
8. See MRI brain image in Figure 3-13.
9. Advantages: Superior visualization of almost all tissue and no exposure to radiation.
10. Disadvantages: Cost, time, and movement artifact if patient moves.
11. Please see Appendix 2B for additional details.

Positron Emission Tomography (PET)

1. Neuroimaging technique in which radioisotopes are inhaled or injected and emissions are measured with a gamma-ray detector system.
2. Advantages: Allows physiological mapping for biochemical analysis; a major clinical research tool for imaging cerebral blood flow and brain metabolism to assist in the screening/diagnosis of tumors, dementia, stroke, and seizure.
3. Disadvantages: Lacks detailed resolution as compared to CT or MRI; less accurate in detecting small or slow-growing tumors; radiation exposure.
4. Please see Appendix 2B for additional details.

Diffuse Tensor Imaging (DTI)

1. A form of MRI imaging.
2. Images microstructural characteristics of water diffusion.
3. Allows visualization of axons and pathways.
4. Advantages: useful for imaging of mild traumatic brain injury and assessing disruption of association/projection fibers; no radiation exposure.
5. Disadvantages: cost and processing time of images.

Functional MRI

1. Examines deoxygenated hemoglobin and contrast agent.
2. Hemodynamics are linked to neural activity and inactivity.
3. Able to introduce various stimuli (e.g., pictures) and measure changes in deoxygenated hemoglobin.
4. Advantages: provides good spatial resolution to identify active areas of the cortex.
5. Disadvantages: poor temporal resolution making it difficult to directly relate timing of events.

Carotid/Vertebral Artery Doppler Ultrasound

1. Commonly used in patients at risk for stroke.
2. Advantages: useful for imaging lumen of carotid or vertebral arteries to analyze flow and detect plaques

in carotid/vertebral arteries; low cost; takes minimal time.

3. Disadvantages: limited visualization of structures surrounding the arteries/veins.

Electrodiagnostic Testing (Nerve Conduction Studies/Electromyography)

1. In combination, nerve conduction and electromyographic studies provide electrophysiologic localization and the degree of involvement for peripheral nervous system, neuromuscular junction, and muscle pathologies.
2. Nerve conduction studies: distal latencies, amplitudes, and nerve conduction velocities are obtained by stimulating peripheral nerves through the skin and recording muscle and sensory nerve action potentials.
   a. Nerve conduction velocity: distance between two points (conduction distance) divided by the difference between the corresponding latencies (conduction time), expressed as meters/second (m/s).
   b. Prolonged distal latencies and decreased conduction velocities are seen in peripheral neuropathies characterized by demyelination (e.g., Guillain-Barré syndrome, chronic demyelinating polyneuropathy, Charcot-Marie-Tooth Type 1 disease, early in compression neuropathies such as carpal tunnel syndrome).
   c. Slowed conduction velocities seen with focal compression/disease of longer segments of peripheral nerve (e.g., Cubitial tunnel, polyneuropathy impacting legs).
   d. Reduced amplitudes are a result of damage to axons (axonopathy) and typically seen in more chronic or severe compression neuropathies (e.g., chronic CTS), radiculopathies, or polyneuropathies that target axons (e.g., Charcot-Marie Tooth Type 2).
   e. Repetitive nerve conduction studies can also be conducted to detect neuromuscular junction disorders. Specific findings include progressive decrements in amplitudes with a series of closely timed stimulations. Patients are also assessed after isometric exercise and rest to determine changes in amplitudes.
3. Electromyography (EMG): detects electrical activity arising from muscles during needle insertion, resting, minimal and maximal muscle recruitment.
   a. Useful in diagnosing anterior horn cell, motor axon, or primary muscle disease (myopathy, myotonia).
   b. Insertional activity (burst of action potentials when EMG needle is inserted into normal muscle) is increased in acute denervated muscle and various muscle diseases. Insertional activity is decreased in more chronic neuropathies/myopathies with significant atrophy and fibrosis of muscle.
   c. At rest the muscle should be quiet. Spontaneous EMG activity (e.g., fibrillation, positive sharp wave potentials, fasciculation) at rest is a hallmark of dennervated or diseased muscles.
   d. Abnormal spontaneous EMG activity typically occurs 14 to 21 days after peripheral nerve injury/compression and correlates with Wallerian degeneration. This is important as EMGs conducted prior to 3 weeks may have to be repeated to avoid false negative results.
   e. Minimal activation allows for assessment in alterations in motor unit frequency and configurations. Rapid firing motor units with multiple phases (polyphasics) are suggestive of reinnervation and collateral sprouting of axons. Large motor units with increased duration are consistent with more chronic neuropathy.
   f. The number of motor unit potentials (MUPs) is decreased in lower motor neuron injury (denervated muscles) with minimal and maximal recruitment.
   g. Myopathy results in specific spontaneous potentials (myopathic potentials) and small amplitude units that rapidly spatially summate on minimal activation (i.e., less muscle fibers requires more motor units to have to fire to produce needed force).

Electroencephalography (EEG)

1. Measures electrical activity of the brain. Specific wave forms are analyzed and correlated to normal, abnormal, or sleep cycles.
2. Provides key information on the timing and firing (temporal resolution) of neurons in the brain.
3. Advantages: provides information that assists in the assessment and localization of seizures and neural activity; often correlated with imaging to localize lesions; noninvasive.
4. Disadvantages: poor spatial resolution for precise localization of lesion; takes time to analyze wave forms.

Evoked Potentials/Evoked Responses

1. External visual, auditory, or somatosensory stimuli are used to evoke potentials in brain; visual evoked potential (VEP), brainstem auditory evoked potential (BAEP), somatosensory evoked potential (SEP).
2. Potentials are recorded from surface electrodes and processed by computer.
3. Delineates conduction times along peripheral and central nervous system sensory pathways.
4. Detects electrophysiologic location and degree of lesions if responses are delayed or absent.

Lumbar Puncture (LP)

1. Insertion of spinal needle below the level of L1–L2.
2. Purposes.
   a. Withdraw CSF for chemical analysis and cytological examination: measurement of protein, glucose, immunoglobulin content, cell count.

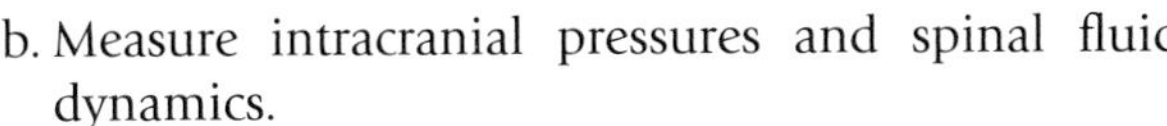

b. Measure intracranial pressures and spinal fluid dynamics.
c. Injection of contrast medium for radiological examination.
d. Injection of therapeutic agents (e.g., treatment of cancer, meningitis).

3. Complications: severe headache caused by CSF leakage (relieved by lying down); more severe complications include infection, epidural hematoma, uncal herniation.
4. Normal CSF.
   a. Appearance: crystal clear and colorless.
   b. Volume: 90–150 mL (adult); 60–100 mL (child).
   c. Pressure: 90–180 mm H_2O (adult); 10–100 mm H_2O (child).
   d. Normal protein: 15–45 mg/dL (adults); 15–100 mg/dL (neonates).
5. Pathological CSF findings.
   a. Increased pressure occurs with intracranial tumors, abscesses, meningitis, inflammatory processes, subarachnoid hemorrhage, cerebral edema, and thrombosis of venous sinuses.
   b. Decreased pressure occurs with leaking CSF, subarachnoid block circulatory collapse, severe dehydration.
   c. Changes in color or appearance occur with inflammatory diseases, hemorrhage, tumors. Red blood cells (RBCs) indicate hemorrhage or traumatic tap; elevated white blood cells (WBCs) indicate significant inflammation and infection.
   d. Elevated proteins may indicate tumors or inflammation.

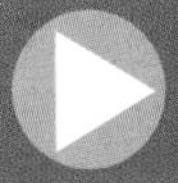

Evaluation, Differential Diagnosis, Prognosis, and Plan of Care

Infectious Diseases

Examine for Meningeal Irritation/Brain Infection

Examine for Increased Intracranial Pressure/Signs of Cerebral Edema and Brain Herniation

Meningitis

1. Inflammation of the membranes of the brain or spinal cord, typically caused by an infection.
2. Etiology: can be bacterial (*Escherichia coli, Haemophilus influenzae, Streptococcus pneumoniae,* other streptococci) or viral; patients with bacterial meningitis are usually sicker with more rapid time course.
3. Symptoms include headache, fever, and stiff neck. Also common: irritability, mental confusion, sensitivity to light, increased heart rate and respiratory rate, sleepiness, and sluggishness.
4. Diagnosis is made by medical history, physical exam (Kernig's sign and symptoms with dural stretch), and laboratory tests (blood cultures, spinal tap, CT imaging).
5. Treat infective organism (bacterial meningitis) with antibacterial therapy (antibiotic, antipyretic); maintain fluid and electrolyte balance.
6. Treatment of viral meningitis is symptomatic: bed rest, fluids, OTC pain medications to reduce fever and body aches. Corticosteriods may be used to reduce brain swelling, anticonvulsant medication to control seizures, and antiviral medication if the herpes virus is the causative agent.
7. Provide supportive symptomatic therapy, including bed positioning, PROM, skin care to prevent complications of immobility; safety measures if confusion is present.

Encephalitis

1. Inflammation of the brain, often due to infection.
2. Etiology.
   a. Primary encephalitis: caused by a virus (e.g., herpes simplex virus, Epstein-Barr virus, coxackievirus, poliovirus) that infects the brain. May also be caused by mosquito-borne viruses (West Nile, western or eastern equine virus), tick-borne viruses (Powassan virus), rabies virus. Effects may be concentrated in one area or widespread.
   b. Secondary encephalitis (postinfection encephalitis): caused by a faulty immune system reaction resulting from an infection in another area of the body (e.g., measles, mumps, German measles). The immune system attacks the healthy brain.
3. Mild inflammation may cause no symptoms or flu-like symptoms: headache, fever, aches in muscles or joints, fatigue or weakness.
4. Severe cases may be life-threatening. Symptoms include: confusion, agitation or hallucinations, seizures, muscle weakness or paralysis, loss of sensation, and loss of consciousness.
5. Diagnosis is made by physical examination, medical history, brain imaging (CT scan), lumbar puncture,

lab tests (blood, urine, throat swab), electroencephalogram, and brain biopsy.
6. Treatment for mild encephalitis includes bed rest, fluids, and anti-inflammatory drugs to relieve headaches and fever. Antiviral medications are used to treat some viruses.
7. Care may include breathing assistance, intravenous fluids, corticosteroids to reduce swelling and pressure, and anticonvulsant medications.
8. Provide supportive symptomatic therapy.

Neurological Complications in COVID-19

1. COVID-19 virus impacts multiple systems to the include the peripheral and central nervous systems.
2. COVID-19 infection can start with headaches, dizziness, decreased alertness, or other neurological symptoms before commonly known respiratory symptoms.
3. Specific COVID-19 neurological symptoms may include loss of smell, impaired taste, fatigue, muscle weakness, numbness or tingling in the hands and feet, dizziness, confusion, and delirium.
4. Although rare, COVID-19 can cause seizures or major strokes.
5. COVID-19 is also associated with disorders of inflammation in the nervous system (e.g., brachial neuritis, Guillain-Barré syndrome, transverse myelitis, and acute necrotizing leukoencephalopathy).
6. In younger children Covid-19 may result in acute disseminated encephalomyelitis (ADEM).
7. Patients who have had COVID-19 may also have long-term effects to include symptoms similar to myalgic encephalomyelitis/chronic fatigue syndrome (ME/CFS).
8. For additional and updated information on COVID-19 and neurologic dysfunction please see the NIH website at: https://www.ninds.nih.gov/Current-Research/Coronavirus-and-NINDS/nervous-system.

Transverse Myelitis (TM)

1. TM is an inflammation of one section of the spinal cord. Myelin is damaged with interruption of signals that the spinal cord sends to the body.
2. Etiology: can be caused by:
   a. Viral infection: e.g., herpes viruses, West Nile virus.
   b. Bacterial infection: e.g., syphilis, tuberculosis, Lyme disease.
   c. Fungal infection: e.g., Aspergillus, Cryptococcus, Blastomyces.
   d. Immune system disorder: postinfection recovery inflammatory disorder.
   e. Autoimmune/inflammatory disorders: e.g., systemic lupus erythematosus, Sjogren's syndrome, scleroderma.
   f. Other myelin disorders such as multiple sclerosis.
3. Symptoms.
   a. Typically develop gradually over hours to days and may progress over weeks.
   b. Usually affects both sides of the body below the level of spinal lesion; may also affect only one side of body.
   c. Symptoms include:
      - Pain: back pain; sharp shooting pains down arms or legs depending on level of lesion.
      - Abnormal sensations (paresthesias) including numbness, tingling, coldness, or burning. May be sensitive to light touch or extreme heat or cold.
      - Weakness in arms or legs; may progress to partial or total paralysis or arms, legs, or both.
      - Stiffness, tightness, or painful muscle spasms and spasticity.
      - Exhaustive fatigue that results in decreased activity levels and lifestyle changes.
      - Bladder and bowel problems, sexual dysfunction depending on lesion level.
4. Diagnosis is based on medical history, signs and symptoms, clinical assessment of nerve function, and test results. Tests can include imaging (MRI), lumbar puncture with analysis of cerebrospinal fluid (CSF), blood tests (positive antibody test).
5. Medical interventions can include intravenous steroids, plasma exchange therapy for patients who don't respond to steroids, antiviral medications, intravenous immunoglobulin (IVG), and medications to treat symptoms and complications.
6. Prognosis: most patient achieve at least a partial recovery; most recovery occurs in the first 3 months and may continue up to two years. About a third of patients are left with permanent disability after the attack, ranging from mild, to moderate, to severe. Recurrent or relapsing transverse myelitis can occur, particularly when MS is found to be the cause.
7. Physical therapy examination, goals, outcomes, and interventions.
   a. Therapists can approach the patient with transverse myelitis and paralysis using examination procedures/outcome measures and interventions similar to those used in spinal cord injury. See section Spinal Cord Injury (SCI) later in this chapter.
   b. Improving strength, coordination, and functional performance are the major goals of treatment. Activity-based rehabilitation with task-specific practice is indicated including weight-bearing exercise and locomotor training.
   c. Training in use of assistive devices (e.g., wheelchairs, crutches, braces) is typically indicated.
   d. The therapist must be mindful of the recovery process; ongoing and periodic examination is indicated in order to modify the plan of care as appropriate.

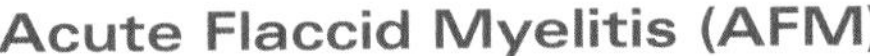

Acute Flaccid Myelitis (AFM)

1. AFM is a rare and polio-like condition that affects the motor neurons in the gray matter of the spinal cord, causing the muscles and reflexes to become weak; occurs mainly in children; seen with increasing frequency over recent years.
2. Specific etiology is unknown; no specific pathogens have been identified but viruses are suspected; most patients have prior history of mild respiratory illness or fever.
3. Symptoms include sudden onset of arm or leg weakness, loss of muscle tone and reflexes. Some individuals experience difficulty moving the eyes or eyelid drooping, facial droop or weakness, and difficulty with swallowing or speech. Pain in the neck, back, or limb may be an early symptom. Some individuals may have inflammation of both gray and white matter (UMN and LMN syndrome) and may experience impaired sensation, bladder, and/or bowel dysfunction.
4. AFM may result in partial or total paralysis of just one limb or all limbs. Weakness most often occurs in the proximal muscles.
5. Severe symptoms can include respiratory failure requiring ventilator support.
6. Diagnosis is based on medical history, signs and symptoms, clinical assessment of nerve function, and test results. Tests can include imaging of the spinal cord (MRI) and lumbar puncture with analysis of CSF.
7. There is no specific medical treatment. Symptomatic treatment may be indicated.
8. Prognosis: most patients regain some strength over time; many do not recover full function. The most affected muscle may be the least likely to recover.
9. Physical therapy examination, goals, outcomes, and interventions.
   a. Early PT and OT is recommended.
   b. See discussion on transverse myelitis.

Myalgic Encephalomyelitis/Chronic Fatigue Syndrome (ME/CFS)

1. ME/CFS is a disabling and complex illness.
2. Specific etiology is unknown; possible multiple triggers; causes currently being studied include infection, immune system changes, stress affecting body chemistry, and changes in energy production. Genetics may also play a role.
3. Symptoms include:
   a. Severe or prolonged fatigue and drop in activity level lasting 6 months or longer.
   b. Post-exertional malaise (PEM) after physical or mental activity; fatigue that is not relieved by rest. Other symptoms may worsen.
   c. Muscle pain (myalgia).
   d. Cognitive impairments: difficulty thinking, concentrating, or with short-term memory.
   e. Difficulty sleeping; sleep that is not refreshing.
   f. Sore throat that is frequent or recurring; tender lymph nodes.
   g. Headaches of a new type, pattern, or severity.
   h. Multi-joint pain (anthralgias) without swelling or redness.
   i. Dizziness and lightheadedness (orthostatic intolerance).
   j. Deconditioning, anxiety, and depression are common.
4. Diagnosis is based on medical history, physical and mental status examination. There are no specific laboratory tests to diagnose ME/CFS.
   a. Must have two major criteria (persistent or relapsing fatigue and reduced physical activity for at least 6 months) and four or more of the eight presenting symptoms.
   b. More common in women than men and in younger ages (20s and 30s).
5. Prognosis: symptoms may persist for months or years; limited recovery in 5%–10% of cases.
6. Medical interventions: no cure or approved treatment.
   a. Some symptoms can be managed with medications.
      - Analgesics and anti-inflammatory nonsteroidal medications for myalgia and arthralgia.
      - Stimulant medications used to treat ADHD to improve concentration.
      - Psychological support, counseling, antidepressants for depression, stress, and anxiety.
      - Nutritional support.
7. Physical therapy examination.
   a. Examine exercise tolerance levels. Vital signs may reveal fluctuations in heart rate and blood pressure; orthostatic hypotension is common. If deconditioned, dyspnea with exercise.
   b. Examine posture. Postural patterns may be abnormal and movement patterns inefficient. Can contribute to chronic pain and fatigue.
   c. Monitor activity levels and degree of fatigue. An activity diary and the Modified Fatigue Impact Scale are useful objective measures.
   d. Examine for depression and degree of emotional support.
8. Physical therapy goals, outcomes, and interventions.
   a. Teach activity pacing, balancing activity with rest. Help patients understand individual limits for mental and physical activity. Avoid "push-and-crash" cycles when a person has a good day and tries to push harder than normal, leading to a crash (worsening of ME/CFS symptoms).
   b. Teach energy conservation techniques based on analysis and modification of daily activities to reduce energy expenditure.

c. Exercise recommendations (ACSM's Exercise Management for Persons with Chronic Diseases and Disabilities, Human Kinetics).
- Overall goal is to prevent deconditioning.
- Aerobic exercise prescription (e.g., walking): low to moderate levels of intensity (RPE 9-12/20) with gradual progression; frequency of 3–5 days/wk; duration to tolerance (5 min/session initially progressing to 40–60 min); distributed practice schedule.
- Maintain flexibility.
- Maintain or improve muscle strength.
- Avoid overexertion. Individuals should understand that they may experience increased fatigue in the first few weeks of an exercise program. Individuals should reduce exercise when symptoms are increased or not feeling well.

d. Teach stress management, relaxation training (e.g., meditation and mindfulness, deep breathing, tai chi chuan, yoga).

e. Refer to a support group or a professional counselor as needed.

Acquired Immunodeficiency Syndrome (AIDS)

1. Viral syndrome characterized by acquired and severe depression of cell-mediated immunity.
2. Symptoms: wide ranging; one-third of patients exhibit CNS or PNS deficits.
   a. AIDS dementia complex (ADC): symptoms range from confusion and memory loss to disorientation.
   b. Motor deficits: ataxia, weakness, tremor, loss of fine motor coordination.
   c. Peripheral neuropathy: hypersensitivity, pain, sensory loss.
3. Treat with anti-HIV drugs (see Chapter 8).
4. Provide rehabilitative, palliative, and supportive therapy as needed.

Cerebrovascular Accident (CVA, Stroke)

Stroke

1. Occurs when the blood supply to the brain is interrupted or reduced.
2. Early diagnosis is critical to minimize brain damage.
3. See Chapter 13 for a discussion of recognizing, assessing, and prioritizing the need for assistance for an individual experiencing a stroke (F.A.S.T.).
4. Stroke syndromes and presenting signs and symptoms depend on the specific location of the insult (see Table 3-12).

Etiological Categories

1. Ischemic stroke: occurs in about 80% of cases.
   a. Cerebral thrombosis: formation or development of a blood clot or thrombus within the cerebral arteries or their branches.
   b. Cerebral embolism: traveling bits of matter (thrombi, tissue, fat, air, bacteria) that produce occlusion and infarction in the cerebral arteries.
2. Hemorrhagic stroke: abnormal bleeding as a result of rupture of a blood vessel (extradural, subdural, subarachnoid, intracerebral). Occurs in about 20% of cases.
3. Transient ischemic attack (TIA): a temporary period of symptoms resulting from decrease blood supply to the brain; there is no permanent damage.

Risk Factors

1. Atherosclerosis.
2. Hypertension.
3. Cardiac disease (rheumatic valvular disease, endocarditis, arrhythmias, cardiac surgery).
4. Diabetes, metabolic syndrome.
5. Transient ischemic attacks: brief warning episodes of dysfunction (<24 hours); a precursor of major stroke in more than one-third of patients.

Pathophysiology

1. Cerebral anoxia: lack of oxygen supply to the brain (irreversible anoxic damage to the brain begins after 4–6 minutes).
2. Cerebral infarction: irreversible cellular damage.
3. Cerebral edema: accumulation of fluids within brain; causes further dysfunction; elevates intracranial pressures, can result in herniation and death.
4. Secondary cell death: death of neurons around the specific area of damage.
   a. Necrotic cells release electrolytes and neurotransmitters (e.g., glutamate) that result in intracellular imbalance in surrounding cells.
   b. The surrounding cells can ultimately undergo programmed cell death (apoptosis).
   c. Controlling secondary cell death is critical for the management of stroke, traumatic brain injury, and spinal cord injuries.
   d. It is important to consider the timing of transfers and exercise and the impact this will have on cranial pressures, blood pressure, respiration, and oxygenation.

Characteristic Signs and Symptoms Associated with Occlusion of Specific Cerebral & Brain Stem Vessels (See Table 3-12)

1. Internal carotid artery (ICA) syndrome: ICA arises off the common carotid artery, gives off an ophthalmic branch, and terminates in the anterior cerebral artery

(ACA) and middle cerebral artery (MCA); occlusions commonly produce signs and symptoms of MCA involvement with reduced levels of consciousness; ACA may also be affected; lesions involving MCA and ACA distributions may produce massive edema, brain herniation, and death.

a. ACA syndrome: ACA supplies anterior two-thirds of the medial cerebral cortex. Occlusions proximal to anterior communicating artery produce minimal deficits due to collateral circulation (circle of Willis).

b. MCA syndrome: MCA supplies lateral cerebral cortex, basal ganglia, and large portions of the internal capsule.

2. Vertebrobasilar artery syndrome: two vertebral arteries arise off the subclavian arteries and supply the ventral surface of the medulla and the posterior inferior aspect of the cerebellum before joining to form the basilar artery at the junction of the pons and the medulla; the basilar artery supplies the ventral portion of the pons and terminates in the posterior cerebral artery (PCA). Syndromes include:

a. Medial medullary syndrome: occlusion of the vertebral anterior branch of the lower basilar artery.

b. Lateral medullary (Wallenberg's) syndrome: occlusion of vertebral, posterior inferior cerebellar, or basilar artery.

Table 3-12

Neurovascular Syndromes: Cerebral and Brain Stem Strokes

LESION LOCATION	CHARACTERISTICS	OTHER LOCALIZING FEATURES (NOT ALWAYS PRESENT)
Hemisphere lesion: cortex and internal capsule 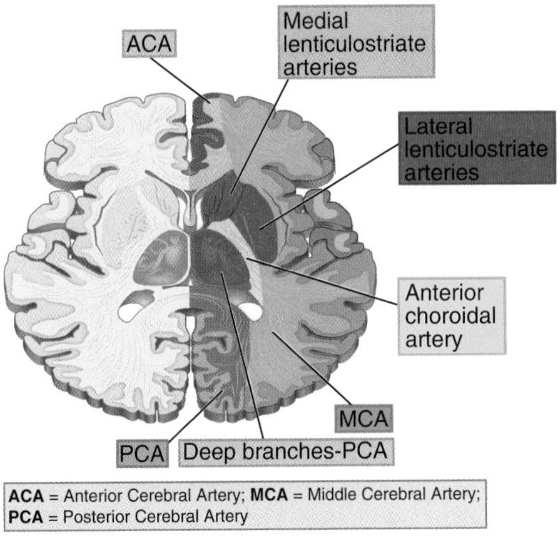 **ACA** = Anterior Cerebral Artery; **MCA** = Middle Cerebral Artery; **PCA** = Posterior Cerebral Artery	*MCA syndrome:* Contralateral hemiplegia face, UE>LE Contralateral hemisensory loss UE>LE Homonymous hemianopsia	Motor speech involvement—fluent, nonfluent global or conduction aphasia (dominant hemisphere) Perceptual deficit (nondominant hemisphere) Loss of conjugate gaze to the opposite side Sensory ataxia
	ACA syndrome: Contralateral hemiplegia LE>UE Contralateral hemisensory loss LE>UE Urinary Incontinence Problems with bimanual tasks Apraxia	Patients may be less mobile (akinetic) Patients may be less verbal (mutism)
Hemisphere lesion: primary visual cortex, occipital lobe	*PCA syndrome:* Contralateral sensory loss Involuntary movements—choreoathetosis, tremor, hemiballismus Transient contralateral hemiparesis Homonymous hemianopsia	Visual agnosia Memory defect Dyslexia Central (thalamic) pain Weber's syndrome Oculomotor n. palsy
Internal capsule lesion-posterior limb	*Lacunar (pure motor)* stroke Contralateral hemiplegia UE and LE	No aphasia Visual field deficit rare

(*Continued*)

Table 3-12

Neurovascular Syndromes: Cerebral and Brain Stem Strokes (Continued)

LESION LOCATION	CHARACTERISTICS	OTHER LOCALIZING FEATURES (NOT ALWAYS PRESENT)
Midbrain lesion 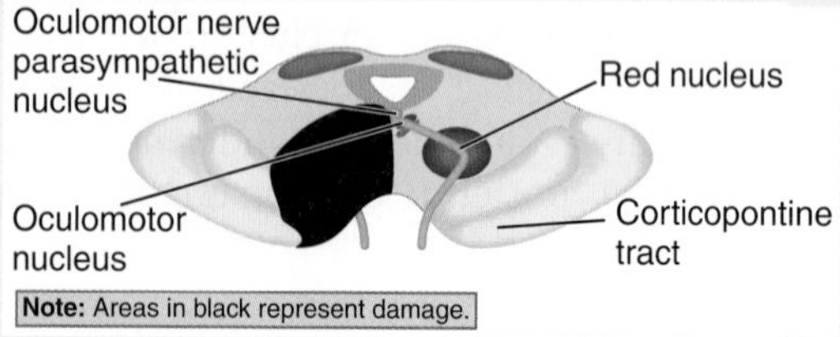 **Note:** Areas in black represent damage.	Contralateral hemiplegia	Contralateral CN III palsy
Pontine lesion 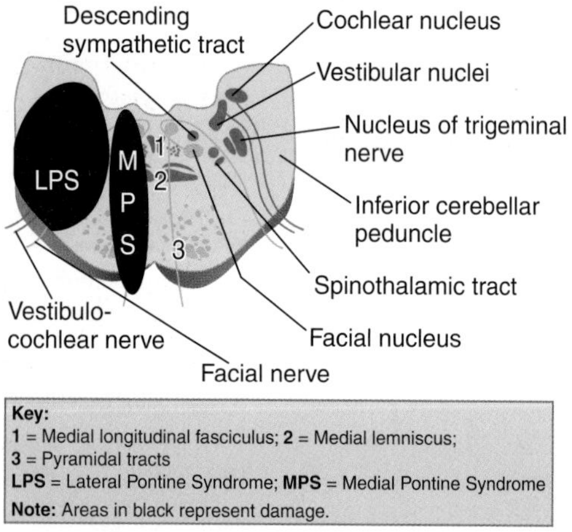 **Key:** **1** = Medial longitudinal fasciculus; **2** = Medial lemniscus; **3** = Pyramidal tracts **LPS** = Lateral Pontine Syndrome; **MPS** = Medial Pontine Syndrome **Note:** Areas in black represent damage.	*Medial pontine syndrome: (occlusion of paramedian branch of basilar artery)* Ipsilateral to lesion: Cerebellar ataxia, nystagmus Paralysis of conjugate gaze to side of lesion Diplopia Contralateral to lesion: Hemiparesis UE, LE Impaired sensation *Lateral pontine syndrome: (occlusion of anterior inferior cerebellar artery)* Ipsilateral to lesion: Cerebellar: ataxia, nystagmus, vertigo Facial paralysis Paralysis of conjugate gaze to the side of the lesion Deafness, tinnitus Impaired facial sensation Contralateral to lesion: Impaired pain and temperature sensation half of body	
Medullary lesion 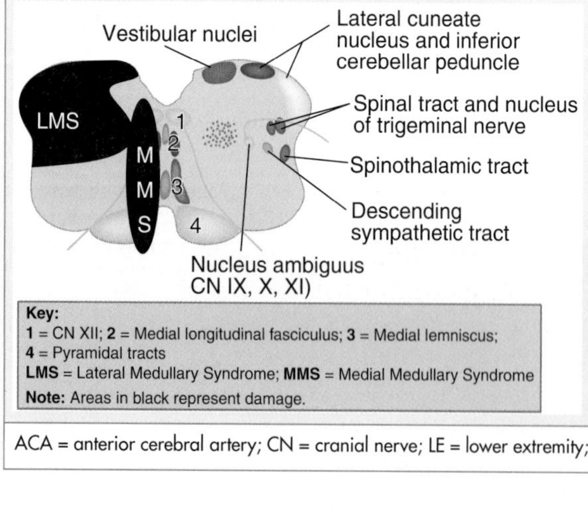 **Key:** **1** = CN XII; **2** = Medial longitudinal fasciculus; **3** = Medial lemniscus; **4** = Pyramidal tracts **LMS** = Lateral Medullary Syndrome; **MMS** = Medial Medullary Syndrome **Note:** Areas in black represent damage.	*Medial medullary syndrome: (occlusion vertebral artery, medullary branch)* Ipsilateral to lesion: paralysis of half of tongue Contralateral to lesion: Hemiplegia UE and LE Impaired sensation *Lateral medullary (Wallenberg's) syndrome: (occlusion of posterior inferior cerebellar artery/vertebral artery)* Ipsilateral to lesion: Cerebellar symptoms (ataxia, vertigo, nystagmus) Loss of pain and temperature to face Sensory loss UE, trunk, or LE Contralateral to lesion: Loss of pain and temperature to body and face	Horner's syndrome (miosis, ptosis, decreased sweating) Dysphagia Impaired speech

ACA = anterior cerebral artery; CN = cranial nerve; LE = lower extremity; MCA = middle cerebral artery; PCA = posterior cerebral artery; UE = upper extremity

c. Basilar artery syndrome: produces brainstem signs and symptoms and PCA signs and symptoms; locked-in syndrome (basilar artery occlusion at the level of the pons).
d. Medial inferior pontine syndrome: occlusion of the paramedian branch of basilar artery.
e. Lateral inferior pontine syndrome: occlusion of the anterior inferior cerebellar artery.
f. PCA syndrome: PCA and posterior communicating arteries supply the midbrain, temporal lobe, diencephalon, and posterior third of cortex; occlusions proximal to posterior communicating artery produce minimal deficits owing to collateral circulation.

3. Lacunar syndromes: seen in small vessel disease in the deep cerebral white matter (penetrating artery disease) and typically impact a small area with distinct symptoms. Types:
   a. Pure motor lacunar stroke: involvement of the posterior limb of the internal capsule, pons, and pyramids.
   b. Pure sensory lacunar stroke: involvement of the ventrolateral thalamus or thalamocortical projections.
   c. Dysarthria/clumsy hand syndrome: involving the base of the pons, genu of anterior limb, or the internal capsule.
   d. Ataxic hemiparesis: involving the pons, genu of internal capsule, corona radiata, or cerebellum.
   e. Sensory/motor stroke: involving the junction of the internal capsule and thalamus.
   f. Dystonia/involuntary movements: hemiballismus with involvement of the subthalamic nucleus; lacunar infarction of the putamen or globus pallidus.
   g. Deficits in consciousness, language, or visual fields are not seen in lacunar strokes because superficial cortical areas are not impacted.

Sequential Recovery Stages

1. Stage 1: initial flaccidity, no voluntary movement.
2. Stage 2: emergence of spasticity, hyperreflexia, synergies (mass patterns of movement).
3. Stage 3: voluntary movement possible, but only in synergies; spasticity strong.
4. Stage 4: voluntary control in isolated joint movements emerging, corresponding decline of spasticity and synergies.
5. Stage 5: increasing voluntary control out of synergy; coordination deficits present.
6. Stage 6: control and coordination near normal.

Examine

1. Generalized signs of increased intracranial pressure.
2. Level of consciousness, cognitive function.
3. Speech and communication.
   a. Examine for aphasia with lesions of parieto-occipital cortex of dominant hemisphere (typically left hemisphere).
   b. Examine for perceptual deficits with lesions of parietal lobe of nondominant hemisphere (typically right hemisphere).

> **RED FLAG:** Perceptual deficits may result in neglect, body scheme impairment, and Pusher's Syndrome. Patients with these conditions are at high risk for falls and traumatic/overuse injuries.

4. Behaviors.
   a. Patients with lesions of the left hemisphere (right hemiplegia) are typically slow, cautious, hesitant, and insecure. They are often aware of their impairments, resulting in frustration.
   b. Patients with lesions of the right hemisphere (left hemiplegia) are typically impulsive, quick, indifferent; often exhibit poor judgment and safety, overestimating their abilities while underestimating their problems.
5. Sensory deficits.
   a. Superficial, proprioceptive and combined sensations of contralateral extremities, trunk, and face.
   b. Hearing, vision; examine for homonymous hemianopsia.
   c. Cranial nerve function with brainstem, vertebrobasilar strokes (pseudobulbar palsy).
   d. Sensory impairments are often diverse and it is important to test various sensory modalities and consider the sensory homunculus, somatotopic organization of the spinal cord (see Figure 3-5), dermatomes (see Figure 3-10), and respective cutaneous peripheral nerves.
6. Motor function.
   a. Presence of abnormal tone and primitive reflexes.
   b. Spasticity (see Table 3-6).
   c. Loss of selective movements, presence of abnormal limb synergies (see Table 3-8).
      - Upper extremity flexion synergy.
      - Upper extremity extension synergy.
      - Lower extremity flexion synergy.
      - Lower extremity extension synergy.
   d. Presence of paresis, incoordination, motor programming deficits (apraxia).
   e. Postural and balance deficits.
   f. Gait: typical deficits.
      - Hip: poor hip position (retracted, flexed); Trendelenburg limp (weak abductors); scissoring (spastic adductors); insufficient pelvic rotation during swing.
      - Weak hip flexors during swing may yield circumducted gait, external rotation with adduction, backward leaning of trunk or exaggerated flexion synergy.

- Knee: weak knee extensors (knee flexes during stance) may result in compensatory locking of knee in hyperextension; spastic quadriceps may also yield a hyperextended knee.
- Ankle: footdrop/plantarflexion spasticity=equinus gait (heel does not touch down); varus foot (weight is borne on lateral side of foot); or equinovarus position (associated with hypertonia of the posterior tibialis).
- Unequal step lengths: leg does not advance through the end of stance into toe-off.
- Decreased cadence, uneven timing.

7. Function: functional mobility skills (FMS), activities of daily living (ADLs).
8. Selected standardized tests and measures for examination of patients with stroke (see Table 3-13 and Appendix 3a).

Physical Therapy Goals, Outcomes, and Interventions

1. Monitor changes associated with recovery and inactivity.
   a. Prevent or minimize indirect impairments/secondary complications.
   - Maintain ROM and prevent deformity through optimal positioning, PROM, and mobilization.
   - Maintain skin integrity.

RED FLAG: Avoid traction or overhead activity with pulleys when patients have flaccid shoulder muscles with risk of subluxation or dislocation.

RED FLAG: Emphasize compensation strategies for patients with sensory and perceptual losses to prevent additional injury and functional losses.

   b. Strengthen all available muscles.
2. Promote awareness, active movement, and use of hemiplegic side (remediation-facilitation approach).
   a. Promote normalization of tone through activities.
   b. Promote selective movement control (out-of-synergy movements) of involved extremities; emphasize functional patterns of movement.
3. Improve postural control, symmetry, and balance.
4. Task-specific training.
   a. Promote active problem-solving independence.
   b. Focus on goal-directed tasks, functional mobility skills (e.g., rolling, supine-to-sit, sitting, sit-to-stand, transfers, wheelchair skills, and locomotion).
   c. Focus on adapting movements to specific environmental demands.
   d. Organize feedback inputs (knowledge of results, knowledge of performance) and practice schedules to facilitate learning.
5. Promote independence in ADL/self-care; compensatory training as appropriate.
6. Improve respiratory and oromotor function; promote functional cardiorespiratory endurance.
   a. Improve chest expansion, diaphragmatic breathing pattern.
   b. Oromotor training.
   c. Aerobic conditioning: cycle ergometry, treadmill, or overground walking.

Table 3-13

APTA Neurology StrokEDGE Task Force Recommended Examination Items for Use by Entry-Level Physical Therapy Students*

EXAMINATION ITEMS	ITEM DESCRIPTION
Fugl-Meyer Assessment of Motor Performance	Includes subtests for upper extremity function, lower extremity function, balance, sensation, range of motion, and pain. Scoring of movements: 0=cannot perform, 1=partially performed, 2=fully performed.
Functional Independence Measure (FIM)-version 4.0	18 items (13 motor, 5 cognitive tasks) that capture function across multiple areas (e.g., feeding, grooming, bathing, dressing, transfers, gait, stairs, cognitive, social interaction, expression, bladder/bowel management).
Postural Assessment Scale for Stroke Patients	12 Items that measure postural control and balance in patients recovering from stroke. Items range from sitting without support to picking up a pencil from the floor. Items scored from 0–3 with higher scores reflecting better postural control.
Trunk Impairment Scale	Evaluates motor impairment of the trunk. Includes 3 subscales (static sitting, dynamic sitting, and coordination). Scores range from 0–23 with higher scores reflecting increased trunk impairment.
Stroke Impact Scale	Self-report measure that evaluates biopsychosocial health and participation following stroke. Measures physical problems, memory, changes in mood, emotions, communication, typical daily activities at home and in the community, participation in activities, and perception of recovery.

*The items above should also be combined with the core examination items in Box 3-1.

Adapted from Recommendations of the American Physical Therapy Association Academy of Neurologic Physical Therapy StrokEDGE Task Force. 2018. Additional information is located at https://www.neuropt.org/practice-resources/neurology-section-outcome-measures-recommendations/stroke

RED FLAG: When treating patients recovering from stroke, it is important to monitor heart rate and blood pressure closely during exercise or activity training; monitor for signs and symptoms of cardiovascular compromise (e.g., extension of stroke, second stroke, myocardial infarction, or deep vein thrombosis); modify or stop the intervention and notify medical and/or nursing staff as appropriate.

7. Isokinetic training: useful to improve timing deficits, velocity control of movement.
8. Locomotor training using body weight-support (BWS) and motorized treadmill training (TT).
9. EMG—biofeedback training: useful to decrease firing in spastic muscles, increase firing in paretic muscles, and improve motor control.
10. Functional electrical stimulation (FES): useful to stimulate muscle action, reduce spasticity, and substitute for an orthosis.
11. Constraint-induced movement therapy (CIMT) for patients with stroke. Patients must meet minimal movement criteria of wrist and finger movement.

Guidelines to Promote Learning with Hemispheric Differences

1. Patients with left hemisphere lesions (right hemiplegia).
   a. Develop an appropriate communication base: words, gestures, pantomime; assess level of understanding.
   b. Give frequent feedback and support.
   c. Do not underestimate ability to learn.
2. Patients with right hemisphere lesions (left hemiplegia).
   a. Use verbal cues; demonstrations or gestures may confuse patients with visuospatial deficits.
   b. Give frequent feedback: focus on slowing down and controlling movement.
   c. Focus on safety (patient may be impulsive).
   d. Avoid environmental (spatial) clutter.
   e. Do not overestimate ability to learn.

Traumatic Brain Injury

Traumatic Brain Injury (TBI)

1. Etiology: mechanism of injury is contact forces to skull and rotational acceleration forces, causing varying degrees of injury to the brain.
2. Signs and symptoms associated with localized lesions of the cortex (see Table 3-14).
3. Pathophysiology.
   a. Primary brain damage.
      - Diffuse axonal injury: disruption and tearing of axons and small blood vessels from shear-strain of angular acceleration; results in neuronal death and petechial hemorrhages.
      - Focal injury: contusions, lacerations, mass effect from hemorrhage, and edema (hematoma).
      - Coup-contracoup injury: injury at point of impact and opposite point of impact.
      - Closed or open injury (with fracture of the skull).
   b. Secondary brain damage/secondary cell death.
      - Hypoxic-ischemic injury: results from systemic problems (respiratory or cardiovascular) that compromise cerebral circulation.
      - Swelling/edema: can result in mass effect, with increased intracranial pressures, brain herniation (uncal, central, or tonsillar), and death.
      - Electrolyte imbalance and mass release of damaging neurotransmitters.
   c. Concussion: loss of consciousness, either temporary or permanent, resulting from injury or blow to head, with impaired functioning of the brainstem reticular activating system (RAS); may see changes in HR, RR, BP.
4. Levels of traumatic brain injury (see Table 3-15).
5. Selected standardized tests/outcome measures for patients with traumatic brain injury (See Table 3-16 and Appendix 3A).
6. Recovery stages from diffuse axonal injury.
   a. Coma: a state of unconsciousness in which there is neither arousal nor awareness; eyes remain closed, no sleep/wake cycles.
   b. Unresponsive Wakefulness Syndrome/vegetative state: marked by the return of sleep/wake cycles and normalization of vegetative functions (respiration, digestion, BP control); persistent vegetative state is determined if patient remains in vegetative state >1 year after TBI.
   c. Mute responsiveness/minimally responsive: state in which patient is not vegetative and does show signs, even if intermittent, of fluctuating awareness.
   d. Confusional state: mainly a disturbance of attention mechanisms; all cognitive operations are affected, patient is unable to form new memories; may demonstrate either hypoarousal or hyperarousal.
   e. Emerging independence: confusion is clearing and some memory is possible; significant cognitive problems and limited insight remain; frequently uninhibited social behaviors.
   f. Intellectual/social competence: increasing independence, although cognitive difficulties (problem solving, reasoning) persist along with behavioral and social problems (enhancement of premorbid traits, mood swings).
   g. Patient can plateau at any stage or regress under conditions of stress or repetitive brain injury.
7. Examine.
   a. For generalized signs of increased intracranial pressure.

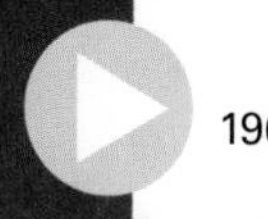

Table 3-14

Signs and Symptoms Associated with Localized Lesions of the Cortex (See Figure 3-1 for anatomical correlation)			
LOBE	**STRUCTURE**	**FUNCTION**	**DESTRUCTIVE LESION**
Frontal	**Precentral area:**		
	Primary motor cortex	Discrete volitional movements	Contralateral paralysis and paresis (most pronounced in distal parts of limbs and lower part of face)
	Premotor area	Motor planning or praxis	Apraxia or motor planning difficulties
	Prefrontal area	Motor association area	Lost of specific motor plans
	Supplementary motor	Bilateral control of posture	Loss of bilateral control of posture
	Middle frontal gyrus	Conjugate eye movements	Transitory paralysis of conjugate eye movements to opposite side
	Motor speech area (Broca)	Language production	Nonfluent (motor) aphasia
	Prefrontal area:		
	Dorsolateral	Motivation, problem-solving, and working memory	Bilateral lesions: Impaired ability to concentrate, memory
	Orbitofrontal	Emotions, behavior	Unstable emotions; unpredictable behaviors
	Orbital Gyri (posterolateral)	Olfaction	Inability to discriminate odors
Parietal	Postcentral gyrus/Primary somatosensory area	Somesthetic sensations	Loss of contralateral stimulus location, intensity
	Secondary somatosensory area	Sensory interpretation	Tactile agnosia: astereognosis, agraphesthesia, loss of two-point discrimination, extinction
	Gustatory cortex	Taste	Impairment of taste in contralateral side of tongue
	Parietal lobe (right hemisphere)	Perceptual function	Visual-spatial disorders, body scheme disorders, apraxias, tactile and auditory perceptual disorders
Temporal	Primary auditory cortex	Hearing	Subtle decrease in hearing and ability to localize sounds, both contralaterally
	Wernicke's speech area	Language understanding and formulation; storage of auditorially presented information	Fluent aphasia
	Superior temporal Gyrus (left hemisphere)		Impairment of learning and memory
	Temporal Cortex (nondominant side)	Storage of visually presented information	Profound memory loss of recent events, no new learning
	Parahippocampal region	Recent memory	
Occipital	Primary visual cortex	Vision	Contralateral homonymous hemianopsia Impairment of vision
	Visual association cortex	Visual understanding	Visual agnosia
	Posterior multimodal area (parietal, occipital, temporal lobes)	Integrates sensory information (somatosensory, visual, auditory)	Perceptual impairment

Table 3-15

Levels of Traumatic Brain Injury (TBI)			
	MILD TBI	**MODERATE TBI**	**SEVERE TBI**
Loss of Consciousness	0–30 minutes	>30 minutes but <24 hours	>24 hours
Alteration of Consciousness	brief; >24 hrs	>24 hours	>24 hours
Posttraumatic Amnesia	<1 day	>1 but <7 days	>7 days
Glasgow Coma Scale	13–15	9–12	<9
Imaging	normal	normal or abnormal	normal or abnormal

Table 3-16

APTA Neurology TBI EDGE Task Force Recommended Examination Items for Use by Entry-Level Physical Therapy Students*

EXAMINATION ITEMS	ITEM DESCRIPTION
Functional Independence Measure (FIM)-version 4.0	See previous discussion in Table 3-13.
Rancho Los Amigos Levels of Cognitive Functioning (LOCF)	Includes 8 general cognitive and behavioral levels for patient management (see Table 3-17).
Coma Recovery Scale—Revised	See previous description in Level of Consciousness Examination Section.
Agitated Behavior Scale	Measures a patient's agitation in acute recovery from an acquired brain injury. Includes items related to aggression, disinhibition, and lability.
Moss Attention Rating Scale	Examines cognition in individuals with moderate to severe impairments with attention.
Modified Ashworth Scale	See previous description in Examine Muscle Tone section.
The Action Research Arm Test (ARAT)	19 items that assess upper extremity performance (coordination, dexterity, and functioning) after CNS injury. Items are categorized into 4 subscales (grasp, grip, pinch, and gross movement).
High-Level Mobility Assessment (Hi-Mat)	See Table 3-11.
Community Balance and Mobility Scale	13-item scale used to detect high level balance and mobility deficient with community related tasks (e.g., Tandem walking, descending stairs, running with a controlled stop, crouch, and walk).
Dizziness Handicap Inventory	25-item questionnaire that examines impairments, activity limitations, and participation restrictions secondary to dizziness.
Community Integration Questionnaire	Examines social role limitations and community interaction in individuals recovering from TBI.

*The items above should also be combined with the core examination items in Box 3-1.

Adapted from McCulloch, KL et al. Outcome measures for persons with moderate to severe traumatic brain injury: Recommendations from the American Physical Therapy Association Academy of Neurologic Physical Therapy TBI EDGE Task Force. *J Neurol Phys Ther.* 2016 Oct; 40(4): 269–80.

Additional information is located at https://www.neuropt.org/practice-resources/neurology-section-outcome-measures-recommendations/traumatic-brain-injury.

b. Level of consciousness (Coma Recovery Scale-Revised), cognitive function (see Table 3-17; LOCF), examine for disorders of learning, attention, memory, and complex information processing.
c. Cranial nerve function.
d. Emotional dysregulation: characterized by poor modulation of emotional responses with environmental and interpersonal challenges, e.g., episodes of crying, anger, emotional outbursts, aggression toward self or others.
e. Changes in behavior: inappropriate physical, verbal, or sexual behaviors; poor judgment, irritability, low frustration tolerance; impulsivity, and safety issues.
f. Speech and communication.
g. Sensory deficits.
h. Motor function: examine for paresis, apraxia (dyspraxia), reflexive behaviors, balance deficits, ataxia, and incoordination (cerebellar damage is common).
i. Functional mobility skills (FMS), ADLs.
j. Level of general deconditioning; after prolonged hospitalization (comatose, vegetative, decreased response levels), patients experience severe deconditioning and effects of prolonged immobilization (disuse atrophy, contractures and deformity, skin breakdown).
k. Sympathetic storming: the result of hypothalamic stimulation of the SNS with an increase in circulating corticoids and catecholamines (stress response).
   - Examine for alterations in level of consciousness, increased posturing, dystonia, hypertension, hyperthermia, tachycardia, tachypnea, diaphoresis, and agitation.
   - Patients generally exhibit minimal alertness, minimal awareness, and reflexive motor response to stimulation.

8. Physical therapy goals, outcomes, and interventions.
   a. Monitor changes associated with recovery and inactivity.
   b. Management based on decreased response levels (LOCF I–III; see Table 3-17).
      - Maintain ROM, prevent contracture development: PROM, positioning, splinting, and serial casting.
      - Maintain skin integrity; prevent development of decubitus ulcers through frequent position changes.
      - Maintain respiratory status, prevent complications: postural drainage, percussion, vibration, suctioning to keep airway clear.

Table 3-17

Rancho Los Amigos Levels of Cognitive Function (LOCF)

LEVEL	RESPONSE	DEFINED
I	No response	Patient does not respond to external stimuli and appears asleep.
II	Generalized response	Patient reacts to external stimuli in nonspecific, inconsistent, and nonpurposeful manner with stereotypic and limited responses.
III	Localized response	Patient responds specifically and inconsistently with delays to stimuli but may follow simple commands for motor action.
IV	Confused, agitated response	Patient exhibits bizarre, nonpurposeful, incoherent or inappropriate behaviors, has no short-term recall, attention is short and nonselective.
V	Confused, inappropriate, nonagitated response	Patient gives random, fragmented, and nonpurposeful responses to complex or unstructured stimuli. Simple commands are followed consistently, memory and selective attention are impaired, and new information is not retained.
VI	Confused, appropriate response	Patient gives context appropriate, goal-directed responses, dependent upon external input for direction. There is carry-over for relearned, but not for new tasks, and recent memory problems persist.
VII	Automatic, appropriate response	Patient behaves appropriately in familiar settings, performs daily routines automatically, and shows carry-over for new learning at lower than normal rates. Patient initiates social interactions, but judgment remains impaired.
VIII	Purposeful, appropriate response	Patient oriented and responds to the environment but abstract reasoning abilities are decreased relative to premorbid levels.

Adapted from Gouvier WD et al. Reliability and validity of the Disability Rating Scale and the Levels of Cognitive Functioning Scale in monitoring recovery from severe head injury. *Arch Phys Med Rehabil.* 1987 Feb; 68(2): 94–7.

- Provide appropriate stimulation for arousal and to elicit movement and function; structure environment to enhance alertness and function.
- Promote early return of FMS: upright positioning for improved arousal, proper body alignment.

c. Management based on mid-level recovery (LOCF IV–VI; see Table 3-17).
- Provide structure and aids as appropriate for patients with cognitive deficits (e.g., posted and written daily schedules, memory logs).

RED FLAG: Prevent overstimulation for the confused and agitated patient; reduce environmental stimulation using a quiet, closed environment; provide calming stimuli.

- Provide consistency: use team-determined behavioral modification techniques, give clear feedback, written contracts.
- Engage the patient in task-specific training; limit activities to familiar, well-liked ones; offer options; break down complex tasks into component parts.
- Provide verbal or physical assistance.
- Control rate of instruction; provide frequent orientation to time, place, your name, and task.
- Emphasize safety, behavioral management techniques.
- Model calm, focused behavior.

d. Management based on high-level recovery (LOCF VII–VIII; see Table 3-17).
- Allow for increasing independence: wean patient from structure (closed to open environments); involve patient in decision-making.
- Assist patient in behavioral, cognitive, emotional reintegration: provide honest feedback, prepare for community reentry.
- Enhance motor learning and promote independence in functional tasks: FMS, ADLs, in real-life environments.
- Improve postural control, symmetry, and balance.
- Encourage active lifestyle, improved cardiovascular endurance.

e. Provide emotional support, encourage socialization, behavioral control, and motivation.
- Reorient and reassure.
- Provide patient and family education.

Concussion

1. The most common and least serious type to traumatic brain injury cause by a sudden direct blow or bump to the head; movement of the brain within the skull can cause bruising, damage to blood vessels, and injury to nerves.
   a. Risk factors: falls, high-risk sports, motor vehicle collision, physical abuse, and combat injuries.

b. Concussion signs observed (source: CDC.gov, HEADS UP):
- Appears dazed or stunned.
- Can't recall events prior to or after a hit or fall.
- Forgets an instruction, appears confused.
- Moves clumsily.
- Answers questions slowly.
- Loses consciousness (even briefly).
- Shows mood, behavior, or personality changes.

c. Concussion symptoms reported (source: CDC.gov, HEADS UP).
- Headache or pressure in head.
- Nausea or vomiting.
- Balance problems, dizziness, blurry vision.
- Bothered by light or noise.
- Feeling sluggish, hazy, foggy, or groggy.
- Confusion, concentration or memory problems.
- Just not "feeling right" or "feeling down."

2. Signs and symptoms typically occur soon after injury but some may be delayed for hours or days. Check for signs and symptoms immediately after injury and a few days after injury. See Chapter 13 for emergency response measures for individuals experiencing a concussion.
3. Grades of concussion:
   a. Mild (grade 1): symptoms last less than 15 minutes; there is no loss of consciousness.
   b. Moderate (grade 2): symptoms last longer than 15 minutes; there is no loss of consciousness.
   c. Severe (grade 3): loss of consciousness lasting seconds to minutes.
4. Physical and cognitive rest are required for the brain to heal. The individual should be closely monitored to include limited screen (phone, TV) time and monitoring of symptoms and slow progression for physical and cognitive activities.

RED FLAG: Seek immediate emergency care if the adult or child experiences any of the following:
- Drowsiness or inability to wake up.
- One pupil larger than the other.
- Repeat vomiting or nausea, convulsions or seizures.
- Loss of consciousness lasting longer than 30 seconds.
- Headache that gets worse over time.
- Slurred speech, numbness, or decreased coordination.
- Changes in behavior: irritability, restlessness, agitation.
- Confusion, disorientation, or amnesia.

5. Concussion occurring during athletic competition requires the individual to stop play; return to play or vigorous activity is contraindicated while signs or symptoms of a concussion persist. Medical clearance is required.
6. Baseline screening: typically done by a team of specialists and consisting of:
   a. Neurocognitive testing: memory, sequencing, speed of mental processing, and executive functions.
   b. Balance and equilibrium testing: the body's reactions to different challenges and positions.
   c. Vision testing: acuity, visual scanning.
7. Teach prevention strategies.
   a. Wear protective gear during sports or recreational activities.
   b. Buckle seatbelt when in an automobile.
   c. Safety proof homes to prevent falls.
   d. Exercise regularly to strength muscles and improve balance.
   e. Educate individuals about concussions.
8. Second-impact syndrome.
   a. A second concussion is experienced before the brain has a chance to heal from the first event.
   b. Can produce severe changes including brain swelling, massive increase in intracranial pressure and brain herniation, resulting in permanent brain damage with long-term disabilities or death.
9. Postconcussion syndrome.
   a. Persistent postconcussion symptoms lasting 3 months or longer; an indicator of concussion severity.
   b. Rare after only one concussion; likely to occur with multiple concussions.
   c. Symptoms may also include post-traumatic seizures, increased risk of depression, and mild-cognitive impairment later in life.
10. Chronic traumatic encephalopathy (CTE).
   a. A progressive neurodegenerative brain disease resulting from repetitive head trauma. Seen in athletes and boxers with a history of multiple concussions and repeated head injury.
   b. Pathological changes: diagnosis only made at autopsy by studying brain sections; brain changes include tau-positive neurofibrillary tangles (NFTs), neuropil threads and neocortical diffuse amyloid plaques, with or without neuritic plaques.
   c. Typical signs and symptoms include:
      - Recurrent headaches and dizziness.
      - Cognitive impairments: memory loss; difficulty thinking, planning, and carrying out tasks eventually progressing to dementia.
      - Mood or behavioral disturbances: depression, apathy, anxiety, suicidal thoughts or behavior, substance abuse.
      - Impaired judgment and impulse control, aggression, irritability, anger.
      - Movement disorders (late): a small subset of individuals with CTE can develop profound weakness, atrophy, spasticity similar to patients with ALS.
   d. Teach concussion prevention strategies.

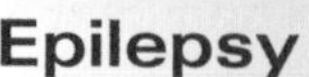

Epilepsy

Characteristics

1. A disorder characterized by recurrent seizures (repetitive abnormal electrical discharges within the brain).
2. Signs and symptoms.
   a. Altered consciousness.
   b. Altered motor activity (convulsion): characterized by involuntary contractions of muscles; tonic activity (stiffening and rigidity of muscles); clonic activity (rhythmic jerking of extremities).
   c. Sensory phenomena: patient experiences somatosensory, visual, auditory, olfactory, gustatory, and vertiginous sensations.
   d. Autonomic phenomena: associated with sudden attack of anxiety, tachycardia, sweating, piloerection, abnormal sensation rising up in upper abdomen and chest.
   e. Cognitive phenomena: sudden failure of comprehension, inability to communicate, intrusion of thought, illusions, hallucinations, affective disturbances (intense feelings of fear, anger, and hate).
3. Common causes of seizures.
   a. Acquired brain disease or trauma, tumor, stroke.
   b. Degenerative brain diseases: Alzheimer's dementia, amyloidosis.
   c. Developmental brain defects, low oxygen at birth.
   d. Drug overdose: cocaine, antihistamines, cholinesterase inhibitors, methylxanthines, tricyclic antidepressants.
   e. Drug withdrawal: alcohol, benzodiazepines.
   f. Electrolyte disorders: hyponatremia, hypernatremia, hypoglycemia, hypomagnesemia.
   g. Hyperthermia.
   h. Infections; brain abscess, meningitis or encephalitis, neurocysticercosis.
   i. Pregnancy complications: eclampsia.
4. Classification of seizures.
   a. Generalized seizures: all areas of the brain (cortex) are involved. Sometimes referred to as *grand mal seizures*.
      - Symptoms include: dramatic loss of consciousness, with stiffening, then rhythmic movements of the arms and legs; eyes are generally open; breathing is altered; loss of urine is common. Typically lasts 2–5 minutes.
      - Postseizure: consciousness is gradually regained; person typically confused, drowsy, and amnesiac after the event; may last several hours.
   b. Absence or petit mal seizures: posture is maintained, repetitive blinking or other small movements may be present. Typically brief, lasting only a few seconds; may occur many times in a day.
   c. Partial or focal seizures: only one part of brain is involved; symptoms are focal (specific area of the body).
      - Complex partial seizure: person appears dazed or confused, not fully alert or unconscious.
      - Temporal lobe seizure: characterized by episodic changes in behavior, with complex hallucinations; automatisms (e.g., lip smacking, chewing, pulling on clothing); altered cognitive and emotional function (e.g., sexual arousal, depression, violent behaviors); preceded by an aura.
   d. Secondarily generalized seizures: simple or complex partial seizures evolving to a generalized seizure.
   e. Status epilepticus: prolonged seizure or a series of seizures (lasting >30 minutes) with very little recovery between attacks; may be life threatening; medical emergency (generalized status epilepticus).

Examine/Determine

1. Time of onset, duration, type of seizure, sequence of events, frequency, duration.
2. Patient activity at onset, presence of aura.
3. Sensory elements, motor activity: type, degree, and location of involvement.
4. Presence of tongue biting, incontinence, respiratory distress.
5. Behavioral elements, changes in mood and perception.
6. Patient responses after the seizure.

Medical Interventions

1. Antiepileptic medications: phenytoin (Dilantin), carbamazepine (Tegretol), phenobarbital; drugs may have significant adverse side effects.
2. Surgical intervention: lobe resection, hemispherectomy.

Physical Therapy Goals, Outcomes, and Interventions

> **RED FLAG:** Recognize signs and symptoms of seizure and protect patient from injury during seizure. Remain with patient, remove potentially harmful nearby objects, loosen restrictive clothing, and do not restrain limbs. Establish airway, prevent aspiration by positioning the patient in sidelying, and wait for tonic-clonic activity to subside. Seek medical and/or nursing assistance ASAP. See Chapter 13, Safety and Protection, for additional discussion.

1. Establish airway, prevent aspiration: turn head to side or side-lying position; check to see if airway is open, wait for tonic-clonic activity to subside before initiating artificial ventilation if needed.
2. Promote regular routines for physical activity and emotional health.

Cerebellar Disorders

Diseases/Lesions of the Cerebellum

1. Hereditary ataxia, Friedreich's ataxia.
2. Neoplastic or metastatic tumors.
3. Infection.
4. Vascular: stroke.
5. Developmental: ataxic cerebral palsy, Arnold-Chiari syndrome.
6. Trauma: TBI.
7. Drugs, heavy metals.
8. Chronic alcoholism.

Cerebellar Lesions

1. Lesions of the archicerebellum (Vestibulocerebellar; flocculonodular lobe).
   a. Central vestibular symptoms: ocular dysmetria, poor smooth pursuit, dysfunctional vestibulo-ocular reflex (VOR), impaired eye-hand coordination.
   b. Gait and trunk ataxia: poor postural control and orientation, wide-based gait.
   c. Little change in tone or dyssynergia of extremity movements.
2. Lesions of the paleocerebellum (spinocerebellum; rostral cerebellum and anterior lobe).
   a. Hypotonia with weakness/fatigue. Key issue is with the timing of muscle activation (mismatch in alpha-gamma motor unit coactivation).
   b. Truncal ataxia: dysequilibrium, static postural tremor, increased sway, wide BOS, and high guard arm position. Posture worse with eyes closed, narrow BOS (Romberg, sharpened Romberg).
   c. Ataxic gait: unsteady, increased falls, uneven/decreased step length, increased step width.
3. Lesions of neocerebellum (hemisphere, posterior lobe). Ipsilateral signs and symptoms are typical.
   a. Intention tremor: irregular, oscillatory voluntary movements.
   b. Dysdiadochokinesia: impaired RAM.
   c. Dysmetria: hypermetria (overshooting), errors or force, direction, amplitude, rebound phenomenon (Holmes).
   d. Dyssynergia: abnormal timing (errors of velocity, onset, and stop), movement decomposition of agonist/antagonist interactions; impairments, of multijoint coordination, movement sequences, complex motor tasks.
   e. Errors in timing related to perceptual tasks.
4. Additional impairments.
   a. Asthenia: generalized weakness (3/5 to 4/5 manual muscle test grades).
   b. Hypotonia: especially in acute cerebellar lesions, difficulty with postural control of proximal (axial) muscles.
   c. Motor learning impairments: decreased anticipatory control, feedback, and learning delays.
   d. Cognition: deficits in information procession, attention deficits.
   e. Emotional dysregulation: changes in emotional behaviors.

Examine

1. Muscle strength, tone.
   a. Patient may have bursts of muscle activation and often misdiagnosed as inconsistent effort. Provide time to build a contraction (use make versus break test).
2. Range of motion.
3. Coordination: determine abnormalities of coordinated movement.
4. Balance: determine abnormalities of postural control and balance.
5. Gait: determine abnormalities of gait (ataxic gait).
6. Motor function: determine abnormalities of motor learning.
7. Functional status.
8. Endurance and fatigue level: fatigue is common with dysmetric patients.
9. Standardized tests/outcome measures for patients with cerebellar disorders (see previous discussions of various tests and also Appendix 3-A).
   a. Scale for Assessment and Rating of Ataxia (SARA).
   b. Dizziness Handicap Inventory (DHI).
   c. Modified Fatigue Impact Scale (MFIS).
   d. Balance tests.
   e. Functional Gait tests.
   f. Functional Independence Measure (FIM) and Functional Assessment Measure (FAM).

Physical Therapy Goals, Outcomes, and Interventions

1. Goals.
   a. Improve accuracy of limb movements.
   b. Improve postural stability and dynamic postural control.
   c. Improve functional mobility and safety: transfers and gait.
   d. Stabilize VOR/vision.
2. Eye-head coordination exercise: slow head movements with visual fixation; active eye and head movements.
3. Stability exercises: use of weight-bearing postures, carefully graded resistance, and approximation to promote steady holding. Use of theraband, weights (ankle and wrist cuffs), weighted waist belts, and walkers to decrease ataxic movements.
4. Dynamic stability exercises: promote small range control, smooth reversals of movements, movement transitions, using carefully graded resistance.

5. Balance training: compensatory training/safety important.
6. Locomotor training: TT with BWS; overground and community training.

RED FLAG: Maintain safety of patient during exercise and activity training; can use a harness and overhead support, parallel bars, weighted walker, or other device. Teach patient to recognize loss-of-balance situations and to utilize fall prevention strategies.

7. Therapeutic pool: water provides graded resistance, decreases ataxic movements and postural instability.
8. Coordination exercises: proprioceptive neuromuscular facilitation (PNF) patterns, ball gymnastics to promote balance.
9. Stationary bike: assists timing of reciprocal movements.
10. Motor learning strategies: low-stimulus environment (closed environment) ideal; focus on practice and repetition; distributed practice (endurance may be low).
11. Biofeedback: augmented feedback to enhance stability and postural control (i.e., balance training platform).
12. Energy conservation techniques, assistive devices as needed.

Central Nervous System Degenerative Disorders

Multiple Sclerosis

1. A chronic, progressive, demyelinating disease of the CNS affecting mostly young adults (age 20–50 years; mean age 34 years at onset).
2. Etiology: unknown; most likely viral, autoimmune (active immune responses detected in CSF). Females are at higher risk than males.
3. Characteristics.
   a. Demyelinating lesions (plaques) impair neural transmission, cause nerves to fatigue rapidly.
   b. Variable symptoms: lesions scattered in time and place; lesions common in pyramidal tract, dorsal columns, optic tract, and periventricular areas of cerebrum, cerebellar peduncles.

RED FLAG: The diverse symptoms, variability, and fluctuating periods of symptoms make the diagnosis of multiple sclerosis challenging. Multiple sclerosis should be part of the differential diagnosis for patients with varying symptoms that do not fit a specific anatomical location, as demyelinating plaques may be in multiple locations within the CNS.

   c. Variable course with fluctuating periods: exacerbations (worsening of symptoms) and remissions, progressing to permanent dysfunction.
   d. Precipitating or exacerbating factors: infections, trauma, pregnancy, stress.
   e. Transient worsening of symptoms: adverse reactions to heat, hyperventilation, dehydration, fatigue.
   f. Major clinical subtypes of MS.
      - Relapsing-remitting MS (RRMS): characterized by discrete attacks of neurological deficits (relapses) with either full or partial recovery (remission) in subsequent weeks or months; periods between relapses are characterized by lack of disease progression. Affects approximately 85% of cases.
      - Primary-progressive MS (PPMS): characterized by disease progression and a deterioration in function from onset; patients may experience modest fluctuations in neurological disability but discrete attacks do not occur.
      - Secondary-progressive MS (SPMS): characterized by an initial relapsing-remitting course, followed by a change to a progressive course with a steady decline in function, with or without continued acute attacks.
      - Progressive-relapsing MS (PRMS): characterized by a steady deterioration in disease from onset (similar to PPMS) but with occasional acute attacks; intervals between attacks are characterized by continuing disease progression.
      - Clinically isolated syndrome (CIS): first episode of inflammatory demyelination in the CNS that could become MS if additional activity occurs; can progress to RRMS.
4. Diagnostic tests: LP/CSF, elevated gamma globulin, CT or MRI, myelogram, EEG.
   a. A brain MRI with gadolinium is recommended for the diagnosis of MS.
   b. A spinal cord MRI is recommended if the brain MRI is nondiagnostic or if the presenting symptoms are referable to the spinal cord (Consortium of MRI Centers, 2018).
5. Examine.
   a. History: symptoms, disease progression, functional deficits.
   b. Cognitive/affective status: mild-to-moderate cognitive impairment common; also euphoria, emotional dysregulation.
   c. Communication: dysarthria and scanning speech common; dysphasia.
   d. ROM, deformity: associated with disuse and inactivity.
   e. Sensation: sensory symptoms common; e.g., paresthesias, hyperpathia (hypersensitivity to sensory stimuli), dysesthesias (abnormal sensations), trigeminal neuralgia, Lhermitte's sign (electric shock-like sensation throughout the body produced by flexing the neck).

f. Vision: diplopia or blurred vision common; also optic neuritis, scotoma (blind spot), nystagmus.
g. Skin integrity and condition.
h. Muscle tone, DTRs: spasticity and hyperreflexia are common (pyramidal tract lesions).
i. Muscle strength and control: paresis is common; if spasticity is severe, MMT may be invalid.
j. Coordination: ataxia is common; intention tremors, dysmetria, dysdiadochokinesia.
k. Balance: vestibular involvement common, with vertigo, dizziness, unsteadiness, paroxysmal or sudden onset of symptoms.
l. Gait: ataxic gait is common.
m. Fatigue: number one complaint; common with high levels of activity and as day progresses.
n. Aerobic capacity and endurance: monitor vital signs (HR, BP, RR) and breathing patterns. Examine for exertional symptoms and perceived exertion.
o. Functional status: FMS, ADLs.
p. General health measures: self report of physical and social function, general health, and vitality (e.g., Health Status Questionnaire—SF-36 or Patient Reported Outcomes Measurement Information System [PROMIS]).
q. Environment: home, community, and work.

6. Selected standardized tests/outcome measures for patients with MS (See Table 3-18 and Appendix 3A).
7. Medical management.
   a. Immunosuppressant drugs: treat acute flare-ups and shorten duration of episode; adrenocorticotropic hormone (ACTH) and steroids (e.g., prednisone, dexamethasone, betamethasone, methylprednisolone).

Table 3-18

APTA Neurology Multiple Sclerosis EDGE Task Force Recommended Examination Items for Use by Entry-Level Physical Therapy Students*

EXAMINATION ITEMS	ITEM DESCRIPTION
Functional Independence Measure (FIM)-version 4.0	See previous discussion in Table 3-13.
Multiple Sclerosis Quality of Life (MSQOL-54)	Multidimensional quality-of-life self-report measure that includes subscales on physical function, role limitations-physical, role limitations-emotional, pain, emotional well-being, energy, health perceptions, social function, cognitive function, health distress, overall quality-of-life, and sexual function.
12-item Multiple Sclerosis Walking Scale	Self-report measure with 12 questions that assess the impact of MS on an individual's perception of mobility (walking, running, and stairs).
2-minute walk test	Tests endurance and the ability to walk as far as possible for 2 minutes.
The Rivermead Mobility Index	14 self-report items and one observed item (sit to stand and stand unsupported) that measure activities from bed mobility to the ability to run.
Dynamic Gait Index	8-items of dynamic gait (e.g., head turns, changes in gait speed, pivot turns, obstacles, and stairs). See Table 3-11.
Timed Up & Go-(TUG) with Cognitive (count backwards by 3's) and Manual (hold a cup of water) tasks	See Table 3-11 for description.
Functional Reach Test	See Table 3-11 for description.
Static Standing Balance Test	5 conditions of static balance: Normal stance feet 10 cm apart, Feet together, Tandem stance 10 cm apart, Tandem stance (heel to toe, single leg stance). Subject completes two 30-second trials.
Dizziness Handicap Inventory (DHI)	See Table 3-16 for description.
Trunk Impairment Scale	See Table 3-13 for description.
Nine-Hole Peg Test (9-HPT)	Measures finger dexterity and ability to move pegs into 9 holes and return them to a container. Measured in seconds.
Fatigue Scale of Motor & Cognitive Function	20 self-report items that examine motor and cognitive fatigue.
Visual Analog Scale (Fatigue)	3 visual analog scales that measure the impact of fatigue on daily life, grooming, and household/occupational activities.

*The items above should also be combined with the core examination items in Box 3-1.
Adapted from recommendations from the American Physical Therapy Association Academy of Neurologic Physical Therapy Multiple Sclerosis EDGE Task Force-2012. Additional information is located at https://www.neuropt.org/practice-resources/neurology-section-outcome-measures-recommendations/multiple-sclerosis.

b. Interferon drugs: slow progression of disease, decrease symptoms (e.g., Avonex, Betaseron, Copaxone).
c. Symptomatic management of spasticity: drugs (e.g., baclofen, diazepam [Valium], dantrolene [Dantrium]), baclofen pump, phenol block surgery.
d. Symptomatic management of urinary problems: anticholinergic drugs.

8. Physical therapy goals, outcomes, and interventions.
   a. Monitor changes associated with disease progression; revise rehabilitation plan accordingly; develop/supervise maintenance program.
      - Examine for signs of urinary tract infection, respiratory infection (common causes of death).
   b. Rehabilitation goals.
      - Restorative: intensive, time-limited rehabilitation services designed to improve/stabilize patient status after a relapse.
      - Functional maintenance: services designed to manage effects of progressive disease and prevent/minimize indirect impairments associated with disuse and inactivity.
   c. Maintain ROM, prevent contracture.
   d. Maintain skin integrity, free of decubitus ulcers and other injury.
   e. Improve respiratory function.
   f. Improve sensory awareness, sensory compensation to prevent injury; consider eye patching with diplopia.
   g. Improve strength.
   h. Improve motor control, coordination: teach tone reduction techniques, compensatory strategies, safety.
   i. Improve postural control, symmetry, and balance; teach compensatory strategies and safety, provide assistive devices for gait.
   j. Locomotor training.
   k. Promote independence in functional mobility skills and ADLs; supervise family/home health aides in assisting patient.
   l. Promote maximum mobility in home and community; provide appropriate mobility aids and adaptive equipment (wheelchair use common); anticipate changes, rate of disease progression.
   m. Teach energy conservation techniques, activity pacing. Education about physical activities and stressors is important to minimize the effects of fatigue. The patient should be instructed in energy conservation and pacing, optimal scheduling, and use of assistive devices as appropriate. An activity diary can be used to assist the patient in identifying and avoiding stressors and highly fatiguing activities.

RED FLAG: For patients who are easily fatigued and/or experience chronic fatigue (e.g., patients with multiple sclerosis, amyotrophic lateral sclerosis, postpolio syndrome, chronic fatigue syndrome) it is important to carefully examine fatigue thresholds and responses to exercise. A distributed practice schedule (discontinuous protocol) should be performed with exercise and rest intervals carefully spaced and rest times exceeding exercise times. Exercises should begin at a low level and increase in duration before intensity. Exercise sessions should be scheduled during optimal times for function (e.g., mid-morning, mid-afternoon).

9. Provide psychological and emotional support.
   a. Emphasize realistic expectations; focus on remaining abilities.
   b. Provide patient, family, and caregiver education.
   c. Teach problem-solving skills, emphasize coping skills.

Parkinson's Disease

1. A chronic progressive disease of the CNS with degeneration of the dopaminergic substantia nigra neurons and nigrostriatal pathways.
2. Etiology: several different causes identified: infectious/postencephalitic, atherosclerosis, idiopathic, toxic, drug induced.
   a. Deficiency of dopamine within the basal ganglia corpus striatum with degeneration of substantia nigra.
   b. Loss of inhibitory dopamine results in excessive excitatory output from cholinergic system (acetylcholine) of basal ganglia.
3. Signs and symptoms.
   a. Classic symptoms: rigidity (leadpipe or cogwheel), bradykinesia (hypokinesia), resting tremor (resting), impaired postural reflexes.
   b. Slowly progressive with emergence of secondary impairments and permanent dysfunction.
   c. Stages (Hoehn and Yahr classification).
      - Stage I-Minimal or absent disability, unilateral symptoms.
      - Stage II-Minimal bilateral or midline involvement, no balance involvement.
      - Stage III-Impaired balance, some restrictions in activity.
      - Stage IV-All symptoms present and severe; stands and walks only with assistance.
      - Stage V-Confinement to bed or wheelchair.
4. Examine.
   a. History: symptoms, disease progression, functional deficits.

- It is important to assess if the patient has taken dopaminergic medication (on period) or not (off period) prior to examination and treatment sessions.

b. Cognitive status: intellectual impairment/dementia occurs in advanced stages; examine for memory deficits, bradyphrenia (slowing of thought processes), and depression.
c. Communication: dysarthria, hypophonia (decreased volume) are common; mutism in advanced stages; mask-like face with infrequent blinking and expression, writing becomes progressively smaller.
d. Oromotor control, nutritional status: dysphagia is common, problems in chewing and swallowing.
e. Cardiorespiratory function: examine for reduced endurance, altered breathing patterns, and chest mobility (decreased thoracic expansion), RR. Examine aerobic capacity (exercise testing, 6- or 12-Minute Walk Test). Orthostatic hypotension with positional change is common.
f. ROM, deformity associated with disuse and inactivity: contractures common in flexors, adductors; persistent posturing in kyphosis with forward head; many patients osteoporotic with high risk of fracture.
g. Sensation/perceptual function: examine for aching and stiffness, abnormal sensations (cramp-like sensations, poorly localized), problems in spatial organization, perception of vertical, extreme restlessness (akathisia).
h. Vision: examine for blurring, cogwheeling eye pursuit, eye irritation from decreased blinking, decreased pupillary reflexes.
i. Skin integrity and condition, edema, and circulatory changes in LE.
j. Autonomic changes: excessive drooling (salivation) or sweating; greasy skin, and abnormalities in thermoregulation.
k. Muscle tone: examine for rigidity, including location, distribution, and symmetry between two sides of body, type (cogwheel or leadpipe).
l. Muscle strength: weakness is associated with disuse and atrophy; assess torque output at varying speeds (isokinetics).
m. Motor function: examine for bradykinesia (slowed movement) or akinesia (absent movement), ability to initiate movement (number of freezing episodes, precipitating factors); assess reaction time versus movement time, overall poverty of movement.
n. Involuntary movements: examine for presence, location of tremor, precipitating factors; resting tremor common, especially pill-rolling of hands; tremors during movement may occur in advanced stages; postural tremors.
o. Balance: impaired postural reactions are common (worse with severe rigidity of trunk, lack of trunk rotation); examine for ability to maintain static and dynamic balance, reactive adjustments and anticipatory adjustments.
p. Gait: characterized by poverty of movements, with generalized lack of extension; festination common (an abnormal, involuntary increase in the speed of walking, often with forward acceleration, but may occur with backward progression). Examine for freezing of gait (FOG) and fall risk.
q. Functional status: functional mobility skills, BADL, IADL, hand function (dexterity a frequent problem).
r. Overall level of fatigue and inability to sustain performance is common; affected by stress and high effort.
s. Psychosocial function: levels of depression, stress and anxiety, and available coping strategies.
t. Patients on levodopa: examine for fluctuations in symptoms related to dosing (end-of-dose deterioration, on-off phenomenon, dyskinesia); common with disease progression and long-term use of levodopa (e.g., 2–3 years).

5. Standardized tests/outcome measures for patients with Parkinson's disease (see Table 3-19 and Appendix 3A).

> **RED FLAG:** Monitor closely for adverse drug effects. Patients taking Sinemet long term may experience nausea and vomiting, orthostatic hypotension, cardiac arrhythmias, involuntary movements (dyskinesias), and psychoses and abnormal behaviors (hallucinations). Monitor closely drug dosing cycles and recognize signs and symptoms of on–off phenomenon (e.g., sudden changes with loss of function, immobility, and severe dyskinetic movements). Notify medical and/or nursing staff as appropriate.

6. Medical management.
   a. Dopamine agonist drugs: enhance the effects of Sinemet therapy (bromocriptine, pergolide mesylate).
   b. Anticholinergic drugs: for control of tremor.
   c. Amantadine: enhances dopamine release.
   d. Selegiline (deprenyl): monoamine oxidase inhibitor increases dopamine; used during early disease to slow progression.
   e. Deep brain stimulation in thalamus or subthalamic nucleus.
7. Physical therapy goals, outcomes, and interventions.
   a. Monitor changes associated with disease progression and pharmacological interventions; revise rehabilitation plan accordingly; develop/supervise maintenance program.

Table 3-19

APTA Neurology Parkinson EDGE Task Force Recommended Examination Items for Use by Entry-Level Physical Therapy Students*

EXAMINATION ITEMS	ITEM DESCRIPTION
The Parkinson's Disease Questionnaire (PDQ-39)	Participation and quality-of-life questionnaire that focuses on the subjective report of the impact of Parkinson's disease on daily life. Measures various domains: Activities of daily living, Memory, Cognition, Communication, Mobility, Quality-of-Life, Social Relationship, and Support.
Montreal Cognitive Assessment	Assesses multiple cognitive domains (visuospatial, executive function, naming, memory, attention, language, abstraction, and orientation). Used to assess mild cognitive impairment.
Sit-to-Stand 5 Times	See Table 3-11.
Functional Gait Assessment	See Table 3-11.
Mini-Balance Evaluation Systems Test (Mini-BEST)	See Table 3-11.
6-minute Walk Test	See Table 3-11.
Nine-hole Peg Test	Measures finger dexterity and ability to move pegs into 9 holes and returns them to a container. Measured in seconds.

*The items above should also be combined with the core examination items in Box 3-1.

Adapted from recommendations from the American Physical Therapy Association Academy of Neurologic Physical Therapy Parkinson EDGE Task Force-2014. Additional information is located at https://www.neuropt.org/practice-resources/neurology-section-outcome-measures-recommendations/parkinson-disease.

b. Prevent or minimize secondary impairments associated with disuse and inactivity (see section on MS).
c. Teach compensatory strategies to initiate movement and unlock freezing episodes, e.g., repetitive auditory stimulation/music.
d. Improve strength: emphasis on improving overall mobility, rotational patterns (consider proprioceptive neuromuscular facilitation patterns, rhythmic initiation technique).
e. Teach relaxation skills.
f. Improve postural control, symmetry, and balance; teach compensatory strategies, safety.
g. Improve gait; locomotor training.
h. Promote independence in FMS and ADLs; supervise family/home health aides in assisting patient.
i. Promote maximum mobility and safety in home and community, improve gait: provide appropriate aids and adaptive equipment; anticipate changes, progression of disease.
j. Improve cardiovascular endurance.
k. Teach energy conservation techniques, activity pacing.
l. Provide psychological and emotional support (see section on MS).

Vestibular Disorders

Signs and Symptoms (See Table 3-20)

1. Dizziness: means different things to different patients. Obtain a precise understanding of symptoms by conducting a thorough subjective examination:
   a. Does the room spin around (external vertigo)?
   b. Do you feel unstable (unsteadiness)?
   c. Do you feel like you may faint (presyncope)?
   d. Do you feel lightheaded?
2. Vertigo: sensation that the visual surrounding is spinning or flowing; can be spontaneous or triggered; if severe, accompanied by nausea and vomiting.
3. Unsteadiness:
   a. Occurs when the brain receives inadequate information about the body's position from the somatosensory, visual, and vestibular systems, may result from peripheral neuropathy, eye disease, or peripheral vestibular disorders.
   b. Patient has ataxia, gait disturbances and increased risk of falls.
4. Presyncope is caused by cardiovascular disorders reducing cerebral perfusion.
5. Lightheadedness is nonspecific and hard to diagnose; it may result from panic attacks with hyperventilation.
6. Visual changes.
   a. Nystagmus: an involuntary, rapid, rhythmic, oscillatory eye movement; e.g., torsional, horizontal, vertical.
   b. Blurred vision: gaze instability secondary to vestibulo-ocular reflex (VOR) dysfunction.
7. Indirect impairments: physical deconditioning, decreased cervical ROM.
8. Reference: Scott DZ et al. (2009). Classification of vestibular signs and examination techniques: Nystagmus and nystagmus-like movements Consensus document of the Committee for the International Classification of Vestibular Disorders of the Bárány Society. *Journal of Vestibular Research*; 29(2-3): 57–87.

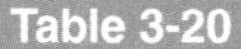

Table 3-20

Terms and Definitions Associated with Vestibular Disorders	
TERM	**DEFINITION**
(Non-vertiginous) dizziness	The sensation of disturbed or impaired spatial orientation without a false or distorted sense of motion
(Internal) vertigo	The sensation of self-motion when no self-motion is occurring or the sensation of distorted self-motion during an otherwise normal head movement
External vertigo	The false sensation that the visual surround is spinning or flowing
Unsteadiness	The feeling of being unstable while seated, standing, or walking without a particular directional preference

Adapted from Bisdorff et al., 2009. Classification of vestibular symptoms: Towards an international classification of vestibular disorders. *Journal of Vestibular Research*; 19(1-2): 1–13.

Etiology: Unilateral Peripheral Vestibular Hypofunction (PVH)

1. Trauma: vestibular symptoms seen in 87% of patients with acute TBI, with PVH occurring in 19%.
2. Vestibular neuronitis, labyrinthitis: an acute infection with prolonged attack of symptoms, persisting for several days or several weeks; caused by viral or bacterial infection.
3. Ménière's disease: an episodic vertigo syndrome associated with low to medium frequency sensorineural hearing loss and fluctuating aural symptoms (hearing, tinnitus and/or fullness) in the affected ear; duration of vertigo episodes is between 20 minutes and 12 hours; etiology unknown, but associated with the accumulation of endolymph.
4. Benign paroxysmal positional vertigo (BPPV): brief attacks of vertigo and nystagmus that occur with a change in head position (looking up, bending, quick head movements, lying down or getting out of bed and rolling over in bed, which comprise the 5-item BPPV score on the Dizziness Handicap Inventory); may be related to degenerative processes, caused by otoconia that are dislodged from the otoliths and are trapped in a semicircular canal (see Table 3-21).
5. Tumor: acoustic neuroma (vestibular schwannoma), gliomas/brainstem, or cerebellar medulloblastoma.
6. References:
   a. Marcus HJ et al. Vestibular dysfunction in acute traumatic brain injury. *J Neurol*. 2019; 266(10): 2430–2433.
   b. Cite: López-Escámez JA et al. (2015). Diagnostic criteria for Meniére's Disease. *Journal of Vestibular Research*; 25(1): 1–7.
   c. Whitney SL et al. (2005). Usefulness of the dizziness handicap inventory in the screening for benign paroxysmal positional vertigo. *Otol Neurotol*. 26(5): 1027–33.
   d. von Brevern M et al. (2015). Benign paroxysmal positional vertigo: Diagnostic criteria. Consensus document of the Committee for the Classification of Vestibular Disorders of the Bárány Society. *Journal of Vestibular Research*; 25(3-4): 105–117.

Etiology: Bilateral Peripheral Vestibular Hypofunction

1. Otoxic drugs
2. Bilateral Meniere's disease
3. Meningitis
4. Other causes: tumors (i.e., bilateral vestibular schwannoma); autoimmune diseases (i.e., neurosarcoidosis, cerebral vasculitis, systemic lupus erythematosus); rarely bilateral labyrinthine concussion.
5. Reference. Strupp M et al. (2017). Bilateral vestibulopathy: Diagnostic criteria Consensus document of the Classification Committee of the Bárány Society. *Journal of Vestibular Research*; 27(4): 177–189.

Examine

1. History: determine type, nature, duration of symptoms, triggering stimuli/activity.
2. ROM: special attention to cervical ROM.
3. VOR function: examine for nystagmus, blurred vision with head and total body movements.

RED FLAG: Down-beating nystagmus or direction-changing gaze-evoked nystagmus are both indicators of central nervous system pathology and need for referral/imaging. Pure torsional nystagmus and inability to walk (even short distances) also raise concerns and suggest the need for further medical work-up.

4. Vertebral artery compression.
   a. Can produce vestibular symptoms.
   b. Patient may have pain in the head and neck; neck stiffness without ROM limitation; dizziness and diplopia, unilateral facial numbness, nausea/vomiting, and ataxia.
   c. Reference. Thiel et al. (2005). Is it time to stop functional pre-manipulation testing of the cervical spine? *Manual Therapy*, 10(2): 154–158.
5. Sensory function.
   a. Examine for intact vision, proprioception, especially of feet/ankles. Important for compensatory postural adjustments with vestibular losses.

b. Examine modified Clinical Test of Sensory Interaction in Balance (mCTSIB).
6. Vestibulospinal Reflex function: examine posture and balance; examine for instability in sitting, standing, during functional activities, and gait.
7. Positional testing: changes in position produce symptoms (e.g., dizziness, vertigo) and often nystagmus.
   a. Dix-Hallpike test or Sidelying test.
   b. Roll test.
8. Diagnostic testing.
   a. Head Impulse test.
   b. Dynamic Visual Acuity test.
9. Standardized tests/outcome measures for patients with vestibular disorders (see previous discussions of various tests and also Appendix 3A).
   a. Dizziness Handicap Inventory (DHI).
   b. Activities-Specific Balance Confidence Scale (ABC).
   c. Postural stability/balance tests (see Table 3-11 for description of selected measures) e.g., Berg Balance Test, MiniBest Test, Four Square Step Test, Romberg and Sharpened Romberg, Functional Reach, and modified Clinical Test for Sensory Interaction in Balance (mCTSIB).
   d. Functional Gait tests: e.g., Functional Gait Assessment, Timed Up and Go, and Gait Velocity (see Table 3-11 for description of selected measures).
   e. Vestibular Disorders Activities of Daily Living Scale (VADL): assesses self-perceived disablement in patients with vestibular impairment.
   f. For additional information regarding recommended examination items from the APTA Neurology Vestibular Edge Task Force please see: https://www.neuropt.org/practice-resources/neurology-section-outcome-measures-recommendations/vestibular-disorders.

Medical Interventions

1. Vestibular suppressant medications; prolonged use may delay recovery.
2. Severe cases may require ablative surgery.

Physical Therapy Goals, Outcomes, and Interventions

> **RED FLAG:** Implement safety measures as appropriate, including effective use of sensory substitution and compensatory strategies; provide ambulatory aids as indicated (e.g., cane or walker).

1. Provide active exercises to promote vestibular adaptation (recalibration of system).
   a. Habituation training: repetition of movements and positions that provoke dizziness and vertigo.
   b. Gaze stability exercises.
      - Head moves horizontally while eyes remain stationary on static target (X1 paradigm) or moving target (X2 paradigm); can also be performed vertically.
      - Head movements up and down, side to side while maintaining eyes focused on a visual target; progressing slow to fast movements, plain to visually complex background, standing on stable to unstable surface to walking.
   c. Postural stability: exercises such as sitting and standing, static and dynamic balance activities (e.g., bending forward, turning); walking, walking and turning, walking with head turns.
   d. Emphasize functional mobility skills: community activities, activities with spatial and timing constraints.
   e. Relaxation training: to decrease anxiety levels.
   f. Begin conservatively, avoid excessive exacerbation of symptoms.
2. Recovery is better, generally faster in unilateral than bilateral vestibular dysfunction.
3. Provide psychological support and reassurance.
4. BPPV treatment techniques (see Table 3-21).
   a. Canalith repositioning maneuver: for debris that is free-floating in the semicircular canal.
   b. Liberatory maneuver: for debris that is adherent to the cupula (cupulolithiasis).
   c. Brandt-Daroff exercises: for residual or mild vertigo.
5. See Chapter 10 for discussion of fall prevention and interventions.
6. See Box 3-2, Clinical Practice Guidelines: Management of Individuals with Peripheral Vestibular Hypofunction.

Spinal Cord Injury (SCI)

1. Etiology: partial or complete disruption of spinal cord resulting in paralysis, sensory loss, altered autonomic and reflex activities.
   a. Traumatic causes: motor vehicle accident (most common cause of SCI), jumps and falls, diving, gunshot wounds.
   b. Mechanisms of injury: flexion (most common lumbar injury), flexion-rotation (most common cervical injury), compression, hyperextension.
   c. Spinal areas of greatest frequency of injury: C5, C7, T12, and L1.
   d. Nontraumatic causes: disc prolapse, vascular insult, cancer, infection.
2. Pathophysiology.
   a. Primary injury, interruption of blood supply.
   b. Secondary sequelae: ischemia, edema, demyelination, and necrosis of axons, progressing to scar tissue formation.

Table 3-21

Diagnosis and Treatment of the Most Common Variants of Benign Paroxysmal Positional Vertigo (BPPV)

LOCATION OF DEBRIS	TEST & POSITIVE FINDING	DIAGNOSIS	COMMON TREATMENT MANEUVERS
Free-floating in posterior semicircular canal	Dix-Hallpike or Sidelying Test: up-beating, ipsitorsional nystagmus of short duration	Posterior canal canalithiasis BPPV	Epley maneuver (starting in the Dix-Hallpike test position for the affected ear, and turning towards the unaffected ear) Semont maneuver (starting with head rotated away from the affected ear, down to the affected ear, and rapidly nose down toward the other side)
Adhered to cupula in posterior semicircular canal	Dix-Hallpike or Sidelying Test: up-beating, ipsitorsional nystagmus of long duration	Posterior canal cupulolithiasis BPPV	Semont maneuver (starting with head rotated away from the affected ear, down to the affected ear, and rapidly nose down toward the other side)
Free-floating in anterior semicircular canal	Dix-Hallpike or Sidelying test: down-beating, ipsitorsional nystagmus of short duration	Anterior canal canalithiasis BPPV	Epley maneuver (starting in the Dix-Hallpike test position for the affected ear, and turning towards the unaffected ear) Semont maneuver (starting with head rotated toward the affected ear, down to the affected ear, and rapidly nose up toward the other side)
Adhered to cupula in anterior semicircular canal	Dix-Hallpike or Sidelying test: down-beating, ipsitorsional nystagmus of long duration	Anterior canal cupulolithiasis BPPV	Semont maneuver (starting with head rotated toward the affected ear, down to the affected ear, and rapidly nose up toward the other side)
Free-floating in horizontal semicircular canal	Roll test: geotropic nystagmus (treat side of greater symptoms/nystagmus)	Horizontal canal canalithiasis BPPV	270° BBQ roll (Lempert maneuver) (starting with head rotated toward the affected ear, and turning towards the unaffected ear) Appiani (Gufoni) maneuver for canalithiasis (down to the unaffected ear for 2 minutes, then rotated nose down for 2 minutes)
Adhered to cupula in horizontal semicircular canal	Roll test: apogeotropic nystagmus (treat side of lesser symptoms/nystagmus)	Horizontal canal cupulolithiasis BPPV	Gufoni maneuver for cupulolithiasis (rapidly down to the affected ear and then rapidly rotated nose up for 2 minutes); must be followed by the Appiani (Gufoni) maneuver for canalithiasis as described above

3. Classification.
   a. Level of injury: UMN injury.
      - Lesion level indicates most distal uninvolved nerve root segment with normal function; muscles must have a grade of at least 3+/5 or fair+ function.
      - Tetraplegia (quadriplegia): injury occurs between C1 and C8, involves all four extremities and trunk.
      - Paraplegia: injury occurs between T1 and T12–L1, involves both lower extremities and trunk (varying levels).
   b. Degree of injury.
      - Complete: no sensory or motor function below level of lesion.
      - Incomplete: preservation of sensory or motor function below level of injury; spotty sensation, some muscle function.
      - American Spinal Injury Association (ASIA) Impairment Scale.
        - A = Complete, no motor or sensory function is preserved in the sacral segments S4–5.
        - B = Incomplete: sensory but no motor function is preserved below the neurological level and includes the sacral segments S4–5.
        - C = Incomplete: motor function is preserved below the neurological level, and most key muscles below the neurological level have a muscle grade of less than 3.
        - D = Incomplete: motor function is preserved below the neurological level, and most key muscles below the neurological level have a muscle grade of 3 or more.
        - E = Normal: motor and sensory function is normal.
4. Clinical Syndromes (see Table 3-22).
   a. Central cord syndrome: loss of more centrally located cervical tracts/arm function, with preservation of more peripherally located lumbar and sacral tracts/leg function; typically caused by hyperextension injuries to the cervical spine.

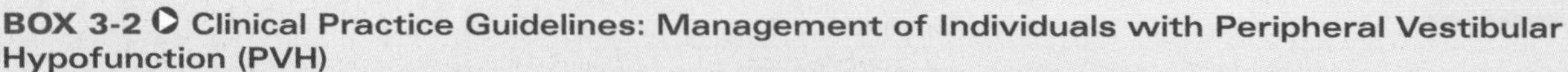

BOX 3-2 Clinical Practice Guidelines: Management of Individuals with Peripheral Vestibular Hypofunction (PVH)

Examination

- Factors that may have a negative impact on recovery from PVH should be identified, including comorbidities (anxiety, migraine, peripheral neuropathy) and vestibular suppressants. Age, gender, and symptom onset time do not affect outcomes. Potential harm exists if rehabilitation is delayed. (A-C-strong to weak recommendation; Levels I-III)

Therapeutic Interventions

- **Vestibular rehabilitation should be offered to people with symptoms due to acute, subacute, and chronic unilateral PVH; and bilateral PVH, including pediatrics. (A – strong recommendation; Level I)**
    - **Benefits include reduced dizziness/vertigo, improved gaze stability, reduced imbalance and falls, improved ADL and quality of life**
- Patient outcomes are improved with supervised and customized vestibular rehabilitation exercises. (B-moderate recommendation; Level I-II)
- **Voluntary saccadic or smooth pursuit eye exercises should not be offered in isolation (i.e., without head movement); should be included in specific exercises for gaze stabilization focusing on adaptation and substitution. (A-strong recommendation; Level I)**
- Targeted exercises for people with PVH (unilateral or bilateral) should address specific goals that focus on identified impairments and functional limitations. (B-moderate recommendation; Level II)
- Optimal exercise dose for people with PVH (unilateral and bilateral) (F-recommendation based on expert opinion; Level V)
    - Acute/Subacute: 3x/day minimum (at least 12 minutes/day)
    - Chronic: 3x/day minimum (at least 20 minutes/day)
- **Quality of life improves and psychological distress is reduced (i.e., improvements in perceived disability and anxiety scores) with vestibular rehabilitation. (A-strong recommendation; Level I)**
- Decision rules for stopping vestibular rehabilitation in persons with PVH (unilateral and bilateral) should be based on goals met, resolution of symptoms, or plateau in progress. (F-recommendation based on expert opinion; Level V)
    - Other factors for stopping may include patient choice or nonadherence, prolonged symptom increase or status deterioration, and/or if comorbidities affect ability to participate
    - General recommendations include
        - Acute/subacute: 1x/week for 2–3 sessions
        - Chronic unilateral: 1x/week for 4–6 weeks
        - Bilateral: 1x/week for 8–12 weeks

Grade = Recommendation Strength; Level = Level of Evidence.

Levels of Evidence and Grades of Recommendation are defined in Table 16-4.

Adapted from: Hall, C, et al. Vestibular rehabilitation for peripheral vestibular hypofunction: An evidence-based clinical practice guideline from the American Physical Therapy Association Neurology Section. *J Neurol Phys Ther.* 2016; 40(2), 124–155.

b. Brown-Séquard syndrome: hemisection of spinal cord typically caused by penetration wounds (gunshot or knife) with asymmetrical symptoms.

c. Anterior cord syndrome: damage is mainly in anterior cord, resulting in loss of motor function, pain, and temperature with preservation of light touch, proprioception and position sense, typically caused by flexion injuries of the cervical spine.

d. Posterior cord syndrome: loss of posterior columns with preservation of motor function, sense of pain and light touch; extremely rare.

e. Cauda equina: injury below L1 results in injury to lumbar and sacral roots of peripheral nerves (LMN) with sensory loss and paralysis and some capacity for regeneration; an LMN lesion with autonomous or nonreflex bladder.

f. Sacral sparing: sparing of tracts to sacral segments, with preservation of perianal sensation, rectal sphincter tone, or active toe flexion.

5. Examine.

a. Vital signs.

b. Respiratory function: action of diaphragm, respiratory muscles, intercostals; chest expansion, breathing pattern, cough, vital capacity; respiratory insufficiency or failure occurs in lesions above C4 (phrenic nerve, C3–5 innervates diaphragm).

Table 3-22

Spinal Cord Injury Syndromes (See also Figure 3-5, spinal cord somatotopic organization)

LESION	CHARACTERISTICS
Complete Cord Lesion: UMN lesion 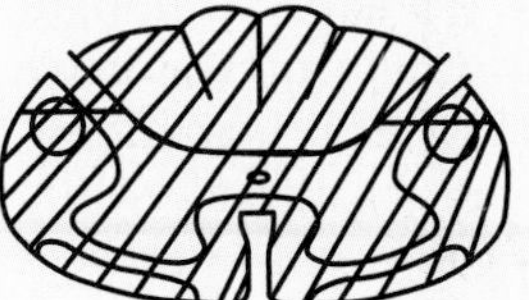	Complete bilateral loss of all sensory modalities Bilateral loss motor function with spastic paralysis below level of lesion Loss of bladder and bowel functions with spastic bladder and bowel
Central Cord Lesion: UMN lesion 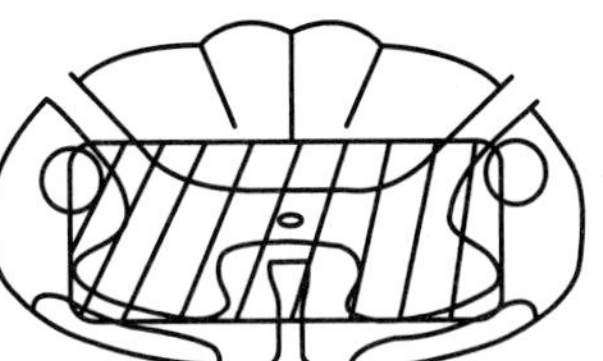	Cavitation of central cord in cervical section Loss of spinothalamic tracts with bilateral loss of pain and temperature Loss of ventral horn with bilateral loss of motor function: primarily upper extremities Preservation of proprioception and discriminatory sensation
Brown-Sequard Syndrome: UMN lesion 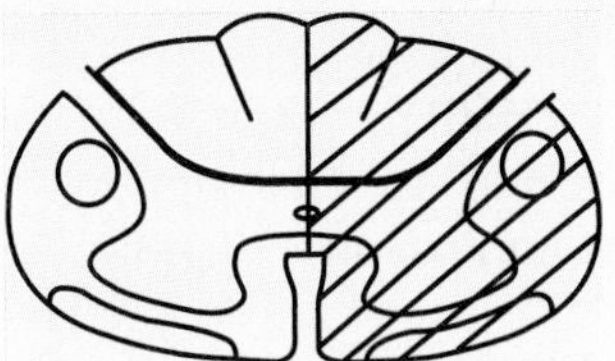	Hemisection of spinal cord Ipsilateral loss of dorsal columns with loss of tactile discrimination, pressure, vibration, and proprioception Ipsilateral loss of corticospinal tracts with loss of motor function and spastic paralysis below level of lesion Contralateral loss of spinothalamic tract with loss of pain and temperature below level of lesion; at lesion level, bilateral loss of pain and temperature
Anterior Cord Syndrome: UMN lesion 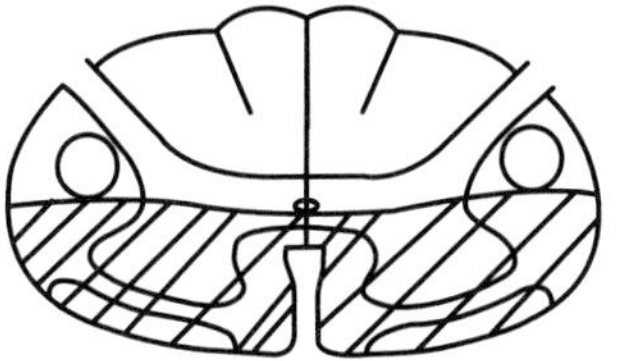	Loss of anterior cord Loss of lateral corticospinal tracts with bilateral loss of motor function, spastic paralysis below level of lesion Loss of spinothalamic tracts with bilateral loss of pain and temperature Preservation of dorsal columns: proprioception, kinesthesia, and vibratory sense
Posterior Cord Syndrome: UMN lesion 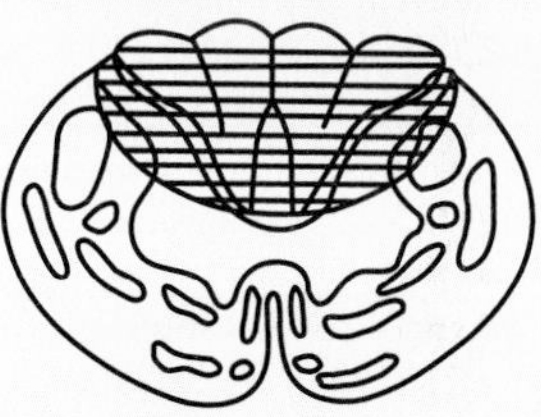	Loss of dorsal columns bilaterally Bilateral loss of proprioception, vibration, pressure, and epicritic sensations (stereognosis, two-point discrimination) Preservation of motor function, pain, and light touch
Cauda Equina Injury: LMN lesion 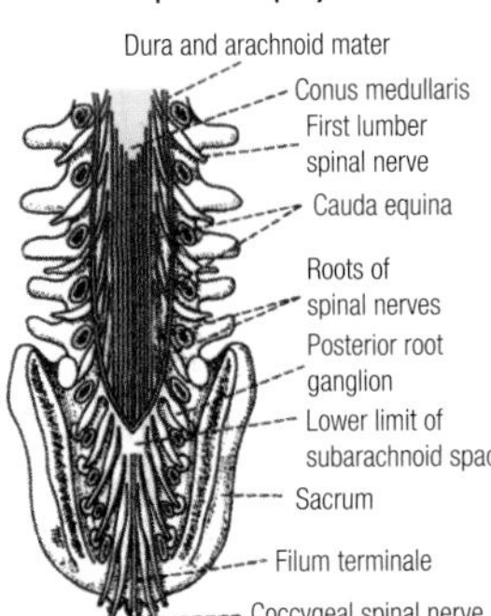	Loss of long nerve roots at or below L1 Variable nerve root damage (motor and sensory signs); incomplete lesions common Flaccid paralysis with no spinal reflex activity Flaccid paralysis of bladder and bowel Potential for nerve regeneration; regeneration often incomplete, slows and stops after about 1 year

LMN = lower motor neuron; UMN = upper motor neuron

c. Skin condition, integrity: check areas of high pressure.
d. Muscle tone, spasms, and DTRs.
e. Sensation/spinal cord level of injury: check to see if sensory level corresponds to motor level of innervation (may differ in incomplete lesions).
f. Muscle strength (MMT)/spinal cord level of injury: lowest segmental level of innervation includes muscle strength present at a fair+ grade (3+/5); use caution when doing MMT in acute phase with spinal immobilization.
g. Functional status: full functional assessment possible only when patient is cleared for activity and active rehabilitation.

6. Standardized tests/outcome measures for patients with spinal cord injury (see Table 3-23 and Appendix 3A).
7. Physical therapy goals, outcomes, and interventions.
   a. Monitor changes associated with spinal cord injury and recovery.
      - Spinal shock: transient period of reflex depression and flaccidity; may last several hours or up to 24 weeks.
      - Spasticity/spasms: determine location and degree of tone. Examine for nociceptive stimuli that may trigger increased tone (e.g., blocked catheter, tight clothing or straps, body position, environmental temperature, infection, decubitus ulcers).

RED FLAG: Examine closely for signs and symptoms of autonomic dysreflexia: hypertension, bradycardia, severe headache, feeling of anxiety, constricted pupils, blurred vision, flushing and piloerection, and increased spasticity. Treat as a medical emergency: if patient is lying flat, bring to an upright position; loosen any tight clothing or restrictive devices; examine/reduce blockage of urinary drainage; monitor blood pressure and heart rate. Notify medical and/or nursing staff ASAP.

      - Heterotopic bone formation (ectopic bone): abnormal bone growth in soft tissues; examine for early changes—soft tissue swelling, pain, erythema, generally near large joint; late changes—calcification, initial signs of ankylosis.
      - Deep venous thrombosis: see discussion in Chapter 4.
   b. Improve respiratory capacity: deep breathing exercises, strengthening exercises to respiratory muscles; assisted coughing, respiratory hygiene (postural drainage, percussion, vibration, suctioning) as needed to keep airway clear; abdominal support.
   c. Maintain ROM, prevent contracture: PROM, positioning, splinting; selective stretching to preserve function (e.g., tenodesis grasp).

Table 3-23

APTA Neurology Spinal Cord Injury EDGE Task Force Recommended Examination Items for Use by Entry-Level Physical Therapy Students*

EXAMINATION ITEMS	ITEM DESCRIPTION
American Spinal Injury Association (ASIA) Impairment Scale.	**A** = Complete, no motor or sensory function is preserved in the sacral segments S4–5; **B** = Incomplete: sensory but no motor function is preserved below the neurological level and includes the sacral segments S4–5; **C** = Incomplete: motor function is preserved below the neurological level, and most key muscles below the neurological level have a grade of less than 3. **D** = Incomplete: motor function is preserved below the neurological level, and most key muscles below the neurological level have a grade of 3 or more. **E** = Normal: motor and sensory function is normal.
Functional Independence Measure (FIM)-version 4.0	See previous discussion in Table 3-13.
10-meter Gait Speed	See Table 3-11.
Timed Up & Go	See Table 3-11.
6-minute Walk Test	See Table 3-11.
Manual Muscle Test (MMT)	Critical measure to support ASIA Impairment Scale.
Handheld dynamometry	Provides a quantitative and more reliable and responsive outcome measure to assess objective strength changes.

*The items above should also be combined with the core examination items in Box 3-1.

Adapted from recommendations from the American Physical Therapy Association Academy of Neurologic Physical Therapy Spinal Cord Injury EDGE Task Force-2013. Additional information is located at https://www.neuropt.org/docs/sci-edge-/sci-edge-entry-level-recommendations.pdf?sfvrsn=71546a8f_2

d. Maintain skin integrity, free of decubitus ulcers and other injury: positioning program, pressure-relieving devices (e.g., cushions, gel cushion, ankle boots), patient education: pressure relief activities (e.g., pushups) and skin inspection; provide prompt treatment of pressure sores.
e. Improve strength: strengthen all remaining innervated muscles; use selective strengthening during acute phase to reduce stress on spinal segments; resistive training to hypertrophy muscles.
f. Reorient patient to vertical position: tilt table, wheelchair; use of abdominal binder, elastic lower extremity wraps to decrease venous pooling; examine for signs and symptoms of orthostatic hypotension (lightheadedness, syncope, mental or visual blurring, sense of weakness).
g. Promote early return of FMS and ADLs: emphasis on independent rolling and bed mobility, assumption of sitting, transfers, sit-to-stand, and ambulation as indicated.
h. Improve sitting tolerance, postural control, symmetry, and balance; standing balance as indicated.

8. Appropriate wheelchair prescription.
   a. Wheelchair prescription varies according to level and extent of injury. Configuring the wheelchair to provide optimal support and mobility requires an individualized prescription. Requirements below address typical needs of patients with ASIA A or B impairments.
   b. Patients with high cervical lesions (C1–4): require electric wheelchair with tilt-in space seating or reclining seat back; microswitch or puff-and-sip controls; portable respirator may be attached.
   c. Patients with cervical lesions, shoulder function, elbow flexion (C5): can use a manual chair with propulsion aids (e.g., projections); independent for short distances on smooth, flat surfaces; may choose electric wheelchair for distances and energy conservation.
   d. Patients with cervical lesions, radial wrist extensors (C6): manual wheelchair with friction surface hand rims; independent.
   e. Patients with cervical lesions, triceps (C7): same as for C6, but with increased propulsion.
   f. Patients with hand function (C8–T1 and below): manual wheelchair, standard hand rims.
   g. Significant changes in lighter, more durable, sports-oriented chairs.
9. Promote wheelchair skills/independence: management of wheelchair parts, turns, propulsion on all surfaces indoors and outdoors, safe fall out of and return to wheelchair.
10. Locomotor training (LT) for individuals with complete injuries.
    a. Patients with midthoracic lesions (T6–9): supervised ambulation for short distances (physiological, limited household ambulator); requires bilateral knee-ankle-foot orthoses (KAFOs) and crutches, swing-to gait pattern; requires assistance; may prefer standing devices/standing wheelchairs for physiological standing.
    b. Patients with high lumbar lesions (T12–L3): can be independent in ambulation on all surfaces and stairs; using a swing-through or four-point gait pattern and bilateral KAFOs and crutches. Patients may also use reciprocating gait orthoses with walker with or without FES system. Typically independent household ambulators; wheelchair use for community ambulation.
    c. Patients with low lumbar lesions (L4–5); can be independent with bilateral AFOs and crutches or canes. Typically independent community ambulators; may still use wheelchair for activities with high-endurance requirements.
    d. High rate of rejection of orthoses/ambulation in favor of wheelchair mobility and energy conservation.
11. Neuromodulation: use of electrical stimulation to replace or improve function of a paralyzed or paretic limb; available to limited number of patients.
    a. Functional electrical stimulation (FES) is used for exercise, walking, and functional use of the UEs.
    b. Robotic-assisted walking.
       - An exoskeletal frame with motorized, fitted braces is used with patients with complete SCI; braces support both LEs and part of upper body.
       - A backpack containing a computer and power supply is worn. Computer program controls hip and knee motions.
       - Crutches or walker are required.
       - High cost, limited availability.
12. Locomotor training for individuals with incomplete injury.
    a. Treadmill training (TT) using body weight support (BWS).
       - Indications: incomplete injuries (ASIA B, C, or D).
       - Promotes spinal cord learning/activation of spinal locomotor pools.
       - Uses body harness to support weight; variable levels of loading, e.g., from 35% unweighting, progressively decreasing to full loading.
       - During early training, therapists can manually assist with foot placement.
       - High-intensity, high-frequency training: 4 to 5 days/wk, 20 to 30 minutes, typically for 8 to 12 weeks.
       - Progression: decrease BWS, increase treadmill speed, eliminate manual assistance.
       - Progression to overground locomotor training for community ambulation.

13. Improve cardiovascular endurance.
    a. Monitor heart rate and blood pressure during all exercise or progressive activity.
    b. Methods (complete injuries): arm crank ergometry; functional electrical stimulation–leg cycle ergometry; hybrid: arm crank ergometry and functional electrical stimulation–leg cycle ergometry; wheelchair propulsion.

RED FLAG: Recognize exercise precautions for individuals with tetraplegia and high-lesion paraplegia; patients may experience blunted tachycardia, lack of pressor response, very low VO2 peak, and substantially higher variability of most responses. Monitor heart rate and blood pressure closely during exercise and activity training.

    c. Trunk stabilization and skin protection important.
    d. Vascular support may be needed (elastic stockings, abdominal binder).
    e. Absolute contraindications to exercise testing and training of individuals with SCI (from American College of Sports Medicine [ACSM]).
        - Autonomic dysreflexia.
        - Severe or infected skin on weight-bearing surfaces.
        - Symptomatic hypotension.
        - Urinary tract infection.
        - Unstable fracture.
        - Uncontrolled hot and humid environments.
        - Insufficient ROM to perform exercise task.
14. Promote maximum independence and mobility in home and community environment; assist patient in community reintegration; ordering of proper equipment, home modification.
15. Provide psychological and emotional support, encourage socialization and motivation.
    a. Reorient and reassure.
    b. Promote independent problem-solving, self-direction.
    c. Provide patient and family education. Focus on strategies to prevent skin breakdown, and maintain ROM, strength, and function.

Central/Peripheral Nervous System and Cranial Nerve Disorders

Amyotrophic Lateral Sclerosis (ALS)

1. ALS (Lou Gehrig's disease) is a degenerative disease affecting both UMNs and LMNs with degeneration of anterior horn cells and descending corticobulbar and corticospinal tracts.
2. Etiology: unknown (viral/autoimmune, toxic); 5%–10% genetic (autosomal dominant).
3. Signs and symptoms (see Table 3-25).
    a. Progressive disease, often leading to death, typically in 2–5 years; highly variable symptoms.
        - Bulbar onset (progressive bulbar palsy) seen in approximately 1/3 of patients.
        - Spinal cord onset (progressive muscular atrophy).
    b. Muscular weakness that spreads over time: early onset involves limbs progressing to whole body; atrophy, cramping, muscle fasciculations, or twitching (LMN signs).
    c. Spasticity, hyperreflexia (UMN signs).
    d. Dysarthria, dysphagia, dysphonia secondary to pseudobulbar palsy and progressive bulbar palsy.
    e. Usually absence of sensory changes; small number may show sensory deficits.
    f. Autonomic dysfunction in about one-third of patients.
    g. Pain due to spasticity, cramping, postural stress syndrome, joint hypomobility, or instability.
    h. Respiratory impairments: weakness > paralysis, nocturnal difficulty, exertional dyspnea, accessory muscle use; paradoxical breathing, ventilator dependent; poor cough, clearance of secretions.
    i. Typical sparing of bowel and bladder function.
    j. Cognition is normal, similar to locked-in syndrome in cerebrovascular accident (CVA).
    k. Depression common.
4. Stages of ALS.
    a. Stage I: early disease, mild focal weakness, asymmetrical distribution; symptoms of hand cramping and fasciculations.
    b. Stage II: moderate weakness in groups of muscles, some wasting (atrophy) of muscles; modified independence with assistive devices.
    c. Stage III: severe weakness of specific muscles, increasing fatigue; mild to moderate functional limitations, ambulatory.
    d. Stage IV: severe weakness and wasting of LEs, mild weakness of UEs; moderate assistance and assistive devices required; wheelchair user.
    e. Stage V: progressive weakness with deterioration of mobility and endurance, increased fatigue, moderate to severe weakness of whole limbs and trunk; spasticity, hyperreflexia; loss of head control; maximal assist.
    f. Stage VI: bedridden, dependent ADLs, FMS; progressive respiratory distress.
5. Examine.
    a. History: varied pattern of onset.
    b. Vital signs, respiratory function.
    c. Cranial nerve function: especially lower cranial nerves (VII, IX, X, XI, XII).
    d. Motor function.
        - Examine for atrophy, widespread weakness; a symmetrical distribution, muscle cramping and muscle twitching.

- Examine for spasticity.
- Coordination tests: manual skills.

e. Sensory function.
f. Reflexes.
- Examine for hypo/hyperreflexia (Unique finding in ALS)
- Examine for pathologic reflexes (Babinski)

g. Gait: timed walk (10-m walk test).
h. Functional status: monitor closely for overwork fatigue, persistent weakness following exercise or activity; e.g., keep activity log.
i. ALS Functional Rating Scale (ALSFRS): assesses disease progression and function across 10 functional categories; scored 0 (loss of function) to 4 (normal function); 40 maximal score.

6. Medical management: there is no effective treatment for this disease.
   a. Riluzole, a glutamate antagonist, may slow progression, prolong survival, especially with bulbar-onset disease.
   b. Symptomatic relief: i.e., spasticity, pain, respiratory failure.
7. Physical therapy goals, outcomes, and interventions.
   a. Maintain respiratory function: may require airway clearance techniques, cough facilitation, breathing exercises, chest stretching, suctioning, incentive spirometry, long-term mechanical ventilation.
   b. Provide for nutritional needs: assist in management of dysphagia; may require nasogastric tube or percutaneous gastrostomy in later stages.
   c. Prevent indirect impairments: maintain activity levels as long as possible, PROM, positioning, skin care.
   d. Provide exercise program.
   - Prevent further deconditioning and disuse atrophy while avoiding overwork damage in weakened, denervated muscle; e.g., mild resistive exercises if muscles are in good to normal ranges; active exercises or functional activities as weakness progresses.
   - Mild aerobic exercise at submaximal levels, as appropriate.

> **RED FLAG:** Exercise precautions: monitor fatigue levels closely; avoid overwork injury (avoid exercise if less than one-third of motor units are functioning); limited positions with decreased pulmonary function.

   - As disease progresses, replace exercise with functional training activities.

   e. Teach energy conservation activity, pacing techniques; e.g., balance activity with rest.
   f. Maintain maximal functional independence: provide appropriate assistive devices, orthotic support, wheelchair, environmental adaptations; anticipate needs.
   g. Symptomatic treatment of pain, spasms, spasticity.
   h. Teach patient, family, caregivers all care, ADLs; assist in utilization of community resources.
   i. Provide psychological support and reassurance, maximum comfort; loss of control is a challenging issue.

Cranial Nerve Disorders

Bulbar Palsy

1. Weakness or paralysis of the muscles innervated by the motor nuclei of the lower brainstem; affects the muscles of the face, tongue, larynx, and pharynx.
2. Etiology: the result of tumors, vascular or degenerative diseases of lower cranial nerve motor nuclei (e.g., amyotrophic lateral sclerosis).
3. Examine/determine.
   a. Glossopharyngeal and vagal paralysis: phonation, articulation, palatal action, gag reflex, swallowing.
   b. Changes in voice quality: dysphonia (hoarseness or nasal quality).
   c. Bilateral involvement: severe airway restriction with dyspnea, difficulty with coughing.
   d. Possible complications: aspiration pneumonia.
4. Pseudobulbar palsy: bilateral dysfunction of corticobulbar innervation of brainstem nuclei; a central or UMN lesion analogous to corticospinal lesions disrupting function of anterior horn cells.
   a. Produces similar symptoms as bulbar palsy.
   b. Examine for hyperactive reflexes: increased jaw jerk, and snout reflex (tapping on lips produces pouting of lips).
5. Medical/surgical treatment of underlying cause.
6. Physical therapy goals, outcomes, and interventions.
   a. Suctioning, oral care.
   b. Maintenance of respiratory function, open airway.
   c. Elevate head of bed.
   d. Dietary changes: soft foods, liquids.

Trigeminal Neuralgia (Tic Douloureux)-CN V

1. Lesion of trigeminal nerve. CN V: etiology unknown or can result from compression (tortuous basilar artery or cerebellopontine tumor); occurs in older population (mean age over 50); abrupt onset.
2. Signs and symptoms: brief paroxysms of neurogenic pain (stabbing and/or shooting pain); reoccurring frequently.
   a. Occurs along the distribution of the trigeminal nerve, mandibular and maxillary divisions (involvement of ophthalmic division is rare); restricted to one side of the face.
   b. There is autonomic instability: exacerbated by stress, cold; relieved by relaxation.
3. Examine/determine.
   a. Pain: location, intensity.
   b. Trigger points: light touch to face, lips, or gums will cause pain.

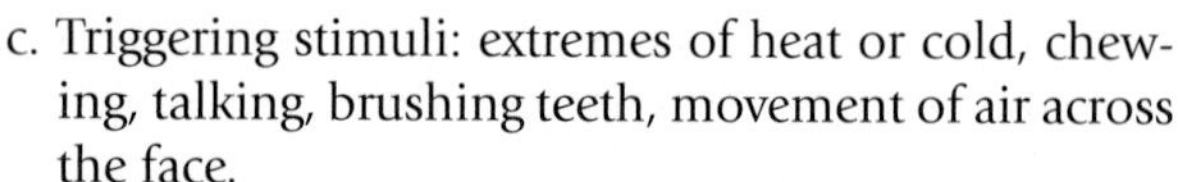

c. Triggering stimuli: extremes of heat or cold, chewing, talking, brushing teeth, movement of air across the face.
d. Motor function: control is normal.

4. Medical: medications (anticonvulsants, vitamin B12); alcohol injections, surgery (sectioning of nerve, permanent anesthesia).
5. Transcutaneous electrical nerve stimulation (TENS) and desensitization may be effective for pain relief.

Bell's Palsy-CN VII

1. Lesion of facial nerve, CN VII, resulting in unilateral facial paralysis (both upper/lower parts of one side of the face).
2. Etiology: acute inflammatory process of unknown etiology (immune or viral disease) resulting in compression of the nerve within the temporal bone.
3. Signs and symptoms.
   a. Muscles of facial expression on one side are weakened or paralyzed.
   b. Loss of control of salivation or lacrimation.
   c. Onset is acute, with maximum severity in a few hours or days; commonly preceded by a day or two of pain behind the ear; most recover fully in several weeks or months.
   d. Sensation is normal.
4. Examine/determine.
   a. Drooping of corner of mouth, eyelids that don't close.
   b. Function of muscles of facial expression: have patient wrinkle forehead, raise eyebrows, frown, smile, close eyes tightly, puff cheeks. The 3 W's (whistle, wink and wrinkle).
   c. Taste of the anterior two-thirds of tongue.
5. Medications: corticosteroids (prednisone); analgesics.
6. Physical therapy goals, outcomes, and interventions.
   a. Protect cornea (artificial tears or temporary patching) until recovery allows for eyelid closure.
   b. Electrical stimulation to maintain tone, support function of facial muscles.
   c. Provide active facial muscle exercises.
   d. May require face sling to prevent overstretching of facial muscles.
   e. Provide functional retraining: foods that can be easily eaten, chewing with opposite side.
   f. Provide emotional support and reassurance.

Peripheral Nerve Disorders

Peripheral Nerve Injury

1. Etiology: Can be a result of acute traumatic or chronic repetitive traction, compression, and/or shear forces.
2. Peripheral nerve injury classification:
   a. Neurapraxia: nerve injury that causes a transient and focal chemical/structural (conduction block/demyelination) loss of function.
      - Often related to compressive forces causing ischemia (e.g., early carpal tunnel syndrome).
      - Nerve dysfunction may be rapidly reversed or persist for weeks or months.
      - Positive prognosis if compression removed in a timely fashion.
   b. Axonotmesis: focal damage to the axon/myelin and varying degrees of peripheral nerve connective tissue (endoneurium, perineurium, and epineurium).
      - Seen with increased duration or larger amplitude compressive(crush injury) or tension (traction injury) forces.
      - With traction injuries (e.g., C5-6 nerve root avulsion), peripheral nerve connective tissue is disrupted from the interior (endoneurium to perineurium) to exterior (epineurium).
      - Results in Wallerian degeneration within disrupted axons.
      - The prognosis for axonal regrow is related to the degree of connective tissue damage. This emphasizes the importance of proper forces/positioning and exercise progression in patients with healing peripheral nerve injuries.
      - Prognosis is also related to the patient's past medical history and overall health.
      - Axonal regrowth in a healthy patient occurs at approximately 1–3 mm day or an inch a month. Delayed in patients with nutritional challenges or health conditions such as diabetes.
   c. Neurotmesis: Severance of axon/myelin and all connective tissue structures to include epineurium.
      - Complete loss of nerve function and Wallerian degeneration with no connective tissue path.
      - Requires surgical intervention.
      - Guarded prognosis even with surgery as axons may not find their terminal target (e.g., muscle fibers or sensory receptor) or have aberrant innervation (e.g., axon that use to innervate sensation to the long finger now innervates thumb).
3. Neuroplasticity and peripheral nerve injuries.
   a. Axonal regeneration: as describe above and important to remember that axons that undergo regeneration often do not remyelinate to their preinjury level. This may impact nerve conduction velocity and speed/coordination of movement.
   b. Collateral sprouting: intact axons can pick up denervated terminal targets (e.g., muscle).
      - In the case of muscle this often results in switching of the muscle fiber type (type 1 becomes

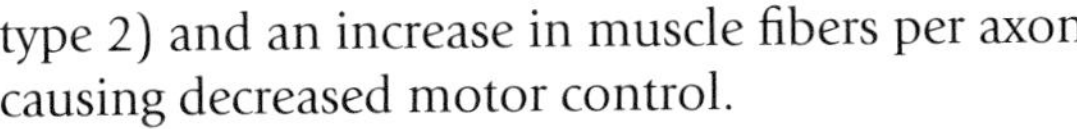

type 2) and an increase in muscle fibers per axon causing decreased motor control.

4. Types of peripheral nerve injuries.
   a. Mononeuropathy: involvement of a single nerve (e.g., cubital tunnel syndrome)
   b. Mononeuropathy multiplex: involvement of 2 or more nerves without a clear pattern of polyneuropathy (e.g., a patient with bilateral carpal tunnel, left cubital tunnel and right tarsal tunnel).
      - This presentation is often related to other health conditions (diabetes, renal disease, or chronic alcohol) and the potential need for additional medical workup/management.
   c. Radiculopathy: involvement of nerve root(s).
   d. Plexopathy: involvement of brachial or lumbosacral plexus.
5. History, examination, diagnostic tests, and intervention (see Chapter 2 for additional information on specific types of mononeuropathies, plexopathies, and radiculopathies).

Peripheral Nerve Disease (Polyneuropathy)

1. Etiology: wide range of factors (more than 100 distinct factors/diseases).
2. Risk Factors (see Table 3-24).
3. Basic pathologic processes. Diseases/factors such as those in Table 3-24 lead to:
   a. Segmental demyelination: disease process primarily impacts myelin; if the disease process can be treated remyelination can occur (e.g., Guillain-Barré syndrome).
   b. Axonal degeneration: disease impacts axons to a greater degree than myelin and progresses from distal to proximal resulting in "dying back" of nerves (e.g., neuropathy secondary to alcohol abuse).
   c. Most polyneuropathic conditions impact both myelin and axons (e.g., diabetic polyneuropathy) and are more chronic in nature.
   d. Acute and rapidly progressing polyneuropathic conditions are typically related to toxins (poison) or autoimmune conditions (e.g., Gullian-Barre).
4. Neuroplasticty and polyneuropathy.
   a. Remyelination, axonal regeneration, and collateral sprouting are all options as long as the causative agent can be treated. This reinforces the importance of identifying polyneuropathy changes early and referring for medical management.
5. History (see Table 3-25).
   a. Sensory, motor, and autonomic (hair loss and vasculature) changes in the extremities occur in a distal to proximal fashion (glove and stocking).
   b. Screen for autonomic dysfunction: vasodilation and loss of vasomotor tone (dryness, warm skin, edema, orthostatic hypotension).
   c. Patients may report problems with balance or falls.
   d. Older age is a key risk factor.
   e. Important to review the medical history and conduct a systems review on potential causes of polyneuropathy (see Table 3-24).
6. Examine.
   a. Neuromuscular screening: see Table 3-25.
   b. Balance/gait/functional testing:
      - Balance: difficulty with static posture and sensitive to looking up or eyes closed conditions (Rhomberg test).
      - Ataxic gait: improved with looking down or cane.
      - Functional testing: difficulty with heel/toe walking and steps (especially if not looking down).

> **RED FLAG:** Important to test both small (pain and temperature) and large (discriminate touch, vibration, proprioception) neural fiber involvement as impairments may vary (pain versus loss of protective sensation versus propriception loss).

   c. Laboratory studies: Initially conduct basic panel to assist in ruling in and out common health conditions (diabetes, renal disease, nutritional deficits). If normal, more extensive labs to include genetic testing.
   d. Nerve conduction/EMG studies: assist in the diagnosis, type (myelinopathy vs. axonopathy vs. combination), acuity (acute vs. chronic) and severity of medium to large fiber polyneuropathy. Also assist

Table 3-24

Common Diseases/Factors Associated with Polyneuropathy
1. Diabetes
2. Renal failure
3. Alcohol abuse
4. Systemic autoimmune disease (Sjogren's, Lupus)
5. Autoimmune disease-nerve (Guillain-Barre syndrome)
6. Nutritional imbalances (e.g., Vitamin B12)
7. Hereditary (e.g., Charcot Marie Tooth I and II)
8. Infections (e.g., Hepatitis B/C, HIV, Lyme disease)
9. Certain cancers
10. Medications (e.g., chemotherapy)
11. Toxins (e.g., radiation, pesticides)
12. Idiopathic: approximately 25% of patients

in ruling out other conditions (radiculopathy, spinal stenosis) with similar symptoms.
 e. Skin punch biopsy: used for the diagnosis of small fiber cutaneous (pain/temperature) neuropathies.
7. Medical management: various interventions based on the caustic agent. Gabapentin is commonly prescribed to treat neuropathic pain and paresthesias.
8. Physical therapy goals, outcomes, and interventions
 a. Maintaining and/or improving balance, gait, strength and endurance, and ADLs to maximize community participation.
 b. Prevention of secondary complications (fall risk, foot deformities, skin ulcers).
 c. Decrease pain associated with small fiber neuropathy (desensitization training, TENs).
 d. Recovery interventions include postural stability exercise (to maximize hip strategy and proximal stability/timing), balance/gait training, sensory reeducation, and strength/endurance training (both involved and uninvolved muscles).
 e. Compensatory strategies/interventions include assistive devices, custom fit orthosis (to prevent foot ulcers/deformities), ankle foot orthosis, check feet/shoes daily to prevent skin breakdown, and fall prevention strategies (use of night light, cane).

Guillain-Barré Syndrome (GBS)

1. Acute inflammatory demyelinating polyradiculoneuropathy presenting with rapid nonsymmetric loss of myelin in both nerve roots and peripheral nerves. Muscle weakness often develops rapidly and accurate diagnosis and medical intervention is paramount.
2. Etiology: unknown; associated with an autoimmune attack, usually occurs after recovery from an infectious illness (respiratory or gastrointestinal).
3. Signs and symptoms (see Table 3-25).
 a. Involves acute demyelination of both cranial and peripheral nerves/nerve roots (LMN disease).
 b. Sensory loss, paresthesias (tingling, burning), pain; sensory loss is typically less than motor loss.
 c. Motor paresis or paralysis: relative symmetrical distribution of weakness; may produce full tetraplegia with respiratory failure.
 d. Dysarthria, dysphagia, diplopia, and facial weakness may develop in severe cases.
 e. Progression evolves over a few days or weeks; recovery usually slow (6 months to 2 years), and although the vast majority of patients return to ADLS and community ambulation, 10%–20% have severe disabilities; 5% mortality.
 f. Complications.
  • Respiratory impairment and failure.
  • Autonomic instability: tachycardia, arrhythmias, BP fluctuations.
  • Pain: myalgia.
  • Risk of pneumonia.
  • Prolonged hospitalizations and immobility: deep venous thrombosis, skin breakdown, contracture.
  • Relapse: if treatment is inadequate.
4. Examine (see Table 3-25).
 a. Cardiac and respiratory status, vital signs.
 b. Cranial nerve function (VII, IX, X, XI, XII).
 c. Motor strength (serial MMTs indicated).
 d. Reflexes: decreased or absent tendon reflexes.
 e. Sensation: changes can include paresthesias, anesthesias, hyperesthesias, pain (muscle aching, burning); may have stocking and glove distribution (anesthesia of distal extremities in a pattern as if the patient were wearing long gloves and stockings) initially but can rapidly progress to diffuse sensory and motor changes impacting all of the extremities and cranial nerves.
 f. Functional status.
5. Medical.
 a. Good nursing care.
 b. Plasmapheresis.
 c. IVIG.
 d. Analgesics for relief of pain.
6. Physical therapy goals, outcomes, and interventions.
 a. Maintain respiratory function: may require endotracheal intubation, tracheotomy, and ventilation; pulmonary physical therapy.
 b. Prevent indirect impairments: PROM within pain tolerance, positioning, and skin care.
 c. Prevent injury to denervated muscles: monitor recovery; splinting, positioning.
 d. Provide muscle reeducation, moderate exercise program (active assistance and active exercise progressing to resistive), functional training as recovery progresses.

RED FLAG: Teach energy conservation techniques and activity pacing: avoid overuse and fatigue, which may prolong recovery.

 e. Improve cardiovascular fitness following prolonged bed rest and deconditioning.
 f. Provide emotional support and reassurance to patient and family.

Postpolio Syndrome (PPS)

1. Slow progressive muscle weakness occurring in individuals with a confirmed history of acute polio; follows a stable period (usually 15 years or more) of functioning.

2. Etiology: unknown; possible hyperfunctioning of motor neurons, long-term overuse at high levels resulting in new denervation.
3. Signs and symptoms.
   a. Gradual (rarely abrupt) onset of new muscle weakness or fatigue, with or without muscle atrophy or muscle/joint pain.
   b. New symptoms >1 year.
   c. Abnormal fatigue: may not be related to activity levels, doesn't recover easily with usual rest periods.
   d. Pain: myalgia, cramping pain, joint pain with repetitive injury, hypersensitivities.
   e. Decreased function with reduced endurance for routine activities.
   f. Slow progression, either steady or stepwise.
   g. Environmental cold intolerance.
   h. Sleep disturbances.
   i. Decreased functional mobility, aerobic capacity, labile exercise blood pressures.
4. Examine.
   a. History: confirm original acute polio illness; document onset of present symptoms, presentation, course, chronology (new symptoms >1 year).
   b. Motor function: strength, atrophy, muscle fatigue, muscle twitching, and/or cramps.
      - Identify problem musculature, weakness found in both new muscles and muscles previously affected by polio.
      - Identify functional contractions (fair grades or above).
      - Look for spotty involvement, asymmetrical paralysis.
   c. ROM and deformity.
   d. Pain.
      - Muscle pain: check tenderness to touch.
      - Skeletal, soft tissue pain: chronic overuse, poor alignment.
   e. Sensory function: any sensory deficit is due to other etiology (sensation is unaffected in PPS).
   f. Respiratory function: examine for dyspnea, difficulty in speaking, weak cough.
   g. Functional status: functional mobility skills, activities of daily living.
   h. Endurance, activity levels: fatigue is a primary symptom.
   i. Aerobic capacity: recommend discontinuous protocol, submaximal exercise test (ACSM recommendation); use whole body movement (e.g., ergometer using upper and lower extremities) to avoid overworking involved muscles.
   j. Critical to rule out other neuromuscular health conditions (radiculopathy, polyneuropathy) as well as the influence of age related changes.
   k. EMG to identify prior anterior horn cell (AHC) disease and new motor unit pathology. See denervation changes, fasciculations, fibrillations, increased motor unit amplitude and duration.
   l. Biopsychosocial measurement in the form of PROMIS or SF-36 maybe helpful to assess the potential influence of pain, fatigue, decreased physical function on mental health, social participation, and sleep disturbance.
5. Medical management.
   a. Antidepressants: e.g., amitriptyline (Elavil), fluoxetine (Prozac).
   b. Neurotransmitter inhibitors: decreases fatigue and sleep disorders; e.g., serotonin, norepinephrine.
6. Physical therapy goals, outcomes, and interventions.
   a. Maintain respiratory function: teach breathing exercises, supportive cough maneuvers, postural drainage as indicated.
   b. Teach energy conservation techniques, activity pacing: balance activity with frequent rest periods to decrease fatigue, prevent overwork damage in weakened, denervated muscle.
      - Teach relaxation techniques to maximize rest.
      - Avoid unnecessary activities to maximize important work.
   c. Preserve or increase muscle strength.
      - Provide moderate exercise program (nonexhaustive exercise): modified strengthening and conditioning; use low-intensity, discontinuous nonfatiguing exercise with increased rest periods.
      - Moderate resistance training recommended for patients with postpolio syndrome who had near-normal muscle strength and no signs of motor unit remodeling on EMG.
      - Submaximumal endurance training recommended for patients with moderate paresis and signs of motor unit remodeling.
      - Patients with severe paresis should avoid muscle training.
      - Foster weight control and reduction.
   d. Aerobic conditioning: moderate to low-level training depending upon class of disease, discontinuous protocol. Similar to testing, use whole body movement (upper/lower extremity ergometer, swimming, aquatic therapy, treadmill walking) to avoid overworking involved muscles.
   e. Foster weight control/reduction programs.
   f. Maintain or increase function: provide recommendations for lifestyle modification; minimize abnormal postures, gait deviations.
   g. Prescribe appropriate orthoses, mobility aids (motorized cart), assistive devices, environmental modifications.
   h. Interdisciplinary pain management and interventions.

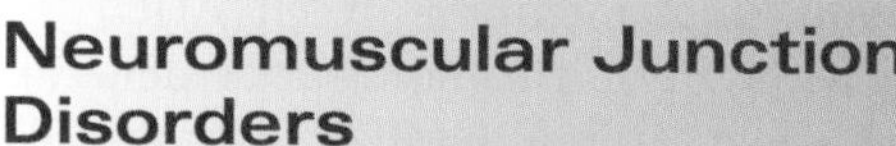

Neuromuscular Junction Disorders

Neuromuscular junction disorders (NMJ) are categorized as acquired or inherited and present with the common features of fatigue and weakness. Congenital myasthenic syndrome is an example of an inherited disorders. Acquired disorders include myasthenia gravis (MG), Lambert-Eaton myasthenic syndrome and botulism. Myasthenia gravis (MG) is the most common NMJ disorder encountered in clinical practice, and botulinum toxin is used for the treatment of hypertonia, dystonia, chronic pain/muscle spasms.

Myasthenia Gravis

1. A postsynaptic neuromuscular junction disorder characterized by progressive muscular weakness and fatigability on exertion.
2. Etiology: autoimmune antibody-mediated attack on acetylcholine receptors at neuromuscular junction.
3. Signs and symptoms. (See Table 3-25.)
   a. Typically seen in females 20–30 years old and equally in men and women 60–80 years of age.
   b. Primary impairment reported by patients is fatigue or weakness with sustained activity.
   c. Muscular strength worse with continuing contraction, improved with rest.
   d. Classified into four types: ocular myasthenia (confined to extraocular muscles), mild generalized myasthenia, severe generalized myasthenia, and crisis.
   e. Generalized myasthenia: usually involves bulbar (extraocular, facial, and muscles of mastication) and proximal limb-girdle muscles.
   f. Course varies: may progress from mild to severe, typically within 18 months.
   g. Myasthenic crisis: myasthenia gravis with respiratory failure; treat as medical emergency.
4. Examine (see Table 3-25).
   a. Cranial nerves: examine for diplopia and ptosis; progressive dysarthria or nasal speech; difficulties in chewing and swallowing; difficulties in facial expression, drooping facial muscles.
   b. Ice pack test: A positive test is decreased ptosis after a 2-minute application of an ice pack to the affected eyelid.
   c. Muscle strength: proximal muscles more involved than distal. Fatigability is characteristic of this disease; repeated muscle use results in rapid weakness.
   d. Functional mobility skills: common difficulties with climbing stairs, rising from chair, or lifting (similar to myopathies).
   e. Nerve conduction studies show abnormal and decremented responses to repetitive nerve stimulation at baseline and 2–4 minutes after isometric exercise.
5. Medical interventions.
   a. Acetylcholinesterase inhibitors: pyridostigmine.
   b. Corticosteroids: prednisone, methylprednisolone.
   c. Immunosuppressants: azathioprine, intravenous immunoglobulin (IVIG).
   d. Alternative treatments: plasmapheresis (removal of blood with filtering and separation of cellular elements from plasma); thymectomy.
6. Physical therapy goals, outcomes, and interventions.
   a. Monitor changes in patient's condition for complications: vital signs, respiration, swallowing.
   b. Promote independence in FMS and ADLs.
   c. Teach energy conservation techniques; activity pacing: promote optimal activity with rest as indicated.
   d. Provide psychological and emotional support.

Botulinum Toxin

1. Binds presynaptically to the high-affinity recognition sites on the cholinergic nerve terminals, thus decreasing the release of acetylecholine.
2. Result in hypotonia and/or flaccid muscle depending on the dose.
3. During the period of hypotonia therapists can work on improving flexibility in contracted muscles (e.g., stretch gastrocnemius to improve dorsiflexion ROM and initial contact phase of gait in a patient with a lower extremity extensor synergy).
4. Treatments usually last 3–4 months.
5. Complications are dependent on the muscle(s) injected and higher risk for muscles in the head/neck and trunk.
6. Adverse events include weakness of unintended muscles, flaccidity, dysphagia, local hemotoma, generalized fatigue, dizziness, dry mouth, pain, and flu-like symptoms.

Myopathic Disorders

Myopathies are usually classified as inherited (e.g., Duchenne's or Becker's muscular dystrophies; see Chapter 9 for additional information) or acquired myopathies. The description below will focus on acquired myopathies.

Acquired Myopathies

1. Aquired myopathies include:
   a. Inflammatory myopathies (e.g., dermatomyositis, polymyositis).
   b. Infectious myopathies (HIV).
   c. Toxic or drug related myopathies (e.g., steriod or cholesterol lowering agents).
   d. Myopathies associated with systemic diseases (e.g., thyroid and parathyroid dysfunction).
2. Etiology: All of the above types of aquired myopathies results in muscle cell structure and/or metabolism dysfunction.

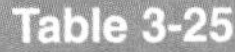

Differential Diagnosis: Comparison of Major Types of Neuromuscular Disorders

DISORDER	AMYOTROPHIC LATERAL SCLEROSIS (ALS)	DIABETIC POLYNEUROPATHY CHRONIC POLYNEUROPATHY	GUILLAIN-BARRE SYNDROME (GBS) ACUTE POLYRADICULO-NEUROPATHY	MYASTHENIA GRAVIS
Location of lesion	Corticospinal Tracts, Anterior Horn Cells, Cranial Motor Nuclei, and Corticobulbar Tracts	Multiple Distal Peripheral Axons/Myelin	Multiple Peripheral Nerves/ Nerve Roots and Cranial Nerves	Post-Synaptic Receptors/ Cleft of the Neuromuscular Junction
Cranial nerve involvement	Yes	No	Yes	Yes; partial ptosis often first sign: Ice Pack Test positive
Sensation	Typically normal May have pain in later stages secondary to immobility	Glove and stocking: often starts as burning pain/ tingling and moves to numbness/loss of proprioception	Sensory impairments typically not as severe as motor impairments	Normal
Strength	Early: asymmetric weakness of hand and leg muscles → to all muscles One-third of patients with initial bulbar weakness (worse prognosis)	Weakness/atrophy of foot muscles → to legs/ fingers hands	Progressive weakness if GBS not treated Rapid progression of nerve roots/nerve/CNs may result in global weakness and need for respiratory support	Fatigue; overt weakness after several repetitions; weakness in ocular/bulbar muscles → proximal extremity → distal muscles
Tone	Mixture of hypo/hypertonia secondary to LMN and UMN involvement	Hypotonia	Hypotonia	Typically, normal at rest May see low tone in severe cases or with repetitive testing
Reflexes	Asymmetric hypo and hyperreflexia	Hyporeflexia	Hyporeflexia	Normal
Involuntary movements	Mixture of fasciculations and spasticity	Periodic fasciculations	Typically, none or limited since initial impact is on myelin	None
Voluntary movements	Absent/delayed (LMN) or dyssynergic (UMN)	Impaired distally and improved with visual feedback	Reduced or absent for multiple movements and typically worse with repetition	Normal with one repetition; reduced with multiple repetitions
Balance	Typically lacks ankle strategy early and progresses to poor hip/trunk control and inability to sit Balance gets worse over time	Difficulty with eyes closed or unlevel surface Uses hip/step strategy	Similar to ALS but a much more rapid progression of sitting/standing impairments if not medically treated	Overall normal but with prolonged standing/ severe disease may demonstrate decreased hip strategy
Gait	Asymmetric foot slap/foot drop and equinus gait deformities Gait deteriorates with repetition secondary to weakness/fatigue	Ataxic; worse on unlevel surfaces or dimly lit areas Foot slap/drop in more severe cases	Initial presentation is often difficulty with running/ jumping that rapidly → inability to walk without assistance	With prolonged walking/ severe disease may demonstrate Trendelenburg
Challenging activity measures	Initially Heel/toe walk and hand dexterity tasks → inability to sit → inability to move in bed → ventilation dependent	Heel/toe walking steps/stairs if looking up	Heel/toe walk; rapidly → to sit to stand → getting out bed May require ventilation support	Vision (secondary to ptosis); prolonged speaking, eating

Cranial nerves = CN; lower motor neuron = LMN; upper motor neuron (UMN); progresses = →

3. Signs and symptoms.
   a. Muscle cramps and pain with exertional fatigue.
   b. Weakness that progresses in a proximal to distal direction.
   c. Patients reports difficulty with overhead activity, getting in and out of chair and stairs.
4. Examine.
   a. Gait/balance: Patients typically have pelvic girdle weakness and associated gait deviations.
   b. Functional test: difficulty with stairs/steps.
   c. Strength testing: weakness in proximal muscles.
   d. Sensory testing: normal (with exception of muscle pain).
   e. Skin changes with dermatomyositis (Butterfly rash: purple-reddish discoloration of the eyelids, cheeks, and bridge of nose; scaling rash on the extensor surface of the fingers).
   f. Joint pain with polymyositis.
   g. Associated symptoms with endocrine disorders (see Chapter 8, Other Systems).
5. Diagnosis.
   a. History/physical examination.
   b. Laboratory tests:
      - Confirm myopathy: elevated creatine phosphokinase (CPK), aldolase, lactate dehydrogenase (LDH) and liver function enzymes.
      - Identify etiology: metabolic panel, thyroid/parathyroid hormone, sedimentation rate and c-reactive protein.
   c. Nerve conduction/EMG studies:
      - Useful to rule out neuropathic conditions.
      - EMG assists in identifying myopathic potentials and muscles for biopsy.
      - EMG can be normal in mild myopathies.
   d. Muscle biopsy: myopathic muscle defined by random areas of connective tissue and/or lipid deposits.
6. Medical management
   a. Targeted at the underlying cause.
7. Physical therapy goals, outcomes and interventions.
   a. Maintain maximal function.
   b. Provide balance exercise program with focus on functional activities that do not overwork or fatigue damaged muscles.
   c. Teach energy conservation techniques that include tracking muscles' pain and activity (e.g., use of pain scale and pedometer).

Pain

The sensory and emotional experience associated with actual or potential tissue damage (International Association for the Study of Pain).

Pain Pathways/Neurophysiology

1. Fast, localized pain (lateral pain system): transmitted over thinly myelinated A delta fibers, processed in spinal cord dorsal horn lamina (I and V), crosses to excite lateral (neo)spinothalamic tract; terminates in brainstem reticular formation and thalamus with projections to cortex; functions for localization, discrimination of pain.
2. Slow pain (divergent pathways): transmitted over small diameter, unmyelinated C fibers; processed in spinal cord lamina (II and III-V), desiccates and travels to all levels of the brainstem to activate the reticular formation (spinoreticular tract); the midbrain to activate the periaqueductal gray and descending pain modulation system (spinomescenphalic tract); and through the medial thalamic nuclei to various areas of the limbic system (spinolimbic tract, which is associated with the emotional component of pain).
3. Intrinsic inhibitory mechanisms.
   a. Gate control theory: transmission of sensation at spinal cord level is controlled by balance between large fibers (A alpha, A beta) and small fibers (A delta, C); temporal summation of large myelinated fibers (70–100 times faster than small fibers) may block activity of small fibers and pain transmission (counterirritant theory).
   b. Descending analgesic systems: endogenous opiates (endorphins, enkephalins) produced throughout CNS (e.g., periaqueductal gray, raphe nuclei, pituitary gland/hypothalamus, SC laminae I and II); can depress pain transmission at various sites through mechanisms of presynaptic inhibition.
   c. Areas of the cortex and limbic system function to upregulate or downregulate the descending pain modulation systems. Various techniques (mediation, counseling, placebo, cognitive behavioral therapy, pain science education) and cultural beliefs are believed to influence these areas.

Acute Pain

1. Pain provoked by noxious stimulation and associated with an underlying pathology (injury or acute inflammation/disease).
2. Signs and symptoms.
   a. Sharp pain.
   b. Sympathetic changes: increased HR, BP, and RR; pupillary dilation, sweating.
   c. Anxiety, protective behaviors.

Chronic Pain

1. Pain that persists beyond the usual course of healing; symptoms that persist for >6 months.
2. An underlying pathology or tissue inflammation is no longer identifiable or may never have been present.

Classification of Pain (See Figure 3-14)

1. Nociceptive pain: response to an immediate noxious stimulus (mechanical, thermal, or chemical) signaling impending tissue damage.
   a. Inflammatory pain occurs after tissue damage and increases sensitivity to pain.
   b. Examples include ankle sprain or osteoarthritis.
2. Neuropathic pain: damage or disease of the somatosensory nervous system.
   a. Evidenced by neural symptoms such as tingling, burning, and/or dysesthesia.
   b. Symptoms evaluated using sensory testing and findings follow a dermatome, cutaneous nerve(s), or central nervous system pattern.
   c. Examples include carpal tunnel syndrome, radiculopathy, and polyneuropathy.
   d. Examination measures may include pain questionnaires (e.g., painDETECT or DN4) and sensory testing.
   e. Possible Diagnosis Neuropathic Pain: History of relevant neurologic lesion or disease and pain distribution neuroanatomically plausible (Body Chart & Screening Questionnaires).
   f. Probable Diagnosis Neuropathic Pain: Clinical examination (sensory, motor, reflex, & neurodynamic testing) and/or quantitative sensory testing.
   g. Definite Diagnosis Neuropathic Pain: Imaging, electrodiagnostic testing, skin biopsy, genetic testing, surgical verification.
3. Nociplastic pain is associated with dysfunction of central pain processing (central sensitization). Nociceptive and neuropathic pain mechanisms can lead to peripheral and central sensitization, ultimately contributing or coexisting with nocioplastic pain.
   a. Nociplastic pain is diffuse and typically persists beyond normal tissue healing/pathology times.
   b. Nociplastic pain includes sustained hyperalgesia (primary and/or secondary) and/or allodynia.
   c. Allodynia-pain due to a stimulus (e.g., brushing or light touch) that does not usually provoke pain.
   d. Primary hyperalgesia—increased pain sensitivity that occurs directly in the area of damaged or inflammed tissues.
   e. Secondary hyperalgesia—pain sensitivity that occurs in surrounding undamaged tissues.
   f. Symptoms maybe widespread and include fatigue, sleep dysfunction, and cognitive disturbances.
   g. Examples include fibromyalgia, traumatic amputation with phantom limb pain, and chronic low back pain.
   h. Examination items/findings include Central Sensitization Inventory questionnaire, diffuse and/or sporadic sensory disturbance, and evidence of sensitization with pain pressure and thermal threshold testing.
4. Identifying the type(s) and source(s) (peripheral vs. central sensitization) of pain, as well as the impact on motor systems/movement, assist in focusing interventions to include potential referrals.
5. Biological pain processes are also influenced by psychosocial factors (fear of movement, anxiety, depression) and emphasize the need for person-centered and holistic assessment and treatment.
6. References:

   a. Chimenti RL et al., A mechanism-based approach to physical therapist management of pain. *Phys Ther*. 2018, 98(5), 302–314.
   b. Cayrol T et al., Stuck in the middle with you: Why a broad-brush approach to defining central sensitization does not help clinicians and patients. *J Orthop Sports Phys Ther*. 2021 May, 51(5), 204–206.

Examination of Pain

1. History: determine chief complaints, description of onset, mechanism of injury, localization (chronic pain is poorly localized, not well defined); nature of pain (constant, intermittent); irritating stimuli/activities.
2. Subjective assessment using pain intensity rating scales.
   a. Simple descriptive scales: verbal report (e.g., select the words that best describe your pain).
   b. Numerical rating scales (rate pain on a scale of 1–10; e.g., 8/10).
   c. Visual analog scale (e.g., bisect line where your pain falls, from mild to severe pain).
   d. Aggravating and easing factors.
   e. Severity, irritability, nature, stage, and stability (SINSS) of pain.
   f. Body chart: using drawings to plot location, type of pain, tingling vs. numbness for neuropathic pain (see Figure 3-14).
   g. Pain response to previous interventions; chronic nociplastic pain is often unresponsive.
   h. Impact of pain on occupational, recreational, and social participation.
3. Self-report questionnaires:
   a. Patient-reported Outcomes Measurement Information System (PROMIS) evaluates biopsychosocial health across multiple domains to include: Pain Behavior, Pain Interference, Physical Function, Social Roles, Fatigue, Depression, and Anxiety. For additional information see: https://www.healthmeasures.net/explore-measurement-systems/promis?
   b. Fear Avoidance Beliefs Questionnaire (FABQ)—see Appendix 2A.
   c. Tampa Scale of Kinesiophobia measures activity avoidance and somatic focus (beliefs that pain is from underlying serious pathology).
   d. Chronic Pain Acceptance Questionnaire evaluates behavioral aspects of pain coping (pain willingness and activity engagement).

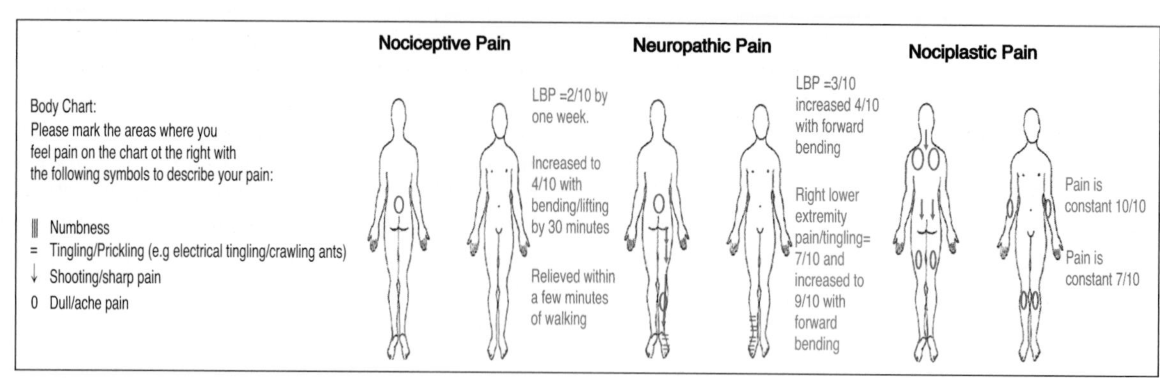

Figure 3-14 **Body Charts Consistent with Nociceptive, Neuropathic, and Nociplastic (Central Sensitization) Pain.**

Nociceptive pain is focal and increases/decreases appropriately with mechanical stress. Neuropathic pain includes radiating, tingling, and burning symptoms with extremity symptoms typically greater than spine pain. Nociplastic pain is often constant with no clear aggravating or easing factors.

4. Systems review to rule in/out potential pain referral sources.
5. Neuromusculoskeletal examination to include pain response to sensory, motor, movement (e.g., posture/transfers/gait), and mechanical (palpation, soft-tissue/joint/neural tension/compression) assessment.
6. Potential referral for additional testing (imaging, NCV/EMG, labs) and/or interdisciplinary treatment.

Physical Therapy Goals, Outcomes, and Interventions

1. Pain science education.
   a. On the initial evaluation/treatment discuss and define safe movements that the patient can complete.
   b. Share the impact of exercise, manual therapy on the nervous system.
   c. Discuss patient's fear of movement and how treatment will assist in regulation of pain.
2. Assist patient in identifying pain behaviors, modify negative behavioral reinforcers, and practice well behaviors.
   a. Establish a behavior contract: establish consistent level of activity.
   b. Provide positive reinforcers, educational support.
   c. Demonstrate change, allow patient to experience success.
3. Provide evidence-based physical therapy treatments that enhance activity and assist pain management.
4. Exercise/Activity: Establish a realistic daily exercise/activity program.
   a. Improve overall level of conditioning: daily walking program, assistive devices as appropriate.
   b. Improve overall functional capacity, independence in functional mobility skills, ADLs: ROM, general strengthening, postural training, motor control training.
5. Interdisciplinary and holistic care.
   a. Pain clinic.
   b. Mental Health—Mindfulness and acceptance based interventions.
   c. Nutrition Care—Diet.
   d. Sleep hygiene.

Complex Regional Pain Syndrome

Overview

1. Complex regional pain syndrome (CRPS) often develops following trauma or disuse.
2. CRPS type 1, also referred to as reflex sympathetic dystrophy, presents with intense pain throughout the limb (upper or lower limb) but does not involve specific damage to the peripheral nervous system.
3. CRPS Type 2, also called causalgia, involves specific damage to the peripheral nervous system (radiculopathy, plexopathy, or mononeuropathies) typically resulting in both overt motor and sensory neuropathic signs and symptoms.
4. It is estimated that 90% of patients with CRPS have type 1.

Signs and Symptoms

1. Intense and diffuse pain.
2. Continuous burning or throbbing pain.
3. Hyperalgesia and allodynia.
4. Decreased movement of the affected area.
5. Cold sensitivity.
6. Edema in the painful area.
7. Changes in skin temperature, color, and texture.
8. Hyperhidrosis.
9. Changes in hair and nail growth.
10. Atrophy and risk of osteoporosis.

Medical Management

1. Diagnosis.
   a. Important to determine type 1 from type 2 as this will determine how aggressive the patient can move.

b. Use of a body chart, neuropathic pain questionnaire, and focused neuromuscular exam helps to determine type 2 with peripheral nervous system involvement in a nerve root, plexus, and/or nerve distribution.
c. Nerve conduction/EMG also helpful if patient is so painful that they will not move.

2. Treatment.
   a. Pharmacology: nonsteroidal anti-inflammatory drugs, corticosteroids, antiseizure and antidepression drugs (gabapentin, pregabalin, amitriptyline, nortriptyline), ketamine, opioids, and lidocaine patches.
   b. Sympathetic nerve block.
   c. Spinal cord stimulator.
   d. Psychotherapy and/or cognitive behavioral therapy.

Physical Therapy Goals, Outcomes, and Interventions

1. Movement is critical for both types of CRPS; patients with type 2 may require more passive/active assistive range of motion and splinting to allow the affected nerve injury to heal.
2. Desensitization training of the affected area.
3. Aerobic exercise to assist with pain management.
4. Manual therapy/modalities as needed for pain relief.
5. Neuroscience pain education.

Fibromyalgia Syndrome (FMS)

Overview

1. A common chronic condition characterized by widespread musculoskeletal pain and fatigue. Affects almost 5 million people in the United States.
2. Etiology is unknown.
   a. Current theories focus on abnormal changes in the brain's processing of painful sensations, including abnormal increases in neurotransmitters and changes in the brain's pain receptors.
   b. FMS tends to run in families.
   c. 80%–90% are females.
3. Symptoms may begin after a physical trauma, surgery, infection, or significant psychological stress.
4. People with conditions such as rheumatoid arthritis, systemic lupus erythematosus, or ankylosis spondylitis are more likely to develop FMS.

Signs and Symptoms

1. Widespread pain described as constant dull ache lasting for at least 3 months.
2. Multiple points (trigger points) on the head, chest, shoulders, elbows, hips, or knees that are tender to a firm touch.
3. Persistent fatigue: both mental and physical.
4. Sleep disturbances: patients often awaken tired with morning stiffness; experience sleep disrupted by pain. Other sleep disorders may be present, including restless legs syndrome and sleep apnea.
5. Cognitive difficulties: impaired ability to focus, pay attention, and concentrate on mental tasks (often referred to as "fibro fog").
6. Sensory changes: atypical patterns of numbness and tingling (sensory amplification).
7. FMS often co-exists with other conditions: irritable bowel or bladder syndrome, migraine and other types of headaches, interstitial cystitis, and temporomandibular joint disorders.
8. Anxiety and depression are common.
9. Stress can make symptoms worse.

Medical Management

1. Diagnosis.
   a. Medical history: widespread pain for more than 3 months with no underlying medical condition.
   b. Physical examination: positive tender point exam. The requirement of 11 positive tender points out of a total of 18 is no longer necessary for the diagnosis.
2. Treatment.
   a. Symptomatic relief of pain: analgesics.
   b. Antidepressants and antiseizure drugs.
   c. Nutritional support.
   d. Psychological support and counseling.

Physical Therapy Goals, Outcomes, and Interventions

1. Regular, moderate exercise to improve strength, flexibility, and endurance.
   a. Patients with FMS typically demonstrate exercise intolerance. Daily exercise is important. The patient is encouraged to start slow, pace themselves, set realistic goals, and modify the program in times of stress.
   b. Aerobic conditioning: mild to moderate intensities, 30-minute durations, 2–3 times/week, slow progression.
   c. Aquatic exercise has been shown to be effective in decreasing pain while increasing cardiovascular conditioning and strength.
   d. Stretching.
   e. Manual therapy techniques and massage to help relieve pain and stiffness.
   f. Strengthening exercise.
   g. Deep breathing, yoga, and tai chi have been shown to be effective.
2. Teach techniques for taking control, managing pain, reducing fatigue, improving function, and quality of life.
   a. Promote self-responsibility for own health management, coping strategies.
   b. Keeping an activity journal may be helpful.
3. Promote energy conservation: work and home environmental adjustments.
4. Refer to support group.

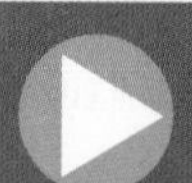

Interventions for Patients with Neurological Dysfunction

Motor Control/Motor Learning Strategies

General Concepts

1. Incorporates theories of motor control and motor learning.
2. Consideration is given to both intrinsic neuromuscular control processes and environmental constraints.

Motor Control Strategies

1. General concepts—motor control.
   a. Motor program: a set of prestructured muscle commands that, when initiated, results in the production of a coordinated movement sequence (learned task); can be carried out largely uninfluenced by peripheral feedback.
   b. Motor plan: an overall strategy for movement; an action sequence requiring the coordination of a number of motor programs.
   c. Feedback: afferent information sent by various sensory receptors to control centers.
      - Feedback updates control centers about the correctness of movement while it progresses; shapes ongoing movement.
      - Feedback allows motor responses to be adapted to the demands of the environment.
   d. Feedforward: readies the system in advance of movement; anticipatory responses that adjust the system for incoming sensory feedback or for future movements; e.g., preparatory postural adjustments.
   e. Motor skill acquisition.
      - Behavior is organized to achieve a goal-directed task.
      - Active problem-solving/processing is required for the development of a motor program/motor plan, motor learning; improves retention of skills.
      - Adaptive to specific environmental demands (regulatory conditions). Closed environment: fixed, nonchanging. Open environment: variable, changing.
   f. CNS recovery/reorganization is dependent upon experience.

Motor Learning Strategies

1. General concepts—motor learning.
   a. A change in the capability of a person to perform a skill; the result of practice or experience.
   b. Measures of motor learning include:
      - Performance: determine overall quality of performance, level of automaticity, level of effort, speed of decision-making.
      - Retention: the ability to demonstrate the skill after a period of no practice.
      - Generalizability: the acquired capability to apply what has been learned to other similar tasks (transfer tests); e.g., transfers wheelchair to mat, to toilet, and to car.
      - Resistance to contextual change: acquired capability to apply what has been learned to other environmental contexts; e.g., clinic, home, work.
   c. Feedback.
      - Intrinsic feedback: sensory information normally acquired during performance of a task.
      - Augmented feedback: externally presented feedback that is added to that normally acquired during task performance; e.g., verbal cueing.
      - Knowledge of results (KR): augmented feedback about the outcome of a movement.
      - Knowledge of performance (KP): augmented feedback about the nature of the movement produced; e.g., movement characteristics.
      - Feedback schedules: feedback given after every trial; feedback summed (after set number of trials), fading (decreasing) or bandwidth (if responses outside a designated range).
   d. Practice.
      - Blocked practice: practice of a single motor skill repeatedly; repetitive practice.
      - Variable practice: practice of varied motor skills in which the performer is required to make rapid modifications of the skill in order to match the demands of the task.
      - Random practice: practice of a group or class of motor skills in random order (no predictable order).
      - Serial practice: practice of a group or class of motor skills in serial or predictable order.
      - Massed practice: relatively continuous practice in which the amount of rest time is small (rest time is less than the practice time).
      - Distributed practice: practice in which the rest time is relatively large (practice time is less than rest time).
      - Mental practice: cognitive rehearsal of a motor skill without overt physical performance.
   e. Transfer: the effects of having previous practice of a skill or skills upon the learning of a new skill or upon performance in a new context; transfer may

be either positive (assisting learning) or negative (hindering learning).
- Part-whole transfer: a learning technique in which a complex motor task is broken down into its component or subordinate parts for separate practice before practice of the integrated whole.
- Bilateral transfer: improvement in movement skill performance with one limb results from practice of similar movements with the opposite limb.

f. Strategies for effective learning (Table 3-26).
- Feedback given after every trial improves performance, while variable feedback improves learning and retention.
- Early training should focus on visual feedback (cognitive phase of learning), while later training should focus on proprioceptive feedback (associative phase of learning).
- Reduce extraneous environmental stimuli early in learning (e.g., closed environment), while later learning focuses on adaptation to environmental demands (e.g., open environment).
- Supportive feedback (reinforcement) can be used to shape behavior, motivate patient.
- Assist learner in recognizing/pairing intrinsic feedback with movement responses.

g. Provide augmented feedback: knowledge of results, knowledge of performance.
- Early in learning, focus feedback on correct aspects of performance.
- Later in learning, focus feedback on errors as they become consistent.
- Feedback after every trial improves performance, useful during early learning.
- Use variable feedback (summed, fading, bandwidth) to improve retention, increase depth of cognitive processing.
- Avoid feedback dependence: reduce augmented feedback as soon as possible; foster active introspection, decision-making by learner.

h. Establish practice schedule: use distributed practice when superior performance is desired, when motivation is low or when the learner has short attention, poor concentration, or fatigues easily.

i. Use variable practice of a group of functional tasks rather than constant practice to improve learning (promotes retention and generalizability).

j. Use random or serial practice order rather than blocked practice to improve learning (retention).

k. Use mental practice to improve learning; have patient verbalize task components, requirements for performance; effective when task has a large cognitive component or to decrease fear and anxiety.

l. Use parts to whole transfer when task is complex, has highly independent parts, or when learner has limited memory or attention, or difficulty with a particular part. Practice both the parts and the integrated whole.

m. Limit information with learners who have attention deficits, mentally fatigue easily; focus on key task elements; give frequent rest periods.

n. Tasks that have highly integrated components should be practiced as a whole; e.g., gait.

o. Transfer of learning is optimized when tasks are highly similar (similar stimuli, similar responses); e.g., bilateral transfer, one arm to the other.

p. Use guided movement early in learning, not late; most effective for slow postural or positioning tasks.

q. Optimal arousal is necessary for optimal learning; low arousal or intense arousal yield poor performance and learning (inverted U theory).

r. Involve learner in goal setting; task should be desirable, functionally relevant, important to learn.

Task-Specific Training

General Concepts

1. Goals: to promote recovery of motor function, the reappearance of motor patterns that were present before CNS injury, or adaptation/compensation, the appearance of new motor patterns resulting from adaptation of remaining motor elements. The involved segments are targeted for practice.
2. Emphasis is on use of the affected body segments/limbs using task-specific activities and experiences.
   a. Patients practice important, functional tasks essential to independence; e.g., stand up and sit down; balance, walking and stair climbing, reaching, and manipulation.
   b. Patients practice tasks in appropriate and safe environments; focus is on anticipated environments for daily function.
   c. Repetition and extensive practice are required, including both in-therapy and out-of-therapy time.
   d. Progressive exercise or activity training requires monitoring of heart rate and blood pressure.
3. Patients practice under therapist's supervision and independently.
   a. Therapists can provide initial assistance through guided movements and verbal cueing; progression is to active, independent movements as soon as possible.
   b. Therapists serve as learning coaches, encouraging correct performance.
   c. Exercise/activity logs help organize the patient's self-monitored practice.
4. Motor learning strategies are utilized, including *behavioral shaping techniques* that use reinforcement and reward to promote skill development.

Table 3-26

Stages of Motor Learning and Training Strategies

COGNITIVE STAGE CHARACTERISTICS	TRAINING STRATEGIES
The learner • develops an understanding of task, *cognitive mapping* • assesses abilities, task demands • identifies stimuli, contacts memory • selects response, performs initial approximations of task • structures motor program • modifies initial responses ***"What to do"*** decision	Highlight purpose of task in functionally relevant terms. Demonstrate ideal performance of task to establish a *reference of correctness.* Have patient verbalize task components and requirements. Point out similarities to other learned tasks. Direct attention to critical task elements **Select appropriate feedback** • Emphasize intact sensory systems, intrinsic feedback systems • Carefully pair extrinsic feedback with intrinsic feedback • High dependence on vision: have patient watch movement • Provide ***Knowledge of Performance (KP):*** focus on errors as they become consistent; do not cue on large number of random errors • Provide ***Knowledge of Results (KR):*** focus on success of movement outcome Ask learner to evaluate performance, outcomes; identify problems, solutions Use reinforcements (praise) for correct performance and continuing motivation **Organize feedback schedule** • *Feedback* after every trial improves performance during early learning • *Variable feedback* (summed, fading, bandwidth designs) increases depth of cognitive processing, improves retention; may decrease performance initially **Organize initial practice** • Stress controlled movement to minimize errors • Provide adequate rest periods using *distributed practice* if task is complex, long, or energy costly or if learner fatigues easily, has short attention, or has poor concentration • Use manual guidance to assist as appropriate • Break complex tasks down into component parts, teach both parts and integrated whole • Use *bilateral transfer* as appropriate • Use *blocked (repeated)* practice of same task to improve performance • Use *variable practice* (serial or random practice order) of related skills to increase depth of cognitive processing and retention; may decrease performance initially • Use *mental practice* to improve performance and learning, reduce anxiety **Assess, modify arousal levels as appropriate** • High or low arousal impairs performance and learning • Avoid stressors, mental fatigue **Structure environment** • Reduce extraneous environmental stimuli, distractors to ensure attention, concentration • Emphasize closed skills initially gradually progressing to open skills
ASSOCIATED STAGE CHARACTERISTICS	**TRAINING STRATEGIES**
The learner • practices movements • refines motor program • spatial and temporal organization • decreases errors • extraneous movements Dependence on visual feedback decreases, increases for use of proprioceptive feedback; cognitive monitoring decreases ***"How to do"*** decision	**Select appropriate feedback** • Continue to provide KP; intervene when errors become consistent • Emphasize proprioceptive feedback, "feel of movement" to assist in establishing an internal reference of correctness • Continue to provide KR; stress relevance of functional outcomes • Assist learner to improve self-evaluation, decision-making skills • Facilitation techniques, guided movements are counterproductive during this stage of learning **Organize feedback schedule** • Continue to provide feedback for continuing motivation; encourage patient to self-assess achievements • Avoid excessive augmented feedback • Focus on use of variable feedback (summed, fading, bandwidth) designs to improve retention **Organize practice** • Encourage consistency of performance • Focus on variable practice order (serial or random) of related skills to improve retention **Structure environment** • Progress toward open, changing environment • Prepare the learner for home, community, work environments

(*Continued*)

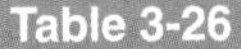

Table 3-26

Stages of Motor Learning and Training Strategies (Continued)

AUTONOMOUS STAGE CHARACTERISTICS	TRAINING STRATEGIES
The learner • practices movements • continues to refine motor responses • spatial and temporal highly organized • movements are largely error-free • minimal level of cognitive monitoring ***"How to succeed"*** decision	Assess need for conscious attention, automaticity of movements **Select appropriate feedback** • Learner demonstrates appropriate self-evaluation, decision-making skills • Provide occasional feedback (KP, KR) when errors evident **Organize practice** • Stress consistency of performance in variable environments, variations of tasks (open skills) • High levels of practice (massed practice) are appropriate **Structure environment** • Vary environments to challenge learner • Ready the learner for home, community, and work environments Focus on competitive aspects of skills as appropriate; e.g., wheelchair sports

From: O'Sullivan S, Schmitz T, Fulk G. Physical Rehabilitation, 7th ed, Philadelphia, FA Davis, 2019, pg 365–366, with permission.

5. Activity-based, task-oriented training effectively counteracts the effects of immobility and the development of indirect impairments such as muscle weakness and loss of flexibility. It prevents *learned nonuse* of the more involved segments while promoting recovery of the central nervous system (neuroplasticity).
6. Box 3-3 presents a summary of Functional, Task-Oriented Training Strategies.

Initial Tasks

1. Focus is on tasks that promote functional independence.
2. Focus is on goals and tasks important to the patient.
3. Focus is on ensuring patient success and motivation.

Progression of Tasks

1. Tasks are varied to improve motor control.
2. Environments are varied to improve generalizability of tasks to home and community environments.
3. Therapists target the functional requirements of the task, e.g., a reciprocal stepping pattern, dynamic equilibrium during propulsion and adaptability.
4. Verbal cueing and manual assistance are provided as needed to assist.
5. Progression is from treadmill walking to overground walking. Community ambulation skills and adaptability are targeted.

Locomotor Training

1. Motorized treadmill training (TT) with partial body weight support (BWS): provides a means of early task training (e.g., for patients with stroke or incomplete spinal cord injury). The activity is continually adjusted to meet the needs of the patient and progress the activity.
   a. Focus is on good stepping and posture.
   b. LE movements are initially manually assisted (e.g., trunk/pelvis, LE stepping); assistance is decreased as skill and control progresses.
   c. Treadmill speeds are increased with focus on achieving normal functional walking speeds.
   d. Progression is from body weight support to no support (e.g., 40% to 30% to 20% to 10% to 0%).
   e. Training is high frequency (3–5 days/week), moderate duration (20–30 minutes), and maximum tolerated intensity (speed and slope).
2. Overground training: using BWS, progressing to no BWS.
3. Overground training with least restrictive device (LRD) to no device, as appropriate.
4. Strategies to vary locomotor task demands: practice walking forward, backward, side-stepping, crossed-stepping (braiding); stopping, starting, and turning on cue; head movements; step-ups, step-up and over, stair climbing, obstacles.
5. Strategies to promote community reintegration: practice walking in open environments; altered support surface; altered speeds; curbs, ramps, walking through doorways, elevators, dual-task walking.
6. See Table 3-27 for clinical practice guidelines to improve locomotor function following chronic neurologic disorders (Hornby TG et al. Clinical practice guideline to improve locomotor function following chronic stroke, incomplete spinal cord injury, and brain injury. *J Neurol Phys Ther*. 2020; 44(1): 49–100).

See Chapter 6, Therapeutic Exercise, for additional information on strength, balance, and gait training interventions.

Constraint-Induced Movement Therapy (CIMT)

1. The less-affected UE is restrained by the use of a protective hand mitt.
2. Task practice is focused on using the more affected UE.
   a. Must meet minimum movement criteria.
   b. Repetitive practice of functional tasks.
   c. Shaping: a functional task is selected and is progressively made more difficult. Goal is for the participant to accomplish the task with effort.

BOX 3-3 Functional, Task-Oriented Training Strategies

Emphasize early training.

- To promote use-dependent cortical plasticity and overcome learned nonuse.

Define the goal of task practice.

- Involve the patient in goal setting and decision-making, thereby enhancing motivation and promoting active commitment to recovery.

Determine the activities to be practiced.

- Consider the patient's history, health status, age, interests, and experience.
- Consider the patient's abilities and strengths, recovery level, learning style, impairments, and activity limitations.
- Determine a set of activities to be practiced for each training goal.
- Select activities that are interesting, stimulating, and important to the patient.
- Choose activities with the greatest potential for patient success and intersperse more difficult tasks with easier tasks.
- Target active movements involving the more involved extremities.
- Limit use of less-involved extremities; set parameters, impose time limits for use of constraints.
- Prevent or limit compensatory strategies.

Determine the parameters of practice.

- Manage fatigue, determine rest and practice times.
- Model ideal performance; establish a *reference of correctness.*
- Establish requirements for intensity, minimal number of repetitions.
- Establish practice schedule of tasks (blocked or variable); shift to variable practice as soon as possible to enhance retention.
- Determine the practice order of tasks (constant, serial, random); shift to random order as soon as possible to enhance retention.
- Control use of instructions and augmented feedback to promote learning.
- Control use of assisted or guided movements to promote initial learning; ensure the patient successfully transitions to active movements as soon as possible.

Utilize behavioral shaping techniques.

- Gradually modify the task to increase the challenge and make it progressively more difficult as patient performance improves.
- Provide immediate and explicit feedback; recognize and acknowledge small improvements in task performance.
- Emphasize positive aspects of performance.
- Avoid excessive effort and fatigue; they degrade performance and dampen motivation.

Promote problem-solving.

- Have the patient evaluate performance, identify obstacles, generate potential solutions.
- Have the patient practice the chosen movement (solution) and evaluate outcome.
- Relate successes to overall goals.

Structure the environment.

- Promote initial practice in a supportive environment, free of distractors (closed environment for highly distractible patients).
- Progress to variable practice in real-world environments (open environments).

Establish parameters for practice outside of therapy.

- Identify specific goals and strategies for unsupervised practice; maximize opportunities.
- Utilize a written behavioral contract, have the patient agree to targeted behaviors to be carried out during the day.
- Have patient document unsupervised practice using an activity log or home exercise diary.

(Continued)

BOX 3-3 Functional, Task-Oriented Training Strategies (Continued)

Maintain focus on active learning.

- Minimize hands-on therapy.
- Maximize therapist's role as *training coach.*

Monitor recovery closely and document progress.

- Use sensitive, valid, and reliable functional outcome measures.

Be cautious about timetables and predictions: recovery is highly individualized and may take longer than expected.

From O'Sullivan S, Schmitz T. Improving Functional Outcomes in Physical Rehabilitation, 2nd ed. FA Davis, 2016, pg 17, with permission.

Table 3-27

APTA Neurology Clinical Practice Guidelines—Recommendations to Improve Locomotion for Chronic (≥6 months) Stroke, ISCI, or Brain Injury

INTERVENTIONS	RECOMMENDATIONS	LEVEL/STRENGTH OF EVIDENCE
Moderate to high intensity (>70% HR max) over ground ambulation	Perform intervention	Level I–II; strong recommendation for individuals ≥6 months post-stroke
Virtual reality treadmill training	Perform intervention	Level I–II; strong recommendation for individuals ≥6 months post-stroke
Strength training multiple sets/ reps at 70% 1RM	Consider intervention	Level I–II; weak recommendation for individuals ≥6 months post-stroke or ISCI
Cycle training (high intensities)	Consider intervention	Level I–II; weak recommendation for individuals ≥6 months post-stroke
Circuit training	Consider intervention	Level I–II; weak recommendation for individuals ≥6 months post-stroke
Virtual reality standing balance exercise	Consider intervention	Level I–II; strong consideration for individuals ≥6 months post-stroke
Sitting/standing balance without visual feedback	Do not perform intervention	Level I–II; strong recommendation for not using for individuals ≥6 months post-stroke
Robotic assistance walking training	Do not perform intervention	Level I–II; strong recommendation for not using for individuals ≥6 months post-stroke or ISCI
Body weight support treadmill training with PT assistance	Do not perform intervention	Level I–II; strong recommendation for not using in individuals ≥6 months post-stroke

ISCI = Incomplete spinal cord injury; HR = heart rate; 1RM = one rep maximum, PT = Physical Therapy

Adapted from Hornby TG et al. Clinical practice guideline to improve locomotor function following chronic stroke, incomplete spinal cord injury, and brain injury. *J Neurol Phys Ther.* 2020; 44(1): 49–100.

3. Adherence-enhancing behavioral strategies are used, including use of:
   a. Daily administration of motor activity log.
   b. Home diary.
   c. Problem-solving to overcome barriers to use of the more-affected UE.
   d. Behavioral contract.
   e. Caregiver contract.
   f. Home skill assignment, home practice, and daily schedule.
4. Therapist provides feedback, coaching, modeling, and encouragement.
5. Training is high intensity (several hours/day), high frequency (daily) for a period of 2–3 consecutive weeks.
6. Modified CI therapy is less intense, using lower intensity and frequency over a longer period of time (e.g., 1 hour/day, 3 days/week for 8 weeks).
7. Progression is to functional skills performed in the home environment.

Remediation-Facilitation Intervention

General Concepts

1. Includes guided movement, neuromuscular facilitation, sensory stimulation; exercises/activities designed to reduce specific impairments, and improve function of *involved* body segments.

2. Goal is to enhance or improve recovery.
3. Emphasis is on progression of postures and activities to improve motor function.

Proprioceptive Neuromuscular Facilitation (PNF)

1. Basic concepts.
   a. Utilizes synergistic patterns of movement (UE, LE, trunk).
   b. Utilizes proprioceptive elements: stretch resistance, overflow, manual contacts, approximation, traction to enhance contraction.
   c. Utilizes motor learning principles: verbal cues, visual guidance of movement, repetition, and practice.
2. PNF techniques.
   a. Rhythmic Initiation.
   b. Rhythmic Rotation.
   c. Stabilizing Reversals (Alternating Isometrics).
   d. Rhythmic Stabilization.
   e. Dynamic Reversals (Slow Reversals).
   f. Combination of Isotonics (Agonist Reversals).
   g. Replication (Hold-Relax-Active Motion).
   h. Contract-Relax Active Contraction (CRAC).
   i. Hold-Relax (HR).
   j. Repeated Stretch (Repeated Contractions).
3. PNF UE patterns of movement: named for motions occurring at the proximal joint (shoulder); intermediate joint (elbow) may be straight, flexing, or extending (intermediate pivot).
   a. Flexion-adduction-external rotation (D1F, diagonal 1 flexion) verbal cues (VC) "Close your hand, turn, and pull your arm across your face."
   b. Extension-abduction-internal rotation (D1E, diagonal 1 extension) VC: "Open your hand, turn, and push your arm down and out."
   c. Flexion-abduction-external rotation (D2F) VC: "Open your hand, turn, and lift your arm up and out."
   d. Extension-adduction-internal rotation (D2E) VC: "Close your hand, turn, and pull your arm down and across your body."
4. PNF LE patterns of movement: named for motions occurring at the proximal joint (hip); intermediate joint (knee) may be straight, flexing or extending (intermediate pivot).
   a. Flexion-adduction-external rotation (D1F) VC: "Bring your foot up, turn, and pull your leg up and across your body."
   b. Extension-abduction-internal rotation (D1E) VC: "Push your foot down, turn, and push your leg down and out."
   c. Flexion-abduction-internal rotation (D2F) VC: "Lift your foot up, turn, and lift your leg up and out."
   d. Extension-adduction-external rotation (D2E) VC: "Push your foot down, turn, and pull your leg down and in."
5. PNF head and trunk patterns of movement:
   a. Sitting, chop: upper trunk flexion with rotation to right or left; lead arm moves in D1E, assist arm holds on top of wrist.
   b. Sitting, lift: upper trunk extension with rotation to right or left; lead arm moves in D2F, assist arm holds beneath the wrist.
   c. Supine, lower trunk flexion with rotation to right or left; knees flexing.
   d. Supine or sitting, head and neck flexion with rotation to right or left.

Neurodevelopmental Treatment (NDT)

1. Basic concepts.
   a. Utilizes individualized therapeutic handling based on movement analysis; utilizes a team approach (PT, OT, speech-language pathologist).
   b. Indicated for individuals with neurological pathophysiology (e.g., stroke or cerebral palsy).
   c. Focus is on optimal sensorimotor processing and promoting movement patterns/synergies, task performance, and skill acquisition. Targets the involved extremities/segments.
   d. Patterns of movement can be facilitated by appropriate handling techniques, a combination of inhibition/facilitation techniques, guided movements, verbal cues, repetition, and experience in the environment.
   e. Anticipated goals and outcomes determined in partnership with the family, client, and the interdisciplinary team.
2. Therapeutic handling: involves dynamic, reciprocal interaction between therapist and client; hands-on treatment using guided or facilitated movements.
3. Focus in on functional activities that are meaningful and goal oriented; e.g., rolling, sitting, standing, walking, UE tasks; for children, appropriate developmental activities.

Sensory Stimulation

1. General concepts.
   a. Indications: patients who demonstrate absent or disordered motor control, i.e., difficulty initiating movement or sustaining movement, who benefit from the use of augmented feedback; most useful in the early stages of motor learning.
   b. Contraindications: patients who will not benefit from a hands-on approach, who demonstrate sufficient motor control to perform active movements, independently practice a motor skill, and self-correct based on feedback mechanisms, e.g., later stages of motor learning.
   c. Response to stimulation is variable and dependent upon a number of multiple factors.
   d. Use of sensory stimulation techniques should be phased out as soon as possible in favor of active

control by the patient; important to avoid feedback/therapist dependence. Can serve as a bridge to active movement control.

e. Spatial summation (multiple techniques) or temporal summation (repeated application of the same technique) may be necessary to produce the desired response in some patients with reduced responses.

f. Consider cumulative effects: the total environment along with the effects of sensory stimulation techniques. Avoid overloading the CNS.

2. Techniques.
   a. Proprioceptive stimulation techniques: quick stretch, resistance, joint approximation and traction.
   b. Tactile/somatosensory techniques: inhibitory pressure, light touch (stimulating), maintained touch (calming).
   c. Vestibular stimulation techniques: slow, repetitive rocking (calming); fast, irregular (stimulating).

Substitution/Compensation

General Concepts

1. Substitution occurs when functions are assumed, replaced, or substituted by different areas of the brain using different effectors or body segments.
2. Indications: to offset or adapt to residual impairments and disabilities.
3. Focus is on resumption of functional independence with reliance on uninvolved segments for function; e.g., the patient with cervical level SCI learns to roll using UEs, the patient with stroke learns to dress using uninvolved segments.
4. Changes are made in the patient's overall approach to tasks.
   a. Patient is made aware of movement deficiencies, alternate ways to accomplish tasks.
   b. Patient relearns functional patterns and habitual ways of moving.
   c. Patient practices functional skills in a variety of environments.

Issues with Substitution

1. Focus on uninvolved segments to accomplish daily tasks (e.g., stroke, traumatic brain injury) may suppress recovery and contribute to *learned nonuse* of the impaired segments.
2. Focus may lead to the development of *splinter skills* in patients with brain damage; skills cannot be easily generalized to other tasks or environmental situations.
3. May be the only approach possible.
   a. If no additional recovery is anticipated (e.g., complete spinal cord injury).
   b. If severe CNS deficits are present.
   c. If patient exhibits extensive comorbidities and poor health.

Strategies

1. Simplify activities.
2. Establish a new functional pattern; identify key task elements, residual segments available for control of movements.
3. Repeated practice; work toward consistency, efficiency.
4. Energy conservation and activity pacing techniques are important to ensure completion of all daily movement requirements.
5. Adapt environment to facilitate relearning of skills, ease of movement.
   a. Simplify; set up for optimal performance.
   b. Use environmental adaptations to enhance performance; e.g., color code stairs, grab bars.

Note: Selected Neuromuscular Outcome Measures can be found in Appendix 3A.

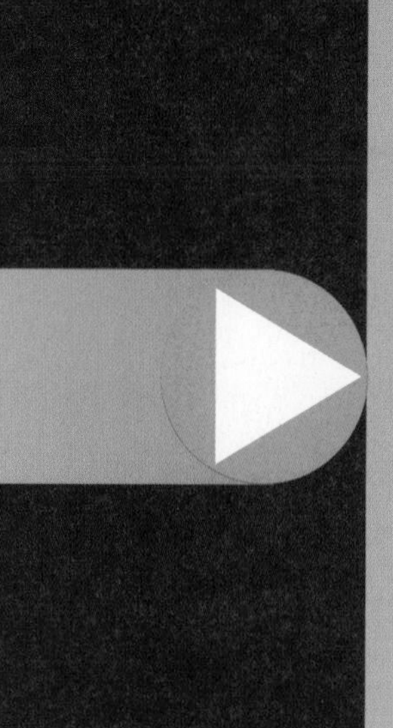

APPENDIX 3A

Selected Neuromuscular Outcome Measures

Table 3A-1

Selected Outcome Measures Organized by the International Classification of Functioning, Disability, and Health (ICF) Categories

BODY STRUCTURE AND FUNCTION MEASURES	REFERENCES
Manual Muscle Test (MMT)	• Hislop HJ, Montgomery J. Daniels and Worthingham's Muscle Testing: Techniques of Manual Examination, 8th ed. Saunders (Elsevier), Philadelphia. 2007. • Kendall, F, McCreary E, Provance P, et al. Muscles Testing and Function with Posture and Pain, 5th ed. Lippincott Williams & Wilkins, Baltimore. 2005.
Joint Motion	• Norkin C, White J. Measurement of Joint Motion: A Guide to Goniometry, 5th ed. FA Davis, Philadelphia. 2016.
Modified Ashworth Scale	• Bohannon RW, Smith MB. Interrater reliability of a modified Ashworth scale of muscle spasticity. *Phys Ther.* 1987; 67: 206–207. • Blackburn M, van Vliet P, Mockett SP. Reliability of measurements obtained with the Modified Ashworth Scale in the lower extremities of people with stroke. *Phys Ther.* 2002; 82: 25–34.
Mini Mental State Exam (MMSE)	• Folstein MF, Folstein SE, McHugh PR. "Mini-mental state." A practical method for grading the cognitive state of patients for the clinician. *J Psychiatr Res.* 1975; 12(3): 189.
Dizziness Handicap Inventory (DHI)	• Jacobson GP, Newman CW. The development of the dizziness handicap inventory. *Arch Otolaryngol Head Neck Surg.* 1990; 16: 424–427.
DISABILITY SPECIFIC MEASURES	**REFERENCES**
STROKE	
Fugl-Meyer Assessment of Motor Performance	• Fugl-Meyer AR, Jaasko L, Leyman I, et al. The post-stroke hemiplegic patient: a method for evaluation and performance. *Scand J Rehabil Med.* 1975; 3: 13–31. • Fugl-Meyer AR. Post-stroke hemiplegia assessment of physical properties. *Scand J Rehabil Med.* 1980; 63: 85–93. • Gladstone DJ, Danells CJ, Black S. The Fugl-Myer assessment of motor recovery after stroke: a critical review of its measurement properties. *Neurorehabil Neural Repair.* 2002; 16: 232.

(*Continued*)

Table 3A-1

Selected Outcome Measures Organized by the International Classification of Functioning, Disability, and Health (ICF) Categories (Continued)

DISABILITY SPECIFIC MEASURES	REFERENCES
STROKE	
National Institutes of Health (NIH) Stroke Scale	• Brott T, Adams HP, Olinger CP, et al. Measurements of acute cerebral infarction: a clinical examination scale. *Stroke.* 1989; 20: 864–870. • Goldstein LB, Bertels C, Davis JN. Interrater reliability of the NIH stroke scale. *Arch Neurol.* 1989; 46: 660–662. • Heinemann A, Harvey R, McGuire JR, et al. Measurement properties of the NIH stroke scale during acute rehabilitation. *Stroke.* 1997; 28: 1174–1180. • The NIH Stroke Scale is available online at: http://www.ninds.nih.gov/doctors/NIH_Stroke_Scale.pdf
Postural Assessment Scale for Stroke Patients (PASS)	• Benaim C, Pérennou DA, Villy J, et al. Validation of a standardized assessment of postural control in stroke patients: the Postural Assessment Scale for Stroke Patients (PASS). *Stroke.* 1999; 30: 1862–1868. • Pyoria O, Talvitie U, Nyrkko H, et al. Validity of the Postural Control and Balance for Stroke Test. *Physiother Res Int.* 2007; 12(3): 162–174.
Motor Activity Log (MAL)	• Uswatte G, et al. The Motor Activity Log-28: assessing daily use of the hemiparetic arm after stroke. *Neurology* 2006: 67: 1189.
Stroke Impact Scale	• Duncan P, et al. The Stroke Impact Scale Version 2.0: Evaluation of reliability, validity, sensitivity to change. *Stroke.* 1999; 30: 2131–2140.
TRAUMATIC BRAIN INJURY (TBI)	
Glasgow Coma Scale (GCS)	• Jennett B, Teasdale G. Management of Head Injuries. FA Davis, Philadelphia. 1981.
Rancho Levels of Cognitive Function (LOCF)	• Hagen C, Malkmus D, Durham P. Levels of cognitive functioning. In: *Rehabilitation of the Head Injured Adult: Comprehensive Physical Management.* Downey, CA: Professional Staff Association of Ranchos Los Amigos Hospital. 1979.
High-Level Mobility Assessment Tool (HiMat)	• Williams GP, Robertson V, Greenwood KM, et al. The high-level mobility assessment tool (HiMAT) for traumatic brain injury. Part 1: Item generation. *Brain Injury.* 2005; 19(11): 925–932. • Williams GP, Robertson V, Greenwood, KM et al. The high-level mobility assessment tool (HiMAT) for traumatic brain injury. Part 2: Content validity and discriminability. *Brain Injury.* 2005; 19(10): 833–843. • Williams GP, Greenwood KM, Robertson VJ, et al. High-Level Mobility Assessment Tool (HiMAT): Inter-rater reliability, retest reliability, and internal consistency. *Phys Ther.* 2006; 86: 395–400. • The HiMat is available online at: http://www.tbims.org/combi/himat/index.html
SPINAL CORD INJURY (SCI)	
ASIA Impairment Scale—Standard Neurological Classification of Spinal Cord Injury	• American Spinal Injury Association (ASIS): International Standards for Neurological Classification of Spinal Cord Injury. ASIS, Chicago. 2006. • American Spinal Injury Association (ASIS): International Standards for Neurological Classification of Spinal Cord Injury. ASIS, Atlanta. 2015. • Spinal Cord Injury Levels & Classification: www.sci-info-pages.com • Kirshblum S, Waring W. Updates for the International Standards for Neurological Classification of Spinal Cord Injury. *Phys Med Rehabil Clin N Am.* 2014; 25(3): 505–17. • Kirshblum S, Burns S, Biering-Sorensen, F, et al. International standards for neurological classification of spinal cord injury. *J Spinal Cord Med.* 2011; 34(6): 535–546.
Multidimensional Pain Inventory-Spinal Cord Version (MPI-SCI)	• Widerstrom-Noga EG, Cruz-Almeida Y, Martinez-Arizala A, Turk DC. Internal consistency, stability, and validity of the spinal cord injury version of the multidimensional pain inventory. *Arch Phys Med Rehabil.* 2006; 87: 516–523.
Penn Spasm Frequency Scale (PSFS)	• Adams MM, Ginis KAM, Hicks AL. The spinal cord injury spasticity evaluation tool: Development and evaluation. *Arch Phys Med Rehabil.* 2007; 88:1185–1192. • Hsieh J, Wolfe D, Miller W, Curt A. Spasticity outcome measures in spinal cord injury: Psychometric properties and clinical utility. *Spinal Cord.* 2008; 46: 86–95.
Quadriplegia Index of Function (QIF)	• Gresham GE, Labi ML, et al. The Quadriplegia Index of Function (QIF): Sensitivity and reliability demonstrated in a study of thirty quadriplegic patients. *Paraplegia.* 1986; 24(1): 38–44.
Spinal Cord Independence Measure (SCIM)	• Ackerman P, Morrison SA, McDowell S, Vazquez L. Using the Spinal Cord Independence Measure III to measure functional recovery in a post-acute spinal cord injury program. *Spinal Cord.* 2010; 48: 380–387. • Anderson K, Aito S, Atkins M, et al. Functional recovery measures for spinal cord injury: an evidence-based review for clinical practice and research. *J Spinal Cord Med.* 2008; 31(2): 133–144.

(*Continued*)

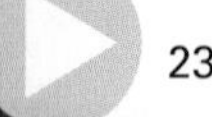

Table 3A-1

Selected Outcome Measures Organized by the International Classification of Functioning, Disability, and Health (ICF) Categories (Continued)

DISABILITY SPECIFIC MEASURES	REFERENCES
SPINAL CORD INJURY (SCI)	
Walking Index for Spinal Cord Injury (WISCI, WISCI II)	• Dittuno PL, Ditunno JF, Jr. Walking index for spinal cord injury (WISCI II): Scale revision. *Spinal Cord.* 2001; 39: 654–656. • Ditunno JF, Jr., et al. Validity of the walking scale for spinal cord injury and other domains of function in a multicenter clinical trial. *Neurorehabil Neural Repair.* 2007; 21: 539–550.
PARKINSON'S DISEASE (PD)	
Freezing of Gait Questionnaire	• Giladi, N., Shabtai, H., et al. Construction of freezing of gait questionnaire for patients with Parkinsonism. *Parkinsonism Relat Disord.* 2000; 6(3): 164–170. • Giladi, N., Tal, J., et al. Validation of the freezing of gait questionnaire in patients with Parkinson's disease. *Mov Disord.* 2009; 24(5): 655–661.
Parkinson's Fatigue Scale	• Brown, et al (2005). The Parkinson fatigue scale. *Parkinsonism and Related Disorders.* 11: 49–55. • Friedman, J et al. (2010). Fatigue rating scales critique and recommendations by the movement disorders society task force on rating scales for parkinson's disease. *Movement Disorders* 25(7): 805–822.
Unified Parkinson's Disease Rating Scale (UPDRS)	• Fahn S, Elton R. Unified Parkinson's Disease Rating Scale. In: Fahn S, et al (eds): *Recent Developments in Parkinson's Disease, Vol 2.* Macmillan Health Care Information, Florham Park, NJ. 1987: 153–167. • Unified Parkinson's Disease Rating Scale available online at: www.etas.ee/wp-content/uploads/2013/10/updrs.pdf • Goetz C, et al. Movement Disorder Society-sponsored revision of the Parkinson's Disease Rating Scale (MDS-UPDRS): Scale presentation and clinimetric testing results. *Mov Disord.* 2008; 23(15): 2129–2170.
MULTIPLE SCLEROSIS (MS)	
Modified Fatigue Impact Scale (mFIS)	• Fisk JD, Pontefract A, Ritvo PG, et al. The impact of fatigue on patients with multiple sclerosis. *Can J Neurol Sci.* 1994; 21(1): 9. • Fisk JD, Ritvo PG, Ross L, et al. Measuring the functional impact of fatigue: Initial validation of the Fatigue Impact Scale. *Clin Infect Dis Suppl.* 1994; 1: S79.
Expanded Disability Status Scale & Kurtzke Functional Systems Score	• Kurtzke JF. Rating neurologic impairment in multiple sclerosis: an expanded disability status scale (EDSS). *Neurology.* 1983; 33(11): 1444–1452.
Scale for the Assessment and Rating of Ataxia (SARA)	• Schmitz-Hubsch T, Tezenas du Montcel S, Baliko L, et al. Scale for the assessment and rating of ataxia: Development of a new clinical scale. *Neurology.* 2006; 66(11): 1717–1720.
Functional Assessment of Multiple Sclerosis (FAMS)	• Cella DF, Dineen K, Armason B, et al. Validation of the functional assessment of multiple sclerosis quality of life instrument. *Neurology.* 1996; 47(1): 129–139.
ACTIVITY MEASURES	**REFERENCES**
Functional Independence Measure (FIM)	• Guide for the Uniform Data Set for Medical Rehabilitation (Adult FIM) version 4.0, State University of New York at Buffalo. 1993. • Dodds TA, Martin DP, Stolov WC, et al. A validation of the functional independence measurement and its performance among rehabilitation in-patients. *Arch Phys Med Rehabil.* 1993; 174: 531–536. • Long WB, Sacco MJ, Coombes SS, et al. Determining normative standards for Functional Independence Measure transitions in rehabilitation. *Arch Phys Med Rehabil.* 1994; 75: 925–932. • The FIM is available online at: http://www.udsmr.org • email: info@udsmr.org
Functional Assessment Measure (FIM + FAM) [TBI]	• Linn RT, et al. Does the Functional Assessment Measure (FAM) extend the Functional Independence Measure (FIM™) Instrument? A Rasch analysis of stroke patients. *J Outcome Measure.* 1999; 3: 339. • Hall KM. The Functional Assessment Measure (FAM). *J Rehabil Outcomes.* 1997; 1(3): 63–65. • Hall KM, Mann N, High WM, et al. Functional measures after traumatic brain injury: Ceiling effects of FIM, FIM+FAM, DRS, and CIQ. *J Head Trauma Rehabil.* 1996; 11(5): 27–39.
Barthel Index (BI)	• Granger CV, Devis LS, Peters MC, et al. Stroke rehabilitation analysis of repeated Barthel Index measures. *Arch Phys Med Rehabil.* 1979; 60: 14–17. • Mahoney FI, Barthel DW. Functional evaluation: The Barthel Index. *Maryland State Med J.* 1965; 14: 61–65.
Physical Performance Test	• Reuben DB, Siu AL. An objective measure of physical function of elderly populations: The Physical Performance Test. *J Am Geriatr Soc.* 1990; 38: 1105.

(*Continued*)

Table 3A-1

Selected Outcome Measures Organized by the International Classification of Functioning, Disability, and Health (ICF) Categories (Continued)

ACTIVITY MEASURES	REFERENCES
Disabilities of the Arm, Shoulder, and Hand Outcome Measure (DASH)	• Beaton DE, Davis AM, Hudak P, McConnell S. The DASH (Disabilities of the Arm, Shoulder and Hand) Outcome Measure: What do we know about it now? *Br J Hand Ther.* 2001; 6(4): 109–118. • Beaton DE, Katz JN, Fossel AH, et al. Measuring the whole or the parts? Validity, reliability & responsiveness of the disabilities of the arm, shoulder, and hand outcome measure in different regions of the upper extremity. *J Hand Ther.* 2001; 14(2): 128. • Bot SDM, Terwee CB, van der Windt DAWM, et al. Clinimetric evaluation of shoulder disability questionnaires: A systematic review of the literature. *Ann Rheum Dis.* 2004; 63(4): 335. • Available online at: http://www.dash.iwh.on.ca/
Lower Extremity Functional Scale (LEFS)	• Wang Y-C, Hart DL, Stratford PW, Mioduski JE. Clinical Interpretation of a Lower-Extremity Functional Scale–derived computerized adaptive test. *Phys Ther.* 2009; 89(9): 957. • Lin CW, Moseley AM, Refshauge KM, Bundy AC. The Lower Extremity Functional Scale has good clinimetric properties in people with ankle fracture. *Phys Ther.* 2009; 89(6): 580. • Binkley JM, Stratford PW, Lott SA, Riddle DL. The Lower Extremity Functional Scale (LEFS): Scale development, measurement properties, and clinical application. *Phys Ther.* 1999; 79(4): 371. • Available online at: www.emoryhealthcare.org
Wheelchair Skills Test (WST)	• Kirby RL, Dupuis DJ, MacPhee AH, et al. The Wheelchair Skills Test (version 2.4): measurement properties. *Arch Phys Med Rehabil.* 2004; 85: 794. • Videotapes for Wheelchair Users and Wheelchair Skills Program (WSP) Version 4.1 Manual available online at: http://www.wheelchairskillsprogram.ca/eng/overview.htm • Additional online resources • The Powered Wheelchair Training Guide: www.wheelchairnet.org • The Manual Wheelchair Training Guide: www.wheelchairnet.org • A Guide to Wheelchair Selection: www.spinalcord.org
Wolf Motor Function Test (WMFT) [CVA]	• Wolf SL, Catlin PA, Ellis M, et al. Assessing Wolf Motor Function Test as outcome measure for research in patients after stroke. *Stroke.* 2001; 32: 1635. • Morris DM, Uswatte G, Crago JE, et al. The reliability of the Wolf Motor Function Test for assessing upper extremity function after stroke. *Arch Phys Med Rehabil.* 2001; 82: 750.
Motor Activity Log (MAL) [CVA]	• Wolf SL, Thompson PA, Morris DM, et al. The EXCITE trial: Attributes of the Wolf Motor Function Test in patients with subacute stroke. *Neurorehabil Neural Repair.* 2005; 19: 194. • Uswatte G, Taub E, Morris D, et al. The Motor Activity Log-28: Assessing daily use of the hemiparetic arm after stroke. *Neurology.* 2006; 67: 1189. • Van der Lee JH, Beckerman H, Knol DL, et al. Clinimetric properties of the motor activity log for the assessment of arm use in hemiparetic patients. *Stroke.* 2004; 35: 1410.
BALANCE AND GAIT MEASURES	**REFERENCES**
Berg Balance Scale (BBS)	• Berg K, Wood-Dauphinee S, Williams J, et al. Measuring balance in the elderly: preliminary development of an instrument. *Physiother Can.* 1989; 41: 304–311. • Berg KO, Maki B, Williams JI, et al. Clinical and laboratory measures of postural balance in an elderly population. *Arch Phys Med Rehabil.* 1992; 73: 1073–1080. • Berg KO, Wood-Dauphinee SL, Williams JI, et al. Measuring balance in the elderly: Validation of an instrument. *Can J Public Health.* 1992; 83: S7–S11. • Berg KO, Wood-Dauphinee S, Williams JI. The balance scale: Reliability assessment with elderly residents and patients with an acute stroke. *Scand J Rehabil Med.* 1995; 27: 27–36.
The Balance Evaluation Systems Test (BESTest); Mini-BESTest	• Horak FB, Wrisley DM, Frank J. The Balance Evaluation Systems Test (BESTest) to differentiate balance deficits. *Phys Ther.* May 2009; 89(5): 484–498. • Franchignoni F, Horak F, Godi M, et al. Using psychometric techniques to improve the Balance Evaluation Systems Test: the mini-BESTest. *J Rehabil Med.* 2010; 42(4): 323–331. • King L & Horak F. On the Mini-BESTest: Scoring and the reporting of total scores. *Phys Ther.* 2013; 93(4): 542–50.
Functional Reach (FR)	• Duncan P, et al. Functional Reach: A new clinical measure of balance. *J Gerontol.* 1990; 45: M192. • Duncan PW, Studenski S, Chandler J, Prescott B. Functional reach: Predictive validity in a sample of elderly male veterans. *J Gerontol.* 1992; 47: M93. • Weiner DK, Duncan PW, Chandler J, Studenski SA. Functional Reach: a marker of physical frailty. *J Am Geriatr Soc.* 1992; 40: 2–3.

(*Continued*)

Table 3A-1

Selected Outcome Measures Organized by the International Classification of Functioning, Disability, and Health (ICF) Categories (Continued)

BALANCE AND GAIT MEASURES	REFERENCES
Multidirectional Functional Reach Test	• Newton R. Validity of the multi-directional reach test: a practical measure for limits of stability in older adults. *J Gerontol Med Sci.* 2001; 56(4): M248–M252. • Newton R. Validity of MDRT. *J Gerontol.* 2001; 56A.4: M248.
Modified Functional Reach (seated)	• Lynch SM, Leahy P, Barker S. Reliability of measurements obtained with a modified functional reach test in subjects with spinal cord injury. *Phys Ther.* 1998; 78(2): 128.
Function in Sitting Test (FIST)	• Gorman SL, Radtka S, Melnick ME, et al. Development and validation of the Function in Sitting Test in adults with acute stroke. *J Neurol Phys Ther.* 2010; 34(3): 150–160.
Stops Walking When Talking (SWWT)	• Lundin-Olsson L, Nyberg L, Gustafson Y. Stops walking when talking as a predictor of falls in elderly people. *Lancet.* 1997; 348: 617.
Timed Up & Go (TUG)	• Ng SS, Hui-Chan CW. The Timed Up & Go test: Its reliability and association with lower-limb impairments and locomotor capabilities in people with chronic stroke. *Arch Phys Med Rehabil.* 2005; 86: 1641–1647. • Podsiadlo D, Richardson S. The Timed "Up & Go": a test of basic functional mobility for frail elderly persons. *J Am Geriatr Soc.* 1992; 39: 142–148.
Performance-Oriented Mobility Assessment (POMA) (Tinetti)	• Tinetti M. Performance-oriented assessment of mobility problems in elderly patients. *J Am Geriatr Soc.* 1986; 34: 119–126.
Clinical Test for Sensory Interaction in Balance (CTSIB)	• Shumway-Cook A, Horak F. Assessing the influence of sensory interaction on balance. *Phys Ther.* 1986; 66(10): 1548–1550.
Modified Clinical Test for Sensory Integration in Balance (mCTSIB)	• Rose DJ. Fallproof: A Comprehensive Balance and Mobility Training Program, 2nd ed. Human Kinetics, Champaign, IL. 2010.
Four Square Step Test	• Dite W, Temple VA. A clinical test of stepping and change of direction to identify multiple falling older adults. *Archives of Physical Medicine & Rehabilitation.* 2002; 83(11): 1566–1571. • Whitney SL, Marchetti GF, Morris LO, Sparto PJ. The reliability and validity of the Four Square Step Test for people with balance deficits secondary to a vestibular disorder. *Archives of Physical Medicine & Rehabilitation.* 2007; 88(1): 99–104.
Functional Gait Assessment (FGA)	• Wrisley DM, Marchetti GF, Kuharsky DK, Whitney SL. Reliability, internal consistency, and validity of data obtained with the functional gait assessment. *Phys Ther.* 2004; 84: 906–918.
Modified Emory Functional Ambulation Profile (mEFAP)	• Baer HR, Wolf SL. Modified Emory Functional Ambulation Profile: an outcome measure for rehabilitation for post stroke gait dysfunction. *Stroke.* 2001; 32: 973. • Wolf SL, Catlin PA, Gage K. Establishing the reliability and validity of measurements using the Emory Functional Ambulation Profile. *Phys Ther.* 1999; 79: 1122. • Nelson, AJ: Functional ambulation profile. *Phys Ther.* 1974; 54: 1059.
Five Times Sit to Stand	• Mong Y, Tilda T, et al. 5-Repetition Sit-to-Stand Test in subjects with chronic stroke: Reliability and validity. *Arch Phys Med Rehabil.* 2010; 91(3): 407–413. • Lord SR, Murr SM, Chapman K, et al. Sit-to-stand performance depends on sensation, speed, balance, and psychological status in addition to strength in older people. *J Gerontol A Biol Sci Med Sci.* 2002; 57: 539–543.
6-Minute Walk Test	• Enright, PL, Sherrill, DL. Reference equations for the six-minute walk in healthy adults. *Am J Respir Crit Care Med.* 1998; 158: 1384–1387. • Liu J, Drutz C, Kumar R, et al. Use of 6-Minute Walk Test post stroke. Is there a practice effect? *Arch Phys Med Rehabil.* 2008; 89: 1686–1692. • Fulk GD, Echternach JL, Nof L, O'Sullivan S. Clinometric properties of the 6-Minute Walk Test in individuals undergoing rehabilitation poststroke. *Physiother Theory and Pract.* 2008; 24: 195–204.
Timed Walk Tests (5 m, 10 m)	• Sullivan KJ, et al: Effects of task-specific locomotor and strength training in adults who were ambulatory after stroke: results of the STEPS randomized clinical trial. *Phys Ther.* 2007; 87: 1580–1602.
Dynamic Gait Index (DGI)	• Shumway-Cook A, Woollacott M. Motor Control—Translating Research into Clinical Practice, 3rd ed. Lippincott Williams & Wilkins. 2007: 395–396. • Jonsdottir J, Cattaneo D. Reliability and validity of the Dynamic Gait Index in persons with chronic stroke. *Arch of Phys Med and Rehabil.* 2007; 88(11): 1410–1415. • Walker ML, Austin G, Banke GM, et al. Reference group data for the Functional Gait Assessment. *Phys Ther.* 2007; 87(11): 1468–1477. • Wrisley D. Functional Gait Assessment. *Phys Ther.* 2007; 84(10): Appendix.

(*Continued*)

Table 3A-1

Selected Outcome Measures Organized by the International Classification of Functioning, Disability, and Health (ICF) Categories (Continued)

BALANCE AND GAIT MEASURES	REFERENCES
Observational Gait Analysis (OGA)	• Pathokinesiology Service and Physical Therapy Department: Observational Gait Analysis Handbook. Los Amigos Research and Education Institute, Inc, Downey, CA, 2001. • Perry JP and Burnfield, JM. Gait Analysis: Normal and Pathological Function, 2nd ed. Thorofare, NJ: Slack. 2010.
Activities and Balance Confidence Scale (ABC)	• Myers AM, Fletcher PC, Myers AN, et al. Discriminative and evaluative properties of the ABC Scale. *J Gerontol.* 1998; 53A: M287–M294. • Powell LE, Myers AM. Activities-specific Balance Confidence (ABC) Scale. *J Gerontol.* 1995; 50A: M28–M34. • The ABC Scale is available online at: www.healthcare.uiowa.edu
PARTICIPATION MEASURES	**REFERENCES**
The MOS SF-36 Health Survey	• Anderson C, Laubscher S, Burns R. Validation of the short-form (SF-36) health survey questionnaire among stroke patients. *Stroke.* 1996; 27: 1812–1816. • Ware JE, Sherbourne CD. The MOS 36-Item Short-Form Health Survey (SF-36), 1: Conceptual framework and item selection. *Med Care.* 1992; 30: 473–483. • The SF-36 Health Survey is available online at: www.rand.org
Satisfaction with Life Scale (SWLS)	• Post MW, Christel M, van Leeuwen CF, Koppenhagen SD. Validity of the Life Satisfaction questions, the Life Satisfaction Questionnaire (LiSat-9) and the Satisfaction with Life Scale (SWLS) in persons with spinal cord injury. *Arch Phys Med Rehabil.* 2012, doi; 10.101/j.apmr.2012.03.025
Participation Objective, Participation Subjective (POPS)	• Brown M, Dijkers MPJ, Gordon W, et al Participation Objective, Participation Subjective: a measure of participation combining outsider and insider perspectives. *J Head Trauma Rehabil.* 2004; 19(6): 459–481. • Mascialino G, Hirshson C, Egan M, et al. Objective and subjective assessment of long-term community integration in minority groups following traumatic brain injury. *NeuroRehabilitation.* 2009; 24(1): 29–36. • The POPS is available online at: http://www.tbims.org/combi/pops/Appendix%20I.doc
Impact of Participation and Autonomy (IPA)	• Cardol M, de Haan RJ, de Jong BA, et al. Psychometric properties of the impact on participation and autonomy questionnaire. *Arch Phys Med Rehabil.* 2001; 82(2): 210–216. • The IPA is available online at: http://www.nivel.nl/pdf/INT-IPA-E.pdf
Outpatient Physical Therapy Improvement in Assessment Log (OPTIMAL)	• Guccione AA, Mielenz TJ, Devellis RF, et al. Development and testing of a self-report instrument to measure actions: Outpatient physical therapy improvement in movement assessment log (OPTIMAL). *Phys Ther.* 2005; 85(6): 515–530. • Optimal is available online at: http://www.apta.org
Craig Handicap Assessment and Reporting Technique (CHART)	• Walker N, Mellick D, Brooks CA, et al. Measuring participation across impairment groups using the Craig Handicap Assessment Reporting Technique. *Am J Phys Med Rehabil.* 2003; 82(12): 936–941. • Hall KM, Dijkers M, Whiteneck G, et al. The Craig Handicap Assessment and Reporting Technique (CHART): Metric properties and scoring. *J Rehabil Outcomes Measure.* 1998; 2(5): 39–49. CHART is available online at: http://www.tbims.org/combi/chart/index.html
Stroke Impact Scale (SIS)	• Duncan PW, Lai SM, Bode RK, et al. Stroke Impact Scale-16: a brief assessment of physical function. *Neurology.* 2003; 60(2): 291. • Duncan PW, Bode R, Lai SM, et al. Rasch analysis of a new stroke specific outcome scale: The Stroke Impact Scale. *Arch Phys Med Rehabil.* 2003; 84(7): 950. • The SIS is available online at: http://www.chrp.org/pdf/HSR082103_SIS_Handout.pdf

Key: TBI: traumatic brain injury; SCI: spinal cord injury; CVA: cerebrovascular accident.
For additional information on outcome measures please see Shirley Ryan Agility Lab. Rehabilitation Measures Database, https://www.sralab.org/rehabilitation-measures and APTA Neurology Section Outcome Measure Recommendations, https://www.neuropt.org/practice-resources/neurology-section-outcome-measures-recommendations

APPENDIX 3B

Review Questions and Case Studies

(Answers to all Review Questions and Case Studies can be found in Chapter 17)

1. Which cranial nerves may play any role in vision? What findings are normal or abnormal?

2. Following a CVA, what are the major considerations when examining the patient for perceptual deficits?

3. When examining deep tendon reflexes, what is the score reported for an obligatory and sustained response?

4. What are the characteristics in terms of communication, gait, tone, balance, and respiratory function in a patient with late Parkinson's disease (Stage IV Hoehn and Yahr)?

5. What are the initial physical therapy goals and interventions upon receiving a referral for a patient recently diagnosed with a unilateral vestibular disorder?

6. Following an MVA, a patient with a complete SCI at the C7 level has been admitted to a rehab facility after a lengthy stay at an acute care hospital. What are the components of the physical therapist's initial examination?

7. What is the common pattern of fatigue in many patients with multiple sclerosis?

Case Scenario/Questions Neuromuscular #1

Patient Profile
- Gender: Male
- Age: 63

Presenting Problem/Current Condition
- Patient is referred to inpatient physical therapy secondary to a right ischemic stroke with left hemiparesis.
- Patient was admitted to the hospital 3 days ago with an intense headache and left upper greater than lower extremity weakness.
- Patient also exhibits neglect of the left side of their body.

Past Medical/Surgical History
- History of hypertension by 10 years.
- Bilateral Knee osteoarthritis,
- Right knee arthroscopy with meniscal debridement.

Other Information
- College basketball coach
- Married and lives in a 2-story home

Question #1
Which of the following arteries is occluded and most closely associated with the patient's presenting symptoms?

1. Anterior cerebral artery
2. Middle cerebral artery
3. Posterior cerebral artery
4. Basilar artery

Question #2
What impairments and/or activity limitations are most consistent with the patient's presenting symptoms and an acute right (non-dominant hemisphere) MCA stroke?

1. Left upper extremity flexor synergy.
2. Non-fluent or motor aphasia.
3. Left hemiplegic gait with standby assistance.
4. Inability to safely roll to the left side.

Question #3
When completing your initial evaluation on this patient, you determine they have significant neglect of the left side with complete paresis/sensory loss of the left upper extremity and moderate hypotonia/weakness of the left lower extremity. What initial intervention is the **BEST** choice for improving this patient's function?

1. Midline orientation and safe weight-bearing (approximation) of the involved upper extremity in assisted static sitting.
2. Constraint induced movement therapy with immobilization of the right upper extremity.
3. Bilateral scapular stabilization and overhead pulley exercises for left upper extremity range of motion.
4. Dynamic sitting with rapid weight shifts to the left to facilitate a quick stretch and increased tone.

Question #4
The patient is making progress with midline orientation in sitting, but once you transition them from sit to stand you notice they forcefully shift weight from the right to the left side. You are concerned about Pusher's syndrome. Which of the following interventions would be **BEST** to maintain a midline posture?

1. Perturbation training with weights shifts in all directions.
2. Visual feedback with a mirror.
3. Use of a cane on the involved side.
4. Cueing the patient to look to the uninvolved side.

Case Scenario/Questions Neuromuscular #2

Patient Profile

- **Gender:** Female
- **Age:** 55

Presenting Problem/Current Condition

- Patient is referred to outpatient physical therapy secondary to an ataxic gait and three falls in the past 6 months.
- Patient also reports consistent burning pain, numbness/tingling, and weakness in the bilateral fingers/thumbs, ankles, feet, and toes by 1 year.
- She denies specific aggravating factors and reports that her numbness and tingling is constant.
- She reports her falls typically happen when she is walking in the dark or on an unlevel surface.

Past Medical/Surgical History

- History of hypertension and diabetes by 15 years. Hypothyroidism by 7 years.
- Obesity (>36 BMI).
- Lumbar and bilateral knee osteoarthritis.
- Past surgeries: bilateral carpal tunnel releases 8 years ago.

Other Information

- Occupation: Information technology manager
- Lives alone.

Question #1

Which of the following health conditions is the most likely cause of the patient's presenting symptoms?

1. Lumbar spinal stenosis
2. Cervical myelopathy
3. Cerebellar disease
4. Polyneuropathy

Question #2

Which of the following examination findings would reinforce both small and large myelinated neural fiber impairments and increased risk for foot ulceration?

1. Impaired monofilament and pinprick sensory testing at the foot and toes.
2. Impaired monofilament and vibration sensory testing at the foot and toes.
3. Hyporeflexia of the Achilles reflexes and impaired vibration sensory testing of the foot/toes.
4. Hyperreflexia of the Achilles reflexes and impaired pinprick sensation of the foot/toes.

Question #3

When completing your initial evaluation on this patient you determine they have significant sensory impairments at the ankles, feet, and toes. They also have atrophy of their intrinsic muscles of the feet/toes, but normal strength at and above the ankles. Which of the following impairments in balance/mobility are most consistent with polyneuropathy and this patient's history and sensory/strength findings?

1. Impaired balance with feet apart eyes open resulting in a hip strategy.
2. Impaired four-square step test.
3. Impaired tandem stance eyes closed requiring a steppage strategy.
4. Impaired 10-meter gait speed that does not improve when the patient looks down.

Question #4

Which of the following compensatory strategies is BEST to enhance this patient's safety when ambulating in the community?

1. Ankle foot orthosis.
2. Use of a cane or walking stick.
3. Use of a rolling walker.
4. Use of supportive footwear.

4

Cardiovascular and Lymphatic Physical Therapy

KELLY MACAULEY, SUSAN O'SULLIVAN,
THOMAS SUTLIVE, AND TODD SANDER

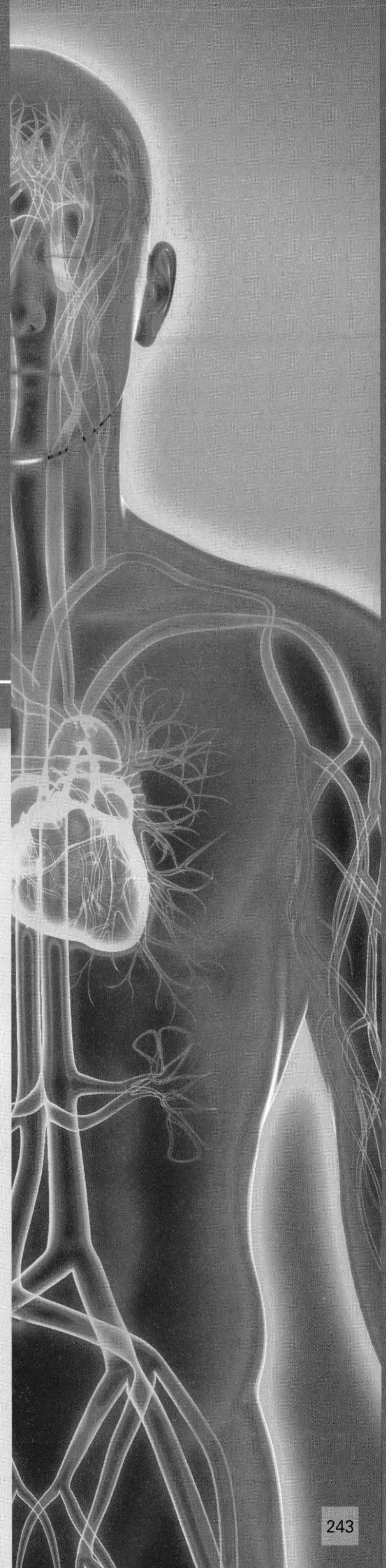

Chapter Outline

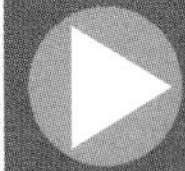

Study Tactics

Questions about the Cardiovascular and Pulmonary Systems comprise 13% of the NPTE, or a total of 23–28 questions. The two systems are grouped together in the NPTE Content Outline. The number of questions for the Cardiovascular System alone is not specified in the Content Outline

The number of questions for the Cardiovascular and Pulmonary Systems by category are:

- Examination of the Patient/Client: 7–9
- Evaluation, Differential Diagnosis, Prognosis: 8–9
- Interventions: 8–10

Questions about the Lymphatic System comprise about 3% of the NPTE, or a total of 3–8 questions

The number of questions for the Lymphatic System by category are:

- Examination of the Patient/Client: 0–2
- Evaluation, Differential Diagnosis, Prognosis: 1–3
- Interventions: 2–3

Examination of the Patient/Client. Focus on:

- Anatomy and physiology of the cardiovascular and lymphatic systems. Comprehensive foundational science knowledge of these systems is critical to understanding components of the examination.
- Tests and measures of the cardiovascular and lymphatic systems, including vital signs, auscultation of heart sounds, ankle/brachial index, capillary refill, girth measurements, and special tests such as the Allen test and Stemmer's sign
- Location of the heart chambers and valves, and relevant surface landmarks as they relate to auscultation points for heart sounds
- Locations of palpation points for distal arterial pulses.
- Pain referral patterns related to cardiovascular diseases such as myocardial infarction, angina pectoris, and aortic aneurysms (abdominal and thoracic)
- Cardiovascular system outcomes measures and their application to effective patient management and interventions

Evaluation, Differential Diagnosis, and Prognosis. Focus on:

- Major cardiovascular disorders seen by physical therapists across the lifespan. These include myocardial infarction, congestive heart failure, angina, electrical conductivity disorders, and coronary artery disease.
- Major lymphatic system disorders seen by physical therapists including lymphedema, lymphangitis, and lymphadenopathy
- The clinical features (signs and symptoms) of these disorders, which serve as the basis for differential diagnosis questions
- Knowledge and interpretation of laboratory tests such as arterial blood gases, red and white blood cells counts, hematocrit, clotting times, and lipid profiles
- Development of a plan of care to include prognosis for common cardiovascular and lymphatic disorders
- Medical management and diagnostic studies of the cardiovascular and lymphatic systems to include imaging, laboratory tests, and surgical procedures (coronary artery bypass graft, valve replacement, etc.)
- Actions and side effects of pharmacological management of cardiovascular problems. Medication categories may include beta blockers, anticoagulants, ACE inhibitors, and diuretics

Interventions. Focus on:

- SAFETY! Safety considerations are of paramount importance, particularly when questions involve management of a patient with a cardiac condition. Recognition of when to stop (or not start) exercise based on the patient's cardiovascular status or response to exercise is critical.
- Phases of cardiac rehabilitation, including goals and exercise guidelines for each phase
- Factors to consider for exercise prescription, such as patient comorbidities, age, obesity, humidity, temperature, and altitude
- Knowledge of physiologic effects and patient response to exercise including perceived exertion, blood pressure, and heart rate changes
- Components of a complex decongestive therapy program for patients with lymphedema, to include manual lymphatic drainage, compression exercise, skin care, and patient education
- Location of lymph nodes and ducts. Knowledge of location of lymph nodes and pathways are fundamental to understanding the principles of treatment with manual lymphatic drainage.
- Potential adverse side effects or complications on the cardiovascular and lymphatic systems from physical therapy interventions

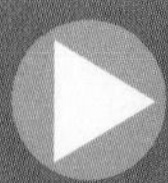

Anatomy and Physiology of the Cardiovascular System

The Heart and Circulation

Heart Tissue

1. Pericardium: fibrous protective sac enclosing heart.
2. Epicardium: inner layer of pericardium.
3. Myocardium: heart muscle, the major portion of the heart.
4. Endocardium: smooth lining of the inner surface and cavities of the heart.

Heart Chambers (See Figure 4-1)

1. Right atrium (RA): receives blood from systemic circulation, from the superior vena cavae (SVC) and inferior vena cavae (IVC).
2. Right ventricle (RV): receives blood from the RA and pumps blood via the pulmonary artery to the lungs for oxygenation; the low-pressure pulmonary pump.
3. Left atrium (LA): receives oxygenated blood from the lungs and the four pulmonary veins.
4. Left ventricle (LV): receives blood from the LA and pumps blood via the aorta throughout the entire systemic circulation; the high-pressure systemic pump. The walls of the LV are thicker and stronger than the RV and form most of the left side and apex of the heart.

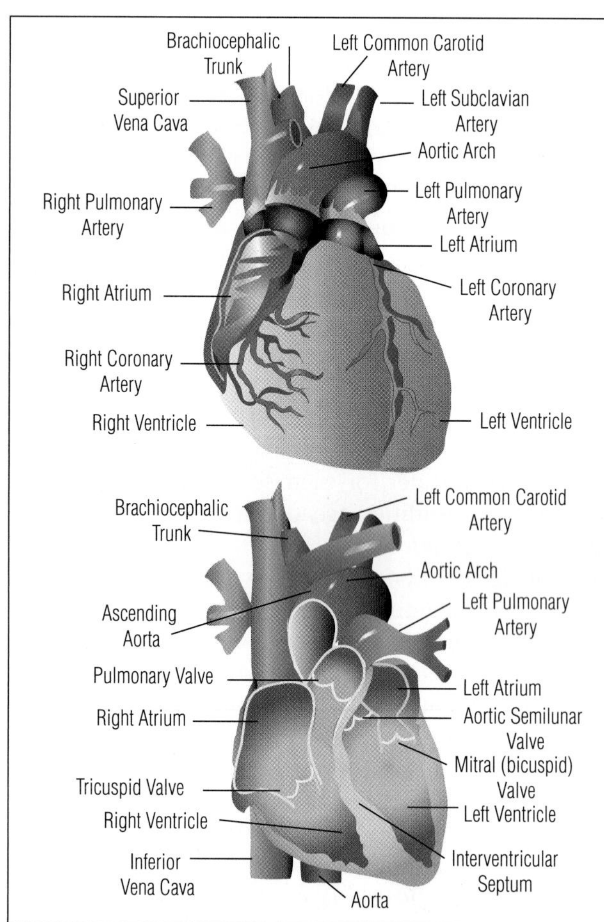

Figure 4-1 The heart.

Valves

1. Valves provide one-way flow of blood.
2. Atrioventricular valves: prevent backflow of blood into atria during ventricular systole; anchored by chordae tendineae to papillary muscles; valves close when ventricular walls contract.
   a. Tricuspid valve (three cusps or leaflets): right heart valve.
   b. Bicuspid or mitral valve (two cusps or leaflets): left heart valve.
3. Semilunar valves: prevent backflow of blood from aorta and pulmonary arteries into the ventricles during diastole.
   a. Pulmonary valve: prevents right backflow.
   b. Aortic valve: prevents left backflow.

Cardiac Cycle (See Figure 4-2)

1. The rhythmic pumping action of the heart.
2. Systole: the period of ventricular contraction. End-systolic volume is the amount of blood in the ventricles after systole; about 50 mL.
3. Diastole: the period of ventricular relaxation and filling of blood. End-diastolic volume is the amount of blood in the ventricles after diastole; about 120 mL.
4. Atrial contraction (atrial kick) occurs during the last third of diastole and completes ventricular filling, comprising last 20%–30% of end diastolic volume.

Coronary Circulation (See Figure 4-3)

1. Arteries: arise directly from aorta near aortic valve; blood circulates to myocardium during diastole.
   a. Right coronary artery (RCA): supplies right atrium, most of right ventricle, and in most individuals, the inferior wall of left ventricle, atrioventricular (AV) node and bundle of His; supplies the sinoatrial (SA) node 60% of the time.
   b. Left coronary artery (LCA): supplies most of the left ventricle; has two main divisions.
      - Left anterior descending (LAD): supplies the left ventricle and the interventricular septum, and in most individuals, the inferior areas of the apex; it may also give off branches to the right ventricle.

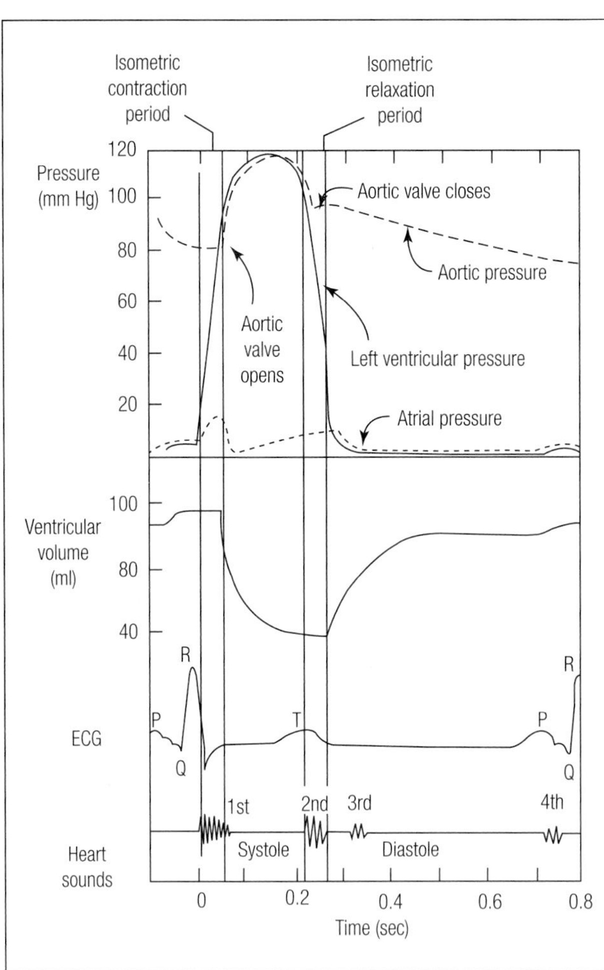

Figure 4-2 **Events of the cardiac cycle.**

- Circumflex (LCx): supplies blood to the lateral and inferior walls of the left ventricle and portions of the left atrium; supplies SA node 40% of the time.

2. Veins: parallel arterial system; the coronary sinus receives venous blood from the heart and empties into the right atrium.
3. Distribution of blood supply is variable from individual to individual.
4. Myocardial oxygen supply and myocardial oxygen demand (MVO_2) should be in balance in order to maintain a given activity level without ischemia.

Conduction (See Figure 4-4)

1. Specialized conduction tissue: allows rapid transmission of electrical impulses throughout the myocardium (normal sinus rhythm, NSR).
2. Sinoatrial (SA) node.
   a. Located at junction of superior vena cava and right atrium.
   b. Main pacemaker of the heart; initiates the impulse at rate of 60–100 beats per minute.
   c. Has sympathetic and parasympathetic innervation affecting both heart rate and strength of contraction.
3. Atrioventricular (AV) node.
   a. Located at the junction of the right atrium and the right ventricle.
   b. Has sympathetic and parasympathetic innervation.
   c. Merges with bundle of His.
   d. Intrinsic firing rate of 40–60 beats per minute.

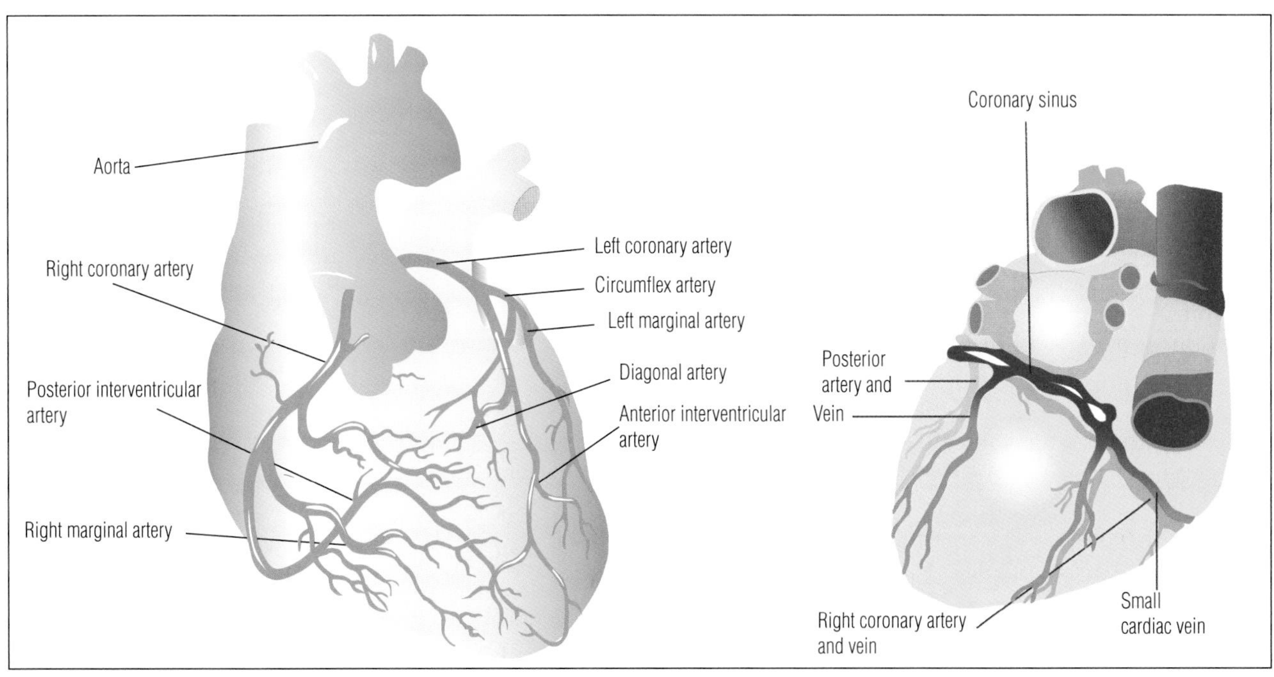

Figure 4-3 **Coronary arteries and veins.**

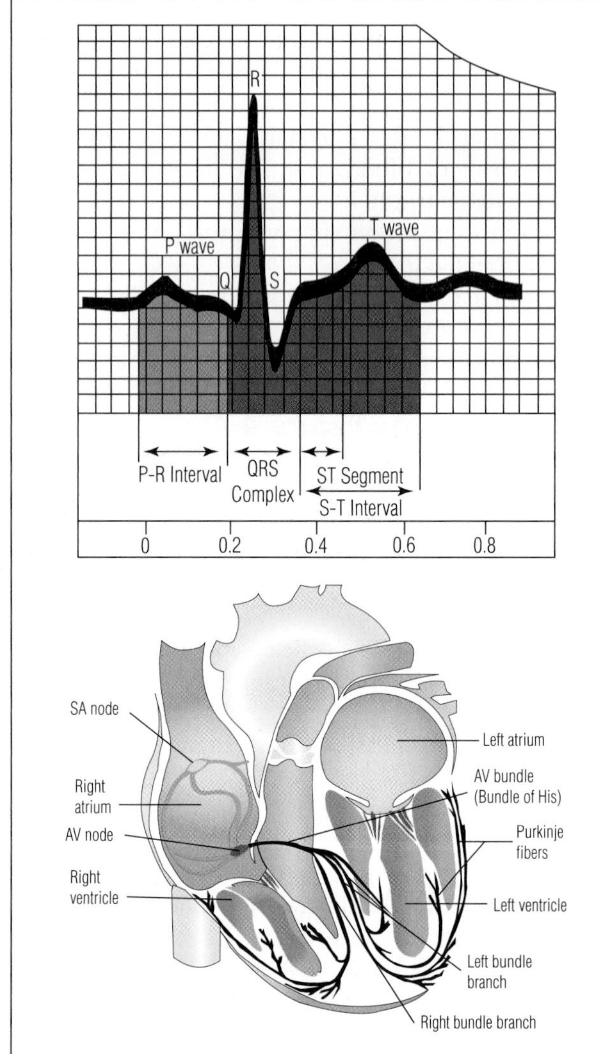

Figure 4-4 **Conduction pathways of the heart.**

4. Purkinje tissue.
   a. Right and left bundle branches of the AV node are located on either side of intraventricular septum.
   b. Terminate in Purkinje fibers, specialized conducting tissue spread throughout the ventricles.
   c. Intrinsic firing rate of 20–40 beats per minute.
5. Conduction of a normal heart beat (normal sinus rhythm).
   a. Origin is in the SA node; impulse spreads throughout both atria, which contract together.
   b. Impulse stimulates AV node, is transmitted down bundle of His to the Purkinje fibers; impulse spreads throughout the ventricles, which contract together.

Myocardial Fibers

1. Muscle tissue: striated muscle fibers with more numerous mitochondria; exhibits rhythmicity of contraction; fibers contract as a functional unit (sliding filament theory of contraction).
2. Myocardial metabolism is essentially aerobic, sustained by continuous O_2 delivery, from the coronary arteries.
3. Smooth muscle tissue is found in the walls of blood vessels.

Hemodynamics

1. Stroke volume (SV): the amount of blood ejected with each myocardial contraction; normal range is 55–100 mL/beat. Influenced by:
   a. Left ventricular end diastolic volume (LVEDV): the amount of blood left in the ventricle at the end of diastole, also known as preload. The greater the diastolic filling (preload), the greater the quantity of blood pumped (Frank-Starling law).
   b. Contractility: the ability of the ventricle to contract.
   c. Afterload: the force the LV must generate during systole to overcome aortic pressure to open the aortic valve.
2. Cardiac output (CO): the amount of blood discharged from the left or right ventricle per minute.
   a. For average adult at rest, normal range is 4–5 L per minute.
   b. Determined by multiplying heart rate (HR) times stroke volume (SV).
   c. Cardiac index is CO divided by body surface area; normal range is 2.5–3.5 L/min.
3. Left ventricular end diastolic pressure (LVEDP): pressure in the left ventricle during diastole. Normal range is 5–12 mmHg.
4. Ejection fraction (EF): percentage of blood emptied from the ventricle during systole; a clinically useful measure of LV function.
   a. EF = stroke volume (SV)/left ventricular end diastolic volume (LVEDV).
   b. Normal EF averages >55%; the lower the EF, the more impaired the LV; <40% indicates heart failure.
5. Atrial filling pressure: the difference between the venous and atrial pressures.
   a. Right atrial filling pressure is decreased during strong ventricular contraction, and atrial filling is enhanced.
   b. Right atrial filling pressure is affected by changes in intrathoracic pressure; decreases during inspiration and increases during coughing or forced expiration.
   c. Venous return increases when blood volume expands and decreases during hypovolemic shock.
6. Diastolic filling time decreases with increased heart rate and with heart disease.
7. Myocardial oxygen demand (MVO_2) represents the energy cost to the myocardium.
   a. Clinically measured by the product of heart rate (HR) and systolic blood pressure (SBP), known as the rate pressure produce (RPP).
   b. MVO_2 increases with activity and with HR and/or BP.

Peripheral Circulation

Arteries (See Figure 4-5)

1. Transport oxygenated blood from areas of high pressure to lower pressures in the body tissues. The only exceptions are the umbilical vein (in utero) and the pulmonary veins.
2. Arterial circulation maintained by heart pump.
3. Influenced by elasticity and extensibility of vessel walls and by peripheral resistance, amount of blood in body.

Arterioles

1. Terminal branches of arteries that attach to capillaries.
2. Primary site of vascular resistance.

Capillaries

1. Include small blood vessels that connect the ends of arteries (arterioles) with the beginning of veins (venules); form an anastomosing network.
2. Function for exchange of nutrients and fluids between blood and tissues.
3. Capillary walls are thin, permeable.

Veins (See Figure 4-6)

1. Transport dark, unoxygenated blood from tissues back to the heart.
2. Larger capacity, thinner walls than arteries, greater number.
3. One-way valves to prevent backflow.
4. Venous system includes both superficial and deep veins (deep veins accompany arteries, while superficial ones do not).
5. Venous circulation is influenced by muscle contraction, gravity, respiration (increased return with inspiration), compliancy of right heart.

Lymphatic System

1. Includes lymphatics (superficial, intermediate, and deep), lymph fluid, lymph tissues, and organs (lymph nodes, tonsils, spleen, thymus, and the thoracic duct).
2. Drains lymph from bodily tissues and returns it to venous circulation.
3. Lymph travels from lymphatic capillaries to lymphatic vessels to ducts to left subclavian vein. Lymphatic contraction occurs by:
   a. Parasympathetic, sympathetic, and sensory nerve stimulation.
   b. Contraction of adjacent muscles.

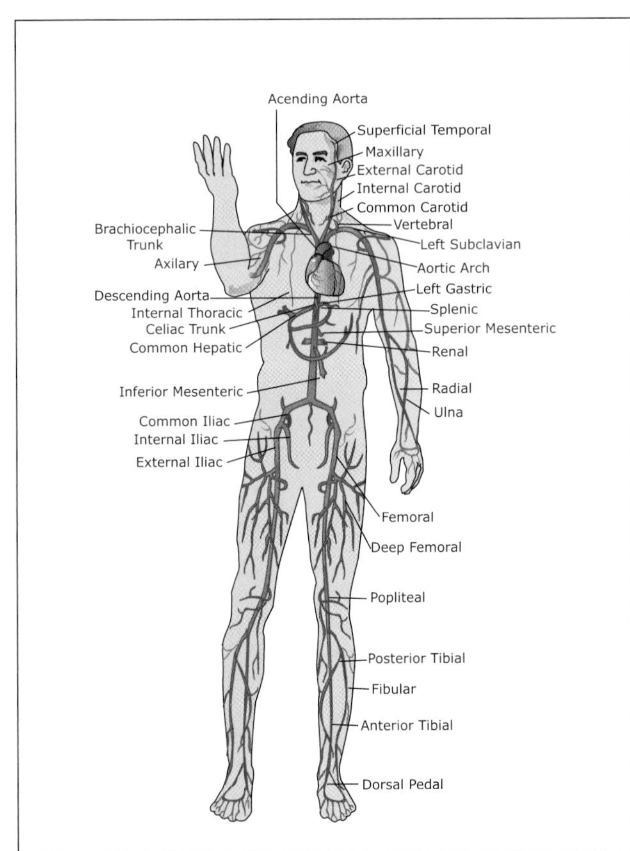

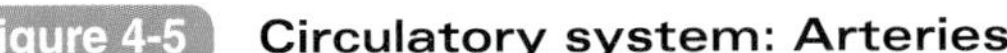
Figure 4-5 Circulatory system: Arteries.

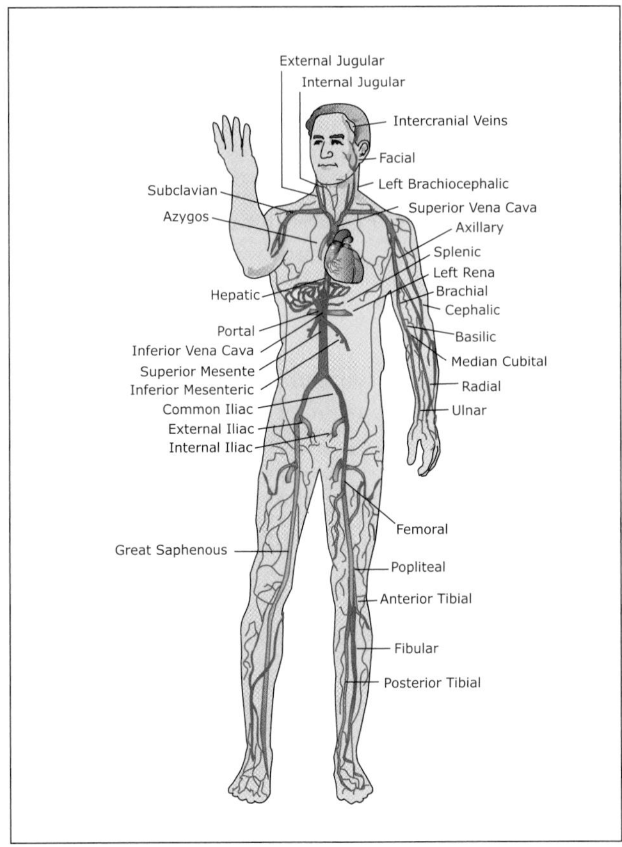

Figure 4-6 Circulatory system: Veins.

c. Abdominal and thoracic cavity pressure changes during normal breathing.
d. Mechanical stimulation of dermal tissues.
e. Volume changes within each lymphatic vessel.
4. Major lymph nodes are submaxillary, cervical, axillary, mesenteric, iliac, inguinal, popliteal, and cubital.
5. Contributes to immune system function: lymph nodes collect cellular debris and bacteria; remove excess fluid, blood waste, and protein molecules; and produce antibodies.

Neurohumeral Influences

Parasympathetic Stimulation (Cholinergic)

1. Control located in medulla oblongata, cardioinhibitory center.
2. Via vagus nerve (CN X), cardiac plexus; innervates the SA node, AV node and sparsely innervates myocardium; releases acetylcholine.
3. Slows rate and force of myocardial contraction; decreases myocardial metabolism.
4. Causes coronary artery vasoconstriction.

Sympathetic Stimulation (Adrenergic)

1. Control located in medulla oblongata, cardioacceleratory center.
2. Via cord segments T1–T4, upper thoracic to superior cervical chain ganglia; innervates SA node, AV node, conduction pathways, and myocytes; releases epinephrine and norepinephrine.
3. Causes an increase in the rate and force of myocardial contraction and myocardial metabolism.
4. Causes coronary artery vasodilation.
5. The skin and peripheral vasculature receive only postganglionic sympathetic innervation. Causes vasoconstriction of cutaneous arteries; sympathetic inhibition must occur for vasodilation.
6. Drugs that increase sympathetic functioning are sympathomimetics (alpha or beta agonists); drugs that decrease sympathetic functioning are sympatholytics (alpha or beta antagonists or blockers).

Additional Control Mechanisms

1. Baroreceptors (pressoreceptors): main mechanisms controlling heart rate.
   a. Located in walls of aortic arch and carotid sinus; via vasomotor center.
   b. Circulatory reflex: respond to changes in blood pressure.
      - Increased BP results in parasympathetic stimulation, decreased rate and force of cardiac contraction; sympathetic inhibition, decreased peripheral resistance.
      - Decreased BP results in sympathetic stimulation, increased heart rate and blood pressure and vasoconstriction of peripheral blood vessels.
      - Increased right atrial pressure causes reflex acceleration of heart rate.
2. Chemoreceptors.
   a. Located in the carotid body.
   b. Sensitive to changes in blood chemicals: O_2, CO_2, lactic acid.
      - Increased CO_2 or decreased O_2, or decreased pH (elevated lactic acid) results in an increase in heart rate.
      - Increased O_2 levels result in a decrease in heart rate.
3. Body temperature.
   a. Increased body temperature causes heart rate to increase.
   b. Decreased body temperature causes heart rate to decrease.
4. Ion concentrations.
   a. Hyperkalemia: increased concentration of potassium ions decreases the rate and force of contraction, produces electrocardiographic (ECG) changes (widened PR interval and QRS, tall T waves).
   b. Hypokalemia: decreased concentrations of potassium ions, produces ECG changes (flattened T waves, prolonged PR and QT intervals); arrhythmias, may progress to ventricular fibrillation.
   c. Hypercalcemia: increased calcium concentration increases heart actions.
   d. Hypocalcemia: decreased calcium concentrations depresses heart actions.
   e. Hypermagnesemia: increased magnesium is a calcium blocker which can lead to arrhythmias or cardiac arrest.
   f. Hypomagnesemia: decreased magnesium causes ventricular arrhythmias, coronary artery vasospasm, and sudden death.

Peripheral Resistance

1. Increased peripheral resistance increases arterial blood volume and pressure.
2. Decreased peripheral resistance decreases arterial blood volume and pressure.
3. Influenced by arterial blood volume: viscosity of blood and diameter of arterioles and capillaries.

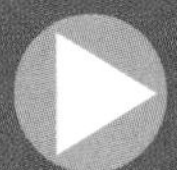

Cardiovascular Examination: History, Systems Review, Tests, and Measures

Patient Interview

History

1. Presenting symptoms. Note onset, progression, nature of symptoms, aggravating and alleviating factors, insight into medical condition, level of activity in increasing or abating the symptoms.
   a. Chest pain, palpitations, shortness of breath.
   b. Fatigue: generalized feeling of tiredness, weakness.
   c. Palpitations: awareness by patient of heart rhythm abnormalities; e.g., pounding, fluttering, racing heartbeat, skipped beats.
   d. Dizziness, syncope (transient loss of consciousness) due to inadequate cerebral blood flow.
   e. Edema: retention of fluid in tissues; swelling, especially in dependent body parts/lower extremities; sudden weight gain.

Past Medical History

1. Other diagnoses, surgeries.
2. Medications.

Social History

1. Current living situation, family/social support.
2. Education level, employment.
3. Lifestyle, risk factors.

Quality-of-Life Issues

1. Functional mobility in home, community.
2. Activities of daily living (ADLs); sleep.

Risk Factors (See Table 4-1)

1. Focus on social habits: smoking, diet.
2. Past and present level of activity.

Table 4-1

Risk Factors for Cardiovascular Disease

Non-Modifiable Risk Factors	
RISK FACTOR	**INCREASED RISK CRITERIA**
Age	Men >45 years and women >55 years
Family History	Cardiac event in 1st degree male relative <55 years or 1st degree female relative <65 years (1.5–2-fold relative risk). Risk increases further with younger age of onset, number of events, and how close genealogically the relative is.
Race	African American
Gender	Men > risk than pre-menopausal women. After menopause, the risk equalizes.
Modifiable Risk Factors	
RISK FACTOR	**GOAL TO REDUCE RISK**
Cholesterol	Total cholesterol: <200 mg/dL LDL cholesterol: <160 mg/dL (if low risk for cardiac disease), <130 mg/dL (if intermediate risk for cardiac disease), <100 mg/dL (if high risk for cardiac disease, have cardiac disease, or diabetes) HDL cholesterol: >40 mg/dL (men) and >50 mg/dL (women) Triglycerides: <150 mg/dL
Diabetes	HgA1C <7%
Diet	Low fat, salt diet with balance of vegetables, fruits, grains, and meats.
Hypertension	Normal blood pressure: less than 120/80 mmHg
Obesity	Body Mass Index (BMI): 18.5–24.9 kg/m2 Waist circumference: <40 inches (men) and <35 inches (women)
Physical inactivity	At least 30 minutes of activity, 5–7 days per week
Tobacco	Smoking cessation, regardless of time smoked, reduces risk.

Adapted from Greenland et al., 2010; World Heart Federation, American Heart Association.

Physical Examination: Cardiovascular System

Examine Skin

1. Observe for possible signs of decreased cardiac output and low oxygen saturation, including:
   a. Cyanosis: bluish color of the skin, nail beds, lips, and tongue.
   b. Pallor: washed out, absence of pink, rosy color.
   c. Diaphoresis: excess sweating and cool, clammy skin.

Examine Pulse

1. Rhythmical throbbing of arterial wall as a result of each heartbeat; note rate and rhythm.
2. Influenced by force of contraction, volume and viscosity of blood, diameter and elasticity of vessels, emotions, exercise, blood temperature, and hormones.
3. Determine pulses; palpate for 30 seconds with regular rhythm, 1–2 minutes with irregular rhythm (Table 4-2).
   a. Apical pulse or point of maximal impulse (PMI): patient is supine, palpate at 5th interspace, midclavicular vertical line (apex of the heart); may be displaced upward by pregnancy or high diaphragm; may be displaced laterally in congestive heart failure, cardiomyopathy, ischemic heart disease.
   b. Radial: palpate radial artery, radial wrist at base of thumb; most common monitoring site.
   c. Carotid: patient is lying down with head of bed elevated; palpate over carotid artery, on either side of anterior neck between sternocleidomastoid muscle and trachea.
      - Assess one side at a time to reduce the risk of bradycardia through stimulation of the carotid sinus baroreceptor, which produces a reflex drop in pulse rate or blood pressure.
   d. Brachial: palpate over brachial artery, medial aspect of the antecubital fossa; used to monitor blood pressure. Best in infants.
   e. Femoral: palpate over femoral artery in inguinal region.
   f. Popliteal: palpate over popliteal artery, behind the knee with the knee flexed slightly.
   g. Pedal: palpate over dorsalis pedis artery, dorsal medial aspect of foot; used to monitor lower extremity circulation.

Table 4-2

Grading Scale for Peripheral Pulses	
0	Absent pulse, not palpable
1+	Pulse diminished, barely perceptible
2+	Easily palpable, normal
3+	Full pulse, increased strength
4+	Bounding pulse

4. Determine heart rate (HR).
   a. Normal HR.
      - Adult and teenagers: 60–100 beats per minute (bpm); 40–60 bpm in aerobically trained.
      - Children: 60–140 bpm.
      - Newborn: average is 127 bpm; normal range 90–164 bpm.
   b. Tachycardia: >100 bpm. Exercise commonly results in tachycardia. Compensatory tachycardia can be seen with volume loss (surgery, dehydration).
   c. Bradycardia: <60 bpm.
5. Postural Tachycardia Syndrome: sustained heart rate increase ≥ 30 beats per minute within 10 minutes of standing (≥ 40 beats per minute in teenagers).
6. Pulse abnormalities.
   a. Irregular pulse: variations in force and frequency; may be due to arrhythmias, myocarditis.
   b. Weak, thready pulse: may be due to low stroke volume, cardiogenic shock.
   c. Bounding, full pulse: may be due to shortened ventricular systole and decreased peripheral pressure; aortic insufficiency.

Examine Heart Sounds

1. Auscultation: the process of listening for sounds within the body; stethoscope is placed directly on chest. Note intensity and quality of heart sounds.
2. Patient position: supine.
3. Auscultation landmarks.
   a. Aortic valve: located at the second right intercostal space at the sternal border.
   b. Pulmonic valve: located at the 2nd left intercostal space at the sternal border.
   c. Tricuspid valve: located at the 4th left intercostal space at the sternal border.
   d. Mitral valve: located at the 5th left intercostal space at the midclavical area.
4. S1 sound ("lub"): normal closure of mitral and tricuspid valves; marks beginning of systole. Decreased in first-degree heart block.
5. S2 sound ("dub"): normal closure of aortic and pulmonary valves; marks end of systole. Decreased in aortic stenosis.
6. Murmurs: extra sounds.
   a. Systolic: falls between S1 and S2. May indicate valvular disease (e.g., mitral valve prolapse) or may be normal.
   b. Diastolic: falls between S2 and S1. Usually indicates valvular disease.
   c. Grades of heart murmurs: grade 1 (softest audible murmur) to grade 6 (audible with stethoscope off the chest).
   d. Thrill: an abnormal tremor accompanying a vascular or cardiac murmur; felt on palpation.

7. Bruit: an adventitious sound or murmur (blowing sound) of arterial or venous origin; common in carotid or femoral arteries; indicative of atherosclerosis.
8. Gallop rhythm: an abnormal heart rhythm with three sounds in each cycle; resembles the gallop of a horse.
   a. S3; associated with ventricular filling; occurs soon after S2; in older individuals may be indicative of congestive (LV) heart failure.
   b. S4: associated with ventricular filling and atrial contraction; occurs just before S1. S4 is indicative of pathology; e.g., coronary heart disease (CAD), myocardial infarction (MI), aortic stenosis or chronic hypertension.

Examine Heart Rhythm

1. Electrocardiogram (ECG): 12-lead ECG provides information about rate, rhythm, conduction, areas of ischemia, and infarct, hypertrophy, electrolyte imbalances, and systemic pathologies (COPD, cerebral T-waves, etc.).
2. Normal cardiac cycle (normal sinus rhythm) (see Figure 4-4).
   a. P wave: atrial depolarization.
   b. P-R interval: time required for impulse to travel from atria through conduction system to Purkinje fibers.
   c. QRS wave: ventricular depolarization.
   d. ST segment: beginning of ventricular repolarization.
   e. T wave: ventricular repolarization.
   f. QT interval: time for electrical systole.
3. Calculate heart rate: count number of intervals between QRS complexes in a 6-second strip and multiply by 10. With irregular heart rates, use the longest strip possible (up to 1 minute) for a more accurate assessment of heart rate.
4. Assess rhythm: regular or irregular.
5. Identify arrhythmias.
   a. Etiology: ischemic conditions of the myocardium, electrolyte imbalance, acidosis or alkalosis, hypoxemia, hypotension, emotional stress, drugs, alcohol, caffeine.
   b. Ventricular arrhythmias: originate from an ectopic focus in the ventricles (outside the normal conduction system).
      - Significant in adversely affecting cardiac output.
      - Premature ventricular contractions (PVCs): a premature beat arising from the ventricle; occurs occasionally in the majority of the normal population. On ECG: no P wave; a bizarre and wide QRS that is premature, followed by a long compensatory pause. Serious PVCs: >6 per minute, paired or in sequential runs, multifocal, very early PVC (R on T phenomena).
      - Ventricular tachycardia (VT): a run of four or more PVCs occurring sequentially; very rapid rate (150–200 bpm); may occur paroxysmally (abrupt onset); usually the result of an ischemic ventricle. On ECG: wide, bizarre QRS waves, no P waves. Seriously compromised cardiac output.
         - NSVT (non-sustained ventricular tachycardia): a run of four or more consecutive beats in duration, terminating spontaneously in less than 30 seconds.
         - VT (sustained ventricular tachycardia): VT >30 seconds in duration and/or requiring termination due to hemodynamic compromise in less than 30 seconds.
      - Ventricular fibrillation (VF): a pulseless, emergency situation requiring emergency medical treatment: cardiopulmonary resuscitation (CPR), defibrillation, medications. Characterized by chaotic activity of ventricle originating from multiple foci; unable to determine rate. On ECG: bizarre, erratic activity without QRS complexes. No effective cardiac output; clinical death within 4–6 minutes.
   c. Atrial arrhythmias (supraventricular): rapid and repetitive firing of one or more ectopic foci in the atria (outside the sinus node).
      - On ECG, P waves are abnormal (variable in shape) or not identifiable (atrial fibrillation).
      - Rhythm may be irregular: chronic or occurring paroxysmally.
      - Rate: rapid with atrial tachycardia (140–250 bpm), atrial flutter (250–350 bpm); fibrillation (>300 bpm).
      - Cardiac output is usually maintained if rate is controlled; may precipitate ventricular failure in an abnormal heart.
   d. Atrioventricular blocks: abnormal delays or failure to conduct through normal conducting system.
      - First-, second-, or third- (complete) degree atrioventricular blocks; bundle branch blocks.
      - If ventricular rate is slowed, cardiac output decreased.
      - Third degree, complete heart block is life threatening: requires medications (atropine), surgical implantation of pacemaker.
6. Metabolic and drug influences on the ECG.
   a. Potassium levels.
      - Hyperkalemia: widens QRS, flattens P wave, T wave becomes peaked.
      - Hypokalemia: flattens T wave (or inverts), produces a U wave.
   b. Calcium levels.
      - Hypercalcemia: widens QRS, shortens QT interval.
      - Hypocalcemia: prolongs QT interval.
   c. Hypothermia: elevates ST segment; slows rhythm.

d. Digitalis: depresses ST segment, flattens T wave (or inverts), QT shortens.
e. Quinidine: QT lengthens, T wave flattens (or inverts), QRS lengthens.
f. Beta blockers (e.g., propranolol [Inderal]): decreases heart rate, blunts heart rate response to exercise.
g. Nitrates (nitroglycerin): increases heart rate.
h. Antiarrhythmic agents: may prolong QRS and QT intervals.

7. Holter monitoring: continuous ambulatory ECG monitoring via recording of cardiac rhythm for up to 24 hours.
   a. Used to evaluate cardiac rhythm, transient symptoms, pacemaker function, effect of medications.
   b. Allows correlation of symptoms with activities (activity diary).

Table 4-4

Pediatric Blood Pressure by Age (mmHg)		
AGE	SYSTOLIC BP	DIASTOLIC BP
Neonate (96 hr)	67–84	35–53
Infant (1–12mo)	72–104	37–56
Toddler (1–2 yr)	86–106	42–63
Preschooler (3–5 yr)	89–112	46–72
School-age (6–9 yr)	97–115	57–76
Preadolescent (10–11 yr)	102–120	61–80
Adolescent (12–15 yr)	110–131	64–83

Novak C and Gill P. Pediatric Vital Signs Reference Chart. PedsCases.com. April 21, 2016.

Examine Blood Pressure (BP) (See Tables 4-3 and 4-4)

1. Determine BP. Brachial BP is measured in right arm using standard measurement practices and an appropriately sized cuff. It is recommended that at least 2 BP readings be taken at a 1-min interval and values averaged.
   a. Hypertension: an increase in BP above normal; see Table 4-3.
      - Under 2017 guidelines, an estimated 46% of US adults have high BP.
      - Medications are prescribed for Stage I hypertension if a patient has already had a heart attack or stroke or is at high risk of heart attack or stroke in the presence of diabetes, chronic kidney disease, or atherosclerotic risk.
      - Individuals without high risk are advised to improve their lifestyles—lose weight, eat healthy, exercise more, limit alcohol, avoid smoking.

Table 4-3

2017 ACC/AHA Blood Pressure Guidelines*			
	BP, mmHg		
	SYSTOLIC		DIASTOLIC
Normal	<120		<80
Elevated	120–129	and	<80
Stage 1	130–139	or	80–89
Stage 2	at least 140	or	at least 90
Hypertensive crisis	>180	and/or	>120

*2017 ACC/AHA Guideline for the Prevention, Detection, Evaluation, and Management of High Blood Pressure in Adults. *J Amer C Cardiology, 71*(19), May 2017.

      - Many people will need two or more types of medication to control their BP.
      - Risk factors for high BP include socioeconomic status and psychosocial stress.
   b. Hypotension: a decrease in BP below normal; blood pressure is not adequate for normal perfusion/oxygenation of tissue (MAP [mean arterial pressure] is <50) may be related to bed rest, drugs, arrhythmias, blood loss/shock, or myocardial infarction.
   c. Orthostatic hypotension: drop in BP that accompanies change from supine to standing position.
      - Initial BP and HR assessment when patient supine, at rest for ≥5 minutes.
      - Patient moves directly to standing position and repeat BP and HR assessment immediately and again at 3 minutes.
      - A patient is orthostatic if the systolic BP drops >20 mmHg or if the diastolic BP drops >10 mmHg.
      - Common symptoms include lightheadedness, dizziness, loss of balance, and leg weakness.
   d. Pediatric BP.
      - BP values in children vary with age, height, and gender.
      - Children should be checked yearly using a pediatric chart: BP levels based on gender, age, and height percentile.
      - After age 13, levels defining high BP are the same as for adults.
2. Mean arterial pressure (MAP): the arterial pressure within the large arteries over time; dependent upon mean blood flow and arterial compliance.
   a. Calculated by taking the sum of the systolic blood pressure (SBP) and twice the diastolic blood pressure (DBP), divided by 3.
   b. An important clinical measure in critical care.
   c. Normal MAP is 70–110 mmHg.

Examine Respiration

1. Determine rate, depth of breathing.
   a. Normal adult respiratory rate (RR) is 12–20 breaths per minute.
   b. Normal newborn RR is 30–40 breaths per minute.
   c. Normal child RR is 20–30.
   d. Tachypnea: an increase in RR ≥ 22 breaths per minute.
   e. Bradypnea: a decrease of RR ≤ 10 breaths per minute.
   f. Hyperpnea: an increase in depth and rate of breathing.
2. Dyspnea: shortness of breath.
   a. Dyspnea on exertion (DOE): brought on by exercise or activity.
   b. Orthopnea: inability to breathe when in a reclining or supine position.
   c. Paroxysmal nocturnal dyspnea (PND): sudden inability to breathe occurring during sleep.
   d. Dyspnea scale (Table 4-5) (Borg, 1982).
3. Auscultation of the lungs: assess respiratory sounds.
   a. Normal breath sounds.
   b. Assess for adventitious sounds.
      - Crackles (rales): rattling, bubbling sounds; may be due to secretions in the lungs.
      - Wheezes (rhonchi): whistling sounds.
4. Assess cough: productive or nonproductive, strong or weak, coordinated or uncoordinated, consistency and color of any secretions.

Examine Oxygen Saturation

1. Use pulse oximetry, an electronic device that measures the degree of saturation of hemoglobin with oxygen (SaO_2). Normal values are 98%–100% oxygen.

Table 4-5

Modified Borg Dyspnea Scale (Borg, 1982)	
0	Nothing at all
0.5	Very, very slight (just noticeable)
1	Very slight
2	Slight
3	Moderate
4	Somewhat severe
5	Severe
6	Severe
7	Very severe
8	Very severe
9	Very, very severe (almost maximal)
10	Maximal

Table 4-6

Anginal Scale	
1+	Light, barely noticeable
2+	Moderate, bothersome
3+	Severe, very uncomfortable
4+	Most severe pain ever experienced

2. Provides an estimate of PaO_2 (partial pressure of oxygen) based on the oxyhemoglobin desaturation curve.
3. Hypoxemia: abnormally low amount of oxygen in the blood (saturation levels below 90% which corresponds to a PaO_2 of 60 mmHg).
4. Hypoxia: low oxygen level in the tissues.
5. Anoxia: complete lack of oxygen.

Examine Pain

1. Chest pain may be cardiac or noncardiac in origin.
2. Ischemic cardiac pain (angina or myocardial infarction): diffuse, retrosternal pain; or a sensation of tightness, achiness, in the chest; associated with dyspnea, sweating, indigestion, dizziness, syncope, anxiety (see anginal descriptions in Acute Coronary Syndromes).
3. Symptoms more likely in women: indigestion or gas-like pain, dizziness or nausea, unexplained weakness or fatigue, discomfort or pain between the shoulder blades, recurring chest discomfort, sense of impending doom.
4. Rate pain using Anginal scale (Table 4-6).
5. Referred pain.
   a. Cardiac pain can refer to shoulders, back, arms, neck, or jaw.
   b. Pain referred to the back can occur from dissecting aortic aneurysm.

Physical Examination: Peripheral Vascular System

Examine Condition of Extremities

1. Examine for diaphoresis: excess sweating can be associated with decreased cardiac output.
2. Examine arterial pulses: decreased or absent pulses associated with peripheral artery disease (PAD); examine bilaterally starting with most distal pulses.
   a. Lower extremity: position patient supine, check femoral, popliteal, dorsalis pedis, posterior tibial pulses.
   b. Upper extremity: check radial, brachial, and carotid pulses.

3. Examine skin color.
   a. Cyanosis: bluish color related to decreased cardiac output or cold; especially lips, fingertips, nail beds.
   b. Pallor: absence of rosy color in light-skinned individuals, associated with decreased peripheral blood flow, PAD.
   c. Rubor: dependent redness with PAD.
4. Examine skin temperature.
5. Examine for skin changes.
   a. Clubbing: curvature of the fingernails with soft tissue enlargement at base of nail: associated with chronic oxygen deficiency, chronic pulmonary disease, or heart failure.
   b. Trophic changes: pale, shiny, dry skin, with loss of hair is associated with PAD.
   c. Fibrosis: tissues are thick, firm, and unyielding.
      - Stemmer's sign: dorsal skin folds of the toes or fingers are resistant to lifting; indicative of fibrotic changes and lymphedema.
   d. Abnormal pigmentation, ulceration, dermatitis, gangrene is associated with PAD.
   e. Temperature: decrease in superficial skin temperature is associated with poor arterial perfusion.
6. Examine for pain.
   a. Intermittent claudication (IC): pain, cramping, and lower extremity fatigue occurring during exercise and relieved by rest, associated with PAD.
   b. IC pain is typically in calf; may also be in thigh, hips, or buttocks.
   c. Patient may experience pain at rest with severe decrease in arterial blood supply; typically in forefoot, worse at night.
7. Examine for edema.
   a. Measure girth measurements using a tape measure at regular intervals, or volumetric measurements using a volumeter (useful with irregular body parts, such as hand or foot).
   b. Pitting edema (indentation): depression is maintained when finger is pressed firmly; grading scale (see Table 4-7).
   c. Peripheral causes of edema include chronic venous insufficiency and lymphedema.
   d. Bilateral edema is associated with congestive heart failure.

Table 4-7

Grading Scale for Edema	
1+	Mild, barely perceptible indentation; <¼ inch pitting
2+	Moderate, easily identified depression; returns to normal within 15 seconds; ¼–½ inch pitting
3+	Severe, depression takes 15–30 seconds to rebound; ½–1 inch pitting
4+	Very severe, depression lasts for >30 seconds or more; >1 inch pitting

Tests of Peripheral Venous Circulation

1. Examine venous system before arterial; venous insufficiency can invalidate some arterial tests.
2. Percussion test: determines competence of greater saphenous vein.
   a. In standing, palpate one segment of vein while percussing vein approximately 20 cm higher.
   b. If pulse wave is felt by lower hand, the intervening valves are incompetent.
3. Trendelenburg test (retrograde filling test): determines competence of communicating veins and saphenous system.
   a. Patient is positioned in supine with legs elevated to 60° (empties venous blood).
   b. Tourniquet is then placed on proximal thigh (occludes venous flow in the superficial veins).
   c. Patient is then asked to stand.
   d. Examiner notes whether veins fill in normal pattern. Should take approximately 30 seconds.
4. Venous filling time: Examine time necessary to refill veins after emptying.
   a. With patient supine, passively elevate lower extremity to approximately 45° for 1 minute, then place in dependent position. Note time for veins to refill.
   b. Delayed filling (>15 seconds) is indicative of venous insufficiency.
5. Doppler ultrasound: examination using an ultrasonic oscillator connected to earphones.
   a. Determines blood flow within a vessel; useful in both venous and arterial diseases.
   b. Doppler probe placed over large vessel; ultrasound signal given transcutaneously; movement of blood causes an audible shift in signal frequency.
   c. Useful in locating nonpalpable pulses and measuring systolic BP in extremities.
6. Air plethysmography (APG): pneumatic device calibrated to measure patency of venous system; volume.
   a. Cuff is inflated around calf, attached to a pressure transducer and microprocessor.
   b. Occludes venous return, permits arterial inflow; recorder registers increasing volume with cuff; time to return to baseline with cuff deflation.
   c. Comparison tests performed in sitting, standing, and up onto toes.

Tests of Peripheral Arterial Circulation

1. Ankle brachial index (ABI): the ratio of lower extremity (LE) pressure divided by upper extremity (UE) pressure.
   a. Pt is positioned supine and at rest for 5 minutes.

b. BP cuff is inflated to occlude blood flow temporarily, then deflated. Examiner listens for return of flow.
c. Performed in UE at brachial artery; LE at posterior tibial and dorsalis pedis arteries.
d. ABI indices (Table 4-8).
e. ABI assists in risk stratification for cardiovascular disease: <0.90 is associated with 2- to 4-fold increased risk for cardiovascular events and death.
f. ABI <0.50: increased risk of progression to severe or critical limb ischemia in 1 year.
g. Clinically significant change in ABI is >0.15 or >0.10 in patients with symptoms.

2. Rubor of dependency. Examine color changes in skin during elevation of foot followed by dependency (seated, hanging position).
   a. With insufficiency, pallor develops in elevated position; reactive hyperemia (rubor of dependency) develops in dependent position.
   b. Changes that take longer than 30 seconds are also indicative of arterial insufficiency.
3. Examine for intermittent claudication: exercise-induced pain or cramping in the legs that is absent at rest. Usually calf pain, but may also occur in buttock, hip, thigh, or foot.
   a. Treadmill test: have patient walk on a level grade, 1 mph; note level of claudication pain (Table 4-9) and time of test pain was experienced.
   b. Higher levels of claudication may be acceptable during the exercise test.
   c. Examine for coldness, numbness, or pallor in the legs or feet; loss of hair over anterior tibial area.
   d. Leg cramps may also result from diuretic use with hypokalemia.

Table 4-8

Significance of Ankle Brachial Index Values

>1.40	Indicates non-compliant arteries
1.00–1.40	Normal
0.91–0.99	Borderline
≤ 0.90	Abnormal
≤ 0.50	Severe arterial disease, risk for critical limb ischemia, may have pain at rest

Table 4-9

Subjective Ratings of Pain with Intermittent Claudication

Grade I	Minimal discomfort or pain
Grade II	Moderate discomfort or pain; patient's attention can be diverted
Grade III	Intense pain; patient's attention cannot be diverted
Grade IV	Excruciating and unbearable pain

Examine Lymphatic System

1. Palpate superficial lymph nodes: cervical, axillary, epitrochlear, superficial inguinal.
2. Examine for edema.
   a. Visual inspection: note swelling, decreased range of motion, loss of functional mobility.
   b. Measure girth.
3. Examine skin.
   a. Changes in skin texture, fibrotic tissue changes.
   b. Presence of papules, leakage, wounds.
4. Changes in function (ADL, functional mobility, sleep).
5. Paresthesias may be present.
6. Lymphangiography and lymphoscintigraphy using radioactive agents (x-ray of lymph vessels); provides information about lymph flow, lymph node uptake, and backflow.

Diagnostic Tests

Chest X-Ray (Figure 4-7)

1. Will reveal abnormalities of lung fluids, overall cardiac shape and size (cardiomegaly), aneurysm.

Myocardial Perfusion Imaging (Figure 4-8)

1. Used to diagnose and evaluate ischemic heart disease, myocardial infarction.
2. Thallium-201 scan: thallium (or other radioisotope) is injected into blood via IV; radioisotopes concentrate in normal tissue but not in ischemic or infarcted tissues (cold spots).
3. Used to identify myocardial blood flow, areas of stress-induced ischemia (exercise test), old infarcts.
4. Thallium stress test: used with exercise test (treadmill or bicycle ergometer); injected at peak exercise.

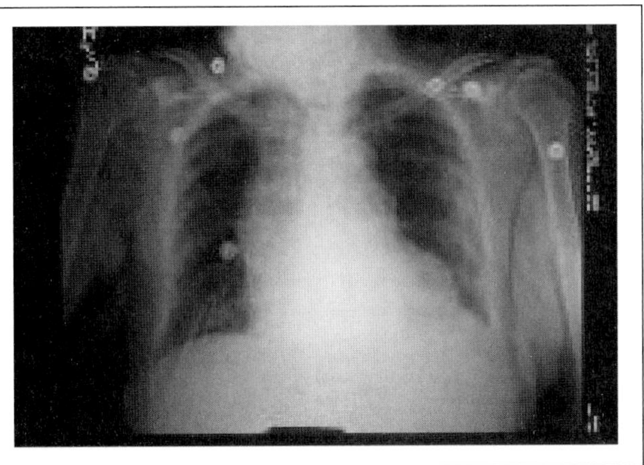

Figure 4-7 Radiographic view: Demonstrates signs of congestive heart failure.

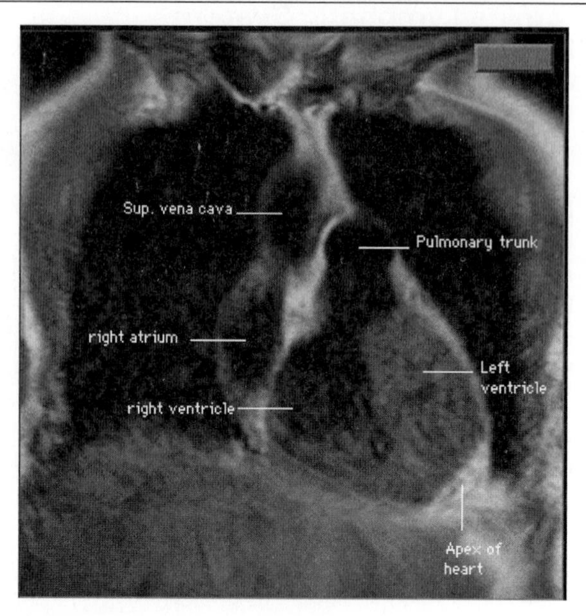

Figure 4-8 **Coronal T1MRI thoracic view of normal female.**

5. Positron emission tomography (PET); uses radioactive marker 18F-fluorodeoxyglucose (FDG).

Echocardiogram

1. Noninvasive test that uses ultrasound to assess internal structures: size of chambers, wall thickness, ejection fraction (EF), movement of valves, septum, abnormal wall movement.

Cardiac Catheterization

1. Passage of a tiny tube from brachial or femoral artery through aorta into blood vessels with introduction of a contrast medium into coronary arteries and subsequent x-ray.
2. Provides information about anatomy of heart and great vessels, ventricular and valve function, abnormal wall movements.
3. Allows determination of ejection fraction (EF).

Central Line (Swan-Ganz Catheter)

1. Catheter inserted through vessels into right side of heart.
2. Measures central venous pressure (CVP), pulmonary artery pressure (PA), pulmonary capillary wedge pressures (PCWP).

Cardiac MRI

1. Creates 3D images of the heart to investigate coronary arteries, aorta, pericardium, and myocardium.

Laboratory Tests and Values

See Table 4-10

1. Enzyme Changes Associated with Myocardial Infarction (Thygesen et al, 2012)
2. Rise and fall of cardiac troponin (I or T) >99th percentile is the primary measure of myocardial infarction. It must accompany one of the following:
   a. Symptoms of ischemia.
   b. New or presumed new ST changes on ECG.
   c. New loss of viable myocardium and/or new wall motion abnormality on imaging.
   d. Evidence of intracoronary thrombus via catheterization or autopsy.
3. Elevation of CK or CPK (serum creatine kinase or creatine phosphokinase) with concomitant elevation of CK-MB (serum creatine kinase MB) can also be assessed, but peaks between 12–24 hours.

Serum Lipids

1. Serum lipid panel: used to determine coronary risk. (See Table 4-1.)

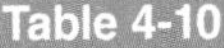

Table 4-10

Laboratory Tests and Values

NORMAL VALUES	CLINICAL SIGNIFICANCE
Arterial Blood Gases (ABGs)	
SpO_2 98%–100%	SaO_2 below 88%–90% usually requires supplemental O_2
PaO_2 90–100 mmHg	↑ in hyperoxygenation ↓ in cardiac decompensation, COPD and some neuromuscular disorders
$PaCO_2$ 35–45 mmHg	↑ in COPD, hypoventilation ↓ in hyperventilation, pregnancy, pulmonary embolism, and anxiety
pH, whole blood 7.35–7.45	<7.35 is acidotic, >7.45 is alkalotic ↑ in respiratory alkalosis: hyperventilation, sepsis, liver disease, fever ↑ in metabolic alkalosis: vomiting, potassium depletion, diuretics, volume depletion ↓ in respiratory acidosis: hypoventilation, COPD, respiratory depressants, myasthenia ↓ in metabolic acidosis (bicarbonate deficit): increased acids (diabetes, alcohol, starvation); renal failure, increased acid intake, and loss of alkaline body fluids
Hemostasis (Clotting/Bleeding Times)	
Prothrombin time (PT) 11–15 sec	↑ in factor X deficiency, hemorrhagic disease, cirrhosis, hepatitis drugs (warfarin)
Partial thromboplastin time (PTT) 25–40 sec	↑ in factor VIII, IX, and X deficiency
International normalized ratio (INR): Ratio of individual's PT to reference range 0.9–1.1 (ratio)	Patients with deep vein thrombosis (DVT), pulmonary embolism (PE), mechanical valves, atrial fibrillation (AF) on anticoagulation therapy will have target INRs 2–3. Patients with these conditions and/or genetic clotting disorders may have a target INR 3.5. Look for active signs of bleeding when treating these patients and use compensatory strategies to reduce fall risk.
Bleeding time 2–10 min C-reactive protein (CRP) <10 mg/L	↑ in platelet disorders, thrombocytopenia ↑ levels associated with ↑ risk of atherosclerosis >100 mg/L associated with inflammation and infection
Complete Blood Cell Count (CBC), Adult Values	
White Blood Cells (WBCs) 4300–10,800 cells/mm^3	Indicative of status of immune system ↑ in infection: bacterial, viral; inflammation, hematologic malignancy, leukemia, lymphoma, drugs (corticosteroids) ↓ in aplastic anemia, B_{12} or folate deficiency With immunosuppression: ↑ risk of infection *Physical therapy considerations:* Consider metabolic demands in presence of fever and use of mask when WBCs <1000–2000 or Absolute Neutrophil Count (ANC) <500–1000
Red Blood Cells (RBCs) Male: 4.6–6.2 10^6/uL Female: 4.2–5.9 10^6/uL	↑ in polycythemia ↓ in anemia
Erythrocyte sedimentation rate (ESR) Male <15 mm/hr Female <20 mm/hr	↑ in infection and inflammation: rheumatic or pelvic inflammatory disease, osteomyelitis used to monitor effects of treatment; e.g., RA, SLE, Hodgkin's disease
Hematocrit (Hct) % of RBC of the whole blood Male 45%–52% Female 37%–48% (age dependent)	↑ in erythrocytosis, dehydration, shock ↓ in severe anemias, acute hemorrhage *Physical therapy considerations:* Can cause ↓ exercise tolerance, ↑ fatigue, and tachycardia.
Hemoglobin (Hgb) Male: 13–18 g/dL Female: 12–16 g/dL (age dependent)	↑ polycythemia, dehydration, shock ↓ in anemias, prolonged hemorrhage, RBC destruction (cancer, sickle cell disease) *Physical therapy considerations:* Can cause ↓ exercise tolerance, ↑ fatigue, and tachycardia
Platelet count 150,000–450,000 cells/mm^3	↑ chronic leukemia, hemoconcentration ↓ thrombocytopenia, acute leukemia, aplastic anemia, cancer chemotherapy *Physical therapy considerations:* Increased risk of bleeding with low levels so monitor for hematuria, petechiae, and other signs of active bleeding. <20,000: AROM, ADLs only 20,000–30,000: light exercise only 30,000–50,000: moderate exercise

Adapted from Hopkins T; *Lab Notes*, 2nd Ed. Philadelphia, FA Davis, 2009.

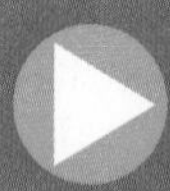

Cardiovascular Disease: Evaluation, Differential Diagnosis, and Prognosis

Atherosclerosis

Characteristics

1. Disease of lipid-laden plaques (lesions) affecting moderate and large-size arteries.
2. Thickening and narrowing of the intimal layer of the blood vessel wall from focal accumulation of lipids, platelets, monocytes, plaque, and other debris.

Risk Factors (See Table 4-1)

Acute Coronary Syndrome (ACS) (Coronary Artery Disease)

Characteristics

1. Involves a spectrum of clinical entities ranging from angina to infarction to sudden cardiac death.
2. An imbalance of myocardial oxygen supply and demand resulting in ischemic chest pain.
3. Symptoms present when lumen is at least 70% occluded.
4. New ST segment changes (>/=1mm) or T wave inversion in multiple leads.

Angina Pectoris

1. Chest pain or pressure due to ischemia; may be accompanied by Levine's sign (patient clenches fist over sternum).
2. Represents imbalance in myocardial oxygen supply and demand; brought on by:
   a. Increased demands on heart: exertion, emotional stress, smoking, extremes of temperature, especially cold, overeating, tachyarrhythmias.
   b. Vasospasm: symptoms may be present at rest.
3. Three major types of angina.
   a. Stable angina: classic exertional angina occurring during exercise or activity; occurs at a predictable rate-pressure product, RPP (HR × BP), relieved with rest and/or nitroglycerin.
   b. Unstable angina (preinfarction, crescendo angina): coronary insufficiency at any time without any precipitating factors or exertion. Chest pain increases in severity, frequency, and duration; refractory to treatment. Increases risk for myocardial infarction or lethal arrhythmia; pain is difficult to control.
   c. Variant angina (Prinzmetal's angina): caused by vasospasm of coronary arteries in the absence of occlusive disease. Responds well to nitroglycerin or calcium channel blocker long term.
4. Women more often describe sensations of discomfort, crushing, pressing, and bad ache when referring to angina.
5. With angina, patients often describe shortness of breath, fatigue, diaphoresis, and weakness as symptoms of ACS.
6. Older adults present more often with atypical symptoms (absence of chest pain): dyspnea, diaphoresis, nausea and vomiting, and syncope.

Myocardial Infarction (MI) (See Figure 4-9)

1. Prolonged ischemia, injury, and death of an area of the myocardium caused by occlusion of one or more of the coronary arteries.
2. Precipitating factors: atherosclerotic heart disease with thrombus formation, coronary vasospasm, or embolism; cocaine use.
3. Zones of infarction.
   a. Zone of infarction: consists of necrotic, noncontractile tissue; electrically inert; on ECG ST-segment deviation >1 mm.
   b. Zone of injury: area immediately adjacent to central zone, tissue is noncontractile, cells undergoing metabolic changes; electrically unstable; on ECG, see elevated ST segments in leads over injured area.
   c. Zone of ischemia: outer area, cells also undergoing metabolic changes, electrically unstable; on ECG, see T wave inversion.

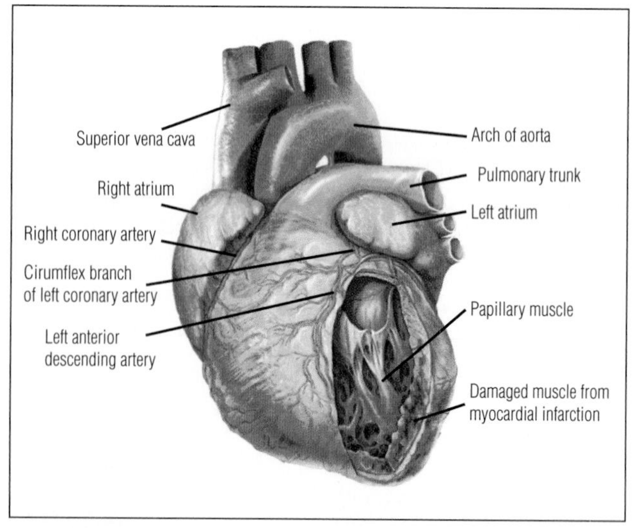

Figure 4-9 **Tissue destruction in myocardial infarction.**

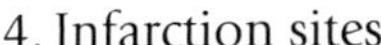

4. Infarction sites.
   a. Transmural: full thickness of myocardium, which is often an ST elevated MI (STEMI).
   b. Nontransmural: subendocardial, subepicardial, intramural infarctions. Non-ST elevated MI (NSTEMI).
   c. Sites of coronary artery occlusion.
      - Inferior MI, right ventricle infarction, disturbances of upper conduction system: right coronary artery.
      - Lateral MI, ventricular ectopy: circumflex artery.
      - Anterior MI, disturbances of lower conduction system: left anterior descending artery.
5. Impaired ventricular function results in:
   a. Decreased stroke volume, cardiac output and ejection fraction.
   b. Increased end diastolic ventricular pressures.
6. Electrical instability: arrhythmias, present in injured and ischemic areas.

Sudden Death Is Usually Due to Significant Ischemia or Ventricular Arrhythmia

Heart Failure (HF) (See Tables 4-11 and 4-12)

Definition and Characteristics

1. A clinical syndrome in which the heart is unable to maintain adequate circulation of the blood to meet the metabolic needs of the body.
2. Types of heart failure.
   a. Left-sided heart failure (congestive heart failure, CHF): is characterized by pulmonary congestion, edema, and low cardiac output due to backup of blood from the left ventricle (LV) to the left atrium (LA) and lungs. Occurs with insult to the left ventricle from myocardial disease; excessive workload of the heart (hypertension, valvular disease or congenital defects); cardiac arrhythmias or heart damage.
   b. Right-sided heart failure: is characterized by increased pressure load on the right ventricle (RV) with higher pulmonary vascular pressures; mitral valve disease, or chronic lung disease (cor pulmonale); produces hallmark signs of jugular vein distention and peripheral edema.
   c. Biventricular failure: severe LV pathology producing back up into the lungs, increased PA pressure and RV signs of HF.
3. Associated symptoms: muscle wasting, myopathies, osteoporosis.
4. Possible clinical manifestations of heart failure (Table 4-11).
5. Compensated heart failure: heart returns to functional status with reduced cardiac output and exercise tolerance. Control is achieved through:
   a. Physiological compensatory mechanisms: SNS stimulation, LV hypertrophy, anaerobic metabolism, cardiac dilatation, arterial vasoconstriction.
   b. Medical therapy.
6. Decompensated heart failure: structural or functional change in heart leads to its inability to eject and/or

Table 4-11

Possible Clinical Manifestations of Cardiac Failure

LEFT VENTRICULAR FAILURE	RIGHT VENTRICULAR FAILURE
Signs and symptoms of pulmonary congestion:	
Dyspnea, dry cough	Dependent edema
Orthopnea	Weight gain
Paroxysmal nocturnal dyspnea (PND)	Ascites
Pulmonary rales, wheezing	Liver engorgement (hepatomegaly)
Signs and symptoms of low cardiac output:	
Hypotension	Anorexia, nausea, bloating
Tachycardia	Cyanosis (nail beds)
Lightheadedness, dizziness	Right upper quadrant pain
Cerebral hypoxia: irritability, restlessness, confusion, impaired memory, sleep disturbances	Jugular vein distension
Fatigue, weakness	Right-sided S_3 heart sounds
Poor exercise tolerance	Murmurs of pulmonary or tricuspid insufficiency
Enlarged heart on chest x-ray	
S_3 heart sound, possibly S_4	
Murmurs of mitral or tricuspid regurgitation	

Table 4-12

Color Zones Associated with Clinical Manifestations of Heart Failure and Physical Therapist Recommendations

ZONE COLOR	SIGNS AND SYMPTOMS	PHYSICAL THERAPIST RECOMMENDATIONS
Green zone	• No shortness of breath • No swelling • No weight gain • No chest pain • No decrease in ability to maintain activity level	Continue activity and therapy as tolerated.
Yellow zone	• Weight gain of 2–3 lbs. in 24 hours • Increased cough • Peripheral edema; increased distal extremity swelling • Increase in shortness of breath with activity • Orthopnea: increase in number of pillows needed	Symptoms may indicate an adjustment in medications, and therefore warrants communication with the physician.
Red zone	• Shortness of breath at rest • Unrelieved chest pain • Wheezing or chest tightness at rest • Paroxysmal nocturnal dyspnea: must sit in chair to sleep • Weight gain or loss of more than 5 lbs. in 3 days • Confusion	Symptoms indicate overt decompensation and warrant an immediate visit to the emergency department or physician's office.

Adapted from Shoemaker MJ, Dias KJ, Lefebvre KM, Heick JD, Collins SM. Physical therapist clinical practice guideline for the management of individuals with heart failure. *Phys Ther.* 2020; 100: 14-43.

accommodate blood within normal physiological levels.

a. Sudden or gradual onset.
b. Can include signs/symptoms of right or left-sided heart failure (dyspnea, fatigue, rales, peripheral edema).
c. Requires immediate medical attention (ER visit, hospitalization, unplanned office visit).

Medical and Surgical Management of Cardiovascular Disease

Medications

1. ACE Inhibitors (e.g., captopril [capoten], enalopril [vasotec], lisinopril [zestril]): inhibit conversion of angiotension I to angiotension II, decreases Na retention and peripheral vasoconstriction in order to decrease blood pressure.
2. Angiotension II receptor blockers (ARBs) (e.g., losartan [cozaar]): blocks binder of angiotension II at the tissue/smooth muscle level, decreasing blood pressure.
3. Nitrates (nitroglycerin): decrease preload through peripheral vasodilation, reduce myocardial oxygen demand, reduce chest discomfort (angina); may also dilate coronary arteries, improve coronary blood flow.
4. Beta-1 adrenergic blocking agents (e.g., atenolol [tenormin], metoprolol [Lopressor, Toprol XL], propranolol [Inderal]): reduce myocardial demand by reducing heart rate and contractility; control arrhythmias, chest pain; reduce blood pressure.
5. Calcium channel blocking agents (e.g., diltiazem [Cardizem, Procardia], amlodipine [Norvasc]): inhibit flow of calcium ions, decrease heart rate, decrease contractility, dilate coronary arteries, reduce BP, control arrhythmias, chest pain.
6. Antiarrhythmics (numerous drugs, four main classes): alter conductivity, restore normal heart rhythm, control arrhythmias, improve cardiac output (e.g., quinidine, procainamide).
7. Digitalis (cardiac glycosides): increases contractility and decreases heart rate; mainstay in the treatment of CHF (e.g., digoxin).
8. Diuretics: decrease myocardial work (reduce preload and afterload), control hypertension, (e.g., furosemide [Lasix], hydrochlorothiazide [Esidrix]).
9. Aspirin: decreases platelet aggregation; may prevent myocardial infarction.
10. Tranquilizers: decrease anxiety, sympathetic effects.
11. Hypolipidemic agents (six major cholesterol-lowering drugs): reduce serum lipid levels when diet and weight reduction are not effective (e.g., cholestyramine [Questran], colestipol [Colestid], simvastatin [Zocor], lovastatin [Mevacor]).

Activity Restriction

1. Acute MI: activity can be increased once the acute MI has stopped (peak in cardiac troponin levels). Activity should be limited to 5 METs or 70% of age predicted HRmax for 4–6 weeks following MI.

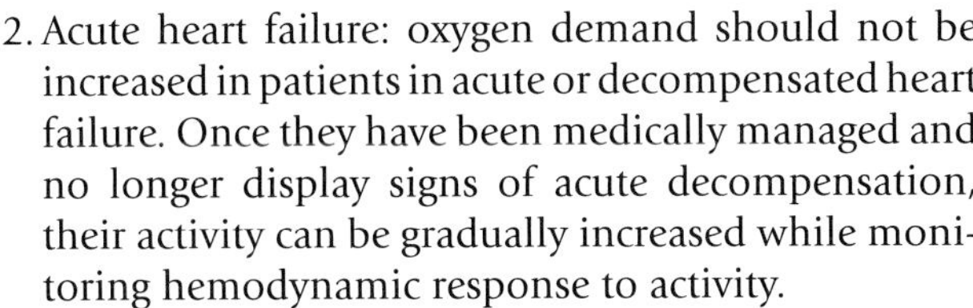

2. Acute heart failure: oxygen demand should not be increased in patients in acute or decompensated heart failure. Once they have been medically managed and no longer display signs of acute decompensation, their activity can be gradually increased while monitoring hemodynamic response to activity.

Surgical Interventions

1. Percutaneous transluminal coronary angioplasty (PTCA): under fluoroscopy, surgical dilation of a blood vessel using a small balloon-tipped catheter inflated inside the lumen; relieves obstructed blood flow in acute angina or acute MI; results in improved coronary blood flow, improved left ventricular function, anginal relief.
2. Intravascular stents: an endoprosthesis (pliable wire mesh) implanted during angioplasty to prevent restenosis and occlusion in coronary or peripheral arteries. May be coated with slow release medication to prevent more plaque buildup (drug-eluting stent, DES).
3. Coronary artery bypass graft (CABG): surgical circumvention of an obstruction in a coronary artery using an anastomosing graft (saphenous vein, internal mammary artery); multiple grafts may be necessary; results in improved coronary blood flow, improved left ventricular function, anginal relief.
4. Transplantation: used in end-stage myocardial disease; e.g., cardiomyopathy, ischemic heart disease, valvular heart disease.
   a. Heteroptics: involves leaving the natural heart and piggybacking the donor heart.
   b. Orthotopic: involves removing the diseased heart and replacing it with a donor heart.
   c. Heart and lung transplantation: involves removing both organs and replacing them with donor organs.
   d. Major problems posttransplantation are rejection, infection, complications of immunosuppressive therapy.
5. Ventricular assist device (VAD): an implanted device (accessory pump) that improves tissue perfusion and maintains cardiogenic circulation; used with severely involved patients; e.g., cardiogenic shock unresponsive to medications, severe ventricular dysfunction.

Thrombolytic Therapy

1. Administered for acute myocardial infarction.
2. Medications activate body's fibrinolytic system, dissolve clot and restore coronary blood flow (e.g., streptokinase, tissue plasminogen activator [TPA], urokinase).

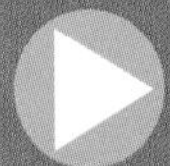

Peripheral Vascular Disease: Evaluation, Differential Diagnosis, and Prognosis

Arterial Disease

Occlusive Peripheral Arterial Disease (PAD)

1. Chronic, occlusive arterial disease of medium- and large-sized vessels, the result of peripheral atherosclerosis.
2. Associated with hypertension and hyperlipidemia; patients may also have CAD, cerebrovascular disease, diabetes, metabolic syndrome, and a history of smoking.
3. Diminished blood supply to affected extremities with pulses decreased or absent.
4. Color: pale on elevation, dusky red on dependency.
5. Early stages: patients exhibit intermittent claudication. Pain is described as burning, searing, aching, tightness, or cramping. Occurs regularly and predictably with walking and is relieved by rest.
6. Late stages: patients exhibit rest pain, muscle atrophy, trophic changes (hair loss, skin and nail changes).
7. Critical stenosis PAD: patients exhibit resting or nocturnal pain, skin ulcers, and gangrene.
8. Affects primarily the lower extremities.

Diabetic Angiopathy

1. An inappropriate elevation of blood glucose levels and accelerated atherosclerosis.
2. Neuropathy a major complication.
3. Neurotrophic ulcers, may lead to gangrene and amputation.

Raynaud's Disease or Phenomenon

1. Episodic spasm of small arteries and arterioles.
2. Abnormal vasoconstrictor reflex exacerbated by exposure to cold or emotional stress; tips of fingers develop pallor, cyanosis, numbness, and tingling.
3. Affects largely females.
4. Occlusive disease is not usually a factor.

Venous Disease

Varicose Veins

1. Distended, swollen superficial veins; tortuous in appearance.
2. May lead to varicose ulcers.

Venous Thromboembolism (VTE)

1. The formation of a blood clot in a deep vein that can lead to complications including deep vein thrombosis (DVT), pulmonary embolism (PE), or postthrombotic syndrome (PTS).
2. Mortality: incidence of 10%–30% within 1 month of diagnosis.
3. Morbidity: 1/3 experiences another VTE within 10 years.
4. Can become chronic: postthrombotic syndrome, leads to diminished quality of life.

Deep Vein Thrombophlebitis

1. Clot formation and acute inflammation in a deep vein.
2. Usually occurs in lower extremity, associated with forced immobilization (bed rest, lack of leg exercise), surgery, trauma, and hyperactivity of blood coagulation or can be unprovoked.
3. Signs and symptoms: may be asymptomatic early; progressive inflammation with tenderness to palpation; dull ache, tightness, or pain in the calf; swelling, warmth, redness, or discoloration in the lower extremity; prominent superficial veins.
4. Standardized risk assessment measure: use Wells Criteria Score for DVT (Table 4-13).

Table 4-13

Wells Criteria Score for DVT

CLINICAL FINDINGS	POINTS
Active cancer (treatment ongoing, or within 6 mo or palliative)	+1
Paralysis, paresis, or recent cast immobilization of the lower extremity	+1
Collateral superficial veins (nonvaricose)	+1
Recently bedridden for >3 days or major surgery <4 wk	+1
Localized tenderness along the distribution of the deep venous system	+1
Entire leg swollen	+1
Calf swelling at least 3 cm larger than asymptomatic side	+1
Pitting edema, confined to the symptomatic leg	+1
Previously documented DVT	+1
Alternative diagnosis to DVT as likely or more likely	−2
Total Criteria Point Count	
Clinical probability of a DVT with score:	
DVT likely	≥2
DVT unlikely	<2

Wells PS, et al. Does this patient have deep vein thrombosis? *JAMA.* 2006; 295(2):199–207

5. Medical management.
   a. Anticoagulation therapy: is used to prevent new clots from forming, prevent the existing clot from getting larger, and stabilize the clot through anti-inflammatory properties (e.g., low-molecular-weight heparin [LMWH]).
   b. LMWH is contraindicated in patients at high risk for bleeding. Patients at high risk are typically treated with unfractionated heparin [UFH].
   c. Both LMWH and UFH are associated with heparin-induced thrombocytopenia (HIT) in a small percent of patients (2%–3%). HIT is associated with a paradoxical increased risk for venous and arterial thrombosis.
   d. Graded compression stockings (GCS).

RED FLAG: Don't use Homan's sign (dorsiflexion sign) to diagnosis DVT; though it still may be in use, it has low sensitivity and specificity and is not diagnostic of DVT.

Pulmonary Embolism

1. Presents abruptly with chest pain and dyspnea, also diaphoresis, cough, and apprehension; requires emergency treatment.
2. Life threatening: 20% with acute PE die almost immediately; 40% die within 3 months.
3. Can result in chronic thromboembolic pulmonary hypertension with reduced oxygenation and pulmonary hypertension.
4. Can lead to right heart dysfunction and failure.

Chronic Postthrombotic Syndrome

1. A combination of clinical signs and symptoms that persists after an LE DVT; thrombosis resolution is incomplete.
2. Symptoms include pain, intractable edema, limb heaviness, skin pigmentation changes, and leg ulcers.
3. Leads to reduced quality of life and impaired functional mobility.

Chronic Venous Stasis/Incompetence

1. Venous valvular insufficiency: from fibroelastic degeneration of valve tissue, venous dilation.
2. Classification:
   a. Grade I: mild aching, minimal edema, dilated superficial veins.
   b. Grade II: increased edema, multiple dilated veins, changes in skin pigmentation.
   c. Grade III: venous claudication, severe edema, cutaneous ulceration.

Differential Diagnosis of Peripheral Vascular Diseases (See Table 4-14)

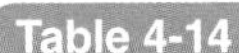
Table 4-14

Differential Diagnosis: Peripheral Vascular Diseases

	CHRONIC ARTERIAL INSUFFICIENCY	CHRONIC VENOUS INSUFFICIENCY
Etiology	Atherosclerosis Thrombosis Emboli Inflammatory process	Thrombophlebitis Trauma Vein obstruction (clot) Vein incompetence
Risk factors	Age: >60 years Smoking Diabetes mellitus Gender: slightly higher in men Dyslipidemia Hypertension Hyperhomocysteinemia Race (African American)	Venous hypertension Varicose veins Inherited trait Gender: female Age Increased BMI Sedentary lifestyle/prolonged sitting Ligamentous laxity
Signs and symptoms: determined by location and degree of vascular involvement		
Pain	Severe muscle ischemia/intermittent claudication Worse with exercise, relieved by rest Rest pain indicates severe involvement Muscle fatigue, cramping, numbness Paresthesias over time	Minimal to moderate steady pain Aching pain in lower leg with prolonged standing or sitting (dependency) Superficial pain along course of vein
Location of pain	Usually calf, lower leg, or dorsum of foot May occur in thigh, hip, or buttock	Muscle compartment tenderness
Vascular	Decreased or absent pulses Pallor of forefoot on elevation Dependent rubor	Venous dilatation or varicosity Edema: moderate to severe, especially after prolonged dependency
Skin changes	Pale, shiny, dry skin Loss of hair Nail changes Coolness of extremity	Hemosiderin deposition: dark, cyanotic, thickened, brown skin Lipodermatosclerosis: fibrosing of the subcutaneous tissue May lead to stasis dermatitis, cellulitis
Acute	Acute arterial obstruction: distal pain, paresthetic, pale, pulseless, sudden onset	Acute thrombophlebitis (deep venous thrombosis, DVT): calf pain, aching, edema, muscle tenderness, 50% asymptomatic
Ulceration	May develop in toes, feet, or areas of trauma; pale or yellow to black eschar, gangrene may develop; regular in shape and may appear punched out	May develop at sides of ankles, especially medial malleolus along the course of veins; gangrene absent; painful, shallow, exudative, and have granulation tissue in the base; irregular borders

Adapted from Bickley L (2016) *Bates' Guide to Physical Examination and History Taking,* 12th ed. Philadelphia, Lippincott Williams & Wilkins.

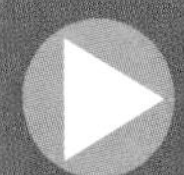

Intervention/Cardiac Rehabilitation

Clinical Exercise Testing

Exercise Tolerance Test, ETT (Graded Exercise Test, GXT)

1. Purpose: to determine physiological responses during a measured exercise stress (increasing workloads); allows the determination of functional exercise capacity of an individual and detects presence of ischemia.
   a. Serves as a basis for exercise prescription. Symptom-limited ETT is typically administered prior to start of Phase II outpatient cardiac rehabilitation program and following cardiac rehabilitation as an outcome measure.
   b. Used as a screening measure for CAD in asymptomatic individuals.
   c. ETT with radionuclide perfusion:
      - A pharmacological stress test is used when patient is unable to perform a regular ETT.
      - Common medications used to increase cardiac demand are adenosine (increases heart rate),

dobutamine (increases contractility), and persantine (vasodilates).
- Imaging is used to detect decreased blood flow to myocardium.

2. Testing modes.
   a. Treadmill and cycle ergometry (leg or arm tests) allow for precise calibration of the exercise workload.
   b. Step test (upright or sitting) can also be used for fitness screening, healthy population.
3. ETT may be maximal or submaximal.
   a. Maximal ETT: defined by target endpoint heart rate. Maximal ETTs should only be completed in settings with ACLS (advanced cardiac life support) trained individuals with appropriate equipment to handle abnormal responses. Risk of abnormal responses increases significantly when working at intensities >85% of heart rate max.
      - Age predicted maximum heart rate.
        - 220 – age: high degree of error associated with it, especially in younger and older adults.
        - 208 – 0.7 × age: less error associated with this across different populations.
      - Heart-rate range (Karvonen's formula): 60%–80% (HR max – resting HR) + resting HR = target HR.
   b. Submaximal ETT: symptom-limited or terminated at 85% of age predicted heart rate max; safe in all settings, used to evaluate the early recovery of patients after MI, coronary bypass, or coronary angioplasty.
4. Continuous ETT: workload is steadily progressed.
   a. Step test: workload increases every 2–3 minutes, allowing the patient to reach steady state.
   b. Ramp test: workload increased every minute so patient is not permitted to reach steady state.
5. Discontinuous (interval) ETT: allows rest in between workloads/stages; used for patients with more pronounced CAD.
6. Positive ETT: indicates myocardial oxygen supply is inadequate to meet the myocardial oxygen demand; positive for ischemia.
7. Negative ETT: indicates that at every tested physiological workload there is a balanced oxygen supply and demand.
8. False-positive ETT: test is interpreted as positive but the patient does not have ischemia.
9. False-negative ETT: test is interpreted as negative but the patient has ischemia.
10. Functional 6-Minute Walk Test (6MWT): patients walk as far as they can in 6 minutes, taking as many rests as needed. Highly correlated to other ETT, submax and maximal VO_2.

Monitoring During Exercise and Recovery

1. Patient appearance, signs and symptoms of excessive effort and exertional intolerance; examine for:
   a. Persistent dyspnea.
   b. Dizziness or confusion.
   c. Anginal pain.
   d. Severe leg claudication.
   e. Excessive fatigue.
   f. Pallor, cold sweat.
   g. Ataxia, incoordination.
   h. Pulmonary rales.
2. Changes in HR: HR increases linearly as a function of increasing workload and oxygen uptake (VO_2), plateaus just before maximal oxygen uptake (VO_2 max).
3. Changes in BP: systolic BP should rise with increasing workloads and VO_2; diastolic BP should remain about the same.
4. Rate pressure product (RPP): the product of systolic BP and HR (the last two digits of a five-digit number are dropped) is often used as an index of myocardial oxygen consumption (MVO_2).
   a. Increased MVO_2 is the result of increased coronary blood flow.
   b. Angina is usually precipitated at a given RPP.
5. Ratings of perceived exertion (RPE): developed by Gunnar Borg. Allows subjective rating of feelings during exercise and impending fatigue. Important to use standardized instructions to reduce misinterpretation.
   a. RPE increases linearly with increasing exercise intensity and correlates closely with exercise heart rates and work rates.
   b. RPE has intra-user reliability over time, but not inter-user reliability. Ratings can be influenced by psychological factors, mood states, environmental conditions, exercise modes, and age.
   c. RPE is an important measure for individuals who do not exhibit the typical rise in HR with exercise (e.g., patients on medications that depress HR, such as beta blockers).
   d. Borg scale: rates exercise intensity using numbers from 6 to 20, with descriptors from very, very light (7) to somewhat hard (13) to very, very hard (19).
   e. Borg CR 10: rates exercise intensity using numbers from 1 to 10 with descriptors from 0 (nothing at all) to very weak (1) to moderate (3) to strong (5) to extremely strong (10).
6. Pulse oximetry: measure arterial oxygen saturation levels (SaO_2) before, during, and after exercise.
7. ECG changes with exercise: healthy individual.
   a. Tachycardia: heart rate increase is directly proportional to exercise intensity and myocardial work.
   b. Rate-related shortening of QT interval.
   c. ST segment depression, upsloping, less than 1 mm.
   d. Reduced R wave, increased Q wave.
   e. Exertional arrhythmias: rare, single PVCs.
8. ECG changes with exercise: an individual with myocardial ischemia and CAD.
   a. Significant tachycardia: occurs at lower intensities of exercise or with deconditioned individuals without ischemia.

b. Exertional arrhythmias: increased frequency of ventricular arrhythmias during exercise and/or recovery.
c. ST segment depression; horizontal or downsloping depression, greater than 1 mm below baseline is indicative of myocardial ischemia.

9. Delayed, abnormal responses to exercise, can occur hours later.
a. Prolonged fatigue.
b. Insomnia.
c. Sudden weight gain due to fluid retention.
d. Hypotension, especially in patients with heart failure.

Ambulatory Monitoring (Telemetry)

1. Continuous 24-hour ECG monitoring.
2. Allows documentation of arrhythmias and of ST segment depression or elevation, silent ischemia (if assessing via 12 leads only).

Transtelephonic ECG Monitoring

1. Used to monitor patients as they exercise at home.

Activity Levels: METs (Metabolic Equivalents)

1. MET: the amount of oxygen consumed at rest (sitting); equal to 3.5 mL/kg per minute.
2. MET levels (multiples of resting VO_2) can be directly determined during ETT: using collection and analysis of expired air; not routinely done.
3. MET levels can be estimated during ETT during steady state exercise; the max VO_2 achieved on ETT is divided by resting VO_2; highly predictable with standardized testing modes.
4. Can be used to predict energy expenditure during certain activities (Table 4-15).

Exercise Prescription

Guidelines for Exercise Prescription

1. The components of aerobic exercise: the FITT principle or Frequency, Intensity, Time, and Type of Exercise.
2. Type (exercise mode).
a. Cardiorespiratory endurance activities: walking, jogging, or cycling recommended to improve exercise tolerance; can be maintained at a constant velocity; very low interindividual variability.
b. Dynamic arm exercise (arm ergometry): uses a smaller muscle mass, results in lower VO_2 max (60%–70% lower) than leg ergometry; at a given workload, HR will be higher, stroke volume lower; systolic and diastolic BPs will be higher.
c. Other aerobic activities: swimming, cross-country skiing; less frequently used due to high interindividual variability, energy expenditure related to skill level.
d. Dancing, basketball, racquetball, competitive activities should not be used with high-risk, symptomatic, and low-fit individuals.
e. Early rehabilitation: activity is discontinuous (interval training), with frequent rest periods; progressing to continuous training. Interval training can also be incorporated in vigorous training

Table 4-15

Metabolic Equivalent (MET) Activity Chart

INTENSITY (70-KG PERSON)	ENDURANCE PROMOTING	ACTIVITY
1.5–2 METs	Too low in energy level	Standing, walking slowly (1 mph)
2–3 METs	Too low in energy level, unless capacity is very low	Level walking (2 mph), level bicycling (5 mph)
3–4 METs	Yes, if continuous and if target heart rate reached	Level walking (3 mph), bicycling (6 mph)
4–5 METs	Recreational activities must be continuous, lasting longer than 2 minutes	Walking (3½ mph), bicycling (8 mph)
5–6 METs	Yes	Walking at brisk pace (4 mph), bicycling (10 mph)
6–7 METs	Yes	Walking at very brisk pace (5 mph), bicycling (11 mph), swimming leisurely (20 yd/min)
7–8 METs	Yes	Jogging (5 mph), bicycling (12 mph)
8–9 METs	Yes	Running (5.5 mph), bicycling (13 mph), swimming (30 yd/min)
>10 METs	Yes	Running 6 mph = 10 METs, 7 mph = 11.5 METs, 8 mph = 13.5 METs, 9 mph = 15 METs, 10 mph = 17 METs; swimming moderate/hard (>40 yd/min)

Adapted from: Fox, Naughton, Gorman. Mod Concepts Cardiovas Dis, 1972, 4:25. American Heart Association.

to allow patient to work at higher percentage of VO_2 max.

f. Warm-up and cool-down activities.
  - Gradually increase or decrease the intensity of exercise, promote circulatory and muscular adjustment to exercise.
  - Type: low-intensity cardiorespiratory endurance activities, flexibility (ROM) exercises, functional mobility activities.
  - Duration: 5–10 minutes.
  - Abrupt beginning or cessation of exercise is not safe or recommended.

g. Resistive exercises: to improve strength and endurance in clinically stable patients.
  - Usually prescribed in later rehabilitation, after a period of aerobic conditioning.
  - Moderate intensities are typically used (e.g., 60%–80% of 1 repetition or 10 repetition maximal voluntary contraction).
  - Monitor responses to resistive training using rate-pressure product (incorporates BP, a safer measure).

RED FLAG: Carefully monitor HR, BP, and breathing during resistive exercise; breath holding can result in a Valsalva's maneuver (forceful exhalation against a closed airway) with a dramatic increase in BP and a reduction of stroke volume and heart output. Proper training during resistance-training is especially important (i.e., exhalation during lifting phase and inhalation during the lowering phase). Resistance training is contraindicated for patients with uncontrolled hypertension or arrhythmias.

h. Relaxation training: relieves generalized muscle tension and anxiety.
  - Usually incorporated following an aerobic training session and cool-down.
  - Assists in successful stress management and lifestyle modification.

3. Intensity: prescribed as percentage of functional capacity revealed on ETT, within a range of 40%–85% depending upon initial level of fitness; typical training intensity is 60%–80% of functional capacity; lower training intensities may necessitate an increase in training duration; most clinicians use a combination of HR, RPE, and METs to prescribe exercise intensity (eliminates problems that may be associated with individual measures).
  a. Heart rate.
    - Percentage of maximum heart rate achieved on ETT; without an ETT, 208 – 0.7 × age. 70%–85% HR max closely corresponds to 60%–80% of functional capacity or VO_2 max.
    - Estimated HR max is used in cases where submaximal ETT has been given.
    - Heart rate range or reserve (Karvonen's formula, see previous description). Can more closely approximate the relationship between HR and VO_2 max, but increased variability in patients on medications. Problems associated with use of HR alone to prescribe exercise intensity.
    - Beta blocking: affects the ability of HR and BP to rise normally in response to exercise.
    - Pacemaker: can affect the ability of HR to rise in response to an exercise stress if it is fixed.
    - Environmental extremes, heavy arm work, isometric exercise, and Valsalva may affect HR and BP responses.
  b. Rating of perceived exertion, the original Borg RPE scale (6–20).
    - Useful along with other measures of patient effort if beta blockers or other HR suppressers are used.
    - Problems with use of RPE alone to prescribe exercise intensity.
      - Individuals with psychological problems (e.g., depression).
      - Unfamiliarity with RPE scale; may affect selection of ratings.
  c. METs, or estimated energy expenditure (VO_2).
    - 40%–85% of functional capacity (maximal METs) achieved on ETT. Without a maximal ETT, this is an estimation of workload.
    - Problems associated with use of METs alone to prescribe exercise intensity.
      - With high-intensity activities (e.g., jogging), need to adopt a discontinuous work pattern: walk 5 minutes, jog 3 minutes to achieve the desired intensity.
      - Varying skill level or stress of competition may affect the known metabolic cost of an activity.
      - Environmental stresses (heat, cold, high humidity, altitude, wind, changes in terrain such as hills) may affect the known metabolic cost of an activity.

4. Time (duration).
  a. Conditioning phase may vary from 10 to 60 minutes, depending upon intensity; the higher the intensity, the shorter the duration.
  b. Average conditioning time is 20–30 minutes for moderate intensity exercise.
  c. Severely compromised individuals may benefit from multiple, short exercise sessions spaced throughout the day (e.g., 3- to 10-minute sessions).
  d. Warm-up and cool-down periods are kept constant; e.g., 5–10 minutes each.

5. Frequency.
  a. Frequency of activity is dependent upon intensity and duration; the lower the intensity, the shorter the duration, the greater the frequency.

b. Average: three to five sessions/week for exercise at moderate intensities and duration, e.g., >5 METs.
c. Daily or multiple daily sessions for low intensity exercise: e.g., <5 METs.

6. Exercise and progressive physical activity regimens require monitoring of heart rate and blood pressure.
7. Progression.
   a. Modify exercise prescription if:
      - HR is lower than target HR for a given exercise intensity.
      - RPE is lower (exercise is perceived as easier) for a given exercise.
      - Symptoms of ischemia (e.g., angina) do not appear at a given exercise intensity.
   b. Rate of progression depends on age, health status, functional capacity, personal goals, preferences.
   c. As training progresses, duration is increased first, then intensity.

RED FLAGS: Consider reduction in exercise/activity with:
- Acute illness: fever, flu.
- Acute injury, orthopedic complications.
- Progression of cardiac disease: edema, weight gain, unstable angina.
- Overindulgence: e.g., food, caffeine, alcohol.
- Environmental stressors: extremes of heat, cold, humidity, air pollution.

RED FLAGS: Adverse responses to inpatient exercise leading to exercise termination (ACSM Guidelines, 2017).
- Diastolic BP equal to or greater than 110 mmHg.
- Decrease in systolic BP >10 mmHg during exercise.
- Significant ventricular or atrial dysrhythmias with or without associated signs/symptoms.
- Second- or third-degree heart block.
- Signs/symptoms of exercise intolerance, including angina, marked dyspnea, and ECG changes suggestive of ischemia.

8. Exercise prescription for post-PTCA (percutaneous transluminal coronary angioplasty).
   a. Wait to exercise vigorously approximately 2 weeks post-PTCA to allow inflammatory process to subside. Walking program can be initiated immediately.
   b. Use post-PTCA ETT to prescribe exercise.
9. Exercise prescription post-CABG (coronary artery bypass grafting).
   a. Limit upper extremity exercise while sternal incision is healing.
   b. Avoid lifting, pushing, pulling for 4–6 weeks post-surgery.

Contraindications for Inpatient and Outpatient Cardiac Rehabilitation (Box 4-1)

BOX 4-1 Contraindications for Inpatient and Outpatient Cardiac Rehabilitation

- Unstable Angina
- Resting SBP >200 mmHg or DBP >110 mmHg
- Orthostatic BP drop of >20 mmHg with symptoms
- Critical aortic stenosis
- Acute systemic illness or fever
- Uncontrolled atrial or ventricular dysrhythmias
- Uncontrolled sinus tachycardia
- Uncompensated CHF
- Third-degree AV block without pacemaker
- Pericarditis or myocarditis
- Recent embolism
- Thrombophlebitis
- Resting ST-segment depression or elevation (>2 mm)
- Uncontrolled diabetes mellitus
- Severe orthopedic conditions that prohibit exercise
- Other metabolic conditions, such as acute thyroiditis, hypokalemia, hyperkalemia, or hypovolemia.

Adapted from ACSM's Guidelines for Exercise Testing and Prescription, 10th ed, 2017.

BOX 4-2 Possible Effects of Physical Training/Cardiac Rehabilitation

- Decreased HR at rest and during exercise; improved HR recovery after exercise
- Increased stroke volume
- Increased myocardial oxygen supply and myocardial contractility; myocardial hypertrophy
- Improved respiratory capacity during exercise
- Improved functional capacity of exercising muscles
- Reduced body fat, increased lean body mass; successful weight reduction requires multifactorial interventions
- Decreased serum lipoproteins (cholesterol, triglycerides)
- Improved glucose tolerance
- Improved blood fibrinolytic activity and coagulability
- Improvement in measures of psychological status and functioning: self-confidence and sense of well-being
- Increased participation in exercise; improved outcomes with adherence to rehabilitation programming
  - Decreased angina in patients with CAD: anginal threshold is raised secondary to decreased myocardial oxygen consumption
  - Reduced total and cardiovascular mortality in patients following myocardial infarction
  - Decreased symptoms of heart failure, improved functional capacity in patients with left ventricular systolic dysfunction
  - Improved exercise tolerance and function in patients with cardiac transplantation

Possible Effects of Physical Training/ Cardiac Rehabilitation (Box 4-2)

Phase 1: Inpatient Cardiac Rehabilitation (Acute)

Length of hospital stay is commonly 3–5 days for uncomplicated MI (no persistent angina, malignant arrhythmias or heart failure).

Exercise/Activity Goals and Outcomes

1. Initiate early return to independence in activities of daily living; typically after 24 hours or until the patient is stable for 24 hours; monitor activity tolerance.
2. Counteract deleterious effects of bed rest: reduce risk of thrombi, maintain muscle tone, reduce orthostatic hypotension, maintain joint mobility.
3. Help allay anxiety and depression.
4. Provide additional medical surveillance of patients.
5. Provide patient and family education.
6. Promote risk factor modification.

Exercise/Activity Guidelines

1. Program components: ADLs, selected arm and leg exercises, early supervised ambulation.
2. Initial activities: low-intensity (2–3 METs) progressing to ≥ 5 METs by discharge.
3. Post-MI: limited to 70% max HR and/or 5 METs until 6 weeks post-MI.
4. Short exercise sessions, two to three times a day; gradually duration is lengthened and frequency is decreased.
5. Postsurgical patients.
   a. Typically are progressed more rapidly than post-MI, unless there was a peri-operative MI.
   b. Lifting activities are restricted, generally for 6 weeks.

Patient and Family Education Goals

1. Improve understanding of cardiac disease, support risk factor modification.
2. Teach self-monitoring procedures, warning signs of exertional intolerance; e.g., persistent dyspnea, anginal pain, dizziness.
3. Teach concepts of energy costs, fatigue monitoring, general activity guidelines, activity pacing, energy conservation techniques; home exercise program (HEP).
4. Provide emotional support and assist with referral to social work as needed.

Home Exercise Program (HEP)

1. Low-risk patients may be safe candidates for unsupervised exercise at home.
   a. Gradual increase in ambulation time: goal of 20–30 minutes, 1–2 times per day at 4–6 weeks post-MI.
   b. Upper and lower extremity mobility exercises.
2. Elderly, homebound patients with multiple medical problems may benefit from a home cardiac rehabilitation program.

3. Patients should be skilled in self-monitoring procedures.
4. Recommend family training in CPR and AED (automated external defibrillator) as indicated; emergency lifeline for some patients.

Phase 2: Outpatient Cardiac Rehabilitation (Subacute)

Eligible Patients

1. MI/acute coronary syndrome.
2. CABG.
3. PCI.
4. Stable angina.
5. Heart valve surgical repair or replacement.
6. Heart or heart/lung transplantation.
7. Heart failure.
8. PAD may not be covered by insurance but this population benefits from a supervised exercise program.

Exercise/Activity Goals and Outcomes

1. Improve functional capacity.
2. Progress toward full resumption of activities of daily living, habitual and occupational activities.
3. Promote risk-factor modification, counseling as to lifestyle changes.
4. Encourage activity pacing, energy conservation; stress importance of taking proper rest periods.

Exercise/Activity Guidelines

1. Outpatient program.
   a. Patients at risk for arrhythmias with exercise, angina, other medical problems benefit from outpatient programs with availability of ECG monitoring, trained personnel, and emergency support.
   b. Group camaraderie and support of program participants may assist in risk-factor modification and lifestyle changes.
   c. Frequency: 2–3 sessions/week.
   d. Duration: 30–60 minutes with 5–10 minutes of warm-up and cool-down.
   e. Programs may offer a single mode of training (e.g., walking) or multiple modes using a circuit training approach (e.g., treadmill, cycle ergometer, arm ergometer); strength training.
   f. Patients are gradually weaned from continuous monitoring to spot checks and self-monitoring.
   g. Suggested exit point: 9 MET functional capacity (5 MET capacity is needed for safe resumption of most daily activities).
2. Strength training in Phase 2 programs.
   a. Guidelines: after 3 weeks cardiac rehab; 5 weeks post-MI, or 8 weeks post-CABG.
   b. Begin with use of elastic bands and light hand weights (1–3 lb).
   c. Progress to moderate loads, 12–15 comfortable repetitions.

Patient and Family Education Goals: Continuation and Progression from Phase 1 Goals

Phase 3: Community Exercise Programs (Postacute, Postdischarge from Phase 2 Program)

Exercise/Activity Goals and Outcomes

1. Improve and/or maintain functional capacity.
2. Promote self-regulation of exercise programs.
3. Promote lifelong commitment to risk-factor modification.

Exercise/Activity Guidelines

1. Location: community centers, YMCA, or clinical facilities.
2. Entry level criteria: functional capacity of 5 METs, clinically stable angina, medically controlled arrhythmias during exercise.
3. Progression is from supervised to self-regulation of exercise.
4. Progression to 50%–85% of functional capacity, 3–4 times/week, 45 minutes or more/session.
5. Regular medical check-ups and periodic ETT generally required.
6. Utilize motivational techniques to maintain compliance with exercise programs, lifestyle modification.
7. Discharge typically in 6–12 months.

Patient and Family Education Goals: Continuation and Progression from Phase 1 Goals

Resistance Exercise Training

Goals and Outcomes

1. Improve muscle strength and endurance.
2. Enhance functional independence.
3. Decrease cardiac demands during daily activities.

Patient Criteria for Resistance Training

1. American Association of Cardiovascular and Pulmonary Rehabilitation Guidelines.
2. Post-MI: resistance training permitted if remain under 70% max HR or 5 METs for 6 weeks post-MI, be cautious of Valsalva with resistance training.

3. Cardiac surgery: lower extremity resistance training can be initiated immediately, in the absence of a peri-operative MI. Upper extremity resistance training should be avoided until soft tissue and bony healing has occurred: 6–8 weeks.
4. Post-transcatheter procedure (PTCA, other): minimum of 3 weeks following procedure and 2 weeks of consistent participation in a supervised CR endurance training program.
5. No evidence of the following conditions: congestive heart failure, uncontrolled dysrhythmias, severe valvular disease, uncontrolled hypertension, and unstable symptoms.

Exercise Prescription

1. Start with low resistance (one set of 10–15 repetitions) and progress slowly.
2. Resistance can include:
   a. Weights, 50% or more of maximum weight used to complete one repetition (1 RM).
   b. Elastic bands.
   c. Light (1- to 5-lb) cuff and hand weights.
   d. Wall pulleys.
3. Perceived exertion (RPE–Borg Scale) should range from 11 to 13 ("light" to "somewhat hard"), but this needs to be correlated to hemodynamic response to activity.
4. Rate-pressure product should not exceed that prescribed during endurance exercise.

Exercise Prescription for Patients Requiring Special Considerations

Heart Failure (HF)

1. Patients demonstrate significant ventricular dysfunction, decreased cardiac output, low functional capacities.
2. Classification Systems (Table 4-16).
3. Criteria for exercise training.
   a. Compensated or chronic HF; no signs of acute HF.
   b. Exercise-induced ischemia and arrhythmias poor prognostic indicators.
4. Exercise training.
   a. General guidelines for physical therapy (see Table 4-17).
   b. Assess for signs of decompensation at each visit: increased SOB; sudden weight gain; increased LE edema or abdominal swelling; increased pain or fatigue; pronounced cough, lightheadedness, or dizziness.
   c. Monitor at rest and during activity.
      - Use RPE that is correlated with objective measures of hemodynamic response (HR, BP, RR, SpO_2) and clinical signs of exertional intolerance.
      - HR response may be impaired (chronotropic incompetence).
      - At risk for persistent post-exercise vasodilation (and hypotension) with later stages of HF.
   d. Use caution exercising in supine or prone positions due to orthopnea.
   e. Avoid breath holding and Valsalva's maneuver.
   f. Respiratory muscle training. Monitoring SaO_2 via pulse oximetry is advisable in some cases.
5. Emphasis on training in energy conservation, self-monitoring techniques.
6. Exercise prescription parameters and guidance for patients with stable, NYHA Class II and III heart failure with reduced ejection fraction (see Tables 4-17 and 4-18).

Table 4-16

Classifications of Heart Failure

NEW YORK HEART ASSOCIATION STAGES	FUNCTION AND SYMPTOMS
Class I: mild HF	No limitation in physical activity (up to 6.5 METs); comfortable at rest, ordinary activity does not cause undue fatigue, palpitation, dyspnea, or anginal pain.
Class II: slight HF	Slight limitation in physical activity (up to 4.5 METs); comfortable at rest, ordinary physical activity results in fatigue, palpitation, dyspnea, or anginal pain.
Class III: marked HF	Marked limitation of physical activity (up to 3.0 METs); comfortable at rest, less than ordinary activity causes fatigue, palpitation, dyspnea, or anginal pain.
Class IV: severe HF	Unable to carry out any physical activity (1.5 METs) without discomfort; symptoms of ischemia, dyspnea, anginal pain present even at rest; increasing with exercise.
AMERICAN COLLEGE OF CARDIOLOGY FOUNDATION (ACCF)/ AMERICAN HEART ASSOCIATION (AHA) STAGES	
Stage A	At high risk for HF but without structural heart disease or symptoms of HF.
Stage B	Structural heart disease but without signs or symptoms of HF.
Stage C	Structural heart disease with prior or current symptoms of HF.
Stage D	Refractory HF requiring specialized interventions.

Cardiac Transplant

1. Patients may present with:
   a. Exercise intolerance due to extended inactivity and deconditioning.

Table 4-17

Key Action Statements for Physical Therapists Treating Patients with Heart Failure with Stable, Class II and III HFrEF (Based on Strength of Evidence Shown in Parentheses)

1. **Advocate for increased total daily physical activity as an essential component of care (A-strong recommendation, Level I).**
2. **Educate on and facilitate chronic disease management behaviors (A-strong recommendation, Level I).**
3. **Prescribe aerobic exercise training (A-strong recommendation, Level I).**
4. **Prescribe high-intensity interval training (A-strong recommendation, Level I).**
5. **Prescribe upper and lower body resistance training (A-strong recommendation, Level I).**
6. Prescribe combined aerobic exercise and resistance training (B-moderate recommendation, Level II).
7. **Prescribe inspiratory muscle training (A-strong recommendation, Level I).**
8. Prescribe combined inspiratory muscle training and aerobic exercise training (B-moderate recommendation, Level II).
9. **Prescribe NMES (A-strong recommendation, Level I).**

HFrEF = heart failure with reduced ejection fraction; NMES = neuromuscular electrical stimulation

Adapted from Shoemaker MJ, Dias KJ, Lefebvre KM, Heick JD, Collins SM. Physical therapist clinical practice guideline for the management of individuals with heart failure. *Phys Ther*. 2020; 100: 14–43.

Level 1 evidence and Grade A recommendations are highlighted in the table with bold font.

   b. Side effects from immunosuppressive drug therapy: hyperlipidemia, hypertension, obesity, diabetes, leg cramps, and proximal muscle weakness.
   c. Decreased lower extremity strength.
   d. Increased fracture risk due to long-term corticosteroid use.
2. Heart rate alone is not an appropriate measure of exercise intensity (heart is denervated and patients tend to be tachycardic). Use combination of HR, BP, RPE, METs, dyspnea scale.
3. Use longer periods of warm-up and cool-down because the physiological responses to exercise and recovery take longer.

Pacemakers and Automatic Implantable Cardioverter Defibrillators (AICDs)

1. Pacemakers are programmed to pace heart rate.
   a. Most are demand pacemakers so that heart will increase as workload increases.
   b. Always have a lower HR limit set, rarely have a upper limit set.
   c. HR will not change with fixed rate pacers, which will impact activity tolerance.
2. AICDs will deliver an electric shock if HR exceeds set limit and/or ventricular arrhythmia is detected.
3. Should know setting for HR limits on AICD.
4. ST segment changes may be common.

Table 4-18

Exercise Prescription Parameters for Patients with Stable, NYHA Class II and III HFrEF

ACTIVITY	EXERCISE PRESCRIPTION
Aerobic exercise	Time: 20–60 minutes Intensity: 50%–90% of peak VO_2 Frequency: 3–5 times/week Duration: 8–12 weeks
High-intensity interval training	Time: >35 minutes Intensity: >90%–95% of peak VO_2 Frequency: 2–3 times/week Duration: 8–12 weeks
Upper and lower body resistance training	Time: 45–60 minute session Intensity: 60%–80% 1 RM Frequency: 3 times per week Duration: 2–3 sets per muscle group, 8–12 weeks
Inspiratory muscle training (IMT)	Time: 30 minutes Intensity: >30% of MIP Frequency: 3 times per week Duration: 8–12 weeks
Neuromuscular electrical stimulation	Biphasic symmetrical pulses 15–50 hertz, on/off time 2/5 seconds, pulse width 200–700 us (large muscles) or 0.5–0.7 ms (small muscles), 20%–30% of MVIC Intensity: to muscle contraction, Frequency: 5–7 days per week Duration: 5–10 weeks

Key: HFrEF = Heart Failure with Reduced Ejection Fraction; MIP/PImax = maximal inspiratory pressure; NYHA = New York Heart Association; VO_2 = oxygen uptake; 1 RM = 1 repetition maximum

Adapted from Shoemaker MJ, Dias KJ, Lefebvre KM, Heick JD, Collins SM. Physical therapist clinical practice guideline for the management of individuals with heart failure. *Phys Ther*. 2020; 100: 14–43.

5. Avoid UE aerobic or strengthening exercises for 4–6 weeks after implant to allow the leads to scar down.
6. Electromagnetic signals may cause devices to fire (defibrillator), or slow down or speed up (pacemaker).
7. With exercise, make sure that the patient's HR remains at least 10 beats below ICD shock and antitachycardia pacing threshold.

Diabetes

1. Patients demonstrate problems controlling blood glucose, with associated cardiovascular disease, renal disease, neuropathy, peripheral vascular disease, and ulceration and/or autonomic dysfunction.
2. Exercise testing.
   a. May need to use submaximal ETT tests; maximal tests can be precluded with autonomic neuropathy.
   b. With PAD/peripheral neuropathy, may need to shift to arm ergometry.
3. Exercise prescription and training. See discussion in Chapter 8 on Diabetes Mellitus.

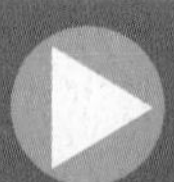

Intervention/Peripheral Vascular Disease

Rehabilitation Guidelines for Arterial Disease

Risk Factor Modification (see Table 4-1)

Limb Protection

1. Avoid excessive strain, protection of extremities from injury, and extremes of temperature.
2. Bed rest may be required if gangrene, ulceration, acute arterial disease are present.

Exercise Training for Patients with PAD

1. May result in improved functional capacity, improved peripheral blood flow via collateral circulation and muscle oxidative capacity.
2. Consider interval training (multistage protocol) with frequent rests.
3. Walking until the patient cannot tolerate pain; it is more effective for collateral circulation to walk at a level of 2 or 3 on the claudication scale, but most patients cannot tolerate this level of pain. An interval program is used with stops until the pain subsides for a total of 30–60 minutes, 3–5 days per week.
4. Record time of pain onset and duration.
5. Non–weight-bearing exercise (cycle ergometry, arm ergometry) may be necessary in some patients; less effective in producing a peripheral conditioning effect.
6. Well-fitting shoes essential; with insensitive feet, teach techniques of proper foot inspection and care.
7. Beta blockers for treatment of hypertension or cardiac disorders may decrease time to claudication or worsen symptoms.
8. Pentoxifylline, dipyridamole, aspirin, and warfarin may improve time to claudication.
9. High risk for CAD.

Lower Extremity Exercise

1. Resistive calf exercises: most effective method of increasing blood flow.
2. Modified Buerger-Allen exercises: postural exercises to promote blood flow.
   a. 3 positions: supine with lower extremities elevated to 45°–90° and supported until feet blanch (turn white), sitting with lower extremities in dependent position until feet turn red/pink, supine for a few minutes.
   b. Can add active plantar and dorsiflexion of the ankle in each position.
   c. Active exercises improve blood flow during and after exercise.
   d. Effects are less pronounced in patients with PAD.

Medical Treatment

1. Medications to decrease blood viscosity, prevent thrombus formation; e.g., heparin.
2. Vasodilators: controversial.
3. Calcium channel blockers in vasospastic disease.

Surgical Management

1. Atherectomy, thromboembolectomy, laser therapy.
2. Revascularization: angioplasty or bypass grafting.
3. Sympathectomy: results in permanent vasodilation, improvement of blood flow to skin.
4. Amputation when gangrene is present.

Rehabilitation Guidelines for Venous Disease

Venous Thromboembolism (VTE)

1. Identification of patients who are at high risk of VTE.
   a. Requires knowledge of signs and symptoms and risk factors.
   b. Use standardized Risk Assessment Measure (e.g., Wells Criteria Score for DVT) (see Table 4-13).
2. Initiate preventive measures: prompt referral to physician, team members.
3. Once therapeutic levels of medication are achieved (e.g., low molecular weight heparin), initiate ambulation and leg exercises (activation of the calf muscle pump).
4. Bed rest is not recommended following diagnosis of VTE once acceptable levels of medication are reached unless there are significant medical concerns.
5. Utilize mechanical compression: graded compression stockings (GCS) with at least 30 mmHg of pressure at the ankle.
6. A trial of intermittent pneumatic compression (IPC) may be appropriate for patients with severe postthrombotic syndrome (PTS) of the leg not adequately relieved with graded compression stockings (GCS).
7. Mobilize patients after IVC filter placement once hemodynamically stable.
8. Provide education to decrease risk of recurring VTE.
9. Assess for fall risk and institute measures to reduce fall risk.

10. See Box 4-3 Synopsis of Clinical Practice Guidelines: Management of Individuals with Venous Thromboembolism (VTE).

Chronic Venous Insufficiency (CVI)

1. Management of edema.
   a. Positioning: extremity elevation, minimum of 18 cm above heart. Encourage patients to elevate leg as much as possible and avoid the dependent position.
   b. Compression therapy.
      - Bandages (elastic, tubular); applied within 20 minutes of rising.
      - Paste bandages (Unna boot). Gauze impregnated with zinc oxide, gelatin, and glycerine; applied for 4–7 days (less with some wounds).
      - Graduated compression stockings with a pressure gradient of 30–40 mmHg.
      - Compression pump therapy, used for a 1- to 2-hour session twice daily.

> **RED FLAG:** Consider contraindications of compression therapy which include an ABI <0.8 in the involved extremity, signs of active cellulitis or infection, systemic arterial pressure <80 mmHg, advanced peripheral neuropathy and uncontrolled congestive heart failure.

   c. Exercise.
      - Active ankle exercises: emphasis on muscle pump exercises (dorsiflexion/plantarflexion, foot circles).
      - Cycle ergometry in sitting or attached to foot of bed.
      - Early ambulation as soon as patient is able to get out of bed, three to four times/day.
2. Patient education: meticulous skin care.
3. Severe conditions with dermal ulceration may require surgery (ligation and vein stripping, vein grafts, valvuloplasty).

BOX 4-3 Synopsis of Clinical Practice Guidelines: Management of Individuals with Venous Thromboembolism (VTE)

Etiology/Diagnosis

- **Screen for risk of VTE (A—strong recommendation; Level I)**
- **Communicate likelihood of LE DVT and recommend further medical testing (A—strong recommendation; Level I)**
- Screen for fall risk (C—weak recommendation; Level III)

Examination

- Identify the likelihood of LE DVT when signs and symptoms are present (B—moderate recommendation; Level II)
- **Communicate the likelihood of LE DVT and recommend further medical testing (A—strong recommendation; Level I)**

Interventions

- **Provide preventive measures for LE DVT (A—strong recommendation; Level I)**
- **Recommend mechanical compression as a preventive measure for DVT (A—strong recommendation; Level I)**
- Recommend mechanical compression for patients with LE DVT (B—moderate recommendation; Level II)
- **Mobilize patients who are at a therapeutic level of anticoagulation (A—strong recommendation; Level I)**
- Verify the patient is taking an anticoagulant (E—theoretical/foundational recommendation; Level V)
- Mobilize patients after IVC filter placement once hemodynamically stable (F—best practice; Level V)
- Consult with medical team when a patient is not anticoagulated and without an IVC filter (F—best practice; Level V)
- Provide management strategies to prevent recurrent VTE and minimize secondary VTE complications (F—best practice; Level V)
- **Advocate for a culture of mobility and physical activity (A—strong recommendation; Level I)**

Adapted from Hillegass E, et al, for the Guideline Development Group: Role of physical therapists in the management of individuals at risk for or diagnosed with venous thromboembolism: Evidence-based clinical practice guideline. *Phys Ther.* 2016; 96(2): 143–166.

See Table 16-4 in Chapter 16 for Levels of Evidence and Grades of Recommendations.

Level 1 evidence and Grade A recommendations are highlighted in the table with bold font.

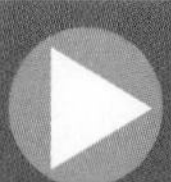

Lymphatic System

The Lymphatic System

1. A network of lymphatic vessels that withdraws excess tissue fluid (lymph) from the body's interstitial spaces, filters it through lymph nodes, and returns it to the bloodstream via the venous system.

Components (See Figure 4-10)

1. Lymphatic vessels (superficial, intermediate, deep) (see Figure 4-11).
2. Lymph fluid.
3. Lymph nodes.
   a. Submandibular.
   b. Cervical.
   c. Upper extremity (see Figure 4-12).
      - Supraclavicular.
      - Axillary.
         - Central.
         - Subscapular.
         - Pectoral.
         - Humeral.
      - Cubital.
   d. Parasternal.
   e. Mesenteric.
   f. Lower extremity.
      - Iliac.
      - Inguinal.
      - Popliteal.
4. Lymph tissues (mucosa associated lymphoid tissue, or MALT).
5. Organs.
   a. Spleen.
   b. Tonsils.
   c. Thymus.
   d. Bone marrow.

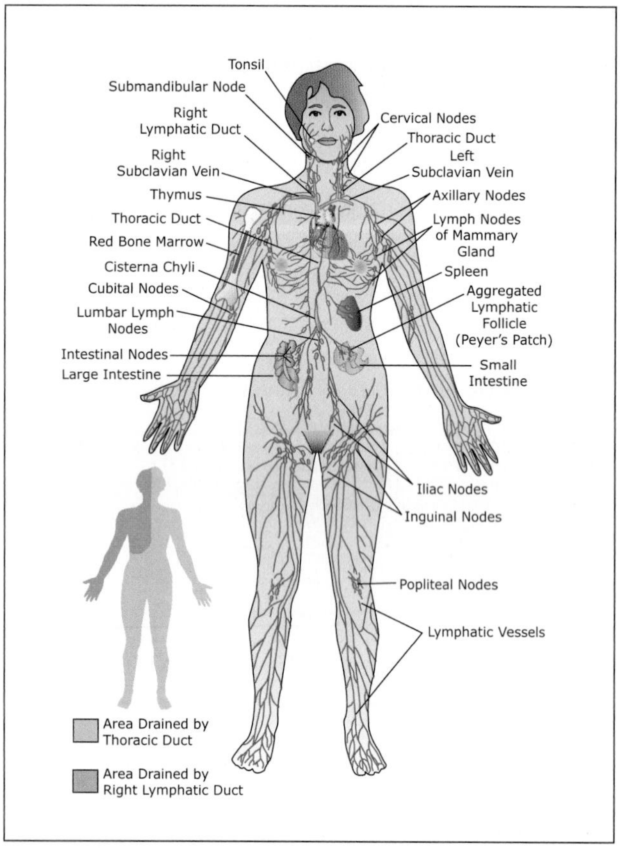

Figure 4-10 **Lymphatic system.**

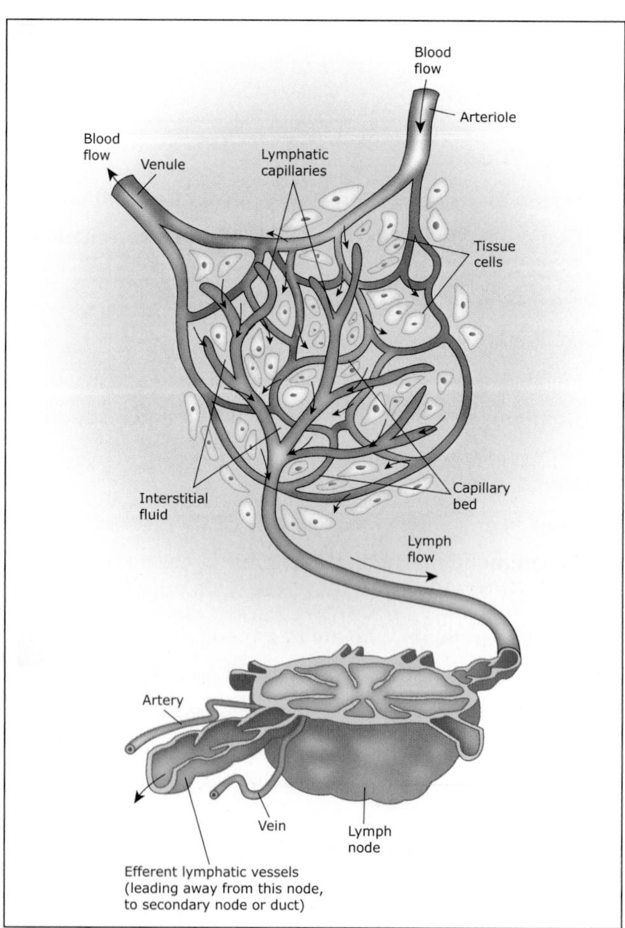

Figure 4-11 **Lymph vessels and nodes.**

Adapted from Moore KM, et al (2014). *Clinically Oriented Anatomy*, 7th ed. Philadelphia, Lippincott, Williams & Wilkins.

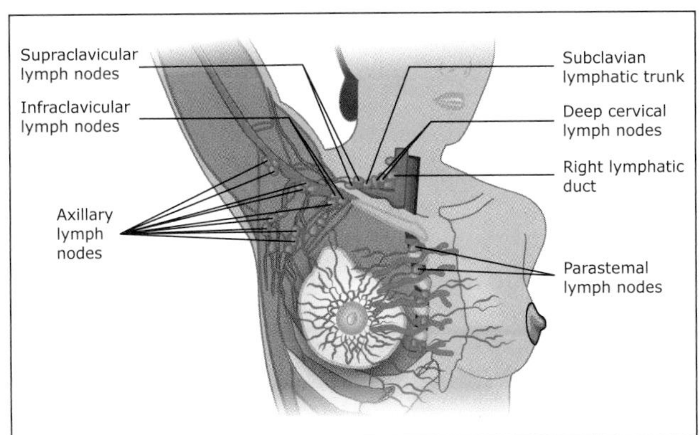

Figure 4-12 Axillary lymph nodes and lymphatic drainage of upper extremity and breast.

Adapted from Moore KM, et al (2014). *Clinically Oriented Anatomy*, 7th ed. Philadelphia, Lippincott, Williams & Wilkins.

Lymph Circulation

1. Lymph travels from the lymphatic capillaries to lymphatic vessels to large lymphatic ducts (right lymphatic duct, thoracic duct to the subclavian veins).

Lymphatic Vessel Contraction Occurs by

1. Autonomic and sensory nerve stimulation.
2. Contraction of adjacent muscles.
3. Abdominal and thoracic cavity pressure changes during normal breathing.
4. Mechanical stimulation of dermal tissues.
5. Volume changes within individual lymphatic vessels.

Pathophysiology/Common Pathologies

Lymphedema

1. Chronic disorder characterized by excessive accumulation of lymph fluid due to mechanical insufficiency of the lymphatic system (obstruction of lymph flow or removal of lymph nodes).
2. Lymph fluid volume exceeds the transport capacity/capability of lymph vessels.
3. Results in swelling of the soft tissues of the upper and lower extremities.
4. Primary lymphedema: a congenital or hereditary disorder with abnormal lymph node or lymph vessel formation.
5. Secondary lymphedema: acquired insult to the lymphatic system. Most commonly seen after surgery for breast or cervical cancer. Possible causes include:
   a. Surgery including lymph node removal.
   b. Tumors, trauma, or infection involving lymphatic system structures.
   c. Radiation therapy.
   d. Chronic venous insufficiency.
   e. Filariasis (parasitic infection of the lymphatic system; seen in tropical and subtropical regions).
6. Stages of lymphedema.
   a. Stage 0: at risk; swelling is not yet evident despite reduced transport capacity of the system. Also called the latent or pre-clinical stage.
   b. Stage 1: reversible; early accumulation of fluid with visible swelling; pitting edema that resolves with elevation (reversible pitting edema); Stemmer's sign is negative.
   c. Stage 2: spontaneously irreversible; increase in swelling; elevation does not reduce the swelling; positive Stemmer's sign.
   d. Stage 3: elephantiasis; fibrotic deep skinfolds; skin may change color; skin changes may limit mobility.
7. Differential diagnosis.
   a. Lipedema (see Figure 4-13).
      - Excessive subcutaneous fat deposition.
      - Appearance may be similar to lymphedema.
      - Normal function of the lymphatic system.
      - Symmetrical swelling of extremities.
      - Negative Stemmer's sign.
      - Seen typically in women (may be seen associated with hormonal changes during pregnancy and puberty).

Lymphadenopathy

1. Enlargement of lymph nodes, with or without tenderness.
2. Typically caused by an infection.
3. Localized lymphadenopathy: enlargement of lymph nodes in just one body region.
4. Generalized lymphadenopathy: enlargement of lymph nodes in two or more body regions.
5. Lymphadenitis describes lymphadenopathy accompanied by signs of inflammation such as redness and tenderness.

Lymphangitis

1. An acute bacterial (often streptococcus) or viral infection that spreads throughout the lymphatic system.
2. Red streaks are often seen in the skin proximal to the infection site.

Examination: History, Tests, and Measures

History

1. Presenting symptoms. In patients who are at risk for secondary lymphedema.
   a. Observable swelling.
   b. Sensation of tightness, heaviness, or fullness in the affected area.

c. Tight fit of clothing or jewelry.
d. Aching sensation.
2. Known risk factors.
   a. Primary (idiopathic): congenital abnormality—hypoplasia, hyperplasia, aplasia.
   b. Secondary (acquired): caused by a known insult to the lymphatic system.
      - Cancer: seen most often in breast and cervical cancer.
         - Lymph node removal.
         - Radiation therapy.
      - Venous disease.
      - Trauma: any condition that may damage or impede lymph flow (e.g., burns, scars, wounds).
      - Cardiac disease: complications from heart failure.
      - Dependent edema.
      - Filariasis: a mosquito-borne illness and the most common cause outside of the United States.

Past Medical History

1. Other diagnoses, surgeries, infections, or cellulitis.
   a. If patient has a history of cancer, then ask:
      - Surgical history (node removal or biopsy).
      - Status of cancer diagnosis.
      - History of radiation, chemo, or hormonal therapy.
2. Medications.
3. Current use of preventive measures for previously asymptomatic patients at risk.
   a. Compressive garments.
   b. Community services and support.
4. Activities that may expose patient to risk.

Social History

1. Family and social support.
2. Living arrangements.
3. Education level/employment.
4. Impact of lifestyle on risk factors.

Quality of Life Issues

1. Impact on functional status.
2. Activities of daily living.
3. Sleep.
4. Past and present level of function.

Physical Examination

1. Assessment of swelling.
   a. Volumetric measurements—in unilateral disease lymphedema is considered present if >10% increase compared to unaffected side.
      - Water displacement.
      - Girth measurement.
      - Bioimpedance—used primarily in bilateral disease and for distinguishing between lipedema and lymphedema.
   b. Pitting edema.
2. Skin assessment: changes in appearance, dryness, scars, wounds, ulcers, skin folds, or fibrotic tissue.
   a. Lymphangiectasia: dilation of lymph vessels, may appear as blister-like protuberances.
   b. Lymphorrhea: leakage of lymph from the skin surface.
   c. Papillomatosis: development of warty growths on the skin that contain dilated lymph vessel and fibrous tissue.
   d. Lipodermatosclerosis: thickening and hardening of the subcutaneous tissue and brown skin discoloration. This is associated with chronic venous insufficiency and, when severe, can damage lymph tissue.
   e. Stemmer's sign. Stemmer's sign is a clinical sign for lymphedema indicated by the presence of a thickened fold of skin at the base of the 2nd toe or 2nd finger. The sign is positive if the skin cannot be lifted but only grasped as a lump of tissue. It is negative if the skin can be normally grasped and pulled away from the underlying tissue.
3. Vascular assessment.
   a. Ankle-Brachial Index (ABI): skin disorders may impact the accuracy of this test.
   b. Alternative assessments may include pulse oximetry, assessment of distal pulses, and tests for arterial and venous insufficiency.
   c. Blood pressure should not be assessed on the affected side.
4. Lymph node palpation.
   a. Soft, moveable, nontender lymph nodes are normal.
   b. Soft, tender lymph nodes that move easily is a sign of inflammation and/or infection. Their presence may correlate with a known illness. If not, patient should be referred to a physician.
   c. Hard, immobile lymph nodes are typically indicative of metastatic cancers and the patient should be referred to a physician.
5. Pain assessment: determine source (e.g., inflammatory, compression, entrapment).
   a. Procedural pain: pain associated with treatment of lymphedema.
   b. Incident pain: pain caused by daily activities.
   c. Background pain: intermittent or continuous pain at rest.
6. Neurological assessment: paresthesia may be present.
7. Postural assessment: changes in limb/body shape and weight may impact posture.
8. Range of motion assessment: changes in limb/body shape and weight may impact active and passive movements.
9. Compensatory movements: changes in limb/body shape and weight may impact movement.

10. Functional assessment.
    a. Changes in mobility. Important to assess suitability of footwear.
    b. Impact on ADLs.
    c. Assessment of sleep quantity and quality.
11. Nutritional status: assessment of body weight.
12. Psychosocial assessment.
    a. Screen for depression.
    b. Anxiety.
    c. Cognitive impairment.
    d. Lack of motivation.
    e. Inability to cope.
    f. Understand disease and treatment.
13. Differential diagnosis.
    a. Lipedema (see Figure 4-13).
14. Differentiate lymphedema from other disorders that affect extremities unilaterally or bilaterally.
    a. Unilateral: acute deep vein thrombosis, post-thrombotic syndrome, arthritis, Baker's cyst.
    b. Bilateral: CHF, chronic venous insufficiency, dependency or stasis edema, renal dysfunction, hepatic dysfunction, lipedema.

Diagnostic Tests

1. Imaging.
    a. Ultrasound: Assess soft tissue for thickening and fibrosis.
    b. Doppler Ultrasound: Used to exclude venous disorders (e.g., DVT).
    c. Lymphoscintigraphy: Identifies lymphatic insufficiency and performed at rest and with exercise.
    d. CT/MRI: evaluates skin thickening and traditional honeycomb patterns in soft tissue. Also differentiates between lipedema and lymphatic obstruction by a foreign mass.
2. Laboratory tests.
    a. Most cases of lymphedema are diagnosed based on the medical history and physical examination.
    b. Other lab tests are used to elucidate the cause of the swelling and to identify comorbidities: CBC, urea and electrolytes, thyroid function tests, liver function tests, fasting glucose, erythrocyte sedimentation rate, plasma total protein, and albumin.
    c. See Table 4-19 for summary.

	Lymphedema	Lipedema
		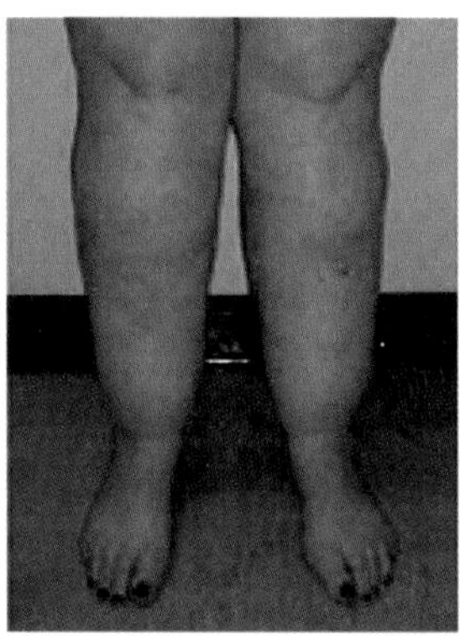
Signs and symptoms	Can involve the legs, arms, trunk, genitalia or head and neck Swelling of limbs affects hands and feet Affects either sex Stemmer sign may be positive; usually not painful on pinching	Usually causes symmetrical bilateral swelling of the lower limbs; can occur in arms Swelling stops at ankles and wrists Pain and bruising are prominent features Affects mainly women In pure lipedema, Stemmer sign is negative; often painful on pinching
Etiology	Result from inadequate lymphatic drainage May be congenital or result from damage to the lymphatic system Not usually associated with hormonal imbalances	Unknown; results in excessive subcutaneous fat deposition Appears to be estrogen-related and starts at the time of hormonal change, e.g., pregnancy, puberty Family history of lipedema often positive

Figure 4-13 **Differential diagnosis: lymphedema vs. lipedema.**

Table 4-19

Lymphedema Summary

ETIOLOGY	Primary lymphedema: congenital Secondary lymphedema: occurs as a result of injury to lymphatic vessels (e.g., cancer surgery and/or radiation, chronic venous insufficiency) or parasitic infection (filariasis)
PROGRESSIVE OVER TIME	Without treatment, may develop into fibrosis, chronic infection (cellulitis, lymphangitis) or loss of limb function
SYMPTOMS	Heaviness, tightness or pain; swelling and persistent edema; loss of ROM and function in an arm or leg
SKIN CHANGES	Hardening and/or discoloration of skin
DIAGNOSIS	History, visual inspection and palpation, girth measurements Tests may include: MRI and CT scans; Doppler ultrasound, radionuclide imaging of the lymphatic system (lymphoscintigraphy)
STAGING	4 stage system: 0 – latent; 1 – spontaneously reversible; 2 – spontaneously irreversible; 3 – lymphostatic elephantiasis (American Society of Lymphology)
TREATMENT	Complete decongestive therapy (CDT): Manual lymph drainage, short-stretch compression bandages, exercises, functional training, skin care, and lymphedema education.

Intervention/Rehabilitation Guidelines for Lymphedema

Intervention for Asymptomatic Patients Who Are at Risk for Lymphedema

1. Meticulous skin and nail care: apply moisturizer regularly, avoid sunburn, and avoid blisters and injuries that could risk infection.
2. Lifestyle management.
   a. Weight management and gradual increases in activity: avoid sports that incorporate centrifugal forces (e.g., golf, tennis).
   b. Avoid sudden heavy lifting.
   c. Mosquito nets for areas where filariasis may be prevalent.
3. Avoid limb constriction.
   a. No blood pressure checks on affected side.
   b. Loose-fitting jewelry and clothing.
4. Compression garments.
   a. Ensure a good fit.
   b. Wear when exercising or flying.
5. Avoid temperature extremes.
   a. No temperatures above 102 degrees in hot tub/saunas.
   b. Avoid extreme cold.
   c. Use high factor sunscreen.

Phase I Management: Edema Secondary to Lymphatic Dysfunction

1. Complete decongestive therapy (CDT).
   a. Manual lymphatic drainage (MLD).
      - Massage (Vodder techniques, modifications by Asdonk, Leduc, and Fodi). Technique requires very low pressure effleurage strokes.
      - Emphasis is on decongesting proximal segments first at the right lymphatic duct (for right upper extremity involvement) and the thoracic duct (for left upper extremity, lower extremities, and the torso).
      - Compression using multilayered padding and short-stretch bandages.
        - Bandages have low resting and high working pressure.
          - Bandages preserve and advance changes associated with MLD and account for 50% of improvement in symptoms.
        - Treatments should be applied by certified specialists: certified lymphedema therapist (CLT).
        - Specialized education resources for MLD and CDT.
          - National Lymphedema Network: http://www.lymphnet.org.
          - Lymphology Association of North America: https://www.clt-lana.org.

RED FLAG: Patients with significant or poorly controlled cardiopulmonary disease may become unstable if they are not able to tolerate the potential increase in plasma volume caused by lymphedema reduction.

   b. Compression bandaging/garments.
      - Short-stretch compression bandages, worn 24 hours per day.
      - Bandages have low resting and high working pressure.
      - Bandages preserve and advance changes associated with MLD and may account for 50% of improvement in symptoms.
      - Must monitor distal symptoms and swelling for excessive pressure in off-the-shelf or customized garments.

RED FLAG: Excessively high pressures will occlude superficial lymph capillaries and restrict fluid absorption.

   c. Exercise.
      - Decongestive exercises work with bandages to compress lymph between the bandage and muscles to move fluid proximally.
      - Walking and cycling program.
      - Water-based programs: water aerobics, swimming.

- Tai chi and balance activities.
- ADL training.

> RED FLAG: Strenuous activities, jogging, ballistic movements, and rotational motions are contraindicated, as they are likely to exacerbate lymphedema.

- Be aware of lymph overload symptoms: discomfort, aching, or pain in proximal lymph areas, change in skin color. If any are present, discontinue activity.

d. Skin care: hygiene, skin care, nail care.
- Protein rich fluids reduce local immune systems.
- Bacterial infections are common: streptococcus, cellulitis.
- Prevention of skin/nail problems.
  - Regular inspection: caregiver assistance if needed.
  - Regular cleansing.
  - Regular moisturizing: Maintain a pH of 5.0 on skin.
  - Protection: Appropriate footwear, use of appropriate socks.

e. Patient education (regarding skin care, garment wear, and other lymphedema self-management principles).

2. Contraindicated modalities.
   a. Modalities that cause vasodilation or increase lymph load (e.g., ice, heat, hydrotherapy, saunas, contrast bath, paraffin).
   b. Electrotherapeutic modalities greater than 30 Hz.

Phase II Management

1. Continue with CDT components/principles.
2. Skin care.
3. Compression garments: may use lymphedema bandaging at night.
4. Exercise: combined with compression garments.
5. Pneumatic compression pumps used with caution.
   a. High pressures can damage lymph nodes.
   b. May move water instead of proteins.
   c. Use on lower extremity increases risk of genital lymphedema.
   d. Low pressure, sequential pumps are preferred.
   e. Use in Stage I lymphedema only: do not use if there is any change in skin or subcutaneous tissue, exacerbation of inflammation and fibrosis can occur in Stage II and Stage III patients.

> RED FLAG: Pressures >45 mmHg are contraindicated.

6. MLD as needed.
   a. Specialized education resources for MLD and CDT.
      - National Lymphedema Network: http://www.lymphnet.org.
      - Lymphology Association of North America: https://www.clt-lana.org.
7. Patient education.
   a. Skin and nail care.
   b. Self-bandaging, garment care.
   c. Infection prevention/management.
   d. Maintain exercise while preventing lymph overload.
8. Surgery to assist in lymph drainage (severe cases).
   a. Surgical reduction: de-bulking subcutaneous tissue and skin in severe cases of those who are considerably symptomatic. Significant risk of postsurgical morbidity.
   b. Restoring lymph flow: lymphovenous anastomoses and lymphatic vessel grafting and lymph node transplantation. Successful in patients with intact distal lymph and proximal lymph obstruction.
   c. Liposuction: may be considered for patients with nonpitting lymphedema and when other conservative measures have failed. Must use compressive garments postsurgically.

Outcome Measures/Self-Report Instruments

1. Lymphoedema Quality of Life (LYMQOL).
2. Lymph-ICF.
3. Lymphedema Life Impact Scale (LLIS).

APPENDIX 4A

Selected Outcome Measures for Cardiac, Pulmonary, and Lymphatic Dysfunction

Table 4A-1

OUTCOME MEASURES	REFERENCES
Chronic Respiratory Questionnaire	• Larson JL, Covey MK, Berry JK, et al: Reliability and validity of the Chronic Respiratory Disease Questionnaire. *Am J Crit Care Med.* 1993; 147: A350. • Guyatt GH, Berman LB, Townsend M, et al: A measure of quality of life for clinical trials in chronic lung disease. *Thorax.* 1987; 42: 773–778. • Jaeschke R, Singer J, Guyatt GH. Measurement of health status ascertaining the minimal clinically important difference. *Controlled Clin Trials.* 1989; 10: 407–415. • Guyatt GH, King DR, Feeny DH, et al: Generic and specific measurement of health-related quality of life in a clinical trial of respiratory rehabilitation. *J Clin Epidemiol.* 1999; 52: 187–192. • Lacasse Y, Wong E, Guyatt G. A systematic overview of the measurement properties of the Chronic Respiratory Questionnaire. *Canadian Respiratory Journal.* 1997; 4(3): 131–139.
St. George's Respiratory Questionnaire	• Jones PW, Quirk FH, Baveystock CM. The St. George's Respiratory Questionnaire. *Resp Med.* 1991; 85(suppl): 25–31. • Jones PW, Quirk FH, Baveystock CM, et al: A self-complete measure of health status for chronic airflow limitation. *Am Rev Respir Dis.* 1992; 145: 1321–1327.
6-Minute Walk Test	• American Thoracic Society: ATS statement: Guidelines for the Six-Minute Walk Test. *Am J Respir Crit Care Med.* 2002; 166: 111–117. • Guyatt GH, Townsend M, Keller J, et al: Measuring functional status in chronic lung disease: conclusions from a random control trial. *Respir Med.* 1991; 85(Suppl B): 17–21. • Rasekaba T, Lee A, Naughton MT, et al: The six-minute walk test: a useful metric for the cardiopulmonary patient. *Internal Medicine Journal.* 2009; 39: 495–501. • Casanova C, Cote CG, Marin MJ, et al: The 6-min walking distance: long-term follow up in patients with COPD. *Eur Respir J.* 2007; 29(3): 535–540. • Casanova C, Cote CG, Marin MJ, et al: Validation and comparison of reference equations for the 6-min walk distance test. *Eur Respir J.* 2008; 31: 571–578.

(*Continued*)

Table 4A-1 (Continued)

OUTCOME MEASURES	REFERENCES
Walking Speed	• Fritz S, Lusardi M: White paper: Walking speed: the sixth vital sign. *J Geriatr Phys Ther.* 2009; 32(2): 46–9. Erratum in: *J Geriatr Phys Ther.* 2009; 32(3): 110. • Andersson M, Moberg L, Svantesson U, et al: Measuring walking speed in COPD: test-retest reliability of the 30-metre walk test and comparison with the 6-minute walk test. *Prim Care Respir J.* 2011; 20: 434–440. • Dolmage TE, Evans RA, Hill K, et al: The effect of pulmonary rehabilitation on critical walk speed in patients with COPD: a comparison with self-paced walks. *Chest.* 2012; 141(2): 413–419. • Afilalo J, Eisenberg MJ, Morin JF et al. Gait speed as an incremental predictor of mortality and major morbidity in elderly patients undergoing cardiac surgery. *J Am Coll Cardiol.* 2010; 56(2): 1668–1676.
10-meter Shuttle Walk Test	• Singh SJ, Morgan MDL, Hardman AE, et al: Comparison of oxygen uptake during a conventional treadmill test and the shuttle walking test in chronic airflow limitation. *Eur Respir J.* 1994; 7: 2016–2020. • Revill SM, Morgan MDL, Singh SJ, et al: The endurance shuttle walk: a new field test for the assessment of endurance capacity in chronic obstructive pulmonary disease. *Thorax.* 1999; 54: 213–222. • Singh SJ, Morgan MDL, Scott S, et al: Development of a shuttle walking test of disability in patients with chronic airways obstruction. *Thorax.* 1992; 47: 1019–1024. • Morales FJ, Martinez A, Mendex M, et al. A shuttle walk test for assessment of functional capacity in chronic heart failure. *Am Heart J.* 1999; 138(2Pt1): 291–298. • Morales FJ, Montemayor T, Martinez A. Shuttle versus six-minute walk test in the prediction of outcomes in chronic heart failure. *Int J Cardiol.* 2000; 76(2–3): 101–105.
BODE Index	• Celli BR, Cote CG, Marin JM, et al: The body-mass index, airflow obstruction, dyspnea, and exercise capacity index in chronic obstructive pulmonary disease. *N Engl J Med.* 2004; 350: 1005–1012. • Mannino DM, Buist AS: Global burden of COPD: risk factors, prevalence, and future trends. *Lancet.* 2007; 370: 765–773. • Cote CG, Pinto-Plata VM, Marin JM, et al: The modified BODE index: validation with mortality in COPD. *Eur Respir J.* 2008; 32: 1269–1274. • Martinez FJ, Han MK, Andrei AC: Longitudinal change in the BODE index predicts mortality in severe emphysema. *Am J Respir Crit Care Med.* 2008; 178: 491–499.
Kansas City Cardiomyopathy Questionnaire	• Garin O, Herdman M, Vialgut G et al. Assessing health related quality of life in patients with heart failure: a systematic, standardized comparison of available measures. *Heart Fail Rev.* 2013. • Green CP, Porter CB, Bresnahan DR, Spertus JA. Development and evaluation of the Kansas City Cardiomyopathy Questionnaire: a new health status measure for heart failure. *J Am Coll Cardiol.* 2000; 35(5): 1245–1255.
Inspiratory/Respiratory Muscle Training	• Cahalin LP, Arena R, Guazzi M et al. Inspiratory muscle training in heart disease and heart failure: a review of the literature with a focus on method of training and outcomes. *Expert Rev Cardiovasc Ther.* 2013; 11(2): 161–177. • Plentz RD, Sbruzzi G, Ribeiro RA, Ferreira JB, Dal Lago P. Inspiratory muscle training in patients with heart failure: meta-analysis of randomized trials. *Arq Bras Cardiol.* 2012; 99(2): 762–771.
Minnesota Living with Heart Failure Questionnaire	• Garin O, Herdman M, Vialgut G et al. Assessing health related quality of life in patients with heart failure: a systematic, standardized comparison of available measures. *Heart Fail Rev.* 2013. • Rector TS. Overview of the Minnesota Living with Heart Failure Questionnaire. 1/1/05. https://docs.google.com/a/umn.edu/viewer?a=v&pid=sites&srcid=dW1uLmVkdXx0bXN8Z3g6MjQxYWMzOTBkMWYwMjAwZA
Walking Impairment Questionnaire	• Jain A, Lui K, Ferrucci L et al. Declining walking impairment questionnaire scores are associated with subsequent increased mortality in peripheral artery disease. *J Am Coll Cardiol.* 2013; 61(17): 1820–1829. • Jain A, Lui K, Ferrucci L et al. The Walking Impairment Questionnaire stair-climbing score predicts mortality in men and women with peripheral artery disease. *J Vasc Surg.* 2012; 55(6): 1662–1673. • Nead KT, Zhou M, Diaz Caceres R, Olin JW, Cooke JP, Leeper NJ. Walking impairment questionnaire improves mortality risk prediction models in high-risk cohort independent of peripheral arterial disease status. *Circ Cardiovasc Qual Outcomes.* 2013; 6(3): 255–261.
Lymphedema Quality of Life Questionnaire (LYMQOL)	• Keeley V, Crooks S, Locke J, et al: A quality of life questionnaire for limb lymphoedema (LYMQOL). *J Lymphoedema* 2010; 5(1): 26–37.
Lymphedema Life Impact Scale (LLIS)	• Weiss J, Daniel T: Validation of the Lymphedema Life Impact Scale Version 2: a condition-specific measurement tool for persons with lymphedema. *Rehab Oncol.* 2018; 36: 28–36.
Lymph-ICF	• Devoogdt N, Van Kampen M, Geraerts I, et al: Lymphoedema functioning, disability and health questionnaire: reliability and validity. *Phys Ther.* 2011; 91: 944–957.

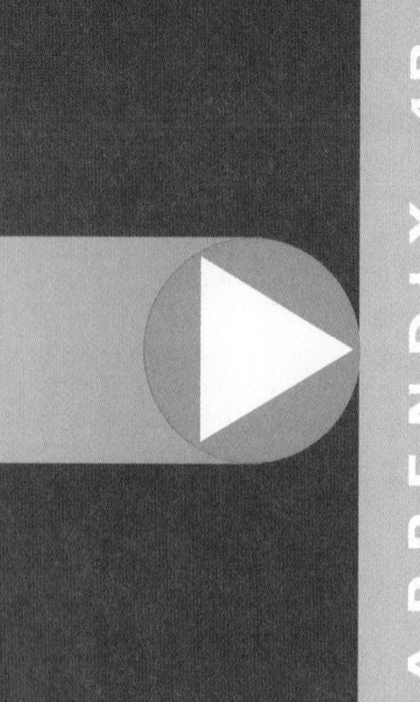

APPENDIX 4B

Review Questions and Case Study

(Answers to all Review Questions and Case Studies can be found in Chapter 17)

1. What risk factors contribute to the development of coronary artery disease?

2. What are the expected ST segment changes following an acute myocardial infarction and with impaired coronary perfusion?

3. How would you instruct your patient regarding possible circumstances that could elicit angina pectoris?

4. When exercising a patient with diabetes and coronary artery disease who is taking beta blockers, what is the best measure to monitor exercise performance?

5. What are the goals of inpatient cardiac rehabilitation in the acute stage or Phase 1?

6. When managing edema secondary to lymphatic dysfunction, use of manual lymph drainage (MLD) emphasizes which directional principles?

Cardiovascular Case Study

Patient Profile

Gender: Male
Age: 84

Presenting Problem/Current Condition

- Seen in emergency room for primary complaint of chest tightness
- Cardiac enzymes were positive for myocardial infarction
- Had surgery for 3-vessel coronary artery bypass graft
- Physical therapy consulted to initiate phase 1 cardiac rehabilitation

Past Medical History

- Hypertension
- Hyperlipidemia
- Smokes 1 pack per day × 60 years

Other Information

- Patient is postoperative day #3 with usual postoperative course
- Patient lives alone and uses a cane to ambulate
- Patient has fallen 3 times in the last month

Question #1

What would the therapist expect on the initial physical therapy examination?

1. Asymmetric breathing pattern.
2. Increased peripheral edema.
3. Effective cough.
4. Normal breath sounds.

Question #2

The first time the patient mobilizes from supine to standing, he demonstrates a drop in blood pressure (supine: 128/72, standing: 106/68). What is the MOST likely explanation for this response?

1. This drop in blood pressure response with position changes is normal and should not be concerning to the physical therapist.
2. The patient has decreased intravascular volume postoperatively and is demonstrating orthostatic hypotension.
3. The workload of the activity was too high, and the patient is unable to maintain their cardiac output.
4. The lack of activity in standing is causing the blood pressure to drop.

Question #3

The physical therapist designs a phase 1 walking program for the patient. What is the MOST appropriate program?

1. Continuous walking for 20 minutes at 80% of HRmax.
2. Continuous walking for 30 minutes at 70% of HRmax.
3. Interval walking for a total of 20 minutes, 1 minute walk at 60% of HRmax, rest 1 minute.
4. Interval walking for a total of 30 minutes, 30 seconds walking at 75% of HRmax, rest 1 minute.

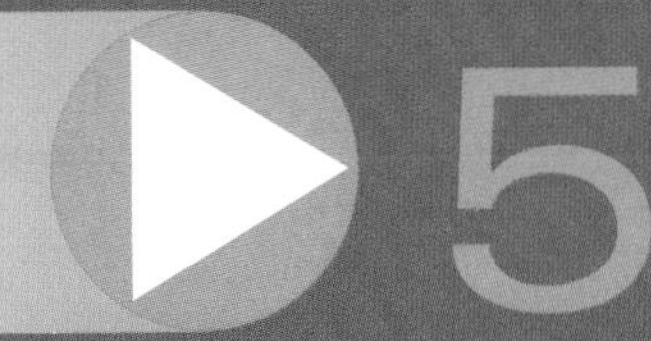

5

Pulmonary Physical Therapy

KELLY MACAULEY

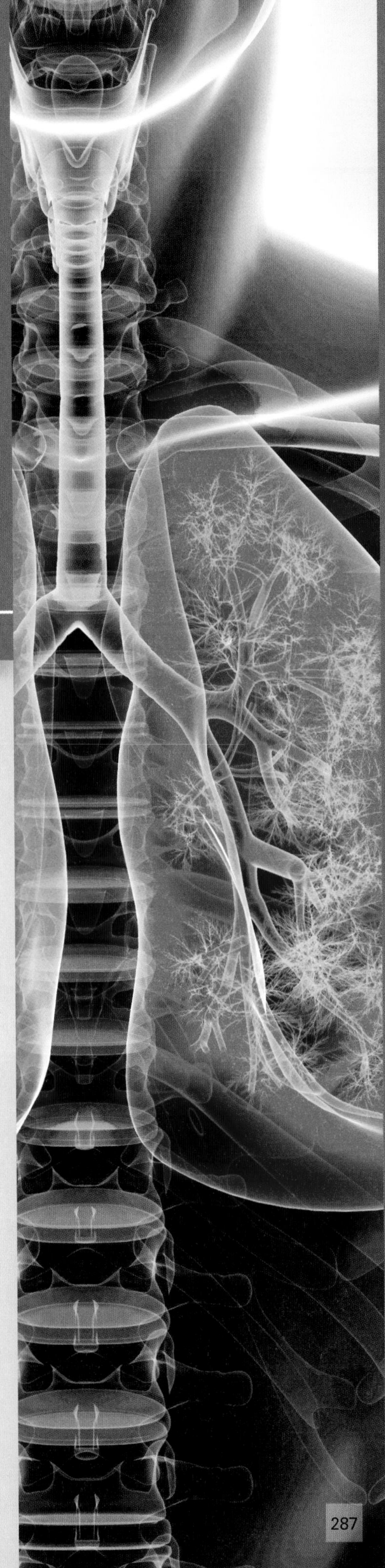

Chapter Outline

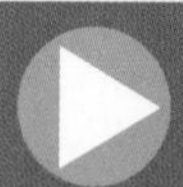

Study Tactics

Questions About the Cardiovascular and Pulmonary Systems Comprise 13% of the NPTE, or a Total of 23–28 Questions. The Two Systems Are Grouped Together in the NPTE Content Outline. The Number of Questions for the Pulmonary System Alone Is Not Specified in the Content Outline

The Number of Questions By Category Are:

- Examination of the Patient/Client: 7–9
- Evaluation, Differential Diagnosis, Prognosis: 8–9
- Interventions: 8–10

Examination of the Patient/Client. Focus on:

- Anatomy and physiology of the pulmonary system. Comprehensive foundational science knowledge of the pulmonary system is critical to understanding components of the examination.
- Movement analysis as related to the pulmonary system. This includes ventilation mechanics such as rib cage excursion and breathing patterns, and the muscles responsible for those actions.
- Locations of the lobes of the lungs and relevant surface landmarks as they relate to auscultation points for lung sounds
- Tests and measures of pulmonary system function. These include respiration rate, spirometry, pulmonary function tests, and ratings of perceived exertion.
- Knowledge of classification of breath sounds (rales, wheezes, crackles, etc.), breathing patterns and observable signs such as sputum color, nail bed and lip color, labored breathing, etc.
- Pain referral patterns related to lung neoplasms such as a Pancoast tumor
- Pulmonary system outcomes measures and their application to effective patient management and interventions

Evaluation, Differential Diagnosis, and Prognosis. Focus on:

- Major pulmonary disorders seen by physical therapists across the lifespan. These include pneumonias (aspiration, bacterial, viral), tuberculosis, emphysema, asthma, cystic fibrosis, pneumothorax, hemothorax, atelectasis, bronchitis, bronchiectasis, and ventilation mechanics problems due to spinal cord injuries, neuromuscular disorders (Parkinson's, multiple sclerosis, stroke), and burns
- Differences between obstructive and restrictive pulmonary disorders. Differential diagnosis questions may test knowledge of these differences, to include interpretation of pulmonary function tests and graphs.
- The clinical features (signs and symptoms) and differential diagnosis of prevalent pulmonary conditions across the lifespan
- Development of a plan of care to include prognosis for common pulmonary disorders
- Medical management and diagnostic studies of the pulmonary systems to include imaging, laboratory tests, and surgical procedures
- Actions and potential side effects of pharmacological management of pulmonary disorders

Interventions. Focus on:

- Physical therapy interventions for pulmonary conditions and their applications for rehabilitation, health promotion, and performance according to current best evidence
- Specific interventions for pulmonary disorders. Intervention questions may also test knowledge of specific techniques such as positioning for postural drainage, breathing exercises, suctioning, percussion, and cough stimulation techniques (autogenic drainage, diaphragmatic breathing, sustained maximal inspiration, pursed-lip breathing, etc.) for a given spinal cord injury level.
- Exercise prescription for patients with pulmonary conditions. Knowledge of the FITT principle (frequency, intensity, time, and type of exercise) may be important.
- Safety considerations. Recognition of when to stop (or not start) exercise based on the patient's pulmonary status or response to exercise is crucial.
- Potential adverse side effects or complications on the pulmonary system from physical therapy interventions

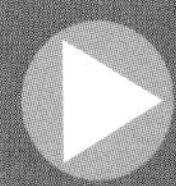

Pulmonary Anatomy and Physiology

Bony Thorax

Anterior Border: The Sternum (Manubrium, Body, Xiphoid Process)

1. The lateral borders of the trachea run perpendicularly into the suprasternal notch.
2. The angle of Louis (sternal angle), the bony ridge between the manubrium and body, is the point of anterior attachment of the second rib and tracheal bifurcation.

Lateral Border: The Rib Cage

1. Ribs 1–6, termed true or costosternal ribs, have a single anterior costochondral attachment to the sternum.
2. Ribs 7–10, termed false or costochondral ribs, share costochondral attachments before attaching anteriorly to the sternum.
3. Ribs 11 and 12 are termed floating or costovertebral ribs, as they have no anterior attachment.

Posterior Border

1. The vertebral column, from T1 through T12.

Shoulder Girdle

1. Can affect the motion of the thorax.
2. Provides attachments for accessory muscles of ventilation.

Internal Structures

Upper Airways (See Figure 5-1)

1. Nose or mouth: entry point into the respiratory system. The nose filters, humidifies, and warms air.
2. Pharynx: common area used for both respiratory and digestive systems.
3. Larynx: connects the pharynx to trachea, including the epiglottis and vocal cords.

Lower Airways

1. The conducting airways, trachea to terminal bronchioles, transport air only. No gas exchange occurs.
2. The respiratory unit: respiratory bronchioles, alveolar ducts, alveolar sacs, and alveoli. Diffusion of gas occurs through all of these structures.

Lung Structures

1. Right lung divides into three lobes by the oblique and horizontal fissure lines. Each lobe divides into segments, totaling 10 segments.
2. Left lung divides into two lobes by a single oblique fissure line. Each lobe divides into segments, totaling eight segments.

Pleura

1. Parietal pleura covers the inner surface of the thoracic cage, diaphragm, and mediastinal border of the lung.
2. Visceral pleura wraps the outer surface of the lung, including the fissure lines.
3. Intrapleural space is the potential space between the two pleurae that maintains the approximation of the rib cage and lungs, allowing forces to be transmitted from one structure to another.

Muscles of Ventilation

Primary Muscles of Inspiration

1. Produce a normal resting tidal volume.
2. Primary muscle of inspiration is the diaphragm. The diaphragm is made of two hemidiaphragms, each with a central tendon. When the diaphragm is at rest, the hemidiaphragms are arched high into the thorax. When the muscle contracts, the central tendon is pulled downward, flattening the dome. The result is a protrusion of the abdominal wall during inhalation.

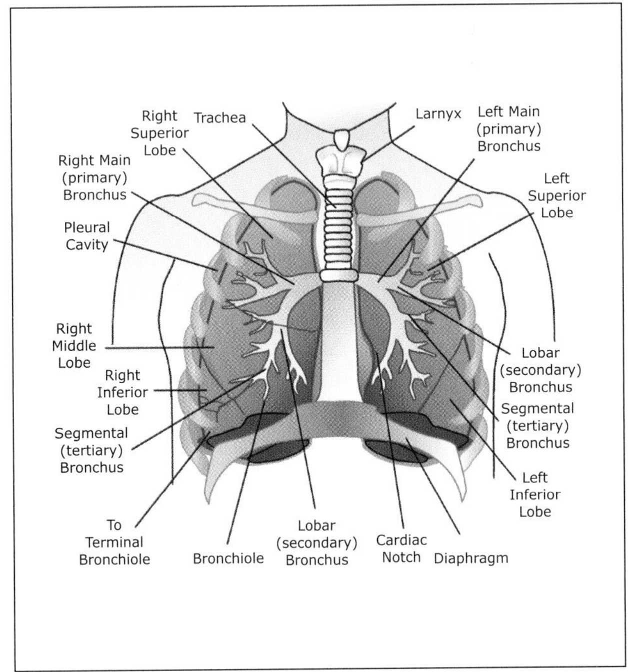

Figure 5-1 Pulmonary anatomy.

3. Additional primary muscles of inspiration are portions of the intercostals.

Accessory Muscles of Inspiration

1. Used when a more rapid or deeper inhalation is required or in disease states.
2. The upper two ribs are raised by the scalenes and sternocleidomastoid. The rest of the ribs are raised by the levator costarum and serratus. By fixing the shoulder girdle, the trapezius, pectorals, and serratus can become muscles of inspiration.

Expiratory Muscles of Ventilation

1. Resting exhalation results from a passive relaxation of the inspiratory muscles and the elastic recoil tendency of the lung. Normal abdominal tone holds the abdominal contents directly under the diaphragm, assisting the return of the diaphragm to the normal high domed position.
2. Expiratory muscles are used when a quicker and/or fuller expiration is desired, as in exercise or in disease states. These are quadratus lumborum, portions of the intercostals, muscles of the abdomen, and triangularis sterni.

Patients Who Lack Abdominal Musculature (e.g., Spinal Cord Injury)

1. Have a lower resting position of the diaphragm, decreasing inspiratory reserve.
2. The more upright the body position, the lower the diaphragm and the lower the inspiratory capacity.
3. The more supine the body position, the more advantageous the position of the diaphragm.
4. An abdominal binder may be helpful in providing support to the abdominal viscera, assisting ventilation. Care must be taken not to constrict the thorax with the abdominal binder.

Mechanics of Breathing

Forces Acting upon the Rib Cage

1. Elastic recoil of the lung parenchyma pulls the lungs and, therefore, visceral pleura, parietal pleura, and bony thorax into a position of exhalation (inward pull).
2. Bony thorax pulls the thorax and, therefore, parietal pleura, visceral pleura, and lungs into a position of inspiration (outward pull).
3. Muscular action pulls either outward or inward, depending on the muscles used.
4. Resting end expiratory pressure (REEP) is the point of equilibrium where these forces are balanced. Occurs at end tidal expiration.

Ventilation

Volumes (See Figure 5-2)

1. Tidal volume (TV): volume of gas inhaled (or exhaled) during a normal resting breath.
2. Inspiratory reserve volume (IRV): volume of gas that can be inhaled beyond a normal resting tidal inhalation.
3. Expiratory reserve volume (ERV): volume of gas that can be exhaled beyond a normal resting tidal exhalation.
4. Residual volume (RV): volume of gas that remains in the lungs after ERV has been exhaled.

Capacities. Two or More Lung Volumes Added Together

1. Inspiratory capacity (IRV + TV): the amount of air that can be inhaled from the resting end-expiratory position (REEP).
2. Vital capacity (IRV + TV + ERV): the amount of air that is under volitional control; conventionally measured as forced expiratory vital capacity (FVC).
3. Functional residual capacity (ERV + RV): the amount of air that resides in the lungs after a normal resting tidal exhalation.
4. Total lung capacity (IRV + TV + ERV + RV): the total amount of air that is contained within the thorax during a maximum inspiratory effort.

Flow Rates

1. Forced expiratory volume in 1 second (FEV1): the amount of air exhaled during the first second of FVC. In the healthy person, at least 70% of the FVC is exhaled within the first second (FEV1/FVC × 100%>70%).
2. Forced expiratory flow rate (FEF 25%–75%) is the slope of a line drawn between the points 25% and

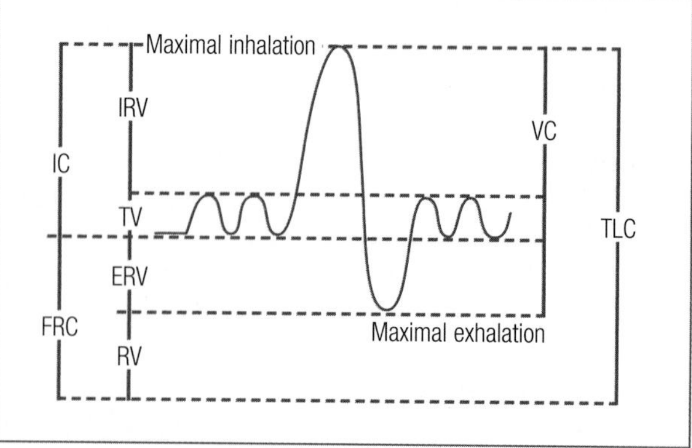

Figure 5-2 Lung volumes and capacities.

IRV = inspiratory reserve volume; TV = tidal volume; ERV = expiratory reserve volume; RV = residual volume; IC = inspiratory capacity; FRC = functional residual capacity, VC = vital capacity; TLC = total lung capacity.

From O'Sullivan S, Schmidt T: Physical Rehabilitation, 7th ed. FA Davis, 2019, p. 435, with permission.

75% of exhaled volume on a forced vital capacity exhalation curve. This flow rate is more specific to the smaller airways and shows a more dramatic change with disease than FEV1.

Pressures

Pressures (See Tables 5-1 and 5-2)

1. Maximal inspiratory pressure (MIP): maximal pressure that is generated during inspiration.
2. Maximal expiratory pressure (MEP): maximal pressure that can be generated during expiration.
3. MIP and MEP are measures of ventilatory muscle strength.
4. MIP values are used as a guide for intubation and are indicative of some disorders including neuromuscular diseases.

Respiration

Diffusion of Gas Across the Alveolar-Capillary Membrane

Arterial Oxygenation

1. Partial pressure of oxygen in the atmosphere (PaO_2) at sea level is 760 mmHg (barometric pressure) × 21% (fraction of inspired oxygen) = 159.6 mmHg.
2. Partial pressure of oxygen in the arterial blood, PaO_2, depends on the integrity of the pulmonary system, the circulatory system, and the PAO_2 (partial pressure of oxygen in the alveolus). Normal PaO_2 at room air is 95–100 mmHg in a young, healthy individual. Hypoxemia: PaO_2 decreases with age, but in a young, healthy individual, mild hypoxemia would be considered at <90 mmHg. Hyperoxemia: PaO_2 >100 mmHg.
3. Fraction of oxygen in the inspired air (FiO_2) is the percentage of oxygen in air, based on a total of 1.00. The FiO_2 of room air, approximately 21% oxygen, is written as 0.21. Supplemental oxygen increases the percentage (>21%) of oxygen in the patient's atmosphere.
4. The PaO_2 is related to pulse oximetry (SpO_2) by the oxyhemoglobin curve. A normal PaO_2 of 90–100 mmHg equates to a SpO_2 of 98%–100%, which is also normal. Between 55–60 mmHg is the point at which oxygen dissociates more quickly from hemoglobin. This corresponds to an SpO_2 of 88%–90%. At this point, supplemental O_2 should be considered.

Alveolar Ventilation

1. Ability to remove carbon dioxide from pulmonary circulation and maintain pH.
2. pH indicates the concentration of free-floating hydrogen ions within the body. Normal range for pH is 7.35–7.45.
3. $PaCO_2$: the normal partial pressure of carbon dioxide within the arterial blood is 35–45 mmHg. Hypercapnea is a $PaCO_2$ >45 mmHg. Hypocapnea is a $PaCO_2$ <35 mmHg. Removal or retention of CO_2 by the respiratory system alters the pH of the body in an inverse relationship. An increase in the $PaCO_2$ decreases the body's pH. A decrease in the $PaCO_2$ raises the body's pH.
4. HCO_3^-: amount of bicarbonate ions within the arterial blood, normally 22–28 mEq/L. Removal or retention of HCO_3^- alters the pH of the body in a direct relationship. An increase in bicarbonate ions increases the body's pH. A decrease in bicarbonate ions decreases the body's pH.

Ventilation (V_E) and Perfusion (Blood Flow or Q)

Optimal Respiration

1. Occurs when ventilation and perfusion (blood flow to the lungs) are matched.
2. Different ventilation and perfusion relationships exist.

Table 5-1

Reference Values for Maximal Inspiratory Pressures (MIP)

AGE	FEMALE cmH_2O	MALE cmH_2O
18–29	97.0	128
30–39	89.0	128.5
40–49	92.9	117.1
50–59	79.7	108.1
60–69	75.1	92.7
70–83	65.3	76.2

Reference: IMB Sclauser Pessoa, V Franco Parreira, GAF Fregonezi, AW Sheel, F Chung, WD Reid. Reference values for maximal inspiratory pressure: a systematic review. *Can Respir J.* 2014; 21(1): 43–50.

Table 5-2

Reference Equations for MIP and MEP in Adults (in cmH_2O)

GENDER	MAXIMAL INSPIRATORY PRESSURE	MAXIMAL EXPIRATORY PRESSURE
Female	108 – (0.61 × age)	131 – (0.86 × age)
Male	120 – (0.41 × age)	174 – (0.83 × age)

Reference: Evans JA, Whitelaw WA. The assessment of maximal respiratory mouth pressures in adults. *Respiratory Care* 2009; 54(10): 1348–1359.

Dead Space

1. Dead space is a space that is well ventilated, but in which no respiration (gas exchange) occurs.
2. Two types of dead space: anatomical (conducting airways) or physiological (diseases such as pulmonary emboli).

Shunt

1. Complete atelectasis of a respiratory unit allows the blood to travel through the pulmonary capillary without gas diffusion.
2. No respiration occurs due to such pathologies as pneumonia, pulmonary edema, or alveolar collapse.

Effects of Body Position on the Ventilation Perfusion Relationship

1. Gravity affects the distribution of ventilation and perfusion.
2. Upright position.
   a. Perfusion is gravity dependent; i.e., more pulmonary blood is found at the base of the lung in the upright position.
   b. Ventilation. At the static point of REEP, the apical alveoli are fuller than those at the base. During the dynamic phase of inspiration, more air will be delivered to the less-filled alveoli at the bases, causing a greater change in V_E (minute ventilation) at the bases.
   c. Ventilation perfusion ratio (V/Q ratio): the ratio of pulmonary alveolar ventilation to pulmonary capillary perfusion. In the upright position, the apices are least effected by gravity (gravity independent), with the lowest perfusion, or Q. Although relatively low, there is still more air than blood, resulting in a high V/Q ratio (dead space). Perfusion and ventilation of the middle zone of the lung are evenly matched. The bases are gravity dependent and therefore have the most Q. Although V_E is relatively high, there is more blood than air, resulting in a (relatively) low V/Q ratio (shunt).
3. Other body positions. Every body position creates these zones: gravity independent, middle, and gravity dependent. The gravity-independent area of the lung, despite the position of the body, acts as dead space. The gravity-dependent area of the lung acts as a shunt. Body positions can be used for a variety of treatment goals: to drain secretions, to increase ventilation, or to optimize ventilation perfusion relationships.

Control of Ventilation

Receptors

1. Baroreceptors, chemoreceptors, irritant receptors, and stretch receptors within the body assist in adjusting the ventilatory cycle by sending information to the controller.

Central Control Centers

1. Cortex, pons, medulla, and autonomic nervous system evaluate the receptors' information.
2. Send a message out to the ventilatory muscles to alter the respiratory cycle in order to maintain adequate alveolar ventilation and arterial oxygenation.

Physical Therapy Examination

Patient Interview

Information from the Patient, the Patient's Family, and the Medical Record

Chief Complaint

1. Usually involves the loss of function (decreased ability to perform activities of daily living [ADLs]) or discomfort (shortness of breath [dyspnea]).

Present Illness

1. Initial onset (sudden vs. insidious) and progression of primary problem.
2. Anything that worsens or improves condition: positions, rest, medications, certain activities, and environmental conditions.

Review the Patient's History

1. Occupational history. Past occupational exposures for diseases such as asbestosis, silicosis, and pneumoconiosis. Present occupational exposure to antigens within the workplace (hypersensitivity pneumonitis).
2. Past medical history that would alter physical exam or treatment plans (e.g., heart disease, long-term steroid use).
3. Current medications that can mask (steroids) or alter (beta blockers, bronchodilators) vital signs.
4. Social habits.
   a. Smoking in pack years (number of packs per day × number of years smoked).
   b. Alcohol consumption.
   c. Recreational drugs.
5. Functional and exertional activity level during periods of wellness, as well as with present illness.

6. Cough and sputum production. Record any changes from baseline because of present illness.
7. Family history of pulmonary disease (e.g., cystic fibrosis).

Tests and Measures

Vital Signs (See Table 5-3 for Normal Values)

1. Temperature: normal (afebrile) 98.6°F (37°C). Core temperature increase indicates infection.
2. Heart rate (HR).
3. Blood pressure.
4. Respiration. See Examination of Respiration in Chapter 4.
   a. Oxygenation: normal SpO_2 98%–100%.
5. Oxygenation.
   a. SaO_2 is the percent saturation of oxygen in the arterial blood. This noninvasive measurement relates to the PaO_2 on the oxyhemoglobin desaturation curve. Normal levels are 98%–100%.
   b. The pulse oximeter utilizes a finger sensor (or an ear, temporal artery, or toe sensor) to obtain a consistent reading.
   c. Error is increased with pulse oximeter in patients with poor circulation, nail deformities, nail polish, or during movement.

Observation

1. Peripheral edema seen in gravity-dependent areas and jugular venous distension indicates possible heart failure. Right ventricular hypertrophy and dilation (cor pulmonale) are common sequelae to chronic lung disease.
2. Body positions: Stabilizing the shoulder girdle (e.g., sitting, hands placed on seat, arms extended, body leaning forward) places the thorax in the inspiratory position and allows the additional recruitment of muscles for inspiration (pectorals).
3. Color: Cyanosis, an acute sign of hypoxemia, is a bluish tinge to nail beds and the areas around eyes and mouth.

Table 5-3

Normal Values for Infants and Adults

PARAMETER	INFANT	ADULT
Heart Rate	120 bpm	60–100 bpm
Blood Pressure	75/50 mmHg	<120/80 mmHg
Respiratory Rate	40 br/min	12–20 br/min
PAO_2	75–80 mmHg	80–100 mmHg
$PaCO_2$	34–54 mmHg	35–45 mmHg
pH	7.26–7.41	7.35–7.45
Tidal Volume	20 ml	500 ml

4. Digital clubbing: a sign of chronic hypoxemia. The configuration of the distal phalanx of fingers or toes becomes bulbous.

Inspection and Palpation

1. Standard precautions should be used when the therapist may come in contact with a patient's body fluids. Gloves are usually all that is needed during a routine physical exam.
2. Neck.
   a. Observe the trachea: it should be in midline, superior to the suprasternal notch.
   b. Note the use of accessory muscles of ventilation.
3. Thorax.
   a. Changes in bony thorax (pectus excavatum, carinatum).
   b. Observe anterior-posterior-lateral dimension. In health, there is a 1:2 ratio. With obstructive pulmonary disease, the lung recoil force is decreased, resulting in a barreled chest and an increase in the A-P dimension.
   c. The right and left thorax should be symmetrical.
      - Symmetry, static and/or dynamic, may be altered by changes in the bony thorax (scoliosis, scapular immobility, pain), changes in the underlying lung and pleura (a patient with pleuritic pain or pneumothorax), or changes in the overlying skin (thoracic burn).
      - (b) Thoracic excursion in healthy adults, measured at the base of the lungs from full inspiration to end tidal volume expiration, is between 2 and 3 inches.
      - Thoracic excursion in health, measured at the base of the lungs from full inspiration to full expiration, is between 2 and 3 inches.
      - Inspect for scars, indicating potential adhesions to underlying soft tissue or surgical removal of structures within the thorax.

Auscultation

1. Intensity of inspiration and expiration is quieter at the bases than the apex.
   a. Vesicular (normal breath sound): a soft rustling sound heard throughout all of inspiration and the beginning of expiration.
   b. Bronchial: a more hollow, echoing sound normally found only over the right superior anterior thorax. This corresponds to an area over the right main stem bronchus. All of inspiration and most of expiration are heard with bronchial breath sounds.
   c. Bronchovesicular: intermediate breath sound between bronchial and vesicular with equal periods of inspiration and expiration.
   d. Decreased: a very distant sound not normally heard over a healthy thorax; allows only some of the inspiration to be heard. Often associated with obstructive lung diseases.

2. Adventitious (extra) sounds. According to the American Thoracic Society, there are only two adventitious breath sounds:
   a. Crackles (also termed rales, crepitations): a crackling sound heard usually during inspiration that indicates pathology (atelectasis, fibrosis, pulmonary edema).
   b. Wheezes: a musically pitched sound, usually heard during expiration, caused by airway obstruction (asthma, chronic obstructive pulmonary disease [COPD], foreign body aspiration). With severe airway constriction, as with croup, wheezes may be heard on inspiration as well.
3. Vocal sounds.
   a. Normal transmission of vocal sounds.
      - As with breath sounds, vocal transmission is loudest near trachea and main-stem bronchi.
      - Words should be intelligible, though softer and less clear at the more distal areas of the lungs.
   b. Abnormal transmission of vocal sounds may be heard through fluid-filled areas of consolidation, cavitation lesions, or pleural effusions.
      - Egophony is a nasal or bleating sound heard during auscultation. "E" sounds are transmitted to sound like "A."
      - Bronchophony, characterized by an intense, clear sound during auscultation, even at the lung bases.
      - Whispered pectoriloquy occurs when whispered sounds are heard clearly during auscultation.

Radiographic Examination

1. See Table 5-4.

Laboratory Tests (See Table 5-3 for Normal Values)

1. Arterial blood gas (ABG) analysis indicates the adequacy of:
   a. Alveolar ventilation by determining pH, bicarbonate ion, and partial pressure of carbon dioxide.

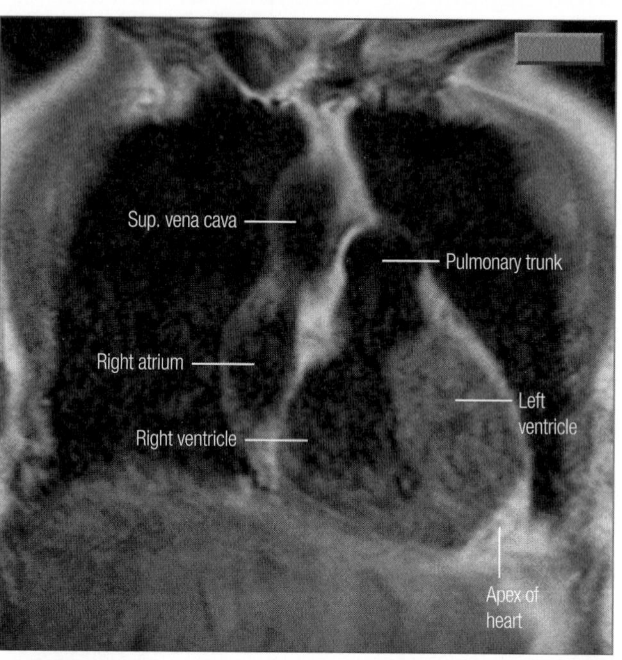

Figure 5-3 **Coronal T1 MRI thoracic view of normal female.**

Table 5-4

Pulmonary Medical Tests and Measures

TEST	USE
IMAGING	
Bronchoscopy	Endoscope used to view, biopsy, wash, suction, dilate, and/or brush the interior aspects of the tracheobronchial tree
Chest film or x-ray (CXR)	Two-dimensional radiographic film to detect the presence of abnormal material (exudate, blood) or a change in pulmonary parenchyma (fibrosis, collapse)
Computed tomography (CT scan)	Computer-generated picture of a cross-sectional plane of the body
Fluoroscopy	Continuous x-ray beam that allows observation of diaphragmatic excursion
Magnetic resonance imaging (MRI)	Provides detailed, sequenced images; especially good for detecting soft tissue issues including lung cancer, perfusion deficits, and interstitial disease (see Figure 5-3)
PET scan	Radioactive tracer is injected or inhaled and images taken. Areas of increased uptake indicate active process. Used often in cancer diagnosis and treatment.
Ventilation-perfusion (V/Q) scan	Assesses airflow and blood flow to match the ventilation pattern of the lung to the perfusion pattern. A mismatch in radioactive tracer identifies the presence of pulmonary emboli.
OTHER	
D-dimer	Assess level of fibrin d-dimer in blood. Elevated levels can indicate PE or DVT.
Thoracentesis	Removal of pleural fluid from intrapleural space for diagnostic (review of cytology) or therapeutic (large volume removal to alleviate dyspnea) purposes

Table 5-5

Interpretation of Abnormal Acid-Base Balance

TYPE	pH	$PaCO_2$	HCO_3^-	CAUSES	SIGNS AND SYMPTOMS
Respiratory alkalosis	↑	↓	WNL	Alveolar hyperventilation	Dizziness, syncope, tingling, numbness, early tetany
Respiratory acidosis	↓	↑	WNL	Alveolar hypoventilation	Early: anxiety, restlessness, dyspnea, headache Late: confusion, somnolence, coma
Metabolic alkalosis	↑	WNL	↑	Bicarbonate ingestion, vomiting, diuretics, steroids, adrenal disease	Vague symptoms: weakness, mental dullness, possibly early tetany
Metabolic acidosis	↓	WNL	↓	Diabetic, lactic, or uremic acidosis, prolonged diarrhea	Secondary hyperventilation (Kussmaul breathing), nausea, lethargy, coma

Roy S, Wolf S, and Scalzitti: The Rehabilitation Specialist's Handbook, 4th ed, Philadelphia, FA Davis, 2013, pg. 520, with permission.

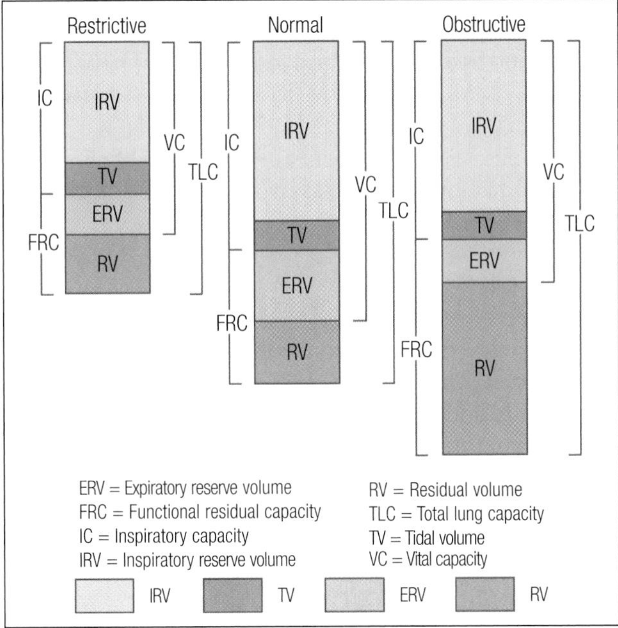

Figure 5-4 **Lung volumes of a healthy pulmonary system compared with lung volumes and capacities found in restrictive and obstructive pulmonary disease.**

From Rothstein J, Roy S, and Wolf S: The Rehabilitation Specialist's Handbook, 4th ed. Philadelphia, FA Davis, 2013, p. 518, with permission.

Table 5-5 presents the four basic conditions of acid-base balance and the $PaCO_2$, pH, and HCO_3^- values that accompany each condition.

b. Arterial oxygenation by determining the partial pressure of oxygen in relation to the fraction of inspired oxygen.

2. Electrocardiogram: see Chapter 4 (Cardiovascular Physical Therapy) for discussion.

Table 5-6

Graded Exercise Test Termination Criteria

1. Maximal shortness of breath.
2. A fall in PAO_2 of greater than 20 mmHg or a PAO_2 less than 55 mmHg.
3. A rise in $PaCO_2$ of greater than 10 mmHg or a $PaCO_2$ greater than 65 mmHg.
4. Cardiac ischemia or arrhythmias.
5. Symptoms of fatigue.
6. Increase in diastolic blood pressure readings of 20 mmHg, systolic hypertension greater than 250 mmHg, decrease in blood pressure with increasing workloads.
7. Leg pain.
8. Total fatigue.
9. Signs of insufficient cardiac output.
10. Reaching a ventilatory maximum.

From Brannon F, et al: Cardiopulmonary Rehabilitation: Basic Theory and Application, 3rd ed. Philadelphia, FA Davis, 1998, p. 300, with permission.

3. Sputum studies.
   a. Gram stain: immediate identification of the category of bacteria (gram-negative or gram-positive) and its appearance (e.g., pairs, chains).
   b. Culture and sensitivity: identifies the specific bacteria as well as the organism's susceptibility to various antibiotics. Results available within a few days.
   c. Cytology: reports the presence of cancer cells in sputum.
4. Pulmonary function tests (PFTs): evaluate lung volumes, capacities, and flow rates. Used to diagnose disease, monitor progression, and determine the benefits of medical management. See Figure 5-4 for changes with disease states. See Table 5-7 for

classification of obstructive lung disease according to the Global Initiative for Obstructive Lung Disease (GOLD), including PFT values for each level of disease severity.
5. Blood values. See Chapter 4 for discussion.

Exercise Tolerance Tests (ETT) or Graded Exercise Test. (See also Chapter 4)

1. Evaluates an individual's cardiopulmonary response to gradually increasing exercise.
2. Determines the presence of exercise-induced bronchospasm by testing pulmonary function, particularly FEV1 before and after ETT.
3. Documents the need for supplemental oxygen during an exercise program by analyzing arterial blood gas values throughout the ETT. ABGs also provide a criterion for test termination. If arterial blood sampling is unavailable, pulse oximetry can be used to monitor the percent saturation of oxygen within the arterial blood. Table 5-6 presents criteria for test termination for patients with pulmonary disease.

See Chapter 4 Appendix: Selected Outcome Measures for Cardiac and Pulmonary Dysfunction

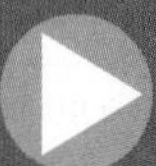

Evaluation and Diagnosis of Pulmonary Pathologies

Common Signs/Symptoms Present in Patients with Pulmonary Pathologies

1. Adventitious breath sounds (crackles, wheezes).
2. Cyanosis and/or clubbing.
3. Hypoxemia and/or hypercapnia.
4. Chest pain or tightness.
5. Shortness of breath at rest and/or with exertion.
6. Cough +/- sputum production.
7. Tachypnea.
8. Fatigue.
9. Weakness.
10. Accessory muscle use at rest.
11. If an infectious pathology, signs and symptoms are consistent with fever, including shaking, chills, sweats, increased white blood cells, and increased temperature.

Obstructive Disorders

1. Clients have difficulty getting air out, as evidenced by decreased expiratory flows (FEV_1, FVC, FEV_1/FVC) and likely increased residual volume (RV) and total lung capacity (TLC). The limitation in expelling air is due to pathology, including alveolar collapse, secretions, and/or bronchoconstriction. CXR findings typically include hyperinflation, flattened diaphragms, and hyperlucency.

Chronic Obstructive Pulmonary Disease (COPD)

1. Slowly progressing, chronic disease that limits expiratory airflow (decreased FEV_1) due to abnormalities in alveoli and/or airways usually from environmental exposure (i.e., smoking or pollutants).
2. Significant evidence supports participation in pulmonary rehabilitation to improve dyspnea, exercise tolerance, and health status, and to reduce hospitalizations.
3. COPD is diagnosed by the Global Initiative for Obstructive Lung Disease (GOLD) criteria, which is a combination of expiratory airflow (see Table 5-7) and functional limitation assessments (modified MRC dyspnea scale and COPD Assessment Test).

Types of COPD

1. Chronic bronchitis.
   a. Chronic inflammation of airways that causes increased mucous production, cough, shortness of breath, and fatigue. Diagnosed after chronic cough is present for at least 3 months for 2 consecutive years.
2. Emphysema.
   a. Progressive alveolar and parenchymal destruction with concomitant enlargement of distal airways, usually leading to severe expiratory airflow limitations. Primary cause is smoking.

Table 5-7

GOLD Classification of Airflow Limitation Severity in COPD (based on post-bronchodilator FEV_1)

IN PATIENTS WITH FEV_1/FVC <0.7		
STAGE	**SEVERITY**	**FEV_1 (PERCENT PREDICTED)**
GOLD 1	Mild	≥80%
GOLD 2	Moderate	50%–80%
GOLD 3	Severe	30%–50%
GOLD 4	Very Severe	<30%

Retrieved May 21, 2019 from https://goldcopd.org/wp-content/uploads/2018/11/GOLD-2019-POCKET-GUIDE-DRAFT-v1.7-14Nov2018-WMS.pdf.

Other Obstructive Disorders

1. Asthma.
   a. Chronic inflammatory disease caused by increased reactivity of the trachea and bronchi to various stimuli (allergens, exercise, cold, viral infections).
   b. Variable symptoms and expiratory airflow limitations from widespread narrowing of the airways due to inflammation, smooth muscle constriction, and increased secretions. Even during remission, some degree of airway inflammation is present. Typical symptoms of asthma include wheezing, shortness of breath, chest tightness, and a cough.
2. Pneumonia.
   a. Aspiration: aspirated material causes an acute inflammatory reaction within the lungs. Usually found in patients with impaired swallowing (dysphagia), fixed neck extension, intoxication, impaired consciousness, neuromuscular disease, or recent anesthesia.
   b. Bacterial: an intra-alveolar bacterial infection.
      - Pneumococcal pneumonia (streptococcal), a gram-positive bacterium, is the most common type of pneumonia and usually acquired in the community.
      - Other common typical infecting organisms are *Haemophilus influenzae* and *Staphylococcus aureus*.
      - Some atypical pneumonia bacteria include Legionella, Mycoplasma pneumonia, and Chlamydia pneumonia.
   c. Viral: an interstitial or intra-alveolar inflammatory process caused by viral agents (influenza, adenovirus, parainfluenza, respiratory syncytial virus [RSV], measles). RSV is the most common viral pneumonia in children.
3. Bronchiectasis.
   a. A chronic congenital or acquired disease characterized by abnormal dilatation of the bronchi and excessive sputum production.
4. Cystic fibrosis (CF).
   a. A genetically inherited disease characterized by thickening of secretions of all exocrine glands, leading to obstruction (e.g., pancreatic, pulmonic, gastrointestinal). CF may present as an obstructive, restrictive, or mixed disease.
   b. Clinical signs include meconium ileus, frequent respiratory infections, especially *Staphylococcus aureus* and *Pseudomonas aeruginosa*, and inability to gain weight despite adequate caloric intake.
   c. Diagnosis is made postnatally by a blood test indicating trypsinogen, or later by a positive sweat electrolyte test.
5. Bronchopulmonary dysplasia.
   a. An obstructive pulmonary disease, often a sequela of premature infants with respiratory distress syndrome; results from high pressures of mechanical ventilation, high fractions of inspired oxygen (FiO_2), and/or infection. Lungs show areas of pulmonary immaturity and dysfunction due to hyperinflation.
6. Respiratory distress syndrome.
   a. Alveolar collapse in a premature infant resulting from lung immaturity, inadequate level of pulmonary surfactant.

Restrictive Disorders

1. Restrictive disorders: clients have decreased vital capacity and normal inspiratory and expiratory flows. A pathology is decreasing the amount of air able to get in and out of the lungs.
2. Interstitial lung disease.
   a. Idiopathic pulmonary fibrosis: chronic, progressive, fibrotic pneumonia that causes irreversible scarring in the lung tissue.
   b. Sarcoidosis: multisystem inflammatory disease consisting of granulomas in multiple organs, most often the lungs, skin, lymph nodes, eyes, and liver.
      - The etiology of sarcoidosis is unknown, peak onset is middle age, and affects persons of color more often than other races.
      - It is most often diagnosed as an incidental finding on chest films. Diagnosis requires radiographic findings, histology with granulomas, and exclusion of all other diagnoses.
      - May have increased secretions if bronchial involvement, which can mimic bronchiectasis and pulmonary fibrosis due to scarring from repeated infections. Patients may exhibit hypoxemia and hypocapnia.
      - Long-term glucocorticoids are used to manage sarcoidosis, but multisystem monitoring is required.
      - PFTs and Six-Minute Walk Test are used to monitor progression of the disease.
      - New symptoms might include skin lesions, visual changes, diaphoresis, palpitations, joint pain, joint swelling, or muscle weakness.
   c. Occupational exposure diseases (pneumoconiosis including asbestosis, byssinosis, silicosis, and coal worker's pneumoconiosis): chronic inflammatory reaction from inhaled causes scarring in lung tissue and interstitial lung disease.
3. Alterations in chest wall (musculoskeletal): restricted motion of bony thorax, with diseases such as ankylosing spondylitis, arthritis, scoliosis, pectus excavatum, arthrogryposis, or the integumentary changes of the chest wall such as thoracic burns or scleroderma.
4. Alterations in neuromuscular apparatus: decreased muscular strength results in an inability to expand the rib cage, seen in disease states such as multiple

sclerosis, muscular dystrophy, Parkinson's disease, spinal cord injury, or cerebrovascular accident (CVA).

5. Trauma.
   a. Rib fracture, flail chest: fracture of the ribs, usually due to blunt trauma. Flail chest is two or more fractures in two or more adjacent ribs.
   b. Pneumothorax: air in the pleural space, usually through a lacerated visceral pleura from a rib fracture or ruptured bullae.
   c. Hemothorax: blood in the pleural space, usually from a laceration of the parietal pleura.
   d. Lung contusion: blood and edema within the alveoli and interstitial space due to blunt chest trauma with or without rib fractures.

Other Pulmonary Pathologies

1. Atelectasis: collapsed or airless alveolar unit, caused by hypoventilation secondary to pain during the ventilatory cycle (pleuritis, postoperative pain, or rib fracture), internal bronchial obstruction (aspiration, mucus plugging), external bronchial compression (tumor or enlarged lymph nodes), low tidal volumes (narcotic overdose, inappropriately low ventilator settings), or neurologic insult.
2. Pleural effusion: excessive fluid between the visceral and parietal pleura, caused mainly by increased pleural permeability to proteins from inflammatory diseases (pneumonia, rheumatoid arthritis, systemic lupus), neoplastic disease, increased hydrostatic pressure within pleural space (congestive heart failure), decrease in osmotic pressure (hypoproteinemia), peritoneal fluid within the pleural space (ascites, cirrhosis), or interference of pleural reabsorption from a tumor invading pleural lymphatics.
3. Pulmonary edema: excessive seepage of fluid from the pulmonary vascular system into the interstitial space; may eventually cause alveolar edema.
   a. Cardiogenic: results from increased pressure in pulmonary capillaries associated with left ventricular failure, aortic valvular disease, or mitral valvular disease.
   b. Noncardiogenic: results from increased permeability of the alveolar capillary membranes due to inhalation of toxic fumes, hypervolemia, or narcotic overdose.
   c. Adult respiratory distress syndrome (ARDS): acute inflammatory response characterized by pulmonary edema in response to systemic pathology (sepsis, pneumonia, trauma, substance abuse).
4. Pulmonary embolism: a thrombus from the peripheral venous circulation becomes embolic and lodges in the pulmonary circulation. Small emboli do not necessarily cause infarction.
5. Pulmonary hypertension: increased arterial pressures within the pulmonary vasculature system due to idiopathic pulmonary hypertension, left heart disease, chronic lung disease/hypoxemia, pulmonary artery obstruction, or multifactorial issues. Exercise consistently has improved quality of life and exercise capacity in patients with pulmonary hypertension.
6. Bronchogenic carcinoma.
   a. Most common type is non–small cell lung cancer (adenocarcinoma > squamous cell carcinoma > large cell carcinoma), and the other is small cell lung cancer.
   b. Smoking is the largest risk factor, followed by radiation, environmental exposure, pulmonary fibrosis, genetics, presence of HIV, and alcohol.
7. Tuberculosis: *Mycobacterium tuberculosis* infection spread by aerosolized droplets from an untreated infected host. Incubation period: 2–10 weeks. Primary disease lasts 10 days to 2 weeks.
   a. Postprimary infection is reactivation of dormant tuberculous bacillus, which can occur years after the primary infection.
   b. Medication is taken for prolonged periods: 3–12 months.
   c. There is an increased incidence of TB in patients with HIV.
   d. Pertinent physical findings of primary disease can go unnoticed, as it causes only mild symptoms: slight nonproductive cough, low-grade fever, and possible CXR changes consistent with primary disease.

RED FLAG: Two weeks on appropriate antituberculin drugs renders the host noninfectious. During the infectious stage, the patient must be isolated from others in a negative-pressure room. Anyone entering the room must wear a protective TB mask and follow universal precautions. If the patient leaves the negative-pressure room, he or she must wear a specialized mask to keep from infecting others.

   e. Pott's disease (tuberculous spondylitis) is a form of spinal TB that primarily affects the thoracic and upper lumbar vertebrae.
      - Arthritic changes often result in kyphosis.
      - Physical therapy interventions can include pain relief, flexibility and strengthening activities, and postural reeducation.

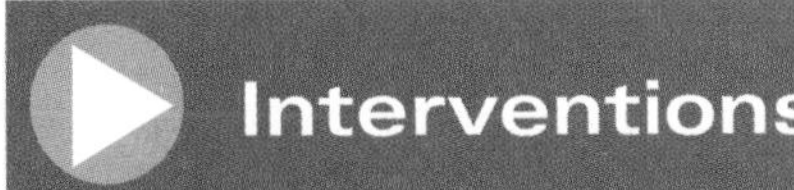

Interventions

Manual Secretion Removal Techniques

Postural Drainage

1. Placing the patient in varying positions for optimal gravity drainage of secretions and increased expansion of the involved segment (see Figure 5-5).
2. Indications for use of postural drainage.
   a. Increased pulmonary secretions.
   b. Aspiration.
   c. Atelectasis or collapse.
3. Considerations prior to use of the postural drainage positions (see Table 5-8). These considerations are not intended to imply absolute danger, but rather a possible need for position modification.
4. Procedure.
   a. Explain procedure to the patient.
   b. Place patient in appropriate postural drainage position.
   c. Observe for signs of intolerance.
   d. Duration of procedure can be up to 20 minutes per postural drainage position. Typically, duration equals the duration of other manual techniques used in conjunction with postural drainage.

Percussion

1. A force rhythmically applied with the therapist's cupped hands to the specific area of the chest wall that corresponds to the involved lung segment.
2. Percussion is used to increase the amount of secretions cleared from the tracheobronchial tree; usually used in conjunction with postural drainage. Indications for use of percussion.
   a. Excessive pulmonary secretions.
   b. Aspiration.
   c. Atelectasis or collapse due to mucous plugging obstructing the airways.
3. Considerations to weigh possible benefits of percussion against possible detriments prior to the application of this technique are listed in Table 5-9. Modification of the technique may be necessary for patient tolerance.
4. Procedure.
   a. Explain procedure to the patient.
   b. Place patient in the appropriate postural drainage position.
   c. Cover the area to be percussed with a lightweight cloth to avoid erythema.
   d. Percuss over area of thorax that corresponds to the involved lung segment. The duration of percussion depends on the patient's needs and tolerance. Three to 5 minutes of percussion per postural drainage position with clinically assessed improvement is a guideline.
   e. The force of percussion causes the patient's voice to quiver.

Shaking (Vibration)

1. Following a deep inhalation, a bouncing maneuver is applied to the rib cage throughout exhalation; to hasten the removal of secretions from the tracheobronchial tree.
2. Commonly used following percussion in the appropriate postural drainage position. Modification may be necessary for patient tolerance.
3. Indications for the use of shaking.
   a. Excessive pulmonary secretions.
   b. Aspiration.
   c. Atelectasis or collapse of an airway from mucous plugging.
4. Considerations prior to the application of shaking are similar to those of percussion (see Table 5-9).
5. Procedure.
   a. Explain procedure to the patient.
   b. Place patient in appropriate postural drainage position.
   c. Perform percussion if appropriate.
   d. As patient inhales deeply, the therapist's hands are placed with fingers parallel to the ribs.
   e. As patient exhales, the therapist's hands provide a jarring, bouncing motion to the rib cage below.
   f. The duration of shaking depends on the patient's needs, tolerance, and clinical improvement. Five to 10 deep inhalations with the shaking technique is generally acceptable practice. Any more than 10 would risk hyperventilation (increased VE resulting in decreased $PaCO_2$), and less than 5 may be ineffective.

Airway Clearance Techniques

1. Cough: patient should be asked to cough in the upright sitting position, if possible, after each area of lung has been treated. Coughing clears secretions from the major central airways.
2. Huffing: more effective in patients with collapsible airways (e.g., chronic obstructive diseases), prevents the high intrathoracic pressure that causes premature airway closure.
   a. Ask patient to inhale deeply.
   b. Immediately, the patient forcibly expels the air, saying "Ha, ha."

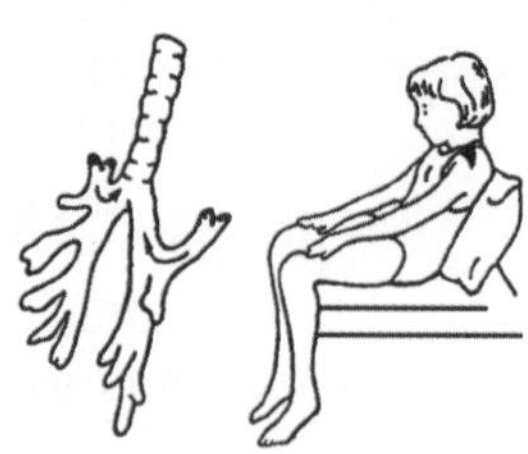

UPPER LOBES Apical Segments

Bed or drainage table flat.

Patient leans back on pillow at 30° angle against therapist.

Therapist claps with markedly cupped hand over area between clavicle and top of scapula on each side.

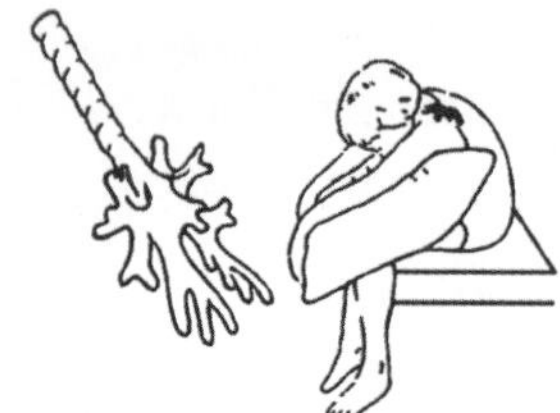

UPPER LOBES Posterior Segments

Bed or drainage table flat.

Patient leans over folded pillow at 30° angle.

Therapist stands behind and claps over upper back on both sides.

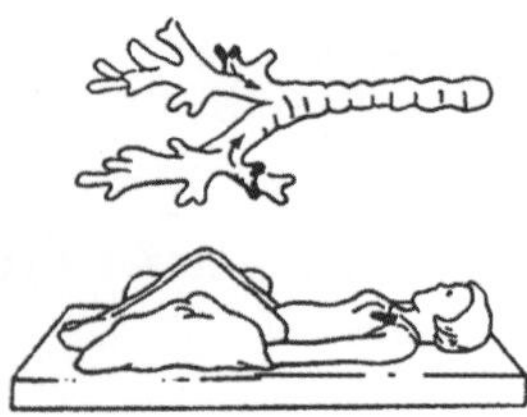

UPPER LOBES Anterior Segments

Bed or drainage table flat.

Patient lies on back with pillow under knees.

Therapist claps between clavicle and nipple on each side.

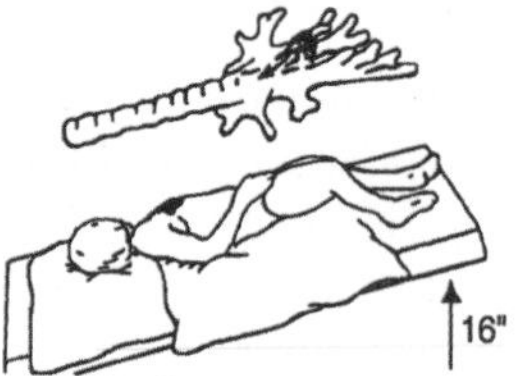

RIGHT MIDDLE LOBE

Foot of table or bed elevated 16 inches.

Patient lies head down on left side and rotates ¼ turn backward. Pillow may be placed behind from shoulder to hip. Knees should be flexed.

Therapist claps over right nipple area. In females with breast development or tenderness, use cupped hand with heel of hand under armpit and fingers extending forward beneath the breast.

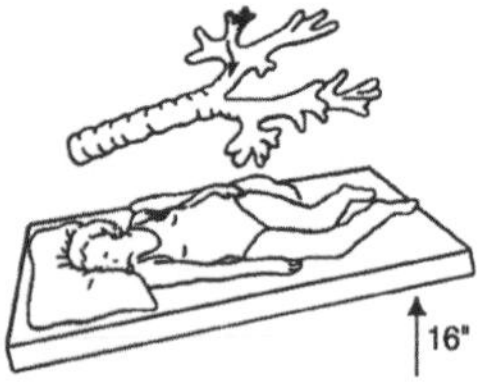

LEFT UPPER LOBE Lingular Segments

Foot of table or bed elevated 16 inches.

Patient lies head down on right side and rotates 1/4 turn backward. Pillow may be placed behind from shoulder to hip. Knees should be flexed.

Therapist claps with moderately cupped hand over left nipple area. In females with breast development or tenderness, use cupped hand with heel of hand under armpit and fingers extending forward beneath the breast.

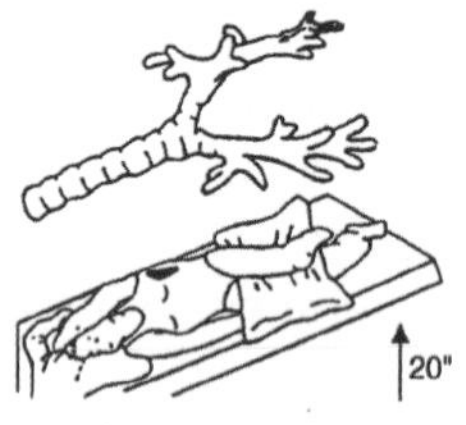

LOWER LOBE Anterior Basal Segments

Foot of table or bed elevated 20 inches.

Patient lies on side, head down, pillow under knees.

Therapist claps with slightly cupped hand over lower ribs. (Position shown is for drainage of left anterior basal segment. To drain the right anterior basal segment, patient should lie on the left side in same posture).

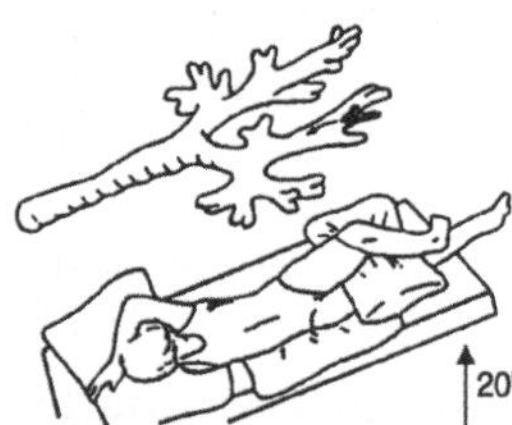

LOWER LOBES Lateral Basal Segments

Foot of table or bed elevated 20 inches.

Patient lies on abdomen, head down, then rotates ¼ turn upward. Upper leg is flexed over a pillow for support.

Therapist claps over uppermost portion of lower ribs. (Position shown is for drainage of right lateral basal segment. To drain the left lateral basal segment, patient should lie on the right side in the same posture).

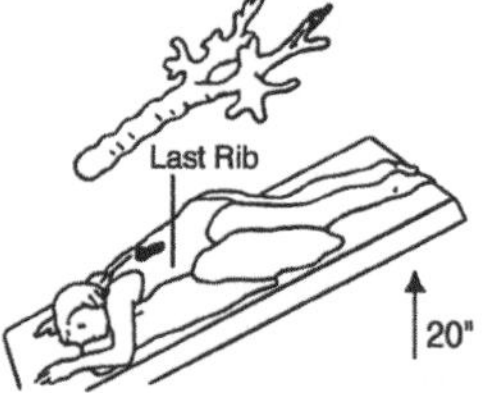

LOWER LOBES Posterior Basal Segments

Foot of table or bed elevated 20 inches.

Patient lies on abdomen, head down, with pillow under hips. Therapist claps over lower ribs close to spine on each side.

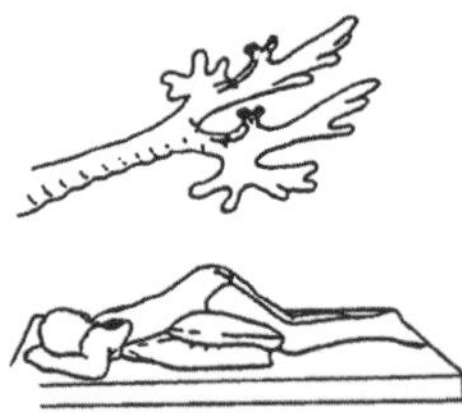

LOWER LOBES Superior Segments

Bed or table flat.

Patient lies on abdomen with two pillows under hips.

Therapist claps over middle of back at tip of scapula on either side of spine.

Figure 5-5 Bronchial drainage.

From Rothstein J, Roy S, and Wolf S: The Rehabilitation Specialist's Handbook, 3rd ed., FA Davis, 2005, p. 444, with permission.

Table 5-8

Considerations Prior to the Use of Postural Drainage	
Precautions to the use of Trendelenburg position (Head of bed tipped down 15° to 18°)	
Circulatory system	Pulmonary edema, congestive heart failure, hypertension
Abdominal problems	Obesity, ascites, pregnancy, hiatal hernia, nausea and vomiting, recent food consumption
Neurologic system	Recent neurosurgery, increased intracranial pressure, aneurysm precautions
Pulmonary system	Shortness of breath
Precautions to the use of sidelying position	
Circulatory system	Axillo-femoral bypass graft
Musculoskeletal system	Humeral fractures, need for hip abduction brace, other situations that make sidelying uncomfortable, e.g., arthritis, shoulder bursitis

3. Assisted cough: the therapist's hand(s) or fist becomes the force behind the patient's exhaled air. Used when the patient's abdominal muscles cannot generate an effective cough (e.g., spinal cord injury). The amount of force by the therapist depends on patient tolerance and abdominal sensation.
   a. Position the patient against a solid surface; supine with head of bed flat or in a Trendelenburg position, or sitting with wheelchair against the wall or against the therapist.
   b. The therapist's hand is placed below the patient's subcostal angle (similar to hand placement for the Heimlich maneuver).
   c. Patient inhales deeply.
   d. As the patient attempts to cough, the therapist's hand pushes inward and upward, assisting the rapid exhalation of air.
   e. Any secretions raised should be removed by a suction catheter if expectoration is problematic.
4. Tracheal stimulation: used with patients who are unable to cough on command, such as infants or patients with brain injury or stroke.
   a. The therapist's finger or thumb is placed just above the suprasternal notch, and a quick inward and downward pressure on the trachea elicits the cough reflex.
5. Endotracheal suctioning: used only when the above airway clearance techniques fail to adequately remove secretions.
   a. Standard precautions are employed, since contact with a patient's body fluid is expected.
   b. Equipment: suction catheters come in sizes of 14 French gauge (Fr), usually for an adult, 10 Fr for older children, 8 and 5–6 Fr for young children and infants. Suction system set at approximately 120 mmHg of suction. Sterile glove/clean glove.
   c. Procedure: a catheter is fed through either an artificial airway, oral airway, or the nares through the pharynx, larynx to the carina. When resistance is felt at the carina, the catheter is rotated and withdrawn. Suction is applied intermittently so as not to damage the inner lining of the trachea. The usual suctioning time is 10 to 15 seconds.

Table 5-9

Considerations Prior to the Use of Percussion and Shaking	
General guidelines	Pain made worse by the technique
Circulatory system	Aneurysm precautions, hemoptysis
Coagulation disorders	Increased partial thromboplastin time (PTT), increased prothrombin time (PT), decreased platelet count (below 50,000), or medications that interfere with coagulation
Musculoskeletal system	Fractured rib, flail chest, degenerative bone disease, bone metastases

RED FLAG: Complications associated with suctioning: hypoxemia, bradycardia or tachycardia, hypotension or hypertension, increased intracranial pressure, atelectasis, tracheal damage, infections.

Independent Secretion Removal Techniques

Active Cycle of Breathing

1. An independent program to assist in the removal of more peripheral secretions that coughing may not clear.
2. Breathe in a controlled, diaphragmatic fashion.
3. Perform thoracic expansion exercises with or without percussion and shaking. These are deep inhalations with a hold at the top, if possible.
4. Controlled diaphragmatic breathing. The patient decides what is needed next. If no secretions seem to be mobilized, patient goes to forced expiratory huffs (#5) and/or coughing (#6). If patient then believes secretions can be cleared, resume controlled diaphragmatic breathing (#7). Repeat as needed (#8).
5. Inhale at a resting tidal volume. Contract the abdominal muscles to produce one or two forced expiratory huffs from mid- to low lung volume to raise secretions.
6. Huff from high lung volume or cough to clear.
7. Controlled diaphragmatic breathing.
8. Repeat these cycles until secretions are in large airways.

Autogenic Drainage

1. An independent program used to sense peripheral secretions and clear them without the tracheobronchial irritation from coughing.
2. Amount of time spent in each of the following phases is determined by where the patient feels the secretions.
   a. Unstick phase: quiet breathing at low lung volumes to affect peripheral secretions.
   b. Collect phase: breathing at mid–lung volumes to affect secretions in the middle airways.
   c. Evacuation phase: breathing from mid- to high lung volumes to clear secretions from central airways; replaces coughing as the means to clear secretions.
   d. Repeat the steps corresponding to the area of retained secretions until all secretions are removed from the airways.

Oscillatory Positive Expiratory Pressure (PEP) Devices

1. The patient uses an external device that vibrates the airways on exhalation to improve airway clearance with intermittent, positive expiratory pressure. Examples include FLUTTER and acapella devices.
2. Patient breathes in a normal tidal volume through the nose or around the mouthpiece of the device.
3. Patient then exhales through the device, setting up a vibration within the airways. Experimentation in the tipped position of the device may provide the most vibration possible with exhalation.
4. Repeat between 5 and 10 times.
5. Patient then breathes in a full inhalation through the nose or around the mouthpiece.
6. This is followed by a 3-second hold at the top of inhalation and rapid, forced exhalations through the device.
7. Repeat 2 or 3 times.
8. Huff or cough to clear secretions.

Low-Pressure Positive Expiratory Pressure (PEP) Mask

1. The patient uses positive expiratory resistance via face mask or mouth piece with nose clips to help remove airway secretions. Low-pressure PEP measures 10–20 cm H_2O.
2. Seated patient breathes at tidal volumes with mask in place.
3. After approximately 10 breaths, the mask is removed for coughing or huffing to clear secretions.
4. The sequence is repeated until all secretions are removed from the airways.

High-Frequency Chest Wall Oscillation

1. Patient wears a vest that fills with air and then rapidly increases/decreases pressure.
2. Pressure oscillation loosens secretions in the airway.
3. Settings: frequency is set to 12–16 Hz (Hertz), and pressure is inflated until snug on patient.
4. Time = 20–30 minutes, with breaks to cough and drink water as needed.
5. Can be completed in postural drainage positions.

Breathing Exercises

Diaphragmatic Breathing

1. Used to increase ventilation, improve gas exchange, decrease work of breathing, facilitate relaxation, and maintain or improve mobility of chest wall.
2. Used with postoperative patients, post-trauma patients, and patients with obstructive or restrictive pulmonary lung diseases.
3. Procedure.
   a. Explain procedure to patient.
   b. Position patient in supine, sitting, or semireclined (e.g., semi-Fowler's position).
   c. Place therapist's hand gently over subcostal angle of the thorax.
   d. Apply gentle pressure throughout the exhalation phase.
   e. Increase to firm pressure at end of exhalation.
   f. Ask patient to inhale against resistance of the therapist's hand.
   g. Release pressure, allowing a full inhalation.
   h. Progress to independence of therapist's hand, in upright sitting, standing, walking, and stair climbing.

Segmental Breathing

1. Used to improve ventilation to hypoventilated lung segments, alter regional distribution of gas, maintain or restore functional residual capacity, maintain or improve mobility of chest wall, and prevent pulmonary compromise.
2. Used for patients with pleuritic, incisional, or post-trauma pain that causes decreased movement in a portion of the thorax (splinting), and those at risk of developing atelectasis.

> **RED FLAG:** Contraindicated with intractable hypoventilation until medical situation is resolved.

3. Procedure.
   a. Explain procedure to patient.
   b. Position patient to facilitate inhalation to a certain segment, such as postural drainage positions, upright sitting.
   c. Apply gentle pressure to the thorax over area of hypoventilation during exhalation.
   d. Increase to firm pressure just prior to inspiration.
   e. Ask patient to breathe in against the resistance of therapist's hands.
   f. Release resistance, allowing a full inhalation.

Sustained Maximal Inspiration (SMI)

1. Used to increase inhaled volume, sustain or improve alveolar inflation, and maintain or restore functional residual capacity.
2. Used in acute situations; e.g., patients with post-trauma pain, postoperative pain, acute lobar collapse.
3. Procedure.
   a. Inspire slowly through nose or pursed lips to maximal inspiration.
   b. Hold maximal inspiration for 3 seconds.
   c. Passively exhale the volume.
   d. Incentive spirometers (devices used to measure and encourage deep inspiration) can help patient achieve maximal inspiration during SMI.

Pursed-Lip Breathing

1. Used to reduce respiratory rate, increase tidal volume, reduce dyspnea, decrease mechanical disadvantages of impaired ventilatory pump, improve gas mixing at rest for patients with COPD, and facilitate relaxation. Primarily used for patients with obstructive disease who experience dyspnea at rest or with minimal activity/exercise, or with ineffective breathing patterns during activity/exercise.
2. Procedure.
   a. Slowly inhale through nose or mouth.
   b. Passively exhale through pursed lips (position mouth as if blowing out candles).
   c. Additional hand pressure from the therapist applied to abdomen can gently prolong expiration.

RED FLAG: Abdominal muscle contraction can be used judiciously to increase exhaled volume. Care must be taken not to increase intrathoracic pressure, which may cause airway collapse.

Abdominal Strengthening

1. Used when abdominal muscles are too weak to provide an effective cough. Abdominal support is used when the abdominal muscles cannot provide the necessary support needed for passive exhalation, e.g., in high thoracic and cervical spinal cord injuries. It is important to ensure that the binder does not restrict inspiration.
2. Glossopharyngeal breathing (air gulping) can also be taught to assist coughing.

Activities for Increasing Functional Abilities

General Conditioning

1. A prescription for exercise using the FITT equation can improve cardiopulmonary fitness based on the results of ETT. (See Chapter 4.)
2. Monitoring of heart rate and blood pressure is required during exercise and progressive physical activity.
3. Frequency: the goal is 20–30 minutes of exercise three to five times per week. With durations of less than 20–30 minutes, exercise should occur more frequently (five to seven times per week).
4. Intensity: patients with mild or moderate lung disease will likely reach their cardiovascular endpoint with an exercise test. Patients with severe and very severe pulmonary disorders will likely reach a pulmonary endpoint before a cardiovascular endpoint. Intensity for these patients should be at or near maximum heart rate. Ratings of Perceived Exertion and Borg Dyspnea on Exertion Scale are used to monitor exercise intensity.
5. Time: with high-intensity exercise, the patient may need an interval exercise program with rest periods for tolerance. Progression is directed first toward a duration of 20–30 minutes of continuous exercise before an increase in intensity is considered.
6. Type: any aerobic activity that allows a graded workload; usually, a circuit program of multiple activities (e.g., bike, walking, arm ergometry) since patients with pulmonary disease may be deconditioned. Patient preference should be considered.

Inspiratory Muscle Training (IMT)

1. Used to load muscles of inspiration by breathing through a series of graded aperture openings on a handheld device. By increasing strength and endurance of muscles of ventilation, the patient will develop more efficient ventilatory muscles, less effort in breathing, and decreased possibility of respiratory muscle fatigue.
2. IMT is appropriate for patients with decreased compliance, decreased intrathoracic volume, resistance to airflow, alteration in length tension relationship of ventilatory muscles, decreased strength of the respiratory muscles. Obese patients would benefit.
3. Procedure.
   a. Explain procedure to patient with emphasis on maintenance of respiratory rate and tidal volume during training sessions.
   b. Determine maximum inspiratory pressure (MIP; see normal values for MIP in Table 5-1).
   c. Choose an aperture opening that requires 30%–70% of MIP (intensity) and allows 10–15 minutes of training per session. With higher intensities, patients can complete 10–20 repetitions similar to other strength training.
   d. Ask patient to inhale through device while maintaining their usual respiratory rate and tidal volume for at least 10–15 minutes.
   e. Progression initially focuses on increasing duration to 30 minutes, then increasing intensity with smaller apertures.

Paced Breathing (Activity Pacing)

1. Used to spread out the metabolic demands of an activity over time by slowing its performance.

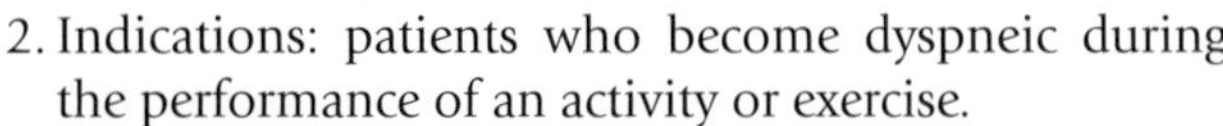

2. Indications: patients who become dyspneic during the performance of an activity or exercise.
3. Procedure.
   a. Break down any activity into manageable components that can be performed within the patient's pulmonary system's abilities.
   b. Inhale at rest.
   c. Upon exhalation with pursed lips, complete the first component of the desired activity.
   d. Stop the activity and inhale at rest.
   e. Upon exhalation with pursed lips, complete next component of activity.
   f. Repeat steps (d) and (e) until activity is accomplished in full without shortness of breath. For example, stair climbing can be done by ascending one or more stairs on exhalation, and then resting, inhaling at rest, then more stairs on exhalation, and so on.

Energy Conservation

1. The energy consumption of many activities of daily living can be decreased with some careful thought and planning, making seemingly impossible tasks possible.
2. For example, showering is difficult for the patient with pulmonary disease, given the activity and the hot, humid environment. With a shower seat, handheld shower, and use of a terry cloth robe after showering, the patient does not have to stand, hold his or her breath as often, or dry off in the humid environment, thus reducing the energy cost of the activity.

Medical and Surgical Management of Pulmonary Disease

Surgical Management

Types of Surgeries to Remove Diseased Lung Portions

1. Pneumonectomy: removal of a lung.
2. Lobectomy: removal of a lobe of a lung.
3. Segmental resection: removal of a segment of a lobe.
4. Wedge resection: removal of a portion of a lung without anatomical divisions.
5. Lung volume reduction surgery (LVRS), or pneumectomy, removes large emphysematous, nonfunctioning areas of the lung to normalize thoracic mobility and improve gas exchange of the remaining lung.

Types of Incisions

1. Midsternotomy: sternum is cut in half lengthwise and rib cage is retracted; used in most heart surgeries. The sternum is wired together at the close of surgery; therefore, physical therapy should encourage full upper-extremity range of motion postoperatively.
2. Thoracotomy: used for most lung resections; incision follows the path of the fourth intercostal space; full range of motion should be encouraged postoperatively.
3. Video-assisted thoracoscopic surgery (VATs): minimally invasive surgical technique used to complete any of above lung resections.

Postsurgical Care

Postoperative Physical Therapy Sessions

1. Decrease the number and severity of pulmonary complications.
2. Prevent postoperative pulmonary complications.
   a. Remove residual secretions.
   b. Improve aeration.
   c. Gradually increase activity.
   d. Return to baseline pulmonary functioning.
3. Pertinent physical findings of postoperative pulmonary complications.
   a. Increased temperature.
   b. Increase in white blood cell count.
   c. Change in breath sounds from the preoperative evaluation.
   d. Abnormal chest x-ray.
   e. Decreased expansion of the thorax.
   f. Shortness of breath.
   g. Change in cough and sputum production.
4. Physical therapy considerations.
   a. Determine need for pain management.
   b. Choose appropriate intervention based on patient's needs.
      - Secretion removal techniques.
      - Breathing exercises to improve aeration, incentive spirometry.
      - Early mobilization.

Medical Management (See Table 5-10)

Table 5-10

Common Pulmonary Medications

CATEGORY	MECHANISM OF ACTION	ADVERSE EFFECTS FOR PTS TO NOTE	EXAMPLES
Rescue/Short-Acting: Used for immediate relief of breakthrough symptoms of tightness, wheezing, and shortness of breath			
Short-acting anticholinergic (muscarinic antagonist)	Bronchodilator (smooth muscle relaxant)	Tachycardia	Atrovent (ipratropium bromide)
Short-acting beta-2 agonists (sympathomimetics)	Bronchodilator (smooth muscle relaxant)	Tachycardia	Ventolin HFA (albuterol), Proventil HFA (albuterol), Xopenex HFA (levalbuterol)
Maintenance: Taken on a regular schedule to maintain optimal airway diameter			
Anti-inflammatory (glucocorticoids)	Reduce airway inflammation (inhibit inflammatory response)	Hyperglycemia, osteoporosis, poor healing, proximal muscle weakness	Flovent HFA (fluicason propionate), Pulmicort (budesonide), prednisone
Long-acting anticholinergic (muscarinic antagonist)	Bronchodilator (smooth muscle relaxant)	Tachycardia	Spirivia (tiotropium bromide)
Long-acting beta-2 agonists (sympathomimetics)	Bronchodilator (smooth muscle relaxant)	Tachycardia	Serevent (salmeterol), Foradil (formoterol)
Cromones	Antiallergen (prevents bronchoconstriction)	None	Cromolyn sodium
Leukotriene antagonist	Prevents bronchospasm and inflammatory response	None	Zafirlukast, motelukast
Mucolytics	Reduces mucus viscosity		Mucomyst (acetylcysteine), Pulmozyme (dornase alfa)
Combination medications: used to treat Asthma and COPD	Combination of a long-acting beta 2-agonist (bronchodilator) and corticosteroid (reduces inflammation)	Tachycardia, hyperglycemia, osteoporosis, poor healing, proximal muscle weakness	Symbicort (budesonide-formoterol), Dulera (mometasone furoate-formoterol), and Advair (fluticasone propionate-salmeterol)
Other			
Antibiotics: Used for the treatment of infection or infectious exacerbation. Antibiotics are dependent upon the culture and sensitivity results.			
Vaccinations: It is recommended that patients with pulmonary disorders routinely receive the influenza and the pneumonia vaccinations to prevent further pulmonary compromise.			

Modifed from: Ciccone, C. D. (2016). Respiratory Drugs. In *Pharmacology in Rehabilitation.* New York: F. A. Davis Company. Panus, P. C., Jobst, E. E., Masters, S. B., Katzung, B., Tinsley, S. L., & Trevor, A. J. (2009). Chapter 35. Drugs Affecting the Respiratory System. In *Pharmacology for the Physical Therapist.* New York: The McGraw-Hill Companies.

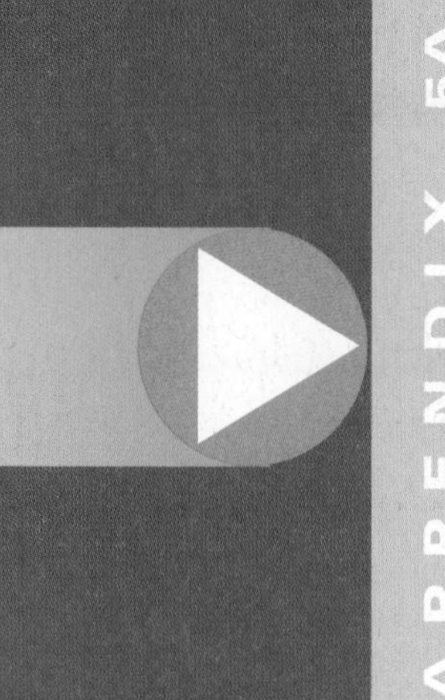

APPENDIX 5A

Review Questions and Case Study

(Answers to all Review Questions and Case Studies can be found in Chapter 17)

1. What are the PAO_2 and FiO_2 normal values in room air?

2. When auscultating the lungs, what are the main characteristics of crackles, wheezes, vesicular, and bronchial breath sounds?

3. What are the expected physical, imaging, PFT, and laboratory findings associated with moderate to severe asthma?

4. What are the precautions when using postural drainage in the Trendelenburg position?

Pulmonary Case Study

Patient Profile

- **Gender:** Female
- **Age:** 72 years

Presenting Problem/Current Condition

- Recent 3-day admission to the hospital with increased shortness of breath and productive cough with yellowish-green sputum
- Treated with high-dose steroids and antibiotics, along with bronchodilators for a chronic obstructive pulmonary disease exacerbation
- Referred to outpatient pulmonary rehabilitation 2 weeks after her hospital discharge

Past Medical History

- Hypertension
- Hyperlipidemia
- Type II diabetes
- Obstructive sleep apnea
- Obesity
- Smoking 1–2 packs per day × 45 years

Other Information

- Patient uses CPAP at night for obstructive sleep apnea.
- She receives assistance from a local agency for house cleaning and grocery shopping.
- She lives alone and uses a rollator for community ambulation.

Question #1

What is the most likely sequelae of the patient's medical treatment in the hospital that the physical therapy should consider during their examination?

1. Cognitive screening due to ongoing delirium.
2. Incontinence due to antibiotic use.
3. Integumentary issue on sacrum due to prolonged immobility.
4. Proximal weakness due to a steroid myopathy.

Question #2

What is one of the primary benefits of pulmonary rehabilitation for patients with chronic obstructive pulmonary disease after an exacerbation of their disease?

1. Decreased dyspnea on exertion.
2. Decreased hospital admissions.
3. Improvement in health-related quality of life.
4. Improved mortality rates.

Question #3

Which intensity of walking program would be the **BEST** option for the patient to start in pulmonary rehabilitation?

1. 20% of maximum, 2 days a week, 5 minutes per day.
2. 30% of maximum, 3 days a week, 10 minutes per day.
3. 50% of maximum, 5 days a week, 20 minutes per day.
4. 85% of maximum, 6 days a week, 40 minutes per day.

6

Therapeutic Interventions

MICHAEL S. CROWELL, KELLY MACAULEY, SCOTT W. SHAFFER, SUSAN O. SULLIVAN, THOMAS SUTLIVE, AND BRADLEY S. TRAGORD

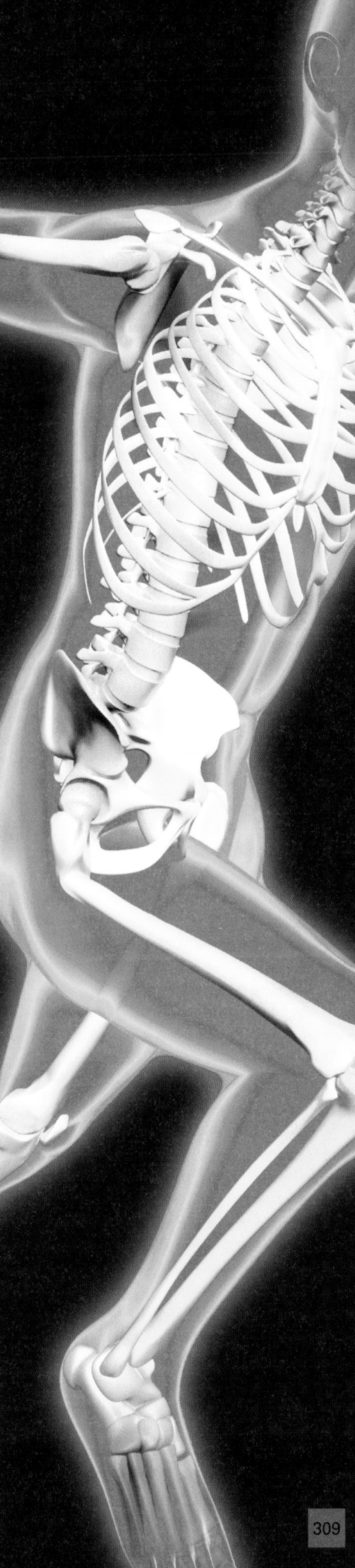

Chapter Outline

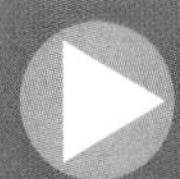

Factors Impacting Therapeutic Intervention Selection

1. Numerous therapeutic interventions are available to the physical therapist, including therapeutic exercise.
2. An essential quality of the therapist is the ability to select, prescribe, and modify effective therapeutic interventions.
3. The therapist must consider many factors when selecting the best therapeutic intervention for their patient. These considerations include:
   a. Current best evidence available based on the diagnosis (e.g., clinical practice guidelines, clinical prediction rules)
   b. Anatomical, physiological, and biomechanical factors
   c. Impairments, activity limitations, and participation restrictions
   d. Acuity of the patient's condition to include tissue healing timelines (See Table 2-35 for a review of tissue healing timelines)
   e. Pain behavior to include Severity, Irritability, Nature, Stage and Stability (SINSS) of the condition
   f. Motor control/motor learning as related to the intervention
   g. Contraindications
   h. Precautions
   i. Potential adverse side effects of the intervention

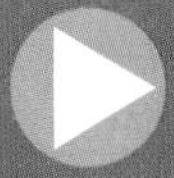

Resistance Training

Concepts of Muscle Function

Basic Muscle Properties and Definitions

1. Contractile elements of muscle.
   a. Muscles are composed of fibers, which are made up of myofibrils. Myofibrils are composed of sarcomeres that are connected in series. The overlapping cross-bridges of actin and myosin make up a sarcomere.
   b. When a muscle contracts, the actin-myosin filaments slide together and the muscle shortens. The cross bridges slide apart when the muscle relaxes and returns to its resting length.
2. Muscle performance.
   a. Muscular strength: the maximum force that a muscle can develop during a single contraction.
   b. Muscular power: the rate of performing work, where work is the magnitude of a force acting on an object multiplied by the distance through which the force acts.
   c. Muscular endurance: the ability of muscle to contract repeatedly or to generate force over a certain period of time.

Motor Units and Muscle Fiber Types (See Table 6-1)

1. A motor unit is an alpha motor neuron (lower motor neuron) and all of the muscle fibers that it innervates.
2. A muscle unit is all of the muscle fibers that are innervated by an individual alpha motor neuron. Table 6-1 lists the most common muscle unit or muscle fiber types.
3. Muscle unit types.
   a. Slow-twitch (ST) fibers (type I).
      - Slow contraction speed.
      - Low force (tension) production.
      - Highly resistant to fatigue.
   b. Fast-twitch (FT) fibers (type IIa).
      - Fast contraction speed.
      - Fatigue resistant.
      - Characteristics can be influenced by the type of training.

Table 6-1

Muscle Fiber Types and Characteristics

CHARACTERISTIC	TYPE I	TYPE IIa	TYPE IIx
Motor neuro size	Small	Large	Large
Conduction velocity	Slow	Fast	Fast
Contraction speed	Slow	Fast	Fast
Relaxation speed	Slow	Fast	Fast
Force production	Low	Moderate	High
Fatigue resistance	High	Moderate	Low
Capillary density	High	Moderate	Low
Energy system	Aerobic	Aerobic	Anaerobic
Diameter	Small	Moderate	Large
Twitch rate	Slow	Fast	Fast
Fiber diameter	Small	Moderate	Large
Color	Red	White/red	White
Myoglobin content and blood supply	High	Low	Low
Mitochondrial density	High	Moderate	Low

Adapted from: Haff and Triplett, Essentials of Strength Training and Conditioning, 4th ed., 2016; Kisner and Colby, Therapeutic Exercise, 7th ed., FA Davis, 2018.

c. Fast-twitch (FT) fibers (type IIx).
- Fast contraction speed.
- High force production.
- Susceptible to quick fatigue.

d. Hereditary influences and fiber type distribution.
- The percentage of either FT or ST fibers in the body is determined by genetics. This ratio cannot be changed via normal exercise.
- Specific training can modify metabolic characteristics of all fiber types; e.g., high-intensity, anaerobic strength training will stimulate optimal FT adaptation.

e. Order of fiber type recruitment.
- Recruitment order depends upon type of activity, force required, movement pattern, and position of the body.
- ST motor units have the lowest functional thresholds and are recruited during lighter, slower efforts such as low-intensity, long-duration endurance activities.
- Higher forces with greater velocity cause the activation of more powerful, higher threshold FT motor units.
- Order of recruitment is ST, followed by FT IIa, and finally followed by FT IIx motor units.

Length-Tension Relationship

1. As the muscle shortens or lengthens through the available range of motion (ROM), the tension it produces varies. Maximum tension is generated at some midpoint in the ROM; less tension is developed in either shortened or lengthened ROM.
2. The weight lifted or lowered cannot exceed that which the muscle is able to control at its weakest point in the ROM.
3. When a muscle is stretched beyond the resting length, there is a mechanical disruption of the cross bridges as the microfilaments slide apart and the sarcomeres lengthen. Releasing the stretch allows the sarcomeres to return to their resting length. This change in ratio of length to tension is called elasticity.
4. Once released, a muscle stretched into the elastic range will contract and produce a force or tension as the muscle returns to its original length.

Adaptations to Resistance Training

Changes in Muscle

1. Hypertrophy is an increase in muscle size as a result of resistance training and can be observed after at least 6–8 weeks of training.
2. Remodeling: individual muscle fibers are enlarged, contain more actin and myosin and have more, larger myofibrils; sarcomeres are increased.
3. An increase in motor unit recruitment and synchronization of firing facilitates contraction and maximizes force production.
4. The average person has a ratio of 50% fast- to slow-twitch motor units. Performing workloads of low intensity will challenge half of the body's muscle mass. High-intensity exercises for shorter durations (less than 20 repetitions) are needed to train the highly adaptable fast-twitch IIa fibers.
5. Disuse atrophy occurs when a muscle loses both size and strength from lack of use or when a limb is immobilized.
6. Cross-section area of a muscle highly correlates with strength gains. The larger the muscle, the greater the strength of that muscle.

Changes in Impairments and Function (See Table 6-2)

1. Positive changes in impairments. Improvement in:
   a. Strength.
   b. Bone mass.
   c. Body composition: fat to lean body composition.
   d. Weight control and weight maintenance; decreased risk of adult-onset diabetes.
   e. Reaction time.
   f. Metabolism, calorie burning during and after exercise.
   g. Cardiovascular status: reduction in resting blood pressure.
   h. Immunological function.
2. Positive changes in function and quality of life.
   a. Improved balance and coordination.
   b. Improved gait and functional mobility.
   c. Improved activities of daily living.
   d. Improved job/recreational/athletic performance.
   e. Improved sense of well-being, posture, and self-image.

Resistance Training Principles (See Table 6-3)

General Principles (See Table 6-4)

1. Principle of individuality: each person is unique and will respond to a training stimulus differently;

Table 6-2

Resistance Training Changes in Muscle and Performance

MUSCULAR STRENGTH TRAINING	MUSCULAR ENDURANCE TRAINING
Muscle fiber hypertrophy	Increased capillary density
Increased motor unit firing rate	Increased mitochondrial density
Decreased capillary density	Increased APT stores
Decreased mitochondrial density	Increased bone density
Increased ATP stores	Decreased body fat percentage
Increased bone density	
Increased lean body mass	

Adapted from: Kisner and Colby, Therapeutic Exercise, 7th ed., FA Davis, 2018.

Table 6-3

Resistance Exercise Evidence-Based Recommendations (FITT-VP) for Healthy Adults	
Frequency	• Each major muscle group should be trained 2–3 days per week.
Intensity	• 60%–70% of 1-RM (one-repetition maximum; moderate to vigorous intensity) for novice to intermediate exercisers to improve strength. • Experienced strength trainers can gradually increase to ≥80% of 1-RM (vigorous to very vigorous intensity) to improve strength. • 40%–50% of 1-RM (very light to light intensity) for older individuals beginning exercise to improve strength. • 40%–50% of 1-RM (very light to light intensity) may be beneficial for improving strength in sedentary individuals beginning a resistance training program. • <50% of 1-RM (light to moderate intensity) to improve muscular endurance. • 20%–50% of 1-RM in older adults to improve power.
Time	• No specific duration of training has been identified for effectiveness.
Type	• Resistance exercises involving each major muscle group are recommended. • Multijoint exercises affecting more than one muscle group and targeting agonist and antagonist muscle groups are recommended for all adults. • Single-joint exercises targeting major muscle groups may also be included in a resistance training program, typically after performing multijoint exercises for those particular muscle groups. • A variety of exercise equipment and/or body weight can be used to perform these exercises.
Repetitions	• 8–12 repetitions are recommended to improve strength and power in most adults. • 10–15 repetitions are effective in improving strength in middle-aged and older individuals starting a resistance training program. • 15–25 repetitions are recommended to improve muscular endurance.
Sets	• 2–4 sets are recommended for most adults to improve strength and power. • A single set of resistance exercise can be effective, especially among older and novice exercisers. • ≤2 sets are effective in improving muscle endurance.
Pattern	• Rest intervals of 2–3 minutes between each set of repetitions are effective. • A rest of ≥48 hours between sessions for any single muscle groups is recommended.
Progression	• A gradual progression of greater resistance, and/or more repetitions per set, and/or increasing frequency is recommended.

Adapted from: Garber CE et al. American College of Sports Medicine position stand. The quantity and quality of exercise for developing and maintaining cardiorespiratory, musculoskeletal, and neuromotor fitness in apparently healthy adults: guidance for prescribing exercise. *Med Sci Sports Exerc.* 2011; 43(7): 1334–59.

NOTE: This table describes exercise guidelines for healthy individuals. For exercise guidelines for individuals with specific diseases, see ACSM's Guidelines for Exercise Testing and Prescription, 10th ed., Williams & Wilkins, 2017; and ACSM's Exercise Management for Persons with Chronic Diseases and Disabilities, 4th ed., Human Kinetics, 2016.

Table 6-4

Progression of Resistance Training Exercise

FACTOR	PROGRESSION
Frequency	Less → more (times per day/week)
Intensity	Submaximal → maximal Low load → high load
Time	Short duration → long duration
Type of muscle contraction	Static → dynamic Concentric and eccentric: variable progression
Body position	Non–weight-bearing → weight-bearing
Repetitions and sets	Low volume → high volume
Range of movement	Short arc → long arc → full arc Stable portion of range → unstable
Velocity of movement	Slow → fast
Plane of movement	Uniplanar → multiplanar
Rest period	Longer rest → shorter

Adapted from: Kisner and Colby, Therapeutic Exercise, 7th ed., FA Davis, 2018.

influenced by biological age, training age, gender, sex, etc.

2. Principle of specificity: adaptations to training are specific to the muscle group trained, metabolic demands of the exercise, and types of movements required.
3. Principle of overload: to achieve adaptation, a stimulus must be applied that is beyond the current capability; may involve changing resistance, terrain, and movement complexity.
4. Principle of progression: to achieve adaptation, a training stimulus must gradually and consistently increase; rest and recovery must be included in the progression.
5. Principle of diminishing returns (neuromuscular adaptation): individuals with less training history will make faster initial gains than individuals with a longer training history.
6. Principle of reversibility: when a training stimulus is not present for a period of time, performance will decrease.

RED FLAG: Common Errors Associated with Resistance or Strength Training:
- Valsalva's maneuver: forcible exhalation with the glottis, nose, and mouth closed while contraction is being held. Valsalva's maneuver increases intrathoracic pressure, slows heart rate (HR), decreases return of blood to the heart, and increases venous pressure and cardiac work.
- Inadequate rest after vigorous exercise. Three to 4 minutes are needed to return the muscle to 90%–95% of preexercise capacity. Most rapid recovery occurs in the first minute.
- Increasing exercise progression too quickly (intensity, duration, frequency) can overwork muscles and cause injuries.
- Substitute motions occur from too much resistance, incorrect stabilization, and when muscles are weak from fatigue, paralysis, or pain.

Exercises to Improve Muscle Strength, Hypertrophy, Endurance, and Power

Resistance Exercise

1. Manual resistance: a type of active exercise in which another person provides resistance.
   a. Advantages.
      - Useful in the early stages of an exercise program when the muscle is weak. The therapist can judge the capability of muscle to safely meet demands of exercise.
      - Can be modified for a painful arc in the joint range of motion.
      - Safe resistance exercise when the joint movement needs to be carefully controlled and the resistance is mild to moderate.
      - Can be easily changed to include diagonal or functional patterns of movement (e.g., proprioceptive neuromuscular facilitation [PNF]) and appropriate facilitation techniques (e.g., quick stretch).

   b. Disadvantages.
      - The amount of resistance cannot be measured quantitatively.
      - It may be difficult to maintain the same resistance during the full joint ROM and to consistently repeat the same resistance.
      - The amount of resistance is limited by the strength of the therapist or caregiver.
2. Mechanical resistance: a type of active exercise in which resistance is applied through the use of equipment or mechanical apparatus.
   a. Advantages.
      - The amount of resistance can be measured quantitatively and increased over time.
      - Can be used when amounts of resistance are greater than the therapist can apply manually.

   b. Disadvantages.
      - Not easily modified to exercise in diagonal or functional patterns.
      - May not be safe if resistance needs to be carefully controlled or maintained at low levels.
3. Goals and indications for resistance exercise.
   a. Increase strength in a muscle group that lifts, lowers, or controls heavy loads for relatively low number of repetitions.
   b. Increase muscular endurance by performing low-intensity repetitive exercise over a prolonged period.
   c. Improve muscular performance related to strength and speed of movement.
4. Precautions.
   a. Local muscle fatigue is a normal response of the muscle from repeated dynamic or static contractions over a period of time. Fatigue is due to depleted energy stores, insufficient oxygen, and build-up of lactic acid. It is characterized by a decline in peak torque and increased muscle pain with occasional spasm and decreased active ROM (AROM).
   b. General muscular fatigue affects the whole body after prolonged activities such as walking or jogging; usually due to low blood sugar, decreased glycogen stores in muscle and liver, depletion of potassium.
   c. General or specific muscle fatigue may be associated with specific clinical diseases; e.g., multiple sclerosis, cardiac disease, peripheral vascular dysfunction, and pulmonary diseases. These patients fatigue more rapidly and require longer rest periods.
   d. Overwork or overtraining causes temporary or permanent loss of strength as a result of exercise. In normal individuals, fatigue causes discomfort, so overtraining and muscle weakness does not usually occur. Patients with lower motor neuron disease who participate in vigorous resistance exercise programs can have a deterioration of strength; e.g., post-polio syndrome, Duchenne muscular dystrophy. Overwork can be avoided with slow progression of the exercise intensity, duration, and progression.
   e. Osteoporosis makes the bone unable to withstand normal stresses and highly susceptible to pathological fracture. May develop as a result of prolonged immobilization, bed rest, inability to bear weight on an extremity, and nutritional or hormonal factors.
   f. Acute muscle soreness develops during or directly after strenuous anaerobic exercise performed to the point of fatigue. Decreased blood flow and reduced oxygen (ischemia) create a temporary build-up of lactic acid and potassium. A cool-down period of low-intensity exercise can facilitate the return of oxygen to the muscle and reduce soreness.

g. Delayed-onset muscle soreness (DOMS) can begin 12–24 hours after vigorous exercise or muscular overexertion. Peaks at 24–48 hours after exercise. Muscle tenderness and stiffness can last up to 5–7 days. Usually greater after muscle lengthening or eccentric exercise. Severity of soreness can be lessened by gradually increasing the intensity and duration of exercises.

RED FLAGS: Contraindications.
- Inflammation: resistance exercises can increase swelling and cause damage to muscles or joints.
- Pain: severe joint or muscle pain during exercise or for more than 24 hours after exercise requires elimination or reduction of the exercise.

5. Types of resistance exercise.
   a. Isometric exercise is static and occurs when a muscle contracts without a length change. Resistance is variable and accommodating. Contractions should be held for at least 6 seconds to obtain adaptive changes in the muscle.
      - Strengthening of muscles is developed at a point in the ROM, not over the entire length of the muscle.
      - This type of resistance exercise can increase blood pressure and should be used cautiously with the patient with a cardiac condition.
      - Monitor for potential Valsalva's maneuver.
   b. Isotonic exercise is dynamic and can have a constant (free weights) or variable (machine) load as the muscle lengthens or shortens through the available ROM. Speed can be variable for this type of exercise.
      - Weight-lifting machines have an oval-shaped cam or wheel that mimics the length-tension curve of the muscle; e.g., Nautilus or Cybex. These machines vary resistance as the muscle goes through the ROM, providing resistance that the muscle can safely complete at various points of the ROM.
      - Free weights do not vary the resistance through the ROM of a muscle. The weakest point along the length-tension curve of each muscle limits the amount of weight lifted.
      - Weight-lifting machines are safer than free weights; used early in a resistance exercise or rehabilitation program.
   c. Isokinetic exercise is dynamic and has a speed control for muscle shortening and lengthening. Resistance is accommodating and variable.
      - Peak torque, the maximum force generated through the ROM, is inversely related to angular velocity (speed) as the body segment moves through ROM; e.g., increasing angular velocity decreases peak torque production.
      - Concentric or eccentric resistance exercise can be performed on isokinetic equipment.
      - Isokinetic exercise provides maximum resistance at all points in the ROM as the muscle contracts.
      - During isokinetic testing, the weight of a body segment creates a torque output around the joint; e.g., the lower leg around the knee joint in sitting knee flexion. This gravity-produced torque adds to the force generated by the muscle when it contracts and gives a higher torque output than is actually created by the muscle. The higher value can affect the testing values of the muscle group and which muscle group needs to be strengthened. Software can correct for the effects of gravity.
   d. Eccentric (lengthening) versus concentric (shortening).
      - Maximum eccentric contraction produces more force than maximal concentric contraction.
      - Resistance training performed concentrically improves concentric muscle strength and eccentric training improves eccentric muscle strength (specificity of training).
      - Eccentric contractions occur in a wide variety of functional activities, such as lowering the body against gravity; e.g., sitting down or descending stairs.
      - Eccentric contractions provide a source of shock absorption during closed-chain functional activities.
      - Eccentric contractions consume less oxygen and fewer energy stores than concentric contractions against similar loads.
6. Range of motion.
   a. Short-arc exercise: resistance exercise performed through a limited ROM; e.g., initial exercise post–knee surgery (anterior cruciate repair), painful full-range movement.
   b. Full-arc exercise: resistance exercise performed through full ROM.
7. Open-chain versus closed-chain exercises.
   a. Open-chain exercise occurs when the distal segment (hand or foot) moves freely in space; e.g., when an arm lifts or lowers a handheld weight.
   b. Resistance exercises usually are open chain, which may be the only option if weight-bearing is contraindicated.
   c. Open-chain exercise does not adequately prepare a patient for functional weight-bearing activities.
   d. Closed-chain exercise occurs when the body moves over a fixed distal segment; e.g., stair climbing or squatting activities.
   e. Closed-chain exercise loads muscles, bones, joints, and noncontractile soft tissues such as ligaments, tendons, and joint capsules.
   f. Mechanoreceptors are stimulated by closed-chain exercises, adding to joint stability, balance, coordination, and agility in functional weight-bearing postures.

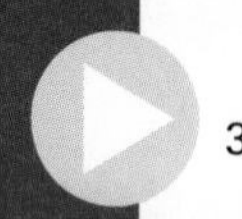

Table 6-5

Recommended Parameters for Developing Muscular Strength, Hypertrophy, Endurance, and Power

FITNESS COMPONENT	RESISTANCE VELOCITY	SETS REPETITIONS	RECOVERY BETWEEN SETS	FREQUENCY
Muscular Strength and Hypertrophy	• 70%–90% 1 RM or 8–12 RM • Slow to moderate velocity	• 2–3 sets • 8–12 reps	2–3 minutes	2–4 times per week
Muscular Endurance	• 50%–70% 1RM or 15+ RM • Moderate to fast velocity Multijoint lifts are optimal for building endurance due to the ability to activate more muscle mass for a given distance moved. Training to increase muscular strength may also increase muscular endurance.	• ≤2 sets • 15–20 reps	60–90 seconds Less than 1 minute for sets of 10–15 reps 1–2 minutes for sets of 15–25 reps	2–4 times per week
Muscular Power	Multijoint, total body exercises combining strength training (as above) with light loads (30%–70% 1RM) moved at fast velocities for upper or lower body Olympic (snatch, clean, and jerk) or component lifts, plyometric, and medicine ball exercises	• 3–5 sets • 3–6 reps	3–5 minutes	2–4 times per week

Exercise sequencing: Perform large muscle group, multijoint, more complex, or higher intensity exercises before small muscle group, single joint, or lower intensity exercises. Consider alternating upper and lower body or opposing muscle group (e.g., push and pull) exercises across the training session for time efficiency.

Volume: In order to accurately track the amount of weight lifted during a resistance training session, routinely calculate volume. One way to determine this parameter is to multiply the total number of sets by the number of repetitions per set by the amount of weight lifted per repetition. For example, the volume for 3 sets of 10 repetitions with 30 pounds would be conveyed as 3 × 10 × 30 pounds, or 900 pounds.

Periodized variation: Systematically change and progress the volume and intensity.

Adapted from: Garber CE et al. American College of Sports Medicine. Position stand: The quantity and quality of exercise for developing and maintaining cadiorespiratory, musculoskeletal, and neuromotor fitness in apparently health adults: Guidance for prescribing exercise. *Med Sci Sports Exerc.* 2011; 43(7): 1334–1359.

Specific Exercise Regimens (See Table 6-5)

Circuit Weight Training

1. A sequence of exercises for total-body conditioning.
2. A rest period of usually 30 seconds to 1 minute is taken between each exercise.
3. Exercises can be done with free weights or weight-machines.

Plyometric Training

1. A stretch-shortening activity using isotonic exercise.
2. Combines speed, strength, and functional activities.
3. Used in later stages of rehabilitation to achieve high level of performance; e.g., jumping off of a platform, then up onto the platform at a rapid pace to improve vertical jumping abilities.

Brief Repetitive Isometric Exercise

1. Occurs with up to 20 maximum contractions held for 5–6 seconds and performed daily.
2. A 20-second rest after each contraction is recommended to prevent increases in blood pressure.
3. Strength gains occur in 6 weeks.

Endurance Training

Training Strategies to Develop Muscular Endurance

Concepts of Muscular Endurance Training

1. Muscular endurance: the ability of an isolated muscle group to perform repeated contractions over time.
2. Muscular endurance is improved by performing low-load resistance exercise for many repetitions. Exercise programs that increase strength also increase muscular endurance.
3. Muscular endurance programs are indicated after injuries to joints and soft tissues. Dynamic exercises at

a high number of repetitions against light resistance are more comfortable and create less joint irritation than heavy resistance exercises.
4. Early in a strength-training program, high repetitions and low-load exercises cause less muscle soreness and reduce the risk of muscle injury.

Training Strategies to Develop Cardiovascular Endurance (See Table 6-6)

Concepts of Cardiovascular Endurance Training

1. Cardiovascular endurance: the ability to perform large-muscle, dynamic exercise, such as walking, swimming, and/or biking, for long periods of time.
2. Overload principle: used to enhance physiological improvement and bring about a training change. Specific exercise overload must be applied.
   a. Training adaptation occurs by exercising at a level above normal.
   b. The appropriate overload for each person can be achieved by manipulating combinations of training frequency, intensity, and duration.
3. Specificity principle: adaptations in the metabolic and physiological systems, depending on the type of overload imposed.
   a. Specific exercise elicits specific adaptations, creating specific training effects; e.g., swim training will increase cardiovascular conditioning only when tested in swimming. There is no crossover for conditioning from swimming to running.
4. Individual differences principle: training benefits are optimized when programs are planned to meet the individual needs and capacities of the participants.
5. Reversibility principle: detraining occurs rapidly, after only 1–2 weeks, when a person stops exercising. If a person has a history of performing regular exercise, the detraining effects are transient and reversible.
6. Exercise and progressive activity regimens require monitoring of heart rate, blood pressure, and other signs and symptoms of exertional intolerance (see Chapter 4).

Exercise Prescription Using the FITT Equation

1. FITT stands for Frequency, Intensity, Time, and Type. Intensity is interrelated with both duration (time) and frequency.
2. Frequency is the number of exercise sessions per week. If training at a lower intensity, then more frequent exercise is indicated.
   a. Recommend 5 days per week at a moderate intensity for most adults. Three days per week is sufficient when exercising at a vigorous intensity or 3–5 days per week at a moderate to vigorous intensity.

Table 6-6

Aerobic (Cardiovascular) Exercise Evidence-Based Recommendations (FITT-VP) for Healthy Adults	
Frequency	• ≥5 days per week of moderate exercise, or ≥3 days per week of vigorous exercise, or a combination of moderate and vigorous exercise of ≥3–5 days per week is recommended.
Intensity	• Moderate and/or vigorous intensity is recommended for most adults. • On a scale of 0–10 for perceived level of physical exertion, 5–6 is moderate intensity and 7–8 is vigorous intensity. • Light to moderate intensity may be beneficial in deconditioned individuals.
Time	• ≥30–60 minutes per day of purposeful moderate exercise, or 20–60 minutes per day of vigorous exercise, or a combination of moderate and vigorous exercise is recommended for most adults. • <20 minutes per day may be beneficial in previously sedentary individuals.
Type	• Regular, purposeful exercise that involves major muscle groups and is continuous and rhythmic in nature is recommended.
Volume	• A target volume of ≥500–1,000 MET-minutes per week is recommended. • Increasing pedometer step counts by ≥2,000 steps per day to reach a daily step count ≥7,000 steps per day is beneficial. • Exercising below these volumes may still be beneficial for individuals unable or unwilling to reach this amount of exercise.
Pattern	• Exercise may be performed in one continuous session, in one interval session, or in multiple sessions of ≥10 minutes to accumulate the desired duration and volume of exercise per day. • Exercise bouts of <10 minutes may yield favorable adaptations in very deconditioned individuals.
Progression	• A gradual progression of exercise volume by adjusting exercise duration, frequency, and/or intensity is reasonable until the desired exercise goal (maintenance) is attained. • This approach of "start low and go slow" may improve adherence and reduce risk of musculoskeletal injury or adverse cardiac incidents.

Adapted from: Garber CE et al. American College of Sports Medicine position stand. The quantity and quality of exercise for developing and maintaining cardiorespiratory, musculoskeletal, and neuromotor fitness in apparently healthy adults: Guidance for prescribing exercise. *Med Sci Sports Exerc.* 2011; 43(7): 1334–1359.

NOTE: This table describes exercise guidelines for healthy individuals. For exercise guidelines for individuals with specific diseases, see ACSM's Guidelines for Exercise Testing and Prescription, 10th ed., Williams & Wilkins, 2017; and ACSM's Exercise Management for Persons with Chronic Diseases and Disabilities, 4th ed., Human Kinetics, 2016.

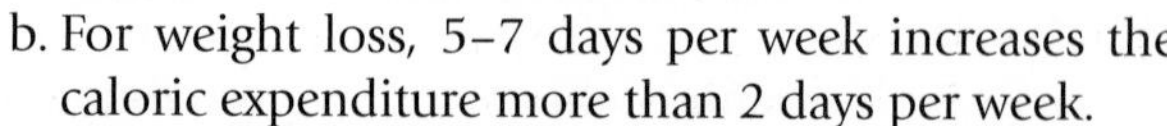

b. For weight loss, 5–7 days per week increases the caloric expenditure more than 2 days per week.
c. Less than 2 days per week does not produce adequate changes in aerobic capacity or body composition.

3. Intensity (creating an overload) is the primary way to improve cardiovascular endurance (aerobic fitness).
   a. Relative intensity for an individual is calculated as a percentage of the maximum function; e.g., maximum oxygen consumption (VO_2 max) or maximum heart rate (HR_{max}).
   b. The VO_2 max or HR_{max} can be measured directly or indirectly based on different methods; e.g., treadmill test 3-minute step, 12-minute run, or treadmill test.
   c. HR_{max} can be estimated using 208–0.7 (age). Training level of target heart rate (THR) can be achieved at 60% of maximum to increase aerobic capacity.
   d. Karvonen's formula is used to predict heart rate reserve (HRR) or HR_{max} minus the resting heart rate (RHR) and correlates directly to VO_2 max. THR = (HR_{max} – RHR) × % of desired training intensity + RHR. The HRR method works best in healthy, unmedicated people.
   e. Rate of perceived exertion (RPE) can be used to evaluate training at submaximal levels. RPE should be coorelated with hemodynamic response to achieve a level that is moderate exercise for each person. The "talk test," or the ability for the exercising person to have a conversation during exercise, usually indicates a moderate level of activity for that person.
4. Duration (time).
   a. Exercise duration is prescribed as the amount of time physical activity is performed (per session).
   b. Duration varies with intensity and frequency of exercise.
      - Moderate exercise performed for at least 30–60 minutes (~150 minutes per week) 3–5 days per week is recommended for most adults with average to good fitness. Vigorous activity for 20–60 minutes per day (~75 minutes per week) is effective.
      - For sedentary individuals (no habitual activity/extremely deconditioned) light to moderate exercise performed for 10–20 min per day 5–7 days per week is recommended.
      - Intensity is decreased, frequency is increased (e.g., 2–4 times per day), and duration is decreased (e.g., 3–5 min) as tolerated for individuals with health conditions (e.g., cardiac or pulmonary disease).
   c. Multiple sessions of short durations are also indicated when intensity is limited by environmental conditions, such as heat and humidity or by medical conditions, such as intermittent claudication or congestive heart failure.
   d. Obese individuals should exercise at longer durations and lower intensities. At this exercise level, the person can speak without gasping and does not have muscle ache or burn from lactic acid accumulation.
5. Type of exercise. Exercises to increase cardiovascular endurance should involve large muscle groups activated in rhythmic aerobic nature. Specificity of training should be considered.
6. See also Chapter 4.

Training Strategies to Develop Pulmonary Endurance

Concepts of Pulmonary Endurance Training

1. Pulmonary endurance is related to the ventilation of the lungs and oxygen consumption.
2. Ventilation is the process of air exchange in the lungs. The volume of air breathed each minute, or minute ventilation ($\dot{V}_E$), is 6 liters. $\dot{V}_E$ = breathing rate × tidal volume. In maximum exercise, increases in breathing rate and depth may produce ventilation as high as 200 liters per minute.
3. Energy is produced aerobically as oxygen is supplied to exercising muscles. Oxygen consumption rises rapidly during the first minutes of exercise, and then levels off as the aerobic metabolism supplies the energy required by the working muscles (steady state).
4. The more fit a person is, the more capable their respiratory system is of delivering oxygen to sustain aerobic energy production at increasingly higher levels of intensity.
   a. Obesity can impair pulmonary function because of the added effort to move the chest wall.
5. In severe pulmonary disease, the cost of breathing can reach 40% of the total exercise oxygen consumption. This decreases the oxygen available to the exercising nonrespiratory muscles and limits exercise capabilities. Obesity can significantly increase the level of impairments.
6. Exercise training makes minimal direct improvements to the pulmonary system and cannot reverse damage to pulmonary tissue. A patient with pulmonary disease who is aerobically conditioned will be able to perform more activities because the overall workload of any activity decreased.

Exercise-Induced Asthma (EIA)

1. EIA can occur when the normal initial bronchodilation is followed by bronchoconstriction. The reduction in airflow from airway obstruction affects the ability of the lungs to provide oxygen to exercising muscles.
2. EIA is an acute, reversible airway obstruction that develops 5–15 minutes after strenuous exercise.

3. In some people who mouth breathe, the air is cold and dry, contributing to the bronchoconstriction.
4. Lowering the intensity level and allowing the person to breathe through the nose can allow prolonged aerobic exercise to continue.
5. The problem is rare in activities that require only short bursts of activity such as baseball, and is more likely to occur in endurance activities such as soccer.
6. When exercising in humid versus dry environments, the exercise-induced asthmatic response is considerably reduced. See Chapter 4.

Aerobic Training

Concepts of Aerobic Training

1. Aerobic training (cardiorespiratory endurance training) can result in higher fitness levels for healthy individuals, slow the decrease in functional capacity in the elderly, and recondition those with illness or chronic disease.
2. Positive effects of aerobic training on the cardiovascular and respiratory systems.
   a. Improve breathing volumes and increase VO_2 max.
   b. Increase heart weight and volume; cardiac hypertrophy is normal with long-term aerobic training.
   c. Increase total hemoglobin and oxygen delivery capacity.
   d. Decrease resting and submaximal exercise heart rates. Can be utilized to measure improvements from aerobic training.
   e. Increase cardiac output and stroke volume.
   f. Improve distribution of blood to working muscles and enhance capacity of trained muscles to extract and use oxygen.
   g. Reduce resting blood pressure.

Types of Aerobic Training

1. Continuous training at a submaximal energy requirement can be prolonged for 20–60 minutes without exhausting the oxygen transport system.
   a. Work rate is increased progressively as training improvements are achieved; overload can be accomplished by increasing the exercise duration.
   b. In healthy individuals, continuous training is the most effective way to improve endurance.
2. Circuit training uses a series of exercise activities that are repeated several times.
   a. Several exercise modes can be utilized, involving large and small muscle groups both statically and dynamically.
   b. Circuit training improves endurance and strength by stressing the aerobic and anaerobic energy systems.
3. Interval training includes an exercise period followed by a prescribed rest interval. It is perceived to be less demanding than continuous training.
   a. The relief interval can be passive or active; its duration ranges from a few seconds to several minutes. Active or work recovery involves doing the exercise at a reduced level. During the relief period, a portion of the adenosine triphosphate (ATP) and oxygen used by the muscles during the work period is replenished by the aerobic system.
   b. The longer the work interval, the more the aerobic system is stressed.
   c. With appropriate spacing of work-relief intervals, a significant amount of high-intensity work can be achieved. The total amount of work completed with interval training is greater than the amount of work accomplished with continuous training.
4. Warm-up and cool-down periods: each exercise session includes a 5- to 15-minute warm-up and a 5- to 15-minute cool-down period.
   a. The warm-up period prevents the heart and circulatory system from being suddenly taxed. It includes low-intensity cardiorespiratory activities and flexibility exercises.
   b. The cool-down period also consists of exercising at a lower intensity. It reduces abrupt physiological alterations that can occur with sudden cessation of strenuous exercise; e.g., venous pooling in the lower extremities, which causes decreased venous return to the heart.
   c. Longer warm-up and cool-down periods may be needed for deconditioned or older individuals.

RED FLAG: Common Errors Associated with Muscular, Cardiovascular, and Pulmonary Endurance Training

- Lack of exercise tolerance testing (ETT) before the exercise prescription is determined could result in a training program set too high or too low for that individual.
- Starting out at too high a level can overly stress the cardiorespiratory and muscular systems and potentially cause injuries.
- Increasing intensity too fast can create a problem for an individual during endurance training.
- Exercising at too intense a level can use the anaerobic energy system, not the aerobic system; this increases strength and power, not endurance.
- Insufficient warm-up or cool-down results in inadequate cardiorespiratory and muscular adaptation; there is inadequate time to prepare for or recover from higher intense activity.
- Inconsistent training frequency, duration, or intensity does not properly stress or overload the aerobic system to create training effects.

Exercise at High Altitude

1. At altitudes of 6,000 feet (1,829 meters [m]) or higher there can be a noticeable drop in performance of aerobic activities.
2. The partial pressure of oxygen is reduced, resulting in poor oxygenation of hemoglobin.
3. This hypoxia at altitude can result in immediate compensatory hyperventilation (stimulation of the baroreceptors) and increased heart rate.
4. Reduction in CO2 from hyperventilation results in more alkaline body fluids.
5. Adjustments or acclimatization to higher altitude. Performance is at risk of decreasing starting at altitudes greater than 3,937 ft (1,200 m).
   a. Takes 2 weeks at 7,545 ft (2,300m) and an additional week for every additional 1,968 ft (600 m) in altitude.
   b. There is a decrease in plasma volume (concentrating red blood cells) and an increase in total red blood cells and hemoglobin improving oxygenation.
   c. Changes in local circulation may facilitate oxygen transport.
   d. Adjustments do not fully compensate for altitude. VO_2 max is decreased 2% for every 984 ft (300 m) above 4,950 ft (1,500 m). Thus, there is a drop in performance for endurance activities.
   e. Training at altitude does not provide any improvement in sea-level performance.
6. The air in mountainous regions tends to be cool and dry.
   a. Body fluids can be rapidly lost through evaporation and result in dehydration.
   b. Ensure adequate hydration for those exercising or engaged in sports at altitude.

Exercise in Hot Weather

1. When exercising in the heat, muscles require oxygen to produce energy.
2. To decrease metabolic heat, blood is shunted to the periphery; thus, working muscles are deprived of needed oxygen.
3. Core temperature increases and sweating increases. Fluids must be continually replaced or core temperatures can rise to dangerous levels.
4. Hot, humid environments diminish the evaporative cooling component, even with profuse sweating. Excess fluid loss can compromise cardiovascular function.
5. Fluid replacement.
   a. Maintain plasma volume.
   b. Colder fluids are emptied from the stomach more rapidly than room-temperature fluids.
   c. Concentrated carbohydrate drinks impair gastric emptying and slow fluid replacement.
   d. Glucose-polymer drinks do not impair physiological functioning. They may also resupply lost electrolytes.
6. Repeated heat stress results in acclimatization in about 10 days of exposure.
   a. Exercise capacity is increased.
   b. Cardiac output is better regulated.
   c. Sweating is more efficient.
   d. Acclimatization to heat stress does not seriously deteriorate with age.
7. Men and women can adapt equally well to heat, even though the mechanisms of thermoregulation differ slightly. The menstrual cycle is not a factor.
8. Obesity is a major consideration when exercising in the heat.
9. Exercise recommendations for individuals with obesity. See Chapter 8.

Mobility and Flexibility Training

Flexibility (See Table 6-7)

1. Flexibility refers to the ability to move a joint through an unrestricted, pain-free ROM; the musculotendinous unit elongates as the body segment moves through the ROM.
2. Dynamic flexibility refers to the active ROM of a joint and is dependent upon the amount of tissue resistance met during active movement.
3. Passive flexibility is the degree to which a joint can be passively moved through the available ROM and is dependent upon the extensibility of the muscle and connective tissue around the joint.

Stretching

1. Stretching involves any therapeutic technique that lengthens shortened soft-tissue structures and increases ROM.

Types of Stretching

1. The type of stretching is determined by the type of force applied, the intensity of stretch, and duration of stretch to contractile and noncontractile tissues.
2. Static stretching takes the structures beyond the free ROM to elongate tissues beyond their resting length.

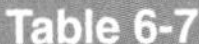
Table 6-7

Flexibility Exercise Evidence-Based Recommendations (FITT-VP) for Healthy Adults

Frequency	• ≥2–3 days per week with daily being most effective.
Intensity	• Stretch to the point of feeling tightness or slight discomfort.
Time	• Holding a static stretch for 10–30 seconds is recommended for most adults. • In older individuals, holding a stretch for 30–60 seconds may result in a greater benefit. • For proprioceptive neuromuscular facilitation (PNF) stretching, a 3- to 6-second light-to-moderate contraction (e.g., 20%–75% of maximum voluntary contraction) followed by a 10- to 30-second assisted stretch is recommended.
Type	• A series of flexibility exercises for each of the major muscle-tendon units is recommended. • Static flexibility, dynamic flexibility, ballistic flexibility, and PNF are each effective.
Volume	• A reasonable target is to perform 60 seconds of total stretching time for each flexibility exercise.
Pattern	• Repetition of each flexibility exercise two to four times is recommended. • Flexibility exercise is most effective when the muscle is warmed through light-to-moderate aerobic activity or passively through external methods such as moist heating packs or warm baths.
Progression	• Methods for optimal progression are unknown.

Adapted from: Garber CE et al. American College of Sports Medicine position stand. The quantity and quality of exercise for developing and maintaining cardiorespiratory, musculoskeletal, and neuromotor fitness in apparently healthy adults: Guidance for prescribing exercise. *Med Sci Sports Exerc.* 2011; 43(7): 1334–1359.

NOTE: This table describes exercise guidelines for healthy individuals. For exercise guidelines for individuals with specific diseases, see ACSM's Guidelines for Exercise Testing and Prescription, 10th ed., Williams & Wilkins, 2017; and ACSM's Exercise Management for Persons with Chronic Diseases and Disabilities, 4th ed., Human Kinetics, 2016.

a. The stretch force is applied for at least 15–30 seconds and repeated several times during a session.
b. Static stretching may be performed by the patient or therapist.
c. Manual stretching (applied by the PT) is considered a short-duration stretch and is maintained statically for less time than mechanical stretching.
d. Intensity and duration depend on patient tolerance and therapist strength and endurance.
e. Low-intensity stretch, applied as long as possible, is better tolerated and results in optimal improvement in tissue length with minimal risk of injury to any weakened tissue.

3. Ballistic stretching is a high-intensity, very short-duration "bouncing" stretch. By contracting the opposite muscle group, the patient uses body weight and momentum to elongate the tight muscle.
   a. It is considered unsafe because of poor control and the potential of rupturing weakened tissues. It should not be performed after an injury or surgery.
   b. Ballistic stretch facilitates the stretch reflex, causing an increase in tension in the muscle that is being stretched. It is contraindicated in spastic muscles.
4. Prolonged low-intensity mechanical stretching.
   a. An external force (5–15 lb to 10% of body weight) is applied by positioning a patient with weighted pulley and traction systems; e.g., to reduce knee flexion contractures in the patient who is bedridden. May be maintained for 20–30 minutes or as long as several hours.
   b. A dynamic splint maintains the limb positioned at end range and is typically applied for 8–10 hours to increase ROM; e.g., to reduce wrist and finger flexion contractures.
   c. A serial cast maintains the limb positioned at end range. Cast is typically applied for 5–7 days. Cast is then removed and a new cast reapplied with the limb positioned in the newly gained range; e.g., to reduce gastrocnemius/soleus contractures.
   d. Low-intensity, prolonged stretching has been shown to be more effective than manual, passive stretching with long-standing flexion contractures.
5. Dynamic stretching occurs when voluntary, unassisted movement by the patient provides the stretch force to a joint. It requires strength and muscular contraction of the prime mover to actively stretch the antagonist muscle group.
   a. The force is controlled by the patient and is considered low intensity (to tolerance). The risk of tissue injury is low.
   b. Duration is equal to passive, manual stretching or about 15–30 seconds and is limited by prime mover muscular endurance.
6. Facilitated stretching (active inhibition) refers to techniques in which the patient reflexively relaxes the muscle to be elongated prior to or during the stretching technique; e.g., PNF (see Table 6-8).
   a. Indications for active inhibition techniques include limitations in ROM caused by muscle tightness or muscle spasm; techniques are not effective with connective tissue changes.
   b. Hold-relax (HR) is indicated for the patient with limited movement and pain.

Table 6-8

Facilitated Stretching Techniques

TECHNIQUE	DESCRIPTION	RATIONALE
Hold-relax (HR)	A relaxation technique usually performed at the point of limited ROM in the agonist pattern; an isometric contraction of the range-limiting antagonist is performed against slowly increasing resistance, followed by voluntary relaxation and passive movement by the therapist into the newly gained range of the agonist pattern.	The muscle relaxes as a result of autogenic inhibition, possibly from the Golgi tendon organ (GTO) firing and decreasing muscular tension.
Hold-relax-active contraction (HRAC)	Following hold-relax technique, active contraction into the newly gained range of the agonist pattern is performed.	Additional muscle relaxation is achieved through active contraction and reciprocal inhibition effects (a spindle response).
Contract-relax-active contraction (CRAC)	A relaxation technique usually performed at a point of limited ROM in the agonist pattern; isotonic movement in rotation is performed followed by an isometric hold of the range-limiting muscles in the antagonist pattern against slowly increasing resistance, voluntary relaxation, and active movement into the new range of the agonist pattern.	Utilizes effects of both autogenic inhibition and reciprocal inhibition.

Adaptive Changes of Contractile Tissue

1. A muscle that is lengthened over a prolonged period will have an increase in the number of sarcomeres in series. The muscle will adjust its length over time.
2. A muscle immobilized in a shortened position will have a decrease in the number of sarcomeres and an increase in connective tissue.
3. The sarcomere adaptation is transient. A muscle allowed to resume its normal length will produce or absorb sarcomeres (lengthen or shorten).

Neurophysiological Properties

1. The muscle spindle monitors the velocity and length changes in muscle.
2. A quick stretch to a muscle stimulates the alpha motoneurons and facilitates muscle contraction via the monosynaptic stretch reflex. This can increase tension in a contracting muscle and provide reciprocal inhibition to the tight muscle.
3. The Golgi tendon organ (GTO) inhibits contraction of the muscle. When excessive tension develops, the GTO fires, inhibiting alpha motoneuron activity and decreasing tension in the muscle.
4. Slow stretching, especially applied at end range, causes the GTO to fire and inhibit the muscle (autogenic inhibition), allowing the muscle to lengthen (stretch-protection reflex).

Noncontractile Tissue Properties

1. Noncontractile connective tissue includes ligaments, tendons, joint capsules, fasciae, and skin; can affect joint flexibility and requires remodeling to increase length.
2. Low-magnitude loads over long periods increase the deformation of noncontractile tissue, allowing a gradual rearrangement of collagen bonds (remodeling). This type of stretch is better tolerated by the patient.
3. 15–20 minutes of low-intensity sustained stretch, repeated on 5 consecutive days, can cause a change in the length of muscles and connective tissue.
4. Intensive stretching is usually not done every day in order to allow time for healing. Without healing time, a breakdown of tissue will occur, as in overuse syndromes and stress fractures.
5. With aging, collagen loses its elasticity and tissue blood supply is decreased, reducing healing capability. Stretching in older adults should be performed cautiously.
6. Overstretch is a stretch well beyond the normal joint ROM, resulting in hypermobility. If the supporting structures of a joint are insufficient and weak, they cannot hold a joint in a stable, functional position during functional activities. This is known as stretch weakness.

Contracture

1. Contracture is the adaptive shortening of muscle or other soft tissues that cross a joint; contracture results in decreased ROM.
2. Myostatic contracture (pertaining to muscle) involves a musculotendinous unit that has adaptively shortened with loss of ROM. Usually occurs without specific tissue pathology and in two-joint muscles such as the hamstrings, rectus femoris, or gastrocnemius. Can typically be resolved in a short time with gentle stretching exercises and active inhibition techniques.
3. Adhesions (an abnormal union of membranous tissue resulting from injury or inflammation) can occur if tissue is immobilized in a shortened position for extended periods of time, resulting in a loss of mobility.

4. Scar tissue adhesions develop due to injury and the inflammatory response. Initially, new fibers develop in a disorganized pattern and will restrict motion unless remodeled along lines of stress; e.g., the patient with burns.
5. Irreversible contracture: a permanent loss of soft tissue extensibility that cannot be released by nonsurgical treatment. Occurs when normal soft tissue is replaced by an excessive amount of nonextensible tissue, such as bone or fibrotic tissue.

Relaxation of Muscles

1. Local relaxation techniques can assist in the lengthening of contractile and noncontractile tissue.
2. Heat increases the extensibility of the shortened tissues. Warm muscles relax and lengthen more easily, reducing the discomfort of stretching. Connective tissue stretches with less force and shorter duration.
   a. GTO sensitivity is increased, making it more likely to fire and inhibit muscle tension.
   b. Low-intensity active exercise performed prior to stretching will increase circulation to soft tissue and warm the tissues to be stretched.
   c. Heat without stretching has little or no effect on long-term improvement in muscle flexibility. The combination of heat and stretching produces greater long-term gains in tissue length than stretching alone.
3. Massage increases local circulation to the muscle and reduces muscle spasm and stiffness.
4. Biofeedback helps the patient reduce the amount of tension in a muscle and improves flexibility while decreasing pain. Increased level of feedback signals (auditory, visual) assists the patient in recognizing tense muscles.

RED FLAG: Common Errors Associated with Mobility and Flexibility Training:
- Passively forcing a joint beyond its normal ROM.
- Aggressively stretching a patient with a newly united fracture or osteoporosis may result in fracture.
- Using high-intensity, short-duration (ballistic) stretching procedures on muscles and connective tissues that have been immobilized over a long time or recovering from injury or surgery.
- Stretching muscles around joints without using strengthening exercises to develop an appropriate balance between flexibility and strength.
- Overstretching of weak muscles, especially postural muscles that support the body against gravity.
- Insufficient warm-up.

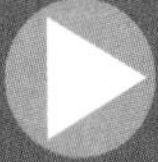

Postural Stability Training

Stability (Static Postural Control)

1. Refers to the synergistic coordination of the neuromuscular system that enables an individual to maintain a stable position in an antigravity, weight-bearing position. The COM is over the BOS, and the body is at rest.
2. Postural stability control involves prolonged holding of core trunk and lower extremity muscles. Postural sway is minimal.

Dynamic Stability

1. Proximal segments and trunk provide a stable base for functional movements.
   a. An individual maintains a stable, nonmoving BOS with the COM within the BOS while parts of the body are moving.
   b. Distal segments are fixed, while proximal segments are moving, e.g., weight shifts in sitting or standing.
   c. Movement normally occurs through increments of range (small range to large range).
   d. Patients with hyperkinetic movement disorders (e.g., ataxia) should be progressed from large range to small range movements, and finally to holding steady (stability control).
2. An individual maintains postural stability of the trunk during dynamic extremity movements (e.g., reaching, kicking a ball).
3. Strength, endurance, flexibility, and coordination are needed for dynamic stability control.

Guidelines to Develop Postural Stability

General Concepts of Stability Training

1. Consider exercise protocols that effectively challenge core muscle groups and create adequate stability to perform functional activities. Stability requires the recruitment of tonic, slow-twitch muscle fibers for sustained periods of time.

2. Start training by teaching safe spinal ROM in a variety of basic postures. Teach chin tucking with axial extension of the cervical spine and pelvic tilting with ROM of the lumbar spine.
3. Incorporate procedures to retrain kinesthetic awareness of postural position.
   a. In sitting, teach optimal posture: head and trunk maintained in midline position, pelvis neutral, weight equally distrubuted over both hips and feet. A neutral pelvis is characterized by:
      - an anterior superior iliac spine (ASIS) that is level or slightly lower than the posterior superior iliac spine (PSIS) (sagittal plane) and
      - a level position of both ASIS (frontal plane).
   b. In standing, teach optimal posture: head and trunk maintained in midline extended position, pelvis neutral, hips and knees extended, feet dorsiflexed, and weight symmetrical over both feet.
   c. Focus patient's awareness on normal alignment of the spine and pelvis, and on muscles required to maintain that position.
   d. Visual, verbal, and proprioceptive cues; e.g., resistance of elastic bands or light manual resistance, can be used to improve postural awareness.
4. To safely develop strength and endurance in the stabilizing muscles, practice maintained holding in a variety of postures. The higher the center of mass (COM) and smaller the base of support (BOS), the greater the degree of postural challenge; e.g., sitting versus standing.
5. Movements of the extremities challenge trunk and neck stabilization; functional position must be maintained as movements are carried out.

Exercise Techniques to Promote Stability

1. Resistance can be applied to the trunk or the moving extremities; functional position must be maintained as resistance is increased.
2. Alternating isometric contractions between antagonists can enhance stabilizing contractions and develop postural control; e.g., PNF techniques of stabilizing reversals and rhythmic stabilization.
   a. Stabilizing reversals: isometric holding is facilitated first on one side of the joint, followed by alternate holding of the antagonist muscle groups. May be applied in a variety of directions; e.g., anterior-posterior, medial-lateral, diagonal.
   b. Rhythmic stabilization (RS): simultaneous isometric contractions of both agonist and antagonist patterns performed without relaxation, using careful grading of resistance; results in cocontraction of opposing muscle groups; RS emphasizes rotational stability control.
3. During early training, emphasize muscles needed for trunk support in the upright posture, for performing basic body mechanics, and for upper extremity lifting.
4. Teach control of functional positions while moving from one position to another. This is called transitional mobilty and requires graded contractions and adjustments of stabilizing muscles. Consider moving out of a posture (eccentric control) before moving into a posture (concentric control).
5. Introduce simple patterns of motion that develop safe body mechanics and movement.
6. Closed-chain tasks are good choices to enhance postural stabilization (e.g., partial squats and controlled lunges); add arm motions and weights as tolerated.
7. More complex patterns of movement (e.g., rotation and diagonal motions) can be added (e.g., PNF trunk patterns of chop/reverse chop, or lift/reverse lift). Postures can be progressed to add difficulty (e.g., supine to sitting to standing).
8. Incorporate stretching into the postural exercise program. Adequate flexibility is necessary for postural muscles to hold body parts in proper alignment.

RED FLAG: Common Errors Associated with Postural Stability Training:
- Inadequate stretching of tight muscles (e.g., tight hip flexors that hold the pelvis in an anterior pelvic tilt or tight hamstrings that hold the pelvis in a posterior tilt); both prevent a stable postural base (neutral pelvis and spine position).
- Inadequate control of core muscles could place excessive stress on proximal structures during functional activities; e.g., the vertebrae and discs of the spine during sitting.
- Progressing too quickly or starting at too high a functional level for the patient to maintain postural stability.
- Exercising past the point of fatigue, which is determined by the inability of the trunk or postural muscles to stabilize in a functional position.
- Attempting to force a patient into a general neutral position instead of finding the proper and safe position for each individual.

Stability Ball Training

Benefits/Uses

1. Promotes balance; provides an unstable base of support, requiring continuous adjustments in balance. Moving the feet and/or the ball changes the base of support and challenges balance. Allows safe practice of falling.
2. Works muscles in functional, synergistic patterns.
   a. Recruits and retrains core muscles (deep spinal and abdominal muscles).
   b. Promotes postural relearning; e.g., neutral position in sitting, cervical or trunk rotation.

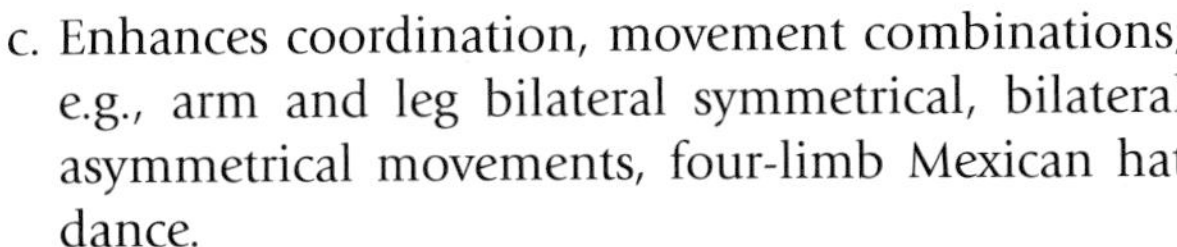

c. Enhances coordination, movement combinations; e.g., arm and leg bilateral symmetrical, bilateral asymmetrical movements, four-limb Mexican hat dance.

3. Heightens proprioception and sensory perception, awareness of the body moving in space.
4. Improves range of motion, allows safe stretching; e.g., total body extension or flexion, upper or lower extremity stretches.
5. Allows relaxation training; e.g., gentle bouncing combined with deep breathing. Gentle rocking can be used to decrease tone in hypertonic patient.
6. Increases strength. Can be combined with resistance training (e.g., lifting a weighted ball), using hand weights or resistive bands while on the ball, or closed-chain exercises (e.g., partial squats using the ball).
7. Advantages: light, portable, durable, and inexpensive.

Precautions

1. Determine appropriate ball size.
   a. Sitting on ball with feet flat, the ball height should place the hips and knees at 90° angles.
   b. Supine with ball under knees, the ball height should equal the distance between the greater trochanter and the knee.
   c. Quadruped, the ball height should equal the distance between the shoulder and the wrist.
2. Ensure proper firmness/inflation.
   a. Ball should be comfortable and have some bounce.
   b. A firm ball moves more quickly.
   c. A soft ball moves more slowly, may make patient feel safer, more secure.
   d. Surface affects movement of the ball: quicker on hard surface, slower on mat or soft surface.
3. Precautions:
   a. Individual weight may exceed ball weight limits.
   b. Sharp belt buckles or other sharp objects may puncture ball.
   c. Lack of foot traction while sitting may result in instability and falls: use bare feet, rubber-soled shoes, yoga sticky mat.
   d. Ensure adequate space around exercising individual.
   e. Sensory overload in patients with heightened sympathetic signs.
   f. Increasing instability with fatigue.
4. Ensure proper foot traction: use bare feet on yoga mat, rubber-soled shoes.
5. Ensure adequate space around exercising individual.
6. Watch for sensory overload: sympathetic signs in children or adults with brain injury.
7. Watch for muscle fatigue, increasing instability.

RED FLAG: Contraindications include dizziness or nausea associated with movement, e.g., the patient with vestibular pathology; extreme anxiety, or fear of being on the ball.

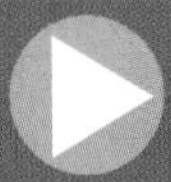

Coordination and Balance Training

Goals and Outcomes

1. Motor function (motor control and learning) is improved.
2. Postural control, biomechanical alignment, and symmetrical weight distribution are improved.
3. Strength, power, and endurance necessary for movement control and balance are improved.
4. Sensory control and integration of sensory systems (somatosensory, visual, and vestibular) necessary for movement control and balance are improved.
5. Performance, independence, and safety are improved in transfers, gait, and locomotion.
6. Performance, independence, and safety are improved in basic activities of daily living (BADL) and instrumental activities of daily living (IADL).
7. Aerobic capacity and endurance are improved.
8. Self-management of symptoms is improved.

Training Strategies to Improve Coordination and Balance (See Table 6-9)

Motor Learning

1. Motor learning strategies are important to assist the central nervous system (CNS) in adaptation for movement control.
2. Learning requires repetition. Practice schedules should be carefully organized.
3. Initial practice may feel threatening to patient; e.g., patient may feel in danger of losing control or balance. Progression should be gradual; the therapist should ensure patient confidence and safety, continuing motivation.
4. Sensory cues are used to enhance motor performance.
5. Feedback should stress knowledge of results (KR). Attention is drawn to the success of the outcome. It is

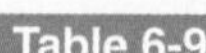

Table 6-9

Neuromotor Exercise Evidence-Based Recommendations (FITT-VP) for Healthy Adults	
Frequency	• ≥2–3 days per week is recommended.
Intensity	• An effective intensity of neuromotor exercise has not been determined.
Time	• ≥20–30 minutes per day is recommended.
Type	• Exercises involving motor skills (e.g., balance, agility, coordination, gait), proprioceptive exercise training, and multifaceted activities (e.g., yoga, tai chi) are recommended for older individuals to improve and maintain physical function and reduce falls in those at risk for falling. • The effectiveness of neuromotor exercise training in younger and middle-aged adults has not been established, but there is probably benefit.
Volume	• The optimal volume (e.g., number of sets and repetitions) is not known.
Pattern	• The optimal pattern of performing neuromotor exercise is not known.
Progression	• Methods for optimal progression are unknown.

Adapted from: Garber CE et al. American College of Sports Medicine position stand. The quantity and quality of exercise for developing and maintaining cardiorespiratory, musculoskeletal, and neuromotor fitness in apparently healthy adults: Guidance for prescribing exercise. *Med Sci Sports Exerc.* 2011; 43(7): 1334–1359.

NOTE: This table describes exercise guidelines for healthy individuals. For exercise guidelines for individuals with specific diseases, see ACSM's Guidelines for Exercise Testing and Prescription, 10th ed., Williams & Wilkins, 2017; and ACSM's Exercise Management for Persons with Chronic Diseases and Disabilities, 4th ed., Human Kinetics, 2016

important to establish a reference of correctness during early, cognitive learning.

6. Feedback should address knowledge of performance (KP). Attention is drawn to missing elements, how to recruit, correct responses, and sequence responses.
7. Feedback schedules: feedback given frequently (after every trial) improves initial performance. Feedback given less frequently (summed after a given number of trials or fading with decreasing frequency) improves retention of skills.
8. A variety of activities and environments should be used to promote adaptability and generalizability of skills. Practice should progress from a closed environment (fixed or controlled) to open variable environments.
9. Patient decision-making skills are promoted. Patients should be encouraged to self-analyze movements and develop strategies to ensure safety and function.

Remedial Strategies

1. Remedial strategies focus on use of involved body segments (e.g., affected extremities in the patient with stroke).
2. Control is first developed in limited movements and progressed to more complex movements. Developmental postures/functional activities can be used to isolate body segments and focus on specific body skills; e.g., weight shifts to improve hip control are practiced first in kneeling before standing.
3. Postural control is first achieved in holding (stability) before moving in a posture (dynamic stability) and skill level function (e.g., gait).
4. Specific techniques can be used to remediate impairments (weakness, incoordination and adaptive shortening, abnormal tone); e.g., tapping to improve responses of a weak quadriceps in standing position.
5. As quality of movement improves, speed of movement and control are increased.
6. Active responses and active learning should be promoted; progression is to unassisted or nonfacilitated movements as soon as possible.

Interventions to Improve Coordination

Functional Training

1. Initial focus is on postural stability activities: holding.
2. A number of different weight-bearing postures can be used; e.g., sitting, quadruped, kneeling, plantigrade, and standing. Progression is to gradually decrease BOS while raising height of COM.
3. Specific exercise techniques to enhance stability previously discussed.

Dynamic Stability Activities

1. Patient practices moving in all directions while maintaining posture.
2. Progression is to increments of range (increasing ROM).
3. Moving in and out of postures (movement transitions); e.g., supine to/from sitting, sitting to/from standing.
4. Specific exercise techniques can include PNF dynamic reversals. Movements can also be resisted using dynamic tubing or resistance bands.
5. PNF patterns can be utilized to challenge dynamic stability control and enhance synergistic and reciprocal action of muscles; e.g., sitting, chop/reverse chop patterns; standing, lift/reverse lift patterns.
6. The patient with ataxia requires the opposite progression: from dynamic stability activities to stabilizing activities: weight shifting through decrements (decreasing) ROM progressing to stability (steady holding).

7. Aquatic exercises: water increases proprioceptive loading of muscles, slows down ataxic movements; provides buoyancy and light resistance assisting core muscles.
8. Stabilization devices; e.g., air splints, splints, soft neck collars, stabilize body segments and eliminate unwanted movement.
9. Environment: patients with ataxia do better in a low-stimulus environment; allows better utilization of cognitive strategies.

Sensory Training

1. Patients with proprioceptive losses benefit from:
    a. Visual training strategies: patient guides movements and postures visually; e.g., use of a mirror and shirt with vertical line taped on it to achieve vertical sitting or standing posture.
    b. Proprioceptive training strategies for patients with some residual proprioceptive sensations: use light weights: wrist cuffs, ankle cuffs, weighted walkers, elastic resistance bands, pool exercises to increase proprioceptive loading.
2. Patients with visual losses benefit from cognitive and proprioceptive training strategies.
3. Patients with vestibular losses benefit from visual and proprioceptive training strategies.
4. Patients with combined losses (two or more systems); e.g., the patient with proprioceptive losses (diabetic peripheral neuropathy) and visual losses (diabetic retinopathy) require compensatory training; e.g., use of environmental adaptations, assistive devices to promote safety.

Interventions to Improve Standing Balance (See Table 6-10)

Exercises to Improve ROM, Strength, and Synergistic Responses

1. "Kitchen sink exercises": heel-cord stretches, heel rises, toe-offs, partial wall squats, single-leg activities (side kicks, back kicks), marching in place, look-arounds

Table 6-10

Interventions to Improve Standing Balance (See Table 3-9: Components of Postural Stability/Balance for matching outcome measures)

COMPONENTS OF BALANCE (GOAL)	EXERCISE RECOMMENDATIONS
Sensory integration (improve ability to stabilize balance/gait with varying degrees of sensory input)	Vision: Practice standing eyes open to eyes closed with wide stance progressing to a narrow stance Vestibular: Practice head turns (up/down/left/right) with standing→ walking on level surface and progress to moving surface Somatosensory: Practice standing and walking on tile floor to carpet to dense foam to un-level surface outside Progress to sensory conflict: Standing on foam with head turns
Motor systems (improve ROM, strength, endurance and movement synergies)	Functional activities (sit to stand; toe raises/heel raises, partial wall squats, and steps/stairs) with focus on minimal sway with initiation/termination of all movements and proper posture
Verticality and orientation in space (maintain proper standing posture with various activities)	Focus for clients with neglect/perception impairments: Standing on level surface with visual feedback (mirror) and proper and safe posture/positioning→ standing without a mirror→ standing on a slope without a mirror→ walking on level surface→ walking hills/slope (proper alignment/safe with all scenarios)
Static stability (improve static stance with variations in the base of support)	Eyes open (EO) feet apart→ EO feet together→ eyes closed (EC) feet apart→ EC feet together→ semi-tandem stance EO/EC→ tandem stance EO/EC→ single leg stance EO/EC with focus on level pelvis and minimal sway
Functional stability limits (improve limits of stability to allow for safe reaching with various foot positions)	Progress stance as listed above but add reaching (arm[s] or leg) in varying directions (anterior/posterior/medial/lateral/diagonals) with attention on appropriate corrective strategies (ankle, hip, stepping) Can progress activity by standing on foam and repeating above conditions
Dynamic stability (improve ability to ambulate, completed transfers, and stairs)	Functional activities of daily living with a focus on postural stability and control of movement in various community settings Start on level surfaces and move to un-level and dimly lit surfaces if safe
Anticipatory postural control	Gait with head turns and/or raising arm; stepping over objects; carrying objects while walking
Reactive postural control	Perturbation training to include random weight shifts, rocker boards, treadmill walking (with harness) with variable speed changes Document corrective strategies (ankle, hip, stepping)
Cognition-multitasking	Balance and gait training while counting backward or answering question

Adapted from Sibley KM et al. Using the systems framework for postural control to analyze the components of balance evaluated in standardized balance measures: a scoping review. *Arch Phys Med Rehabil.* 2015; 96(1): 122–132.

(head and trunk rotation), and hip circles. Progression from bilateral upper extremity (UE) touch-down support to unilateral UE support to no UE support.
2. Postural awareness training: focus on control of body position, centering the COM within the limits of stability (LOS).
3. Weight shifts (postural sway): training of ankle strategies, hip strategies. Can include postural sway biofeedback; e.g., Balance Master.
4. Training of change-of-support strategies: stepping strategies (forward, backward, sideward, crossed-step); UE reaching and protective extension.

Functional Training Activities

1. Sit-to-stand (STS) and sit-down (SIT) activities. Practice moving body mass forward over BOS, extending lower extremities (LEs), and raising body mass over feet and reverse. Focus on balance control while pivoting body mass over feet.
2. Floor-to-standing rises. Practice rising from floor to standing in the event of a fall; e.g., side-sit to quadruped to kneeling to half-kneeling to standing transitions.
3. Elevation activities: practice step-ups, lateral step-ups.
4. Dual-task training.
   a. In standing, practice simultaneous UE activities (e.g., holding a tray with a glass of water; catching/throwing a ball).
   b. In standing, practice simultaneous LE activities (e.g., kicking a ball).
   c. In standing, practice simultaneous cognitive activities (e.g., counting backwards from 100 by 3's).

Disturbed Balance Activities

1. Include manual perturbations, use of moveable BOS devices (stability ball, wobble board, split foam roller, dense foam mat).
2. Carefully grade force of perturbations, range and speed of movements.
3. Stability ball training. Practice sitting, active weight shifts (e.g., pelvic clock), UE movements (e.g., arm circles, reaching), LE movements (e.g., stepping, marching), trunk movements (e.g., head and trunk turns).
4. Wobble board/equilibrium boards. Practice both self-initiated and therapist-initiated shifts in sitting or standing. Gradually increase range and speed of shifts.

Interventions to Improve Locomotor Control

Functional Gait Activities

1. Practice walking forward, backward, sideways.
2. Progress from slow speeds to normal walking speeds to fast walking speeds.
3. Progress from normal BOS to narrowed BOS.
4. Practice wide turns to small-based turns; to the right and left; 360° turns.
5. Practice head turns right and left, up and down.
6. Practice PNF braiding (grapevine stepping).
7. Practice over and around obstacles, through doorways.
8. Practice elevation activities: practice step-ups, lateral step-ups, stair climbing, and ramps.
9. Practice simultaneous UE activities, LE activities, and cognitive activities.
10. Community activities. Practice walking in open (variable) environments; e.g., pushing or pulling doors, car transfers, grocery shopping.
11. Practice anticipatory timing activities; e.g., getting on/off elevator, escalator.

Treadmill Training

1. Focus is on velocity control, moving from slow to fast walking.
2. Progression is from slow to fast walking.
3. Safety harness is worn to provide partial body weight support (BWS) if the patient is unstable (e.g., the patient with ataxia or stroke).
4. Progression is achieved by decreasing BWS, increasing the treadmill incline and distance walked (total time).

Cycle Ergometers

1. Pedaling on cycle ergometer is paced.
2. Progression is from slow to fast.
3. Resistance and distance can also be modified.
4. Can include both LE and UE training.

Exercise Training

1. Strength training.
   a. Active/active assistive exercise.
   b. Manual resistance; PNF patterns can be used to promote synergistic control, improve timing.
   c. Weights, pulleys, hydraulics, elastic resistance bands, mechanical or electromechanical devices.
2. Stretching exercises.

Compensatory Strategies

1. Compensatory strategies are used as appropriate to promote safety and early resumption of functional skills; e.g., the patient with delayed or absent recovery, multiple comorbidities.
2. Compensatory strategies may lead to learned nonuse of impaired extremities and delay recovery in those patients with recovery potential; e.g., the patient with stroke.
3. Safety is improved by substitution: intact segments (sound limbs) for impaired segments; cognitive control for impaired motor control; e.g., the patient with ataxia.

4. Safety is improved by altering postural strategies; e.g., widening the BOS and lowering the COM.
5. Safety is improved by use of appropriate assistive devices and shoes; e.g., overhead support harness, walker, athletic shoes.
6. Safety is improved through environmental adaptations; e.g., handrails, adequate lighting, contrast tape on stairs, and removal of throw rugs.

Activity Pacing and Energy Conservation

1. The patient with debilitating fatigue (e.g., cerebellar ataxia, multiple sclerosis, chronic fatigue syndrome, fibromyalgia) will need to conserve energy.
2. Activity-based intervention refers to selection of activities and adaption of tasks so they will be easier and safer for the patient to complete (primary role of the occupational therapist).
3. Energy conservation refers to guidelines that allow for successful task completion, e.g., increased time for task completion; taking frequent, short rest breaks; avoiding complicated tasks; using energy-saving equipment.

Safety Education/Fall Prevention

1. Assist patient in identification of fall risk factors; e.g., effect of medications, postural hypotension, environmental factors at home or work.
2. Lifestyle counseling: assist patient in recognizing unsafe activities, harmful effects of a sedentary lifestyle.

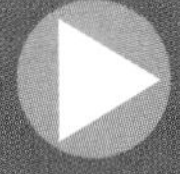

Aquatic Exercise

Goals and Outcomes

1. Motor function and motor learning are enhanced.
2. ROM and flexibility are improved.
3. Postural control, biomechanical alignment, and symmetrical weight distribution are improved.
4. Strength, power, and endurance are improved.
5. Sensory control and integration of sensory systems (somatosensory, visual, and vestibular) are improved.
6. Performance, independence, and safety in balance, gait, and locomotion are improved.
7. Aerobic capacity and endurance are improved.
8. Relaxation, reduction of pain, and decreased muscle spasm are enhanced.

Strategies

1. Immersion in pools or tanks is used to facilitate movement and exercise. Water buoyancy, buoyant devices, and various depths of immersion decrease body weight and enhance movement; similar movements on land may be more difficult or impossible to perform.
2. Pools or tanks with a walking track, with or without a treadmill, are used to enhance gait and endurance.

Physics Related to Aquatic Exercise

1. Buoyancy: the upward force of water on an immersed or partially immersed body or body part. Equal to the weight of the water that it displaces (Archimedes' principle). This creates an apparent decrease in the weight and joint unloading of an immersed body part, allowing easier movement in water.
2. Cohesion: the tendency of water molecules to adhere to each other. The resistance encountered while moving through water is due to cohesion; some force is needed to separate water molecules.
3. Density: the mass per unit volume of a substance. The density of water is proportional to its depth; deeper water must support the water above it.
4. Hydrostatic pressure: the circumferential water pressure exerted on an immersed body part. A pressure gradient is established between the surface water and deeper water, due to the increase in water density at deeper levels.
   a. Pascal's law states that the pressure exerted on an immersed body part is equal on all surfaces.
   b. Increased pressure counteracts effusion and edema, and enhances peripheral blood flow.
5. Turbulence: movement of a body part through water creates circular motion of the water (eddy current) near the surface of the part, producing frictional drag.

a. As speed of movement increases, greater resistance is encountered.
b. Moving through turbulent water creates greater resistance as compared to calm water.
c. Use of equipment (e.g., paddle or boot) increases resistance and drag as the patient moves through water.

6. Physiologic considerations: Water immersion influences multiple systems.
   a. Decreases weight-bearing.
   b. Increases venous return and stroke volume.
   c. Reduces inspiratory reserve volume and may reduce forced vital capacity.

Thermodynamics

1. Water temperature affects body temperature and performance.
2. Water temperature is determined by specific needs of patient and intervention goals.
   a. Cooler temperatures are used for higher intensity exercise.
   b. Warmer temperatures are used to enhance mobility, flexibility, and relaxation; e.g., patients with arthritis.
   c. Ambient air temperature should be close to water temperature (e.g., ±3°C or ±4°F).
3. There is decreased heat dissipation through sweating with immersion.
4. At temperatures > 37°C (98.6°F), patients have increased cardiovascular demands at rest and during exercise.
5. At temperatures < 25°C (77°F), patients have difficulty maintaining core temperature.

Special Equipment

1. Buoyancy assistance devices: inflatable cervical collar, flotation rings, buoyancy belt or vest, kickboard.
2. Buoyant dumbbells (swimmers): used for upright or horizontal support.
3. Webbed gloves and hand paddles: used to increase resistance to upper extremity movement.
4. Fins and boots: used to increase resistance to lower extremity movement.

Exercise Applications

1. Movement horizontal to or upward toward the water surface (active assistive exercise) is made easier due to the buoyancy of water. A flotation device may be needed to support very weak patients.
2. Movement downward into the water is more difficult because of the buoyancy of water.
   a. A flotation device or handheld paddle can be used to increase resistance.
   b. A paddle turned to slice through the water decreases resistance.
3. Resistance exercise can be controlled by the speed of the movement.
   a. Resistance increases with increased velocity of movement due to the cohesion and turbulence of the water.
   b. Slower movements meet less resistance.
   c. Ataxic movements are slower and more controlled against the resistance of water.
4. Stretching exercises can be assisted by the buoyancy of water.
5. The amount of weight-bearing on the lower extremities is determined by the height of the water/level of immersion (buoyancy) relative to the upright patient.
   a. The greater the water depth, the less the weight/loading on extremities.
   b. Can be used for partial weight-bearing (PWB) gait training.
6. Lower extremity reciprocal movements are enhanced by use of a kickboard and using kicking movements.
7. Aerobic conditioning is enhanced with deep-water walking or running, high-step marching, or other calisthenics. Progresses to reduced water levels and then to land walking/running.
   a. Immersed equipment (e.g., cycle ergometer, treadmill, or upper body ergometer) can be used to enhance conditioning. Hand floatation weights can be used to increased UE resistance.
   b. Swimming is an excellent aerobic training activity.
   c. Regular monitoring of exercise responses (e.g., ratings of perceived exertion) is required.
8. Treatment time varies with the type of activity, patient tolerance, and level of skill.

RED FLAG: Contraindications include bowel or bladder incontinence, severe kidney disease, severe epilepsy, severe cardiac or respiratory dysfunction; e.g., cardiac failure, unstable angina, severely reduced vital capacity, unstable blood pressure, severe peripheral vascular disease, large open wounds, skin infections, colostomy, bleeding or hemorrhage, water and airborne infections; e.g., influenza, gastrointestinal infections.

Precautions

1. Fear of water, inability to swim. Floatation supports can be used.
2. Patients with heat intolerance; e.g., patients with multiple sclerosis.
3. Patients with cold intolerance: e.g., hypothyroidism, Raynaud's disease, peripheral artery disease, anemia.
4. Use waterproof dressing on small open wounds.
5. Buoyancy unweights bones and joints; bone health requires weight-bearing impact exercise on land and resistance/strengthening exercise to counteract low bone density and osteoporosis.

Acknowledgment to Thomas Bianco PT, MSPT for his original contribution in formulating this chapter.

APPENDIX 6A

Review Questions and Case Study

(Answers to all Review Questions and Case Studies are found in Chapter 17)

1. During strength training, what is the influence of the Valsalva maneuver regarding intrathoracic pressure, heart rate, venous pressure, and cardiac work?

2. What are the implications of the FITT equation in terms of strategies to develop cardiovascular endurance?

3. When exercising a patient in an aquatic environment, what are the factors that can make the activity easier to perform? More difficult to perform?

4. What is the main principle being employed when using the PNF-facilitated stretching technique of contract-relax?

5. What are the most common errors associated with training a patient to improve postural stability?

Therapeutic Interventions Case Study

Patient Profile:

- Gender: Male
- Age: 35

Presenting Problem/Current Condition

- Referred to physical therapy with a diagnosis of right biceps brachii Grade II muscle strain
- Sustained injury playing recreational softball 3 weeks ago
- Initially placed in sling for a suspected rotator cuff tear
- Now has full range of motion of RUE but weakness of biceps brachii muscle due to inactivity (MMT = 3+/5 or Fair+)
- No current pain with ADLs

Past Medical History

- No prior medical history or prior surgical history involving the RUE

Other Information

- Denies neck pain
- Denies any neurologic symptoms of the RUE

Question #1

What is the typical healing timeline for a Grade II muscle injury?

1. 0–4 weeks.
2. 3–12 weeks.
3. 4 weeks to 6 months.
4. 6 to 12 months.

Question #2

Which set of exercise parameters should be used to initiate a resistance training program for this patient?

1. Three days per week, 12–15 repetitions of 3 sets at 50% of the 1RM weight.
2. Seven days per week, 2–3 repetitions of 3 sets at 3RM weight.
3. Five days per week, 10 repetitions of 3 sets at 10RM weight.
4. Three days per week, 6–8 repetitions of 5 sets at 10RM weight.

Question #3

Which adjustment should be made to progress the rehabilitation program and increase strength of the affected muscle?

1. Increase the number of repetitions to 10–15.
2. Increase the days per week to 5.
3. Increase the intensity to 60%–70% of the 1RM.
4. Increase the number of sets to 5.

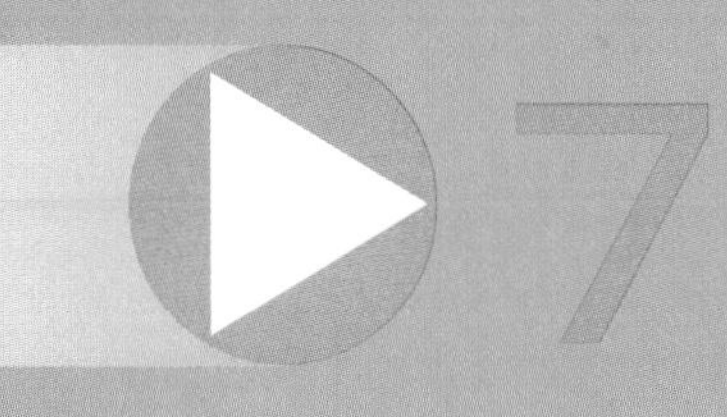

Integumentary Physical Therapy

SUSAN B. O'SULLIVAN AND VINCENT LEPAK

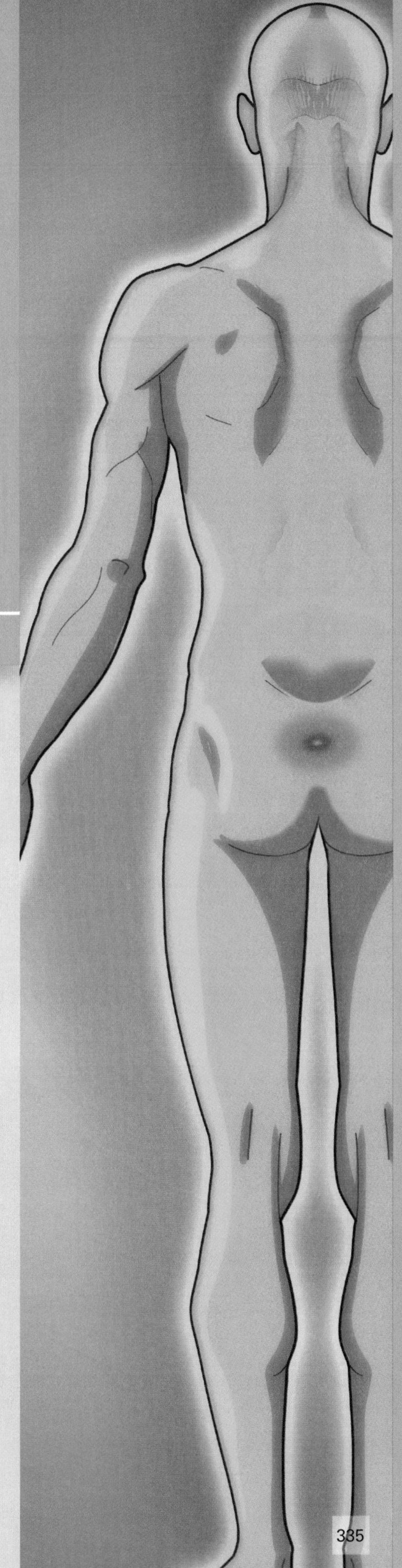

Chapter Outline

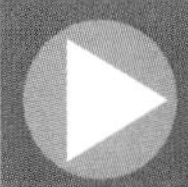

Study Tactics

Questions About the Integumentary System Comprise 5.5% of the NPTE, or a Total of 9–12 Questions

The Number of Questions by Category Are

- Examination of the Patient/Client: 3–4
- Evaluation, Differential Diagnosis, Prognosis: 3–4
- Interventions: 3–4

Examination of the Patient/Client. Focus on

- Anatomy and physiology. Specifically, layers of the skin and associated structures, body temperature regulation, healing processes
- Recognition of various kinds of ulcers (arterial, venous, pressure, diabetic), burns, and the appearance of other skin lesions
- Measurement and description of skin lesions and burns
- Screening for common skin cancers (melanoma, basal and squamous cell carcinoma)

Evaluation, Differential Diagnosis, and Prognosis. Focus on

- Characteristic of various types of skins lesions to include ulcers, burns, skin cancer, dermatitis, wounds, and skin infections (such as staph infections and MRSA)
- Differentiation and description of various kinds of ulcers (arterial, venous, pressure, diabetic), burns, and the appearance of other skin lesions
- Development of a plan of care to include prognosis for common integumentary disorders
- Actions and side effects of pharmacological management used to treat common integumentary problems

Interventions. Focus on

- Wound and burn care, including types and selection of dressings, topical agents, and debridement techniques
- Pressure garments and pressure dressings for wound care (hypertrophic scarring) and venous ulcers (Unna boot)
- Best interventions for the management of venous, arterial, and pressure ulcers
- Positions and procedures to reduce pressure, shear, friction, scar formation, or contractures
- Potential adverse side effects or complications on the integumentary or other systems from physical therapy interventions

Chapter 7 ITG

Integumentary System

Skin or Integument

Organ System

1. Skin is an organ of the integumentary system and is the largest organ system of the body (15%–20% of body weight).
2. Thickness of skin varies by location; skin on the palms and soles of the feet is the thickest skin of the body.

Functions of Skin

1. Protection against injury or invasion and ultraviolet radiation.
2. Insulation of body.
3. Maintenance of homeostasis: fluid balance, regulation of body temperature.
4. Assists in metabolism: vitamin D production, aids in elimination of metabolic waste (e.g., urea and salt are excreted in sweat).
5. Attachment of muscles (e.g., erector pili, frontalis).
6. Receptors in dermis give rise to cutaneous sensations.
7. Communication: skin plays a role in expressions, identification, and self-image.

Structure of Skin

1. Layers of skin: see Table 7-1.
2. Age-related changes: see Table 7-2.
3. Cross section of the skin: see Figure 7-1.

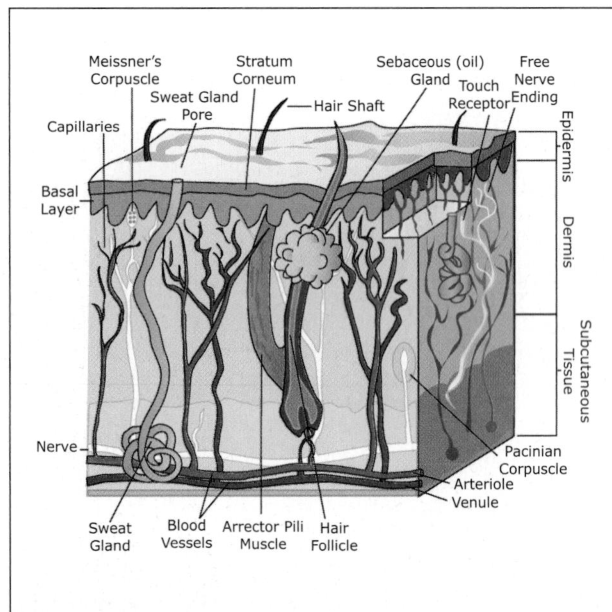

Figure 7-1 **Cross section of the skin.**

Table 7-1

Layers of Skin	
Epidermis	Outer, most superficial layer; contains no blood vessels Composed of five layers: 1. Stratum corneum: outermost layer, shingle-like dead cells are filled with keratin 2. Stratum lucidum: formed from dead cells and only occurs in thick portions of the palms and soles of feet 3. Stratum granulosum: contains live keratinocytes (differentiate from epidermal stem cells in basal layer and eventually form outermost layer of epidermis) and Langerhans (immunity) cells 4. Stratum spinosum (spiny layer): also contain keratinocytes and Langerhans cells 5. Stratum basale (stratum germinativum): deepest layer of epidermis, contains epidermal cells, melanocytes (produce melanin), and Merkel cells (associated with light touch sensory discrimination)
Dermis (corium)	Inner layer composed primarily of collagen and elastin fibrous connective tissues Mucopolysaccharide matrix and elastin fibers provide elasticity, strength to skin Contains lymphatics, blood vessels, nerves and nerve endings, hair follicles, sebaceous and sweat glands Cells include fibroblasts, macrophages, lymphocytes, and mast cells
Subcutaneous tissues (hypodermis)	Underneath dermis Consists of loose connective and fat tissues Provides insulation, support, and cushion for skin; stores energy for skin Muscles and fascia lie underneath subcutaneous layer

Appendages of the Skin

1. Hair.
   a. Terminal hair: coarse, thick, pigmented; e.g., scalp, eyebrows.
   b. Vellus hair: short, fine; e.g., arms, chest.
   c. Hair follicle density and metabolism decreased in older adults.
2. Nails: nail plate, lunula (whitish moon), proximal nail fold/cuticle, lateral nail folds.
3. Sebaceous glands: exocrine glands that secrete fatty substance (sebum) through hair follicles; on all skin surfaces except palms and soles. Sebum lubricates skin and defends against bacteria and fungus.
4. Sweat glands.
   a. Eccrine glands: widely distributed, open on skin; help control body temperature.

b. Apocrine glands: found in axillary and genital areas, open into hair follicles; stimulated by emotional stress.

Circulation

Blood Flow to Capillaries of the Skin

1. Increased blood flow with an increase in oxyhemoglobin to skin capillaries causes reddening of the skin.
2. Peripheral cyanosis is due to reduced blood flow to skin and loss of oxygen to tissues (changes to deoxyhemoglobin) and results in a darker, somewhat blue color.
3. Central cyanosis is due to reduced oxygen level in the blood; causes include advanced lung disease, congenital heart disease, and abnormal hemoglobins.

Table 7-2

Integumentary Age-Related Changes

	NEWBORN	MIDDLE AGED	OLDER ADULT
Skin Thickness	~70% of full thickness	Full thickness	~70% of full thickness
Skin Layers	Thinner	Mature	Thinner
Vascularity	Maturing	Mature	Reduced
Metabolism	Similar to adults	Mature	Reduced
Thermoregulation	Reduced	Mature	Reduced
Immunity Cells (i.e., Langerhans and mast cells)	Reduced	Mature	Reduced

Reference: Wysocki, AB. Anatomy and physiology of skin and soft tissue. In: Bryant RA, Nix DP, ed. *Acute and chronic wounds: current management concepts*. Fifth edition. St. Louis, Missouri: Elsevier; 2016: 40–62.

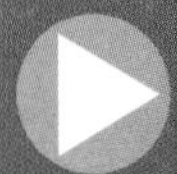

Wound Healing

1. Types of tissue union.
   a. Primary (first intention): No major loss of connective tissue, wound is not contaminated, closure within 3–7 days.
   b. Secondary: full thickness, little epithelialization—Chronic wounds, pressure injuries, venous ulcerations, and other open wounds heal through secondary intention.
   c. Tertiary (delayed primary)—used for contaminated tissue (risk of infection), closure will result in too much tension, usually closed within 5–7 days of initial injury.
2. Epidermal (superficial or partial-thickness).
   a. Heals through regeneration.
   b. Epithelial cells proliferate and migrate from the wounds margin. They detach from the basal layer and require a wound border that is free of scaring or necrotic tissues to migrate. This type of wound usually heals without scarring.
   c. If dermal tissue is involved then granulation occurs simultaneously.
   d. Moist wounds epithelize much quicker than wounds left open to air.
3. Dermal (full-thickness) has four overlapping phases.
   a. Homeostasis (after growth factors released): Vasoconstriction initially to reduce loss and prevent infection. A fibrin plug is formed. This happens within 10–15 minutes to contain the area. Growth factors released.
   b. Inflammation (24–48 hours): The cardinal signs of inflammation (i.e., rubor [redness], calor [increased heat], tumor [swelling], dolor [pain], and functiolaesa [loss of function]) become apparent due to the vasodilation of the noninjured vessels to allow leukocytes and growth factors into the area. Phagocytosis and neovascularization began at the end of this cycle. Key cells in this phase include platelets, leukocytes, macrophages, and mast cells. Conditions such as diabetes may impair this phase.
   c. Granulation, proliferation, or fibroblastic phase (names are synonymous). The four primary events are angiogenesis, granulation formation, wound

contraction, and epithelialization. The primary cells associated with this phase include myofibroblasts for wound contraction; fibroblasts for collagen, elastin, and glycosaminoglycan production; epithelial cells for epithelialization.

d. Maturation and matrix formation (begins 2–4 weeks and may last for years). Collagen synthesis and alignment. Normal scar formation; bright pink for 6–12 weeks, then becomes lavender to a soft pink from 12–15 months, and finally flattens, becoming white and flat. Abnormal scar formation includes hypotrophic, hypertrophic, and keloid scar formation. Compression garments, silicone gels, or sheets are used to reduce hypertrophic or keloid scarring.

4. Factors that delay wound healing (Table 7-3).

Table 7-3

Factors That Delay Wound Healing

Advanced age ↓ metabolism and proliferation of important cellular and growth factors for healing	**Medications** Chemotherapy, corticosteroids (add vitamin A to improve healing), NSAIDS
Impaired Oxygenation ↓ angiogenesis, cell differentiation and migration, re-epithelialization, and collagen synthesis ↑ risk of infection	**Disease** Diabetes, kidney disease, hypertension, cardiopulmonary and vascular disease, hyperlipidemia
Poor nutrition ↓ protein, vitamins/minerals and wound healing requires ↑ demand for caloric intake	**Stress** ↓ proinflammatory cytokines ↑ wound hypoxia ↑ risk of infection
Comorbidities Diabetes, obesity, ↓ perfusion and/or oxygenation due to cardiovascular or pulmonary disorders (e.g., COVID-19)	**Cool Temperatures** ↓ cellular metabolism (Note: Normothermic 37–38°C [98.6–100.4°F] temperatures improve wound healing)
Wound Bioburden ↑ bacterial load/pathogenic organism and ↓ bacterial diversity leading to inflammatory state and impaired keratinocyte proliferation	**Iatrogenic** Excessive pressure, shear, wound desiccation, and moisture
Infection ↑ bacteria and endotoxins cause prolonged inflammatory phase; bacteria form of biofilms that lead to antibiotic resistance	**Smoking** ↑ rates of infection, impaired immune response, ↓ fibroblast activity

Reference: Bryant, RA, Nix, DP, ed. *Acute and chronic wounds: current management concepts.* 5th ed. St. Louis, Missouri: Elsevier; 2016: 40–62.

Examination of Integumentary Integrity

Patient/Client History

Complete History

1. Age, gender, race/ethnicity, social/health habits, work, living, general health status, previous ulcer, previous treatment of ulcers, allergies, medical/surgical.
2. Current condition(s)/chief complaint(s).
3. Functional status/activity level.
4. Current medications.
5. Clinical tests.
6. Risk factor assessment.

Examination of Skin

Components

1. Observation.
2. Palpation.
3. Photographic assessment.
4. Thermography.

Pruritus

1. Itching.
2. Common in diabetes, drug hypersensitivity, hyperthyroidism.

Urticaria

1. Smooth, red, elevated patches of skin, hives.
2. Indicative of an allergic response to drugs or infection.

Rash

1. Local redness and eruption on the skin, typically accompanied by itching.
2. Seen in inflammation, skin diseases, chronic alcoholism, vasomotor disturbances, fever, and diaper rash, heat rash, drug rash.

Xeroderma

1. Excessive dryness of skin with shedding of epithelium.
2. Can indicate deficiency of thyroid function, diabetes.

Edema

1. Can indicate anemia, venous or lymphatic obstruction, inflammation; cardiac, circulatory, or renal decompensation.
2. Determine activities and postures that aggravate or relieve edema.
3. Palpation, volume, and girth measurements.

Changes in Nails

1. Clubbing: thickened and rounded nail end with spongy proximal fold.
   a. Indicative of Crohn's disease, cardiac-related cyanosis, lung (cancer, chronic hypoxia), ulcerative colitis, biliary cirrhosis, neoplasm, GI involvement.
   b. Present at birth (harmless).
   c. Schamroth's window test is often positive (loss of diamond-shaped space when nails from opposite hands are placed back to back).
2. White spots seen with trauma to nails.
3. Splinter hemorrhages: small areas of bleeding under nails that look like splinters (potential cardiac or renal signs).
4. Changes in nails (e.g., koilonychias [concave shape], leukonychia [whiteness]) often indicate systemic issues unless it is congenital.

Changes in Skin Pigmentation, Tissue Mobility, Turgor, and Texture

1. Wrinkling may be due to aging or prolonged immersion in water, dehydration.
2. Blistering.
3. Stemmer's sign. A thickened fold of skin at the base of the second toe or second finger that can be pinched or lifted; an early diagnostic indication of primary lymphedema.

Changes in Skin Color

1. Cherry red: palmar erythema could indicate liver or renal issues.
2. Cyanosis: slightly bluish, grayish, slate-colored discoloration.
   a. Indicative of lack of oxygen (hemoglobin); can indicate congestive heart failure, advanced lung disease, congenital heart disease, venous obstruction.
   b. Examine lips, oral mucosa, tongue for blue color (central causes) or nails, hands, feet (peripheral causes).
3. Pallor (lack of color, paleness).
   a. Can indicate anemia, internal hemorrhage, lack of exposure to sunlight.
   b. Temporary pallor seen with arterial insufficiency and syncope, chills, shock, vasomotor instability, or nervousness.
4. Yellow: indicates jaundice, liver disease; look for yellow color in sclera of eyes, lips, skin. Orange-yellow occurs with increased carotene intake (carotenemia), look for orange-yellow color of palms, soles, and face.
5. Liver spots: brownish yellow spots may be due to aging, uterine and liver malignancies, pregnancy.
6. Brown: increased pigmentation sometimes associated with venous insufficiency (i.e., hemosiderinosis).
7. Vitiligo: immune disorder that causes white patches of skin to develop due to melanocytes destruction. Affects all races and skin types but is more noticeable in people with darker skin; individuals with vitiligo are at greater risk for sunburn, skin cancer, hearing loss, and eye problems.

Changes in Skin Temperature

1. Correlate with internal temperature, unless skin is exposed to local heat or cold.
2. Examine with backs of fingers for generalized warmth or coolness.
   a. Abnormal heat can indicate febrile condition, hyperthyroidism, mental excitement, excessive salt intake.
   b. Abnormal cold can indicate poor circulation or obstruction; e.g., vasomotor spasm, venous or arterial thrombosis, hypothyroidism.
3. Examine temperature of reddened areas: local warmth may indicate inflammation or cellulitis.

Hidrosis

1. Moist skin (hyperhidrosis), increased perspiration: can indicate fevers, pneumonic crisis, drugs, hot drink ingestion, exercise.
2. Dry skin (hypohidrosis): can indicate dehydration, ichthyosis, or hypothyroidism. Seen in later stages of diabetes mellitus.
3. Cold sweats: can indicate great fear, anxiety, depression, or disease (AIDS).

Changes in Hair

1. Examine quality, texture, distribution.
2. Alopecia: hair loss.
3. Hypothyroidism: thinning hair; hyperthyroidism sees silky hair.
4. Hirsutism: male pattern hair growth (facial and body) in women; may indicate polycystic ovary syndrome, Cushing's syndrome, tumor, or an inherited trait.

Presence of Lesions, Unusual Growths

1. Determine anatomical location and distribution; i.e., generalized or localized, exposed or nonexposed surface, symmetrical or asymmetrical.
2. Type.
   a. Flat spot: macule (small, up to 1 cm), patch (1 cm or greater).
   b. Palpable elevated solid mass: papule (small, up to 1 cm), plaque (elevated, 1 cm or larger), nodule (marble-like lesion), wheal (irregular, localized skin edema; e.g., hives).
   c. Elevated lesions with fluid cavities: vesicle (up to 1 cm, contains serous fluid; e.g., herpes simplex); bulla or blister (1 cm or larger, contains serous fluid; e.g., second-degree burn); pustule (contains pus; e.g., acne).
3. Color.

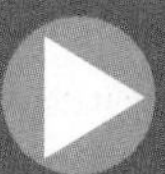

Examination of Wounds

Risk Factors and Clinical Examination

1. Determine location of wound: use anatomical landmarks.
2. Assess size: (length, width, depth, wound area).
   a. Use clear film grid superimposed on wound for size.
   b. Insert sterile cotton tip applicator into deepest part of wound for depth; indicate gradations of depth from shallow to deep.
3. Examine for tunneling (rimming or undermining): underlying tissue destruction beneath intact skin.
   a. Evaluate for sinus tracts (communication with deeper structures); associated with unusual or irregular borders.
4. Determine wound exudate (drainage).
   a. Type: serous (watery serum), purulent (containing pus), sanguineous (containing blood).
   b. Amount: dry, moderate, or high exudate.
   c. Odor.
   d. Consistency: e.g., macerated ulcer (softened tissues due to high fluid environment).
5. Identify color and tissues involved.
   a. Clean red wounds: healthy granulating wounds (in need of protection); absence of necrotic tissue.
   b. Yellow wounds: include slough (necrotic or dead tissue), fibrous tissue.
   c. Black wounds: covered with eschar (dried necrotic tissue).
   d. Indolent ulcer: ulcer that is slow to heal; is not painful.
   e. Check to see if fascia, muscle, tendons, or bone involved.
   f. Record if epithelialization or granulation is present.
6. Determine temperature: indicative of inflammation. Use temperature probe (thermistor) to detect surface temperature.
7. Determine girth.
   a. Use circumferential measurements of both involved and noninvolved limbs; referenced to bony landmarks.
   b. Use volumetric measurements: measure water displacement from filled volumeter. Reliable and valid for girth (edema) measurements, but unreliable for wound volume measurements.
8. Examine viability of periwound tissue.
   a. Halo of erythema, warmth, and swelling may indicate infection (cellulitis).
   b. Maceration of surrounding tissues due to moisture (urine, feces) or wound drainage increases risk for wound deterioration and enlargement.
   c. Trophic changes may indicate poor arterial nutrition.
   d. Cyanosis may indicate arterial insufficiency.
9. Determine sensory integrity, risk for trauma or pressure breakdown.
10. Examine for signs of infection.
    a. Bacterial culture: to identify colonization and infection; culture wound site only.
    b. Observations, palpation.
11. Wound scar tissue characteristics: banding, pliability, texture.
12. Photographic records of wound appearance aid narrative descriptions. Use marker pen to outline wound edges on transparent dressing with a calibrated grid to provide a measuring scale.
13. Pain: use a valid tool.
14. Selected imaging in wound care:
    a. Arterial system: arteriogram, Doppler US, magnetic resonance angiography, CT angiography.
    b. Venous system: Doppler US, magnetic resonance venography, CT venography.

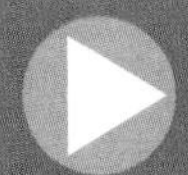

Evaluation, Differential Diagnosis, Prognosis, and Intervention of Integumentary Disorders

Dermatitis (Eczema)

Inflammation: Causes Itching, Redness, Skin Lesions

Causes

1. Allergic or contact dermatitis; e.g., poison ivy, harsh soaps, chemicals, adhesive tape.
2. Actinic: photosensitivity, reaction to sunlight, ultraviolet.
3. Atopic: etiology unknown, associated with allergic, hereditary, or psychological disorders.

Stages

1. Acute: red, oozing, crusting rash; extensive erosions, exudate, pruritic vesicles.
2. Subacute: erythematous skin, scaling, scattered plaques.
3. Chronic: thickened skin, increased skin marking secondary to scratching; fibrotic papules, and nodules; postinflammatory pigmentation changes. Course can be relapsing.

Precautions or Contraindications

1. Some physical therapy modalities.
2. Avoid use of alcohol.

Medical Management

1. Target inflammation and eliminate triggers (e.g., allergens, skin irritants, stress).
2. Topical or systemic therapy: corticosteroids, immunosuppressants, antihistamines.
3. Daily care: Use mild nonfragrant soaps; apply emollients (lotions) within 5 minutes of bathing.

Bacterial Infections

Etiology

1. Bacteria enter through portals in the skin, e.g., abrasions, punctures, open wounds.
2. Some may be antibiotic resistant (e.g., methicillinresistant *Staphylococcus aureus*, MRSA).

Impetigo

1. Superficial skin infection caused by staphylococci or streptococci.
2. Associated with inflammation, small pus-filled vesicles, itching.
3. Highly contagious; common in children and the elderly.

Cellulitis

1. Suppurative inflammation of cellular or connective tissue in or close to the skin.
2. Tends to be poorly defined and widespread.
3. Streptococcal or staphylococcal infection common; can be contagious.
4. Skin is hot, red, and edematous.
5. Management: antibiotics; elevation of the part; cool, wet dressings.
6. If untreated, lymphangitis, gangrene, abscess, and sepsis can occur.
7. The elderly and individuals with diabetes, wounds, malnutrition, or on steroid therapy are at increased risk.

Abscess

1. A cavity containing pus and surrounded by inflamed tissue.
2. The result of a localized infection.
3. Commonly a staphylococcal infection.
4. Healing typically facilitated by draining or incising the abscess.

Viral Infections

Herpes 1 (Herpes Simplex)

1. Itching and soreness, followed by vesicular eruption of the skin on the face or mouth; a cold sore or fever blister.
2. Spread by contact.
3. Treatment includes antiviral therapy and no close contact until there are no new lesions, and lesions are dry for several days.

Herpes 2

1. Common cause of vesicular genital eruption.
2. Spread by sexual contact.
3. In newborns, may cause meningoencephalitis; may be fatal.

Herpes Zoster (Shingles)

1. Caused by varicella-zoster that causes chickenpox; the virus is reactivated after lying dormant for years in cerebral ganglia or ganglia of the posterior nerve roots.
2. Pain and tingling affecting spinal or cranial nerve dermatome; progresses to red papules along distribution of infected nerve; red papules progressing to vesicles develop along a dermatome.

3. Usually accompanied by fever, chills, malaise, gastrointestinal (GI) disturbances.
4. Ocular complications with cranial nerve (CN) III involvement: eye pain, corneal damage; loss of vision with CN V involvement.
5. Postherpetic neuralgic pain: may be intermittent or constant; lasts weeks; occasionally, intractable pain lasts months or years.
6. Management: no curative agent, antiviral drugs slow progression; symptomatic treatment for itching and pain; e.g., systemic corticosteroids.
7. Contagious to individuals who have not had chickenpox.
8. Heat or ultrasound contraindicated: can increase severity of symptoms.
9. Vaccine is recommended for healthy adults 50 years and older.

Warts

1. Common, benign infection by human papilloma viruses (HPVs).
2. Transmission is through direct contact; autoinoculation is possible.
3. Common warts: on skin, especially hands and fingers.
4. Plantar wart: on pressure points of feet.
5. Management: cryotherapy, acids, electrodessication, and curettage; over-the-counter medications.

Fungal Infections

Ringworm (Tinea Corporis)

1. Fungal infection involving the hair, skin, or nails.
2. Forms ring-shaped patches with vesicles or scales.
3. Itchy; transmission is through direct contact.
4. Treated with topical or oral antifungal drugs (e.g., griseofulvin). Treatment lasts from weeks to months even as symptoms subside. Systemic antifungal side effects may include headache, GI issues, fatigue, insomnia, and photosensitivity. Liver function is monitored.

Athlete's Foot (Tinea Pedis)

1. Fungal infection of foot, typically between the toes.
2. Causes erythema, inflammation, pruritus, itching, and pain.
3. Treated with antifungal creams.
4. Can progress to bacterial infections, cellulitis if untreated.

Transmission

1. Person-to-person or animal-to-person.
2. Observe standard precautions.

Yeast (Candidiasis)

1. Common in skin folds due to excessive moisture. Immunocompromised are more susceptible.
2. Symptoms.
   a. Oral symptoms (thrush) include oral patches, redness and soreness, and pain.
   b. Genital symptoms include erythema, inflammation, itching, burning with urination, pain with sex, and a white discharge.
   c. Topical symptoms include redness, rash, and soreness.
3. Treated with skin care (reduce moisture), antifungal ointment, and potentially silver-infused dressing for skin folds.

Parasitic Infections

Caused by Insect and Animal Contacts

Scabies (Mites)

1. Burrow into skin, causing inflammation, itching, and possibly pruritus or urticaria (hives).
2. Treated with scabicide.

Lice (Pediculosis)

1. A parasite that can affect head, body, genital area with bite marks, redness, and nits.
2. Treatment with special soap or shampoo.

Transmission

1. Person-to-person or sexually transmitted.
2. Avoid direct contact; observe standard precautions.

Immune Disorders of the Skin

Psoriasis

1. Chronic autoimmune disease of skin characterized by erythematous plaques covered with a silvery scale; common on ears, scalp, knees, elbows, and genitalia (see Figure 7-2).
2. Common complaints: itching and pain from dry, cracked lesions.
3. Variable course: exacerbations and remissions are common.
4. May be associated with psoriatic arthritis, joint pain, particularly of small distal joints.
5. Etiological factors: hereditary, associated immune disorders, certain drugs.
6. Precipitating factors: trauma, infection, pregnancy, and endocrine changes; cold weather, smoking, anxiety, and stress.
7. Management: no cure; topical preparations (corticosteroids, occlusive ointments, coal tar); immunosuppressive drugs (methotrexate).
8. Daily skin care: Use mild nonfragrant soaps; apply emollients (lotions) within 2–4 minutes of bathing (maintains skin hydration). Avoid irritants such as brisk drying, excessive sun light exposure, and remove chlorine from skin after swimming in a pool.

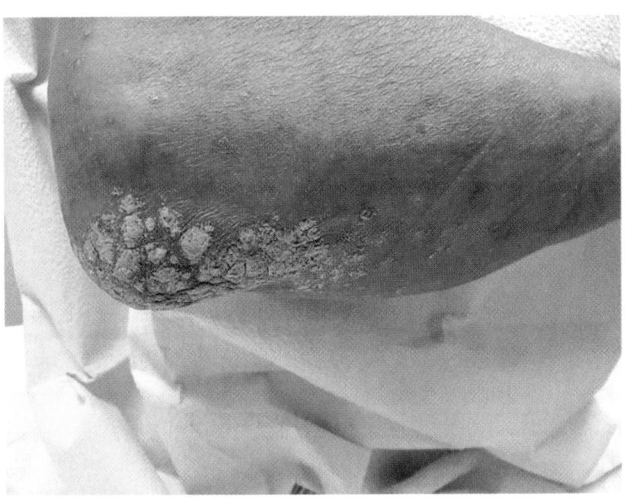

Figure 7-2 Psoriasis at the Elbow.

Lupus Erythematosus

1. Chronic, progressive autoimmune inflammatory disorder of connective tissues; characteristic red rash with raised, red, scaly plaques.
2. Discoid lupus erythematosus (DLE): affects only skin; flare-ups with sun exposure; lesions can resolve or cause atrophy, permanent scarring, hypopigmentation, or hyperpigmentation.
3. Systemic lupus erythematosus (SLE): chronic, systemic inflammatory disorder affecting multiple organ systems, including skin, joints, kidneys, heart, nervous system, mucous membranes; can be fatal; commonly affects young women. Symptoms can include fever, malaise, characteristic butterfly rash across bridge of nose, skin lesions, chronic fatigue, arthralgia, arthritis, skin rashes, photosensitivity, anemia, hair loss, Raynaud's phenomenon.
4. Medical management: no cure; topical treatment of skin lesions (corticosteroid creams), aspirin, acetaminophen, and NSAIDS for fever and joint pain; immunosuppressive agents (e.g., corticosteroids, biologics) are used to manage systemic inflammation.
5. Observe for side effects of corticosteroids: edema, weight gain, acne, hypertension, bruising, purplish stretch marks. Long-term use of corticosteroids is associated with increased risk of Cushing's syndrome, diabetes, osteoporosis, and myopathy (see Chapter 8 and Table 8-2 for additional information).
6. Physical therapy management: skin care, prevention of deconditioning and secondary musculoskeletal impairments, joint pain relief, fatigue management, and healthy lifestyle principles.

Systemic Sclerosis (Scleroderma)

1. Chronic, autoimmune diffuse disease of connective tissues causing fibrosis of skin, joints, blood vessels, and internal organs (GI tract, lungs, heart, kidneys). Usually accompanied by Raynaud's phenomenon.
2. Skin is taut, firm, edematous, firmly bound to subcutaneous tissues.
3. Limited systemic sclerosis/scleroderma: symmetrical skin involvement of distal extremities and face; slow progression of skin changes; late visceral and pulmonary hypertension involvement. Associated with CREST syndrome (Calcinosis, Raynaud's phenomenon, Esophageal dysfunction, Sclerodactyly, Telangiectasias).
4. Diffuse systemic sclerosis disease/scleroderma: symmetrical, widespread skin involvement of distal and proximal extremities, face, trunk; rapid progression of skin changes with early appearance of visceral involvement. Important internal organs that are frequently involved include kidneys, heart, and lungs.
5. Management: no specific therapy; supportive therapy can include corticosteroids, vasodilators, analgesics, immunosuppressive agents.
6. Physical therapy management: slow development of contractures and deformities, skin management (hydration and prevention of excessive pressure/shear), exercise, and joint protection.
7. Precautions with sclerosed skin, sensitive to pressure; acute hypertension may occur, stress regular blood pressure checks and vital sign monitoring. Pulmonary hypertension can lead to right-sided heart failure in severe cases.

Polymyositis (PM) and Dermatomyositis (DM)

1. PM: autoimmune myopathies characterized by edema, inflammation, and degeneration of proximal muscles. Affects primarily proximal muscles: shoulder and pelvic girdles, neck, pharynx; symmetrical distribution.
2. DM is the term used if PM has the characteristic skin rash (distinguishing feature). Immunologically PM and DM are different, but by presentation they are similar. Sclerodactyly and interstitial lung disease are commonly associated with this disease, but they are nonspecific to these disorders.
3. Etiology unknown; autoimmune reaction affecting muscle tissue with degeneration and regeneration, fiber atrophy; inflammatory infiltrates; drug induced.
4. Onset is variable. It can be rapid and severe, requiring ventilatory assistance and tube feeding.
5. Cardiac or pulmonary involvement may be fatal.
6. Medical management: medication (corticosteroids and immunosuppressants).

> **RED FLAG:** Additional muscle fiber damage (e.g., rhabdomyolysis) may result with too much exercise; contractures and pressure injuries (ulcers) may result from prolonged bed rest and inactivity.

7. Physical therapy includes:
   a. Fatigue management and conservation of energy principles.
   b. Exercise: aerobic and resistance exercise at low levels are appropriate provided fatigue and overload are avoided.

c. Skin care and positioning to prevent contractures and pressure injuries.
d. Monitoring for side effects of steroid induced pathologies (e.g., myopathy, neuropathy, diabetes).

8. See Chapter 3 for additional information on acquired myopathies.

Skin Cancer

Benign Tumors

1. Seborrheic keratosis: proliferation of basal cells leading to raised lesions, typically multiple lesions on trunk of older individuals; untreated unless causing irritation, pain; can be removed with cryotherapy.
2. Actinic keratosis: flat, round, or irregular lesions, covered by dry scale on sun-exposed skin. Precancerous: can lead to squamous cell carcinoma.
3. Common mole (benign nevus): proliferation of melanocytes, round or oval shape, sharply defined borders, uniform color, <6 mm, flat or raised. Can change into melanoma: signs include new swelling, redness, scaling, oozing, or bleeding.

Malignant Tumors

1. Basal cell carcinoma: slow-growing epithelial basal cell tumor, characterized by raised patch with ivory appearance or as a reddened area of eczema; has rolled border with indented center or presents as a thickened area of skin. Rarely metastasizes, common on face in fair-skinned individuals. Associated primarily with prolonged sun exposure although can occur in non–sun-exposed areas.
2. Squamous cell carcinoma (SCC): has poorly defined margins; presents as a flat red area, ulcer, or nodule. Grows more quickly, common on sun-exposed areas, face and neck, back of hand. Can be confined (in situ) or invasive to surrounding tissues; much higher risk than basal cell carcinoma to metastasize. Mucosal and lingual SCC are often related to alcohol and tobacco use.
3. Malignant melanoma: tumor arising from melanocytes (cells that produce melanin); superficial spreading melanoma (SSM) most common type.
   a. Clinical manifestations of melanoma. (See Table 7-4.)
   b. Melanoma risk factors: family history, intense year-round sun exposure, fair skin and freckles, nevi that are changing or atypical, especially if >50 years of age.

Table 7-4

Clinical Examination of Malignant Melanoma "ABCDEs"	
Asymmetry	Uneven edges, lopsided
Border	Irregular, poorly defined edges, notching
Color	Variations, especially mixtures of black, blue, or red
Diameter	Larger than 6 mm
Elevation (or Evolving)	Usually elevated, but may be flat; moles that changed over time

   c. Lesions may have swelling or redness beyond the border, oozing or bleeding, or sensations of itching, burning, or pain.

RED FLAG: Early detection requires skill and expertise since melanomas may look identical to a harmless mole. Suspicious lesions are referred immediately to a dermatologist for further evaluation and biopsy.

   d. Treatment depends on stage and may include surgery, radiation, medication, or chemotherapy. Prognosis depends on early diagnosis and the extent of invasion.
   e. Skin Cancer prevention **AWARE** guidelines: **A**void unprotected sun exposure (no tanning devices), **W**ear protective clothing, **A**pply sunscreen, **R**outinely examine your skin, and **E**ducate others.

4. Kaposi's sarcoma (KS): lesions of a vascular endothelial cell origin that became prominent in the United States due to human herpes virus 8. This angioproliferative tumor presents with red or dark purple/blue macules that progress to nodules or ulcers; associated with itching and pain.
   a. Common on lower extremities; may involve internal structures producing lymphatic obstruction.
   b. Increased incidence in individuals of central European descent and with AIDS-associated immunodeficiency.
   c. Physical therapy management: wound care (whirlpool may be appropriate if there are multiple lesions all over the body), pulsed lavage with suction for local lesions, skin care. Avoid interventions or positions that cause edema, shearing, or contractures.

Skin Trauma

Contusion

1. Injury in which skin is not broken; a bruise.
2. Characterized by pain, swelling, and discoloration.
3. Immediate application of cold may limit effects.

Ecchymosis

1. Bluish discoloration of skin caused by extravasation of blood into the subcutaneous tissues.
2. The result of trauma to underlying blood vessels or fragile vessel walls.

Petechiae

1. Tiny red or purple hemorrhagic spots on the skin.

Abrasion

1. Scraping away of skin due to injury or mechanical abrasion (e.g., dermabrasion).

Laceration

1. An irregular tear of the skin that produces a torn, jagged wound.

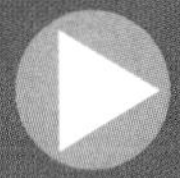

Skin Ulcers

Venous Ulcer

Etiology

1. Associated with chronic venous insufficiency, valvular incompetence, deep vein thrombosis (DVT), venous hypertension, calf muscle pump failure. See discussion in Chapter 4 on Venous Disease.
2. Recurrence is high.
3. Arterial insufficiency may coexist.

Clinical Features

1. Can occur anywhere in lower leg; common over area of medial malleolus, sometimes lateral.
2. Pulses: normal.
3. Pain: none to aching pain in dependent position.
4. Color: normal or cyanotic in dependent position. Dark pigmentation (hemosiderosis) may appear, liposclerosis or lipodermatosclerosis (thick, tender, indurated, fibrosed tissue).
5. Temperature: normal.
6. Edema: present, often marked.
7. Skin changes: pigmentation, stasis dermatitis may be present; thickening of skin as scarring develops; Atrophie blanche lesions (ivory white plaques with hemosiderin borders) in about a third of those with significant LE valvular incompetence.
8. Ulceration: may develop, especially medial ankle; wet, with large amount of exudate.
9. Gangrene: absent.

Staging for Venous, Arterial, and Diabetic Ulcers: Uses Partial- and Full-Thickness Classifications

Differential Diagnosis of Venous and Arterial Ulcers (See Table 7-5)

Examination

1. See section on examination of wounds.
2. Venous ulcers are typically shallow and irregular and located over bony prominences.

Table 7-5

Differential Diagnosis: Arterial versus Venous Ulcers

	ARTERIAL	VENOUS
Etiology	Arteriosclerosis obliterans, Atheroembolism	Valvular incompetence, Venous hypertension
Appearance	Irregular, smooth edges, Minimum to no granulation Usually deep	Irregular: dark pigmentation, sometimes fibrotic Good granulation, Usually shallow
Location	Distal lower leg: toes, feet, Lateral malleolus Anterior tibial area	Distal lower leg, Medial malleolus
Pedal Pulses	Decreased or absent	Usually present
Pain	Painful, especially if legs elevated	Little pain, comfortable with legs elevated
Drainage	Not present	Moderate to large amounts of exudate
Associated Gangrene	May be present	Absent
Associated Signs	Trophic changes Pallor on foot elevation, Dusky rubor on dependency	Edema Stasis dermatitis Possible cyanosis on dependency

3. Associated findings: edema, venous dermatitis, hyperpigmentation, varicosities, and chronic cellulitis.
4. Subjective reports of venous insufficiency: burning, throbbing, cramping, aching, and leg fatigue.
5. Duplex ultrasound used to examine perfusion.
6. Indications for DVT assessment discussed in Chapter 4.

Interventions

1. See section on wound care interventions.
2. Inelastic or short-stretch compression bandages (Unna boot, Profore, CircAid): worn during the day and night.
3. Compression pumps are an adjunct: 45–60 mmHg at ankle, 1–2 hours, potentially several times a day.
4. Inconvenient, requires secondary compression to prevent edema when not in pump.
5. Limb elevation
6. Other adjunct treatments if wound shows no signs of healing in 30 days:
   a. Ultrasound.
   b. Biological or bioengineered dressings, or pharmacological options.
   c. Surgery or radiofrequency vein ablation may be necessary if conservative measures fail.
7. Lifelong disorder, some form of compression garment, exercise, and weight control are necessary to prevent reoccurrence.
8. Compression garments: most garment pressures range from 20–55 mmHg at the ankle. Goal is to use the lowest level of effective pressure possible.

> **RED FLAG:** High compression is contraindicated with ABI <0.7. All sustained compression is contraindicated with ABI <0.6 or active DVT.

Arterial Ulcer

Etiology

1. Associated with chronic arterial insufficiency, arteriosclerosis obliterans, Thromboangiitis obliterans (Buerger's disease), and atheroembolism (cholesterol embolization syndrome). See discussion in Chapter 4 on Arterial Disease.
2. History of minor nonhealing trauma.

Clinical Features

1. Can occur anywhere in lower leg; common on small toes, feet, bony areas of trauma (shin).
2. Preceded by signs and symptoms of arterial insufficiency; pulses poor or absent, intermittent claudication.
3. Pain: often severe, intermittent, progressing to pain at rest, exacerbated with limb elevation.
4. Color: pale or cyanotic; pale on elevation; dusky rubor on dependency.
5. Temperature: cool.
6. Skin changes: trophic changes (thin, shiny, atrophic skin); loss of hair on foot and toes; nails thickened.
7. Ulceration: of toes or feet; can be deep.
8. Gangrene: black, gangrenous skin adjacent to ulcer can develop.

Examination

1. See section on examination of wounds.
2. Examine peripheral pulses, temperature, segmental BP (>20 mmHg drop between segments is significant).
3. Ankle brachial index (ABI); toe brachial index (TBI) indicated with elevated ABI since calcification of toe arteries is less likely.
4. Arterial Doppler studies: transcutaneous partial pressure of oxygen (TcPO2): values >40 mmHg are good while values <20 mmHg are unlikely to heal; laser Doppler skin perfusion pressure <30 mmHg unlikely to heal.
5. Outcome measure: Walking Impairment Questionnaire.

Interventions

1. See section on wound care interventions.
2. Manage BP, cholesterol, triglyceride, and glucose levels.
3. Exercise: walking 3–5 times a week. Try to accumulate 30–60 minutes, if claudication pain occurs, stop and rest until pain has abated, then resume. Contraindicated with chronic ischemic rest pain, ulcerations, gangrene, or ABI <0.4.
4. Patient education for limb care:
   a. Skin care: emollients after bathing, dry carefully.
   b. Avoid mechanical trauma, wear properly fitting closed toe shoes, nail care.
   c. Avoid thermal and chemical trauma, inspect feet daily and report minor injuries.

Diabetic Ulcer

Etiology

1. Diabetic ulcer is associated with atherosclerotic peripheral artery disease and peripheral neuropathy.
2. Caused by loss of protective sensation, loss of muscle coordination, mechanical trauma, and autonomic dysfunction.

Clinical Features

1. Occurs where arterial ulcers usually appear; or where peripheral neuropathy appears (plantar aspect of foot).

2. Pain: typically not painful; sensory loss usually present.
3. Pulses: may be present or diminished.
4. Absent ankle jerks with neuropathy.
5. Infection is more common; sepsis and/or gangrene may develop.

Examination

1. See section on examination of wounds.
2. Examine general condition of extremity.
3. Examine for vascular insufficiency.
4. Examine for peripheral neuropathy: 10-g (5.07 Semmes-Weinstein) monofilament testing at multiple sites in the plantar/dorsal feet and toes. Vibration testing (tuning fork) is helpful to detect early sensory loss.
5. Classify neurotrophic ulcers with the Wagner Classification System
   a. Grade 0 – No open lesions, foot deformity, or cellulitis may be present; high-risk for ulcer development
   b. Grade 1 – Superficial ulcer
   c. Grade 2 – Tendon, capsule, or bone exposed
   d. Grade 3 – Ulcer with abscess, osteomyelitis, or joint infection
   e. Grade 4 – Localized gangrene
   f. Grade 5 – Gangrene not localized

Intervention

1. See section on wound care interventions.
2. Off-loading the wound by using protective therapeutic footwear.
3. Provide support for patient education on nutritional guidelines for glycemic control.
4. Patient education for bathing (avoid soaking feet, dry between toes); skin, callus, and nail care (see patient education for skin care with arterial ulcers); avoid lotion between toes to help prevent maceration.

Pressure Injuries (Pressure or Decubitus Ulcers)

Etiology

1. Lesions caused by unrelieved pressure resulting in ischemic hypoxia and damage to underlying tissue.

Risk Factors

1. Prolonged pressure, shear forces, friction, repetitive stress.
2. Nutritional deficiency.
3. Maceration (softening associated with excessive moisture).

Table 7-6

Staging of Pressure Injury

STAGE	CHARACTERISTICS	EXAMPLE
Stage I	Nonblanchable erythema of intact skin. May include changes in skin temperature (warm or cool), tissue consistency (firm or boggy), and/or sensation (pain, itching). More difficult to distinguish with darker skin, redness may not be visible in darker skin (dark blue-purple tint).	
Stage II	Partial-thickness skin loss: involves epidermis, dermis, or both. Ulcer is superficial. Presents clinically as an abrasion, blister, or shallow crater.	
Stage III	Full-thickness skin loss: involves damage to or necrosis of subcutaneous tissue. May extend down to, but not through, underlying fascia. Presents clinically as a deep crater.	
Stage IV	Full-thickness skin loss: involves extensive destruction, tissue necrosis, or damage to muscle, bone, or supporting structures. Undermining and sinus tracts may be present.	
Unstageable	Tissue depth is obscured due to slough or eschar and extent of damage cannot be determined.	
Deep Tissue Injury	Discolored area of tissue (e.g., bruise) that is not reversible and will likely progress to a full-thickness injury.	

Adapted from National Pressure Ulcer Advisory Panel: NPUAP 2016 Staging Consensus Conference.
The National Pressure Ulcer Advisory Panel 2016 pressure injuries definitions, www.npuap.org.

4. Common in:
   a. Elderly, debilitated, or immobilized individuals.
   b. Decrease blood flow from hypotension or microvascular disease: diabetes, atherosclerosis.
   c. Neurologically impaired skin: decreased sensation.
   d. Cognitive impairment.

Clinical Features

1. Location: occurs over bony prominences; i.e., sacrum, heels, trochanter, lateral malleoli, ischial areas, elbows.
2. Color: red, brown/black, or yellow.
3. Localized infection.
4. Pain: can be painful if sensation intact.
5. Inflammatory response with necrotic tissue: hyperemia, fever, increased white blood cell count (WBC).
6. If left untreated, will progress from superficial simple erosion to involvement of deep layers of skin and underlying muscle and bone.
7. Graded by stages of severity (tissue damage). (See Table 7-6.)

Examination

1. See section on examination of wounds.
2. Use a standardized pressure injury assessment instrument (e.g., Bates-Jensen Wound Assessment Tool, Pressure Ulcer Scale).
3. Examine circulation, sensory integrity, and pain level.
4. Utilize a risk assessment instrument for individuals at risk for development of pressure injuries (e.g., Gosnell, Braden, or Norton Scales: see Appendix 7A).

Interventions

1. See section on wound care interventions.

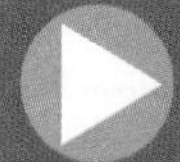

Burns

Pathophysiology

Burn Injury

1. Can result from heat, chemicals, electricity, sunlight, or radiation.
2. Most common causes are scalds from hot liquids and steam, fires, and flammable liquids and gases.
3. Inhalation injuries are caused by breathing smoke and create significant risk for morbidity and mortality.

Burn Wound, Consists of Three Zones

1. Zone of coagulation: cells are irreversibly injured, cell death occurs.
2. Zone of stasis: cells are injured; may die without specialized treatment, usually within 24–48 hours. Sensitive to infection and trauma (e.g., pressure and shearing during transfers).
3. Zone of hyperemia: minimal cell injury; cells should recover.

Degree of Burn

1. Burns are classified by severity, layers of skin damaged (Table 7-7).
2. Extent of burned area.
   a. Rule of Nines for estimating burn area (estimates are for adult patients).
      - Head and neck: 9%.
      - Anterior trunk: 18%.
      - Posterior trunk: 18%.
      - Arms: 9% each.
      - Legs: 18% each.
      - Perineum: 1%.

   b. Percentages vary by age (growth): use Lund-Browder charts for estimating body areas. It is the most accurate method to account for age and development.
3. Classification by percentage of body area burned.
   a. Critical: children or older adults with >10% of body with full-thickness burns or 20% or more with partial-thickness burns; any patient >25% total body surface area (TBSA). Any patient with burns to the face, eyes, ears, hands, or perineum, or if impairment exists. Respiratory complications.
   b. Moderate: Children or older adults with <10% with full-thickness burns and 10%–20% TBSA with partial-thickness burns or adults with <15%–25% TBSA mixed partial/full-thickness. Burns cannot involve face, hands, feet, genitalia, perineum, or major joints.
   c. Minor: Children or older adults <2% TBSA full-thickness burns or <10% with partial-thickness burns or adults with <15% TBSA partial-thickness burns. Burns cannot involve face, hands, feet, genitalia, perineum, or major joints.

Complications of Burn Injury

Infection

1. Loss of skin's protective barrier leads to infection.
2. Can progress to sepsis, gangrene, and even death.

Table 7-7

Burn Wound Classification

DEPTH OF BURN	CHARACTERISTICS	HEALING/SCARRING	EXAMPLE
Epidermal Burn (first degree)	• Damage is to epidermis only • Pink or red appearance; no blistering (dry surface) Minimal edema • Tenderness, delayed pain	• Spontaneous healing in 3–7 days No scarring	
Superficial Partial-thickness Burn (second degree)	• Epidermis and upper layers of dermis are damaged • Bright pink or red appearance • Blanching with brisk capillary refill Blisters, moist surface, weeping • Moderate edema • Painful, sensitive to touch, temperature changes	• Spontaneous healing, typically in 7–21 days • Minimal or no scarring; discoloration	
Deep Partial-thickness Burn (second degree)	• Severe damage to epidermis and dermis with injury to nerve endings, hair follicles, and sweat glands • Mixed red or waxy white appearance Blanching with slow capillary refill Broken blisters, wet surface • Marked edema • Sensitive to pressure but insensitive to light touch or soft pin prick	• Healing is slow and occurs through scar formation and re-epithelialization • Excessive scarring without preventive treatment	
Full-thickness Burn (third degree)	• Complete destruction of epidermis, dermis, and subcutaneous tissues, may extend into muscle • White (ischemic), charred, tan, or black appearance • No blanching; poor distal circulation • Parchment-like, dry leathery surface; depressed area • Little pain; nerve endings are destroyed	• Removal of eschar and skin grafting are necessary due to destruction of dermal and epidermal tissue • Risk of infection is increased • Hypertrophic scarring and wound contracture are likely to develop without preventive measures	
Subdermal Burn (fourth degree)	• Complete destruction of epidermis, dermis, with involvement of subcutaneous tissues and muscle • Charred appearance • Destruction of vascular system, may lead to additional necrosis from electrical burns; prolonged contact with flame • Additional complications likely with electrical burns: ventricular fibrillation, acute kidney damage, spinal cord damage	• Heals with skin grafting and scarring • Requires extensive surgery; amputation may be necessary	Fourth degree burn Epidermis Dermis Hypodermis (fat) Muscle Bone

Pulmonary Complications

1. Smoke inhalation injury from breathing hot gases; results in pulmonary edema and airway obstruction; suspicious signs include burns to the face and/or singed nose hairs.
2. Restrictive lung disease may also occur from burns to the trunk.
3. Pneumonia and/or pulmonary edema.

Metabolic Complications

1. Increased metabolic and catabolic activity results in weight loss, negative nitrogen balance, and decreased energy.
2. Hypermetabolic state may persist for months or years after a major burn.

Cardiac, Renal, and Circulatory Complications

1. Fluid and blood loss can result in shock and death.
2. Burns greater than 30% of total body surface area result in decreased renal perfusion and increased risk for acute kidney failure.
3. With severe burns can see hypothermia, hypovolemia, edema, hypoproteinemia, tachycardia, and decreased urinary output.

Keloid and Hypertrophic Scars

1. Hypertrophic scar. A raised scar that stays within the boundaries of the burn wound and is characteristically red, raised, and firm.
2. Keloid scar. A raised scar that extends beyond the boundaries of the original burn wound and is red, raised, and firm. More common in young women and those with dark skin.
3. Hypotrophic scar. Flat and depressed below the surrounding skin.

Burn Management

Emergency Local Burn Care

1. Immersion in cold water. If less than half the body is burned and injury is immediate, cold compresses may also be used.
2. Cover burn with sterile bandage or clean cloth; no ointments or creams.

Medical Management

1. Asepsis and wound care.
   a. Removal of charred clothing.
   b. Wound cleansing.
   c. Topical medications (antibacterial agents): reapplied one to three times daily.
      - Ointments: bacitracin, polymyxin B, and neomycin.
      - Silver sulfadiazine: common topical agent. Avoid at term pregnancy, on infants <2 months, and those with sulfa drug allergies.
      - Sulfamylon (mafenide acetate): penetrates through eschar. Avoid with sulfa drug allergies.
   d. Dressings (see Table 7-8).
      - Prevents bacterial contamination, prevents fluid loss, and protects the wound.
      - May additionally limit ROM.
      - Dressings include silver-impregnated, hydrogels, petroleum-impregnated, and gauze dressing.
2. Establish and maintain airway, adequate oxygenation, and respiratory function.
3. Monitor.
   a. Arterial blood gases, serum electrolyte levels, urinary output, vital signs.
   b. Gastrointestinal function: provide nutritional support.
4. Pain relief and psychological support: pharmaceutical (e.g., morphine) and psychological interventions (e.g., reframing, distraction, virtual reality, relaxation, and cognitive behavioral therapy).
5. Prevention and control of infection.
   a. Tetanus prophylaxis.
   b. Antibiotics.
   c. Standard precautions (see Chapter 13).
6. Fluid replacement therapy and nutrition management.
   a. Prevention and control of shock.
   b. Postshock fluid and blood replacement.
   c. Nutritional support should begin as soon as possible.
7. Surgery.
   a. Primary excision: escharotomies, fasciotomies may be required to prevent tourniquet effects. As the patient is stabilized, surgical removal of eschar begins.
   b. Grafts: closure of the wound.
      - Allograft (homograft): use of other human skin; e.g., cadaver skin; temporary grafts for large burns, used until autograft is available.
      - Xenograft (heterograft): use of skin from other species; e.g., pigskin; a temporary graft.
      - Biosynthetic grafts: combination of collagen and synthetics.
      - Cultured skin: laboratory grown from patient's own skin.
      - Autograft: use of patient's own skin.
      - Split-thickness graft: contains epidermis and upper layers of dermis from donor site.
      - Full-thickness graft: contains epidermis and dermis from donor site.
   c. Emergency escharotomy and fasciotomy is necessary with circumferential burns of the extremities when compression from increased tissue edema and massive fluid retention occur within confined anatomic spaces (compartment syndrome). Circulation is compromised.

RED FLAG: Monitor closely for signs and symptoms of acute compartment syndrome in both burned and nonburned limbs.

   d. Surgical resection of scar contracture; e.g., Z-plasty (surgical incision in the form of the letter "Z" used to lengthen a burn scar).

Other Considerations

1. Factors that affect healing include nutrition, infection, associated illnesses (e.g., diabetes, malignancy, vascular insufficiency, cytotoxic treatments).
2. Significant burn injury more likely in very young or the elderly who have very thin skin.
3. Loss of sebaceous glands can result in drying and cracking of wound; protection with moisturizing creams is important for healed burns and any donor sites.

Burn Wound Cleansing and Debridement

1. Use infection control techniques at all times.
2. Maintain temperature of burn wound by warming cleansing solutions, maintaining ambient temperature, and avoiding lengthy exposure of wet wound surfaces.
3. Cleansing with disinfectant soap and warm water.
   a. Some wounds or dressings benefit from soaking, wet removal of dressings.
   b. Excessive immersion is contraindicated. Risks include auto-contamination and electrolyte imbalance.

4. Wound debridement: removal of loose, charred, dead skin (see Table 7-8).
   a. Autolytic dressings: use of moist dressings such as hydrogels or hydrocolloids to help remove eschar.
   b. Surgical or sharp debridement: excision of eschar using sterilized surgical instruments (forceps, scalpel, scissors).
   c. Enzymatic: e.g., fibrinolysins.
   d. Mechanical: wet to dry dressings, pulsed lavage, gentle washing.

Rehabilitation

1. Overall goals: limit loss of ROM, reduce edema, prevent predictable contractures through positioning and splinting, and prevent or reduce complications of immobilization.
2. Typically includes twice-daily therapy sessions timed with planned pain medication.
3. Exercises to promote deep breathing and chest expansion.
4. Anticontracture positioning and splinting: starts from day one and continues for many months.
   a. Anterior neck: common deformity is flexion; stress hyperextension; position with firm (plastic) cervical orthosis.
   b. Shoulder: common deformity is adduction and internal rotation; stress abduction, flexion, and external rotation; position with an axillary splint (airplane splint).
   c. Elbow: common deformity is flexion and pronation; stress extension and supination; position in extension with posterior arm splint.
   d. Hand: common deformity is a claw hand (intrinsic minus position); stress wrist extension (15°), MP flexion (70°), PIP, and DIP extension, thumb abduction (intrinsic plus position); position in intrinsic plus position with resting hand splint.
   e. Hip: common deformity is flexion and adduction; stress hip extension and abduction; position in extension, abduction, neutral rotation.
   f. Knee: common deformity is flexion; stress extension; position in extension with posterior knee splint.
   g. Ankle: common deformity is plantar flexion; stress dorsiflexion; position with foot–ankle in neutral with splint or plastic ankle–foot orthosis.
5. Edema control: elevation of extremities, active ROM.
6. Stretching and early mobilization, taking all joints through full passive ROM.

RED FLAGS: Schedule therapy to coincide with optimal pain medication (30–45 minutes before session), and dressing changes/wound cleansing.
- Postgrafting: discontinue exercise for 3–5 days to allow grafts to heal.
- Compression wraps may be necessary initially to prevent edema.
- Avoid shearing and avoid prolonged dependent positioning.

Rehabilitation (Post-Acute)

1. Continued passive ROM, increasing active ROM.
2. Progressive strengthening to correct loss of muscle mass and strength.
3. Minimize edema. Elastic supports to control edema.
4. Scar management.
   a. Massage and application of moisturizer.
   b. Regular massage and touching of scars to desensitize hypersensitive scars.
   c. Pressure garments to help prevent hypertrophic scarring or keloid formation.
5. Progressive ambulation to improve cardiovascular endurance and activity tolerance.
6. Training in activities of daily living (ADL) and functional mobility skills.
7. Preparation for home, work, play, or school.
8. Management of chronic pain.
9. Provide education and emotional support.

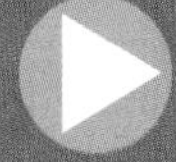

Physical Therapy Interventions for Impaired Integumentary Integrity

Wound Bed Preparation (TIME Principles)

1. Wound bed preparation is essential for proper tissue healing. Moist wound healing and the removal of bioburden is critical for optimal healing. The mnemonic TIME is a method for remembering proper wound bed preparation.
2. Tissue – Is the tissue viable or nonviable
   a. Viable – choose dressing that promotes moist wound healing and fills dead space
   b. Nonviable – choose the best type of debridement to remove necrotic tissues, slough, or bioburden.
3. Infection/Inflammation – Address infection (local or systemic), excessive colonization, or edema.
4. Moisture balance – promotes optimal wound healing
   a. Dry or desiccated wounds – choose a dressing that hydrates and/or promotes a moist wound environment.

b. Excessive moisture (maceration is present) – choose a dressing that absorbs moderate to heavy drainage.
5. Edge of Wound – healthy wound edges promote healing. Edges that are not contracting impedes healing and factors such as scarring, necrotic tissue, undermining, or tunneling must be addressed for proper epithelial migration.

Wound Care Interventions

Infection Control

1. Wounds are cultured; antibiotic treatment regimen prescribed.
   a. Topical antimicrobial agents: e.g., silver nitrate, silver sulfadiazine, erythromycin, gentamicin, neomycin, triple antibiotic.
   b. Wound cleansing.
   c. Remove bio-burden and nonviable tissue.
2. Hand washing of health care practitioners.
3. Sterile technique is most appropriate with invasive procedures and collecting specimens. Clean technique is most appropriate for chronic wounds, home care, long-term care facilities, outpatient, and routine procedures.
4. Negative-pressure wound therapy (vacuum-assisted closure).
   a. An open-cell foam dressing placed into the wound.
   b. Controlled subatmospheric pressure (typically 125 mmHg below ambient pressure) is applied via specialized device.
   c. Helps to maintain a moist wound environment, control edema, increases localized blood flow, removes exudate, and reduces infectious material.
   d. Indicated in wounds of all shapes and sizes from many various conditions.
   e. Contraindications include malignancy in wound, exposed nerve or vascular structure, exposed organ, untreated osteomyelitis, and significant eschar.

Surgical Intervention

1. Indicated for excising of ulcer, enhancing vascularity, resurfacing wound (grafts), and preventing sepsis and osteomyelitis.
2. May be indicated for stages III and IV pressure injuries.

Hyperbaric Oxygen Therapy (HBO)

1. Patient breathes 100% oxygen in a sealed, full-body chamber with elevated atmospheric pressure (usually around 2.4 atmospheres).
2. Hyperoxygenation reverses tissue hypoxia and facilitates wound healing due to enhanced solubility of oxygen in the blood.
3. Indicated with compromised skin grafts, acute ischemia, osteomyelitis, necrotizing infections, thermal burns, and other wounds that are not healing due to hypoxia.
4. Contraindicated in untreated pneumothorax and with patients on antineoplastic medications (e.g., doxorubicin, disulfiram, cisplatin, mafenide acetate).

Wound Cleansing

1. Removal of loose cellular debris, metabolic wastes, bacteria, and topical agents that retard wound healing.
2. Cleanse wounds initially and at each dressing change.
3. Normal saline (0.9% NaCl) recommended for most ulcers; nontoxic effects in wound.
4. Cleansing topical agents: contain surfactants that lower surface tension. Limited use, may be toxic to healing tissues; e.g., povidone-iodine solution, sodium hypochlorite solution, Dakin's solution, acetic acid solution, hydrogen peroxide.
5. Mechanical delivery systems.
   a. Minimal mechanical force: cleansing with gauze, cloth, or sponge.
   b. Irrigation: recommend pressures range from 4–15 psi. These pressures are sufficient to remove debris and bacteria without harming granulating tissues.
      - Squeeze bottle, bulb syringe, or piston syringe.
      - Pulsed lavage: delivery of irrigating solution under pressure that is produced by an electrically powered device. Pulsed lavage with vacuum (PLWV) assists in removal of wound debris.

RED FLAG: Whirlpool therapy (WP) is *not* supported for wound care. Adverse events with WP can include contamination and infection associated with pathogens found in WP equipment, higher and unregulated pressures can damage fragile granulation tissue, and limbs placed in a dependent position experience increased venous hypertension and vascular congestion. PLWV is a more effective treatment alternative.

- Burn care is one area that WP is occasionally used to treat patients with burns in need of extensive debridement.

RED FLAG: Do not use harsh soaps, alcohol-based products, or harsh antiseptic agents; may erode skin.

Wound Debridement

1. Removal of necrotic or infected tissue and biofilms that interfere with wound healing. (See Table 7-8.)
2. Purposes:
   a. Allows examination of ulcer, determination of extent of wound.

Table 7-8

Methods of Debridement

METHOD	DEFINITION	INDICATIONS	CONTRAINDICATIONS
Autolytic	A selective method of natural debridement promoted under occlusive or semiocclusive moisture-retentive dressings that results in solubilization of necrotic tissue only by phagocytic cells and by proteolytic and collagenolytic enzymes inherent in the tissues.	• Individuals on anticoagulant therapy • Individuals who cannot tolerate other forms of debridement • All necrotic wounds in people who are medically stable	• Infected wounds • Wounds of immunosuppressed individuals • Dry gangrene or dry ischemic wounds
Enzymatic	A selective method of chemical debridement that promotes liquefaction of necrotic tissue by applying topical preparation of collagenolytic enzymes to those tissues.	• All moist necrotic wounds • Eschar after cross-hatching • Homebound individuals • People who cannot tolerate surgical debridement	• Ischemic wounds unless adequate vascular status has been determined • Dry gangrene • Clean, granulated wounds
Mechanical	A nonselective method of debridement that removes foreign material and devitalized or contaminated tissue by physical forces (wet-to-dry gauze dressing, dextranomers, pulsatile lavage with suction), and may remove healthy tissue as well.	• Wounds with moist necrotic tissue or foreign material present	• Clean, granulated wounds
Sharp	A selective method of debridement using sterile instruments (scalpel, scissors, forceps, and silver nitrate stick) that sequentially removes only necrotic wound tissue without anesthesia and with little or no bleeding induced in viable tissue.	• Scoring and/or excision of leathery eschar • Excision of moist necrotic tissue • Biofilm removal	• Clean wounds • Advancing cellulitis with sepsis • When infection threatens the individual's life • Individual on anticoagulant therapy or has coagulopathy
Surgical	For deep (stage III or IV) or complicated pressure ulcer, the most efficient method of debridement. It is selective and is performed by a physician or surgeon using sterile instruments (scalpel, scissors, forceps, hemostat, silver nitrate sticks) in a one-time operative procedure. The procedure usually removes most, if not all, necrotic tissue, but may also remove some healthy tissue in what is termed wide excision. Because there may be associated pain and/or bleeding, the individual may require anesthesia, and the procedure will likely require an operating or special procedures room.	• Advancing cellulitis with sepsis • Immunocompromised individuals • When infection threatens the individual's life • Clean wounds as a preliminary procedure to surgical wound closure line • Granulation and scar tissue may be excised • Biofilm removal	• Cardiac disease, pulmonary disease, or diabetes • Severe spasticity • Individuals who cannot tolerate surgery • Individuals with a short life expectancy • Quality of life cannot be improved
Kilohertz Ultrasound (e.g., MIST, Sonoca 180, Misonix devices)	This long-wave low-frequency ultrasound typically operates between 20 and 50 kHz. This is a selective form of debridement. Autoclaving of contact probe is usually required (not all devices make direct contact with wound).	• Selective removal of necrotic tissue and biofilm desired • Reduces bioburden • Increase angiogenesis • Wound bed preparation for grafting or flap closure	• Contraindications include vascular abnormalities (DVT, emboli, advanced PVD), irradiated areas, tumors, organs, or electrical devices • Precautions over nerves, infections, anesthetic areas
Biological (rarely used)	The use of maggots to debride nonviable tissue. They produce enzymes and phagocytize necrotic tissue and bacteria (e.g., MRSA, group A and B *streptococcus, Pseudomonas*). They may stimulate granulation formation and epithelialization.	• Individuals who cannot tolerate other forms of debridement • All nonhealing necrotic wounds in people who are medically stable	• Psychological stress arises from having living creatures in wounds • Reports of pain increasing • Poor perfusion or exposed blood vessels

Adapted from Consortium for Spinal Cord Medicine: Pressure Ulcer Prevention and Treatment Following Spinal Cord Injury, Paralyzed Veterans of America, August 2000.

b. Promotes wound healing, decreases bacterial concentration in wound; and decreases spread of infection; i.e., cellulitis or sepsis.
c. Improves patients' outcomes.
3. More than one type of debridement is typically used as part of the patient's plan of care as wound healing progresses.
4. Types of debridement:
a. Autolytic: uses the body's own enzymes and moisture beneath a dressing; nonviable tissue becomes liquefied. Dressing type, frequency, and absorbency are important. Dressing types include hydrocolloids, hydrogels, and transparent films (semiocclusive and occlusive). Promotes fast wound healing with less pain.
b. Enzymatic: involves the application of a topical agent that chemically liquefies necrotic tissue. May be used in conjunction with surgical and sharp debridement. Common in the long-term setting because there is less pain and can be applied daily.
c. Biological: involves the use of maggots grown in a sterile environment. A dressing is used to confine the maggots to the wound.
d. Mechanical: involves irrigation (pulsed-lavage), hydrotherapy, or wet-to-dry dressings.
e. Surgical sharp debridement: performed by a skilled practitioner using surgical instruments such as a scalpel, curette, scissors, and forceps to remove biofilm and devitalized tissue.

RED FLAG: Special consideration with heel pressure injuries (ulcers): Do NOT debride *if* the heel pressure injury (ulcer) is dry without edema, erythema, fluctuance, or drainage. If complications arise, then debridement may be necessary.

Wound Dressings

1. Ideal wound dressings maintain a moist environment and control excessive exudate, facilitate gaseous exchange (oxygen, carbon dioxide, water), insulates, prevent contamination from microorganisms, and are nontraumatic to the wound. (See Table 7-9.)
2. Dressing selections are generally based on wound bed color, depth, and exudate production.
a. Wound Bed Color
- Red: Support moist wound healing and prevent trauma to granulating tissues
- Yellow/Black: Indicates the presences of slough or necrotic tissue and needs debridement.

b. Depth: Wound beds, tunneling, and undermining will need to be filled with dressing.
c. Exudate production
- Select dressing that promotes moist wound healing and prevents maceration.

3. Common dressings:
a. Alginate and hydrofiber gelling dressings: e.g., AlgiSite, Sorbsan, Kaltostat, Aquacel Hydrofiber.
b. Transparent film dressings: e.g., Bioclusive, OpSite, Tegaderm.
c. Foam dressings: e.g., LYOfoam, Flexzan, Hydrocell
d. Hydrogel dressings: e.g., Carrasyn gel, Vigilon, Second Skin, Clearsite.
e. Hydrocolloid dressings: e.g., DuoDerm, Exuderm, Curaderm, 3M Tegasorb.
f. Gauze dressings.
- Standard gauze (not impregnated): e.g., Kerlix, 4 × 4 s, Nugauze, Telfa.
- Impregnated gauze: e.g., silver-, iodine-, or Vaseline (petroleum)-impregnated gauze, e.g., Adaptic, Xeroform.

g. Silver dressings: common antimicrobial agent found in foams, films, alginates, hydrocolloids, hydrogels, and other types of dressings.
h. Composite: e.g., Tegaderm absorbent clear acrylic, Covaderm Plus. Combine components of other dressing categories into one dressing (alginate and a semiocclusive film barrier).
i. Contact layer: Adaptic, impregnated gauze dressings. Serves as a porous barrier layer to protect wound bed from direct trauma from other dressings.
j. Specialty dressings: wound matrix dressings: provide a scaffolding for cellular deposit. Typically, collagen or hyaluronan-based dressings (e.g., Prisma); skin substitutes: epidermal, dermal, or both, e.g., Epicel, Dermagraft, Apligraf. Most are expensive and used when standard wound care has failed.
4. Topical agents: used to manage nonhealing or infected wounds. Includes wound cleanser and antiseptics (e.g., acetic acid, Dakin's solution, providone-iodine), antimicrobials (e.g., antifungals [nystatin] and antibacterials [bacitracin, neosporin, polymyxin B]), anesthesia and analgesia agents (e.g., topical lidocaine), and enzymatic debridement (e.g., Santyl).

Edema Management

1. Leg elevation and exercise (ankle pumps).
2. Compression therapy: to facilitate movement of excess fluid from lower extremity.
a. Compression wraps: elastic or tubular bandages.
b. Paste bandages; e.g., Unna boot is a pliable, nonstretchable dressing impregnated with zinc or calamine and gelatin.
c. Compression stockings; e.g., Jobst.
d. Compression pump therapy (see Chapters 4 and 11)

Electrical Stimulation for Wound Healing Therapy (See Chapter 11)

1. Used to improve circulation, facilitate debridement, and enhance tissue repair.
2. Continuous waveform application with direct current.
3. High-voltage pulsed current.
4. Pulsed biphasic current.

Nutritional Considerations

1. Delayed wound healing associated with malnutrition and poor hydration.
   a. Albumin: normal is 3.5–5.5 mg/dl; <3.5 = malnutrition.
   b. BMI ≤21 with weight loss increased risk for pressure injury.
2. Provide adequate hydration.
   a. Individuals with wounds require approximately 3 or more liters of water a day.
   b. Patients on air-fluidized beds require greater hydration (40–60 ml/Kg a day).
3. Provide adequate nutrition: frequent high-calorie/high-protein meals; energy intake (25–35 kcal/kg/body weight) and protein (1.5–2.5 gm/kg body weight).
4. Patients with trauma stress and burns require higher intakes.

Injury Prevention or Reduction

1. Daily, comprehensive skin inspection.
   a. Pay particular attention to bony prominences (e.g., sacrum, coccyx, trochanter, ischial tuberosities, medial or lateral malleolus).
   b. In darkly pigmented skin, observe changes in skin tone, skin temperature, and tissue consistency compared to surrounding skin. Moistening the skin assists in identifying changes in color.
2. Therapeutic positioning to relieve pressure and allow tissue reperfusion. Avoid positioning on an area of erythema or pressure injury.
   a. In bed: turning or repositioning every 2 hours during acute and rehabilitation phases.
   b. In wheelchair: wheelchair push-ups every 15 minutes.
3. Use techniques to ensure skin protection, avoid friction, shear, or abrasion injury, use of sheepskin.
   a. Lifting, not dragging.
   b. Use of turning and draw sheets; trapeze, manual, or electric lifts.
   c. Use of cornstarch, lubricants, pad protectors, thin film dressings, or hydrocolloid dressings over friction risk sites.
   d. Use of transfer boards for sliding wheelchair transfers.
4. Pressure-relieving devices (PRDs).
   a. Reduce tissue interface pressures.
   b. Static devices: use if patient can assume a variety of positions; examples include foam, air, or gel mattress overlays; water-filled mattresses; pillows or foam wedges, protective padding (heel relief boots).
   c. Dynamic devices: use if patient cannot assume a variety of positions; examples include alternating pressure air mattresses, fluidized air or high-air-loss bed.
   d. Seating supports: use for chair-bound or wheelchair-bound patients; examples include cushions made out of foam, gel, air, or some combination.
5. Avoid restrictive clothing, e.g., with rough textures, hard fasteners, and studs. Avoid tight-fitting shoes, socks, splints, and orthoses.
6. Avoid maceration injury.
   a. Prevent moisture accumulation and temperature elevation where skin contacts support surface.
   b. Incontinence management strategies:
      - Cleanse skin immediately after incontinence. Use cleansers that are pH balanced for the skin.
      - Use absorbent pads, brief, or panty pad as needed.
      - Schedule toileting and use of prompted voiding techniques.
      - Use ointments and creams on dry skin and as skin barriers prophylactically in perineal and perianal areas.
7. Patient and caregiver education.
   a. Mechanisms of pressure injury development.
   b. Daily skin inspection and hygiene.
   c. Avoidance of prolonged positions.
   d. Repositioning, weight shifts, lifts.
   e. Safety awareness during self-care.
   f. Safety awareness with use of devices and equipment.
   g. Importance of ongoing activity/exercise program.

Special Considerations Populations

1. Obesity.
   a. More perspiration for proper thermoregulation, pressure injuries over the buttocks versus sacrum, pressure between skin folds, and moisture-associated skin damage.
   b. Prevention: properly sized bariatric equipment and support surfaces; repositioning larger areas such as breasts and panniculus formations (dense layers of fatty tissue) along with normal repositioning every 2 hours; Burrow's solution (aluminium triacetate) as an astringent to reduce skin irritation, allergic reactions, and for its antibacterial properties; monitor and prevent moisture-associated damage.

Table 7-9

Characteristics of Some Major Dressing Categories

DRESSING CATEGORY AND DEFINITION	INDICATIONS	ADVANTAGES
Transparent Films Clear, adhesive, semipermeable membrane dressings. Permeable to atmospheric oxygen and moisture vapor yet impermeable to water, bacteria, and environmental contaminants.	• Stages I and II pressure ulcers • Secondary dressing in certain situations • For autolytic debridement • Skin donor sites • Cover for hydrophilic powder and paste preparations and hydrogels	• Visual evaluation of wound without removal • Impermeable to external fluids and bacteria • Transparent and comfortable • Promote autolytic debridement • Minimize friction
Hydrocolloids Adhesive wafers containing hydroactive/absorptive particles that interact with wound fluid to form a gelatinous mass over the wound bed. May be either occlusive or semiocclusive. Available in paste form that can be used as a filler for shallow cavity wounds.	• Protection of partial-thickness wounds • Autolytic debridement of necrosis or slough • Wounds with mild exudate	• Maintain a moist wound environment • Nonadhesive to healing tissue • Conformable • Impermeable to external bacteria and contaminants • Support autolytic debridement • Minimal to moderate absorption • Waterproof • Reduce pain • Easy to apply • Time-saving • Thin forms diminish friction
Hydrogels Water- or glycerine-based gels. Insoluble in water. Available in solid sheets, amorphous gels, or impregnated gauze. Absorptive capacity varies.	• Partial- and full-thickness wounds • Wounds with necrosis and slough • Burns and tissue damaged by radiation	• Soothing and cooling • Fill dead space • Rehydrate dry wound beds • Promote autolytic debridement • Provide minimal to moderate absorption • Conform to wound bed • Transparent to translucent • Many are nonadherent • Amorphous form can be used when infection is present
Foams Semipermeable membranes that are either hydrophilic or hydrophobic. Vary in thickness, absorptive capacity, and adhesive properties.	• Partial- and full-thickness wounds with minimal to moderate exudate • Secondary dressing for wounds with packing to provide additional absorption • Provide protection and insulation	• Insulate wounds • Provide some padding • Most are nonadherent • Conformable • Manage minimal to heavy exudate • Easy to use • Some newer products are designed for deep cavities
Alginates and Hydrofibers Alginates are soft, absorbent, nonwoven dressings derived from seaweed that have a fluffy cotton-like appearance. React with wound exudate to form a viscous hydrophilic gel mass over the wound area. Available in ropes and pads. Hydrofibers (Aquacel) are similar to alginates but are composed of a polymer.	• Wounds with moderate to large amounts of exudate • Wounds with combination exudate and necrosis • Wounds that require packing and absorption • Infected and noninfected exuding wounds	• Absorb up to 20 times their weight in drainage • Fill dead space • Support debridement in presence of exudate • Easy to apply
Gauze Dressings Made of cotton or synthetic fabric that is absorptive and permeable to water and oxygen. May be used wet, moist, dry, or impregnated with petrolatum, antiseptics, or other agents. Come in varying weaves and with different size interstices.	• Exudative wounds • Wounds with dead space, tunneling, or sinus tracts • Wounds with combination exudate or necrotic tissue WET TO DRY • Mechanical debridement of necrotic tissue and slough CONTINUOUS DRY • Heavily exudating wounds CONTINUOUS MOIST • Protection of clean wounds • Autolytic debridement of slough or eschar • Delivery of topical needs	• Readily available • Can be used with appropriate solutions such as gels, normal saline, or topical antimicrobials to keep wounds moist • Can be used on infected wounds • Good mechanical debridement if properly used • Cost-effective filler for large wounds • Effective delivery of topicals if kept moist
Specialty Dressings (Cellular or Tissue-based, Bioengineered, Growth Factors)	Used when conventional approaches failed or unlikely to succeed. Full-thickness should show signs of healing in 2–4 weeks; partial-thickness should show signs of healing in 1–2 weeks.	Promotes or reduces abnormal biological activity and scaffolding in recalcitrant wounds. Example: Collagen matrix reduces abnormal amounts of proteases (matrix metalloproteinases) in chronic wounds.

(*Continued*)

Table 7-9

Characteristics of Some Major Dressing Categories (Continued)

DISADVANTAGES	CONSIDERATIONS
Transparent Films • Nonabsorptive • Application can be difficult • Channeling or wrinkling occurs • Not to be used on wounds with fragile surrounding skin or infected wounds	• Allow 1- to 2-inch wound margin around bed • Shave surrounding hair • Secondary dressing not required • Dressing change varies with wound condition and location • Avoid in wounds with infection, copious drainage, or tracts
Hydrocolloids • Nontransparent • May soften and change shape with heat or friction • Odor and yellow drainage on removal (melted dressing material) • Not recommended for wounds with heavy exudate, sinus tracts, or infections; wounds that expose bone or tendon; or wounds with fragile surrounding skin • Dressing edges may curl	• Characteristic odor with yellow exudate similar to pus; normal when dressing is removed • Allow 1- to 1½-inch margin of healthy tissue around wound edges • Taping edges will help prevent curling • Frequency of changes depends on amount of exudate • Change every 3–7 days and as needed with leakage • Avoid in wounds with infection or tracts
Hydrogels • Most require a secondary dressing • Not used for heavily exudating wounds • May dry out and then adhere to wound bed • May macerate surrounding skin	• Sheet form works well on partial-thickness ulcers • Do not use sheet form on infected ulcers • Sheet form can promote growth of *Pseudomonas* and yeast • Dressing changes every 8–48 hours • Use skin barrier wipe on surrounding intact skin to decrease risk of maceration
Foams • Nontransparent • Nonadherent foams require secondary dressing, tape, or net to hold in place • Some newer foams have tape on edges • Poor conformability to deep wounds • Not for use with dry eschar or wounds with no exudate	• Change schedule varies from 1–5 days or as needed for leakage • Protect intact surrounding skin with skin sealant to prevent maceration
Alginates and Hydrofibers • Require secondary dressing • Not recommended for dry or lightly exudating wounds • Can dry wound bed	• May use dry gauze pad or transparent film as secondary dressing • Change schedule varies (with type of product used and amount of exudate) from every 8 hours to every 2–3 days
Gauze Dressings • Delayed healing if used improperly • Pain on removal (wet to dry) • Labor-intensive • Require secondary dressing • Avoid direct contact with granulating tissue • Increase infection rates compared to semiocclusive dressings	• Change schedule varies with amount of exudate • Pack loosely into wounds; tight packing compromises blood flow and delays wound closure • Use continuous roll of gauze for packing large wounds (ensures complete removal) • If too wet, dressings will macerate surrounding skin • Use wide mesh gauze for debridement and fine mesh gauze for protection • Protect surrounding skin with moisture barrier ointment or skin sealant as needed
Specialty Dressings (Cellular or Tissue-based, Bioengineered, Growth Factors) • Expensive • May not be readily available	• Application, precautions, and contraindications are specific to product

Adapted from Consortium for Spinal Cord Medicine: Pressure Ulcer Prevention and Treatment Following Spinal Cord Injury, Paralyzed Veterans of America, August 2000 and Bryant, RA, Nix DP. Principles of wound healing and topical management. In: Bryant RA, Nix DP, ed. *Acute and chronic wounds: current management concepts.* Fifth edition. St. Louis, Missouri: Elsevier; 2016: 306–324.

2. Neonate to pediatrics.
   a. Age integumentary differences: see Table 7-2. Integumentary age-related changes.
   b. Use mild cleansers and less-frequent bathing. Poor thermoregulation with preterm. Skin is thinner so avoid friction with toweling off. Moistening creams or ointments to prevent drying. Be careful of topical agents since they are more readily absorbed, leading to potentially systemic effects (Cushing's syndrome with excessive use of topical corticosteroids). Additionally, infants are generally more sensitive to irritants.
   c. Diaper rash is moisture-associated skin damage. Prevent through proper cleansing (avoid vigorous rubbing) and skin protectants and barriers. If candidiasis develops, see yeast infections earlier in chapter.
   d. Pressure injuries more common on head.

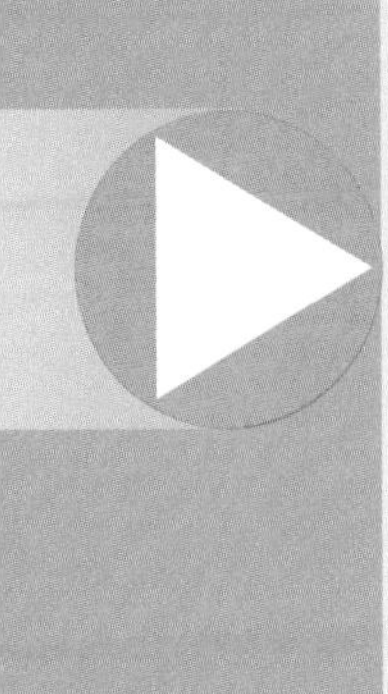

APPENDIX 7A

Selected Wound-Related Assessment and Outcome Measures

Table 7A-1

MEASUREMENT TOOLS	TARGET POPULATION AND INTENDED USE	REFERENCES
Activity Measure for Post-Acute Care (AM-PAC™) "6-Clicks" Inpatient Short Forms	Assess functional outcomes in the post-acute care setting. It measures difficulty, assistance, and limitations in ADLs. Cognition is only included in the longer form.	Andres PL, Haley SM, Ni PS. Is patient-reported function reliable for monitoring postacute outcomes? *Am J Phys Med Rehabil.* 2003; 82(8): 614–621.
Neuropathic Pain Scale	Intended for measuring qualities associated with chronic neuropathic pain. The 10 items are intensity, sharp, hot, dull, cold, sensitive, itchy, unpleasant, intense deep, and intense surface.	Lavoie Smith EM, Cohen JA, Pett MA, Beck SL. The validity of neuropathy and neuropathic pain measures in patients with cancer receiving taxanes and platinums. *Oncol Nurs Forum.* 2011; 38(2): 133–142.
Rapid Eating and Activity Assessment for Patients (REAP)	This measures diet and physical activity habits.	Gans KM, Ross E, Barner CW, Wylie-Rosett J, McMurray J, Eaton C. REAP and WAVE: new tools to rapidly assess/discuss nutrition with patients. *J Nutr.* 2003; 133(2): 556S–562S.
Pressure Ulcer Scale for Healing	Primarily used to assess and monitor the healing of pressure ulcers. Valid to use for monitoring the healing of venous leg ulcers and diabetic foot ulcers.	Thomas DR, Rodeheaver GT, Bartolucci AA, et al. Pressure ulcer scale for healing: Derivation and validation of the PUSH tool. The PUSH Task Force. *Adv Wound Care.* 1997; 10(5): 95–101.
Bates-Jensen Wound Assessment Tool (formerly, the Pressure Sore Status Tool)	Designed to assess and monitor healing rates in pressure ulcers and various other chronic wounds.	Harris C, Bates-Jensen B, Parslow N, Raizman R, Singh M, Ketchen R. Bates-Jensen wound assessment tool: Pictorial guide validation project. *JWOCN.* 2010; 37(3): 253–259.
Pressure Sore Status Tool	Developed as both a research and clinical tool to assess and monitor tissue changes in pressure ulcers. In 2001, this tool was modified and formally renamed as the Bates-Jensen Wound Assessment Tool (see above).	Bates-Jensen BM, Vredevoe DL, Brecht ML. Validity and reliability of the Pressure Sore Status Tool. *Decubitus.* 1992; 5(6): 20–28.

(Continued)

Table 7A-1 (Continued)

MEASUREMENT TOOLS	TARGET POPULATION AND INTENDED USE	REFERENCES
Sussman Wound Healing Tool	Monitors tissue status, wound size, and phases of wound healing. Can be used with various wounds, but was primarily developed to monitor healing of pressure ulcers.	Sussman C, Swanson G. Utility of the Sussman Wound Healing Tool in predicting wound healing outcomes in physical therapy. *Adv Wound Care.* 1997; 10(5): 74–77.
Spinal Cord Impairment Pressure Ulcer Monitoring Tool	Used to monitor pressure ulcer healing in people with spinal cord injuries.	Thomason SS, Luther S, Nelson A, Palacios P, Harrow J. Pressure ulcer healing in SCI: a novel evidence-based tool: 2435. *JWOCN.* 2008; 35(3): S70.
Photographic Wound Assessment Tool	This tool was designed to examine the photograph of various wounds versus the actual wound. It is intended to be used when the expert clinician cannot be present to physically examine the wound (e.g., rural areas, home health, telemedicine).	Thompson N, Gordey L, Bowles H, Parslow N, Houghton P. Reliability and validity of the revised photographic wound assessment tool on digital images taken of various types of chronic wounds. *Adv Skin Wound Care.* 2013; 26(8): 360–373.
The Wound Bed Score	Used to monitor wound bed preparation prior to the application of advance technologies. Does not monitor healing rates.	Falanga V, Saap LJ, Ozonoff A. Wound bed score and its correlation with healing of chronic wounds. *Dermatol Ther.* 2006; 19(6): 383–390.
Wagner Classification System	Designed to assess the depth and tissue involvement of diabetic foot ulcers.	Oyibo SO, Jude EB, Tarawneh I, Nguyen HC, Harkless LB, Boulton AJ. A comparison of two diabetic foot ulcer classification systems: the Wagner and the University of Texas wound classification systems. *Diabetes Care.* 2001; 24(1): 84–88.
University of Texas Wound Classification System	Designed to assess the depth and tissue involvement of diabetic foot ulcers. This scheme goes further than the Wagner Classification System by incorporating the presence or absence of infection and ischemia.	Armstrong DG, Lavery LA, Harkless LB. Validation of a diabetic wound classification system. The contribution of depth, infection, and ischemia to risk of amputation. *Diabetes Care.* 1998; 21(5): 855–859.
Braden	Six-item pressure sore risk assessment scale (score range 6–23; 18 and lower scores indicate progressive risk).	Braden BJ, Bergstrom N. Clinical utility of the Braden Scale for Predicting Pressure Sore Risk. *Decubitus.* 1989; 2(3): 44–46, 50–51.
Glamorgan	Pressure ulcer risk assessment scale. Higher score equals higher risk. 10+ at risk, 20+ very high risk. Birth to 18 years old.	Nix DR, Best M, Bryant RA. Skin care needs of the neonatal and pediatric patient. In: Bryant RA, Nix DP. *Acute and chronic wounds: current management concepts.* Fifth edition. ed. St. Louis, Missouri: Elsevier; 2016: 516-530.
Braden Q Scale (pediatric population)	Braden + Tissue perfusion and oxygenation. Pressure sore risk assessment scale for the pediatric population (score range 7–28; 16 and lower scores indicate progressive risk). 21 days to 8 years old.	Curley MA, Razmus IS, Roberts KE, Wypij D. Predicting pressure ulcer risk in pediatric patients: the Braden Q Scale. *Nursing Research.* 2003; 52(1): 22–33.
Norton	Five-item pressure sore risk assessment scale (score range 5–20; 16 or lower indicate progressive risk).	Norton D. [Norton scale for decubitus prevention]. *Krankenpflege (Frankf).* 1980; 34(1): 16.
Gosnell	Five-item pressure sore risk assessment scale (score range 5–20; *higher* score indicates progressive risk—opposite Braden and Norton).	Gosnell DJ. Pressure sore risk assessment: a critique. Part I. The Gosnell scale. *Decubitus.* 1989; 2(3): 32–38.
Rule of Nines	Estimates the size of burn injury using a percentage of total body surface area (TBSA) with partial- and full-thickness burns. Does not account for variations in age and body sizes.	Knaysi GA, Crikelair GF, Cosman B. The rule of nines: its history and accuracy. *Plast Reconstr Surg.* 1968; 41(6): 560–563.
Lund-Browder Charts (pediatric and adult population)	Estimates the size of burn injury using a percentage of total body surface area (TBSA) with partial- and full-thickness burns. Designed for infants and adults to account for variations in age and body sizes. Preferred for the pediatric population.	Lund CC, Browder NC. The estimation of areas of burns. *Surg Gynecol Obstet.* 1944; 79: 352–358.
Palmar Method for TBSA	Size of a person's palm is approximately 1% of their TBSA.	Nagel TR, Schunk JE. Using the palm to estimate the surface area of a burn in children. *Pediatr Emerg Care.* 1997; 13(4): 254–255.
Walking Impairment Questionnaire	Self-reported tool to examine treatment effects on walking impairments and symptoms in patients with peripheral arterial disease with claudication. It examines pain, distance, walking speed, and stair climbing.	McDermott MM, Liu K, Guralnik JM, Martin GJ, Criqui MH, Greenland P. Measurement of walking endurance and walking velocity with questionnaire: Validation of the walking impairment questionnaire in men and women with peripheral arterial disease. *J Vasc Surg.* 1998; 28(6): 1072–1081.

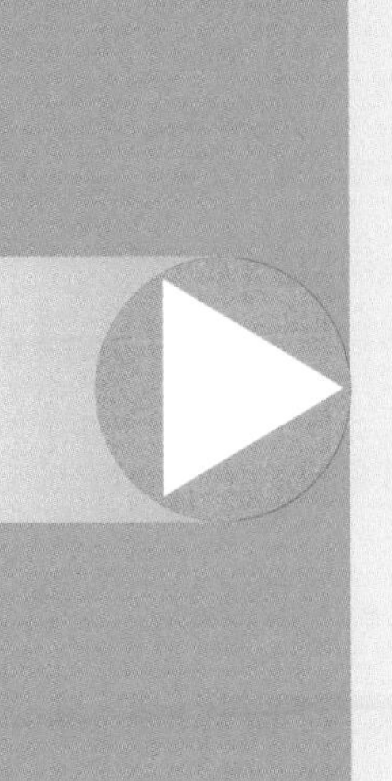

APPENDIX 7B

Review Questions and Case Study

(Answers to all Review Questions and Case Studies are found in Chapter 17)

1. Differentiate between the viral infections herpes simplex and herpes zoster in terms of expected symptoms.

2. When performing a physical examination of pressure injury (ulcer), what elements should be part of the physical therapist's examination?

3. Differentiate between a superficial partial-thickness burn and a full-thickness burn.

4. Differentiate between venous and arterial ulcers in terms of expected clinical presentation.

5. Which categories of wound dressings can be used for exudative wounds?

6. What are the important clinical changes affecting prognosis for a patient with diffuse systemic sclerosis?

Case Study Chapter 7-Integumentary

Patient Profile

- Gender: Male
- Age: 75

Presenting Problem/Current Condition

- Patient referred to physical therapy for management of wound at amputated site
- Digits 1–3 on the right foot were amputated 2 months ago due to gangrene
- The amputation site has not healed. The patient has been using a silver-based wound gel with a gauze dressing cover changed twice a day
- The wound bed is pale and dry. The skin below the knees is dry, hairless, atrophied, and shiny
- Patient is experiencing numbness in the legs, feet, and toes

Past Medical History

- 15-year history of diabetes (Most recent A1C = 7.3%); takes Metformin once a day with meals
- 20-year history of hypertension and peripheral vascular disease
- Smoked one-half a pack of cigarettes for 60 years (30 pack-years), stopped smoking last year
- Raynaud's disease

Other Information

- Retired respiratory therapist
- Regular consumption of alcohol (2–3 drinks a day)
- BMI = 20

Question #1

What is the most likely reason the wound is not healing?

1. The nutritional intake is inadequate.
2. The patient is not managing their diabetes properly.
3. The wound is infected.
4. There is inadequate blood flow to allow for healing.

Question #2

Which of the following diagnostic tests is **BEST** to establish the ideal level for future amputation of this limb?

1. Ankle-brachial index (ABI)
2. Capillary refill times
3. Semmes-Weinstein monofilament (SWM) testing
4. Transcutaneous oximetry (TcPO2)

Question #3

Which of the following interventions are important to implement in a person with a gangrenous toe due to ischemia?

1. Hydrogel dressing changed twice a day.
2. Instruct the patient to keep the limb in a dependent position.
3. Normothermic hydrotherapy.
4. Sharp debridement of the gangrenous toe.

8

Other Systems

SUSAN B. O'SULLIVAN, SCOTT SHAFFER, AND JODI CUSACK

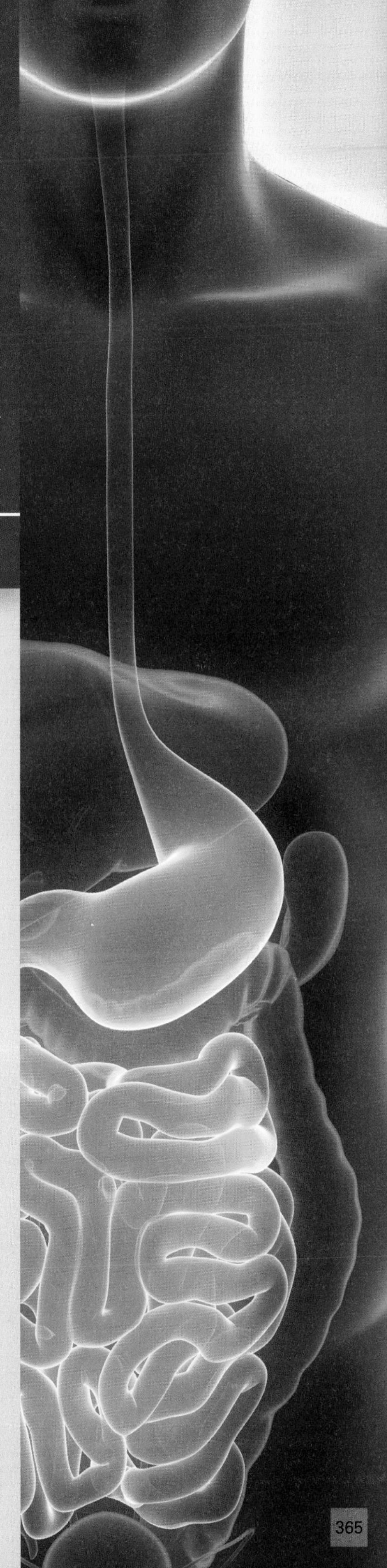

Chapter Outline

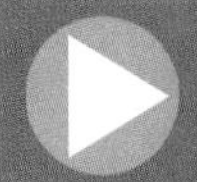

Study Tactics

Questions About Other Systems (Those Not Listed in Chapters 2–5 and 7) Comprise 13.5% of the NPTE, or a Total of 20–33 Questions

The Number of Questions by System Are:

- System Interactions: 8–12 questions (5% of the NPTE)
- Metabolic and Endocrine: 5–7 questions (3%)
- Genitourinary: 4–7 questions (3%)
- Gastrointestinal: 3–7 questions (2.5%)

Additional Systems on the NPTE Covered in Earlier Chapters Include:

- Lymphatics: 3–8 questions (3%; see Study Tactics in Chapter 4)
- Integumentary: 9–12 questions (5.5%; see Study Tactics in Chapter 7)

System Interactions. Focus on:

- **Evaluation, Differential Diagnosis, and Prognosis. There will be no questions based on Examination or Interventions in this category**
- The interaction between more than one body system. This is a broad category covering an indeterminate coupling of comorbidities (e.g., diabetes and cardiac disease, obesity and hypertension, dementia and fractures), and the effects of conditions such as cancer, pregnancy, obesity, infectious/autoimmune diseases, and psychological disorders (depression, schizophrenia, functional neurologic disorder) on various systems. Know the diseases and the possible PT ramifications:
  - Can you diagnose the problems and establish management priorities? What information might be available related to lab or imaging results?
  - Are there any overriding psychosocial or psychiatric conditions that will temper PT management decisions?
  - How is the patient being managed medically? The PT should be familiar with potential for multiple medications or interventions (e.g., surgery, chemotherapy, radiation) affecting various systems. What are the implications for the PT?
  - Sorting out diagnoses/prognoses and setting treatment priorities for patients with multiple physical and/or mental health conditions that affect various systems can be extremely challenging.

Metabolic and Endocrine Systems. Focus on:

- Evaluation, Differential Diagnosis, and Prognosis, and Interventions. **There will be no questions based on Examination in this category**
- Common metabolic/endocrine disorders such as diabetes (Type I and II), Cushing's syndrome, Graves' disease, hypothyroidism, parathyroid disorders, Paget's disease, osteomalacia, osteoporosis, obesity, and metabolic syndrome. Know the disease and the possible PT ramifications:
  - What are the characteristics, signs, symptoms of a given disorder and the relevant laboratory findings? Awareness of the laboratory values for diabetes and laboratory tests for other major endocrine deficiencies is worthwhile.
  - How is the patient being managed medically?
  - Can you implement an appropriate plan of care?
  - Intervention questions will likely emphasize diabetes and its related comorbidities (peripheral polyneuropathies, retinopathies, cardiovascular issues), exercise considerations, foot care, frequency or time of treatment related to insulin management or blood glucose levels.

Gastrointestinal System. Focus on:

- Quadrant examination and correlating organs to be specific quadrant(s) and pain referral patterns
- Special tests that will assist in the diagnosis of insidious GI disorders. Knowledge of the following tests is worthwhile: Murphy's sign, McBurney test, rebound tenderness, psoas, obturator and Rovsing tests
- Signs, symptoms, and related issues of common GI disorders to include constipation, gastroesophageal reflux disease (GERD), ulcers, appendicitis, inflammatory bowel disease such as Crohn's disease, diverticular disease, irritable bowel syndrome, celiac disease, gallbladder disorders, and cancer. Bowel disorders and bowel programs associated with SCI or developmental disorders in children are worth a look.
- Consider the following questions as you prepare for this portion of the NPTE:
  - Can you identify various GI problems?
  - What are pain referral patterns of GI organs?
  - How will a GI disorder impact treatment planning and prognosis for the PT?

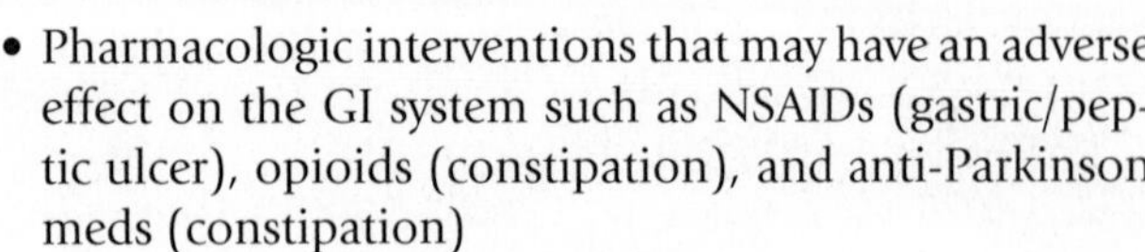

- Pharmacologic interventions that may have an adverse effect on the GI system such as NSAIDs (gastric/peptic ulcer), opioids (constipation), and anti-Parkinson meds (constipation)
- Positioning and activity for a patient with GERD or bowel dysfunction are worthwhile
- Potential adverse effects of PT interventions on the GI system such as strenuous exercise resulting in diarrhea

Genitourinary System. Focus on:

- Basic anatomy and physiology of the urinary and reproductive systems
- Quadrant examination and correlating organs to be specific quadrant(s) and pain referral patterns
- Examination techniques such as pelvic floor muscle assessment and special tests such as Murphy's percussion or punch sign
- Historical questions such as pain behavior and location, bleeding, difficult urination, signs of infection (fever, chills), and sexual dysfunction
- Characteristics, referred pain patterns, signs and symptoms of common genitourinary disorders to include kidney stones, bladder infections, women's health issues, prostate cancer, and emergent conditions such as ectopic pregnancy
- Effective intervention plans and a realistic prognosis for a given diagnosis to include bladder programs for individuals with spinal cord injuries
- Pelvic floor exercises and biofeedback for treatment of incontinence

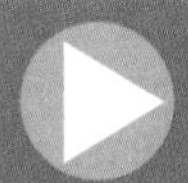

System Interactions—Immune System

Overview

Anatomy and Physiology of the Immune System

1. The immune system consists of immune cells, central immune structures where immune cells are produced (the bone marrow and thymus), and the peripheral immune structures (lymph nodes, spleen, and other accessory structures).
2. There are several different types of immune cells.
   a. An antigen (immunogen) is a foreign molecule that elicits the immune response. Antibodies or immunoglobulins are the proteins that are engaged to tag antigens.
   b. Lymphocytes (T and B lymphocytes) are the primary cells of the immune system.
   c. Macrophages are the accessory cells that process and present antigens to the lymphocytes.
   d. Cytokines are molecules that link immune cells with other tissues and organs. Cytokines assist in homeostasis for normal cellular processes and in response to disease, infection, or cellular damage.
   e. CD molecules (e.g., CD4 helper cells) serve as master regulators of the immune response by influencing the function of all other immune cells.
   f. Recognition of foreign threat from self (autoimmune responses) is mediated by major histocompatibility complex (MHC) membrane molecules.
3. The thymus is the primary central gland of the immune system. It is located behind the sternum above the heart and extends into the neck region to the lower edge of the thyroid gland.
   a. It is fully developed at birth and reaches maximum size at puberty. It then decreases in size and is slowly replaced by adipose tissue.
   b. It produces mature T lymphocytes.
4. The lymph system is a vast network of capillaries, vessels, valves, ducts, nodes, and organs that function to produce, filter, and convey various lymph and blood cells. (See Figures 4-10 and 4-11.)
   a. Lymph nodes are small areas of lymphoid tissue connected by lymphatic vessels throughout the body. High concentrations are found in the axillae, in the groin, and along the great vessels of the neck, thorax, and abdomen.
   b. Lymph nodes function to filter the lymph and trap antigens. Lymphocytes, monocytes, and plasma cells are formed in lymph nodes.
5. The spleen is a large lymphoid organ located in the upper left abdominal cavity between the stomach and the diaphragm.
   a. It functions to filter antigens from the blood and produce leukocytes, monocytes, lymphocytes, and plasma cells in response to infection.
   b. In the embryo, the spleen produces red and white blood cells; after birth, only lymphocytes are produced unless severe anemia exists.

The Immune Response

1. A coordinated response of the body's cells and molecules that provides protection from infectious disease (bacteria, viruses, fungi, parasites) and foreign substances (plant pollens, poison ivy resin, insect venom, transplanted organs). It also defends against abnormal cells produced by the body (cancer cells).
2. Provides natural resistance to disease and consists of rapidly activated phagocytes (macrophages, neutrophils, natural killer cells, dendritic cells). Barriers also provide a natural defense (skin, mucous membranes) as do inflammation and fever (antimicrobial molecules).
3. The adaptive immune response includes the slower acting defenses mediated by the lymphocytes.
4. Repeat exposure activates immunological memory, producing more rapid and efficient responses.
5. Excessive immune response causes allergies or autoimmune reactions.

Immunodeficiency Diseases

1. Characterized by depressed or absent immune responses.
2. Primary immunodeficiency disorders result from a defect in T cells, B cells, or lymphoid tissues.
   a. Congenital disorders are a failure of organs to develop and produce mature lymphocytes.
   b. Severe combined immunodeficiency disease (SCID).
3. Secondary immunodeficiency disorders are caused by underlying pathology or treatment that depresses the immune system, resulting in failure of the immune response.
   a. Diseases include leukemia, bone marrow tumor, chronic diabetes, renal failure, cirrhosis, cancer treatment (chemotherapy, radiation therapy).
   b. Organ transplant, graft-versus-host disease.

Autoimmune Diseases

1. Characterized by immune system responses directed against the body's normal tissues; self-destructive processes impair body function.

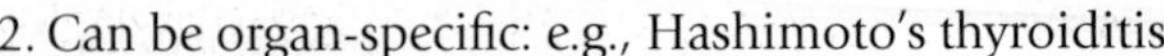

2. Can be organ-specific: e.g., Hashimoto's thyroiditis.
3. Can be systemic (non–organ specific): e.g., systemic lupus erythematosus (SLE), rheumatoid arthritis, or Guillain-Barré syndrome.
4. Etiology often unknown; possible factors include genetic predisposition, hormonal changes, environment, viral infection, and stress.

Human Immunodeficiency Virus (HIV) and Acquired Immunodeficiency Syndrome (AIDS)

Characteristics
1. Caused by a virus (HIV-1 or HIV-2) that weakens the immune system.
2. Cells that fight disease and infection are destroyed.

Pathophysiology
1. Reduction of $CD4^+$ helper T cells, resulting in $CD4^+$ T lymphocytopenia; a major defect in the immune system.
2. A retrovirus: replicates in reverse fashion; the RNA code is transcribed into DNA.

Stages of HIV
1. Stage 1 acute HIV infection: flu-like illness within 2–4 weeks after infection.
2. Stage 2 clinical latency: asymptomatic HIV infection or chronic HIV infection; can last a decade or longer.
3. Stage 3 AIDS: the most severe phase; over time, HIV destroys so many cells that the body can't fight off infections and disease, resulting in opportunistic illnesses.

Transmission
1. Through contact with certain body fluids (blood, semen, pre-seminal fluid, rectal fluids, vaginal fluids, and breast milk) from a person who has HIV. Fluid must come in contact with a mucous membrane, damaged tissue, or be directly injected into the blood stream (needle or syringe).
2. High-risk behaviors for HIV transmission.
   a. Unprotected anal or vaginal sex with someone who has HIV.
   b. Sharing needles or syringes, rinse water, or other equipment used to prepare drugs for injection with someone who has HIV.
   c. Less commonly, HIV can be spread from mother to child during pregnancy, birth, or breastfeeding.
   d. By being stuck with an HIV-contaminated needle or other sharp object (risk is mainly for health care workers).
3. In rare cases HIV can be transmitted by:
   a. Oral sex.
   b. Receiving blood transfusions, blood products, or organ/tissue transplants contaminated with HIV.
   c. Being bitten by a person with HIV.
   d. Eating food that has been pre-chewed by an HIV-infected person.
   e. Contact between broken skin, wounds, or mucous membranes with HIV-infected blood or bodily fluids.
   f. Deep open-mouth kissing if both partners have sores or bleeding gums.
4. HIV is not spread by saliva, tears, or sweat that is not mixed with the blood of an HIV-positive person; touching; hugging; shaking hands; sharing toilets; sharing dishes; or closed-mouth "social" kissing.
5. AIDS cannot be contacted through respiratory inhalation, skin contact, or human waste (urine, feces, sweat, or vomit).

Diagnosis of HIV. Requires Positive Results from Two HIV Tests
1. CD4 cell count: 500–1200 cells/mm.
2. Testing with HIV-1/HIV-2 antigen/antibody combination immunoassays.
3. Medical evaluation and laboratory evaluation including plasma HIV viral load, blood cell and CD4 count, antiretroviral resistance assay, drug-resistance testing, and testing for sexually transmitted infections (STDs).

Diagnosis of AIDS
1. CD4 cell count drops below 200 cells/mm or if they develop certain opportunistic illnesses. People with AIDs have a high viral load and are very infectious.
2. AIDS-related complex (ARC): presence of acute symptoms secondary to immune system deficiency.

HIV Signs and Symptoms
1. Includes flu-like symptoms: recurrent fever and chills, night sweats, swollen lymph glands, sore throat, rash, and muscle aches. Symptoms usually disappear after a few weeks.
2. Getting tested is the only way to tell if HIV is present.

AIDS Signs and Symptoms
1. Infected person exhibits some or all of the symptoms along with a general failure to thrive.
2. Opportunistic infections: AIDS-defining conditions include pneumocystis pneumonia, candidiasis, cytomegalovirus, and toxoplasmosis.
3. Malignancies: most common is Kaposi's sarcoma; also non-Hodgkin's lymphoma; primary brain lymphoma.

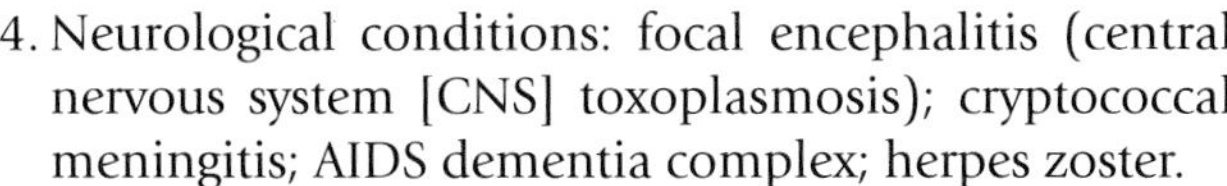

4. Neurological conditions: focal encephalitis (central nervous system [CNS] toxoplasmosis); cryptococcal meningitis; AIDS dementia complex; herpes zoster.
5. Deconditioning, anxiety, and depression are common.

Clinical Course

1. May exhibit brief, early, nonspecific viral HIV infection, and then remain asymptomatic for many years.
2. There is no cure for HIV infection. Without treatment nearly every person will progress to AIDS.

Medical Interventions HIV

1. Antiretroviral therapies (ARTs): antiviral drugs (ARVs) are used to reduce the amount of virus (viral load) in the system and are always given in combination (usually three or more drugs); recommended for everyone infected with HIV, starting immediately.
2. ART does not not cure HIV, but does keep people with HIV healthy for many years if taken consistently and correctly.

> **RED FLAG:** common adverse effects of ART include rash, nausea and vomiting, diarrhea, headaches, dizziness, fatigue, and pain.

3. Symptomatic treatment.
   a. Education to prevent the spread of infection and disease.
   b. Treat opportunistic infections; prophylactic vaccinations.
   c. Maintain nutritional status.
   d. Provide supportive care for management of fatigue, e.g., energy-conservation techniques, self-care.
   e. Respiratory management as needed.
   f. Provide skin care.
   g. Maintain functional mobility and safety; prevent disability.
   h. Provide supportive care, e.g., emotional support for patients and families.

Physical Therapy Goals, Outcomes, and Interventions

1. Observe standard precautions: CDC Guidelines reviewed in later section in this chapter and discussed more fully in Chapter 13.
2. Exercise has a positive effect on the immune system; reduces stress level and pain; improves cardiovascular endurance and strength (disuse effects common).
3. Exercise: a moderate exercise program is recommended to improve body composition and minimize health risks (ACSM's Exercise Management for Persons with Chronic Diseases and Disabilities, Human Kinetics, 2016).
   a. Postpone exercise testing during acute infections.
   b. Aerobic exercise: at least 20 minutes three times a week working up to 45 minutes to an hour, 3–4 times per week.
   c. Resistance exercise: moderate levels—weights that can be lifted 8–10 times.
   d. Avoid exhaustive exercise with symptomatic individuals. Possible immune suppression can occur with more intense exercise.
   e. Day to day variations in health affect participation. During acute stages of opportunistic infections, reduce exercise to mild levels.
   f. Avoid contact sports due to increased risk with bleeding.
4. Teach activity pacing: balancing rest with activity; scheduling strenuous activities during periods of high energy.
5. Teach energy conservation: analysis and modification of daily activities to reduce energy expenditure.
6. Teach stress management, relaxation training (e.g., meditation and mindfulness, tai chi chuan, yoga).
7. Neurological rehabilitation for patients with involvement of the CNS. (See Chapter 3.)

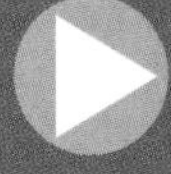

System Interactions—Infectious Diseases

Staphylococcal Infections

Staphylococcus Aureus (SA)

1. A common bacterial pathogen.

Pathophysiology

1. Typically begins as localized infection; entry is through skin portal, e.g., wounds, ulcers, burns.
2. Bacterial invasion and spread is through bloodstream or lymphatic system to almost any body location, e.g., heart valves, bones (acute staphylococcal osteomyelitis), joints (bacterial arthritis), skin (cellulitis, furuncles and carbuncles, ulcers), respiratory tract (pneumonia), and bowel (enterocolitis).
3. Infection produces suppuration (pus formation) and abscess.

Medical Interventions

1. Laboratory diagnosis to confirm pathogen.
2. Antibiotic therapy; determine antibiotic sensitivity. Antibiotic resistance is common.
3. Drainage of abscesses.
4. Skin infections that are untreated can become systemic; sepsis can be lethal.

Methicillin-Resistant *Staphylococcus Aureus* (MRSA)

1. A type of staph bacteria that has become resistant to many of the antibiotics used to treat ordinary staph infections.
2. Symptoms typically include swollen, painful red bumps that can quickly progress to deep abscesses full of pus or other drainage. The area is warm to the touch and fever is present.
3. Can result in life-threatening infections in the bloodstream, heart valves, lungs, bones, joints, or surgical wounds.
4. Risk factors for health care–associated MRSA (HA-MRSA) include:
   a. Hospitalization: affects older adults and patients with weak immune systems.
   b. Invasive medical devices such as medical tubing.
   c. Individuals residing in long-term care facilities.
5. Risk factor for community-associated MRSA (CA-MRSA) include:
   a. Participants in contact sports with cuts and abrasions.
   b. Unsanitary and crowded living conditions, sharing of personal items.
   c. Persons injecting intravenous drugs.
6. MRSA can be treated and reappear in the same individual; persons can also carry MRSA bacteria on the skin or in the nose.

Vancomycin-Resistant *Staphylococcus Aureus* (VRSA)

1. Resistant to vancomycin.
2. Can be a life-threatening infection.

> **RED FLAGS:** MRSA is contagious staph infection that can spread from person-to-person contact or indirect contact. Standard precautions and disinfection procedures should be strictly adhered to.

Streptococcal Infections

Characteristics

1. A common bacterial pathogen.
2. Types.
   a. Group A streptococcus (*S. pyogenes*): pharyngitis, rheumatic fever, scarlet fever, impetigo, necrotizing fasciitis (gangrene), cellulitis, myositis.
   b. Group B streptococcus (*S. agalactiae*): neonatal and adult streptococcal B infections.
   c. Group C streptococcus (*S. pneumoniae*): pneumonia, otitis media, meningitis, endocarditis.

Medical Interventions

1. Laboratory diagnosis to confirm pathogen.
2. Antibiotic therapy; antibiotic resistance common.
3. Skin infections that are untreated can become systemic.

Tick Borne Illnesses

Lyme Disease

1. Caused by bacterium *Borrelia burgdorferi* and transmitted to humans through the bite of infected blacklegged ticks. Most infections occur in endemic areas: northeast and mid-Atlantic, north central states (Wisconsin and Minnesota), and west coast (Northern California).
2. Early symptoms (3–30 days) include fever, chills, swollen lymph nodes, headache, muscle and joint aching, fatigue, and characteristic skin rash called erythema migrans (bull's-eye rash).
3. Later symptoms if left untreated (days to months after tick bite):
   a. Severe headaches and neck stiffness.
   b. Arthritis with severe joint pain and swelling; intermittent pain in muscles, joints, and bones.
   c. Heart palpitations or irregular heartbeat (Lyme carditis).
   d. Nervous system changes: inflammation of the brain and spinal cord; nerve pain, shooting pains, numbness, or tingling in the hands and feet; facial palsy; problems with short-term memory.
   e. Episodes of dizziness or shortness of breath.
4. Diagnosis is made by signs and symptoms, history of exposure to blacklegged ticks, and laboratory blood tests.
5. Most cases successfully treated with a short course of antibiotics in the early stages of Lyme disease.
6. Post-Lyme disease syndrome (PLDS) or post-treatment Lyme disease syndrome. Symptoms linger for months or years after a treated acute infection (estimated 10% of cases).
   a. Use of the term *chronic Lyme disease* is not recommended by the CDC due to confusion in how the term is used.

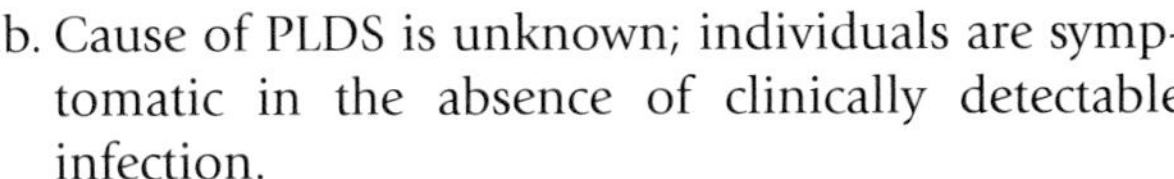

b. Cause of PLDS is unknown; individuals are symptomatic in the absence of clinically detectable infection.
c. Symptoms may include persistent musculoskeletal pain (arthralgia, myalgia), fatigue, impaired cognitive function, difficulty sleeping, and unexplained numbness.
d. Extended course of antibiotics has not been shown to be beneficial.
e. Treatment is symptomatic and can include antidepressants, analgesics, and psychotherapy.
f. Most patients recover with time.

Rocky Mountain Spotted Fever

1. Caused by rickettsia group bacteria transmitted by the bite of a tick. A rash may be present and skin at site of tick bite may be crusted or black. Most infections occur in endemic areas: Rocky Mountains and southeastern United States.
2. Symptoms include high fever and chills, severe headache, rash, muscle aches, confusion or other neurological changes, and nausea or vomiting.
3. Complications can include inflammation of the brain (encephalitis); inflammation of the heart and lungs that can lead to heart failure, kidney failure; serious infection in fingers and toes that can lead to amputation and death if untreated.
4. Treatment includes a course of antibiotics. Complications can be avoided if started within 5 days of developing symptoms.

> RED FLAG: Recognition of symptoms and early treatment using antibiotics is critical to successful treatment and avoiding long-term complications.

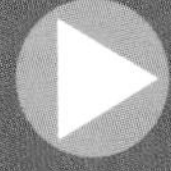

System Interactions—Hematological System

Overview

Composition of Blood (See Table 4-10 for Normal Values)

1. Plasma makes up about 55% of total blood volume and is the liquid part of blood and lymph; it carries the cellular elements of blood through the circulation.
   a. Plasma is composed of about 91% water, 7% proteins, and 2%–3% other small molecules.
   b. Electrolytes in plasma determine osmotic pressure and pH balance and are important in the exchange of fluids between capillaries and tissues.
   c. Carries nutrients, waste products, and hormones.
   d. Plasma proteins include albumin, globulins, and fibrinogen.
   e. Serum is plasma without the clotting factors.
2. Erythrocytes, or red blood cells (RBCs), make up about 45% of the total blood volume and contain the oxygen-carrying protein hemoglobin responsible for transporting oxygen.
   a. RBCs are produced in the marrow of the long bones and controlled by hormones (erythropoietin). RBCs are time-limited, surviving for approximately 120 days.
   b. RBC count varies with age, activity, and environmental conditions.
3. Leukocytes, or white blood cells (WBCs), make up about 1% of total blood volume and circulate through the lymphoid tissues.
   a. Leukocytes function in immune processes as phagocytes of bacteria, fungi, and viruses. They also aid in capturing toxic proteins resulting from allergic reactions and cellular injury.
   b. Leukocytes are produced in the bone marrow.
   c. There are five types of leukocytes: lymphocytes, monocytes (agranulocytes), neutrophils, basophils, and eosinophils (granulocytes).

Hematopoiesis

1. The normal function and generation of blood cells in the bone marrow.
2. Production, differentiation, and function of blood cells is regulated by cytokines and growth factors (chemical messengers) acting on blood-forming cells (pluripotent stem cells).
3. Disorders of hematopoiesis include aplastic anemia and leukemias.

Blood Screening Tests

1. Complete blood count (CBC) determines the number of red blood cells, white blood cells, and platelets per unit of blood.

2. White cell differential count determines the relative percentages of individual white cell types.
3. Erythrocyte sedimentation rate (ESR) is the rate of red blood cells that settle out in a tube of unclotted blood; expressed in millimeters per hour.
   a. Elevated ESR indicates the presence of inflammation.
   b. Normal values (see Table 4-10).

Hemostasis

1. The termination or arrest of blood flow by mechanical or chemical processes. Mechanisms include vasospasm, platelet aggregation, and thrombin and fibrin synthesis.
2. Blood clotting requires platelets produced in bone marrow, von Willebrand's factor produced by the endothelium of blood vessels, and clotting factors produced by the liver using vitamin K.
3. Fibrinolysis is clot dissolution that prevents excess clot formation.

Hypercoaguability Disorders

1. Results in thrombosis secondary to certain inherited, molecular, or environmental factors.
2. Increased platelet function as seen in atherosclerosis, diabetes mellitus, elevated blood lipids, and cholesterol.
3. Accelerated activity of the clotting system as seen in congestive heart failure, malignant diseases, pregnancy and use of oral contraceptives, immobility.

Hypocoagulopathy (Bleeding) Disorders

1. Platelet defects as seen in bone marrow dysfunction, thrombocytopenia, thrombocytopathia.
2. Coagulation defects as seen in hemophilia and von Willebrand's disease.
3. May be the result of certain medications over a short (e.g., heparin, coumadin) or long (steroids, NSAIDs) duration.
4. Vascular disorders as seen in hemorrhagic telangiectasia, vitamin C deficiency, Cushing's disease, senile purpura.
5. Signs/Symptoms:
   a. Easy bruising with spontaneous petechiae, purpura, or hematomas.
   b. Anemia.

RED FLAGS: Physical therapy interventions.
- Use extreme caution with manual therapy (e.g., vigorous soft tissue mobilization, dry needling) and use of some modalities (e.g., mechanical compression).
- Strenuous exercise is contraindicated due to the risk of increased hemorrhage.

Shock

1. An abnormal condition of inadequate blood flow to the body tissues. It is associated with hypotension, inadequate cardiac output, and changes in peripheral blood flow resistance.
2. Hypovolemic shock is caused by hemorrhage, vomiting, or diarrhea. Loss of body fluids also occurs with dehydration, Addison's disease, burns, pancreatitis, or peritonitis.
3. Orthostatic changes may develop, characterized by a drop in systolic blood pressure of 10–20 mmHg or more. Pulse and respiration increase to maintain cardiac output and oxygenation.
4. Progressive shock is associated with restlessness and anxiety; weakness; lethargy; pallor with cool, moist skin; and fall in body temperature.
5. Please see Chapter 13 for recommended management of shock.

Anemia

Characteristics

1. Decrease in hemoglobin levels in the blood.
2. Normal range. (See Table 4-10.)

Etiology

1. Decrease in RBC production: nutritional deficiency (iron, vitamin B, folic acid); cellular maturation defects, decreased bone marrow stimulation (hypothyroidism), bone marrow failure (leukemia, aplasia, neoplasm), and genetic defect.
2. Destruction of RBCs: autoimmune hemolysis, sickle cell disease, enzyme defects, parasites (malaria), hypersplenism, chronic diseases (rheumatoid arthritis, tuberculosis, cancer).
3. Loss of blood (hemorrhage): trauma, wound, bleeding, peptic ulcer, excessive menstruation.

Signs and Symptoms

1. Fatigue and weakness with minimal exertion.
2. Dyspnea on exertion.
3. Pallor or yellow skin of the face, hands, nail beds, and lips.
4. Tachycardia.
5. Bleeding of gums, mucous membranes, or skin in the absence of trauma.
6. Severe anemia can produce hypoxic damage to liver and kidney, heart failure.

Medical Intervention

1. Variable, depends on causative factors.
2. Transfusion.
3. Nutritional supplements.

Physical Therapy Intervention

RED FLAGS: Patients with anemia exhibit decreased exercise tolerance.
- See Table 8.1.
- Exercise should be instituted gradually with physician approval.
- Close monitoring of vital signs to include O_2 saturation.
- Use rate of perceived exertion (RPE) ratings.

Sickle Cell Disease

Characteristics

1. Group of inherited, autosomal recessive red blood cell (RBC) disorders; erythrocytes, specifically hemoglobin (Hb), are abnormal. RBCs are crescent or sickle-shaped instead of biconcave.
2. Types include HbSS (most severe); HbSC, HbS beta thalassemia, HbSD, HbSE, and HbSO.
3. Sickle cell trait: heterozygous form of sickle cell anemia characterized by abnormal red blood cells. Individuals are carriers and do not develop the disease. Counseling is important, especially if both parents have the trait.
4. Chronic hemolytic anemia (sickle cell anemia): hemoglobin is released into plasma with resultant reduced oxygen delivery to tissues; results from bone marrow aplasia, hemolysis, folate deficiency, or splenic involvement.
5. Vasoocclusion from misshapen erythrocytes: results in ischemia, occlusion, and infarction of adjacent tissue.
6. Chronic illness that can be fatal.

Sickle Cell Crisis

1. Acute episodic condition occurring in individuals with sickle cell anemia.
2. Signs and symptoms.
   a. Pain: acute and severe from sickle cell clots formed in any organ, bone, or joint.
      - Acute abdominal pain from visceral hypoxia.
      - Painful swelling of soft tissue of the hands and feet (hand-foot syndrome).
      - Persistent headache.

   b. Bone and joint crises: migratory, recurrent joint pain; extremity and back pain.
   c. Neurological manifestations: dizziness, convulsions, coma, nystagmus.
   d. Pulmonary (acute chest syndrome): chest pain, coughing, dyspnea, tachypnea may occur.

Complications

1. Vascular: stroke, chronic leg ulcers, bone infarcts, avascular necrosis of femoral head, hand-and-foot syndrome (dactylitis).
2. Pulmonary hypertension.
3. Neurologic: paresthesias, cranial nerve palsies, blindness, hemiplegia.
4. Renal: enuresis, nocturia, hematuria, renal failure.
5. Anemic crisis: characterized by rapid drop in hemoglobin levels.
6. Aplastic crisis: characterized by severe anemia; associated with acute viral, bacterial, or fungal infection. Increased susceptibility to infection.
7. Splenic: liver and spleen enlargement, spleen atrophy.

Medical Interventions

1. Exchange transfusions of packed red cells in acute anemic crisis or severe anemia.
2. Medications that stimulate hemoglobin production (e.g., hydrooxyurea).
3. Analgesics or narcotics as needed for pain.
4. Short-term oxygen therapy in severe anoxia.
5. Hydration, electrolyte replacement.
6. Antibiotics for infection control.
7. Oral anticoagulants to relieve pain of vasoocclusion; associated with increased risk of bleeding.
8. Splenectomy may be considered.
9. Bone marrow transplant in severe cases.
10. Uremia may require renal transplantation or hemodialysis.
11. Stem cell transplant.

Physical Therapy Goals, Outcomes, and Interventions

1. During sickle cell event, pain control.
   a. Application of warmth is soothing (e.g., hydrotherapy).
   b. Relaxation techniques.

RED FLAG: Cold is contraindicated, as it increases vasoconstriction and sickling.

2. Exercise and activity training: appropriate for developmental level and patient status.
   a. Exercise intolerance common: exaggerated heart rate response to exercise, limited peak performance in patients with anemia.
   b. Low- to moderate-level exercise indicated.
   c. Ensure adequate fluid intake.
   d. High-level exercise and dehydration may increase risk of sickle cell crisis.

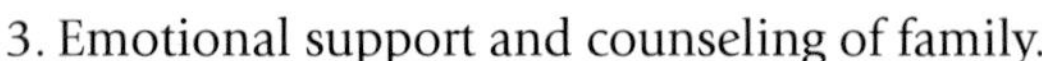

3. Emotional support and counseling of family.
4. Patient and family education: avoidance of stressors that can precipitate a crisis; teach joint protection strategies.

Hemophilia

Characteristics

1. A group of bleeding disorders inherited as a sex-linked recessive disorder; affects males; females are carriers.
2. Clotting factor VIII deficiency (hemophilia A) is most common; classic hemophilia.
3. Clotting factor IX deficiency (hemophilia B or Christmas disease).
4. Level of severity and rate of spontaneous bleeds varies by percentage of clotting factor in blood: mild, moderate, severe.
5. Bleeding is spontaneous; maybe atraumatic or traumatic (to include microtrauma); may result in internal hemorrhage and hematuria.
6. Hemarthrosis (bleeding into joint spaces) most common in synovial joints: knees, ankles, elbows, hips.
   a. Joint becomes swollen, warm, and painful with decreased range of motion (ROM).
   b. Long-term results can include chronic synovitis and arthropathy leading to bone and cartilage destruction.
7. Hemorrhage into muscles often affects forearm flexors, gastrocnemius/soleus, and iliopsoas; results in pain and decreased movement.

Medical Interventions

1. Blood infusion, factor replacement therapy.
2. Use of acetaminophen (Tylenol), not aspirin, for pain management.
3. Rest, ice, elevation, functional splinting, and no weight-bearing during an acute bleed.

Complications

1. Joint contractures.
   a. Hip, knee, elbow flexion; ankle plantar flexion.
2. Muscle weakness around affected joints.
3. Leg length discrepancies.
4. Postural scoliosis.
5. Decreased aerobic fitness.
6. Gait deviations.
   a. Equinus gait.
   b. Lack of knee extensor torque.
7. Activities of daily living (ADL) deficiencies, e.g., elbow contractures could affect dressing ability.

Physical Therapy Examination

1. Clinical signs and symptoms of acute bleeding episodes: decreased ROM, stiffening, pain, swelling, tenderness, heat, prickling or tingling sensations.
2. Pain.
3. Range of motion.
   a. Care should be taken to not increase bleeding (intra or extra-articular).
   b. Pain free active or active assist range of motion preferred over passive range of motion.
4. Joint deformities, e.g., genu valgum, rearfoot/forefoot.
5. Muscle strength; girth.
6. Functional mobility skills, gait; activity limitations dependent on specific joint versus diffuse multijoint involvement which can occur with uncontrolled bleeding disorders.
7. Participation restrictions.

Physical Therapy Interventions. Acute Stage

1. RICE: rest, ice, compression, elevation.
2. Maintain position, prevent deformity.

Physical Therapy Interventions. Subacute Stage After Hemostasis

1. Factor replacement best done just before treatment.
2. Isometric exercise and aquatic therapy early.
3. Pain management: transcutaneous electrical nerve stimulation (TENS), massage, relaxation techniques, ice, biofeedback.
4. Active assistive exercise progressing to active, isokinetic, and open chain resistive exercises.
   a. Closed chain exercise may put too much compressive force through joint.
   b. Important to strengthen hip, knee, elbow extensors, and ankle dorsiflexors.
5. Contracture management.
   a. Manual traction, mobilization techniques, serial casting, dynamic splinting during the day, resting splints at night.

> **RED FLAG:** Passive stretching is rarely used, due to risk of myositis ossificans.

6. Functional and gait training as needed.
   a. Protective use of helmets or pads for very young boys during ambulation and play.
   b. Temporary use of ambulatory aids as needed.
   c. Foot orthoses, shoe inserts, and adhesive taping for ankle or foot problems.

Physical Therapy Interventions. Chronic Stage

1. Daily home exercise program to maintain or increase joint function, aerobic fitness, and strength.
2. Outpatient physical therapy as necessary.
3. Appropriate recreational activities or adaptive physical education if at school.
4. Emotional support for patients and families.

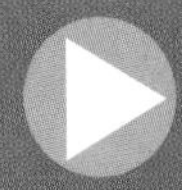

System Interactions—Cancer

Overview

Characteristics

1. A broad group of diseases characterized by rapidly proliferating anaplastic cells.
2. Can involve all body organs; invasive.
3. Etiology: multiple causative factors are implicated.
   a. Environmental carcinogens: asbestos, smoking oral tobacco, ionizing radiation (e.g., x-rays, sun exposure, petrochemicals, or solvants).
   b. Viral carcinogens: herpes simplex, AIDS.
   c. Genetic factors: hereditary.
   d. Dietary factors: obesity, high-fat diet, diet low in vitamins A, C, E.
   e. Psychological factors: chronic stress.
4. Early warning signs.
   a. Unusual bleeding or discharge.
   b. A lump or thickening of any area, e.g., breast.
   c. A sore that does not heal.
   d. A change in bladder or bowel habits.
   e. Hoarseness or persistent cough.
   f. Indigestion or difficulty swallowing.
   g. Change in size or appearance of a wart or mole.
   h. Unexplained weight loss.
5. Classification (staging): delineates extent and prognosis of disease.
6. Incidence: second leading cause of death in United States.
7. Prognosis: aggressive treatments have resulted in higher cure rates, increased survival times.
8. Quality of life (maintaining normal function and lifestyle) is an important issue.

Pathophysiology

1. Tumor or neoplasm: an abnormal growth of new tissue that is nonfunctional and competes for vital blood supply and nutrients.
2. Benign tumor (neoplasm): localized, slow-growing, usually encapsulated; not invasive.
3. Malignant tumor (neoplasm): invasive, rapid growth giving rise to metastasis; can be life-threatening.
   a. Carcinoma: a malignant tumor originating in epithelial tissues, e.g., skin, stomach, colon, breast, rectum. Carcinoma in situ is a premalignant neoplasm that has not invaded the basement membrane.
   b. Sarcoma: a malignant tumor originating in connective and mesodermal tissues, e.g., muscle, bone, fat.
   c. Lymphoma: affecting the lymphatic system, e.g., Hodgkin's disease, lymphatic leukemia.
   d. Leukemias and myelomas: affecting the blood (unrestrained growth of leukocytes) and blood-forming organs (bone marrow).
4. Metastasis: movement of cancer cells from one body part to another; spread is via lymphatic system or bloodstream.

Cancer Staging

1. Stages describe the extent or severity of a person's cancer. Based on primary tumor (T), regional lymph node involvement (N), and metastasis (M).
   a. Stage 0: carcinoma in situ.
   b. Stage I: tumor is localized, equal to or less than 2 cm; has not spread to lymph nodes.
   c. Stage II: tumor is locally advanced; 2 cm to 5 cm with or without lymph node involvement.
   d. Stage III: tumor is locally more advanced; spread to lymph nodes; cancer is designated stage II or III depending upon specific type of cancer.
   e. Stage IV: the tumor has metastasized, or spread to other organs throughout the body.
2. Cancer grades.
   a. Grade I (low-grade): cancer cells resemble normal cells (well differentiated) and are slow growing.
   b. Grade II (intermediate-grade): cancer cells look more abnormal (moderately differentiated) and are slightly faster growing.
   c. Grade III (high-grade): cancer cells are abnormal (poorly differentiated); grow or spread more aggressively.
   d. Grade IV (high-grade): cancer cells are abnormal (undifferentiated).

Medical Interventions

1. Curative versus palliative (relief of symptoms, e.g., pain); can be used singly or in combination. May be considered cured if patient does not have a reoccurrence within 5 years after treatment.
2. Surgery.
   a. Can be curative (tumor removal following biopsy) or palliative (to relieve pain, correct obstruction).
   b. Often used in combination with chemotherapy or radiation therapy.
   c. Can result in significant functional deficits and weakness; edema.
3. Radiation therapy.
   a. Destroys cancer cells, inhibits cell growth and division.
   b. Can be used preoperatively to shrink tumors, prevent spread.
   c. Can be used postoperatively to kill/prevent residual cancer cells from metastasizing.
4. Chemotherapy.
   a. Drugs can be given orally, subcutaneously, intramuscularly, intravenously, intrathecally (within the spinal canal).

b. Usually intermittent doses to allow for bone marrow recovery.
5. Immunotherapy.
a. Strengthens host's ability to fight cancer cells.
b. Agents can include interferons, interleukin-2, and cytokines.
c. Bone marrow (stem cell) transplant; follows high doses of chemotherapy or radiation that destroys both cancer cells and bone marrow cells.
d. Monoclonal antibodies.
e. Hormonal therapy.

RED FLAGS: Local and systemic effects of cancer therapy.
- With radiation therapy, can see pain and fatigue, radiation sickness, immunosuppression, fibrosis, burns, delayed wound healing, edema, hair loss, nervous system effects (radiation encephalopathy, neuropathy with unique feature of rapid motor weakness that can occur several years after radiation).
- With chemotherapy, can see fatigue, gastrointestinal symptoms (anorexia, nausea, vomiting, diarrhea, ulcers, hemorrhage), bone marrow suppression (anemia, leukopenia, thrombocytopenia), skin rashes, neuropathies, phlebitis, and hair loss.
- With immunotherapy, can see fatigue, weight loss, flu-like symptoms (fever, chills), nausea, vomiting, anorexia, fluid retention.
- With hormonal therapy, can see gastrointestinal symptoms, hypertension, steroid-induced diabetes and myopathy, weight gain, hot flashes and sweating, altered mental status, impotence.

Palliative and Hospice Care
1. Palliative care is specialized medical care for people living with a serious illness. Focus is on relief from symptoms and the stress of illness.
2. Hospice care is designed to give supportive care to people in the final phase of a terminal illness. Focus is on comfort and quality of life.
3. Both include provision of multidisciplinary and supportive services.

Physical Therapy Examination

Detailed Assessment Based on the Patient's
1. Type and stage of cancer.
2. Past medical/surgical history.
3. Medical interventions (e.g., surgery, chemotherapy, radiation) and side effects.
4. Comorbidities and impairments.
a. Pain (nociceptive, neuropathic, nociplastic/central sensitization)
b. Weakness and fatigue (muscular and aerobic).
c. Mental Health–Anxiety and Depression.
5. Past and current levels of activity (function) and participation.

Pain
1. Cancer pain syndrome: cancer-related pain is a common experience, e.g., nerve or nerve root compression, ischemic response to blockage of blood supply, bone pain. Sympathetic signs and symptoms may accompany moderate to severe pain, e.g., tachycardia, hypertension, tachypnea, nausea, vomiting.
2. Pain at site distal to initial tumor site may suggest metastasis.
3. Iatrogenic pain may result from surgery, radiation, or chemotherapy.

Cancer-Related Fatigue
1. Most common symptom reported by patients with all cancers.
2. Multiple causative factors: physical and emotional. Can use brief fatigue inventory (BFI).
3. Need to assess impact on quality of life (QOL).

RED FLAGS: Adverse side effects of cancer treatment.
- With immunosuppressed patient, monitor vital signs, physiological responses to exercise carefully; may see elevated HR and BP, dyspnea, pallor, sweating, fatigue. Patient is easily fatigued with minimal exertion.
- Muscle atrophy and weakness: secondary to high doses of steroids in many chemotherapy protocols; radiation; disuse; or tumor compression/invasion.
- ROM deficits: particularly with high-dose radiation around joints.
- Hematological disruptions.
  - White blood suppression (leukopenia).
  - Platelet suppression and increased bleeding (thrombocytopenia).
  - Red blood cell suppression (anemia) with diminished aerobic capacity.

Physical Therapy Goals, Outcomes, and Interventions

Educate Patient and Family About Disease Process, Rehabilitation Goals, Process, and Expected Outcomes

Educate and Support Patient and Family
1. Educate about disease process, rehabilitation process, interventions, and expected outcomes.
2. Assist in coping mechanisms.

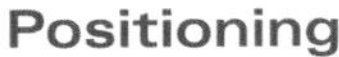

Positioning

1. Provide for proper positioning to prevent or correct deformities, maintain skin integrity.
2. Provide for overall patient comfort.

Edema Control

1. Elevation of extremities, active ROM.
2. Postoperative compression (elastic bandages, pressure garments).

Pain Control

1. Pain assessment and education.
2. Manual therapy.
3. Activity/Exercise as tolerated.

Maintain or Correct Loss of ROM

1. Active-assisted/stretching.
2. Active ROM exercises.

Maintain or Improve Strength

1. Resistance exercise prescription and programs should be individualized and based on examination/evaluation findings to include detailed review of red flags and precautions/contraindications to resistance exercise (see Red Flag Box and Chapter 6).
2. Isometric and lightweight isotonic strengthening is typically safe for most patients with cancer.
3. Resistance exercise prescription/evidence (see ACSM Exercise Guidelines for Cancer Patients and Survivors, 2019).
   a. 2 times a week for 2 sets of 12–15 repetitions at moderate intensity for patients with reports of cancer-related fatigue **(Strong Evidence)**.
   b. 2 times a week for 2 sets of 8–15 repetitions at moderate to vigorous intensity for patients with a goal to improve health-related quality of life **(Strong Evidence)**.
   c. 2–3 times a week for 2 sets of 8–15 repetitions at moderate to vigorous intensity for patients with a goal to improve physical function **(Strong Evidence)**.
   d. 2–3 times a week of progressive, supervised program for major muscle groups that does not exacerbate lymphedema **(Strong Evidence)**.
   e. 2–3 times a week of moderate to vigorous resistance training plus high-impact training (generates ground reaction force of 3–4 times body weight) for ≥ 1 year **(Moderate Evidence)**.
4. References.
   a. ACSM Exercise Guidelines for Cancer Patients and Survivors, 2019 at https://www.acsm.org/read-research/newsroom/news-releases/news-detail/2019/11/27/new-infographic-available-exercise-guidelines-cancer-patients-survivors.
   b. Campbell KL et al. Exercise Guidelines for cancer survivors: consensus statement from international multidisciplinary roundtable. *Med Sci Sports Exerc.* 2019 Nov; 51(11): 2375–2390.
   c. See Chapter 6, Table 6-5 for additional information on resistance exercise.

> **RED FLAGS:** Patients with significant bony metastases, osteoporosis, or low platelet counts (<20,000).
> - AROM, ADL exercise only.
> - Weight-bearing may be restricted secondary to primary/secondary bone tumors or osteopenia; provide appropriate ambulatory aids, orthoses.
> - High risk of vertebral compression and other fractures with metastatic disease. Use light exercise only and avoid movements that force overpressure at end range.

Improve Aerobic Capacity

1. Formal aerobic exercise testing is important for patients with a current or past history of cancer.
2. Exercise prescription should be individualized and matched to the patient's level of function and desired goals (See ACSM Exercise Guidelines for Cancer Patients and Survivors, 2019).
   a. 3 times a week, 30 minute sessions at moderate intensity (40%–59% heart rate reserve or VO_2R) for patients with cancer-related fatigue **(Strong Evidence)**.
   b. 2–3 times a week, 30–60 minute sessions at moderate to vigorous intensity (60%–80% heart rater or VO_2R) for patients with the goal to improve health-related quality of life **(Strong Evidence)**.
   c. 3 times a week, 30–60 minute sessions at moderate to vigorous intensity (60%–80% heart rater or VO_2R) for patients with the goal to improve physical function, anxiety, and depression **(Strong Evidence)**.
   d. 3–4 times a week, 30–40 minute sessions at moderate intensity (40%–59% heart rate reserve or VO_2R) for patients' with the goal of improving sleep (Moderate Evidence).
   e. Intensity—Start at low to moderate intensities (40%–59% heart rate reserve or VO_2R) and progress to vigorous intensity (60%–80% heart rate or VO_2R) based on patient's tolerance and goals.
   f. Monitor exertion (Borg rating of perceived exertion) and fatigue levels closely. Start slowly, progress incrementally, avoid exhaustion.
3. References.
   a. ACSM Exercise Guidelines for Cancer Patients and Survivors, 2019 at https://www.acsm.org/read-research/newsroom/news-releases/news-detail/2019/11/27/new-infographic-available-exercise-guidelines-cancer-patients-survivors.
   b. Campbell KL et al. Exercise Guidelines for Cancer Survivors: Consensus Statement from International

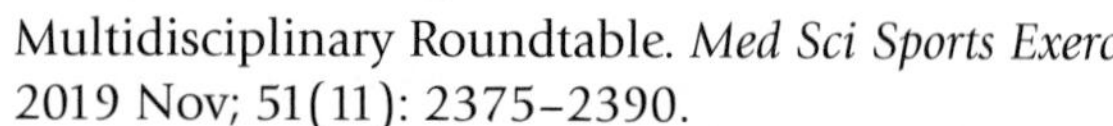

Multidisciplinary Roundtable. *Med Sci Sports Exerc.* 2019 Nov; 51(11): 2375–2390.

c. See Chapter 6, Table 6-6 for additional information on aerobic exercise.

Exercise Contraindications/Precautions

1. Exercise recommendations will vary based on individual patients and their past and present medical history.
2. Review lab values prior to beginning each examination or treatment session. Table 8-1 presents exercise guidelines based on lab values.

Table 8-1

Exercise Guidelines Based on Lab Values

NORMAL RANGE	ABNORMAL RANGE	EXERCISE RECOMMENDATIONS
Platelet count		
150,000–450,000 cells/mm^3		Normal activity, unrestricted
	50,000–150,000	Some limitations
	30,000–50,000	Moderate exercise
	20,000–30,000	Light exercise
	<20,000	ROM, ADLs, walking with physician approval
Complete Blood Count		
White Blood Cell Count (WBC)		
4800–10,800 cells/mm^3		
	>5000	Light or regular exercise
	<5000 with fever	No exercise
	<1000	No exercise; protective mask required
Hemoglobin (Hgb)		
Women 12–16 g/dL Men 13–18 g/dL		Normal activity, unrestricted
	>10	Regular exercise
	<8–10	Light exercise
	<8	No exercise
Hemtocrit (HCT) % of RBC of whole blood		
Women 37%–48% Men 45%–52%		Normal activity, unrestricted
	>25%	Light or regular exercise
	<25%	No exercise

Adapted from Goodman C, Fuller K. Pathology: Implications for the Physical Therapist, 4th ed. St Louis, Elsevier, 2014.

RED FLAGS: Contraindications to exercise:

- Day of intravenous chemotherapy or within 24 hours of treatment.
- Severe reaction to radiation therapy.
- Acute infection or febrile illness (temp. >100 °F).
- Severe nausea, vomiting, or diarrhea within 24–36 hours, dehydration, poor nutrition.
- Unusual or extreme fatigue, muscular weakness, recent bone pain.
- Chest pain, rapid or slow HR, elevated BP, swelling of ankles.
- Severe dyspnea, pain on deep breath, cough/wheezing.
- Dizziness/lightheadedness, disorientation, confusion, blurred vision, ataxia.

3. Patients with low platelets (PLT) may experience shortness of breath, excessive fatigue, possibly angina. Patients may develop petechiae, purpura, ecchymoses, hematuria, anemia, and hematochezia. Patients with critically low PLT (<10,000/mm) may experience spontaneous bleeding.
4. Patients with neutropenia (decreased neutrophils in blood) are at increased risk for infection. Adhere to infection control guidelines.
5. Patients with bony metastases have increased risk of pathological fractures. Manual muscle testing, progressive resistive exercises, and high-stress activities should be avoided.
6. Recognize cancer-specific emergencies (sudden loss of limb function, spinal cord compression, fever in immune-compromised patients, superior vena cava syndrome). Initiate plan for emergency situation.

Specific Considerations for Exercise Programs

1. Postmastectomy.
   a. Focus is on restoration of pain-free full ROM of the shoulder, prevention/reduction of edema, restoration of function.
   b. Early postoperative exercise is stressed: some protocols as early as Day 1.
2. Post–bone marrow transplant.
   a. Experience prolonged hospitalization and inactivity: average is 30 days; prolonged chemotherapy and radiotherapy, strict isolation.
   b. Focus is on restoration of function, overcoming the effects of deconditioning.

RED FLAG: Exercise is contraindicated in patients with platelet counts 20,000 or less; use caution with counts 20,000–50,000.

Physical Agents (See Chapter 11)

RED FLAGS: Thermal agents (hot packs, paraffin baths, fluidotherapy), deep heating agents (ultrasound, diathermy), and hydrotherapy may be contraindicated.
- Do not use directly over tumor.
- Do not use over dysvascular tissue: tissue exposed to radiation therapy.
- Do not use with individuals with decreased sensitivity to temperature or pain in affected area.
- Do not use in areas of increased bleeding or hemorrhage, typically the result of corticosteroid therapy.
- Do not use with acute injury, inflammation, open wounds.

RED FLAGS: Cryotherapy.
- Do not use with patients with insensitivity to cold or delayed wound healing.
- Do not use over dysvascular tissue: tissue exposed to radiation therapy.

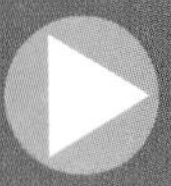

Systems Interaction—Psychological/ Psychiatric Conditions

Mental Health Conditions (https://www.nimh.nih.gov/health/topics/)

Anxiety Disorders

1. Anxiety is often a normal response to tension, conflict, or stress, and may temporarily result in feelings of apprehension, worry, or uneasiness.
2. The degree of anxiety is related to degree of perceived threat and capacity to engage behaviors that can reduce anxiety.
3. Anxiety can be constructive and stimulate an individual toward purposeful activity or it may lead to ongoing anxiety disorders in the form of generalized anxiety, pain attacks, phobias, or obessive-complusive disorders.
4. Generalized anxiety disorder results in ongoing symptoms of restlessness, difficulty concentrating, irritability, muscle tension, and difficulty controlling feelings of worry.
5. Panic attacks: acute, intense anxiety or terror; may be uncontrollable, accompanied by sympathetic signs (e.g., increased heart rate, dyspnea, hyperventilation, dry mouth, nausea, palpitations), loss of mental control, sense of impending death.
6. Phobias: excessive and unreasonable fear leads to avoidance behaviors, e.g., agoraphobia (fear of being alone or in public places).
7. Obsessive-compulsive behavior: persistent anxiety is manifested by repetitive, stereotypic acts; behaviors interfere with social functioning, e.g., hand washing, counting, and touching.

Depression (Mood Disorder)

1. Altered mood characterized by morbid sadness, dejection, sense of melancholy. Can be a chronic, relapsing disorder.
2. Management.
   a. Treatment: pharmacologic (e.g., tricyclic antidepressant drugs) and/or cognitive behavior therapy

RED FLAG: Patients on antidepressant medications may exhibit disturbed balance, postural hypotension, increased risk for falls and fractures, increased HR and risk of dysrhythmias, and seizures.

3. Physical therapy interventions.
   a. Maintain a positive attitude, consistently demonstrate warmth and interest.
   b. Acknowledge depression, provide hope.
   c. Use positive reinforcement, build in successful treatment experiences.
   d. Involve the patient in treatment decisions.
   e. Avoid excessive cheerfulness.
   f. Take all suicidal thoughts and actions seriously.
   g. NIH 5 steps for someone in emotional pain (https://www.nimh.nih.gov/health/topics/suicide-prevention):
      - Ask–"Are you thinking about hurting or killing yourself"
      - Keep Them Safe–Remove access to unsafe items or places.
      - Be There–Listen and acknowledge the individual's thoughts and feelings.
      - Help Them Connect–Critical to make contact with a trusted individual and professional (National Suicide Prevention Lifeline at 1-800-273-TALK [8255]).
      - Stay Connected–Research shows suicide deaths goes down when someone follows up an at-risk person.

Bipolar Disorder (Mood Disorder)

1. A disorder characterized by mood swings from depression to mania.
2. Often intense outbursts, high energy and activity, excessive euphoria, decreased need for sleep, unrealistic beliefs, distractibility, poor judgment, denial.

3. Followed by extreme depression (see depression symptoms).
4. Treatment is pharmacological (e.g., lithium carbonate).

Personality Disorders

1. Antisocial personality disorder: individual has a long-term pattern of manipulating, exploiting, or violating the rights of others. This behavior is often criminal.
2. Borderline personality disorder: individual has varying moods, impulsive actions and problems with relationships; may experience intense episodes of anger, depression, and anxiety that can last from a few hours to days.
3. Narcissistic personality disorder: individual has inflated sense of their own importance, troubled relationships, a deep need for excessive admiration, and a lack of empathy for others.
4. Avoidant personality disorder: individual has feelings of extreme social inhibition and sensitivity to negative criticism and rejection.

Post-Traumatic Stress Disorder (PTSD)

1. Exposure to a traumatic event produces a variety of stress-related symptoms.
2. PTSD symptoms.
   a. Reexperiencing the traumatic event.
   b. Psychic numbing with reduced responsiveness.
   c. Detachment from the external world; survival guilt.
   d. Exaggerated autonomic arousal, hyperalertness.
   e. Disturbed sleeping.
   f. Ongoing irritability.
   g. Impaired memory and concentration.
3. PTSD can be acute (symptoms last <3 months) or chronic (3 months or longer); onset can also be delayed.
4. Symptoms should not be ignored. A mental health consultation is indicated.

Schizophrenia (Psychotic Disorder)

1. A group of disorders characterized by disruptions in thought patterns; of unknown etiology; a biochemical imbalance in the brain.
2. Symptoms.
   a. Disordered thinking: fragmented thoughts, errors of logic, delusions, poor judgment, memory.
   b. Disordered speech: may be coherent but unintelligible, incoherent, or mute.
   c. Disordered perception: hallucinations and delusions.
   d. Inappropriateness of affect: withdrawal of interest from other people and from the outside world; loss of self-identity, self-direction; disordered interpersonal relations.
   e. Functional disturbances: inability to function in daily life and work.
   f. Little insight into problems and behavior.
3. Paranoia: a type of schizophrenic disorder characterized by feelings of extreme suspiciousness, persecution, grandiosity (feelings of power or great wealth), or jealousy; withdrawal of all emotional contact with others.
4. Catatonia: a type of schizophrenic disorder characterized by mutism or stupor; unresponsiveness; catatonic posturing (remains fixed, unable to move or talk for extended periods).

Psychosomatic Disorders (Somatoform Disorders)

1. Physical signs or diseases that are related to emotional causes, e.g., psychosocial stress.
2. Characteristics.
   a. Cannot be explained by identifiable disease process or underlying pathology.
   b. Not under voluntary control; provides a means of coping with anxiety and stress.
   c. Patient is frequently indifferent to symptoms.
3. Types.
   a. Functional neurologic symptom disorder (aka functional neurologic syndrome; functional neurologic disorder; conversion disorder [past terminology]): patient experiences neurological symptoms (e.g., weakness, paralysis, sensory symptoms) without evidence of specific neurological disease or other medical condition.
      - Symptoms are real and can cause significant loss of function and emotional distress; symptoms can vary in severity and fluctuate or be persistent.
      - Cause is unknown; may be triggered by psychological or physical trauma, or stress.
      - Treatment involves PT or OT for movement and functional symptoms; psychiatric treatment (e.g., cognitive behavioral therapy).
4. Functional neurologic symptom disorder management.
   a. Physical symptoms are real: treat the patient as you would any other patient with similar symptoms.
   b. Provide a supportive environment.
   c. Identify primary gain (internal conflicts); assist patient in learning new, alternative methods of stress management.
   d. Identify secondary gains (additional advantages, e.g., attention, sympathy); do not reinforce.
   e. Provide encouragement and support for the total person.
5. Reference: Perez DL et al. (2021). Decade of progress in motor functional neurological disorder: continuing the momentum. *J Neurol Neurosurg Psychiatry*, 15, 323–953.

Grief Process

Characteristics

1. An emotional process by which an individual deals with a loss, e.g., of a significant loved one, body part, or function.

2. Somatic symptoms: e.g., fatigue, sighing, hyperventilation, anorexia, insomnia.
3. Psychological symptoms: e.g., sorrow, discomfort, regret, guilt, anger, irritability, depression.
4. Resolution may take months or years.

Stages

1. Shock and disbelief; inability to comprehend loss.
2. Increased awareness and anguish; crying or anger is common.
3. Mourning.
4. Resolution of loss.
5. Idealization of lost person or function.

Management

1. Provide support and understanding of the grief process.
2. Encourage expression of feelings, memories.
3. Respect privacy, cultural or religious customs.

Death and Dying

End of Life Changes

1. Decreasing activity and physical functioning.
2. Emotional and spiritual concerns.
3. Withdrawal from the social and physical world.
4. Disorientation and confusion common.
5. Terminal agitation may occur; individual becomes restless and agitated.
6. Many become unconscious in last few hours or days before death.

Five Stages of Death and Dying (Kubler-Ross and Colleagues)

1. Denial: patients insist they are fine, joke about themselves, are not motivated to participate in treatment.
   a. Allow denial: denial is a protective compensatory mechanism necessary until such time as the patient is ready to face his/her illness.
   b. Provide opportunities for patient to question, confront illness and impending death.
2. Anger, resentment: patients may become disruptive, blame others.
   a. Be supportive: allow patient to express anger, frustration, resentment.
   b. Encourage focus on coping strategies.
3. Bargaining: patients bargain for time to complete life tasks; turn to religion or other individuals, make promises in return for function.
   a. Provide accurate information, honest, truthful answers.
4. Depression: patients acknowledge impending death, withdraw from life; demonstrate an overwhelming sense of loss, low motivation.
   a. Observe closely for suicidal ideation.
   b. Allay fears and anxieties, especially loneliness and isolation.
   c. Assist in providing for comfort of the patient.
5. Acceptance and preparation for death: acceptance of their condition; relate more to their family, make plans for the future.

Management

1. Support patient and family during each stage.
2. Maintain hope without supporting unrealistic expectations.

Interventions

Physical Therapist's Role

1. Motivate patients, manage the human side of rehabilitation.
2. Establish boundaries of the professional relationship: identify problems, expectations, purpose, roles, and responsibilities.
3. Provide empathic understanding: the capacity to understand what your patient is experiencing from that patient's perspective.
   a. Recognize losses; allow opportunity to mourn "old self."
   b. Ask open-ended questions that reflect what the patient is feeling.
      - Empathetic response; e.g., "It sounds like you are worried and anxious about your pain and are trying your best."
4. Set realistic, meaningful goals; involve the patient and family in the goal-setting process; self-determination is important.
5. Set realistic time frames for the rehabilitation program; recognize symptoms, stages of the grief process or death and dying and adjust accordingly.
6. Recognize and reinforce healthy, positive, socially appropriate behaviors; allow the patient to experience success.
7. Recognize secondary gains, unacceptable behaviors; do not reinforce (e.g., malingering behaviors such as avoidance of work).
8. Provide an environment conducive to the patient's emotional state, learning, and optimal function.
   a. Provide a message of hope tempered with realism.
   b. Keep patients informed.
   c. Lay adequate groundwork or preparation for expected changes or discharge.
   d. Help to reestablish personal dignity and self-worth; acknowledge whole person.
9. Help patients identify feelings, successful coping strategies, recognize successful conflict resolution and rehabilitation gains.
   a. Stress ability to overcome major obstacles.
   b. Stress that the process is unique and highly individualized.

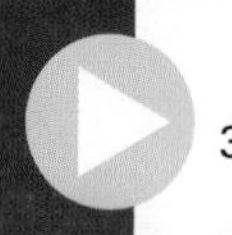

Gastrointestinal System

Overview

Anatomy/Physiology (See Figure 8-1)

1. The gastrointestinal (GI) tract is a long, hollow tube extending from the mouth to the anus. Ingested foods and fluids are broken down into molecules that are absorbed and used by the body, while waste products are eliminated.
   a. The upper GI tract consists of the mouth, esophagus, and stomach and functions for ingestion and initial digestion of food.
   b. The middle GI tract is the small intestine (duodenum, jejunum, and ileum). The major digestive and absorption (nutrients) processes occur here.
   c. The lower GI tract consists of the large intestine (cecum, colon, and rectum), with primary functions that include absorption of water and electrolytes, storage, and elimination of waste products.

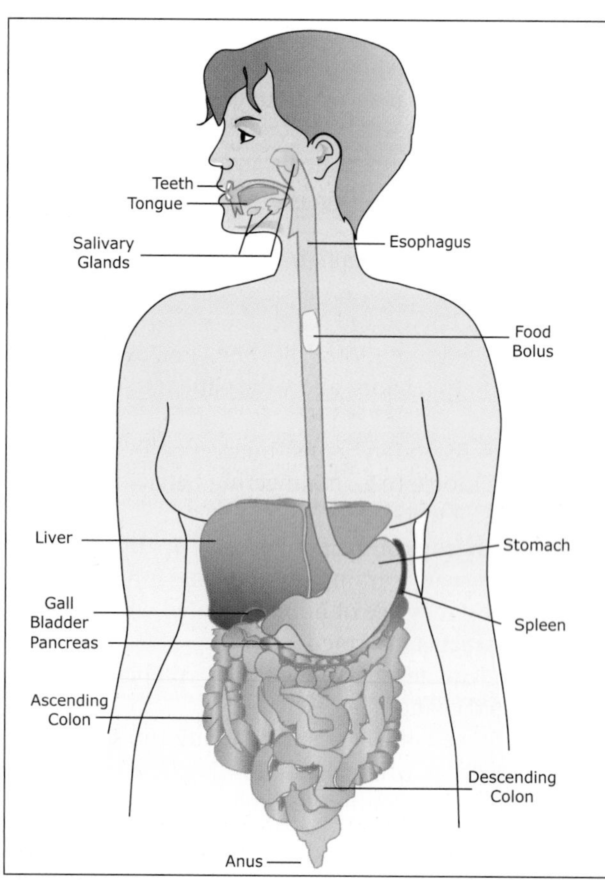

Figure 8-1 **Gastrointestinal system anterior view.**

   d. Accessory organs aid in digestion by producing digestive secretions and include the salivary glands, liver, and pancreas.
2. GI motility propels food and fluids through the GI system and is provided by rhythmic, intermittent contractions (peristaltic movements) of smooth muscle (except for pharynx and upper one-third of the esophagus).
3. Neural control is achieved by the enteric nervous system, a division of the autonomic nervous system (ANS). Both sympathetic and parasympathetic plexuses extend along the length of the GI wall. Vagovagal (mediated by the vagus nerve) reflexes control the secretions and motility of the GI tract.
4. Major GI hormones include cholecystokinin, gastrin, and secretin.

Abdominal Quadrants and Associated Organs

1. Figure 8-2 shows location of organs within the various quadrants.
2. Correlating organ location with pain referral patterns (Figure 2-47) is required for accurate differential diagnosis.

Signs and Symptoms Common to Many Types of GI Disorders

1. Dysphagia refers to difficulty in swallowing.
   a. Patients experience choking, coughing, or abnormal sensations of food sticking in the back of the throat or esophagus.
   b. Numerous conditions can cause dysphagia, including lesions of the CNS (stroke, Alzheimer's disease, Parkinson's disease), esophageal and gastric disorders (GERD, cancer), arthritis of cervical spine, swelling and scleroderma.
   c. Achalasia is a condition in which the lower esophageal sphincter fails to relax and food is trapped in the esophagus.
2. Heartburn is a painful burning sensation felt in the esophagus in the midepigastric area behind the sternum or in the throat.
   a. It is typically caused by reflux of gastric contents into the esophagus.
   b. Certain foods (fatty foods, citrus foods, chocolate, peppermint, alcohol, coffee, caffeine), increased abdominal pressure (food, tight clothing, back supports, pregnancy), and certain positions/ movements (bending over or lying down after a large meal) can aggravate heartburn.

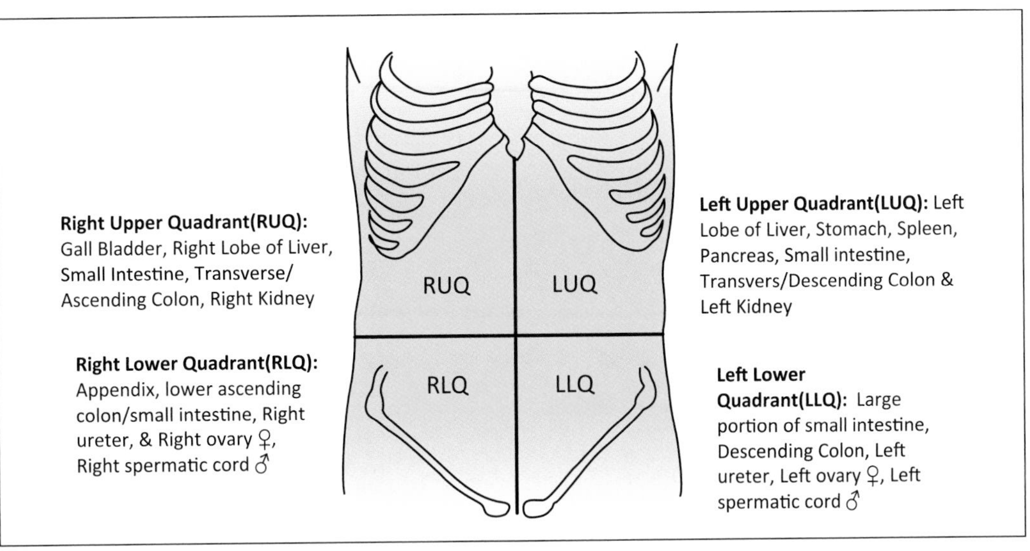

Figure 8-2 **Quadrants and respective organs.**

3. Nausea and vomiting. Nausea is an unpleasant sensation that signals stimulation of medullary vomiting center and often precedes vomiting. Vomiting is the forceful oral expulsion of abdominal contents.
   a. Nausea and vomiting can be triggered by many different causes including food, drugs, hypoxia, shock, inflammation of abdominal organs, distention, irritation of the GI tract (virus, blood), and motion sickness.
   b. Prolonged vomiting can produce fluid and electrolyte imbalance and can result in pulmonary aspiration and mucosal or GI damage.
4. Diarrhea is the passage of frequent, watery, unformed stools. The amount of fluid loss determines the severity of the illness.
   a. Dehydration, electrolyte imbalance, dizziness, thirst, and weight loss are common complications of prolonged diarrhea.
   b. Numerous conditions can trigger diarrhea, including infectious organisms (*Escherichia coli*, rotavirus, *Salmonella*), dysentery, diabetic enteropathy, irritable bowel syndrome, hyperthyroidism, neoplasm, and diverticulitis. Diet, medications, and strenuous exercise can also cause diarrhea.
   c. *Clostridium difficile* (C. diff) is an infectious bacteria that can result in life-threatening diarrhea. Symptoms include watery diarrhea, fever, loss of appetite, nausea, and belly pain and tenderness.
      - Very prevalent in hospitals and long-term care facilities among the elderly following antibiotic treatment.
      - Can spread from person-to-person on contaminated equipment and on the hands of health care providers.
      - Can also affect others that are neither high-risk nor on antibiotics.
      - Single rooms are used whenever possible.
      - Contact precautions are mandatory including hand washing, gown, and gloves.
      - Any equipment or device used by the therapist that is not disposable or patient-dedicated must be thoroughly cleaned with chlorine bleach or E.P.A.-approved spore-killing disinfectant. This might include stethoscopes, goniometers, ambulatory aids, exercise devices, etc.
      - C. diff can be treated with antibiotics; in severe cases, surgery may be required.
5. Constipation is a decrease in normal elimination with excessively hard, dry stools and difficult elimination.
   a. Constipation causes increased bowel pressure and lower abdominal discomfort.
   b. Many different factors can trigger constipation, including a diet lacking in bulk and fiber, inadequate consumption of fluids, sedentary lifestyle, increasing age, and drugs (opiates, antidepressants, calcium channel blockers, anticholinergics).
   c. Numerous conditions can cause constipation including hypothyroidism, diverticular disease, irritable bowel syndrome, Parkinson's disease, spinal cord injury, tumors, bowel obstruction, and rectal lesions.
   d. Obstipation is intractable constipation with resulting fecal impaction or inability to pass gas and the retention of hard, dry stools in the rectum and colon. Impaction can cause partial or complete bowel obstruction. The patient may exhibit a history of watery diarrhea, fecal soiling, and fecal incontinence. Removal of the fecal mass is indicated. Can be seen in postsurgical patients, those taking long-term opiates, or individuals with spinal cord injuries.

RED FLAG: Constipation can cause abdominal pain and tenderness in the anterior hip, groin, or thigh regions.

e. Constipation may develop as a result of muscle guarding and splinting; e.g., in the patient with low back pain.

6. Anorexia is the loss of appetite with an inability to eat. It is associated with anxiety, fear, and depression along with a number of different disease states and drugs.
   a. Anorexia nervosa is a disorder characterized by prolonged loss of appetite and inability to eat. Individuals exhibit emaciation, emotional disturbance concerning body image, and fear of gaining weight. It is common in adolescent girls, who may also exhibit amenorrhea. Key concerns include nutritional and electrolyte imbalances leading to multisystem issues (neuropathy, arrhythmias).
7. Abdominal pain.
   a. Abdominal pain is common in GI conditions. Can result from inflammation, ischemia, or mechanical stretching. Visceral pain can occur in the epigastric region (T3–T5 sympathetic nerve distribution), the periumbilical region (T10 sympathetic nerve distribution), and the lower abdominal-hypogastric region (T10–L2 sympathetic nerve distribution).
   b. Abdominal pain is generally aggravated by coughing, sneezing, or straining.

RED FLAGS: Referred GI pain patterns (see Figure 2-47, Pain referred from viscera).
- Visceral pain from the esophagus can refer to the midback.
- Midthoracic spine pain (nerve root pain) can appear as esophageal pain.
- Visceral pain from the liver, diaphragm, or pericardium can refer to the shoulder.
- Visceral pain from the gallbladder, stomach, pancreas, or small intestine can refer to the midback and scapular regions.
- Visceral pain from the colon, appendix, or pelvic viscera can refer to the pelvis, low back, or sacrum.

8. GI bleeding is evidenced by blood appearing in vomitus or feces.
   a. It can result from erosive gastritis, peptic ulcers, prolonged use of NSAIDs, and chronic alcohol use.
   b. Blood in vomit is consistent with oral or acute esophageal bleeding.
   c. Vomit that looks like coffee grounds is consistent with gastric ulcers, gastritis, or esophageal cancer.
   d. Small amount of blood in feces requires stool testing.
   e. Stool: bright red blood is more consistent with lower colon/rectum disorders; tarry or black stools are more consistent with upper digestive tract disorders.

Hepatobiliary System

Liver

1. Hepatitis.
   a. Characteristics.
      - Inflammation of the liver; may be caused by viral or bacterial infection; chemical agents (alcohol, drugs, toxins, herbals); autoimmune hepatitis; biliary cirrhosis and metabolic disorders such as Wilson's disease.
      - Types.
        - Hepatitis A virus (HAV, acute infectious hepatitis).
          - Transmission is primarily through fecal-oral route; contracted through contaminated food or water, or person-to-person contact (infected food handlers).
          - An acute illness (not chronic): can range in severity from mild to severe.
          - Prevention: good personal hygiene, hand washing, sanitation; immunization (vaccine).
        - Hepatitis B virus (HBV, serum hepatitis).
          - Transmission from blood, body fluids, or body tissues, through blood transfusion, oral or sexual contact with a person infected with HBV or contaminated needles.
          - Can range in severity from mild (acute, lasting a few weeks) to severe (chronic, lifelong).
          - Prevention: education, use of disposable needles, screening of blood donors; precautions for health care workers; immunization (vaccine).
        - Hepatitis C virus (HCV).
          - Transmission is same as for HBV (post-transfusion or needle sharing are the most common routes).
          - Can be acute or chronic.
        - Hepatitis D (HDV).
          - Hepatitis D is dependent upon having Hepatitis B.
          - The prognosis is poor, and patients often present with fulminant liver failure.
   b. Clinical signs and symptoms.
      - Initial (preicteric phase): low-grade fever, anorexia, nausea, vomiting, diarrhea, fatigue, malaise, headache, abdominal tenderness, and myalgia and arthralgia.
      - Jaundice (icteric) phase: fever, jaundice, enlarged liver with tenderness; abatement of earlier symptoms. Amber-colored or dark urine.
      - Elevated lab values: hepatic transaminases and bilirubin.
      - Course: variable.
        - Acute: may last from several weeks to months.
        - Chronic: HBV and HCV may lead to chronic liver infection, including necrosis, cirrhosis, and liver failure.

c. Medical interventions.
- No specific treatment for acute viral hepatitis; treatment is symptomatic, e.g., IV fluids, analgesics.
- Chronic hepatitis: direct acting antivirals are the main therapy.
- Viral hepatitis is the leading cause of liver cancer and common reason for liver transplantation.

2. Cirrhosis.
   a. Irreversible chronic injury of the hepatic parenchyma as a result of chronic hepatitis.
   b. Clinical manifestations include jaundice, peripheral edema, Dupuytren's contracture, palmar erythema, angiomas, hepatomegaly, splenomegaly, and ascites (accumulation of fluid in the peritoneal cavity).
   c. Pharmacotherapy includes furosemide (Lasix) or spironolactone (potassium-sparing diuretic).
   d. Paracentesis drainage can be used to remove peritoneal fluid.
   e. Late complication may be hepatic encephalopathy.
   - Neuropsychiatric abnormalities with personality changes, intellectual impairment, depressed levels of consciousness, slurred speech, and slowed movement.
   - Asterixis ('liver flap") is myoclonus of the hand with the wrist in extension. A result of the liver unable to convert ammonia to urea. It is a characteristic of hepatic encephalopathy as well as other disorders such as drug overdose and Wilson's disease.
   - Lactulose can be used to increase bowel movements and excrete ammonia in the stool.

Gallbladder

1. Cholelithiasis or gallstones present in the gallbladder.
   a. Often asymptomatic and no intervention needed.
   b. If gallstones block the common bile duct, biliary colic can result. Characterized by pain in the RUQ with radiation to the right scapula. Can worsen after a fatty meal.
2. Cholecystitis is a partial or complete obstruction of the common bile duct resulting in inflammation of the gallbladder.
   a. Severe RUQ pain radiating to the right scapula. Nausea, vomiting, or low grade fever possible.
   b. Positive Murphy's sign. Palpate near right subcostal margin as patient takes a deep breath. Pain is elicited.
   c. Interventions include both nonsurgical and surgical (cholecystectomy) options.

Pancreas

1. Acute pancreatitis.
   a. Caused by gallstones, alcoholism, substance abuse, and more.
   b. Characterized by acute "bandlike" pain, which can radiate to the back and is worse in supine position.
   c. May be accompanied by hypotension, tachycardia, nausea, vomiting.
   d. Intervention is IV fluids, pain control, NPO, and occasionally surgery.
2. Chronic pancreatitis.
   a. Epigastric and LUQ pain.
   b. Characterized by anorexia, nausea, vomiting, constipation, flatulence, weight loss, and steatorrhea (greasy stools).
   c. Intervention consists of dietary modification, pain control, and supplemental pancreatic enzymes.
3. Pancreatic cancer.
   a. Often minimal or no symptoms until the disease is advanced.
   b. Later symptoms include abdominal pain that radiates to the back, unexplained weight loss, jaundice, dark-colored urine, light-colored stool, and fatigue.

Esophagus

Gastroesophageal Reflux Disease (GERD)

1. Caused by reflux or backward movement of gastric contents of the stomach into the esophagus, producing heartburn.
2. Results from failure of the lower esophageal sphincter to regulate flow of food from the esophagus into the stomach and increased gastric pressure.
3. The diaphragm that surrounds the esophagus and oblique muscles also contributes to antireflux function.
4. Over time, acidic gastric fluids (pH <4) damage the esophagus, producing reflux esophagitis.
5. Heartburn commonly occurs 30–60 minutes after eating and at night when lying down (nocturnal reflux).

RED FLAGS: Esophageal Pain
- Atypical pain may present as head, neck, or chest pain.
- Esophageal pain is sometimes mistaken for heart attack; it is unrelated to activity.

   a. Respiratory symptoms can occur, including wheezing and chronic cough due to microaspiration, laryngeal injury, and vagus-mediated bronchospasm. Hoarseness can also result from chronic inflammation of the vocal cords.
6. Complications include strictures and Barrett's esophagus (a precancerous state).
7. Physical therapy interventions.
   a. Positional changes from full supine to modified, more upright positions are indicated.
   b. Avoid positions (supine or declined) or exercises (jogging, jumping) that exacerbate symptoms.
8. Lifestyle modifications include avoiding large meals and certain foods; sleeping with head elevated; medications include acid-suppressing proton pump inhibitors (PPIs) (e.g., Prilosec), H2 blockers (e.g., famotidine [Pepcid], cimetidine [Tagamet]), and antacids (e.g., Tums). In severe cases, surgery is an option.

Hiatal Hernia

1. Protrusion of the stomach upward through the diaphragm (rolling hiatal hernia) or displacement of both the stomach and gastroesophageal junction upward into the thorax (sliding hiatal hernia).
2. May be congenital or acquired.
3. Symptoms include heartburn from GERD.
4. Conservative or symptomatic treatment is the same as for GERD. Surgery may be indicated.

Esophageal Cancer

1. Risk factors: history of GERD, smoking, alcohol, Barrett's esophagus, diet, males.
2. Symptoms: dysphagia, unexplained weight loss, chest pain/pressure, worsening indigestion, coughing/hoarseness.

Stomach

Gastritis

1. Inflammation of the stomach mucosa. Gastritis can be acute or chronic.
2. Acute gastritis is caused by severe burns, aspirin or other NSAIDs, corticosteroids, food allergies, or viral or bacterial infections. Hemorrhagic bleeding can occur.
3. Symptoms include anorexia, nausea, vomiting, and pain.
4. Chronic gastritis occurs with certain diseases such as peptic ulcer, bacterial infection caused by *Helicobacter pylori*, stomach cancer, pernicious anemia or with autoimmune disorders (thyroid disease, Addison's disease).

> **RED FLAG:** Patients taking NSAIDs long term should be monitored carefully for stomach pain, bleeding, nausea, or vomiting.

5. Management is symptomatic and includes avoiding irritating substances (caffeine, nicotine, alcohol), dietary modification, and medications that include acid-suppressing PPIs, H2 blockers, and antacids.

Peptic Ulcer Disease

1. Refers to ulcerative lesions that occur in the upper GI tract in areas exposed to acid-pepsin secretions. It can affect one or all layers of the stomach or duodenum.
2. Caused by a number of factors, including bacterial infection (*H. pylori*), acetylsalicylic acid (aspirin) and NSAIDs, excessive secretion of gastric acids, stress, and heredity.
3. Symptoms include epigastric pain, which is described as a gnawing, burning, or cramplike. Pain is aggravated by change in position and absence of food in the stomach and relieved by food or antacids.
4. Complications include hemorrhage. Bleeding may be sudden and severe or insidious with blood in vomitus or stools. Symptoms can include weakness, dizziness, or other signs of circulatory shock.
5. Management includes use of antibiotics for treatment of *H. pylori* along with acid-suppressing drugs (PPIs, H2 blockers, and antacids). Dietary modification including avoidance of stomach irritants is indicated. Surgical intervention is indicated for perforation and uncontrolled bleeding.

> **RED FLAGS:**
> - Pain from peptic ulcers located on the posterior wall of the stomach can present as radiating back pain. Pain can also radiate to the right shoulder.
> - Stress and anxiety can increase gastric secretions and pain.

Intestines

Malabsorption Syndrome

1. A complex of disorders characterized by problems in intestinal absorption of nutrients (fat, carbohydrates, proteins, vitamins, calcium, and iron).
2. Can be caused by gastric or small bowel resection (short-gut syndrome) or a number of different diseases including cystic fibrosis, celiac disease, Crohn's disease, chronic pancreatitis, and pernicious anemia. Malabsorption can also be drug-induced (NSAID gastroenteritis).
3. Deficiencies of enzymes (pancreatic lipase) and bile salts are contributing factors.
4. Symptoms can include anorexia, weight loss, abdominal bloating, pain and cramps, indigestion, and steatorrhea (abnormal amounts of fat in feces). Diarrhea can be chronic and explosive.

> **RED FLAGS:** Can produce iron-deficiency anemia and easy bruising and bleeding due to lack of vitamin K.

   a. Muscle weakness and fatigue due to lack of protein, iron, folic acid, and vitamin B.
   b. Bone loss, pain, and predisposition to develop fractures from lack of calcium, phosphate, and vitamin D.
   c. Neuropathy including tetany, paresthesias, numbness and tingling from lack of calcium, vitamins B and D, magnesium, potassium.
   d. Muscle spasms from electrolyte imbalance and lack of calcium.
   e. Peripheral edema.

Inflammatory Bowel Disease (IBD)

1. Refers to two related chronic inflammatory intestinal disorders: Crohn's disease (CD) and ulcerative colitis (UC). Both diseases result in inflammation of the bowel and are characterized by remissions and exacerbations.

2. Symptoms include abdominal pain, frequent attacks of diarrhea, fecal urgency, and weight loss.
3. Stunted growth is common in pediatric patients with CD and UC.

RED FLAGS:
- Joint pain (reactive arthritis) and skin rashes can occur. Pain can be referred to the low back.
- Complications can include intestinal obstruction and corticosteroid toxicity (low bone density, increased fracture risk).
- Intestinal absorption is disrupted and nutritional deficiencies are common.
- Chronic IBD can lead to anxiety and depression.

4. Crohn's disease involves a granulomatous type of inflammation that can occur anywhere in the GI tract. Areas of adjacent normal tissue called skip lesions are present.
5. Ulcerative colitis involves an ulcerative and exudative inflammation of the large intestine and rectum. It is characterized by varying amounts of bloody diarrhea, mucus, and pus. Skip lesions are absent.

Irritable Bowel Syndrome (IBS)

1. Characterized by abnormally increased motility of the small and large intestines. IBS is also known as spastic, nervous, or irritable colon.
2. IBS is associated with emotional stress and certain foods (high fat content or roughage, lactose intolerance). No structural or biochemical abnormalities have been identified.
3. Symptoms include persistent or recurrent abdominal pain that is relieved by defecation. Patients may experience constipation or diarrhea, bloating, abdominal cramps, flatulence, nausea, and anorexia.
4. Stress reduction and medications to reduce anxiety or depression are important components of treatment.
5. Regular physical activity is effective in reducing stress and improving bowel function.

Diverticular Disease

1. Characterized by pouchlike herniations (diverticula) of the mucosal layer of the colon through the muscularis layer.
2. Diverticulosis refers to pouchlike herniations of the colon, especially the sigmoid colon.
   a. Symptoms are minimal but can include rectal bleeding.
   b. Dietary factors (lack of dietary fiber), lack of physical activity, and poor bowel habits contribute to its development.
   c. Diverticulosis can lead to diverticulitis.
3. Diverticulitis refers to inflammation of one or more diverticula. Fecal matter penetrates diverticula and causes inflammation and abscess.
   a. Symptoms include pain and cramping in the lower left quadrant, nausea and vomiting, slight fever, and an elevated WBC.
   b. Complications include bowel obstruction, perforation with peritonitis, and hemorrhage.

RED FLAG: Patients may complain of back pain.

4. Regular exercise is an important component of treatment.

Appendicitis

1. An inflammation of the vermiform appendix. As the condition progresses, the appendix becomes swollen, gangrenous, and perforated. Perforation can be life threatening and lead to the development of peritonitis.
2. Pain is abrupt at onset, localized to the epigastric or periumbilical area, and increases in intensity over time.
3. Rebound tenderness (Blumberg's sign) is present in response to depression of the abdominal wall at a site distant from the painful area.
4. Point tenderness is located at McBurney's point, a point one-third of the distance from the anterior superior iliac spine and umbilicus.
5. Rovsing's sign elicits pain in the right lower quadrant with pressure exerted on the left lower quadrant.
6. Pain in the right lower quadrant occurs with hip extension from inflammation of the peritoneum overlying the psoas muscle (psoas sign; please see Figure 8-3a and 8-3b).
7. Obturator sign (please see Figure 8-4): right lower quadrant pain with external rotation and flexion to 90 degrees of the right hip with 90 degrees of knee flexion. Indicative of inflammation of the sheath of the obturator nerve.
8. Markle's sign: pain elicited in the RLQ when a patient drops from standing on toes to the heels with a jarring landing.

RED FLAG: Immediate medical attention is required with positive signs. Elevations in WBC count (>20,000/mm^3) are indicative of perforation; surgery is indicated.

Peritonitis

1. Inflammation of the peritoneum, the serous membrane lining the walls of the abdominal cavity.
2. Peritonitis results from bacterial invasion and infection of the peritoneum. Common agents include *E. coli*, *Bacteroides*, *Fusobacterium*, and streptococci.

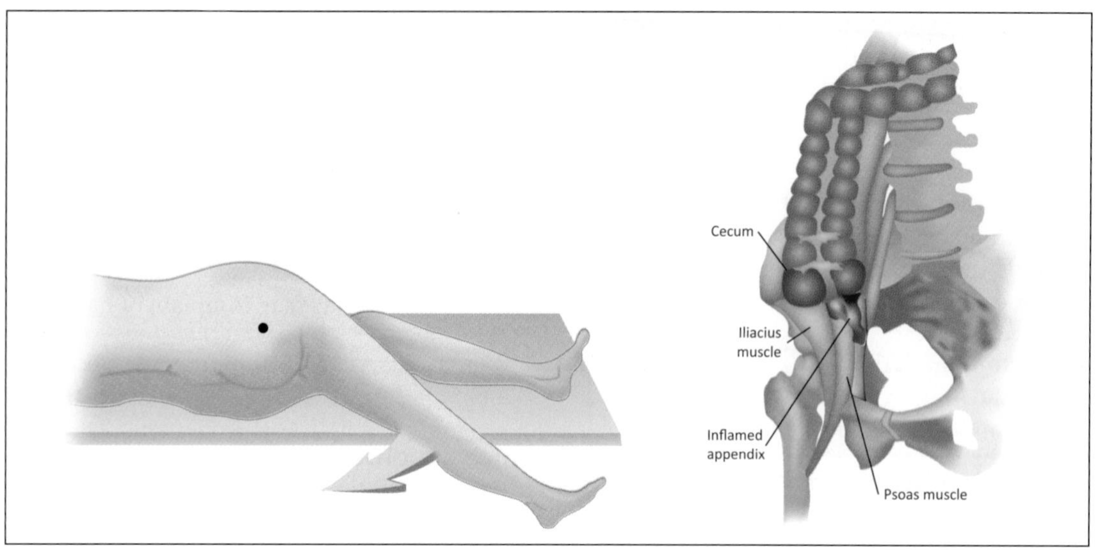

Figure 8-3 **(a) Psoas test position (b) Psoas muscle impacting inflamed appendix.**
Adapted from Floyd E. Hosmer, 1999.

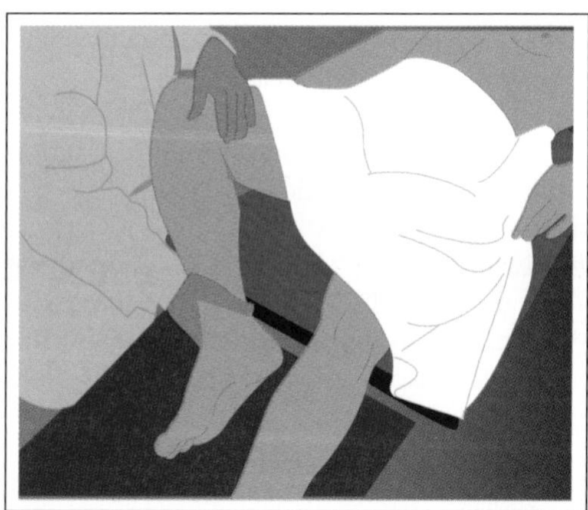

Figure 8-4 **Obturator test position.**
Adapted from Mosby's Medical Dictionary, 9th edition, 2009, Elsevier.

3. A number of different factors can introduce infecting agents, including penetrating wounds, surgery, perforated peptic ulcer, ruptured appendix, perforated diverticulum, gangrenous bowel, pelvic inflammatory disease, and gangrenous gallbladder.
4. Symptoms include abdominal distension, severe abdominal pain, rigidity from reflex guarding, rebound tenderness, decreased or absent bowel sounds, nausea and vomiting, and tachycardia.
5. Elevated WBC count, fever, electrolyte imbalance, and hypotension are common.
6. Peritonitis can lead to toxemia and shock, circulatory failure, and respiratory distress.
7. Treatment is aimed at controlling inflammation and infection and restoring fluid and electrolyte imbalances. Surgical intervention may be necessary to remove an inflamed appendix or close a perforation.

Rectum

Rectal Fissure

1. A tear or ulceration of the lining of the anal canal.
2. Constipation and large, hard stools are contributing factors.

Hemorrhoids (Piles)

1. Varicosities in the lower rectum or anus caused by congestion of the veins in the hemorrhoidal plexus.
2. Hemorrhoids can be internal or external (protruding from the anus).
3. Symptoms include local irritation, pain, rectal itching.
4. Prolonged bleeding can result in anemia.
5. Straining with defecation, constipation, and prolonged sitting contribute to discomfort.
6. Pregnancy increases the risk of hemorrhoids.
7. Treatment includes topical medications to shrink the hemorrhoid, dietary changes, sitz baths, local hot or cold compresses, and ligation or surgical excision.

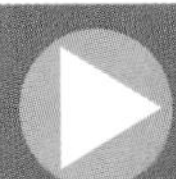

Genital/Reproductive System

Overview: Female Reproductive System

Anatomy/Physiology (See Figure 8-5)

1. External genitalia, located at the base of the pelvis, consist of the mons pubis, labia majora, labia minora, clitoris, and perineal body.
2. The urethra and anus are in close proximity to the external genital structures, and cross-contamination is possible.
3. The internal genitalia consist of the vagina, the uterus and cervix, the fallopian tubes, and paired ovaries.

Sexual and Reproductive Functions

1. The ovaries store female germ cells (ova) and produce female sex hormones (estrogens and progesterone) under control of the hypothalamus (gonadotropin-releasing hormone) and the anterior pituitary gland (gonadotropic follicle-stimulating and luteinizing hormones).
2. Sex hormones influence the development of secondary sex characteristics, regulate the menstrual cycle (ovulation), maintain pregnancy (fertilization and implantation, gestation), and influence menopause (cessation of the menstrual cycle).
   a. Estrogens decrease the rate of bone resorption.

> **RED FLAG:** Osteoporosis and risk of bone fracture increase dramatically after menopause.

   b. Estrogens increase production of the thyroid and increase high-density lipoproteins (a protective effect against heart disease).

> **RED FLAG:** Heart disease and stroke risk increase after menopause.

Breasts

1. Mammary tissues located on the anterior chest wall between the 3rd and 7th ribs.
2. Breast function is related to production of sex hormones and pregnancy, producing milk for infant nourishment.

Pregnancy: Normal

Pregnancy Weight Gain. Average 20–30 Lb

Physical Therapists Teach Childbirth Education Classes

1. Relaxation training: e.g., Jacobsen's progressive relaxation, relaxation response, mental imagery, yoga.

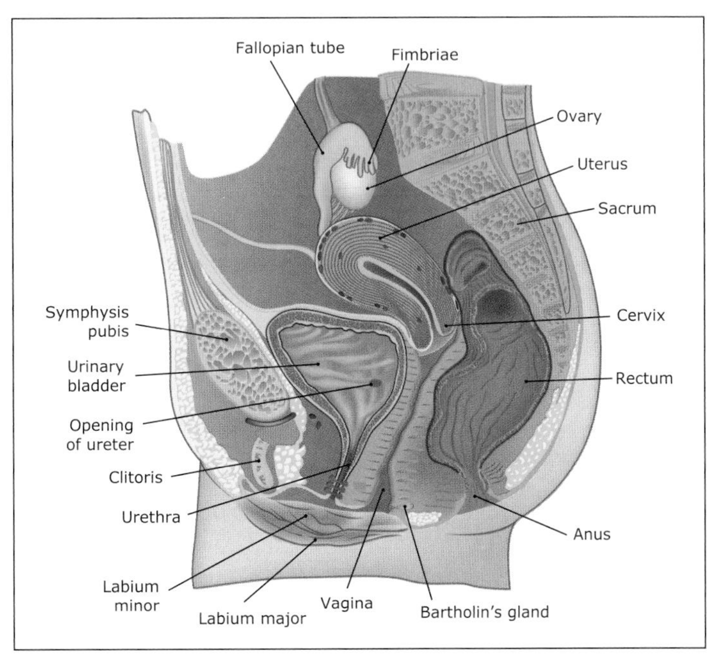

Figure 8-5 Female reproductive system.

2. Breathing management: slow, deep, diaphragmatic breathing; Lamaze techniques; avoidance of Valsalva's maneuver.
3. Provide information about pregnancy and childbirth.

Common Changes with Pregnancy and Physical Therapy Interventions

1. Postural changes: kyphosis with scapular protraction, cervical lordosis, and forward head; lumbar lordosis; postural stress may continue into postpartum phase with lifting and carrying the infant.
   a. Postural evaluation.
   b. Teach postural exercises to stretch, strengthen, and train postural muscles.
   c. Teach pelvic stabilization exercises, e.g., posterior pelvic tilt.
   d. Teach correct body mechanics, e.g., sitting, standing, lifting, ADLs.
   e. Limit certain activities in the third trimester, e.g., supine position to avoid inferior vena cava compression, bridging.
2. Balance changes: center of gravity shifts forward and upward as the fetus develops; with advanced pregnancy, there will be a wider base of support, increased difficulty with walking and stair climbing, rapid challenges to balance.
   a. Teach safety strategies.
3. Ligamentous laxity secondary to hormonal influences (relaxin).
   a. Joint hypermobility (e.g., sacroiliac joint), pain.
   b. Predisposition to injury especially in weight-bearing joints of lower extremities and pelvis.
   c. May persist for some time after delivery; teach joint protection strategies.
4. Muscle weakness: abdominal muscles are stretched and weakened as pregnancy develops; pelvic floor weakness with advanced pregnancy and childbirth. Stress incontinence secondary to pelvic floor dysfunction (experienced by 80% of women).
   a. Teach exercises to improve control of pelvic floor, maintain abdominal function.
   b. Stretching exercises to reduce muscle cramping.
   c. Avoid Valsalva's maneuver: may exacerbate condition.
5. Urinary changes: pressure on bladder causes frequent urination; increased incidence of reflux, urinary tract infections.
6. Respiratory changes: elevation of the diaphragm with widening of thoracic cage; hyperventilation, dyspnea may be experienced with mild exercise during late pregnancy.
7. Cardiovascular changes: increased blood volume; increased venous pressure in the lower extremities; increased heart rate and cardiac output, decreased blood pressure due to venous distensibility.
   a. Teach safe progression of aerobic exercises.
      - Exercise in moderation, with frequent rests.
      - Stress use of familiar activities; avoidance of unfamiliar.
      - Postpartum: emphasize gradual return to previous level of activity.
   b. Stress gentle stretching, adequate warm-ups and cool-downs.
   c. Teach ankle pumps for lower extremity edema (late-stage pregnancy); elevate legs to assist in venous return.
   d. Wear loose, comfortable clothing.
8. Altered thermoregulation: increased basal metabolic rate; increased heat production.

Pregnancy-Related and Pelvic Floor Pathologies

Diastasis Recti Abdominis

1. Lateral separation or split of the rectus abdominis; separation from midline (linea alba) greater than 2 cm is significant; associated with loss of abdominal wall support, increased back pain.
2. Physical therapy interventions.
   a. Teach protection of abdominal musculature: avoid abdominal exercises, e.g., full sit-ups or bilateral straight leg raising.
   b. Resume abdominal exercises when separation is less than 2 cm: teach safe abdominal strengthening exercises, e.g., partial sit-ups (knees bent), pelvic tilts; utilize hands to support abdominal wall.

Pelvic Floor Disorders

1. The result of weakening of pelvic floor muscles (pubococcygeal [PC] muscles).
2. PC muscles normally function to support the vagina, urinary bladder, and rectum and help maintain continence of the urethra and rectum.
3. Weakness or laxity of PC muscles typically results from overstretching during pregnancy and childbirth. Further loss of elasticity and muscle tone during later life can result in partial or total organ prolapse. Examples include:
   a. Cystocele: the herniation of the bladder into the vagina.
   b. Rectocele: the herniation of the rectum into the vagina.
   c. Uterine prolapse: the bulging of the uterus into the vagina.
4. PC muscles can also go into spasm.
5. Symptoms include pelvic pain (perivaginal, perirectal, lower abdominal quadrant), urinary incontinence, and pain with sexual intercourse.

RED FLAG: Pain can radiate down the posterior thigh.

6. Surgical correction may be indicated with prolapse.

Pelvic Floor Exercises

1. Indications: women and men with urinary and/or bowel incontinence; women who have started menopause or have cancer treatments causing early menopause; women who are pregnant or who have previously given birth, middle aged, and older women.
2. Contraindications: individuals with recent surgery, urinary catheter in place, or excessive pelvic pain.
3. Teaching pelvic floor exercises (Kegel exercises).
   a. Patient assumes comfortable position, typically lying down with knees bent to start; can also be progressed to sitting or standing; make sure bladder is empty before beginning.
   b. Tighten pelvic floor muscles: imagine sitting on a toilet and peeing. Then imagine stopping the flow of urine midstream. The muscles around the vaginal/anal area should tighten. Hold for 5–10 seconds. Relax for 10 seconds.
   c. Repeat 5 times to start, progress to 10 times, 3 times/day.
   d. Finding the pelvic muscles can be facilitated by briefly stopping the flow of urine midstream once while urinating.

> RED FLAG: Stopping and starting urine while emptying the bladder is not part of Kegel exercises and can be harmful; can interfere with urinary reflexes and contribute to bladder infection.

4. Postural education and muscle reeducation, pelvic mobilization, and stretching of tight lower extremity (LE) muscles are also important components.

Low Back and Pelvic Pain

1. Physical therapy interventions.
   a. Teach proper body mechanics.
   b. Balance rest with activity.
   c. Emphasize use of a firm mattress.
   d. Manual therapy (soft-tissue and joint mobilization).
   e. Joint mobilization is a precaution in the third trimester secondary to ligamentous laxity.
   f. Having the patient in sidelying (left side better than right) for treatment techniques is best to maximize blood flow to the fetus.

Sacroiliac Dysfunction

1. Secondary to postural changes, ligamentous laxity.
2. Symptoms include posterior pelvic pain; pain in buttocks, may radiate into posterior thigh or knee.
3. Associated with prolonged sitting, standing, or walking.
4. Physical therapy interventions.
   a. External stabilization, e.g., sacroiliac support belt, may help reduce pain.
   b. Avoid single-limb weight-bearing: may aggravate sacroiliac dysfunction.

Varicose Veins

1. Physical therapy interventions.
   a. Elevate extremities; avoid crossing legs, which may press on veins.
   b. Use of elastic support stockings may help.

Preeclampsia

1. Pregnancy-induced, acute hypertension after the 24th week of gestation.
2. May be mild or severe.
3. Evaluate for symptoms of hypertension, edema, sudden excessive weight gain, headache, visual disturbances, or hyperreflexia.
4. Initiate prompt physician referral.

Postcesarean Complications

1. Surgical delivery of the fetus by an incision through the abdominal and uterine walls; indicated in pelvic disproportion, failure of the birth process to progress, fetal or maternal distress, or other complications.
2. Physical therapy interventions.
   a. Postoperative TENS can be used for incisional pain; electrodes are placed parallel to the incision.
   b. Prevent postsurgical pulmonary complications: assist patient in breathing, coughing.
   c. Postcesarean exercises.
      - Gentle abdominal exercises; provide incisional support with pillow.
      - Pelvic floor exercises: labor and pushing is typically present before surgery.
      - Postural exercises; precautions about heavy lifting for 4–6 weeks.
   d. Ambulation.
   e. Prevent incisional adhesions: friction massage.

Disorders of the Female Reproductive System

Endometriosis

1. Characterized by ectopic growth and function of endometrial tissue outside of the uterus. Common sites include ovaries, fallopian tubes, broad ligaments, uterosacral ligaments, pelvis, vagina, or intestines.
   a. The ectopic tissue responds to hormonal influences but is not able to be shed as uterine tissue during menstruation.

b. Endometrial tissue can lead to cysts and rupture, producing peritonitis and adhesions as well as adhesions and obstruction.
2. Symptoms include pain, dysmenorrhea, dyspareunia (abnormal pain during sexual intercourse), and infertility.

RED FLAG: Patients may complain of back pain. Endometrial implants on muscle (e.g., psoas major, pelvic floor muscles) may produce pain with palpation or contraction.

3. Treatment involves pain management, endometrial suppression, and surgery.

Endometrial Carcinoma (Uterine Cancer)

1. Most common cancer of the female reproductive organs.
2. Causes: imbalance in progesterone and estrogen; ovarian tumor; hormone therapy for breast cancer; never been pregnant; older age; obesity.
3. Symptoms: Pelvic pain; bleeding between periods; vaginal bleeding despite menopause; Central LBP, posterior thigh pain, and/or abdominal pain.
4. Diagnosis: Pelvic exam; imaging (ultrasound, CT scan, Positron emission tomography); biopsy.
5. Medical intervention: Surgery when caught early; Later stages with metastasis often require chemotherapy/radiation.

Pelvic Inflammatory Disease (PID)

1. An inflammation of the upper reproductive tract involving the uterus (endometritis), fallopian tubes (salpingitis), or ovaries (oophoritis).
2. PID is caused by a polymicrobial agent that ascends through the endocervical canal.
3. Symptoms include lower abdominal pain that typically starts after a menstrual cycle, purulent cervical discharge, and painful cervix. Fever, elevated WBC count, and increased ESR are present.
4. Complications can include pelvic adhesions, infertility, ectopic pregnancy, chronic pain, and abscesses.
5. Treatment involves antibiotic therapy to treat the infection and prevent complications.

Overview: Male Reproductive System

Anatomy/Physiology (See Figure 8-6)

1. The male reproductive system is composed of paired testes, genital ducts, accessory glands, and penis.
2. The testes, or male gonads, are located in the scrotum, paired egg-shaped sacs located outside the abdominal cavity. They produce male sex hormones (testosterone) and spermatozoa (male germ cells).

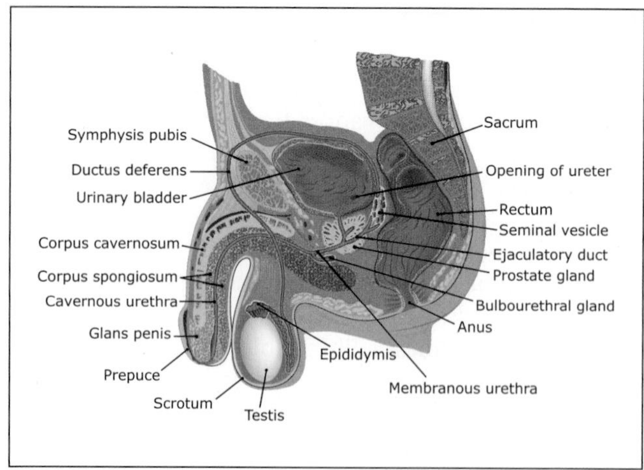

Figure 8-6 Male reproductive system.

3. The accessory glands (seminal vesicles, prostate gland, and bulbourethral glands) prepare sperm for ejaculation.
4. The ductal system (epididymides, vas deferens, and ejaculatory ducts) stores and transports sperm.
5. The urethra, enclosed in the penis, functions in the elimination of urine and semen.
6. Sperm production requires an environment that is 2°C–3°C lower than body temperature.
7. Testosterone and other male sex hormones (androgens).
   a. During development, induce differentiation of the male genital tract.
   b. Stimulate development of primary and secondary sex characteristics during puberty and maintain them during life.
   c. Promote protein metabolism, musculoskeletal growth, and subcutaneous fat distribution (anabolic effects).
8. The hypothalamus and anterior pituitary gland maintain endocrine via gonadotropic hormones (follicle-stimulating hormone [FSH] and luteinizing hormone [LH]).
   a. FSH initiates spermatogenesis.
   b. LH regulates testosterone production.

Disorders of the Male Reproductive System

Erectile Dysfunction (ED) (Impotence)

1. The inability to achieve and maintain erection for sexual intercourse.
2. Organic causes.
   a. Neurogenic causes: stroke, cerebral trauma, spinal cord injury, multiple sclerosis, Parkinson's disease.

b. Hormonal causes: decreased androgen levels with hypogonadism, hypothyroidism, and hypopituitarism.
c. Vascular causes: hypertension, coronary heart disease, hyperlipidemia, cigarette smoking, diabetes mellitus, pelvic irradiation.
d. Drug-induced: antidepressants, antipsychotics, antiandrogens, antihypertensives, amphetamines, alcohol.
e. Aging increases risk of ED.
3. Psychogenic causes.
a. Performance anxiety.
b. Depression and psychiatric disorders (schizophrenia).
4. Surgical causes.
a. Transurethral procedures.
b. Radical prostatectomy.
c. Proctocolectomy.
d. Abdominoperineal resection.
5. Treatment requires accurate identification and remediation of specific causes of ED.
6. Medications are available to improve function (e.g., sildenafil [Viagra]).

Testicular Cancer

1. Most common between the ages of 15–35 years of age.
2. Symptoms: lump or enlargement in testicle; ache in the groin or abdomen; enlargement of the breasts, low back pain that may or may not radiate to the groin.
3. Diagnosis: ultrasound; labs.
4. Medical intervention: Surgery is usually very successful (especially if diagnosed early).

Prostatitis

1. Infection and inflammation of the prostate gland.
2. Types include acute bacterial, chronic prostatitis, and nonbacterial.
a. Acute bacterial prostatitis involves bacterial urinary tract infection (UTI) and is associated with catheterization and multiple sex partners. Symptoms include urinary frequency, urgency, nocturia, dysuria, urethral discharge, fever and chills, malaise, myalgia and arthralgia, and pain.

> RED FLAG: Prostrate referral pain may include dull, aching pain in the low back, sacral, genital, and rectal regions.

b. Chronic prostatitis can also be bacterial in origin and is associated with recurrent UTI. Symptoms include urinary frequency and urgency, myalgia and arthralgia, and pain in the low back or perineal region.
c. Nonbacterial inflammatory prostatitis produces pain in the penis, testicles, and scrotum; painful ejaculation; low back pain or pain in the inner thighs; urinary symptoms; decreased libido; and impotence.
3. Because the prostate encircles the urethra, obstruction of urinary flow can result.

Benign Prostratic Hyperplasia (BPH)

1. Age-related nonmalignant enlargement of the prostate gland.
2. Risk factors: Age (1/3 of men have moderate to severe symptoms by age 60, 1/2 by age 80); obesity; diabetes and heart disease.
3. Symptoms: Frequent urination; nocturia; difficulty starting urination; weak stream; inability to completely empty the bladder with risk of developing UTIs, bladder stones, or damage.
4. Diagnosis: rectal exam; Labs-Prostate-specific antigen (PSA); urine flow test; ultrasound (pre/post-void).
5. Medical intervention: Medications; Minimally invasive surgery.

Prostrate Cancer

1. 2nd most common cause of male death from cancer; cancer that metastasizes to bone.
2. Risk Factors: Age (50% of men over 80 years); obesity; family history.
3. Symptoms: Early there are often no signs/symptoms; later stages symptoms similar to BPH but may also have blood in the urine/semen, bone and night pain, weight loss without trying; erectile dysfunction.
4. Diagnosis: similar to BPH but elevated PSA; ultrasound; biopsy; genomic testing; if concerns of metastasis bone scan/CT Scan/MRI/PET imaging.
5. Medical intervention: Surgery, radiation therapy; heating/freezing tissue; chemotherapy; immunotherapy.
6. Complications (from cancer and/or surgery): metastatis (often to the spine); erectile dysfunction, incontinence.

Renal and Urological Systems

Overview

Anatomy (See Figure 8-7)

1. Kidneys are paired, bean-shaped organs located outside of the peritoneal cavity (retroperitoneal) in the posterior upper abdomen on each side of the vertebral column at the level of T12–L2.
2. Each kidney is multilobular; each lobule is composed of more than 1 million nephrons (the functional units of the kidney).
3. Each nephron consists of a glomerulus that filters the blood and nephron tubules. Water, electrolytes, and other substances vital for function are reabsorbed into the bloodstream, while other waste products are secreted into the tubules for elimination.
4. The renal pelvis is a wide, funnel-shaped structure at the upper end of the urethra that drains the kidney into the lower urinary tract (bladder and urethra).
5. The bladder is a membranous sac that collects urine and is located behind the symphysis pubis.
6. The ureter extends from the renal pelvis to the bladder and moves urine via peristaltic action.
7. The urethra extends from the bladder to an external orifice for elimination of urine from the body.
8. In females, proximity of the urethra to vaginal and rectal openings increases the likelihood of UTI.

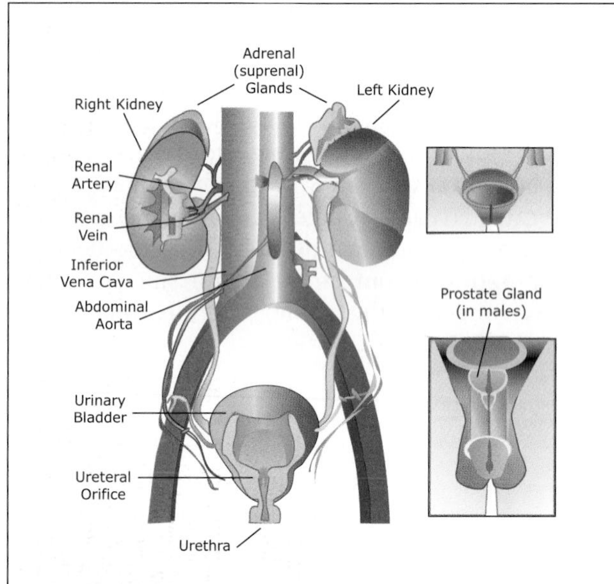

Figure 8-7 Renal and urological system anterior view.

Functions of the Kidney

1. Regulates the composition and pH of body fluids through reabsorption and elimination; controls mineral (sodium, potassium, hydrogen, chloride, and bicarbonate ions) and water balance.
2. Eliminates metabolic wastes (urea, uric acid, creatinine) and drugs/drug metabolites.
3. Assists in blood pressure regulation through rennin-angiotensin-aldosterone mechanisms and salt and water elimination.
4. Contributes to bone metabolic function by activating vitamin D and regulating calcium and phosphate conservation and elimination.
5. Controls the production of red blood cells in the bone marrow through the production of erythropoietin.
6. The glomerular filtration rate (GFR) is the amount of filtrate that is formed each minute as blood moves through the glomeruli and serves as an important gauge of renal function.
   a. Regulated by arterial blood pressure and renal blood flow.
   b. Measured clinically by obtaining creatinine levels in blood and urine samples.
   c. Normal creatinine clearance is 115–125 mL/min.
7. Blood urea nitrogen (BUN) is urea produced in the liver as a by-product of protein metabolism that is eliminated by the kidneys.
   a. BUN levels are elevated with increased protein intake, gastrointestinal bleeding, and dehydration.
   b. BUN-creatinine ratio is abnormal in liver disease.

Normal Values of Urine (Urinalysis Findings)

1. Color: yellow-amber.
2. Clarity: clear.
3. Specific gravity: 1.010–1.025 with normal fluid intake.
4. pH: 4.6–8.0; average is 6 (acid).
5. Protein: 0–8 mg/dL.
6. Sugar: 0.

Urinary Regulation of Fluids and Electrolytes

Homeostasis

1. Regulated through thirst mechanisms and renal function via circulating antidiuretic hormone (ADH).

Fluid Imbalances

1. Daily fluid requirements vary based on presence or absence of such factors as sweating, air temperature, and fever.

2. Dehydration: excessive loss of body fluids; fluid output exceeds fluid intake.
   a. Causes: poor intake; excess output: profuse sweating, vomiting, diarrhea, and diuretics; closely linked to sodium deficiency.
   b. Observe for poor skin turgor, dry mucous membranes, headache, irritability, postural hypotension, incoordination, lethargy, disorientation.
   c. May lead to uremia and hypovolemic shock (stupor and coma).
   d. Decreased exercise capacity, especially in hot environments.
3. Edema: an excess of body fluids with expansion of interstitial fluid volume.
   a. Causes.
      - Increased capillary pressure: heart failure, kidney disease, premenstrual retention, pregnancy, environmental heat stress; venous obstruction (liver disease, acute pulmonary edema, venous thrombosis).
      - Decreased colloidal osmotic pressure: decreased production or loss of plasma proteins (protein-losing kidney disease, liver disease, starvation, malnutrition).
      - Increased capillary permeability: inflammation, allergic reactions, malignancy, tissue injury, burns.
      - Obstruction of lymphatic flow.
   b. Observe for swelling of the ankles and feet, weight gain; headache, blurred vision; muscle cramps and twitches.
      - Edema can be restrictive, producing a tourniquet effect.
      - Tissues are susceptible to injury and delayed healing.
      - Pitting edema occurs when the amount of interstitial fluid exceeds the absorptive capacity of tissues.

Potassium

1. Normal serum level is 3.5–5.5 mEq/L.
2. Hypokalemia.
   a. Causes: deficient potassium or excessive loss due to diarrhea, vomiting, metabolic acidosis or alkalosis, renal tubular disease.
   b. Observe for muscle weakness, aches, fatigue; abdominal distention; nausea; and vomiting.
   c. ECG changes: increased size of P wave, flattened or inverted T wave, ST depression, prominent U waves; can progress to supraventricular and life-threatening ventricular arrhythmias.
3. Hyperkalemia.
   a. Causes: inadequate secretion with acute renal failure, kidney disease, metabolic acidosis, diabetic ketoacidosis, sickle cell anemia, SLE.
   b. Often symptomless until very high levels. Observe for muscle weakness.
   c. ECG changes: tall T wave, prolonged P-R interval and QRS duration, arrhythmias.

Sodium

1. Normal serum level is 135–146 mEq/L.
2. Hyponatremia.
   a. Causes: water intoxication (excess extracellular water) associated with excess intake or excess ADH (tumors, endocrine disorders).
   b. Observe for confusion; decreased mental alertness can progress to convulsions; signs of increased intracerebral pressure; poor motor coordination; sleepiness; anorexia.
3. Hypernatremia.
   a. Causes: occurs with water deficits (not salt excesses) with dehydration, insufficient water intake.
   b. Observe for circulatory congestion (pitting edema, excessive weight gain); pulmonary edema with dyspnea; hypertension, tachycardia; agitation, restlessness, convulsions.

Calcium

1. Normal total calcium in blood is 8.4–10.4 mg/dL.
2. Hypocalcemia.
   a. Causes: reduced albumin levels, hyperphosphatemia, hypoparathyroidism, malabsorption of calcium and vitamin D, alkalosis, acute pancreatitis, vitamin D deficiency.
   b. Observe for muscle cramps, tetany, spasms; paresthesias; anxiety, irritability, twitching convulsion; arrhythmias, hypotension.
3. Hypercalcemia.
   a. Causes: hyperparathyroidism, tumors, hyperthyroidism, vitamin A intoxication.
   b. Observe for fatigue, depression, mental confusion, nausea/vomiting, increased urination, occasional cardiac arrhythmias.

Magnesium

1. Normal serum level is 1.8–2.4 mg/dL.
2. Hypomagnesemia.
   a. Causes: hemodialysis, blood transfusions, chronic renal disease, hepatic cirrhosis (alcoholism), chronic pancreatitis, hypoparathyroidism, malabsorption syndromes, severe burns, excess loss of body fluid.
   b. Observe for hyperirritability, confusion; leg and foot cramps.
3. Hypermagnesemia.
   a. Causes: renal failure, diabetic acidosis, hypothyroidism, Addison's disease, with dehydration and with use of antacids.
   b. Observe for hyporeflexia, muscle weakness, drowsiness, lethargy, confusion, bradycardia, hypotension.

Acid-Base Balance

1. Balance of acids and bases in the body (normally a ratio of 20 base to 1 acid; normal serum pH is 7.35–7.45 [slightly alkaline]); regulated by blood buffer systems (the lungs and the kidneys).

2. Metabolic acidosis: a depletion of bases or an accumulation of acids; blood pH falls below 7.35.
   a. Causes: diabetes, renal insufficiency or failure, diarrhea.
   b. Observe for hyperventilation (compensatory), deep respirations; weakness, muscular twitching; malaise, nausea, vomiting, and diarrhea; headache; dry skin and mucous membranes, poor skin turgor.
   c. May lead to stupor and coma (death).
3. Metabolic alkalosis: an increase in bases or a reduction of acids; blood pH rises above 7.45.
   a. Causes: excess vomiting, excess diuretics, hypokalemia; peptic ulcer, and excessive intake of antacids.
   b. Observe for hypoventilation (compensatory), depressed respirations; dysrhythmias; prolonged vomiting, diarrhea; weakness, muscle twitching; irritability, agitation, convulsions and coma (death).
4. Respiratory acidosis: CO2 retention, impaired alveolar ventilation.
   a. Causes: hypoventilation, drugs/oversedation, chronic pulmonary disease (e.g., emphysema, asthma, bronchitis, pneumonia) or hypermetabolism (sepsis, burns).
   b. Observe for dyspnea, hyperventilation cyanosis; restlessness, headache.
   c. May lead to disorientation, stupor and coma, death.
5. Respiratory alkalosis: diminished CO2, alveolar hyperventilation.
   a. Causes: anxiety attack with hyperventilation, hypoxia (emphysema, pneumonia), impaired lung expansion, congestive heart failure (CHF), pulmonary embolism, diffuse liver or CNS disease, salicylate poisoning, extreme stress (stimulation of respiratory center).
   b. Observe for tachypnea, dizziness, anxiety, difficulty concentrating, numbness and tingling, blurred vision, diaphoresis, muscle cramps, twitching or tetany, weakness, arrhythmias, convulsions.

Renal and Urological Disorders

Urinary Tract Infections (UTIs)

1. Infection of the urinary tract with microorganisms.
2. Lower UTI: cystitis (inflammation and infection of the bladder) or urethritis (inflammation and infection of the urethra).
   a. Usually secondary to ascending urinary tract infections; may also involve kidneys and ureters.
   b. Associated with symptoms of urinary frequency, urgency, burning sensation during urination. Urine may be cloudy and foul smelling. Pain is noted in suprapubic, lower abdominal, or groin area, depending on site of infection.
3. Upper UTI: pyelonephritis (inflammation and infection of one or both kidneys).
   a. Associated with symptoms of systemic involvement: fever, chills, malaise, headache, tenderness and pain over kidneys (back pain), tenderness over the costovertebal angle (Murphy's sign). Symptoms also include frequent and burning urination; nausea and vomiting may occur.
   b. Palpitation or percussion over the kidney typically causes pain.
   c. Can be acute or chronic; generally more serious than lower UTI.
4. Increased risk of UTI in persons with autoimmunity, urinary obstruction and reflux, neurogenic bladder and catheterization, diabetes, and kidney transplantation. Older adults and women are also at increased risk for UTI.

Renal Cystic Disease

1. Renal cysts are fluid-filled cavities that form along the nephron and can lead to renal degeneration or obstruction.
2. Types include polycystic, medullary sponge, acquired, and simple renal cysts.
3. Symptoms can include pain, hematuria, and hypertension. Fever can occur with associated infection. Cysts can rupture, producing hematuria. Simple cysts are generally asymptomatic.

Obstructive Disorders

1. Developmental defects, renal calculi, prostatic hyperplasia or cancer, scar tissue from inflammation, tumors, and infection.
2. Pressure build-up backward from site of obstruction; can result in kidney damage. Dilation of ureters and renal pelves may be used to reduce obstruction. Observe for pain, signs and symptoms of UTI and hypertension.
3. Renal calculi (kidney stones): crystalline structures formed from normal components of urine (calcium, magnesium ammonium phosphate, uric acid, and cystine).
   a. Etiological influences include concentration of stone components in urine and a urinary environment conducive to stone formation.
   b. Symptoms include renal colic pain (pain from a stone lodged in the ureter made worse by stretching the collecting system). Pain may radiate to the lower abdominal quadrant, bladder area, and perineal area (scrotum in the male and labia in the female). Nausea and vomiting are common and the skin may be cool and clammy.
   c. Extracorporeal shock wave lithotripsy (ESWL) is used to break up stones into fragments to allow for easy passage.
   d. Treatment/prevention can also include increased fluid intake, thiazide diuretics, dietary restriction of foods high in oxalate, acidification or alkalinization of urine depending on type of stone.

Renal Failure

1. Acute renal failure: sudden loss of kidney function with resulting elevation in serum urea and creatinine.
   a. Etiology: may be due to circulatory disruption to kidneys, toxic substances, bacterial toxins, acute obstruction, rhabdomyolysis, or trauma.
2. Chronic renal failure: progressive loss of kidney function leading to end-stage failure.
   a. Etiology: may result from prolonged acute urinary tract obstruction and infection, diabetes, SLE, uncontrolled hypertension.
   b. Uremia: an end-stage toxic condition resulting from renal insufficiency and retention of nitrogenous wastes in blood; symptoms can include anorexia, nausea, and mental confusion.
3. Dialysis: process of diffusing blood across a semipermeable membrane for the purposes of removal of toxic substances; maintains fluid, electrolyte and acid-base balance in presence of renal failure; peritoneal, or renal (hemodialysis).
   a. Dialysis disequilibrium: symptoms of nausea, vomiting, drowsiness, headache, and seizures; the result of rapid changes after beginning dialysis.
   b. Dialysis dementia: signs of cerebral dysfunction (e.g., speech difficulties, mental confusion, myoclonus, seizures, eventually death); the result of long-standing years of dialysis treatment.

> RED FLAG: Taking BP on the vascular access arm of a dialysis patient is contraindicated. Avoid trauma to the area of peritoneal catheter (peritoneal dialysis is used with patients in kidney failure).

   c. Examine for multisystem dysfunction: vital signs, strength, sensation, ROM, function, and endurance.
4. Transplantation is a major treatment choice (renal allograft).

Renal Cancer

1. Risk factors: smoking, high blood pressure, males, African-Americans, family history of renal cancer, advanced kidney disease.
2. Symptoms: flank pain, hematuria, fatigue, unexplained weight loss.

Bladder Cancer

1. Risk factors: smoking, work place exposures (textiles, rubber, leather, paint), not drinking enough fluid, older than 55 years old, males, previous radiation/chemotherapy, family history.

Urinary Incontinence

1. Inability to retain urine; the result of loss of sphincter control; may be acute (due to transient causes, e.g., cystitis) or persistent (e.g., stroke, dementia).
2. Types.
   a. Stress incontinence: sudden release of urine due to:
      - Increases in intra-abdominal pressure, e.g., coughing, laughing, exercise, straining, obesity.
      - Weakness and laxity of pelvic floor musculature, sphincter weakness, e.g., postpartum incontinence, menopause, damage to pudendal nerve.
   b. Urge incontinence: bladder begins contracting and urine is leaked after sensation of bladder fullness is perceived; an inability to delay voiding to reach toilet due to:
      - Detrusor muscle instability or hyperreflexia, e.g., stroke.
      - Sensory instability: hypersensitive bladder.
   c. Overflow incontinence: bladder continuously leaks secondary to urinary retention (an overdistended bladder or incomplete emptying of bladder) due to:
      - Anatomical obstruction, e.g., prostate enlargement.
      - Acontractile bladder, e.g., spinal cord injury, diabetes.
      - Neurogenic bladder, e.g., multiple sclerosis, suprasacral spinal lesions.
   d. Functional incontinence: leakage associated with inability or unwillingness to toilet due to:
      - Impaired cognition (dementia); depression, e.g., Alzheimer's type dementia.
      - Impaired physical functioning, e.g., stroke.
      - Environmental barriers.
3. Management.
   a. Dietary management: control of food and beverages that aggravate the bladder or incontinence (e.g., citrus fruit or juices, caffeine, chocolate); control fluid intake.
   b. Medical management.
      - Identify and treat acute, reversible problems, e.g., cystometry.
      - Drug therapy for urge, stress, and overflow incontinence, e.g., estrogen with phenylpropanolamine.
      - Control of medications that may aggravate incontinence, e.g., diuretics for CHF, anticholinergic or psychotropic drugs.
      - Catheterization: used for overflow incontinence and other types if unresponsive to other treatments and skin integrity is threatened; associated with high rates of urinary tract infection.
      - Surgery: bladder neck suspension, removal of prostate obstructions; suprapubic cystostomy.
   c. Bladder training: prompted voiding to restore a pattern of voiding.
      - Involves toileting schedule: taking patient to bathroom at regular intervals.
      - May also include intermittent catheterization, e.g., for patients with overdistention, persistent retention (e.g., multiple sclerosis).
4. Examination.
   a. Symptoms of incontinence: onset and duration, urgency, frequency, timing of episodes/causative factors.

b. Strength of pelvic floor muscles using a perineometer.
c. Functional mobility, environmental factors.

5. Physical therapy goals, outcomes, and interventions for stress and urge incontinence.
   a. Teach pelvic floor muscle exercises (pubococcygeus muscle): used to treat stress incontinence.
      - Kegel's exercises: active, strengthening exercises; type 1 works on holding contractions, progressing to 10-second holds, rest 10 seconds between contractions; type 2 works on quick contractions, 10–80 repetitions a day. Avoid squeezing buttocks or contracting abdominals (bearing down).
      - Functional electrical stimulation: for muscle reeducation if patient is unable to initiate active contractions.
      - Biofeedback: uses pressure recordings to reinforce active contractions, relax bladder.
      - Progressive strengthening: use of weighted vaginal cones for home exercises or pelvic floor exerciser.
      - Incorporating Kegel's exercise into everyday life: e.g., with lifting, coughing, changing positions.
   b. Provide behavioral training.
      - Record keeping: patients are asked to keep a history of their voiding (voiding diary).
      - Education: regarding anatomy, physiology, reasons for muscle weakness, incontinence; avoidance of Valsalva's maneuver, heavy resistance exercises.
   c. Functional mobility training as needed. Ensure independence in sit-to-stand transitions, ambulation and safe toilet transfers.
   d. Environmental modifications as needed: e.g., toilet rails, raised toilet seat or commode.
   e. Maintain adequate skin condition.
      - Teach appropriate skin care, maintain toileting schedule.
      - Adequate protection: adult diapers, underpads.
   f. Provide psychological support: emotional and social consequences of incontinence are significant.

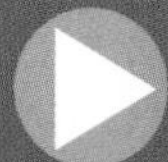

Endocrine and Metabolic Systems

Overview of the Endocrine System (See Table 8-2)

Hormonal Regulation (See Figure 8-8)

1. The endocrine system uses hormones (chemical messengers) to relay information to cells and organs and regulate many of the body functions (digestion, use of nutrients, growth and development, electrolyte and water balance, and reproductive functions).
2. The hypothalamus and pituitary gland, along with the nervous system, make up the central network that exerts control over many other glands in the body with wide-ranging functions. Endocrine functions are also closely linked with the immune system.
3. Hormones bind to specific receptor sites that are linked to specific systems and functions.
4. The hypothalamus controls release of pituitary hormones (corticotropin-releasing hormone [CRH], thyrotropin-releasing hormone [TRH], growth hormone–releasing hormone [GHRH], and somatostatin).
5. The anterior pituitary gland controls the release of growth hormone (GH), adrenocorticotropic hormone (ACTH), follicle-stimulating hormone (FSH), luteinizing hormone (LH), and prolactin.
6. The posterior pituitary gland controls the release of antidiuretic hormone (ADH) and oxytocin.

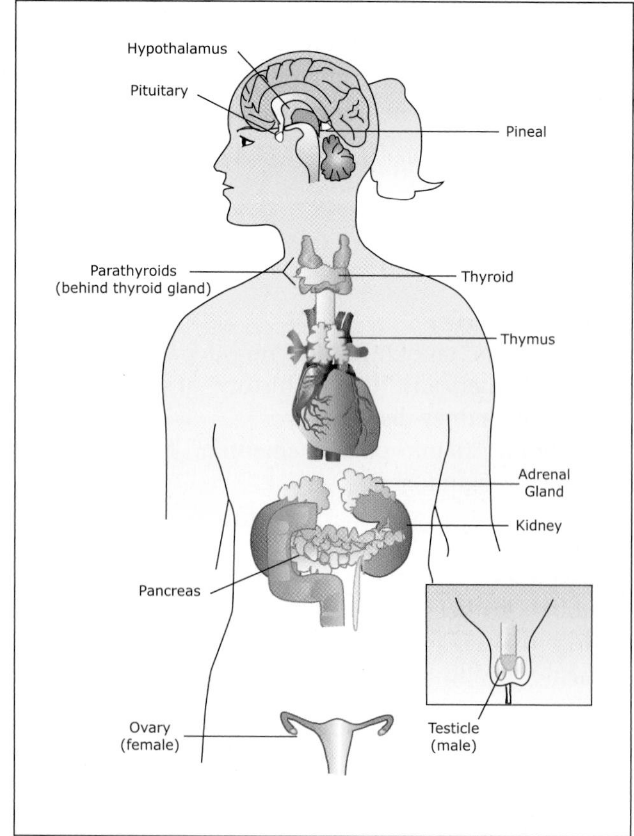

Figure 8-8 **Endocrine system anterior view.**

Table 8-2

Common Endocrine Disorders, Findings, and PT Implications

ENDOCRINE DISORDER-PATHOLOGY	SIGNS/SYMPTOMS/SECONDARY HEALTH CONDITIONS	PT IMPLICATIONS
Diabetes Mellitus Deficient or defective insulin action leading to hyperglycemia	• See Boxes 8-1 and 8-2 • Acute: excessive thirst/urination, fatigue, weight loss, vision problems, headaches/dizziness • Chronic: neuropathy, retinopathy, nephropathy, atherosclerosis (small and large vessels)	Exercise-related complications (see Box 8-3) • >300 mg/dl: postpone exercise session; adjust insulin • <100 mg/dl: snack and retest before exercising • Closely monitor blood pressure if retinopathy, hypertension • Distal sensory screening for neuropathy
Hyperthyroidism ↑ secretion of thyroid hormones Grave's Disease: 85% of cases; autoimmune with autoantibodies, thyroid-stimulating immunoglobulins (TSIs) ↑ T4 production ↑ sympathetic activity	• Female, age 20–40 years • Weight loss, fatigue, excessive sweating, diarrhea, palpitations, hyperreflexia, tremor, and exophthalmos • Atrial fibrillation, congestive heart failure, and myocardial infarction	Exercise intolerance and reduced exercise capacity Thyrotoxicosis can aggravate preexisting heart disease
Hypothyroidism ↓ secretion of thyroid hormones Type 1 (↓ hormone secretion with gland dysfunction); vast majority of cases Type 2 (↓ release of thyroid stimulating and releasing hormones)	• Female; age 30–60 years • Weight gain, hair loss, fatigue, bradycardia, constipation, anemia, carpal tunnel syndrome, fibromyalgia, depression • Chronic: forgetfulness, myxedema (excessive swelling of the body), coma/death	Exercise intolerance with fatigue, weakness, myalgias, and risk of rhabdomyolysis if excessive progression of exercise After long-term medication at risk for pseudogout, osteoporosis, and atrial fibrillation
Hyperparathyroidism ↑ secretion of parathyroid hormone -> hypercalcemia (in blood/urine) impacts multiple systems (musculoskeletal, kidneys, GI, and central nervous system [CNS])	• Female, >60 years of age • Bone decalcification-pain/pathologic fractures • Weakness/fatigue • Joint hypermobility • Peptic ulcers, pancreatitis • Renal calculi, renal failure • CNS: Memory, depression, personality changes	Bone pain (especially spine) Appropriate weight-bearing secondary fracture risk Care with joint mobilization Proper hydration and monitor for fatigue
Hypoparathyroidism ↓ secretion of parathyroid hormone -> hypocalcemia (in blood/urine) results in pronounced neuromuscular, CNS, and cardiac impairments	• Muscle weakness, pain, and tetany • Trousseau sign (carpal spasm) • Chvostek sign (facial spasm) • Cardiac arrythmias • Seizures	Acute: Life threatening; immediate emergency care Chronic: Hyperventilation may worsen tetany; focus on breathing during exercise Cardiac complications may occur; careful monitoring of vital signs
Hypercortisolism **Cushing's Syndrome:** ↑ cortisol production by adrenal gland or an excess of corticosteroid medication. **Cushing's Disease:** Pituitary tumor results in ↑ adrenocorticotropic hormone (ACTH)	• Sxs: Moon-shaped face; dorsocervical fat pad; truncal obesity, slender limbs; thinning of the skin-striae, hair loss, bruise easily • Myopathy • Hyperglycemia (see Box 8-2) • Hypertension and edema • Osteoporosis	Caution secondary to impaired wound healing/bruise easily Closely monitor resistance exercise for muscle pain or increased weakness Slow progressive weight-bearing and precautions with mobilization secondary to osteoporosis
Adrenal Insufficiency ↓ or absent adrenocortical function with ↓ cortisol/aldosterone **Primary: Addison's Disease** (dysfunction in the gland); autoimmune, infection, neoplasm **Secondary:** ↓ in releasing or trophic hormones; hypothalamic or pituitary tumor or rapid withdrawal corticosteroid drugs	• Cortisol Sxs: Personality changes; bronze skin pigmentation; hypoglycemia with associated symptoms (see Box 8-1), susceptible to infections • Aldosterone Sxs: ↑ Na^{++} excretion-dehydration, hypotension, diarrhea, abdominal pain	Slow progression of exercise and monitor vitals Fall risk secondary to hypoglycemia and orthostatic hypotension

Reference: Goodman C, Fuller K. Pathology: Implications for the Physical Therapist, 5th ed. St Louis, Elsevier, 2020.

7. The adrenal cortex controls the release of mineral corticosteroids (aldosterone), glucocorticoids (cortisol), adrenal androgens (dehydroepiandrosterone [DHEA]), and androstenedione.
8. The adrenal medulla controls the release of epinephrine and norepinephrine.
9. The thyroid controls the release of triiodothyronine and thyroxine. Thyroid C cells control the release of calcitonin.
10. The parathyroid glands control the release of parathyroid hormone (PTH).
11. The pancreatic islet cells control the release of insulin, glucagons, and somatostatin.
12. The kidney controls the release of 1,25-dihydroxyvitamin D.
13. The ovaries control the release of estrogen and progesterone.
14. The testes control the release of androgens (testosterone).

Overview of the Metabolic System

Glucose Control

1. Normal glucose control is the result of nutrient, neural, and hormonal regulation.

Hormones. Released by Islets of Langerhans in Pancreas

1. Insulin: allows uptake of glucose from the bloodstream; suppresses hepatic glucose production, lowering plasma glucose levels. Secreted by the beta cells.
2. Glucagon: stimulates hepatic glucose production to raise glucose levels, especially in fasting state. Secreted by the alpha cells.
3. Amylin: modulates rate of nutrient delivery (gastric emptying); suppresses release of glucagon. Secreted by the beta cells.
4. Somatostatin: acts locally to depress secretion of both insulin and glycogen; decreases motility of stomach, duodenum, and gallbladder; decreases secretion and absorption of GI tract. Secreted by the delta cells.

Metabolic Syndrome (Syndrome X)

Characteristics

1. The name for a group of risk factors that raises the risk for heart disease, stroke, and diabetes.

Metabolic Risk Factors

1. Diagnosis requires presence of three or more of the following:
2. Abdominal obesity: large waist size: For men: 40 inches or larger; for women: 35 inches or larger.
3. High triglyceride level: 150 mg/dl or higher or using a cholesterol medicine.
4. Cholesterol: low HDL cholesterol; for men, less than 40 mg/dL; for women: less than 50 mg/dL or using a cholesterol medicine.
5. High blood pressure: systolic BP 135 mmHg or higher and/or diastolic pressure 85 mmHg or higher.
6. Blood sugar: fasting plasma glucose level 100 mg/dL or higher.

Etiology

1. No one cause, due to a collection of risk factors.
2. Unhealthy lifestyle: diet high in fats; low levels of physical activity.
3. Occurs with certain diseases and hormonal imbalance.

Incidence

1. May affect as many as one in four adults.
2. More common in older adults and individuals prone to blood clots and inflammation.
3. May run in families.

Treatment: Management of Risk Factors

1. Lifestyle changes can reverse or reduce the chance of developing metabolic syndrome: healthy diet, weight loss, exercise, smoking cessation.
2. Medications to control cholesterol, blood pressure, or diabetes (glucose intolerance).

Diabetes Mellitus (DM)

Characteristics

1. A complex disorder of carbohydrate, fat, and protein metabolism caused by deficiency or absence of insulin secretion by the beta cells of the pancreas or by defects of the insulin receptors. Causes an abnormally high level of sugar or glucose in the blood.
2. May be acquired, familial, idiopathic, neurogenic, or nephrogenic. Possible viral/autoimmune and genetic etiology.

Types

1. Type 1 diabetes mellitus (T1DM); also known as insulin-dependent, juvenile-onset diabetes. Affects about 1% of the population and 10% of all people with diabetes. Characteristics include:
   a. Decrease in size and number of islet cells resulting in absolute deficiency in insulin secretion.
   b. Initially occurs in children and young adults. Long preclinical period, often with abrupt onset of symptoms around the age of puberty.

c. Etiology: caused by autoimmune abnormalities, genetic causes, or environmental causes.
d. Insulin-dependent: requires insulin delivery by injection, insulin pump, or inhalation.
e. Prone to ketoacidosis. Presence of ketone bodies in the urine, the by-products of fat metabolism (ketonuria).

2. Type 2 diabetes mellitus (T2DM) results from inadequate utilization of insulin (insulin resistance) and progressive beta cell dysfunction; also known as non-insulin dependent or adult-onset diabetes. Represents 90%–95% of DM cases. Characteristics include:
   a. Gradual onset.
   b. Usually not insulin dependent.
   c. Individual is not prone to ketoacidosis (may form ketones with stress).
   d. Etiology: a progressive disease caused by a combination of factors, including:
      - Insulin resistance in muscle and adipose tissue.
      - Progressive decline in pancreatic insulin production.
      - Excessive hepatic glucose production.
      - Inappropriate glucagon secretion.
   e. Risk factors.
      - Linked to obesity and older adults (significant risk factor over the age of 45). Increased incidence in obese children. Can occur in nonobese individuals with increased percentage of body fat in the abdominal region.
      - Family history of diabetes.
      - Unhealthy eating patterns.
      - Lack of physical activity.
3. Secondary diabetes: associated with other conditions (pancreatic disease or removal of pancreatic tissue), endocrine disease (e.g., acromegaly, Cushing's syndrome, pheochromocytoma), drugs (e.g., some diuretics, diazoxide, glucocorticoids, levodopa), and chemical agents.
4. Gestational diabetes mellitus (GDM): glucose intolerance (high blood sugar) associated with pregnancy; most likely in third trimester. Affects approximately 4% of pregnancies.
5. Prediabetes: impaired glucose tolerance (IGT) with abnormal response to oral glucose test; 10%–15% of individuals will convert to type 2 diabetes within 10 years.

Signs and Symptoms

1. Elevated blood sugar (hyperglycemia).
2. Elevated sugar in urine (glycosuria).
3. Excessive excretion of urine (polyuria).
4. Excessive thirst (polydipsia), dry mouth.
5. Excessive hunger (polyphagia) especially after eating.
6. Unexplained weight loss.
7. Fatigue.
8. Blurred vision, headaches.

Complications of DM

1. Microvascular disease.
   a. Retinopathy.
   b. Renal disease.
   c. Polyneuropathy.
2. Macrovascular disease: dyslipidemia (accelerated atherosclerosis).
   a. Cerebrovascular accident (CVA, stroke).
   b. Myocardial infarction (MI).
   c. Peripheral arterial disease (PAD).
3. Integumentary impairments: including degenerative connective tissue changes; slow healing of sores or cuts, anhidrosis; increased risk of ulcers and infections.
4. Musculoskeletal impairments.
   a. Joint stiffness and increased risk of contractures.
   b. Increased risk of adhesive capsulitis of shoulder, tenosynovitis, plantar fasciitis.
   c. Increased risk of osteoporosis.
5. Neuromuscular impairments.
   a. Diabetic polyneuropathy.
      - Symmetrical numbness and tingling of the hands and feet (stocking and glove distribution).
      - Distal (long nerves first) progressing to proximal.
      - Altered sensations; paresthesias, shooting pain; loss of protective sensations.
      - Motor weakness: foot/ankle weakness initially with balance and gait impairments.
   b. Diabetic autonomic neuropathy (DAN).
      - Cardiovascular autonomic neuropathy (CAN): resting tachycardia; exercise intolerance with abnormal HR, BP, and cardiac output responses; exercise-induced hypoglycemia; postural hypotension.
      - Integumentary: anhidrosis, abnormal sweating, dry skin, heat intolerance.
      - Gastrointestinal: gastroparesis, GERD, diarrhea, constipation.
      - Metabolic: abnormal or delayed responses to hypoglycemia; lack of awareness of hypoglycemia.
   c. Mononeuropathies: focal nerve damage resulting from vasculitis with ischemia and infarction.
   d. Entrapment neuropathies: resulting from repetitive trauma to superficial nerves.
6. Kidney impairments, including kidney failure.
7. Vision impairments, including diabetic retinopathy (associated with chronic hyperglycemia) and diabetic macular edema.
8. Liver impairments, including fatty liver disease (steatosis).

Diagnostic Criteria for DM

1. Symptoms of diabetes plus casual plasma glucose concentration ≥200 mg/dL (11.1 mmol/L). Casual is defined as nonfasting any time of day, without regard to time since last meal.

Chapter 8 OTH

2. Fasting plasma glucose (FPG) ≥126 mg/dL (7 mmol/L). Fasting is defined as no caloric intake for at least 8 hours.
3. 2-hour postload glucose ≥200 mg/dL (11.1 mmol/L) during an oral glucose tolerance test (OGTT). OGTT, as described by the World Health Organization, uses a glucose load containing the equivalent of 75 g anhydrous glucose dissolved in water.
4. The A1c test measures average blood glucose for the past 2–3 months. Normal is less than 5.7%; prediabetes is 5.7% to 6.4%; diabetes is diagnosed at an A1c of greater than or equal to 6.5%.

Medical Goals and Interventions

1. Maintain insulin glucose homeostasis.
   a. Frequent monitoring of blood glucose levels.
   b. Dietary control: weight reduction, control of carbohydrate, protein, fat, and calorie intake.
   c. Oral hypoglycemic agents to lower blood glucose; indicated for type 2 diabetes.
   d. Insulin to lower blood glucose via injections, infusion pump, or intraperitoneal dialysis for patients with renal failure. Indicated for type 1 diabetes or for more severe type 2 diabetes.
   e. Maintenance of normal lipid levels.
   f. Control of hypertension.
2. Exercise and physical fitness.
3. Health promotion.

Physical Therapy Goals, Outcomes, and Interventions

1. Exercise.
   a. Outcomes of regular exercise include improved glucose tolerance, increased insulin sensitivity, decreased glycosylated hemoglobin, and decreased insulin requirements. Additional outcomes include improved lipid profiles, BP reduction, weight management, increased physical work capacity, and improved well-being.
   b. Response to exercise is dependent upon adequacy of disease control.
2. Exercise testing is recommended prior to exercise due to increased cardiovascular risk.
3. Exercise prescription—Cardiovascular training—ACSM Guidelines for Exercise Testing and Prescription, 2021.
   a. Intensity: 50%–80% of maximal oxygen uptake (VO2 max) or heart rate reserve (HRR) corresponding to rating of perceived exertion (RPE) of 12–16 on the 6–20 Borg scale.
   b. Frequency: 3–7 days/week.
   c. Duration: 20–60 minutes.
   d. Type: rhythmic, large muscle activity: biking, treadmill walking, overground walking.
4. Exercise prescription: resistance training (ACSM Guidelines for Exercise Testing and Prescription, 2021).
   a. Frequency: 2–3 days/week.
   b. Intensity: resistance 60%–80% of one repetition max, 2–3 sets of 8–12 repetitions.
   c. Type: multijoint exercises of major muscle groups.
   d. Proper technique: minimize sustained gripping, static work, and Valsalva's maneuver (essential to decrease risk of hypertensive response).
5. Flexibility exercises.
6. Balance exercises.

See Boxes 8-1, 8-2, and 8-3 for Signs or Symptoms of Hypoglycemia, Hyperglycemia, and Exercise Precautions

1. With peripheral neuropathy emphasize proper diabetic foot care: good footwear, hygiene.
2. Patient and family education.
   a. Control of risk factors (obesity, physical inactivity, prolonged stress, and smoking).
   b. Dietary intervention strategies.
   c. Injury prevention strategies.
   d. Self-management strategies.

Obesity

Obesity

1. A condition characterized by excess body fat.

Body Mass Index (BMI)

1. Formula for determining obesity.
2. BMI is calculated by dividing an individual's weight in kilograms by the square of the person's height in meters.
3. Criteria: World Health Organization classification (adopted by National Institutes of Health):
   a. Overweight is defined as a BMI ranging from 25 to 29.9.
   b. Obesity is defined as a BMI ≥30.
   c. Morbid obesity is defined as a BMI >40.
4. Measurement by skin calipers using a fold of skin and subcutaneous fat from various body locations (midbiceps, midtriceps, and subscapular or inguinal areas). Greater than 1 inch is indicative of excess body fat.

Scope of Problem

1. A national health problem: 39.8% of U.S. adults are obese; for children and adolescents age 2–19, the prevalence of obesity is 18.5% (CDC Obesity Facts, 2017).
2. Health risks associated with obesity: hypertension, hyperlipidemia, type 2 diabetes, cardiovascular disease, stroke, glucose intolerance, gallbladder disease, menstrual irregularities and infertility, and cancer (endometrium, breast, prostate, colon).

BOX 8-1 Signs and Symptoms of Hypoglycemia (Low Blood Sugar)

Glucose is low: <70 mg/dL or a rapid drop in glucose
Onset is rapid (minutes)

Early signs and symptoms:

Pallor

Shakiness/trembling

Sweating

Excessive hunger

Tachycardia and palpitations

Fainting or feeling faint

Dizziness

Fatigue and weakness

Poor coordination and unsteady gait

Late signs and symptoms:

Nervousness and irritability

Headache

Blurred or double vision

Slurred speech

Drowsiness

Inability to concentrate, confusion, delusions

Loss of consciousness and coma

Response: If patient is awake, provide sugar (juice, candy bar, glucose tablets, and gel).

If patient unresponsive, seek immediate medical treatment; glucagon injection or intravenous glucose is required.

BOX 8-2 Signs and Symptoms of Hyperglycemia (Abnormally High Blood Sugar)

Glucose is high: >300 mg/dL. Gradual onset (days).

Weakness

Increased thirst

Dry mouth

Frequent, scant urination

Decreased appetite, nausea/vomiting, abdominal tenderness

Dulled senses, confusion, diminished reflexes, paresthesias

Flushed, signs of dehydration

Deep, rapid respirations

Pulse: rapid, weak

Fruity odor to the breath (acetone breath)

Hyperglycemic coma

Response: Seek immediate medical treatment.

BOX 8-3 Exercise Precautions for Individuals with Diabetes Mellitus

Monitor glucose levels prior to and following exercise.

Hypoglycemia is the most common problem for patients with diabetes who exercise.

- Observe for signs and symptom of hypoglycemia (Box 8-1). Do not exercise if blood glucose is <70 mg/dL. Provide carbohydrate snack initially (15 g of carbohydrate); have readily available during exercise (15 g carbohydrate for every hour of intense activity).
- Hypoglycemia associated with exercise may last as long as 48 hours after exercise. To prevent postexercise hypoglycemia, monitor plasma glucose levels and ingest carbohydrates as needed.

Hyperglycemia: Do not exercise when blood glucose levels are high (fasting glucose >300 mg/dL) or poorly controlled (ketosis is present with urine test) (Box 8-2).

Do not exercise without eating at least 2 hours before exercise.

Do not exercise without adequate hydration. Maintain hydration during exercise session.

Do not exercise alone. Exercise with a partner or under supervision.

Do not inject short-acting insulin in exercising muscles or sites close to exercising muscles as insulin is absorbed more quickly. Abdominal injection site is preferred.

Use caution or do not exercise patients with poorly controlled complications.

- Cardiovascular disease, hypertension. May see chronotropic incompetence, blunted HR and systolic BP response, blunted oxygen uptake, and anhidrosis. RPE may be used to regulate exercise intensity.
- Retinopathy. Avoid activities that dramatically increase BP (>170 mmHg systolic BP); avoid pounding or jarring activities.
- Neuropathy, nephropathy. Limit weight-bearing exercise for patients with significant neuropathy. There is increased fall risk with balance and gait abnormalities.
- Autonomic neuropathy is associated with sudden death and silent ischemia. Monitor for signs and symptoms of silent ischemia due to patient's inability to perceive angina.
- Nephropathy. Limit exercise to low to moderate intensities; discourage strenuous intensities.

Do not exercise in extreme environmental temperatures (very hot or cold due to impaired thermoregulation).

3. Waist circumference is used to determine distribution of body fat. Abdominal obesity (central accumulation of fat) is an independent predictor of morbidity and mortality.

Causes
1. An imbalance when energy intake exceeds energy consumption. Excess calories are consumed, exceeding those expended through exercise and activity.
2. Interaction of psychological and environmental factors (behavioral, cultural, social, economic factors). Observe for depression, smoking, yo-yo dieting with fluctuations in weight.
3. Genetic factors (biochemical defects): may account for 30%–40% of BMI.
4. Medical causes: endocrine and metabolic disorders (e.g., metabolic syndrome); hypothyroidism, Cushing's syndrome.

Prevention and Management
1. Lifestyle modification: combination of dietary changes to reduce body weight combined with increased physical activity.
   a. Personalized diet with reduced caloric intake: fat intake of <30% of total energy intake, emphasis on fruits, vegetables, whole grains, and lean protein.
   b. Personalized exercise program, including stretching exercises, resistance exercises, and aerobic exercises.
   c. Instruction in self-monitoring of exercise responses (heart rate, perceived exertion).
2. Behavior therapy: self-monitoring of eating habits and physical activity (use of a food and exercise diary); stress management, relapse prevention, and social support.
3. Pharmacology: over-the-counter (OTC) and prescriptive weight loss therapy (e.g., sibutramine, orlistat).
4. Surgery (bariatric surgery): usually limited to persons with BMI over 40 (or individuals with comorbid conditions and BMI over 35). Procedures include gastric banding and gastric bypass.

Exercise Evaluation (ACSM Guidelines for Exercise Testing and Prescription, 2021)
1. Individuals are typically sedentary with low physical work capacities.
2. Interviews should include goals, past exercise history, perceived barriers to exercise participation, and exercise likes and dislikes.
3. Exercise testing: submaximal, low initial workload (typically 2–3 METs), small workload increments per test stage (0.5–1.0 METs).
4. Use of leg or arm ergometry may enhance testing performance.
5. Use of proper size equipment: wide seat ergometer, large-size BP cuff.

Exercise Prescription (ACSM Guidelines for Exercise Testing and Prescription, 2021)
1. Start slowly, provide adequate warm-ups and cooldowns. Initial exercise intensity should be moderate (40%–60% oxygen uptake reserve [VO2R] or HRR).
2. Increase intensity gradually in order to prevent injury: moderate-intensity activity (50%–70% VO2R or HRR).
3. Frequency: 5–7 days/week.
4. Duration: 30–60 minutes.
5. Type: aerobic physical activities. Use of circuit training in order to combine resistive training with aerobic training activities. Provide with short rests between activities/exercise bouts.
6. Involve the patient in activity selection, incorporating individual preferences.
7. Select adequate footwear and orthotic devices as needed.
8. Aquatic exercise programs can assist in reducing musculoskeletal strain and injury.
9. Use of special bariatric equipment: wide seats on ergometers, bariatric lifts.
10. See Chapter 6, Table 6-6, Aerobic exercise for additional information.

See Box 8-4 for Exercise Precautions

BOX 8-4 Exercise Precautions for Individuals Who Are Overweight or Obese

Typically exhibit cardiopulmonary compromise: shortness of breath, elevated blood pressure, and angina.

Typically exhibit altered biomechanics affecting hips, knees, ankle/foot; back and joint pain; and increased risk of orthopedic injury.

Increased risk of skin breakdown due to shear forces.

Increased heat intolerance, risk of hyperthermia and heat exhaustion.

Increased risk of therapist injury: poor body mechanics, inadequate assistance during transfers and lifts.

Thyroid Disorders

Hypothyroidism
1. An underactive thyroid gland with deficient thyroid secretion (thyroxine); lower than normal T4 levels.
2. Results in slowed metabolic processes, affecting body temperature, heartbeat, and slowing of body processes.
3. Etiology: decreased thyroid-releasing hormone secreted by the hypothalamus or by the pituitary gland; atrophy of the thyroid gland; chronic autoimmune thyroiditis (Hashimoto's disease); overdosage with antithyroid medication.
4. Symptoms may include constipation, depression, dry hair and hair loss, dry skin, fatigue, slow heart rate,

swelling of the thyroid gland (goiter), unexplained weight gain or difficulty losing weight, carpal tunnel syndrome.
5. If untreated, leads to myxedema (severe hypothyroidism) with symptoms of swelling of hands, feet, face. Can lead to coma and death.
6. Treatment: lifelong thyroid replacement therapy.

RED FLAG: Can result in exercise intolerance, weakness, apathy; exercise-induced myalgia; reduced cardiac output.

Hyperthyroidism

1. Hyperactivity of the thyroid gland.
2. Etiology unknown.
3. Thyroid gland is typically enlarged and secretes greater than normal amounts of thyroid hormone (thyroxine), e.g., Graves' disease, thyroid storm, thyrotoxicosis.
4. Metabolic processes are accelerated.
5. Symptoms include nervousness, hyperreflexia, tremor, hunger, weight loss, fatigue, heat intolerance, palpitations, tachycardia, goiter, and diarrhea.
6. Treatment: antithyroid drugs.
7. Radioactive iodine may also be prescribed; surgical ablation may be necessary.

RED FLAG: Can result in exercise intolerance; fatigue is associated with hypermetabolic state.

Adrenal Disorders

Primary Adrenal Insufficiency (Addison's Disease)

1. Partial or complete failure of adrenocortical function; results in decreased production of cortisol and aldosterone.
2. Etiology: autoimmune processes, infection, neoplasm, or hemorrhage.
3. Signs and symptoms.
   a. Increased bronze pigmentation of skin.
   b. Weakness, decreased endurance.
   c. Anorexia, dehydration, weight loss, gastrointestinal disturbances.
   d. Anxiety, depression.
   e. Decreased tolerance to cold.
   f. Intolerance to stress.
4. Medical interventions.
   a. Replacement therapy: glucocorticoid, adrenal corticoids.
   b. Adequate fluid intake, control of sodium and potassium.
   c. Diet high in complex carbohydrates and protein.

Secondary Adrenal Insufficiency

1. Can result from prolonged steroid therapy (ACTH); rapid withdrawal of drugs; and hypothalamic or pituitary tumors.

Cushing's Syndrome/Cushing's Disease

1. Cushing's syndrome: Metabolic disorder resulting from chronic and excessive production of cortisol by the adrenal cortex.
   a. Etiology: Over-administration of corticosteroids; benign or malignant adenomas.
2. Cushing's disease:
   a. Etiology: Pituitary tumor with increased secretion of ACTH. Patients may exhibit headaches and visual changes (bitemporal hemianopsia) secondary to compression of the optic chiasm.
   b. Note: Pituitary tumors (adenoma or maligant) often results in hyper- or hypopituitarism with increase/decrease of multiple hormones and subsequent endocrine disorders/sxs.
3. Signs and symptoms of hypercortisolism (Cushing's syndrome/disease).
   a. Decreased glucose tolerance.
   b. Round "moon" face.
   c. Obesity: rapidly developing fat pads on chest and abdomen; buffalo hump.
   d. Decreased testosterone levels or decreased menstrual periods.
   e. Muscular atrophy.
   f. Edema.
   g. Hypokalemia.
   h. Emotional changes.
4. Medical interventions.
   a. Goal is to decrease excess ACTH: irradiation or surgical excision of pituitary tumor or control of medication levels.
   b. Monitor weight, electrolyte and fluid balance.

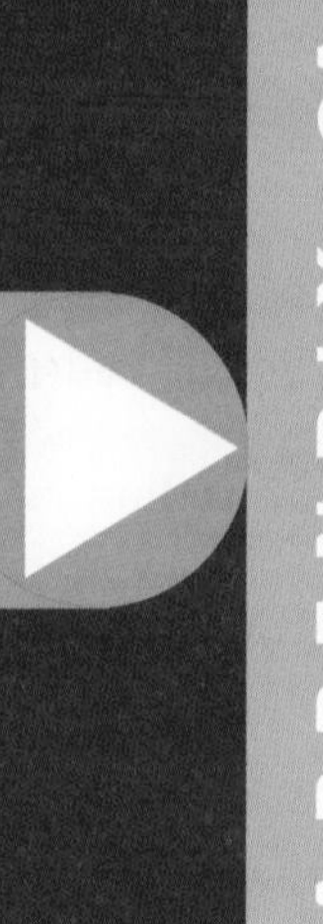

APPENDIX 8A

Review Questions and Case Study

(Answers to all Review Questions and Case Studies are found in Chapter 17)

1. What are the adverse side effects of cancer treatment that can impact physical therapy intervention?

2. What are the typical medications that may be prescribed for a patient diagnosed with GERD?

3. What are three possible interventions a physical therapist might use in the management of stress incontinence?

4. What are some of the long-term complications of diabetes that a physical therapist needs to consider during examination and treatment?

5. Differentiate between hypothyroidism and hyperthyroidism in terms of expected symptoms.

Case Scenario/Questions—Other Systems

Gender: Male
Age: 64

Presenting Problem/Current Condition:

- Patient referred to outpatient physical therapy with low back pain X 5 years with increased symptoms over the past year. No known mechanism of injury.
- Rates pain as a constant 4/10 with no consistent aggravating or easing factors
- Denies numbness, tingling, or weakness in either lower extremity
- Denies bowel or bladder incontinence but reports frequent urination, nocturia, and difficulty starting urination

Past Medical/Surgical History:

- Well-controlled hypertension for 7 years
- Well-controlled high cholesterol for 8 years

Other Information

- Mechanic
- Married
- Does not smoke and has 1–2 drinks a week

Question #1

Which of the following questions is BEST for determining if prostate dysfunction is contributing to the patient's low back pain?

1. Does the patient have pain in the suprapubic region?
2. Does the patient have foul-smelling urine?
3. Does the patient have blood in their stool?
4. Does the patient have genital and sacral pain?

Question #2

The patient shares that he has noticed periodic blood in his urine, increased pain at night, and erectile dysfunction over the past 6 months. These symptoms are most consistent with which medical diagnosis?

1. Prostatitis.
2. Benign prostratic hyperplasia.
3. Prostrate cancer.
4. Bladder cancer.

Question #3

The patient is diagnosised with prostrate cancer and undergoes surgery and radiation. The patient is referred for evaluation and treatment secondary to significant pelvic floor dysfunction. What is the BEST option for initially starting pelvic floor exercises?

1. Perform Kegel exercises while voiding.
2. Perform Kegel exercises in supine with knees bent.
3. Perform Kegel exercises in sitting.
4. Perform Kegel exercises everytime they move from sit to stand.

9

Pediatric Physical Therapy

SUZANNE M. GIUFFRE

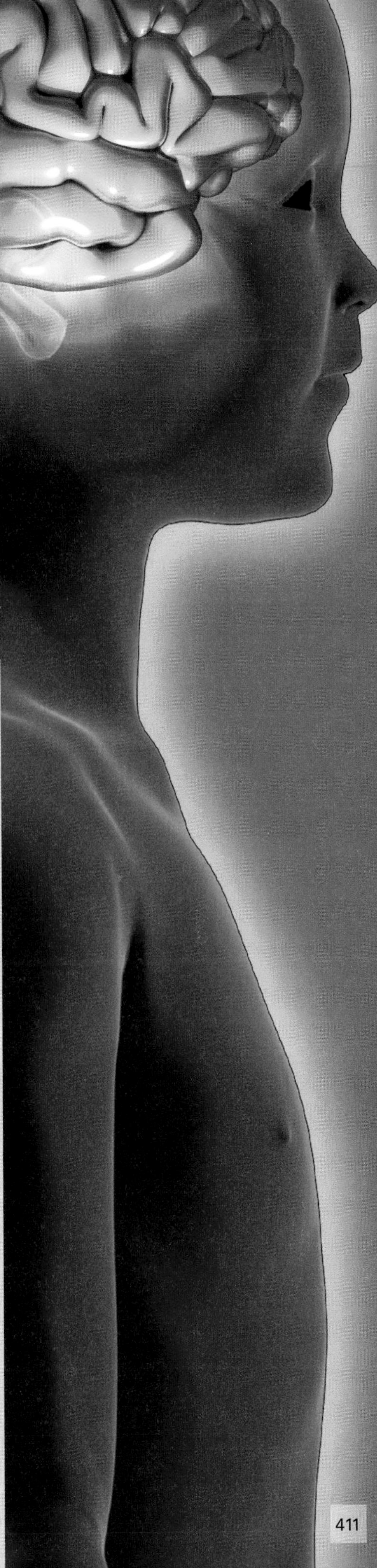

Chapter Outline

Chapter 9 PED

Theories of Development, Motor Control, and Motor Learning

Development

The Sequence of Events Through Which the Individual Grows, Changes, Evolves, and Matures (See Tables 9-1 and 9-2)

Theories of Development

1. Maturationist Hierarchical theory.
   a. Individual genetically and biologically determined.
   b. Aspects of human behavior are preformed and innate.
2. Empiricist theory.
   a. Source of human behavior is the environment.
3. Behaviorist theory.
   a. Environmental reinforcement motivates and shapes cognitive and motor behavior.
   b. Used in behavior modification treatment where desired behaviors are positively reinforced and unwanted behaviors are ignored.
4. Interactionist theory.
   a. Child is an active social being who contributes to his or her development.
5. Piagetian theory.
   a. Interaction of environment and neural maturation results in spiraling of development, with equilibrium and disequilibrium resulting.

Table 9-1

Developmental Sequence Summary

Age	Milestones
1 Month	• Decreased flexion • Momentary head elevation with minimal forearm support • Tracks a moving object with head rotation • Head usually to side • Reciprocal and symmetrical kicking • Positive support and primary walking reflexes in supported standing • Hands fisted with indwelling thumb most of the time • Neonatal reaching • Alert, brightening expression
2 Months	• Head elevation to 45° in prone, prone on elbows with elbows behind shoulders • Head bobs in supported sitting • Does not accept weight on lower extremities (astasia-abasia) • Responds to friendly handling
3 Months	• Prone on elbows, weight-bearing on forearms • Elbows in line with shoulders, head elevated to 90° • Head in midline in supine, hands on chest • Increased back extension with scapular adduction in supported sitting • Takes some weight with toes curled in supported standing • Coos, chuckles • Optical and labyrinthine head-righting present
4 Months	• Rolls prone to side, supine to side • Sits with support • No head lag in pull-to-sit • Bilateral reaching with forearm pronated when trunk supported • Ulnar-palmar grasp • Laughs out loud
5 Months	• Rolls from prone to supine • Weight shifting from one forearm to the other in prone • Head control in supported sitting
6 Months	• Prone on hands with elbows extended, weight shifting from hand to hand • Rolls supine to prone • Independent sitting • Pulls-to-stand with hands held, bounces

(Continued)

Table 9-1

Developmental Sequence Summary (Continued)

Age	Milestones
7 Months	• Can maintain quadruped • Pivots on belly; moves body in circle while prone • Assumes sitting from quadruped • Trunk rotation in sitting • Recognizes tone of voice • May show fear of strangers • Belly crawls
8–9 Months	• Quadruped creeping • Side-sitting • Pulls-to-stand through kneeling at furniture • May stand independently for 1–2 seconds • Reaches with closest arm, radial digital grasp, radial palmar, three-jaw chuck grasp, and inferior pincer grasp with thumb and forefinger • Can transfer objects from one hand to the other
10–15 Months	• Begins to walk unassisted • Transitions in/out of squatting • Creeps up/down steps • Transitions floor to stand • Begins self-feeding • Reaches with supination, neat pincer grasp, can release, build a tower of two cubes • Searches for hidden toys • Suspicious of strangers • Plays patty-cake and peekaboo • Imitates others
20 Months	• Ascends stairs step-to pattern (2 feet on each step-non-reciprocal pattern) • Immature running pattern more coordinated • Jumps off bottom step • Plays make-believe • Throws ball overhand a few feet
2 Years	• Immature running with increased speed • Can go upstairs foot-over-foot (reciprocal stair climbing) • Active, restless, tantrums • Catches large ball
3 Years	• Jumps with two feet • Rides tricycle • Stands on one foot briefly • Jumps off step • Hops on one foot • Gallops • Kicks ball • Understands sharing • Climbs on playground equipment • Mature/true run
4 years	• Hops on one foot several times • Stands on tiptoes • Relates to friends
5 years	• Skips • Kicks ball well • Dresses self • Swings self on playground swing (pumps legs independently)

Table 9-2

Development of Gait	
Birth–9 months	• Antigravity strength is obtained. Hip flexor strength by kicking, hip extensor strength by crawling on hands and knees and kneeling. Hip ABD strength by cruising. Extremities and trunk lengthen.
9–15 months	• Fat decreases. Initial gait consists of flexion, ABD and ER of hips, genu varum, eversion of the calcaneus, absent longitudinal arches, excessive femoral anteversion, and internal tibial torsion. Myelination of nerves completed (by 12 months).
18–24 months	• Gait characterized by decreased base of support, heel remains everted, less co-contraction of muscles, genu varum resolved, knee in neutral, and longitudinal arches (seen at 24 months or 1 year after started walking).
3–3.5 years	• More mature gait: genu valgum, heel eversion decreasing, consistent heel strike, femoral anteversion decreasing, arm swing noted.
6–7 years	• Fully mature gait: knees and heels in neutral position. Excessive femoral anteversion almost resolved.

Motor Control

The Study of Postures and Movement, and the Parts of the Mind and Body That Control Them

Theories of Motor Control

1. Neuromaturationist theory.
   a. Cortex is command center, with descending control and inhibition of lower centers by higher one in central nervous system (CNS).
2. Dynamic Systems theory.
   a. Command center changes from cortex to other levels, depending on the task.
   b. Stresses interaction between brain, body, and environment, including biomechanics and body geometry.
   c. Sensory systems mature, become integrated and connected to muscle coordination patterns, starting with the visual system.
   d. Immature postures involve cocontraction of agonists and antagonists; cocontraction decreases with maturation.
3. Neuronal group selection theory.
   a. Genetic code of species outlines limits of neural network formation.
   b. Actual network formation results from individual experience.
   c. Cell death of unexercised synaptic and strengthening of synaptic connections selectively activated.

Early Motor Learning

Motor Skill

1. Any motor activity that becomes better organized, more effective, and more efficient as a result of practice.

Enhancement of Early Motor Skills Development

1. Use of goal-oriented tasks.
2. Internal feedback via corollary discharge and effector organ feedback (i.e., visual, somatosensory vestibular feedback).
3. External feedback through knowledge of results and knowledge of performance feedback from instructor; i.e., every other time and after a delay.
4. Practice of high intensity and duration as tolerated.

Principles of Motor Development

1. Occurs in cephalocaudal and proximal to distal directions.
2. Unrefined to refined movement.
3. Stability to controlled mobility.
4. Occurs in spiraling manner, with periods of equilibrium and disequilibrium.
5. Sensitive periods occur when infant/child is especially affected by environmental input.

Fetal Sensorimotor Development

Gestational Age (GA)

1. Age of fetus or newborn, in weeks, from first day of mother's last normal menstrual period.
2. Normal gestational period is 38–42 weeks. Infant considered premature if born at <37 weeks GA. In calculating prematurity or corrected age, 40 weeks is typically used.
3. Gestational period is divided into three equal trimesters (see Table 9-3).

Conceptional Age

1. Age of a fetus or newborn in weeks since conception.

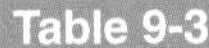

Table 9-3

Fetal Sensorimotor Development

	FIRST TRIMESTER	SECOND TRIMESTER	THIRD TRIMESTER
Muscle Spindle	• Muscle starts to differentiate • Tissue becomes specialized	• Motor endplate forms • Clonus response to stretch	• Some muscles are mature and functional, others still maturing
Touch and Tactile System	• First sensory system to develop • Response to tactile stimulus	• Receptors differentiate	• Touch functional • Actual temperature discrimination at end of third trimester • Most mature sensory system at birth
Vestibular System	• Functioning at the end of the first trimester (not completely developed)		
Vision	• Eyelids fused • Optic nerve and cup being formed	• Startle to light • Visual processing occurs	• Fixation occurs • Able to focus (fixed focal length)
Auditory		• Turns to auditory sounds	• Debris in middle ear, loss of hearing
Olfactory			• Nasal plugs disappear, some olfactory perception
Taste	• Taste buds develop		• Responds to different tastes (sweet, sour, bitter, salt)
Movement	• Sucking, hiccupping • Fetal breathing • Quick, generalized limb movement • Positional changes • 7½ weeks: bends neck and trunk	• Quickening • Sleep states • Grasp reflex • Reciprocal and symmetrical limb movements	At 28 weeks, the following primitive reflexes present: • Rooting, sucking, swallowing • Palmar grasp • Plantar grasp • Moro away from perioral stroke • Crossed extension

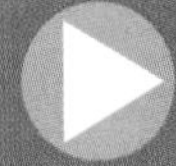

Examination

Patient Interview

Mother's Pregnancy and Birth History

1. Prematurity, fetal distress, difficult labor, umbilical cord around neck.
2. High-risk pregnancy can include many things (drug use, multiple births, gestational diabetes, etc.).

Medical History

1. Special care unit admission, diagnoses, intubated or on ventilator, surgeries, medications.

Family History

1. Caretakers, current home situation, support to family, socioeconomic status.

Review of Systems

Determine Corrected Age if Premature. Example

1. If chronological age of child is 6 months old (24 weeks), but they were born at 32 weeks gestational age (GA) [8 weeks early as 40 is typical]. Thus, their correct age is 4 months (16 weeks).
2. Calculate prematurity (40 weeks-child's GA), then subtract prematurity from chronological age to get corrected age.

Preterm Infant Examination

Neurological Assessment. Preterm and Full-Term Newborn Infants

1. Neurological items include newborn reflexes, infant states of alertness.
2. Neurobehavioral items from Neonatal Behavioral Assessment Scale (NBAS).
3. Assessment of gestational age by evaluation of muscle tone, physical characteristics.

Assessment of Premature Infant Behavior (APIB)

1. Refinement and extension of NBAS.
2. Assesses the organization and balance of infant's physiological, motor, and behavioral states.
3. Test is lengthy, used mainly for research.

Newborn Individualized Developmental Care and Assessment of Progress (NIDCAP)

1. Systematic behavioral observation of preterm or full-term infant in nursery or home during environmental input, caretaking, and treatments.
2. An interventional model developed with the aim of providing adequate sensory stimulation to premature infants at a level that is adapted to the degree of neurological maturity of the infant.
3. Note what stresses, consoles infant.

Test of Infant Motor Performance (TIMP)

1. Developed for infants from 32 weeks postconceptual age to 3½ months post-term.
2. Evaluates spontaneous and elicited movements to analyze postural alignment and selective control for functional movements.

Full-Term Newborn, Infant, and Child Examination

Apgar Screening Test

1. Administered to newborn at 1, 5, 10 minutes after birth.
2. Continues every 5 minutes if infant is having difficulties.
3. Appearance (color), Pulse, Grimace (reflex irritability), Activity, Respirations, each scored 0, 1, or 2.
4. Score of 7–10 is considered good.

Neurological Examination of the Newborn

1. Assigns states of consciousness.
2. Tests newborn reflexes.

Neonatal Behavioral Assessment Scale

1. Tests interactive, self-organizational abilities and newborn reflexes and muscle tone.

Skeletal System Examination

1. Clavicle, as it may fracture during birth.
2. Dislocated hip: asymmetrical gluteal folds, hip click.
3. Spine: at birth is normal for the spine to be kyphotic. Abnormal would be scoliosis, spina bifida occulta with dimple, patch of hair, and pigmentation visible.
4. Talipes equinovarus (clubfoot): ankle in plantar flexion, forefoot adduction and supination.

Range of Motion (ROM)

1. Newborn has decreased ROM into extension due to physiological flexion, but increased dorsiflexion of ankles and flexion at wrists.

Posture

1. Physiological flexion of all four limbs due to position in utero.
2. Head to one side.

Movements

1. Spontaneous and reflexive.
2. Occasional tremulousness normal.

Neonatal Reflexes. Primary Motor Patterns and Infant Reflexes and Postural Reactions (See Table 9-4)

1. Present at birth and become "integrated" or inhibited, or not evident later in development.
2. In CNS lesions, they may persist and interfere with motor milestone attainment or cause deformities.

Postural Reactions (Once Thought to Be Reflexes)

1. Protective extension: quick displacement of trunk in downward direction while held or while sitting in forward, sideward, or backward direction results in extension of legs downward and extension of arms in sitting position to catch weight. Downward begins at 4 months, sideward sitting at 6 months, forward sitting at 7 months, backward sitting at 9 months; these reactions persist through life.
2. Body-righting reaction acting on the head (BOH): contact of body with solid surface results in head righting with respect to gravity, interacts with labyrinthine righting reaction on head to maintain orientation of head in space. Begins at 4–6 months and persists through life.
3. Body-righting reaction acting on the body (BOB): rotation of head or thorax results in rolling over, with rotation between trunk and pelvis. Begins at 6–8 months and persists.
4. Tilting reactions: slow shifting of base of support or slow displacement of body in space will result in lateral flexion of spine toward elevated side of support, abduction of extremities on elevated side, and sometimes trunk rotation toward elevated side. Prone begins at 5 months; supine begins at 7 months; sitting at 8 months; quadruped at 12 months. These reactions persist throughout life.

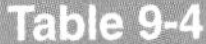

Table 9-4

Selected Neonatal or Primitive Reflexes

REFLEX NAME	TIME FRAME	STIMULUS	RESPONSE	IF PERSISTS INTERFERES WITH:
Crossed Extension	28 weeks gestational age (GA) to 1–2 months	Noxious stimulus to the sole of one foot	Flexes stimulated lower limb and then extend and adduct the opposite lower limb	Crawling, standing balance, and gait (all upright motor skills).
Flexor Withdrawal	28 weeks GA to 1–2 months	Noxious stimulus to the sole of one foot	Flexes stimulated lower limb (hip and knee flexes, ankle DF)	Standing balance and gait (especially walking on uneven surfaces such as on gravel) due to hypersensitivity to stimuli on sole of feet. This may lead to abnormal gait patterns.
Positive Support Reflex (primary standing reaction)	35 weeks GA to 1–2 months	Stand infant up on balls of feet in contact with a firm surface	Extends lower limbs to support weight	Standing balance, gait (movement of lower extremities, esp. LE flexion and all upright motor skills). Can cause plantar flexion contractures. Squatting/sitting from a standing position. May have a rigid gait pattern.
Galant	28 weeks GA to 3 months	In prone position, stroke paraspinals on one side	Lateral flexion of the lumbar spine to the side of the stimulus	Sitting balance, crawling, creeping, gait, could lead to scoliosis. Could lead to fidgeting and an inability to sit still causing issue with concentration; hypersensitive to wearing clothes.
Rooting	28 weeks GA to 3 months	Stroke cheek toward mouth	Head rotates toward stimulus and mouth opens	Controlling head movements for visual purposes, ADLs (e.g., washing face), speech (often due to tongue lying too far forward) Hypersensitivity to stimuli on the face.
Stepping Reflex (Primary Walking or Dancing Reflex)	37 weeks GA to 3–4 months	Holds infant upright with their feet on the support surface and lean forward	Infant exhibits high stepping movements with regular rhythm (robotic looking)	Standing balance, walking volitionally (all upright motor skills).
Tonic Labyrinthine (classic reflex)	32 weeks GA to 4 months	Prone (neck usually flexed) or supine position (neck usually extended)	Prone: infant goes into overall flexion Supine: infant goes into overall extension	Affects anti–gravity control for developing mobility. Prone propping, rolling, belly crawling, creeping, transition to sit. Negatively affects ability to orient the head and control posture.
Moro	28 weeks GA to 3–5 months	Allow infant's head to drop backward when in reclined sitting position (quickly catch head)	Abduction and extending of B UEs and splaying of fingers. Followed by flex and adduct their arms, pulling them close to their chest.	Sitting Balance, standing balance, oversensitive/reactive to sensory stim, supine to sit, potential issues in adults include driving, playing sports, drinking (if neck extends quickly).
Startle	28 weeks GA to 3–5 months	Loud noise or sudden movement or bright light	Abduction and extending of B UEs and splaying of fingers. Followed by flex and adduct their arms, pulling them close to their chest.	Oversensitive and overreactive to sensory stimuli (hypersensitivity and hyperreactivity), easily startled/distracted (could led to poor interaction and attention and/or performing fine motor tasks in loud environment), sitting balance, standing balance, potential issues in adults include driving, playing sports.
Asymmetrical Tonic Neck (ATNR)	20 weeks GA to 4–5 months	Rotation of head/neck in supine actively or passively to one side	Upper limb on face side will extend and hand will open, while the contralateral upper limb will flex, and hand will make a fist. More known as upper limb reflex, may see flexion of the lower limb on the face side and extension of the lower limb on the opposite side	Prone propping, rolling, belly crawling, creeping, sitting balance, gait, hand eye coordination and visual tracking, difficulty crossing mid-line, bimanual activities, ALL fine motor skills, could lead to torticollis.

(Continued)

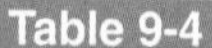

Table 9-4

Selected Neonatal or Primitive Reflexes (Continued)

REFLEX NAME	TIME FRAME	STIMULUS	RESPONSE	IF PERSISTS INTERFERES WITH:
Palmar Grasp Reflex	28 weeks GA to 4–7 months	Apply pressure to palm of a hand	Finger flexion to grasp object in palm	Intentional grasp and release of objects (fine motor skills), ability to bear weight on open hands for prone propping, belly crawling and creeping, pull to stand.
Sucking	28–34 weeks GA to 5 months	Place gloved finger, pacifier, bottle nipple in mouth	Rhythmically sucking (tongue rides up and down with jaw)	Eating, drinking, speech impairments, drooling, risk for choking. Tendency to suck thumb.
Head/Neck on Body	34 weeks GA to 4–6 months	Passively rotate head in supine	Body follows head by trunk rotating into side-lying	Complete voluntary rolling.
Body on Head/ Neck	7 months to 5 years	Passively rotate trunk/body into side-lying	Head follows trunk and rotates to the same side	Complete voluntary rolling.
Gag	19 weeks GA to 6 months	Stimulates back of the throat	Tongue thrusts forward	Intraoral hypersensitivity, difficulties in eating, drinking, risk for choking. Can lead to impaired speech. Leads to poor nutrition.
Symmetrical Tonic Neck (STNR)	Appears at 5 months but not present in most children; disappears at 8–9 months	Flexion or extension of head/neck (actively or passively)	With neck flexion, arms flex and hips extend With head extension, arms extension and hips flexion	Prone propping, belly crawling, creeping, sitting balance (slumped posture), sit to stand, standing balance, gait (independent movement of lower limbs), hand-eye coordination, inability to dissociate between lower limbs. Can lead to W-sitting.
Plantar Grasp	28 weeks GA to 9 months	Apply pressure to the sole of the foot just distal to the metatarsal heads	Toes will flex	Standing balance, walking, running.
Landau	3–12 months	1. Support in prone 2. Flex neck	1. Infant will extend head and hips above horizon 2. Hips flex	N/A
Babinski	0–24 months	Firmly stroke sole of the foot heel to toes, in lateral to medial curve	Great toe extends and other toes splay (spread apart)	Standing balance and walking.

Pediatric Screening Tools and Outcome Measures (See Appendix 9A for a summary table and description of selected pediatric screening tools and outcome measures)

Screening Tests

1. Denver Developmental Screening Test II.
   a. To screen for developmental delay.
   b. Tests social, fine, gross motor, and language skills from birth to 6 years of age.
2. Alberta Infant Motor Scale (AIMS): observational scale for assessing gross motor milestones in infants from birth through independent walking.

Standardized Motor Tests

1. Movement Assessment of Infants.
   a. Identifies motor dysfunction and changes in the status of motor dysfunction and establishes an intervention program for infants from birth to 1 year.
   b. Criterion-referenced exam of muscle tone, reflexes, automatic reactions, and volitional movements.
2. Peabody Developmental Motor Scales.
   a. Assesses gross and fine motor development from birth to 72 months.
   b. Includes spontaneous, elicited reflexes and automatic reactions.
3. GMFM-88.
   a. Developed to measure change in gross motor function over time; now validated for use in children with cerebral palsy, TBI, and children with Down syndrome.

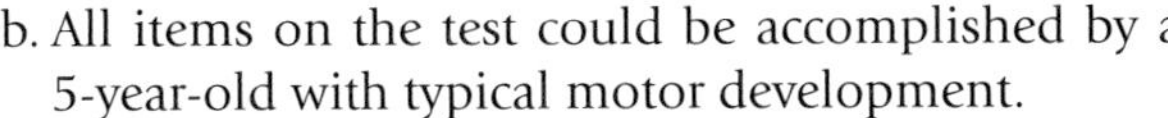

b. All items on the test could be accomplished by a 5-year-old with typical motor development.
c. Focuses on voluntary movement in five developmental dimensions: prone and supine, sitting, crawling and kneeling, standing, walking and jumping.

4. Bruininks-Oseretsky Test of Motor Proficiency (BOT-2).
   a. Developed to measure gross motor and fine motor abilities from 4–21 years of age.
   b. Norm-referenced on typical children.
   c. Can use full battery or a short form for screening.

Sensory Integration and Praxis Test

1. Sensorimotor assessment for children between ages of 4 and 9 years with mild to moderate learning impairment.
2. Includes tests of balance, proprioceptive and tactile sensation, and control of specific movements.

Comprehensive Developmental Assessments

1. Bayley Scales of Infant Development III revision: norm-referenced motor and mental scales for children from birth to 42 months of age.
2. Battelle Developmental Inventory (BDI-2). It is for children 0–7 years. It includes assessment of adaptive, personal-social, communication, motor, and cognitive domains.
3. HELP (Hawaii Early Learning Profile), a comprehensive tool for 0–36 months and includes 7 domains: cognitive, gross motor, fine motor, communication, social-emotional, self-help, sensory regulation. Typically used in early intervention.

Pediatric Functional Assessments

1. Pediatric Evaluation of Disability Inventory (PEDI): interview or questionnaire scale of activities of daily living (ADL), with or without modification completed by caregiver.
2. Functional Independence Measure for children (WeeFIM): assesses function in self-care, mobility, locomotion, and communication and social cognition.
3. School Functional Assessment (SFA): measures participation, task supports, activity performance, physical tasks, and cognitive/behavioral tasks within the school setting.
   a. For children in grades K–6 (5–12 years of age).
   b. Criterion-referenced.

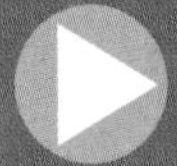

Overview of Pediatric Physical Therapy Intervention

Roles of the Pediatric Physical Therapist

Direct Care Provider

1. In children's hospital settings.
2. In special care nurseries, neonatal intensive care units.
3. Pediatric rehabilitation settings.
4. In Early Intervention Programs (EIPs) (0–3 years).
5. In educational settings.

Consultant/Indirect Care Provider

1. Pediatric PT may be consultant in educational settings, instructing teachers and teachers' assistants in facilitating attainment of educational goals.
2. Pediatric PT may work with physical therapist assistant in delivery of care in many settings.

Parent Education

1. Key intervention in providing pediatric physical therapy.

Goals, Outcomes, and Intervention

Primary Prevention of Disability Through Education and Treatment

Prevention and/or Improvement of Secondary Disabilities (e.g., Contractures/Deformities)

Attainment of Maximal Functional Goals of Child and Family

Obtaining Positioning Equipment, Orthoses, Assistive Devices, and Wheelchairs as Needed

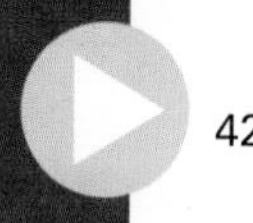

Pediatric Therapies

Developmental Activities to Facilitate Development of Functional Motor Skills

1. These activities use postures and movements from the developmental sequence to increase strength, ROM, coordination.
2. Play is the work of the child; make activities fun.

Neurodevelopmental Treatment (NDT)

1. Sets anticipated outcomes and impairment goals in partnership with the family, the client, and the interdisciplinary team.
2. Encourages active, goal-directed functional movements appropriate for the developmental level of the child.
3. Utilizes therapeutic handling as the primary intervention strategy.
4. Provides specific sensory input using careful grading of the intensity, rhythm, and duration of somatosensory inputs.
5. Focuses on important components of motor learning.
   a. Practice of task components as well as practice of the whole task.
   b. Repetition.
   c. Structuring an environment conducive to client participation and support.

Motor Control/Motor Learning Approaches

1. Utilize principles of motor control and early motor learning appropriate for individual child.

Sensory Integration

1. Goal is to facilitate child's organization and processing of proprioceptive, tactile, and vestibular input.
2. Facilitation will influence postural responses, environmental awareness, and motor planning.

Prematurity Physical Therapy Practice

A Subspecialty of Pediatrics. Requires Advanced Didactic and Supervised Practical Experience

Definition and Categories

1. Birth of infant before 37 weeks gestation.
2. Categorized by birth weight.

Preterm Postural and Movement Profile

1. Preterm infant does not develop the physiological flexion of full-term newborn.
2. May exhibit hyperextended neck and trunk (may be partially a result of supine and intubation positions).
3. Shoulders may be elevated, abducted, extended with scapular retraction.
4. Hips abducted and extended.
5. Pelvis tipped anteriorly (increased lumbar lordosis).
6. Decreased midline arm movement.
7. May bear weight on toes when in supported standing position.

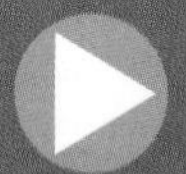

Conditions and Interventions

Prematurity Medical Complications

Complications Depend on Severity of Prematurity and Birth Weight

1. Meconium Aspiration syndrome.
   a. Due to bowel movement in utero (meconium) that mixes with amniotic fluid.
   b. Near-term or term infant inhales substance and can develop respiratory distress.
   c. Infants are hypersensitive to environmental stimuli—treat in quiet environment.
   d. 20% present with developmental delays, some up until 3 years of age.
2. Respiratory distress syndrome (RDS) or hyaline membrane disease.
   a. Surfactant does not develop in the lungs until 24 weeks GA and lungs are not ready for air exchange until 26 weeks GA. Atelectasis is caused by insufficient surfactant in premature lungs.
   b. May lead to acute respiratory failure and death.
   c. Treatment includes oxygen supplementation, assisted ventilation, and surfactant administration.
   d. Chronic RDS may lead to bronchopulmonary dysplasia.
3. Bronchopulmonary dysplasia.
   a. Chronic lung disease as a result of damage to lungs from mechanical ventilation, oxygen administration, and chronic RDS.

b. Predisposes child to frequent respiratory infections and developmental disability.
c. Treatment includes respiratory support, infection control, and bronchodilator administration.
4. Periventricular leukomalacia (PVL).
a. Necrosis of white matter adjacent to ventricles of brain due to systemic hypotension or ischemia.
b. May result in cerebral palsy.
5. Periventricular-intraventricular hemorrhage.
a. Bleeding into immature vascular matrix.
b. Bleeds graded I–IV; grades II–IV may result in cerebral palsy.
6. Retinopathy of prematurity (ROP).
a. Due to combination of low birth weight and high oxygen levels.
b. Sequelae may range from nonsignificant to detachment of retinas and blindness.
c. In NICU premature infants eyes are covered to prevent exposure to bright light.
7. Necrotizing enterocolitis.
a. Ischemia results in inflammatory, infected bowel.
8. Patent Ductus Arteriosus (PDA).
a. Ductus arteriosus (temporary vessel between aorta and the pulmonary artery) should close soon after birth.
b. Non-oxygenated blood is circulated.
c. PT should monitor O_2 saturation, signs of cyanosis, shortness of breath, and respiratory rate.
9. Failure to thrive.
a. Infant lacks adequate nutritional intake.
b. Infant can present with developmental delays.
10. Increased fragility of skin.
11. Premature infants lack adipose tissue and the CNS is unable to control body temperature prior to 32 weeks GA. Need to keep infant warm; otherwise, they shiver and expend energy needed for other vital body functions such as respiration.
12. Feeding problems.
13. Interaction/attachment problems with caregivers.

Physical Therapy Examination in Prematurity

1. Medical history review.
2. Autonomic functions.
3. Neurobehavioral organization (interactive items after infant is 32 weeks conceptional age).
4. Muscle tone.
5. Postural control.
6. Spontaneous movements.
7. Reflexes including feeding.
8. Musculoskeletal evaluation.
9. Family needs.

Intervention/Activities to Teach Parents

1. Play activities and positioning to facilitate shoulder protraction and adduction such as supported side-lying while doing visual (use black, white, and red objects 9 inches away) and auditory tracking, and reaching.
2. Midline positioning of head.
3. Encourage reaching for toys, parent's face if infant is over 32 weeks conceptional age.
4. Avoid activities that may increase extensor tone, such as use of infant jumpers and walkers.
5. Positioning goals/principles:
a. Supervised side-lying and prone positioning ("tummy time") for periods during the day. These positions promote physiologic flexion.
b. Academy of Pediatrics recommends sleeping in the supine position ("Safe to Sleep" or "Back to Sleep") to decrease the possiblity of sudden infant death syndrome (SIDS).
c. Place hand close to face to help children self-regulate or soothe/comfort themselves (e.g., thumb-sucking).
d. Provide barriers to push against (end of crib, firm bumpers).
e. Prevent skin breakdown.
f. Prevent musculoskeletal issues such as plagiocephaly and torticollis.

Cerebral Palsy (CP)

Pathology

1. Group of disorders that are prenatal, perinatal, or postnatal in origin (up to 2 years of age).
2. Nonprogressive encephalopathy: major causes include hemorrhage below lining of ventricles, hypoxic encephalopathy, malformations, and trauma of CNS.
3. Preterm birth associated with CP.

Classifications of CP

1. By area of body showing impairment.
a. One limb: monoplegia.
b. Two lower limbs: diplegia.
c. Upper and lower limbs of one side of the body: hemiplegia.
d. All four limbs: quadriplegia.
e. Trunk can be involved in all types.
2. Movement disorders are the most obvious impairment.
a. Spastic: increased tone, lesion of motor cortex, or projections from motor cortex.
b. Athetosis: fluctuating muscle tone, involuntary slow writhing movements, lesion of basal ganglia.
c. Ataxia: instability of movement, lesion of cerebellum.
d. Dystonia: involuntary movements with sustained contractions.
e. Hypotonia: decreased muscle tone.
f. Mixed: can present with a multiple/mixture of movement disorders.
3. Gross motor function classification system for CP (see Table 9-5).

Table 9-5

Gross Motor Classification for Cerebral Palsy	
Level I	• Walk without restrictions; limitations in more-advanced gross motor skills.
Level II	• Walk without assistive devices; limitations walking outdoors and in the community.
Level III	• Walk with assistive mobility devices; limitations walking outdoors and in the community.
Level IV	• Self-mobility with limitations; children are transported or use power mobility outdoors and in the community.
Level V	• Self-mobility is severely limited, even with the use of assistive technology.

Impairments for All Classifications of CP

1. Insufficient force generation.
2. Tone abnormality.
3. Poor selective control of muscle activity.
4. Poor regulation of muscle activity in anticipation of postural changes.
5. Decreased ability to learn unique movements.
6. Abnormal patterns of movement in total flexion and extension.
7. Persistence of primitive reflexes.
   a. Interfere with normal posture and movement.
   b. May cause contractures and deformities.

Impairments by Classification of CP

1. Spastic cerebral palsy.
   a. Increased muscle tone in antigravity muscles.
   b. Abnormal postures and movements with mass patterns of flexion/extension.
   c. Imbalance of tone across joints may cause contractures and deformities, especially of hip flexors, adductors, internal rotators, and knee flexors, ankle plantarflexors in lower extremities; scapular retractors, glenohumeral extensors and adductors, elbow flexors, forearm pronators.
   d. Visual, auditory, cognitive, and oral motor deficits may be associated with spastic CP.
   e. Crouching gait: walks with hip flexion, adduction, internal rotation, and knee flexion. May also toe walk.
2. Athetoid cerebral palsy.
   a. Characterized by involuntary, slow writhing movements, with generalized decreased muscle tone (floppy baby syndrome). This is a result of basal ganglion involvement.
   b. Poor functional stability especially in proximal joints.
   c. Ataxia and incoordination when child assumes upright position, with decreased base of support and muscle tone fluctuations.
   d. Poor visual tracking, speech delay, and oral motor problems.
   e. Tonic reflexes such as asymmetrical tonic neck reflex (ATNR), symmetrical tonic neck reflex (STNR), and tonic labyrinthine reflex (TLR) may be persistent, blocking functional postures and movement.
3. Ataxic cerebral palsy.
   a. Low postural tone with poor balance.
   b. Stance and gait are wide based.
   c. Intention tremor of hands.
   d. Uncoordinated movement.
   e. Ataxia follows initial hypotonia.
   f. Poor visual tracking, nystagmus.
   g. Speech articulation problems.
   h. May occur with spastic or athetoid CP.

Functional Limitations

1. Dependent on classification and severity of CP.
2. Spasticity may lead to decreased ROM, which may limit mobility. Special attention to ROM needed during growth spurts.
3. Ambulation.
   a. Ambulation without use of assistive devices may be attained by children with hemiplegia, and by some with diplegia and ataxia.
   b. Ambulation may be attained with use of rollator walkers or crutches by some children with diplegia, athetosis, and a few with mild quadriplegia.

Interventions and Goals in CP

1. Very individualized, depending on abilities, age, type of CP. Incorporate child and family in intervention planning, implementation, and goal-setting.
2. Focus on prevention of disability by minimizing effects of impairment, preventing or limiting secondary impairment such as contractures, scoliosis.
   a. Utilize static positioning and dynamic patterns of movement opposite to habitual abnormal spastic patterns.
   b. Facilitate symmetry in postures.
   c. Elongate spastic hamstrings and heel cords.
   d. Serial casting may be used to increase length of muscle and decrease tone.
3. Maximize the gross motor functional level.
   a. Use principles of motor learning and motor control; facilitate functional motor skills, including voluntary movement, anticipatory and reactive postural adjustments. Use toys, fun activities, balls, and bolsters to facilitate postural control and developmental activities.

b. Use weight-bearing and postural challenge to increase muscle tone and strength.
c. Incorporate orthoses as necessary.
- Ankle-foot orthosis (AFO) most commonly used; may be rigid or with articulated ankle.
- Submalleolar orthosis for forefoot and midfoot malalignment; e.g., pronated foot.

d. Utilize adaptive equipment as necessary.
- Seating should maintain head in neutral position; trunk upright; hips, knees, and ankles at 90° flexion (hips in abduction if spastic adductors). Wheelchair or seat may be tilted posteriorly to decrease extensor tone and maintain hip flexion.
- Prone or supine standers and parapodium will promote weight-bearing through lower extremities and encourage bone mineralization (requires minimum of 5 hours/week in weight-bearing), gastrointestinal function, tone, strengthening of lower extremity muscles, and social interaction. TLR will elicit more extensor tone in supine, more flexor tone in prone.
- Side-lying will help decrease effect of TLR.
- Rollator walkers often used. Posterior rollator walker helps child maintain upright position, and arm position helps decrease extensor tone.

Prognosis for CP

1. Prognosis depends on severity of brain lesion.
2. Most children with spastic hemiplegia, mild to moderate spastic CP, and mild ataxia will be able to ambulate.
3. Good prognosis for ambulation if child can sit independently by 2 years of age.
4. If child is going to walk, most will walk by 8 years of age.

Medical, Surgical and Pharmacological Interventions for CP

1. Management of spasticity (see Table 9-6).
   a. Oral medications—presynaptic inhibition of acetylcholine release.
   b. Intrathecal baclofen (ITB) pump.
   - GABA b-agonist; GABA is an inhibitory CNS neurotransmitter. Catheter delivers drug to the intrathecal (subarachnoid) space in the spinal cord,

Table 9-6

Medical Treatment for Spasticity

ORAL MEDICATIONS

MOST COMMON	SITE OF ACTION	PROS OF ORAL MEDS	CONS OF ORAL MEDS
Baclofen (Lioresal)	CNS	Decreases spasticity and spasms	Decreased strength, may lose postural control
Diazepam (Valium)	CNS	Improves motor control	Difficult to maintain steady state
Tizanidine (Zanaflex)	CNS	Noninvasive, not permanent	Following dosage schedule may be difficult
Dantrolene Sodium (Dantrium)	Muscle	Can be effective for some patients	Side effects: drowsiness, hypotonia, weakness

*Oral meds are systemic and may be suggested for patients that have widespread areas of spasticity.

INJECTION THERAPY

	PROS	CONS
Anesthetic/Diagnostic Nerve Blocks (Procaine, Lidocaine)	Decreases local spasticity and dystonia Not permanent Decreases contractures Improves motor control Not systemic	Not permanent
Neurolytic Nerve Blocks (Ethanol, Phenol)	Decreases local spasticity and dystonia Not permanent Decreases contractures Improves motor control Not systemic	Not permanent Ethanol and Phenol—great skill needed to inject; risk of paresthesias
Botulinum Toxin [Botox] (Clostridium Botulinum)—injected into muscles, interferes with release of acetylcholine at the neuromuscular junction. EMG used for guidance if needed.	Decreases local spasticity and dystonia Not permanent Decreases contractures Improves motor control No systemic effect Can be administered without anesthesia Lasts 4–6 months	Not permanent Expensive Hypotonia

*Injections are used for specific muscles and are better for patients with focal spasticity.

producing muscle relaxation with less medication. Intrathecal baclofen (ITB) is delivered to a specific segment of the spine and controls spasticity below that segment. Pump is implanted subcutaneously in abdomen with catheter to spinal cord. Programmable to allow for precise dosage and easily adjusted.

- Pros: longer lasting, decrease spasticity/spasm, improves motor control, reversible, noninvasive dose, fewer side effects, reservoir holds 1–4-month supply.
- Cons: side effects can include hypotonia, nausea, headaches, surgical complications, catheter kink/malfunction, overdose, and withdrawal. Refills needed approximately every 3 months.

> **RED FLAGS:** Adverse reactions of oral baclofen: drowsiness, dizziness, fatigue, weakness, ataxia, confusion, depression.
> Abrupt withdrawal may result in exaggerated rebound spasticity, fever, mental status changes, and muscle rigidity.

c. Neurosurgery.
- Neurectomy, anterior rhizotomy, selective dorsal rhizotomy, corectomy, thalmotomy, deep brain stimulation.
  - Selective dorsal rhizotomy (SDR).
    - Common procedure: dorsal sensory nerve rootlets are stimulated; those responding abnormally are severed. Usually done between 4 and 10 years of age.
    - Pros: decrease spasticity, improved motor control, and not reversible.
    - Cons: Possible sensory loss, not reversible, not effective for dystonia, anesthesia risks.
- Intensive strengthening program after surgery when ambulation is goal.

d. Peripheral nerve block.
- Injection of phenol/alcohol into peripheral nervous system from nerve root to motor end-plate.
- Lasts 3–6 months.

e. Botox.
- Minute amounts of botulinum toxin injected into muscle paralyzing it for 4–6 months.
- There is a maximum amount of botox that can be given at one time, so if spasticity is widespread, injections will have to prioritize selective muscles, and intrathecal infusion may be a better option.

Orthopedic Management of CP (See Table 9-7)

1. Lengthening procedures.
   a. Muscle/tendon lengthening is typically used to correct moderate to severe deformities or those that do not respond to pharmacological and/or rehabilitation.
   b. Muscles/tendons most often lengthened include Achilles, hamstrings, iliopsoas, and hip adductors.
   c. Tendon lengthening decreases contactility of muscles and is used less now since spasticity can be reduced by medication.
2. Muscle transfers.
   a. Muscle attachments moved to change direction of force in order to increase function and decrease spasticity.
   b. Most often done with hip adductors transferred to hip abductor.
3. Osteotomies.
   a. Cutting, removing, or repositioning bone to facilitate normal alignment, prevent subluxation/dislocation.
   b. Most often performed in lower extremities (femoral, tibial, or pelvic osteotomy).

Myelodysplasia/Spina Bifida

Pathology

1. Neural tube defect resulting in vertebral and/or spinal cord malformation. Elevated serum or amniotic alpha-fetoprotein, amniotic acetylcholinesterase in prenatal period and sonogram are used for detection.
2. Spina bifida occulta: no spinal cord involvement, may be indicated by a tuft of hair, dimple, or sinus.

Table 9-7

Orthopedic Surgery
Soft tissue operations (tendon or muscle lengthening, muscle releases, tendon transfers). Bone-related (osteotomies, fusions).

PROS	CONS
Decrease contracture	Anesthesia risks
Decrease abnormal bony alignment	Non–weight-bearing after bony procedures for several weeks
Improve motor control	Risk of weakness and decreased function
Effects last a few years or more	

3. Spina bifida cystica/asperta: visible or open lesions but cystica means contained in a cyst.
   a. Meningocele: cyst includes cerebrospinal fluid; cord intact.
   b. Myelomeningocele: cyst includes cerebrospinal fluid (CSF) and herniated cord tissue.
4. Neural tube defects linked to maternal decreased folic acid, infection, hot tub soaks, and exposure to teratogens such as alcohol and valproic acid.
5. Hydrocephalus significantly related to closure of neural tube defect. Shunting relieves pressure of hydrocephalus. May develop Arnold-Chiari malformation Type II: cerebellum and brain stem are pushed through the foramen magnum.
6. Meningitis common if defect not closed soon after birth.
7. Foot deformities such as talipes equinovarus (clubfoot) common, especially with L4, L5 level.
8. Tethered cord may lead to increased severity of problems as child grows.
9. Latex sensitivity/allergy.

Impairments

1. Depends on level of lesion and amount of malformation of cord.
2. Muscle paralysis and imbalance resulting from spinal and lower limb deformities and joint contractures.
   a. Kyphoscoliosis.
   b. Shortened hip flexors and adductors.
   c. Flexed knees.
   d. Pronated feet.
3. L4, L5 lesion results in bowel and bladder dysfunction.
4. Sensory loss.
5. Developmental delays.
6. Abnormal tone: may have low tone, leading to poor strength and/or spasticity in upper extremities.
7. Osteoporosis.
8. Cognitive impairments including mental retardation, learning and perceptual disabilities, language disorders.

Functional Limitations

1. Highly variable, depending on level of lesion.
2. Weakness or paralysis of hip flexors (high lumbar level lesion) makes ambulation possible only with reciprocating gait orthosis (RGO).
3. Problems with learning, communication.

Medical-Surgical Management of Spina Bifida

1. If an open (aperta) defect, surgical closure within 24–48 hours postnatally. Lesion can also be closed in utero.
2. Ventriculoperitoneal (VP) shunt performed for hydrocephalus. Ventriculoatrial (AV) shunts can also be used.
3. Orthopedic surgeries similar to cerebral palsy.

Physical Therapy Examination for Spina Bifida

1. Physiological homeostasis in infants, breathing, oxygenation.
2. Gross and fine motor development including reflex and behavioral examination of infant.
3. Communicate with parents, family members about concerns, goals for intervention.
4. Functional abilities using PEDI or WeeFIM.
5. Active and passive ROM.
6. Muscle strength: may observe developmental abilities if child under 3 years of age.
7. Sensation: stroke skin and note response; record by dermatome.
8. Skin: check for skin breakdown, suture of closure, skin over shunt line.

Interventions, Goals, and Prognosis for Spina Bifida

1. Teach parents proper positioning, handling, and exercise, keeping physiological flexion of the newborn. Include prone positioning to avoid shortening of hip flexors, as well as hip ROM, low tone, and osteoporosis.
2. Use adaptive equipment/orthoses, such as spinal orthoses for alignment, adaptive chairs for sitting (if needed), parapodium for early standing, lower extremity (LE) orthoses and ambulation assistive devices and/or wheelchair as needed.
3. Facilitate functional motor development, including appropriate developmental activities, primary or voluntary movement as well as reactive and anticipatory postural adjustments.
4. Educate parents regarding shunt malfunction. Signs include increased irritability, decreased muscle tone, seizures, vomiting, bulging fontanels, headache, and redness along shunt tract.
5. See Table 9-8.

Brachial Plexus Injury

Pathology

1. Traction or compression injury to unilateral brachial plexus during birth process or due to cervical rib abnormality.
   a. Erb's paralysis (also known as Erb-Duchenne paralysis) involves C5–6, upper arm paralysis, may involve rhomboids, levator scapulae, serratus anterior, deltoid, supraspinatus, infraspinatus, biceps brachii, brachioradialis, brachialis, supinator, and long extensors of wrist, fingers, and thumb.
   b. Klumpke's paralysis involves C8–T1, lower arm paralysis, involves intrinsic muscles of hand, and finger flexors and extensors (also weakness of the flexor carpi ulnaris).

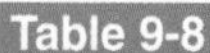

Table 9-8

Myelodysplasia Orthotics and Functional Prognosis by Spinal Cord Level

LEVEL	MUSCLE ACTIVITY	ORTHOSES	ASSISTIVE DEVICE	WHEELCHAIR	FUNCTIONAL PROGNOSIS
Thoracic	No hip flexion	THKAFO or RGO Parapodium/stander	Walker	Typically manual W/C potential power W/C for long distances	W/C for all mobility; standing and walking for physiologic benefits only
L1-2	Have some hip flexion: • L1:psoas major (<3/5) • L2:psoas major, iliacus, sartorius, pectineus (>3/5)	KAFO	Walker/forearm crutches	Manual W/C	W/C for most mobility; ambulation for short/household distances
L3	Strong hip flexion, weak hip rotators, at least antigravity knee extension Partial innervation of sartorius, gracilis and quadriceps	KAFO if quadriceps <4/5; AFO if quadriceps >4/5.	Walker/forearm crutches	Manual W/C	W/C for community; ambulation primary means if using AFO
L4	Partial innervation of tibialis anterior and peroneus tertius, tensor fascia lata, gluteus medius and gluteus minimus	AFO with posterior stop	Forearm crutches/ canes	No W/C	Community ambulation
L5	Partial innervation of hamstrings Partial innervation of tibialis posterior, peroneus longus and brevis, extensor hallucis longus, flexor digitorum longus and flexor hallucis longus Near full innervation peroneus tertius and extensor digitorum longus	AFO with posterior stop	Canes	No W/C	Community ambulation
S1	Near full innervation of hamstrings Partial innervation of gluteus maximus, gastrocnemius, soleus	FO, maybe AFO	No device	No W/C	Community ambulation
S2	Good strength for gait	No orthosis	No device	No W/C	Community ambulation

c. Total or whole arm paralysis (formerly known as Erb-Klumpke palsy), C5–T1.

2. Brachial plexus injuries may range from minor neuropraxic involvement of myelin to complete nerve root avulsions.

Impairments

1. Sensory deficits of upper extremity.
2. Paralysis or paresis of upper extremity.
3. Characteristic position for Erb's paralysis of upper extremity is adduction, internal rotation of shoulder with extension of elbow, pronation of forearm, and flexion of wrist. Waiter's tip deformity.

Functional Limitations

1. Dependent on severity of injury.
   a. Erb's paralysis results in decreased shoulder girdle function with 1:1 humeroscapular movement. Only have use of the hand.
   b. Klumpke's paralysis results in decreased wrist and hand function.
2. Traction injuries resolve spontaneously.
3. Avulsion injuries may require surgical nerve repair if not resolved within 3 months.
4. Shoulder subluxation and contractures of muscles may develop.

Physical Therapy Examination for Brachial Plexus Injury

1. Observe infant posture, as well as arm position and movement.
2. Test reflexes: Moro, biceps, radial reflexes are not present; grasp is intact.
3. Sensory testing of affected upper extremity (UE).

Physical Therapy Intervention and Prognosis

1. Partial immobilization of limb across upper abdomen for 1–2 weeks to avoid further injury.
2. Gentle ROM after initial immobilization to avoid contractures and traction on healing neural fibers.
3. Elicit muscle activity with age-appropriate functional movements of UE.

4. May use gentle constraint of unaffected arm to facilitate use of affected UE. This can be done with positioning.
5. Prognosis depends on severity of nerve injury, favorable in most instances. If recovery does not occur, surgery is indicated.

Down Syndrome (Trisomy 21)

Pathology

1. Chromosomal abnormality caused by breakage and translocation of a piece of chromosome onto normal chromosome. Three types: Standard (95% of cases), translocation (normal number of chromosomes), and mosaic (rare).
2. Those with mosaic can have normal cognition and less impairment. There may be less disability as not all cells are impacted by the extra chromosome.
3. Brain weight less than normal.
4. Cerebellum and brain stem lighter than normal.
5. Smaller convolutions of cortex.

Impairments

1. Hypotonia.
2. Decreased force generation of muscles.
3. Congenital heart defects, especially septal defects.
4. Visual and hearing losses.
5. Atlantoaxial subluxation/dislocation could be due to laxity of transverse odontoid ligament.
   a. Signs include decreased strength, decreased ROM, hyporeflexic deep tendon reflexes (DTRs) and decreased sensation in extremities, persistent head tilt, and increase in muscle tone.
6. Cognitive deficit can be mild to severe.

Functional Limitations

1. Gross motor developmental delay.
2. Difficulties in eating and speech development due to low tone.

RED FLAG: Forceful neck flexion and rotation activities should be limited, due to atlantoaxial ligament laxity. Children should not do somersaults, dive into water, participate in contact sports.

3. Cognitive and perceptual deficits may result in delay of fine motor and psychosocial development.

Physical Therapy Examination for Down Syndrome

1. Developmental test of gross and fine motor skills.
2. Test of tone by passive ROM.
3. Active and passive ROM.
4. Muscle testing; may use observation of developmental postures and movements if child under 3 years of age.
5. Functional level.

Physical Therapy Interventions, Goals, and Prognosis for Down Syndrome

1. Minimize gross motor delay.
   a. Facilitate gross and fine motor development through appropriate positioning, posture, and movement activities.
   b. Increase strength and stability by manipulating gravity and resistance in a graded manner.
2. Encourage oral motor function.
   a. Facilitate lip closure and tongue retrusion.
   b. Short, frequent feeding sessions for energy conservation.
3. Avoid hyperextension of elbows and knees during weight-bearing activities.
4. Avoid all traction on extremities or spine due to ligamentous laxity and low muscle tone.
5. Prognosis may be correlated with tone: the lower the tone, the more significant the motor delay. Most children will walk by age 2 and all will walk by age 5.

Medical-Surgical Management of Down Syndrome

1. Yearly radiographs to rule out atlantoaxial subluxation starts at age 3. X-ray is unable to detect subluxation prior to 3 years of age, so assume and treat as if child has AA instability.
2. Medical-surgical correction of cardiac problems.

Plagiocephaly (Flat Head Syndrome)

Pathology

1. A type of cranial deformation that is classified based on severity.
2. Described as a parallelogram-shaped skull with ipsilateral occipital flattening and contralateral bulging.
3. Positional left plagiocephaly typically develops due to congenital right muscular torticollis (CMT) or supine positioning that results in excessive pressures on a malleable skull with "floating" plates.
4. May result, if unresolved, in facial, mandible, ear asymmetries, and protrusion of the frontal bone.
5. Was regarded as a cosmetic problem, but now known to be associated with gross motor delays.

Physical Therapy Examination

1. History of onset, pregnancy, delivery, postural preferences, or positions throughout the day including asymmetries in movement, family history, developmental milestones.
2. Review of systems: musculoskeletal, visual, gastrointestinal, cardiopulmonary, and integumentary issues.
3. Cervical range of motion (ROM) and strength.
4. Gross motor function and prone tolerance.
5. Pain.

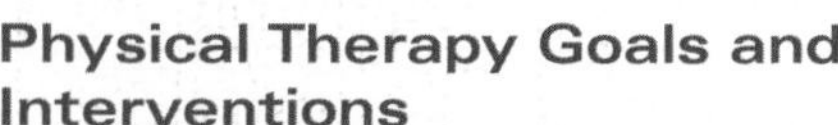

Physical Therapy Goals and Interventions

1. Prevention by educating about prolonged supine positioning and CMT.
   a. More successful with early intervention (before 3 months of age).
   b. Caregiver education including use of positioners, seats and swings, neck PROM exercises, facilitation of AROM of neck and trunk, gross motor development.

Cranial Remolding

1. If severe flattening or no progress with PT intervention, a helmet is prescribed made of thermoplastic material lined with high-density foam.
2. Typically custom made.
3. Helmet provides a symmetrical shape. As brain grows it pushes the skull into the helmet for molding.
4. Worn 20–23 hours per day for 2–7 months.
5. Best outcomes if helmet is started at 4–6 months of age.
6. Once child is 18 months of age and sutures of plates in the skull fuse, helmets are no longer useful.
7. Surgery is only considered in very severe cases.

Traumatic Brain Injury (TBI)

Pathology

1. Primary brain injury due to mechanical forces of initial impact.
   a. Acceleration-dependent injuries when force is applied to movable head such as coup-contrecoup and rotational injury.
   b. Nonacceleration-dependent injuries include skull depression into brain tissue and vibration.
   c. May be accidental or due to child abuse such as "shaken baby syndrome."
2. Secondary brain injury due to processes initiated as a result of initial trauma.
   a. Cerebral edema increases intracranial pressure and may lead to herniation, cerebral infarctions, brain stem injury, and coma.
   b. Epidural hematoma due to bleeds of middle meningeal artery, vein or venous sinus bleeds into epidural space.
   c. Subdural hematoma due to lacerated cortical blood vessels.
3. Evaluation of traumatic brain injury.
   a. Imaging such as computed tomography (CT) scan and magnetic resonance imaging (MRI) to determine extent of initial and secondary injury.
   b. Monitoring intracranial pressure.
   c. Behavioral scales such as the Glasgow Coma Scale and the Rancho Los Amigos Coma Scale (see Appendix 3A) assess the child's orientation to time and place and the ability to respond to various stimuli. Infant coma scale used for nonverbal infants.

Impairments

1. Depend on the severity and location of the initial and secondary injuries.
2. Level of consciousness and cognitive level may be temporarily or permanently impaired.
3. Spasticity, loss of functional ROM, contractures, and deformities.
4. Weakness, balance and coordination problems.
5. Heterotopic ossification—pathological bone formation around joint due to increased tone around joint, immobility and coma.

Functional Limitations

1. Decreased mobility skills.
2. Cognitive and perceptual difficulties.
3. Developmental process may be affected, resulting in abnormal development or developmental delay.

Physical Therapy Examination of Traumatic Brain Injury

1. History, MRI, CT, electroencephalogram (EEG) results, current medications.
2. Level of consciousness (Pediatric Coma Scale, Rancho Los Amigos Coma Scale).
3. Active and passive ROM.
4. Muscle strength: observe spontaneous movements if manual muscle test (MMT) is not possible.
5. Sensory testing.
6. Balance and coordination testing, developmental testing if appropriate.
7. Determination of muscle tone (modified Ashworth Scale; see Appendix 3A).
8. Cranial nerve testing.
9. Functional level testing.
10. Integumentary examination to check for pressure sores.

Interventions, Goals, and Prognosis

1. Maintain or improve joint flexibility by positioning, serial casting, ROM.
2. Stimulate/arouse level of consciousness through sensory stimuli.
3. Minimize gross and fine motor delay.
   a. Facilitate gross and fine motor development through appropriate positioning, postures, and movement activities.
   b. Increase strength and stability by manipulating gravity and resistance in a graded manner.
4. Parent/family or caregiver education.
5. Prognosis depends on severity of injury, rate of recovery, social and physical supports available.

Medical-Surgical Management for TBI

1. Mechanical ventilation, if needed.
2. Pharmacological agents to control intracranial pressure, including sedatives, paralytics, diuretics, and barbiturates.

3. Intracranial pressure monitored by intracranial pressure bolt.
4. Surgical evacuation of hematoma.

Duchenne's Muscular Dystrophy (DMD)* (Pseudohypertrophic Muscular Dystrophy)

Pathology

1. X-linked recessive, inherited by boys, carried by recessive gene of mother. Diagnosis confirmed by clinical examination, EMG, muscle biopsy, DNA analysis, and blood enzyme levels.
2. Dystrophin gene missing results in increased permeability of sarcolemma and destruction of muscle cells.
3. Collagen, adipose laid down in muscle leading to pseudohypertrophic calf muscles.

Impairments

1. Diagnosis is usually made between 3–6 years of age. Early signs include progressive weakness, delay in walking, difficulty rising from supine or sitting. Frequent falls. Proximal shoulder or pelvic muscle weakness occurs before distal weakness.
2. Positive Gower's sign due to weak quadriceps and gluteal muscles; child must use upper extremities to "walk up legs" and rise to standing.
3. Cardiac tissue also involved.
4. Contractures and deformities develop due to muscle imbalance, especially of heel cords and tensor fascia latae, as well as lumbar lordosis and kyphoscoliosis.

Functional Limitations

1. Developmental milestones may be delayed.
2. Ambulation ability will be lost, necessitating eventual use of wheelchair.
3. Progressive cardiopulmonary limitations.

Examination for Muscular Dystrophy

1. Muscle strength—MMT, dynamometer.
2. Active and passive ROM.
3. Functional testing.
4. Skeletal alignment (check for lordosis, scoliosis, kyphosis).
5. Respiratory function, chest excursion during breathing or spirometer.
6. Assess need for adaptive equipment.

*See Chapter 2, Musculoskeletal Physical Therapy, for additional pediatric conditions, e.g., torticollis, arthrogryposis multiplex congenita, osteogenesis imperfecta, and other deformities; disorders of the hip, knee, ankle/foot, and spine.

Interventions, Goals, and Prognosis

1. Maintain mobility as long as possible by encouraging recreational and functional activities to maintain strength and cardiopulmonary function.
2. Maintain joint ROM with active and passive ROM exercises, and positioning devices, such as prone standers or standing frames. Gastrocnemius and tensor fascia lata shorten first. Night splints may be used.
3. Electrical stimulation of muscles for younger children may increase contractile ability.
4. Educate and support parents and family in a sensitive manner.

> RED FLAG: Do not exercise at maximal level; may injure muscle tissue (overwork injury).

5. Supervise use of adaptive equipment as needed.
6. Disease is progressive, leading to respiratory insufficiency and death in young adulthood.

Medical-Surgical Management

1. Palliative and supportive, treating symptoms as they occur.
2. Steroids (prednisone) increase life expectancy by decreasing pulmonary dysfunction. Antibiotics for pulmonary infections.
3. Orthopedic surgery for scoliosis (spinal instrumentation), muscle lengthening of gastrocnemius.

Autism Spectrum Disorder

Pathology

1. Developmental disorder that appears in the first 3 years of life and affects the brain's normal development of social and communication skills.
2. Linked to abnormal biology and chemistry in the brain.
3. Exact causes are unknown. It is probably a combination of factors that lead to autism. However, there seems to be a genetic link in some cases as it can "run in the family."
4. Difficulties with verbal and nonverbal communication, social interaction, and atypical play skills.
5. Sensory integration issues: hyposensitive (sensory-seekers) or hypersensitive (sensory-avoiders).
6. Complex condition that varies greatly in severity. 40% have average to above average intelligence.
7. Seen more in boys (1:54 boys versus 1:252 girl births).
8. Diagnosis can now be made in some cases as early as 6 months of age.

Impairments

1. Decreased coordination.
2. High-level balance impairments.
3. Occasional strength and ROM deficits.
4. Sensory impairments.

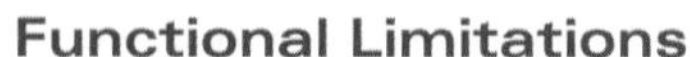

Functional Limitations

1. Delayed gross motor skills.

Physical Therapy Examination

1. Functional testing: age appropriate gross motor skills.
2. Muscle strength: MMT, dynamometer.
3. Coordination.
4. High-level balance activities.
5. Active and passive ROM.
6. Sensory examination often uses Sensory Profile 2.

Interventions, Goals, and Prognosis

1. Gross motor skill training to promote age-appropriate abilities.
2. Strengthening.
3. Coordination training.
4. Balance training.
5. Sensory integration.
6. Children tend to appear high functioning and age appropriate because they are independent ambulators. Many have delay in high-level skills such as coordinated running, skipping, riding a bike, standing on one leg, etc. Some will demonstrate toe walking.
7. Child with autism tends to have difficulty with new people and situations. They prefer a consistent routine and schedule.
8. Aggressive behaviors or passive behaviors are seen.

Other Interventions

1. Speech and occupational therapy is common.
2. Medications for attention deficits and anxiety disorders that can exist.
3. Some children are on special diets.

Pediatric Adaptive Equipment

Positioning Equipment

1. Used to maintain skeletal alignment, prevent or reduce development of contractures and deformities, and facilitate functional abilities.
2. Standers give the child weight-bearing experience, which maintains hips, knees, ankles, and trunk in optimal position, facilitates formation of acetabulum and aids bowel and bladder function.
3. Side-lyers decrease effects of TLR, put hands in visual field.
4. Adaptive seating is customized to meet the specific support and posture needs of the individual.
5. Abductor pad at hips often used in positioning equipment to decrease scissoring extension pattern of hip extension, adduction, with knee extension and plantar flexion of ankles.

Equipment for Therapeutic Exercise

1. Balls of different sizes to promote strengthening, balance, and coordination, and make motor learning fun.
2. Wedges to facilitate or increase muscle contraction needed, depending on position of wedge.
3. Bolsters combine characteristics of ball and wedge.
4. Swings to promote sensory integration.
5. Scooter boards for prone stability/mobility work.
6. Others include toys, modified tricycles, music, pets, and family members.

Lower Extremity Orthotics

1. AFOs to provide support to foot, ankle, and knee, to provide a stable base of support, and to reduce the effects of spasticity and hypoextensibility of muscles.
   a. Ankle set at 5°–10° dorsiflexion to decrease genu recurvatum.
   b. Articulating-ankle AFO controls amount of dorsiflexion and plantar flexion.
   c. Tone-reducing AFO. Made of polypropylene.
      - Decreases effects of spasticity, including scissoring by maintained stretch.
      - Stretches and maintains length of heel cord to prevent or lessen contracture.
      - Provides good mechanical base of support for standing and ambulation.
      - Floor reaction AFO to decrease "crouched gait" by preventing the tibia from moving too far forward in stance. This limits dorsiflexion and decreases knee flexion during ambulation.
2. Knee-ankle-foot orthosis (KAFO).
   a. For standing or ambulation.
   b. Reciprocal or swing-through gait.
   c. Knee may be solid at 0°–5° flexion or hinged.
   d. Used by children with spina bifida or muscular dystrophy.
3. Hip-knee-ankle-foot orthosis (HKAFO).
   a. For standing and ambulation.
   b. Swing-through gait.
   c. Used by children with spina bifida or spinal cord injuries.
4. Reciprocating gait orthosis (RGO).
   a. HKAFO with molded body jacket.
   b. Cable system allows forward step with lateral weight shift.
   c. Used by children with thoracic level spinal bifida or spinal cord injuries.
5. Pavlik harness.
   a. For infants with congenital hip dysplasia.
   b. Hips held in flexion and abduction to maintain femoral head in acetabulum.

Mobility Aids

1. Wheelchairs.
   a. Must be the correct size for the child.
   b. Posture, movement, strength, endurance, abnormal tone, contractures are important in determining custom features of a wheelchair, including method of mobility, seating stability.
   c. Stroller-type chairs limit independence of child.
   d. Scooter/three-wheelers require fair (3/5) sitting balance and upper extremity control.
   e. Power wheelchairs can be used as early as 18 months of age, depending on the specific child.
2. Walkers.
   a. Rollator walkers with wheels usually used.
   b. Forward walker (anterior rollator walker).
      - Encourages forward trunk leaning.
      - Provides maximum anterior stability.
   c. Posterior walker (posture control walker).
      - Encourages trunk extension.
      - Encourages shoulder depression, elbow extension, neutral wrist, which may decrease scissoring in lower extremities.
   d. Gait trainers offer maximum support to upper extremities and trunk.
3. Crutches.
   a. Require more postural control than walkers.
   b. Axillary and Lofstrand crutches available.

Family, Early Intervention, and the Education Setting

Family. The Single Most Important Constant and Environmental Factor

1. PT must collaborate with child and family.
2. Family-centered approach begins with child's and family's strengths, needs, and hopes, and results in a service plan that responds to the needs of the whole family. Role of PT is to support, encourage, and enhance the competence of parents or caretakers in their role as caregivers.
3. Parents of children with developmental disabilities often suffer from chronic sorrow due to the loss of the typical potential of their child.

Early Intervention Programs (EIPs)

1. Mandated by public law (IDEA or Individuals with Disabilities Act).
   a. To provide comprehensive, multidisciplinary EIP.
   b. For infants and children from birth to 3 years.
   c. Multidisciplinary assessment.
   d. Individual Family Service Plan (IFSP) developed.
   e. Family is a member of the team.

School System: Individual Education Plan (IEP)

1. Mandated by public law (IDEA or Individuals with Disabilities Act).
   a. Free and appropriate public education for all children with disabilities.
   b. For children 3 to 21 years.
   c. Multidisciplinary assessment.
   d. Right to related services such as PT is related to educational need.
   e. Least restrictive environment.

The authors would like to acknowledge Linda Kahn-D'Angelo, PT, ScD for her original contributions in formulating this chapter.

APPENDIX 9A

Selected Pediatric Screening Tools and Outcome Measures

Table 9A-1

Selected Pediatric Screening Tools and Outcome Measures

SCREENING TOOL OR OUTCOME MEASURE	NORM/CRITERION REFERENCED	DOMAINS TESTED	MODE	AGES
Alberta Infant Motor Scale (AIMS)	Norm	Gross motor	Observational	0–18 months or until independent walking
Assessment of Premature Infant Behavior (APIB)	Norm	Refinement and extension of NBAS (see below). Assesses the organization and balance of physiological, motor, and behavioral states (lengthy and used mainly for research).	Physical	Birth to 1 month after expected due date
Battelle Developmental Inventory (BDI-2)	Norm	Comprehensive (adaptive, personal-social, communication, motor, cognitive)	Interview and Physical	0–7 years, 11 months
Bayley Scale of Infant Development III	Norm	Comprehensive (cognitive, communication, motor, social, emotional, adaptive behavior)	Physical (for gross motor part)	0–42 months
Bruininks-Oseretsky Test of Motor (BOT-2)	Norm	Fine and gross motor	Physical	4–21 years
Denver Developmental Screening Test II	Norm	Screens for developmental delay in areas of social, fine motor, gross motor, and language skills	Physical	0–6 years
Functional Independence Measure for Children (WeeFIM)	Norm	Self-care, mobility, and cognition	Physical	6 months to 12 years of age with a disability without cognitive impairment, or for any child with a mental age below 7

(*Continued*)

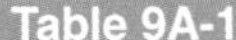

Table 9A-1

Selected Pediatric Screening Tools and Outcome Measures (Continued)				
SCREENING TOOL OR OUTCOME MEASURE	**NORM/CRITERION REFERENCED**	**DOMAINS TESTED**	**MODE**	**AGES**
Gross Motor Function Measure (GMFM-88)	Criterion	Gross motor	Physical	Best suited for 2–5 years of age, but can be used at any age
Hawaii Early Learning Profile (HELP)	Criterion	Comprehensive (7 domains: cognitive, gross, fine, communication, social-emotional, self-help, sensory regulation)	Physical	0–36 months
Movement Assessment of Infants (MAI)	Criterion	Identifies motor dysfunction and changes in the status of motor dysfunction and establishes an early intervention program.	Physical	0–12 months
Neonatal Behavioral Assessment Scale (NBAS), also known as the Brazelton Neonatal Assessment Scale (BNAS)	Norm	Comprehensive exam of newborns (reflexes, state of alertness, muscle tone, and physical characteristics)	Physical and Observational	3 days to 4 weeks of age
Peabody Developmental Motor Skills (PDMS)	Norm	Fine and gross motor	Physical	0–72 months
Pediatric Evaluation of Disability Index (PEDI)	Criterion	Self-care, mobility and social function	Physical	6 months to 7.5 Years (can go higher if child not functioning at 7.5 or with cognitive delay)
Routines-Based Interview (RBI)	Criterion	Comprehensive (cognitive, motor, adaptive, communication, social skills)	Interview	0–5 years
School Function Measure (SFM)	Criterion	Participation, task support, and activity performance	Observational, Physical and Professional Judgment	K to 6th grade (5–12 years of age)
Sensory Integration and Praxis Test	Norm	Sensory integration processes that underlie learning and behavior	Physical	4 years to 8 years, 11 months
Sensory Profile-2	Norm	Sensory processing patterns in the context of home, school, and community-based activities	Physical	3 years–14 years, but Infant and Toddler versions also available
Test of Infant Motor Performance (TIMP)	Criterion	Gross motor	Observational and Physical	34 weeks gestational age to 4 months

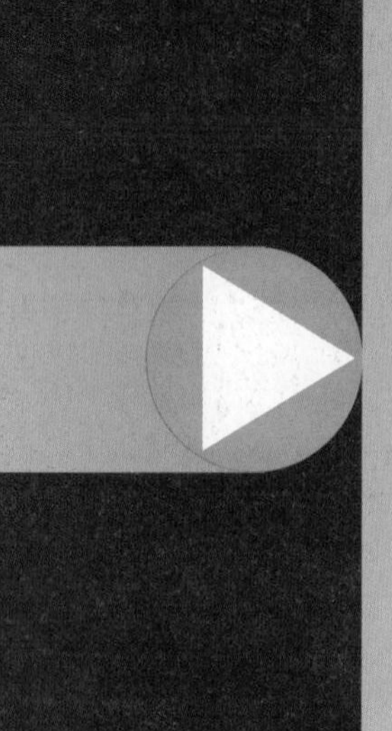

APPENDIX 9B

Review Questions and Case Study

(Answers to all Review Questions and Case Studies are found in Chapter 17)

1. In the developing infant, what are the differences in terms of age of onset and response between the asymmetrical tonic neck reflex (ATNR) and the symmetrical tonic neck reflex (STNR)?

2. When performing an examination of the skeletal system in a full-term neonate, what possible abnormal bony conditions should be part of the screening process?

3. What are the typical lower extremity contractures seen with the child with spastic cerebral palsy?

4. What is a realistic expectation for functional mobility in the community and in the household for a patient with myelodysplasia affecting the midlumbar levels (about L3)?

Case Study

Patient Profile

- Gender: Male
- Age: 12 months

Presenting Problem/Current Condition

- The infant has been referred to physical therapy for early intervention services
- Diagnosis is Down syndrome (Trisomy 21)

Past Medical/Surgical History

- Born at full term via Cesarean section
- Pediatric cardiologist hopes a ventricular septal defect will close as he gets older
- Receiving speech therapy due to delays in expressive communication skills

Other Information

- Child is currently in foster care due to neglect and is awaiting adoption
- Foster care provider is unfamiliar with Down syndrome and has many questions about the condition and prognosis
- Child is pleasant and smiles at everyone
- Fine motor skills are age-appropriate
- Child can belly crawl, sit independently, get into the quadruped position, and is starting to pull to stand
- Prefers to sit in a W-sitting position and sleep in prone with hips in abduction, ER, and flexion
- Transitions into sitting from prone by pushing up on hands and maximally abducting hips
- Very little interest in toys

Question #1

Which of the following would be the **GREATEST** priority for the PT when planning education with the foster care provider?

1. Low muscle tone and potential joint laxity.
2. Prognosis of gross motor skills, especially ambulation.
3. Precautions and contraindications associated with atlantoaxial joint instability (AA instability).
4. Potential causes and interventions for his ventricular septal defect.

Question #2

Which of the following is potentially **MOST** problematic with the preferred W-sitting posture?

1. Development of a kyphosis of the spine.
2. Further laxity of lateral collateral ligaments in the knees.
3. Development of bilateral femoral retroversion.
4. Developing a "toeing-in" posture when standing.

Question #3

What is the prognosis for children with Down syndrome in terms of independent ambulation?

1. Most will walk by 5 years of age but will typically require an assistive device.
2. All children with Down syndrome will walk, likely by 2 years of age.
3. It is highly variable, and some children will not acquire this skill.
4. Children with Down syndrome typically walk "on time."

10

Geriatric Physical Therapy

SUSAN B. O'SULLIVAN, ANNE L. HARRISON, AND SCOTT W. SHAFFER

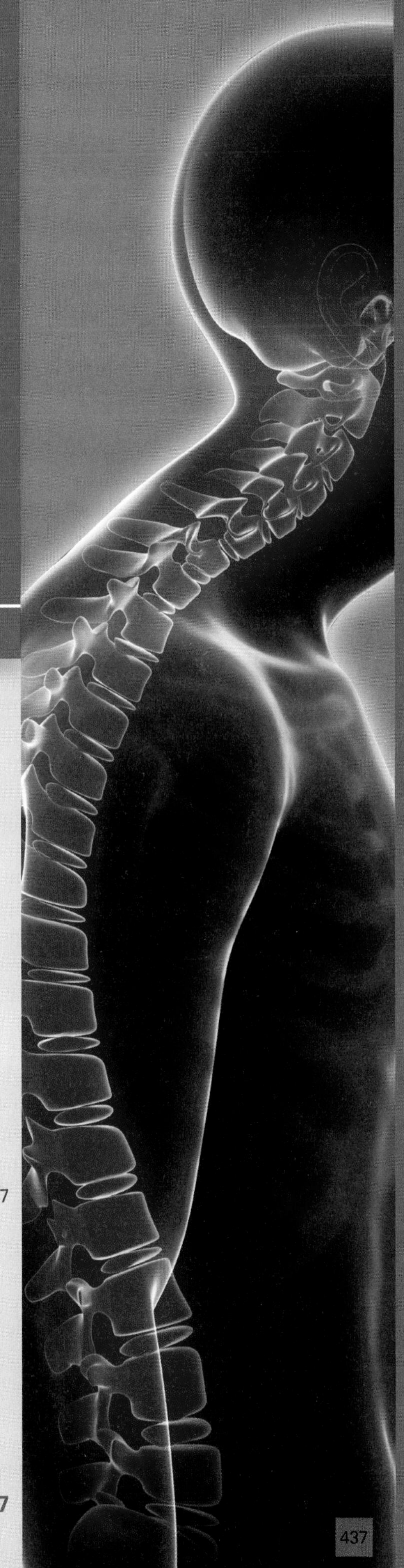

Chapter Outline

Foundations of Geriatric Physical Therapy

General Concepts and Definitions of Aging

Aging

1. The process of changing over time, or growing older.
2. Common to all members of a given species.
3. Characterized by:
   a. Declining ability to respond to stress and increasing homeostatic imbalance.
   b. Increasing probability of disease with decreasing ability to successfully respond to insult.
4. Varies among and within individuals.

Gerontology

1. The scientific study of all aspects of aging (biological, psychosocial, cultural, and cognitive aspects).

Geriatrics

1. The branch of medicine that addresses health, health care, and wellness of older adults.

Life Span

1. Maximum survival potential, the inherent natural life of the species.
2. In humans, 110–122 years.

Life Expectancy

1. The number of years of life expectation from year of birth.
2. In the United States, the average life expectancy is 78.8 years (CDC National Center for Health Statistics).
3. Life expectancy for women is approximately 5 years longer than men.

Categories of Elderly

1. Young elderly: ages 65–74 (60% of elderly population).
2. Old elderly: ages 75–84.
3. Old, old elderly, or old and frail elderly: ages ≥85.
4. Centenarians: 100 years or older.
5. Supercentenarians: 110 years or older.

Ageism

1. Discrimination and prejudice leveled against individuals on the basis of their age.

Demographics, Mortality, and Morbidity

Persons Over 65

1. A rapidly growing segment of the population with lengthening of life expectancy; the number of Americans aged 65 and older is projected to double from 46 million (15% of population in 2017) to more than 98 million (24% of population by 2060).
2. Older women outnumber older men; 145 women for every 100 men.

Increased Life Expectancy

1. Aging of the population due to:
   a. Advances in health care, improved infectious disease control.
   b. Advances in infant/child care, decreased mortality rates.
   c. Improvements in nutrition and sanitation.

Leading Causes of Death (Mortality) in Persons Over 65, in Order of Frequency (2018 Data, CDC)

1. Heart disease.
2. Cancer.
3. Chronic obstructive pulmonary disease.
4. Cerebrovascular disease (stroke).
5. Alzheimer's disease.
6. Diabetes.
7. Pneumonia and influenza.
8. Accidents.
9. Nephritis.
10. Septicemia.

*For 2020, COVID was the leading cause of death in adults >65 years old.

Health Factors (in Noninstitutionalized Older Adults; 2018 Data, CDC)

1. Approximately 20% of those 65 years and older are in fair or poor health.
2. Approximately 9% of those 65 years and older smoke.
3. Obesity:
   a. Approximately 40% of those 65 to 74 years old.
   b. Approximately 30% of those 75 years or older.
4. Physical activity: defined as 150 minutes of moderate-intensity exercise, 75 minutes of vigorous exercise, or a combination of both.
   a. Approximately half of those aged 65 to 74 years old met the standard.
   b. Approximately a third of those 75 years or older met the standard.
5. Hypertension:
   a. Approximately 61% of males 65 to 74 years old; 67% for males >75 years old.
   b. Approximately 67% of female 65 to 74 years old; 78% for males >75 years old.
6. Diabetes: Approximately 25% those 65 years and older.

Socioeconomic Factors

1. Half of all older women are widows; older men are twice as likely to be married as older women.
2. Most live on fixed incomes: Social Security is the major source of income; poverty rate for persons over 65 is 9%; another 26% of older persons have low annual incomes.
3. About half of older persons have completed high school.
4. Noninstitutionalized elderly: most live in family settings (7.0% of older adults >65 years need help with personal care from other persons).
5. Institutionalized elderly: about 5% of persons over 65 reside in nursing homes; percentage increases dramatically with age (22% of persons over 85).

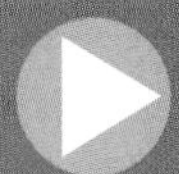

Physiological Changes and Clinical Implications for the Older Adult

Health-Related Pathology versus Age-Related Changes

1. Figure 10-1 shares the impact that pathology (aka structural and functional impairments) associated with health conditions (e.g., diabetes, hypertension, osteoarthritis), age-related changes, and optimal aging has on older adults' activity and participation.
2. PTs need to identify expected age-related changes from more progressive pathological health conditions and refer older adults for additional care or workup when needed.
3. Additionally, PTs need to target treatment options that enable a positive shift toward age-related and/or optimal activity and participation for older adults.

Muscular (See Table 10.1)

Age-Related Changes

1. Changes are due to both decreased activity levels and age-related physiological changes.
2. Muscle strength: peaks at around 30 years old, remains fairly constant until age 50, after which there is an accelerated loss of strength (20%–40% loss by age 65 in the nonexercising adult).
3. Loss of power (force/unit time): significant declines due to losses in speed of contraction, changes in nerve conduction and synaptic transmission.
4. Loss of skeletal muscle mass (atrophy): both size and number of muscle fibers decrease; by age 70, loss of 33% of skeletal muscle mass.
5. Changes in muscle fiber composition: selective loss of type II, fast-twitch fibers, with increase in proportion of type I fibers.
6. Changes in muscular endurance: muscles fatigue more readily.
   a. Decreased muscle tissue oxidative capacity.
   b. Decreased peripheral blood flow, oxygen delivery to muscles.
   c. Altered chemical composition of muscle: decreased myosin adenosine triphosphatase (ATPase) activity, glycoproteins, and contractile protein.
   d. Collagen changes: denser, irregular due to cross-linkages, loss of water content and elasticity; affects tendons, bone, cartilage.

Figure 10-1 A continuum representing the influence of health conditions and typical age-related changes on older adults' activity and participation.

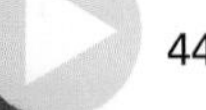

Table 10-1

Potential Age-Related Musculoskeletal and Neuromuscular Physiological Changes, Impairments, Activity Limitations, and Participation Restrictions

SYSTEM/PHYSIOLOGICAL CHANGES	IMPAIRMENTS	ACTIVITY LIMITATIONS	PARTICIPATION RESTRICTIONS
Muscular: ↓ muscle fibers, muscle fiber diameter, preferentially affecting type 2 fibers	↓ muscle strength, power, and force production; Impaired trunk/pelvic stability and balance	Affects sit to stand, steps/stairs, gait speed, postural stability, upper extremity strength (e.g., grip); ↑ fall risk	↓ efficiencies in IADLS,* ADLs,** leisure, work; self-restrictions outside of home secondary to weakness and/or kinesiophobia
Skeletal: Imbalance in bone remodeling, with bone resorption outpacing bone formation	↓ bone density (gms/cm^2), potential vulnerability to fracture (e.g., compression fractures), ↑ fracture healing time, ↑ risk of postural deviations (e.g., kyphosis)	Dependent on fracture type, site and corresponding non-surgical and/or surgical treatment (e.g., plate/compression screw/intermedullary rod)	↓ efficiencies in IADLS,* ADLs,** leisure, work; self-restrictions outside of home secondary to pain, disuse weakness, weight-bearing status and kinesiophobia
Connective tissue: ↓ hydration; ↓ nutrition; ↓ ability to repair	Cartilage thins with ↑ prevalence of osteoarthritis; tendon and ligaments weaken at insertion sites; ↑ prevalence of tendinopathy, ligament/capsular sprains	Pain with weight-bearing in gait and transitional postures, and/or pain in hands, spine with ADLs	↓ efficiencies in IADLS,* ADLs,** leisure, work; self-restrictions outside of home secondary to pain, disuse weakness, weight-bearing status and kinesiophobia
Sensory: ↓ numbers of sensory receptors, ↓ speed of sensory neuronal firing; changes (smudging) of primary/association sensory cortices	↓ sensory processing (vision, cutaneous, proprioception, vestibular, hearing); impaired balance; intermittent dizziness/vertigo; Fear of falling	Ataxia; inability to turn head while walking (visual/vestibular); ↓ hand/eye coordination; ↑ reaction time; ↑ fall risk	Difficulty walking in low light conditions and on unlevel surfaces; ↓ ability to multitask; difficulty reading (e.g., medication labels); self-restrictions outside of home secondary to fall risk and/or kinesiophobia
Central Nervous System: ↓ myelin, neurons and neurotransmitter synthesis in the CNS (cortex, basal ganglia, hippocampus, cerebellum). ↓ blood flow ↓ nerve conduction velocity	↓ speed and efficiency of processing in sensory, motor, and autonomic nervous systems	Occasional memory or word finding problems; potential challenges with organization; occasional slowing of psychomotor speed and coordination; challenge with multiple tasks (e.g., walk and talk test)	Normal changes do not typically restrict participation; self-restrictions may occur secondary to challenges with dual/multitask activities

↑=increased; ↓=decreased/reduced; *IADLS=Instrumental Activities of Daily Living including shopping, housekeeping, money management, food prep, transportation, phone, laundry; **ADLs=Activities of Daily Living including toileting, grooming, bathing, dressing, transferring.

References: Guccione A, Wong R, Avers D (2019). Guccione's Geriatric Physical Therapy, 4th ed. St Louis, Elsevier and Goodman C, Fuller K (2014). Pathology: Implications for the Physical Therapist, 4th ed. Elsevier.

Clinical Implications

1. Weakness/fatigue is often related to disuse and not disease.
   a. Stresses importance of determining what activities the client typically performs and correlating these to physical performance and strength testing.
   b. If weakness/decreased power fit patterns of inactivity, these have a positive prognosis for recovery.
   c. If weakness does not fit with disuse and aging, consider additional pathology (e.g., peripheral neuropathy, osteoarthritis, etc.).
2. Movements become slower in part as a result of loss of strength and power. Declines in power emphasize the importance of using timed outcome measure (e.g., timed up and go, sit to stand) in addition to independence level and quality of movement.
3. Movements fatigue more easily. Important to measure the client's perception of fatigue (Fatigue Severity Scale) and physical activity (e.g., Physical Activity Scale for the Elderly) and compare it to objective physical performance tests with multiple repetitions (e.g., 5 Times Sit-to-Stand Test).
4. Connective tissue becomes denser and stiffer.
   a. Increased risk of muscle sprains, strains, tendon tears.
   b. Loss of range of motion (ROM): highly variable by joint and individual; activity level.

c. Increased tendency for fibrinous adhesions, contractures.
5. Decreased functional mobility, limitations to movement.
6. Gait changes.
   a. Stiffer, fewer automatic movements: Older adults often sacrifice speed of movement for stability, resulting in cocontraction of knee extensors/flexors during midstance.
   b. Decreased amplitude and speed, slower cadence.
   c. Shorter steps, wider stride, increased double support to ensure safety, compensate for decreased balance.
   d. Decreased trunk rotation, arm swing.
   e. Gait may become unsteady due to changes in balance, strength; increased need for assistive devices.
7. Clinical risk of falls is evident in many older adults.

Interventions to Slow or Reverse Changes

1. Improve health.
   a. Correction of medical problems that may cause weakness: hyperthyroidism, excess adrenocortical steroids (e.g., Cushing's disease, steroids); hyponatremia (low sodium in blood).
   b. Improve nutrition.
      - Correction of hyponatremia.
      - Increased fatigue associated with diarrhea, prolonged use of diuretics.
2. Increase levels of physical activity, stress functional activities and activity programs.
   a. Gradual increase in intensity of activity to avoid injury.
   b. Adequate warm-up and cool-down; appropriate pacing and rest periods.
3. Provide strength training.
   a. Significant increases in strength noted in older adults with isometric and progressive resistive exercise programs.
   b. High-intensity and power training programs (70%–80% of one-repetition maximum) produce quicker and more predictable results than moderate-intensity programs; both have demonstrated success with older adult populations.
   c. Even small improvements in strength correlate to improved functional abilities.
4. Provide flexibility, ROM exercises.
   a. Utilize slow, prolonged stretching, maintained for 20–30 seconds.
   b. Tissues heated prior to stretching are more extensible; e.g., warm pool.
   c. Maintain newly gained range: incorporate into functional activities.
   d. Mobility gains are slower with older adults.
5. Provide balance training.
   a. Significant increases in balance noted in older adults with balance training programs.
   b. Improvements in balance correlate to increased function and a reduction in falls.

Skeletal System (See Table 10.1)

Age-Related Changes

1. Cartilage changes: decreased water content, becomes stiffer, fragments, and erodes; by age 60, more than 60% of adults have degenerative joint changes, cartilage abnormalities.
2. Bone mass and density: peak bone mass in the late 20s; between ages 45 and 70, bone mass decreases (in women, by about 25%; in men, by 15%); decreases another 5% by age 90.
   a. Loss of calcium and bone strength, especially trabecular bone.
   b. See discussion of osteoporosis under Pathological Conditions Associated with Older Adults.
   c. Decreased bone marrow red blood cell production.
3. Intervertebral discs: flatten, less resilient due to loss of water content (30% loss by age 65) and loss of collagen elasticity; trunk length, overall height decreases.
4. Postural changes associated with aging (Figures 10-2 and 10-3).
   a. Forward head.
   b. Kyphosis of thoracic spine.
   c. Flattening of lumbar spine.
   d. With prolonged sitting, tendency to develop hip and knee flexion contractures.
   e. Foot deformities: hallux valgus, pes planus, and pes cavus.

Clinical Implications

1. Increased risk of fractures associated with aging.
2. Increased age-related arthritis.

Interventions to Slow or Reverse Changes

1. Postural exercise should focus on strengthening postural extensors and scapular stabilizers (see Figure 10-4).
2. Weight-bearing (gravity-loading) exercise may decrease bone loss in older adults; e.g., walking, stair climbing, weight belts can increase load.
3. Resistance exercise may decrease the rate of bone loss among older adults.
4. Nutritional, hormonal, and medical therapies are critical (for additional information see the section on osteoporosis).

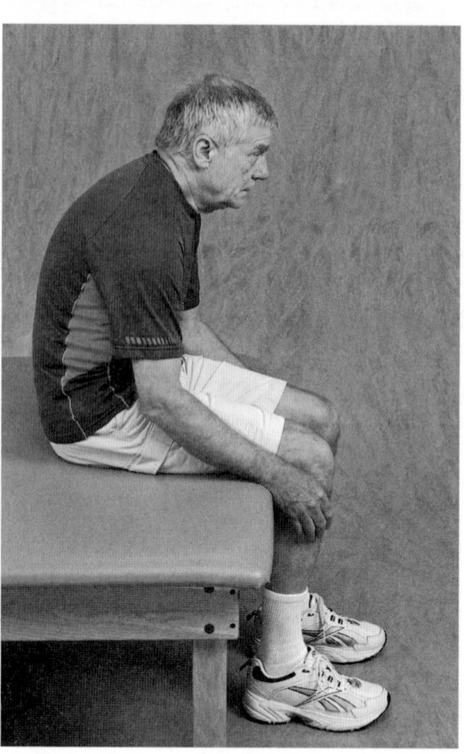

Figure 10-2 Postural changes associated with aging (sitting posture). This patient exhibits a forward head position, dorsal kyphosis, flattening of the lumbar spine, and a posterior pelvic tilt.

From O'Sullivan, S, and Bezkor, E. Interventions to Improve Sitting and Sitting Balance Skills, Ch 5. In O'Sullivan, S, and Schmitz T. Improving Functional Outcomes in Physical Rehabilitation, 2nd ed. F A Davis, Philadelphia, 2016, with permission.

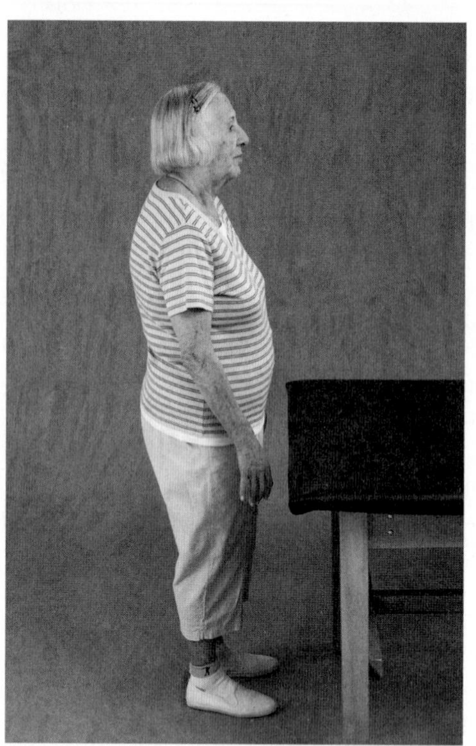

Figure 10-3 Postural changes associated with aging in standing. This patient exhibits a slight forward head position and dorsal kyphosis. Increased hip and knee flexion is also typical.

From O'Sullivan, S, and Moriarity-Baron, J. Interventions to Improve Standing and Standing Balance Skills, Ch. 9. In O'Sullivan, S, and Schmitz T. Improving Functional Outcomes in Physical Rehabilitation, 2nd ed. F A Davis, Philadelphia, 2016, with permission.

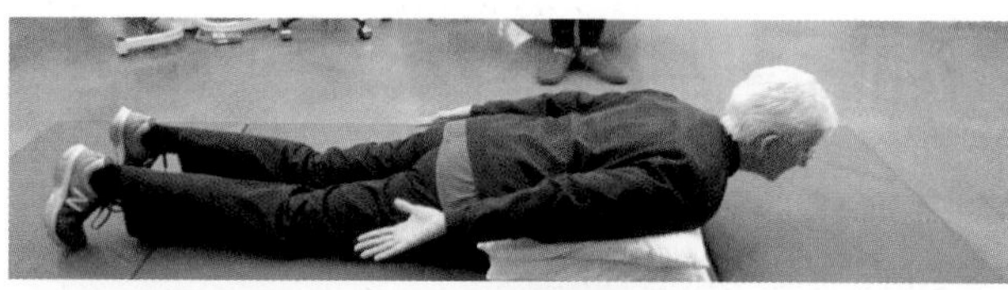

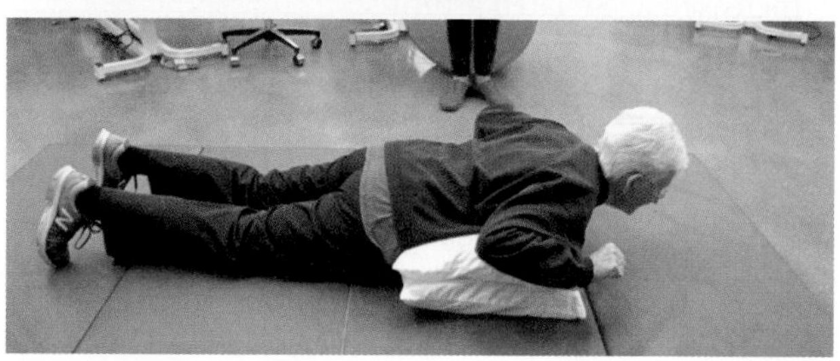

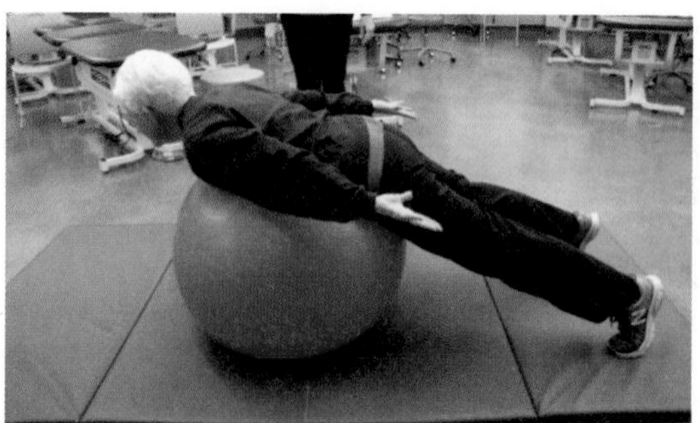

Figure 10-4 Postural exercise to strengthening postural extensors and scapular stabilizers.

Neurological System (See Table 10.1)

Age-Related Changes

1. Atrophy of nerve cells in cerebral cortex: overall loss of cerebral mass/brain weight of 6%–11% between ages of 20 and 90; accelerating loss after age 70.
2. Changes in brain morphology.
   a. Gyral atrophy: narrowing and flattening of gyri with widening of sulci.
   b. Ventricular dilation.
   c. Generalized cell loss in cerebral cortex: especially frontal and temporal lobes, association areas (prefrontal cortex, visual).
   d. Presence of lipofuscins, senile or neuritic plaques, and neurofibrillary tangles (NFT): significant accumulations associated with pathology; e.g., Alzheimer's dementia.
   e. More selective cell loss in basal ganglia (substantia nigra and putamen), cerebellum, hippocampus, locus coeruleus; brainstem minimally affected.
3. Decreased cerebral blood flow and energy metabolism.
4. Changes in synaptic transmission.
   a. Decreased synthesis and metabolism of major neurotransmitters; e.g., acetylcholine, dopamine.
   b. Slowing of many neural processes, especially in polysynaptic pathways.
5. Changes in spinal cord/peripheral nerves.
   a. By age 90, 30%–50% loss of anterior horn cells and 30% loss of posterior roots (sensory fibers).
   b. Loss of motoneurons results in increase in size of remaining motor units (development of macromotor units).
   c. Slowed nerve conduction velocity.
   d. Loss of sympathetic fibers: may account for diminished, autonomic stability, increased incidence of postural hypotension in older adults.
6. Age-related tremors (essential tremor, ET).
   a. Occur as an isolated symptom, particularly in hands, head, and voice.
   b. Characterized as postural or kinetic, rarely resting.
   c. Benign, slowly progressive; in late stages, may limit function.
   d. Exaggerated by movement and emotion.

Clinical Implications

1. Effects on movement.
   a. Overall speed and coordination are decreased; increased difficulty with fine motor control.
   b. Slowed recruitment of motoneurons contributes to loss of strength.
   c. Both reaction time and movement time increase.
   d. Older adults are affected by the speed/accuracy tradeoff.
      - The simpler the movement, the less the change.
      - More complicated movements require more preparation, longer reaction and movement times.
      - Faster movements result in decreased accuracy and increased errors.
   e. Older adults demonstrate increased reliance on visual feedback for movement.
   f. Older adults may become error averse and develop fear of movement.
2. General slowing of neural processing: learning and memory may be affected.
3. Autonomic nervous system dysfunction (see Reg Flag box).

> **RED FLAG:** Older adults may exhibit impairments in homeostatic regulation; stressors (heat, cold, excess exercise); can be harmful, even life-threatening; emphasizes the importance of consistent vital sign checks when working with older adults.

Interventions to Slow or Reverse Changes

1. Correction of medical problems: improve cerebral blood flow.
2. Improve health behaviors: diet, smoking cessation, and address alcohol use (risk factor for polyneuropathy and cerebellar disease); consider interprofessional referrals.
3. Increase levels of physical activity to encourage neuronal branching, slow rate of neural decline, improve central and peripheral nervous system circulation.
4. Provide effective strategies to improve motor learning and control.
   a. Allow for increased reaction and movement times to improve motivation, accuracy of movements.
   b. Allow for limitations of memory by avoiding long sequences of movements.
   c. Allow for increased cautionary behaviors: provide adequate explanation, demonstration when teaching new movement skills.
   d. Focus on meaningful functional activities to enlist implicit procedural memory.
   e. Emphasize repetition (i.e., practice) to facilitate transition from "performance" effect to "motor learning" effects.
   f. Gradually introduce dual task activities (e.g., cognitive and motor tasks performed simultaneously) in order to facilitate adaptation.
   g. Use mental imagery practice during periods of rest and between activities.

Sensory Systems (See Table 10.1)

Collective Sensory Systems Age-Related Changes

1. Often leads to sensory integration issues to include sensory deprivation, isolation, disorientation, and confusion.
2. May challenge social interactions and community participation.
3. The combination of age-related sensory impairments may lead to decreased coordination, impaired motor control, and postural instability that is not attributed to a medical diagnosis (e.g., polyneuropathy, retinopathy, vestibular dysfunction).
4. May lead to increased injury risk (falls, skin ulcers) and decreased activity/participation.

Vision

1. Aging changes: there is a general and gradual decline in visual acuity until sixth decade; increased decline between 60 to 90 years of age with rapid loss after age 75.
   a. Presbyopia: visual loss in middle and older ages characterized by inability to focus properly and blurred images due to loss of accommodation, elasticity of lens.
   b. Decreased ability to adapt to dark and light.
   c. Increased sensitivity to light and glare, increased difficulty with night driving.
   d. Loss of color discrimination, especially for blues and greens.
   e. Decreased pupillary responses, size of resting pupil increases.
   f. Decreased sensitivity of corneal reflex: less sensitive to eye injury or infection.
   g. Oculomotor responses diminished: restricted upward gaze, reduced pursuit eye movements; ptosis may develop.
2. Additional vision loss with pathology.
   a. Cataracts: opacity, clouding of lens due to changes in lens proteins; results in gradual loss of vision: central first, then peripheral; increased problems with glare; general darkening of vision; loss of acuity, distortion; often correctable with surgery.
   b. Glaucoma: increased intraocular pressure, with degeneration of optic disc, atrophy of optic nerve; results in early loss of peripheral vision (tunnel vision), progressing to total blindness if not managed medically.
   c. Senile macular degeneration: loss of central vision associated with age-related degeneration of the macula, compromised by decreased blood supply or abnormal growth of blood vessels under the retina; initially, patients retain peripheral vision; may progress to total blindness; if not managed medically.
   d. Diabetic retinopathy: damage to retinal capillaries, growth of abnormal blood vessels and hemorrhage leads to retinal scarring and finally retinal detachment; central vision impairment; complete blindness is rare.
   e. Cerebrovascular accident (CVA), homonymous hemianopsia: loss of half of visual field in each eye (nasal half of one eye and temporal half of other eye); produces an inability to receive information from right or left side; corresponds to side of sensorimotor deficit.
   f. Medications: impaired or fuzzy vision may result with antihistamines, tranquilizers, antidepressants, steroids.
3. Clinical implications/compensatory strategies.
   a. Examine vision: acuity, peripheral vision, light and dark adaptation, depth perception, diplopia, eye fatigue, eye pain.
   b. PT vision exam should include visual acuity, eye tracking, peripheral vision, and cranial nerve testing (to include pupillary light reflex).
   c. Maximize visual function: assess for use and accessibility of glasses, cleanliness of glasses, need for environmental adaptations, and prescription updates.
   d. Sensory thresholds are increased: allow extra time for visual discrimination and response.
   e. Work in adequate light, reduce glare; avoid abrupt changes in light; e.g., light to dark.
   f. Decreased peripheral vision may limit social interactions, physical function: stand directly in front of patient at eye level when communicating with patient.
   g. Assist in color discrimination: use warm colors (yellow, orange, red) for identification and color coding.
   h. Provide other sensory cues when vision is limited; e.g., verbal descriptions to new environments, touching to communicate you are listening.
   i. Provide safety education; reduce fall risk.
   j. Refer to optometry and/or ophthalmologist as needed.

Hearing

1. Aging changes: occur as early as fourth decade; affect a significant number of elderly (23% of individuals aged 65–74 have hearing impairments and 40% over age 75 have hearing loss; rate of loss in men is twice the rate of women, also starts earlier).
   a. Outer ear: build-up of cerumen (earwax) may result in conductive hearing loss; common in older men.
   b. Middle ear: minimal degenerative changes of bony joints.
   c. Inner ear: significant changes in sound sensitivity, understanding of speech, and maintenance of equilibrium may result with degeneration and atrophy of cochlea and vestibular structures, loss of neurons.

2. Types of hearing loss.
   a. Conductive: mechanical hearing loss from damage to external auditory canal, tympanic membrane, or middle ear ossicles; results in hearing loss (all frequencies); tinnitus (ringing in the ears) may be present.
   b. Sensorineural: central or neural hearing loss from multiple factors; e.g., noise damage, trauma, disease, drugs, arteriosclerosis.
   c. Presbycusis: sensorineural hearing loss associated with middle and older ages; characterized by bilateral hearing loss, especially at high frequencies at first, then all frequencies; poor auditory discrimination and comprehension, especially with background noise; tinnitus.
3. Additional hearing loss with pathology.
   a. Otosclerosis: immobility of stapes results in profound conductive hearing loss.
   b. Paget's disease.
   c. Hypothyroidism.
4. Clinical implications/compensatory strategies.
   a. Examine hearing: acuity, speech discrimination/comprehension, tinnitus, dizziness, vertigo, pain.
   b. Measure air and bone conduction: Rinne's test, Weber's test. See Chapter 3.
   c. Determine use of hearing aids; check for proper functioning.
   d. Minimize auditory distractions: work in quiet environment.
   e. Speak slowly and clearly, directly in front of patient at eye level; don't assume you have to speak loudly.
   f. Use nonverbal communication to reinforce your message; e.g., gesture, demonstration.
   g. Orient person to topics of conversation they cannot hear to reduce paranoia, isolation.

Vestibular/Balance Control

1. Aging changes: degenerative changes in otoconia of utricle and saccule; loss of vestibular hair-cell receptors; decreased number of vestibular neurons; vestibular ocular reflex (VOR) gain decreases, begins at age 30, accelerated decline at ages 55–60 results in diminished vestibular sensation.
   a. Diminished acuity, delayed reaction times, longer response times.
   b. Reduced function of VOR; affects retinal image stability with head movements, produces blurred vision.
   c. Altered sensory organization: older adults more dependent on somatosensory inputs for balance.
   d. Less able to resolve sensory conflicts when presented with conflicting visual or proprioceptive inputs due to vestibular losses.
   e. Postural response patterns for balance are disorganized: characterized by diminished ankle torque, increased hip torque, increased postural sway.
2. Additional loss of vestibular sensitivity with pathology.
   a. Ménière's disease: episodic attacks characterized by tinnitus, dizziness, and a sensation of fullness or pressure in the ears; may also experience sensorineural hearing loss.
   b. Benign paroxysmal positional vertigo (BPPV): brief episodes of vertigo (<1 minute) associated with position change; the result of degeneration of the utricular otoconia that settle on the cupula of the posterior semicircular canal; common in older adults.
   c. Medications: antihypertensives (postural hypotension), anticonvulsants, tranquilizers, sleeping pills, aspirin, nonsteroidal anti-inflammatory drugs (NSAIDs).
   d. Cerebrovascular disease: vertebrobasilar artery insufficiency (transient ischemic attack [TIA], stroke); cerebellar artery stroke, lateral medullary stroke.
   e. Cerebellar dysfunction: hemorrhage, tumors (acoustic neuroma, meningioma); degenerative disease of brainstem and cerebellum; progressive supranuclear palsy.
   f. Migraine.
   g. Cardiac disease.
3. Clinical implications/compensatory strategies.
   a. Increased incidence of falls in older adults.
   b. May benefit from vestibular rehabilitation.
   c. See section on falls and instability for additional information.

Somatosensory

1. Aging changes.
   a. Decline in the numbers and morphology of muscle spindles, joint receptors, cutaneous receptors, and corresponding myelinated axons contribute to decreased distal > proximal extremity vibration, discriminate touch, and proprioception.
   b. Loss of lower extremity proprioception and discriminate touch may contribute to impaired balance, ataxic gait, difficulty walking on unlevel surfaces, and increased fall risk.
   c. Distal upper extremity changes may contribute to decreased fine motor control in the upper extremities.
   d. Cutaneous pain thresholds increased: greater changes in upper body areas (upper extremities, face) than in lower extremities.
   e. Impairments with pain thresholds may also contribute to loss of protective sensation, but also raises concerns of associated health conditions (e.g. diabetic polyneuropathy, spinal stenosis, cervical myelopathy).
2. Additional loss of sensation with pathology (see Chapter 3).
   a. Polyneuropathy.
   b. CVA, central sensory losses.
   c. Peripheral vascular disease, peripheral ischemia.

3. Clinical implications/compensatory strategies.
   a. Examine sensation: check for increased thresholds to stimulation, sensory losses by modality (e.g., light touch, pinprick, vibration, proprioception, and temperature), area of body.
   b. Allow extra time for responses with increased thresholds. Delays in recognition of sensory stimuli (monofilament, vibration, sharp/dull) of >1 second are typically considered abnormal.
   c. Use touch to communicate: maximize physical contact; e.g., rubbing, stroking.
   d. Provide augmented feedback through appropriate sensory channels; e.g., walking on carpeted surfaces may be easier than on smooth floors.
   e. Teach compensatory strategies to prevent injury to anesthetic limbs; e.g., bathing.
   f. Provide assistive devices as needed to prevent falls.
   g. Provide biofeedback devices as appropriate (e.g., limb-load monitor).
   h. Focus on functional activities which facilitate adaptation through compensation. For example, use a treadmill at varying speeds and combined with cognitive activity to facilitate compensatory sensorimotor strategies for balance and stability.
   i. Exercise to retain/challenge proprioception as appropriate and safe.

Taste and Smell

1. Aging changes.
   a. Gradual decrease in taste sensitivity.
   b. Decreased smell sensitivity.
2. Additional loss of sensation.
   a. Smokers.
   b. Chronic allergies, respiratory infections.
   c. Dentures.
   d. CVA, involvement of hypoglossal nerve.
3. Clinical implications/compensatory strategies.
   a. Examine ability to identify odors, tastes (sweet, sour, bitter, salty); somatic sensations (temperature, touch).
   b. Decreased taste, enjoyment of food leads to poor diet and nutrition.
   c. Older adults frequently increase use of taste enhancers; e.g., salt or sugar.
   d. Decreased home safety; e.g., gas leaks, smoke.

Cognition (See Table 10.1, Nervous System)

Age-Related Changes

1. No uniform decline in intellectual abilities throughout adulthood.
   a. Changes do not typically show up until mid-60s; significant declines affecting everyday life do not show up until early 80s.
   b. Most significant decline in measures of intelligence occurs in the years immediately preceding death (termed terminal drop).
2. Tasks involving perceptual speed (e.g., reaction time) may show early declines (in some individuals by age 40); require longer times to complete tasks.
3. Numeric ability (tests of adding, subtracting, multiplying) and verbal abilities well maintained in active individuals.
4. Memory.
   a. Impairments typically noted in short-term memory; long-term memory retained.
   b. Impairments are task-dependent; e.g., deficits primarily with novel conditions, new learning.
5. Learning. All age groups can learn; learning in older adults affected by:
   a. Increased cautiousness.
   b. Anxiety.
   c. Pace of learning: fast pace is problematic.
   d. Interference from prior learning.

Clinical Implications

1. Older adults utilize different strategies for memory (context-based strategies) than young adults (memorization).
2. Trust in the therapeutic relationship is important for optimal cognitive function.

Interventions to Slow or Reverse Changes

1. Improve health.
   a. Correction of medical problems: imbalances between oxygen supply and demand to central nervous system (CNS); e.g., cardiovascular disease, hypertension, diabetes, hypothyroidism.
   b. Pharmacological changes: drug reevaluation; decreased use of multiple drugs; monitor closely for drug toxicity.
   c. Reduction in chronic use of tobacco and alcohol.
   d. Correction of nutritional deficiencies.
2. Increase physical activity.
3. Increase mental activity.
   a. Keep mentally engaged—"Use it or Lose it"; e.g., chess, crossword puzzles, high level of reading.
   b. Engaged lifestyle: socially active; e.g., clubs, travel, work.
   c. Cognitive training activities.
4. If auditory processing is decreased, provide written instructions.
5. Provide stimulating, "enriching" environment; avoid environmental dislocation; e.g., hospitalization or institutionalization may produce depression, disorientation, and agitation in some older adults.
6. Stress support systems for remaining active: family and friends, senior groups supporting participation, activity, travel, and sports.

Cardiovascular System (See Table 10.2)

Age-Related Changes

1. Changes due to inactivity and disease, combined with age-associated changes.
2. Degeneration of heart muscle with accumulation of lipofuscins (characteristic brown heart); mild cardiac hypertrophy, left ventricular wall.
3. Decreased coronary blood flow.
4. Cardiac valves thicken and stiffen.
5. Changes in conduction system: loss of pacemaker cells in sinoatrial node (SA) node.
6. Changes in blood vessels: arteries thicken, less distensible; slowed exchange through capillary walls; increased peripheral resistance.
7. Decline in neurohumoral control: decreased responsiveness of end-organs to beta-adrenergic stimulation of baroreceptors.
8. Decreased blood volume, hemopoietic activity of bone.
9. Increased blood coagulability.

Clinical Implications

1. Changes at rest are minor: resting heart rate and cardiac output relatively unchanged; resting blood pressures typically increases with age but in some older adults blood pressure may be chronically low.
2. Cardiovascular responses to exercise: blunted; decreased heart rate acceleration, maximal oxygen uptake and heart rate; reduced exercise capacity; increased recovery time.

Table 10-2

Potential Age-Related Cardiopulmonary, Integumentary, Gastrointestinal, and Renal/Urologic Physiological Changes, Impairments, Activity Limitations, and Participation Restrictions

SYSTEM/PHYSIOLOGICAL CHANGES	IMPAIRMENTS	ACTIVITY LIMITATIONS	PARTICIPATION RESTRICTIONS
Cardiovascular: ↓ sympathetic nerve response; ↓ functional capacity; ↓ coronary blood flow; thickening of arteries	↑ risk of orthostatic hypotension ↓ max heart rate ↓ functional capacity	↓ endurance (e.g., 6-minute walk tests) ↑ fatigue	↓ engagement due to fatigue in IADLS,* ADLs,** leisure & work
Pulmonary: Stiffening of chest wall; ↓ lung recoil; fewer capillaries; ↓ respiratory muscle strength/endurance	↓ in vital & inspiratory capacity ↓ homeostatic responses Prolonged recovery time following respiratory illness	↓ endurance (e.g., 6-minute walk tests) ↑ fatigue Reduced responses to exercise at higher intensities (VO_2 max, O_2 saturation)	↓ engagement due to fatigue or breathlessness in IADLS,* ADLs,** leisure and work
Integumentary: dehydration; ↓ immune response; ↓ #'s and efficiency of sweat glands, nerve endings, and hair follicles	Dry skin ↓ elasticity/↑ wrinkles ↓ ability to resist infection; ↓ inflammatory reaction ↓ sweat capacity ↓ sensitivity to touch, temperature, and pain	Insensate feet may contribute to reduced balance and mobility	↓ engagement in leisure and work due to ↑ risk of infection, reduced thermal regulation, and frail skin
Gastrointestinal (GI): ↓ GI tract tone & motility; ↓ acid production	↓ peristalsis (constipation) ↓ acid production Malabsorption (e.g., vitamin D and B_{12}) GI impairments may impact multiple systems		↓ engagement in leisure and work due to ↑ risk of reflux, constipation, diverticulitis, diarrhea, weight loss, and malnutrition
Renal/Urologic: ↓ mass of kidneys; ↓ #'s of nephrons; ↓ renal blow flow; ↓ pelvic floor muscle fibers	Sodium dysregulation ↓ bladder capacity and/or control ↑ pelvic floor weakness & impaired motor control		↓ engagement in leisure and work due to ↑ risk of electrolyte imbalance, frequent urination, urinary tract infections, or urinary incontinence

↑=increased; ↓=decreased/reduced; *IADLS=Instrumental Activities of Daily Living including shopping, housekeeping, money management, food prep, transportation, phone, laundry; **ADLs=Activities of Daily Living including toileting, grooming, bathing, dressing, transferring.

References: Guccione A, Wong R, Avers D (2019). Guccione's Geriatric Physical Therapy, 4th ed. St Louis, Elsevier and Goodman C, Fuller K (2014). Pathology: Implications for the Physical Therapist, 4th ed. Elsevier.

3. Decreased stroke volume due to decreased myocardial contractility.
4. Maximum heart rate declines with age (HR max = 220 – age).
5. Cardiac output decreases 1% per year after age 20 due to decreased heart rate and stroke volume.
6. Orthostatic hypotension: common problem in elderly due to reduced baroreceptor sensitivity and vascular elasticity.
7. Increased fatigue; anemia common in elderly.
8. Systolic ejection murmur common in elderly.
9. Possible electrocardiographic (ECG) changes: loss of normal sinus rhythm; longer PR and QT intervals; wider QRS; increased arrhythmias.

Pulmonary System (See Table 10.2)

Age-Related Changes

1. Chest wall stiffness. Declining strength of respiratory muscles results in increased work of breathing.
2. Loss of lung elastic recoil, decreased lung compliance.
3. Changes in lung parenchyma: alveoli enlarge, become thinner; fewer capillaries for delivery of blood.
4. Changes in pulmonary blood vessels: thicken, less distensible.
5. Decline in total lung capacity: residual volume increases, vital capacity decreases.
6. Forced expiratory volume (airflow) decreases.
7. Altered pulmonary gas exchange: oxygen tension falls with age, at a rate of 4 mm Hg/decade; PaO_2 at age 70 is 75, compared to 90 at age 20.
8. Blunted ventilatory responses of chemoreceptors in response to respiratory acidosis: decreased homeostatic responses.
9. Blunted defense/immune responses: decreased ciliary action to clear secretions, decreased secretory immunoglobulins, alveolar phagocytic function.

Clinical Implications

1. Respiratory responses to exercise: similar to younger adults at low and moderate intensities; at higher intensities, responses include increased ventilatory cost of work, greater blood acidosis, increased likelihood of breathlessness, and increased perceived exertion.
2. Clinical signs of hypoxia are blunted; changes in mentation and affect may provide important cues.
3. Cough mechanism is impaired.
4. Gag reflex is decreased, increased risk of aspiration.
5. Recovery from respiratory illness: prolonged in the elderly.
6. Significant changes in function with chronic smoking, exposure to environmental toxic inhalants.

Interventions

1. To slow or reverse changes in cardiopulmonary systems.
2. Important to complete a thorough cardiopulmonary examination before starting an exercise program as the incidence of cardiopulmonary pathologies in older adults is increased.
   a. Selection of appropriate exercise tolerance testing (ETT) protocol is important.
   b. Limited (2- or 3-minute walk, step test, seated step test) standardized test batteries and norms for older adults.
   c. Many older adults cannot tolerate maximal testing; submaximal testing commonly used.
3. Individualized exercise prescription essential.
   a. Rating of perceived exertion (RPE) is helpful (see Chapter 4).
   b. Choice of training program based on fitness level, presence or absence of cardiovascular disease, musculoskeletal limitations, individual's goals and interests.
   c. Prescriptive elements (frequency, intensity, time, type-FITT equation) for older adults (see Table 10-4).
   d. Walking, chair and floor exercises, modified strength/flexibility well tolerated by most elderly.
   e. Consider pool programs (exercises, walking, and swimming) with bone and joint impairments.
   f. Consider multiple modes of exercise (circuit training) on alternate days to reduce likelihood of muscle injury, joint overuse, pain, and fatigue.
4. Aerobic training programs can significantly improve cardiopulmonary function in older adults.
   a. Reduced max heart rate at a given submaximal power output.
   b. Improve maximal oxygen uptake (VO_2 max).
   c. Greater improvements in peripheral adaptation, muscle oxidative capacity than central changes; major difference from training effects in younger adults.
   d. Improves recovery heart rates.
   e. Decreases systolic blood pressure, may produce a small decrease in diastolic blood pressure.
   f. Increases maximum ventilatory capacity: vital capacity.
   g. Reduces breathlessness, improves perceived exertion.
   h. Psychological gains: improved sense of well-being, self-image.
   i. Improves functional capacity.
5. Improve overall daily activity levels for independent living.
   a. Lack of exercise is an important risk factor in the development of cardiopulmonary diseases.
   b. Lack of exercise contributes to problems of immobility and disability in the elderly.

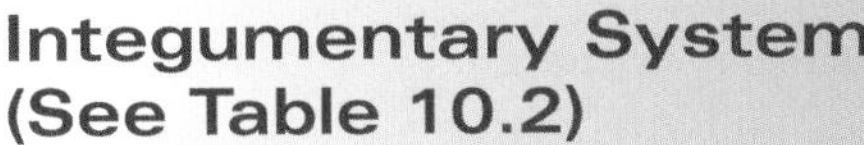

Integumentary System (See Table 10.2)

Changes in Skin Composition

1. Dermis thins with loss of elastin.
2. Decreased vascularity; vascular fragility results in easy bruising (senile purpura).
3. Decreased sebaceous activity and decline in hydration.
4. Appearance: skin appears dry, wrinkled, yellowed, and inelastic; age spots appear (clusters of melanocyte pigmentation); increase with sun exposure.
5. General thinning and graying of hair due to vascular insufficiency and decreased melanin production.
6. Nails grow more slowly, become brittle and thick.

Loss of Effectiveness of Skin as Protective Barrier

1. Skin grows and heals more slowly, less able to resist injury and infection.
2. Inflammatory response is attenuated.
3. Decreased sensitivity to touch, perception of pain and temperature; increased risk for injury from concentrated pressures or excess temperatures.
4. Decreased sweat production with loss of sweat glands results in decreased temperature regulation and homeostasis.

Gastrointestinal System (See Table 10.2)

Age-Related Changes

1. Decreased salivation, taste, and smell. Along with inadequate chewing (tooth loss, poorly fitting dentures), poor swallowing reflex may lead to poor dietary intake, nutritional deficiencies.
2. Esophagus: reduced motility and control of lower esophageal sphincter; acid reflux and heartburn, hiatal hernia common.
3. Stomach: reduced motility, delayed gastric emptying; decreased digestive enzymes and hydrochloric acid; decreased digestion and absorption; indigestion common.
4. Decreased intestinal motility; constipation common.

Renal System (See Table 10.2)

Age-Related Changes

1. Kidneys: loss of mass and total weight with nephron atrophy, decreased renal blood flow, decreased filtration.
   a. Blood urea rises.
   b. Decreased excretory and reabsorptive capacities.
2. Bladder: muscle weakness; decreased capacity, causing urinary frequency; difficulty with emptying, causing increased retention.
   a. Urinary incontinence common (affects over 10 million adults; over half of nursing home residents and one-third of community-dwelling elders); affects older women with pelvic floor weakness and older men with bladder or prostate disease.
   b. Urinary incontinence may be due to urinary stress (USI), urge incontinence (UI), or both. USI is related to weakness of the pelvic floor muscles, and UI is related to bladder problems.
   c. USI can be managed through pelvic floor strengthening/motor control exercise. UI may be managed with medications, behavioral change, and pelvic floor exercise.
   d. Urinary incontinence is a risk factor for urinary tract infections.
   e. USI can be managed through pelvic floor strengthening/motor control exercise. UI may be managed with medications, behavioral change, and pelvic floor exercise.

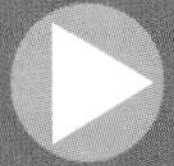

Pathological Conditions Associated with Aging

Musculoskeletal Disorders and Diseases

Osteoporosis

1. Disease process that results in reduction of bone mass; a failure of bone formation (osteoblast activity) to keep pace with bone reabsorption and destruction (osteoclast activity).
2. World Health Organization diagnostic criteria.
   a. Osteoporosis is defined by bone mineral density (BMD) at the hip or spine that is ≥2.5 standard deviations (SD) below the young, normal mean reference population.
   b. Osteopenia is defined by a BMD between 1.0 and 2.5 SD below the reference population (adults in their late 20s).

3. Etiological factors.
   a. Hormonal deficiency associated with menopause and hypogonadism: loss of estrogens or androgens.
   b. Age-related deficiencies.
   c. Nutritional deficiency: decreased calcium, vitamin B_{12}, and vitamin D; often associated with impaired absorption.
   d. Decreased physical activity: Low levels of mechanical loading (weight-bearing) across the life span.
   e. Diseases that affect bone loss: hyperthyroidism, diabetes, hyperparathyroidism, rheumatic disease (lupus), celiac disease, gastric bypass, pancreatic disease, multiple myeloma, sickle cell disease, end-stage renal disease, Paget's disease, cancer, and chemotherapeutic drugs.
   f. Medications that affect bone loss: corticosteroids, thyroid hormone, anticonvulsants, catabolic drugs, some estrogen antagonists, chemotherapy.
   g. Additional risk factors: family history, Caucasian/Asian race, late menopause, thin/small build, smoking.
4. Characteristics.
   a. Approximately 12% (19% female/4.4% males) and 43% (51% females/33% males) of adults over age 50 in the United States will have osteoporosis and/or low bone mass, respectively (CDC, 2018).
   b. Bone loss is about 1% per year (starting at ages 30–35 in women and at ages 50–55 in men), accelerating loss in postmenopausal women, approximately 5% per year for 3–5 years.
   c. Structural weakening of bone.
   d. Decreased ability to support loads.
   e. High risk of fractures.
   f. Trabecular bone more involved than cortical bone; common areas affected:
      - Vertebral column.
      - Femoral neck.
      - Distal radius/wrist, humerus.
5. Examination.
   a. Medical record review.
      - History, physical exam, nutritional history.
      - BMD testing.
      - X-rays for known or suspected fractures.
      - Check for secondary causes.
   b. Physical activity/fall history.
   c. Assess dizziness: Dizziness Handicap Inventory.
   d. Sensory integrity: vision, hearing, somatosensory, vestibular; sensory integration.
   e. Motor function: strength, endurance, motor control.
   f. ROM/flexibility.
   g. Postural deformity.
      - Feet: hammer toes, bunions lead to antalgic gait.
      - Postural kyphosis, forward head position.
      - Hip and knee flexion contractures.
   h. Postural hypotension.
   i. Gait and balance assessment.
6. Goals, outcomes, and interventions.
   a. Medications that may be prescribed work to slow bone breakdown; some may rebuild bone.
      - Biphosphonates: alendronate (Fosamax); risedronate (Actonel); ibandronate (Boniva); zoledronic acid (Reclast).
      - Raloxifene (Evista).
      - Denosumab (Prolia, Zgeva).
      - Terparatide (Forteo).
      - Abaloparatide (Tymlos).
   b. Promote healthy behaviors; provide counseling on risk of osteoporosis, fall-related injuries, the impact of fear of falling, and falls prevention.
      - Recommended daily calcium intake (National Osteoporosis Foundation):
        - Women: 50 and younger, 1000 mg/day; 51 and older, 1200 mg/day.
        - Men: 70 and younger, 1000 mg/day; 71 and older, 1200 mg/day.
      - Recommended daily vitamin D intake: 50 and younger 400–800 IU; 51 and older 800–1000 IU daily.
      - Avoid tobacco smoking and excessive alcohol intake.
      - Diet: low in salt; avoid excess protein, since it inhibits body's ability to absorb calcium.
   c. Maintain bone mass: regular weight-bearing exercise.
      - Walking (30 minutes/day); stair-climbing; use of weight belts to increase loading.
      - Muscle-strengthening (resistance) exercises to reduce risk of falls and fractures.
   d. Postural/balance training.
      - Postural reeducation, postural exercises to reduce kyphosis, forward head position.
      - Strengthening exercise for postural extensors, scapular stabilizers.
      - Flexibility exercises.
      - Functional balance exercises; e.g., chair rises, standing/kitchen sink exercises (e.g., toe raises, unilateral stance, hip extension, hip abduction, partial squats).
      - Tai chi.
      - Gait training.
   e. Safety education/fall prevention (see Falls Prevention Section).

RED FLAG: Advise individuals with osteoporosis/low bone mass or risk factors for these health conditions to avoid movements that can result in spinal fractures, including forward bending, twisting motions, lifting heavy objects, sudden forceful movements involving spinal stability.

Fractures

1. High risk of fractures in the elderly: associated with low bone density and multiple risk factors; e.g., age, comorbid diseases, dementia, psychotropic medications.
2. Hip fracture: each year more than 300,000 older people 65 and older are hospitalized with hip fracture (CDC).
   a. More than 95% are caused by falling, usually falling sideways.
   b. Women experience three-quarters of all hip fractures.
   c. Chances of hip fracture increase as individuals get older.
   d. Mortality rate: 20%, associated with complications.
   e. About 50% will not resume their premorbid level of function; e.g., walk independently.
   f. May result in dependency; continued institutionalization occurs in as many as one-third of patients with hip fractures.
   g. Majority of hip fractures are treated surgically: 95% are femoral neck or intertrochanteric fractures; remaining 5% are subtrochanteric fractures.
   h. Intensive interdisciplinary rehabilitation program with early mobilization may improve outcome.
   i. Treatment protocols based on type of fracture and surgical procedure used: internal fixation versus prosthetic replacement.
3. Vertebral compression fractures.
   a. Vertebral compression fractures are usually caused by osteoporosis and range from mild to severe. They affect approximately 25% of all postmenopausal women and 40% of women 80 years of age. Older men are also affected to a lesser degree.
   b. Severe fractures typically cause significant pain and a reduction of the ability to perform daily living activities.
   c. Fractures can occur anywhere in the spine; common in the lumbodorsal junction, T8-T12 and L4.
   d. Typically result from routine activity: bending, lifting, rising from chair.
   e. Chief complaints: immediate, severe local spinal pain, increased with trunk flexion.
   f. Lead to shortening of spine, progressive loss of height, spinal deformity (kyphosis); can progress to respiratory compromise.
   g. Goals, outcomes, and interventions: acute phase.
      - Horizontal bed rest, out of bed 10 minutes every hour.
      - Emphasis on proper posture, extension in sleeping, sitting, and standing.
      - Isometric extension exercises in bed.
   h. Goals, outcomes, and interventions: chronic phase.
      - Strengthening regimen for postural extensors and scapular stabilizers.
      - Avoid flexion activities.
      - Safety education and injury prevention.
      - Environmental modifications, reduce home hazards.
      - Decrease vertebral loading; rest lying down for 15–30 minutes after prolonged upright activities; wear shock-absorbing shoes.
      - Spinal orthotics: may provide pain relief; long-term use may lead to muscle weakness and further deconditioning.

> **RED FLAG:** Pain medications can cause disorientation or sedation and increase fall risk.

   i. Surgery: Kyphoplasty or vertebroplasty can be performed for individuals with painful vertebral fractures.
4. Stress fractures: fine, hairline fracture (insufficiency fracture) without soft tissue injury.
   a. In older adults, common in pelvis, proximal tibia, distal fibula, metatarsal shafts, foot.
   b. May be unsuspected source of pain.
   c. Observe for signs of local tenderness and swelling; e.g., postexercise.
   d. Goals, outcomes, and interventions.
      - Correction of exercise excesses or faulty exercise program.
      - Reduction of repetitive stresses such as vertical loading.
5. Upper extremity fractures: humeral head, Colles' fractures are common and are usually the result of a fall.
6. For discussion of fracture assessment and management, see Chapter 2.
7. Clinical implications of fracture management among older adults.
   a. Fractures heal more slowly.
   b. Older adults are prone to complications; e.g., pneumonia, decubitus ulcers, mental status complications with hospitalization.
   c. Rehabilitation may be complicated or prolonged by lack of support systems, comorbid conditions, decreased vision, poor balance.

Degenerative Arthritis (Osteoarthritis)

1. Osteoarthritis (OA) is a chronic condition that can affect any joint; occurs most often in knees, hips, lower back and neck, fingers, bases of thumb and big toe.
   a. Cartilage in the joint breaks down, causing pain, swelling, and problems with joint movement.
   b. Bone spurs may develop and chips of bone or cartilage may break off and cause additional inflammation and damage.
   c. In the final stages, bone contacts bone with resulting frictional forces.

2. Over 22% (over 54.4 million) of US adults had doctor-diagnosed arthritis, with increased prevalence with age (CDC).
   a. It is more common in women (26%) than men (19%).
   b. OA is the most common cause of disability in adults; 43% report functional activity limitations.
   c. Arthritis is strongly associated with major depression (18%).
3. Characteristics.
   a. Pain, swelling, and stiffness, worse early morning or with overuse; e.g., knee pain, hip pain.
   b. Muscle inhibition due to pain progressing to weakness secondary to disuse.
   c. Loss of ROM and mobility; crepitus.
   d. Bony deformity.
4. Goals, outcomes, and interventions.
   a. Reduction of pain and muscle inhibition/weakness: modalities, muscle reeducation.
   b. Manual Therapy (soft tissue/joint mobilization).
   c. Exercises.
      - Maintain or improve ROM via progressive ROM and flexibility.
      - Correct muscle imbalances: strengthening exercises to support joints, improve balance and ambulation.
      - Aerobic conditioning: walking programs are associated with decreased joint symptoms, improved function, and sense of well-being.
      - Aquatic programs; e.g., pool walking, Arthritis Foundation program: produces beneficial effects similar to aerobic conditioning; enhances ease of movement.
   d. Patient education and empowerment.
      - Teach patients about disease, taking an active role in care.
      - Teach joint protection, energy conservation strategies.
   e. Provide assistive devices for ambulation and activities of daily living; e.g., canes, walkers, shoe inserts, reachers.
   f. Promote healthy lifestyle: weight reduction to relieve stress on joints.
5. Medical management.
   a. Medications: NSAIDS (if tolerated), analgesics (e.g., acetaminophen).
   b. conservative management including physical therapy (e.g., manual therapy, exercise, bracing, education).
   c. Injections: corticosteroid; viscosupplementation.
   d. Surgery
      - Arthroscopic lavage and debridement.
      - Articular cartilage repair (e.g., osteochondral autograft [OATS] or allograft [OCA]).
      - Total joint replacement: indicated with moderate to severe arthritis and pain that limits participation.

Cachexia

1. A multifactorial degenerative illness characterized by extreme weight loss and malnutrition, muscle atrophy, fatigue, and weakness.
2. Loss of body mass that cannot be reversed nutritionally.
3. Associated with severe chronic disease: e.g., cancer, HIV/AIDS, COPD, CHF, and kidney failure.

Neurological Disorders and Diseases

Stroke (CVA)

1. Sudden, focal neurological deficit resulting from ischemic or hemorrhagic lesions in the brain.
2. Most common cause of adult disability in the United States.
   a. Incidence of stroke increases dramatically with age; most strokes (43%) occur in persons over the age of 74.
   b. Approximately 30% die during the acute phase, and another 30%–40% will have severe disability.
3. Early warning signs of stroke (F.A.S.T.) are discussed in Chapter 13.
4. Clinical signs and symptoms, examination, and intervention of persons with stroke are discussed in Chapter 3.

Degenerative Diseases

1. Parkinson's disease: chronic, progressive disease of nervous system.
   a. Parkinson's symptoms afflict about 20% of individuals over the age of 65; frequency of symptoms increases with age, affecting 50% of individuals over the age of 85.
   b. Parkinson's disease affects about 1% of individuals over age 55, reaching proportions of 2.6% by age 85 in the United States. Affects approximately 1.5 million individuals, with 50,000 new cases annually; mean age of onset is between 59 and 62.
2. Clinical signs and symptoms, examination, and intervention of persons with Parkinson's disease are discussed in Chapter 3.

Clinical Implications

1. Older adults are prone to complications/indirect impairments related to immobility and inactivity (e.g., contracture and deformity, decubitus ulcers).
2. Rehabilitation may be complicated or prolonged by lack of support systems, comorbid conditions, decreased sensorimotor function, poor balance.
3. With irreversible neurological disease, it is important to address the impairments and activity limitations responsive to interventions; overall focus should be on improved function, quality-of-life, and patient safety.

4. Compensatory treatment strategies should be considered when disability is severe, there are multiple comorbidities, and impairments cannot be remediated; strategies can include environmental modifications, assistive devices, mobility devices, use of home health aides.

Cognitive Disorders

Delirium

1. Fluctuating attention state causing temporary confusion and loss of mental function; an acute disorder, potentially reversible.
2. Etiology: drug toxicity and/or systemic illness, oxygen deprivation to brain; environmental changes and sensory deprivation; e.g., recent hospitalization, general anesthesia, and institutionalization. One in four older adults experience delirium after major surgeries.
3. Characteristics.
   a. Acute onset, often at night; fluctuating course with lucid intervals; worse at night.
   b. Duration: hours to weeks.
   c. May be hypoalert or hyperalert, distractible; fluctuates over course of day.
   d. Orientation usually impaired.
   e. Delusions/hallucinations, periods of agitation.
   f. Memory deficits: immediate and recent.
   g. Disorganized thinking, incoherent speech.
   h. Sleep/wake cycles always disrupted.

Dementia (Neurocognitive Disorders)

1. An acquired disorder of cognitive and behavioral impairment causing dysfunction in daily living (see Table 10-3).
2. Characteristics of Dementia (within the category of Neurocognitive Disorders in the Diagnostic and Statistical Manual of Mental Disorders-DSM-5).
   a. Deterioration of intellectual functions: impoverished thinking, impaired judgment; disorientation, confusion; impaired social functioning.
   b. Disturbances in higher cortical functions: language (aphasia), motor skills (apraxia), perception (agnosia).
   c. Memory impairment.
   d. Personality changes: alteration or accentuation of premorbid traits; behavioral changes.
   e. Alertness (consciousness) usually normal.
   f. Sleep often fragmented.
3. Reversible Dementia (Neurocognitive Disorders): 10%–20% of dementias; multiple causes.
   a. Drugs: sedatives, hypnotics, antianxiety agents, antidepressants, antiarrhythmics, antihypertensives, anticonvulsants, antipsychotics, drugs with anticholinergic side effects.
   b. Nutritional disorders: vitamin B_6 deficiency, thiamine deficiency, vitamin B_{12} deficiency/pernicious anemia, folate deficiency.
   c. Metabolic disorders: hyper-/hypothyroidism, hypercalcemia, hyper-/hyponatremia, hypoglycemia, kidney or liver failure, Cushing's syndrome, Addison's disease, hypopituitarism, carcinoma.
   d. Psychiatric disorders: depression, anxiety, psychosis.
   e. Toxins: air pollution, alcohol.
4. Alzheimer's type dementia (Alzheimer's disease) (AD): 60%–80% of dementias.
   a. Most common cause of dementia; affects more than 6 million Americans; 2/3 are women, primarily explained by the fact that women live longer than men and greatest risk is in the oldest age category.
   b. Costliest disease in United States; 6th leading cause of death.
   c. One in three seniors dies with AD or another dementia; leading cause of institutionalization; affects up to 50% of nursing home population.
   d. Etiology unknown.
      - An incurable disease with a long and progressive preclinical course.
      - Evidence of chromosomal abnormalities.
      - Potential predisposing factors: family history, Down syndrome, and traumatic brain injury.
   e. Pathophysiological changes.
      - Generalized atrophy of brain (hippocampus, entorhinal cortex, other cortical areas).
      - Moderately enlarged ventricules.
      - Decreased synthesis of neurotransmitters.
      - Histopathological changes: accumulation of neurofibrillary tangles (protein tau) and beta-amyloid plaques eventually accompanied by damage and death of neurons.
   f. Risk factors for AD.
      - Advanced age.
      - Family history.
      - Apolipoprotein E (APOE)-$_E$4 gene.
      - Cardiovascular disease risk factors.
      - Fewer years of formal education.
      - Limited social and cognitive engagement.
   g. Types.
      - Alzheimer's disease: onset after the age of 60 (average age 75).
      - Early Onset Alzheimer's disease: onset between ages of 40–60.
   h. Diagnosis.
      - Medical history and clinical examination: signs and symptoms.
      - Cognitive tests.
      - Biomarker tests: on lumbar puncture (CSF) see elevated levels of tau and phosphorylated tau; low amyloid levels.

Chapter 10 GER

Table 10-3

Differences Among the Most Prevalent Types of Dementia (Neurocognitive Disorders)				
	ALZHEIMER'S DISEASE (AD)	VASCULAR DEMENTIA (VAD)	(DIFFUSE) LEWY BODY DISEASE (DLBD)	FRONTOTEMPORAL LOBE DEMENTIA (FTD)
Age at Onset (typically)	65+ (40–65 for early onset/familial)	55–75	50+	45–65
Gender Distribution	Women > Men: 3:2	Men > Women: 3:1	Men slightly more than women	Men slightly more than women (mixed evidence)
Prevalence Among Dementia	50%–75%	20%–30% (often occurs mixed with AD, or DLB)	10%–25% (often co-exists with AD or VaD)	10%–15%
Course	Insidious onset, gradual progression, more rapid progression in early onset (40–60, familial type)	Intermittent stepwise decline	Insidious onset, gradual progression	Insidious onset, gradual progression
Prevalence Among Dementia	50%–75%	20%–30%	10%–25%	10%–15%
Presentation	Memory loss, impaired learning. With progression, visuospatial and language impairments, disorientation, apraxia, delusions/hallucinations. Late stages: severe impairments in mobility, sleep, eating, insight, dysphagia, incontinence.	Dependent on location of cardiovascular impairment in brain; usually memory loss. Episodes of confusion with lucid intervals, insight may be preserved.	Changes in attention, executive functions (planning, sequencing, organizing), fluctuating cognition.	Behavioral variant: Altered social abilities/executive abilities (planning, sequencing, organizing); disinhibition, apathy, compulsivity. Language variant: loss of word recall or understanding, incoherent speech, grammar altered. May have elements of both behavioral and language.
Associated Components	Depression (early); psychotic features (later); agitation, wandering. Late stage: gait/mobility impairment, dysphagia, incontinence.	Cardiovascular event history (e.g., stroke, MI). Personality/mood changes. Mild to moderate gait impairments.	Sleep disorders; falls, syncope, autonomic dysfunction, intermittent delirium, hallucinations, delusions.	Extrapyramidal symptoms may be present. Often mistaken for depression, bipolar disorder, schizophrenia.
Imaging	Hippocampal and temporoparietal cortical atrophy; more diffuse global atrophy with progression.	Infarct evidence or white hyperintensities; areas of preserved function.	Lewy bodies found in cortex.	Brain atrophy varies.
Neuromuscular	Occasional tremors, generalized weakness, unsteady gait, increased tone; increased fall risk; repetitive behaviors; with progression, mobility impairments increase, rigid postures, contractures.	Dependent on history of infarcts; may see hemiparesis.	Parkinsonian like gait, shuffling, difficulty initiating movement, poor balance, rigidity, fall risk.	Less common subtypes result in Parkinsonian type motor symptoms.

DSM-5=Diagnostic and Statistical Manual of Mental Disorders

- MRI scan to identify brain changes and rule out other causes of dementia (e.g., subdural hematoma, stroke, tumor, normal-pressure hydrocephalus).

i. Stages of AD.
- AD is classified into stages (Box 10-1):
  - Preclinical AD: individuals have measurable changes in brain CSF and blood biomarkers without noticeable symptoms.
  - Mild Cognitive Impairment: characterized by mild but measurable changes in cognitive abilities noticeable to person affected and family members; able to carry out everyday activities.
  - Mild AD: measurable changes in more than one cognitive domain with interference in completing work and some usual functions, still able to complete ADLs.
  - Moderate AD: characterized by noticeable memory, thinking, and behavioral symptoms that impair a person's ability to function in daily life.

BOX 10-1 Signs/Symptoms and Corresponding Communication Strategies for Patients with Alzheimer's Type Dementia

Signs/Symptoms	Communication Strategies
Minimal Cognitive Impairment (MCI): • Mild memory changes may be noted by family and individual • Difficulty in complex planning or multitasking • Daily life not generally affected • May not have diagnosis yet • May not progress to dementia • Important time for neurological examination	• Increased repetition in demonstration and teaching • Multimodal instruction (see, hear, read, practice)
Mild AD: • Memory loss • Short-term (working) memory loss • Difficulty with word finding • Confusion about the location of familiar places • Taking longer to accomplish normal, daily tasks • Trouble handling money and paying bills • Compromised judgment, often leading to bad decisions • Loss of spontaneity and sense of initiative • Mood and personality changes; increased anxiety	• Speak directly to the individual rather than their companion or caregiver. • Take time in asking questions and give the person time to respond. • Ask the person what form of communication is most comfortable (face-to-face, email, or phone calls).
Moderate AD: • Increasing memory loss and confusion • Shortened attention span • Problems recognizing friends and family members • Difficulty with language; problems with reading, writing, and numbers • Difficulty organizing thoughts and thinking logically • Difficulty learning new things • Difficulty coping with new or unexpected situations • Restlessness, agitation, anxiety, tearfulness • Wandering, especially in the late afternoon or at night (sundowning) • Repetitive statements or movement; occasional muscle twitches • Hallucinations, delusions, suspiciousness or paranoia, irritability • Loss of impulse control (e.g., taking clothes off, vulgar language) • Perceptual-motor problems: trouble getting out of a chair or setting the table	• Communicate in a quiet space with minimal distractions. • Speak slowly and maintain eye contact. • Be patient and ask one question at a time. • Allow them to complete their thoughts and avoid correcting them if possible. • Ask yes or no questions. • Give clear step-by-step instructions for tasks. • Give visual cues. Demonstrate a task to encourage participation. • Written notes may be helpful. • Use procedural memory to engage in physical activity.
Severe AD: • Often unable to communicate • May be unable to recognize family or significant others • Complete dependence on others for ADL and care • Loss of sense of self Other symptoms can include: • Weight loss • Diffculty swallowing • Lack of bladder and bowel control	• Approach from the front and introduce yourself. • Encourage nonverbal communication (pointing or gestures). • Use various senses (sight, touch, sounds, smells, and tastes) to communicate. • Treat the person with dignity and avoid talking down to the person.

End-stage AD, patients are restricted to bed; death results from other illnesses (e.g., aspiration pneumonia)

Adapted from: 1) Alzheimer Disease. Medscape. Retrieved April 17, 2014 from http://emedicine.medscape.com/article/1134817-overview and 2) Alzheimer's Association. Alzheimer's and Communication. Retrieved June 1, 2021 from: https://www.alz.org/help-support/caregiving/daily-care/communications.

   - Severe AD: characterized by loss of ability to communicate, recognize others, and complete dependence.
 - Rate of progression varies from individual to individual.

j. Signs and symptoms of AD (Box 10-1).
 - Signs and symptoms vary by stage and presentation from patient to patient.

k. Pharmacologic treatment.
 - Currently there is no cure for Alzheimer's.
 - Disease-modifying drugs may help lessen cognitive and behavioral symptoms (memory loss and confusion), behavioral changes (irritability, anxiety, confusion), and sleep disturbances.
 - Individual responses to drugs variable, based on age, overall health, and severity of symptoms.

5. Vascular dementia (includes multi-infarct dementias), approximately 5%–10% of dementias.
   a. Etiology: large and small vascular infarcts in both gray and white matter of brain, producing loss of brain function.
   b. Characteristics.
      - Sudden onset rather than insidious; stepwise progression.
      - Spotty and patchy distribution of deficits: areas of preserved ability along with impairments.
      - Focal neurological signs and symptoms; e.g., gait and balance abnormalities, weakness, exaggerated deep tendon reflexes (DTRs).
      - Pseudobulbar affect common.
      - Associated with history of stroke, cardiovascular disease, hypertension.
6. Other types of dementia.
   a. Parkinson's disease (PD): symptoms include movement problems (slowness, rigidity, tremor, gait changes); dementia estimated in 10%–35% of cases, in late stages of the disease.
   b. Dementia with Diffuse Lewy Body Disease (DLBD): some symptoms of AD along with sleep disturbances, visual disturbances, slowness, and other PD movement features.
   c. Frontotemporal dementia: Insidious onset with gradual progression; results in behavioral problems with diminished executive function and/or significant impairments with language.
   d. Creutzfeldt-Jakob disease: rare and rapidly fatal disorder with memory, behavior changes, and incoordination; results from protein (prion) disorder.
   e. Normal pressure hydrocephalus: symptoms include memory loss, difficulty walking, inability to control urination; results from impaired reabsorption of CSF with build-up of fluid in the brain and increased brain pressures.
   f. Down syndrome: individuals demonstrate accelerated aging and AD; symptoms typically in late 40s or 50s.
   g. Chronic alcoholism with prolonged nutritional (vitamin B_{12}) deficiency; e.g., Korsakoff's psychosis.
7. Physical therapy examination.
   a. History: determine onset of symptoms, progression, triggering events, common problems, social history.
   b. Examine cognitive functions: orientation, attention, calculation, recall, language.
   c. Standardized screening test for dementia (moderate to severe cognitive impairment). Mini-Mental State Examination (MMSE); score of <24 out of possible 30 is indicative of mental decline/dementia. Limited ability to detect mild cognitive impairment and influenced by education level/literacy (some items test the ability to read and write).
   d. Examine for impairments in higher cortical functions: inability to communicate, perceptual dysfunction.
   e. Examine for behavioral changes: restless, agitated, distracted, paranoid, wandering, inappropriate social behaviors, repetitive behaviors.
   f. Examine self-care: ability to carry out activities of daily living; e.g., limitations in grooming and hygiene, continence.
   g. Examine motor function: dyspraxia, gait, balance instability.
   h. Examine environment for safety, optimal function.
   i. Standardized scales for AD: Blessed Performance of Everyday Activities; Alzheimer's Type Dementia Assessment Scale.
8. Goals, outcomes, and interventions.
   a. Environment.
      - Provide safe environment: prevent falls, injury, or further dysfunction, safety from wandering; utilize safety monitoring devices as needed; e.g., alarm device.
      - Provide soothing environment with reduced environmental distractions: reduces agitation, increases attention.
      - Assistive and supportive devices to enhance self-care, effective positioning.
   b. Support individual's highest level of cognitive function.
      - Approach the patient in a friendly, supportive manner; model calm behavior.
      - Use consistent, simple commands; speak slowly.
      - Use nonverbal communication as appropriate: sensory cues and demonstration.
      - Provide reorienting information: use prompts; e.g., wall calendars, daily schedules, memory aids whenever possible.

- Avoid stressful tasks; emphasize familiar, well-learned skills; provide redirection.
- Approach learning in a simple, repetitious way; proceed slowly; and provide adequate rest time.
- Provide mental stimulation: utilize simple, well-liked activities, games.

c. Provide regular physical activity, maintain physical fitness.
- Utilize functionally directed activities.
- Active assistive and passive ROM exercises to maintain ROM.
- Low-intensity strengthening exercises.
- Safe daily walking program.
- Balance activities for fall prevention.
- Enhance body awareness and sensory stimulation; touch and light massage can be effective in promoting relaxation.

d. Participate in restraint reduction program.
e. Educate/support family, caregivers, significant others.
f. Present a realistic, consistent team approach to management.

Depression

1. A disorder characterized by depressed mood and lack of interest or pleasure in all activities, and other associated symptoms, lasting for at least 2 weeks.
2. Incidence.
   a. Community-dwelling elderly: 5% have clinically diagnosed major depression (exhibit at least five symptoms); another 10%–20% have depressive symptoms.
   b. Institutionalized elderly: 12% have major depression; another 15%–20% have depressive symptoms.
3. Determine predisposing factors.
   a. Family history, prior episodes of depression.
   b. Illness, drug side effects; hormonal.
   c. Chronic condition: loss of physical functions, pain; e.g., stroke.
   d. Sensory deprivation (loss of vision or hearing).
   e. History of losses: death of family and friends, job, income, independence.
   f. Social isolation: lack of family support.
   g. Psychological losses: memory, intellectual functions.
4. Examine for depressive symptoms.
   a. Nutritional problems: significant weight loss or weight gain; dehydration.
   b. Sleep disturbances: insomnia or hypersomnia.
   c. Psychomotor changes: inactivity with resultant functional impairments, weakness or agitation.
   d. Fatigue or loss of energy.
   e. Feelings of worthlessness, low self-esteem, guilt.
   f. Inability to concentrate, slowed thinking, impaired memory, indecisiveness.
   g. Withdrawal from family and friends, self-neglect.

RED FLAG: Recurrent thoughts of death and threats of suicide should be taken seriously, documented, and reported to medical staff immediately.

   h. Decline in cognitive function; i.e., document with Mini Mental State Examination (MMSE).
   i. Standardized test: Geriatric Depression Scale; 30-item yes/no scale; score >8 indicates depression.
5. Goals, outcomes, and interventions.
   a. Medical treatment.
      - Pharmacotherapy; tricyclic antidepressants (e.g., Chlorpromazine, fluoxetine [Prozac]) widely used.
      - Psychotherapy.
      - Electroconvulsive shock therapy (ECT) may be used if drug treatment is unsuccessful or contraindicated.
   b. Avoid excessive cheerfulness; provide support and encouragement.
   c. Assist patient in adjustment process to losses, coping strategies.
   d. Encourage activities, exercise program: aerobic training is associated with increased feelings of well-being.
   e. Assist in improving/maintaining independence; emphasize mastery by patient, achievement of short-term rather than long-term goals.

Cardiopulmonary and Integumentary Disorders and Diseases

Cardiovascular Diseases

1. Hypertension.
   a. Significant risk factor in cardiovascular disease, stroke, renal failure, and death.
2. Coronary artery disease (CAD)
   a. Affects 40% of individuals aged 65–74 and 50% over age 75.
   b. Angina.
      - Angina pain not always a consistent indicator of ischemia in elderly; shortness of breath, ECG ST segment depression may be more reliable indicators.
   c. Acute myocardial infarction.
      - Clinical presentation may vary from younger adults: may present with sudden dyspnea, acute confusion, syncope.
      - Clinical course often more complicated in the elderly, mortality rates twice that of younger adults.
   d. Congestive heart failure.
   e. Conduction system diseases: pacemaker dysfunction results in low cardiac output.

3. Peripheral vascular disease.
4. Clinical signs and symptoms; examination and intervention are discussed in Chapter 4.

Pulmonary Diseases

1. Chronic bronchitis.
2. Chronic obstructive pulmonary disease (COPD).
3. Asthma.
4. Pneumonia.
   a. Initial symptoms may vary: instead of high fever and productive cough, may see altered mental status, tachypnea, dehydration.
5. Lung cancer.
6. Clinical signs and symptoms; examination and intervention are discussed in Chapter 5.

Integumentary Conditions

1. Pressure ulcers (decubitus ulcers).
   a. Characteristics.
      - Affects 10%–25% of hospitalized, ill elderly patients.
      - Risk factors: immobility and inactivity, sensory impairment, cognitive deficits, decreased circulation, poor nutritional status, incontinence, and moisture.
      - Common over bony prominences: ischial tuberosities, sacrum, greater trochanter, heels, ankles, elbows, and scapulae.

RED FLAG: If not treated promptly ulcers can progress to infection and damage of deep tissues; can be potentially fatal in the frail elderly and chronically ill.

   b. Clinical signs and symptoms; examination and intervention are discussed in Chapter 7.

Metabolic Pathologies

Diabetes Mellitus

1. Aging is associated with deteriorating glucose tolerance; type 2 diabetes affects as many as 10%–20% of individuals over age of 60.
2. Associated with obesity and sedentary lifestyle.
3. Clinical signs and symptoms; examination and intervention are discussed in Chapter 8.

Hypothyroidism

1. Estimated that 1/4 of older adults in nursing home care may have undiagnosed hypothyroidism.
2. Correlated with memory loss in older adults and important to rule out with progressive cognitive decline.
3. Clinical signs and symptoms; examination and intervention. See Chapter 8.

Gastrointestinal (GI) Pathologies

See Chapter 8 for Clinical signs and symptoms; examination and interventions for GI pathologies below.

Gastroesophageal Reflex

1. Approximately 20% of older adults.
2. Complications (Barrett's esophagus, severe ulcerations or strictures) more common in older adults.

Peptic and Duodenal Ulcers

1. Approximately 10% of older adults.
2. Ulcers typically larger and higher rate of mortality in older adults.
3. Clinical presentation is often atypical (only 30% have epigastric pain).
4. Long-term use of proton-pump inhibitors (PPIs) in elderly associated with osteoporosis and pneumonia.

Diverticulitis

1. Most common large intestine disease in older adults.
2. Increased risk with age and 70% of adults >80 years and older.

Genitourinary (GU) Pathologies

See Chapter 8 for Clinical signs and symptoms; examination and interventions for GU pathologies below.

Urinary Tract Infections

1. 10% of females 65 to 84 year olds; 30% of females ≥85 years old.
2. Increased risk with use of catheters.

Urinary Incontinence (UI)

1. Up to 35% of community dwelling adults ≥60 years old.
2. UI in older adults associated with fall risk, depression, and cognitive impairment.
3. Urinary stress (USI) and urge incontinence (UI) are common with aging.
4. See Chapter 8 for additional information regarding the types and management of incontinence.

Chronic Renal Failure

1. Approximately 10% of older adults.
2. Risk factors: Hypertension, diabetes, obesity, smoking, and high-protein diet.
3. Treatment is focused on managing risk factors and dialysis as needed.

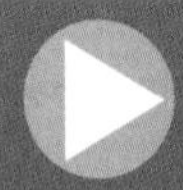

Patient Care Concepts

General Principles of Geriatric Rehabilitation

Recognize Variability of Older Adults

1. Increased heterogeneity of the population with aging.
2. Developmental issues unique to older adults.

Focus on Careful and Accurate Clinical Examination

1. Identify remediable problems.
2. Determine capacity for safe function.
3. Determine effects of inactivity versus activity.
4. Determine effects of disease pathologies and inactivity versus normal aging.

Focus on Functional Goals

1. Determine priorities, remediable problems.
2. Develop goals, plan of care in conjunction with the patient and the caregiver.
3. Determine therapies needed to promote recovery (e.g., exercise) versus those that utilize compensatory (e.g., bracing, assistive device) methods to enhance independence.

Promote Optimal Health (See Table 10-4)

RED FLAG: Strength training programs yield positive results with older adults; failure to prescribe adequate frequency, intensity, and duration of exercise matched to the individual's abilities and strengths will negate the impact on functional abilities and outcomes.

Table 10-4

FITT Recommendations for Older Adults

	AEROBIC	RESISTANCE	FLEXIBILITY
Frequency	• ≥5 days per week for moderate intensity. • ≥3 days per week for vigorous intensity. • 3–5 days per week for a combination of moderate and vigorous intensity.	• ≥2 days per week.	• ≥2 days per week.
Intensity	• On a scale of 0–10 for level of perceived physical exertion, 5–6 for moderate intensity and 7–8 for vigorous intensity.	• Light intensity (i.e., 40%–50% of 1-RM [one-repetition maximum]) for beginners and frail older adults. • Progress to moderate-to-vigorous intensity (60%–80% of 1-RM). • Alternatively, moderate (5–6) to vigorous (7–8) intensity on a 0–10 perceived exertion scale.	• Stretch to the point of feeling tightness or slight discomfort.
Time	• 30–60 minutes per day of moderate intensity exercise. • 20–30 minutes per day of vigorous intensity exercise. • Or an equivalent combination of moderate and vigorous intensity exercise (may be accumulated in bouts of at least 10 minutes each).	• 8–10 exercises involving the major muscle groups • 1–3 sets of 8–12 repetitions each.	• Hold stretch for 30–60 seconds.
Type	• Any modality that does not impose excessive orthopedic stress such as walking. Aquatic exercise and stationary cycling exercise may be advantageous for those with limited tolerance for weight-bearing activity.	• Progressive weight-training programs or weight-bearing calisthenics, stair climbing, and other resistance activities that use major muscle groups.	• Any physical activities that maintain or increase flexibility using slow movements that terminate in static stretches for each muscle group rather than rapid ballistic movements.

Adapted from: Riebe D, et al. ACSM's Guidelines for Exercise Testing and Prescription. 9th ed. Philadelphia: Wolters Kluwer/Lippincott Williams & Wilkins Health, 2018.

1. Monitor patient's heart rate and blood pressure during exercise or progressive physical activity regimens.
2. Focus on increasing health-conducive behaviors, prevention of disability.
3. Minimize and compensate for health-related losses and impairments of aging.

Restore/Maintain

1. Individual's highest level of function and independence within the care environment.
2. Determine how patient autonomy can be maximized by appropriate assistance and environmental manipulations.
3. Empower elders: ensure they are in control of their own decisions whenever possible.
4. Be sensitive to cultural and ethnicity issues; losses, fears, and insecurities; provide comfort and sustenance.
5. Enhance coping skills.
6. Recognize functional abilities, limitations of caregivers; enhance function and support caregivers.

Holism

1. Consider the whole person; integrate all facets of an individual's life.
2. Determine social support systems, effects of social isolation.
3. Determine effects of losses.
4. Determine effects of depression, dementia.

Recognize Demands

1. Enhance continuity of care, interactions in a complex health care delivery system.
2. Advocate for needed services.
3. Provide effective documentation.

Reimbursement Issues

Benefits from Government Programs

1. Cover about two-thirds (63%) of health care expenditures of older persons.
2. Medicare: federal government–sponsored insurance for persons over age 65, disabled persons of all ages. See discussion of government programs in Chapter 14.
3. Medicaid (federal-state funding): covers care of adults with little income and assets before Medicare age, and children from low-income families.
   a. Individuals must spend down or exhaust income to qualify for low-income status.
   b. Administered by individual states that set qualification guidelines; specific requirements vary by state.

Supplemental Private Health Insurance

1. See discussion of insurance plans, managed health care systems, health savings accounts, and the Affordable Care Act in Chapter 14.

Documentation and Reimbursement

1. Requirements specific to type of insurance program.
   a. Medicare requirements for physical therapy services.
      - Must be under the care of a physician; plan of care established and reviewed regularly by M.D.
      - Must include a determination of need: reasonable and necessary for individual's illness or injury according to acceptable standards of practice.
      - Requires the skilled services of a licensed physical therapist.
         - Condition must be expected to improve in a reasonable and generally predictable period of time.
         - A skilled therapist is needed to safely and effectively establish the plan of care (POC) for a patient.
         - A skilled therapist is needed to safely and effectively establish and supervise maintenance therapy for a patient's chronic condition.
      - The physician should review and sign and date the POC (certification). The POC should be certified for the first 30 days of treatment and recertified every 30 days (signed and dated).
      - If the service is not covered under Medicare statutes (e.g., exceeds the therapy cap), the patient can be billed directly.
   b. Private insurance requirements: vary by specific carrier; most adopt Medicare requirements (e.g., physician certification).
2. See Chapter 14 for discussion of defensible documentation.

Ethical and Legal Issues

Professional Practice

1. Affirms patient rights and dignity (professional ethical standards, APTA Code of Ethics).

Informed Consent

1. Respect for personal autonomy; competent patients have the right to refuse treatment; e.g., do not resuscitate (DNR) orders.
2. Legal right to self-determination. Information must be provided to patient that outlines:
   a. The nature and purpose of treatment.
   b. Treatment alternatives.
   c. Risks and consequences of treatment.
   d. Likelihood of success or failure of treatment.
3. Consent must be obtained from a legal guardian if the individual is judged incompetent.
   a. Older adults with fluctuating mental abilities must be carefully evaluated for periods of lucidity.
   b. Documentation with a mental status exam is essential.

Advance Care Medical Directive (Living Will)

1. Established by Federal Patient Self-Determination Act of 1990.
2. Health Care Proxy (aka health care surrogate or medical durable power of attorney): identifies a valid agent who is granted authority to make health care decisions for an individual, should that individual become incapacitated.
3. Requirements.
   a. Regulated by individual states; specific requirements vary by state.
   b. Must be in writing, signed by principal, witnessed by two adults.
   c. Empowers health care agent: includes specific guidelines on which treatment options will and will not be allowed; e.g., artificial life support, feeding tubes.
   d. Defines conditions/scope of agent's authority.

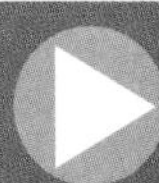

Common Problem Areas for Geriatric Clients

Immobility and Disability

Impaired Mobility and Disability

1. Can result from a host of diseases and conditions.
2. Prolonged inactivity is a significant factor in impaired mobility and disability.

Limitations in Function

1. Increase with age in persons over age 65.
2. 23% report difficulty with one or more personal care activities.
3. 27% report difficulty with one or more home management activities.

Immobility

1. Can result in additional problems.
2. Can lead to complications in almost every major organ system; e.g., pressure sores, contractures, bone loss, muscular atrophy, deconditioning.
3. Metabolic changes can include negative nitrogen and calcium balance, impaired glucose tolerance, decreased plasma volume, altered drug pharmacokinetics.
4. Psychological changes can include loss of positive self-image, depression.
5. Behavioral changes can include confusion, cognitive decline secondary to sensory deprivation, egocentricity.
6. Loss of independence and increased dependency.

Examination and Evaluation (See Appendix 10A)

1. To identify the source of immobility or disability.
2. Determine which impairments (e.g., strength, balance) and activity limitations are modifiable, which require compensatory strategies (e.g., peripheral neuropathy, joint degeneration, some balance disorders, irreversible cognitive decline), and which require interprofessional referral (e.g., vision, hearing, depression, medication adjustment).

Goals, Outcomes, and Interventions

1. Establish a supportive relationship and promote self-determination of goals.
2. Focus on optimal function, gradual progression of daily physical activity and exercise.
3. Prevent further complications or injury.
4. A team approach of health professionals to address all aspects of the patient's problems; patient participation in decision-making.

Falls and Instability

Falls and Fall Injury

1. Falls are a major public health concern for the elderly.
2. One in three Americans aged 65+ falls each year.
3. One out of five falls causes a serious injury (fractures, traumatic brain injury); falls are the most common cause of hospital admissions among older adults.
4. Falls are the leading cause of fatal injury in older adults.
5. Additional consequences of a fall include:
   a. Increased caution and fear of falling.
   b. Loss of confidence to function independently.
   c. Reduced motivation and levels of activity.
   d. Increased risk of recurrent falls.

Fall Etiology (See Tables 10.5 and 10.6 for Common Intrinsic/Extrinsic Fall Risk Factors)

1. Most falls are multifactorial, the result of multiple intrinsic and extrinsic factors and their cumulative effects on mobility; e.g., disease states, age-related changes.
2. Biological risk factors.
   a. Age: incidence of falls increases with age.
   b. Sensory changes.
      - Reduced vision, hearing, cutaneous proprioceptive, and vestibular function.
      - Altered sensory organization for balance, reduced resolution of sensory conflict situations, increased dependence on support surface somatosensory inputs.

Table 10-5

Most Common Intrinsic Fall Risk Factors	
INPATIENT/RESIDENTIAL	**OUTPATIENT/COMMUNITY DWELLING**
Reduced balance/Gait instability	Reduced balance/Gait instability
Lower extremity weakness	Lower extremity weakness
Previous fall history	Previous fall history
Impaired judgment	Impaired judgment
Psychoactive meds: narcotic, hypnotics	Psychoactive meds: narcotic, hypnotics
Vision loss	Vision loss
Orthostatic hypotension	Orthostatic hypotension
Urinary incontinence	

Table 10-6

Most Common Extrinsic Fall Risk Factors	
INPATIENT/RESIDENTIAL	**OUTPATIENT/COMMUNITY DWELLING**
Room: floor not clean/dry	Home: rugs with edges protruding
Bathroom inaccessible/bedside commode not available, low toilet seat	Bathroom lacks rails, bath inaccessible, low toilet seat
Clutter	Clutter: in home or in driveway/yard
Nightlight not available	Lighting poor in/out of home
Call light, water, and light not easily accessible	Stair rails missing or broken in/out of home
Footwear	Footwear
Glasses not available	Glasses not updated

c. Musculoskeletal changes.
- Weakness.
- Decreased ROM.
- Altered postural synergies.

d. Neuromuscular changes:
- Dizziness, vertigo common.
- Timing and control problems: impaired reaction and movement times; slowed onset.

e. Cardiovascular changes.
- Orthostatic hypotension.
- Hyperventilation, coughing, arrhythmias.

f. Medications.
- Strong evidence linking psychotropic drugs: antidepressants, benzodiazepines, sedatives, and hyponotics.
- Evidence linking neuroleptics and antipsychotics.
- Evidence linking cardiovascular drugs that reduce blood pressure or slow the heart rate resulting in hypotension and syncope.
- Fall risk increases with the number of drugs used per day and polypharmacy.

3. Psychosocial/behavioral risk factors.
   a. Mental status/cognitive impairment.
   b. Depression.
   c. Risky behaviors; denial of physical limitations.
   d. Fear of falling: associated with self-imposed activity restriction.
   e. Alcohol abuse.
4. Environmental risk factors.
   a. Setting: three times as many falls for institutionalized or hospitalized older adults than for community dwelling older adults.
   b. Consider ground surfaces, lighting, doors/doorways, stairs.
   c. At home, most falls occur in bedroom (42%); bathroom (34%).
   d. In facilities, consider slippery floor, inaccessibility of call light, lack of bedside commode if needed, and need for more frequent bathroom checks.
5. Activity-related risk factors.
   a. Most falls occur in the home during normal daily activity: getting up from bed/chair, turning head/body, bending, walking, climbing/descending stairs.
   b. Only a small percentage (5%) occur during clearly hazardous activities; e.g., climbing on ladder.
   c. Improper use of assistive device; e.g., walker, cane, wheelchair.
   d. In facilities, many falls occur on the way to the bathroom, or while individual is transferring from bed or chair unattended.

Fall Risk Screening and Prevention (See Table 10.7)

1. Examination.
   a. Accurate fall history: location, activity, time, symptoms, previous falls, past medical/surgical history, and medications.
   b. Physical examination of patient: cognitive, sensory, neuromuscular, and cardiopulmonary.

Table 10-7

Evidence-Based Falls Reduction Interventions for Community Dwelling Older Adults
INTERVENTIONS
Exercise with focus on balance, strength, gait*
Adaptation of environment and reduction of home hazards
Managing vision
Management of foot problems
Management of orthostatic hypotension
Withdrawal/minimizing of psychoactive meds
Additional medication management

Above interventions may reduce the rate of falls.[1,3]
*Evidence also supports that exercise reduces the number of people who fall.[2]

References:

1. Hopewell S, et al. Multifactorial and multiple component interventions for preventing falls in older people living in the community. *Cochrane Database Syst Rev*. 2018 Jul 23; 7(7): CD012221.
2. Sherrington C, et al. Exercise for preventing falls in older people living in the community. *Cochrane Database Syst Rev*. 2019 Jan 31; 1(1): CD012424.
3. Gillespie LD, et al. Interventions for preventing falls in older people living in the community. *Cochrane Database Syst Rev*. 2012 Sep 12; 2012(9): CD007146.

   c. Standardized tests and measures for functional balance and instability (see Figure 10-5, Appendix 10A, and Chapter 3 for additional information).
2. Identify fall risk: determine all intrinsic and/or extrinsic factors.
3. Goals, outcomes, and interventions.
   a. Eliminate or minimize all fall risk factors; stabilize disease states, medications.
   b. Exercise to increase strength, flexibility.
   c. Sensory compensation strategies.
   d. Balance and gait training (see Chapters 3 and 6 for additional information on balance and gait training).
   e. Functional training.
      - Focus on sit-to-stand transitions, turning, walking, and stairs.
      - Modify activities of daily living for safety; provide assistive devices, adaptive equipment as appropriate.
      - Allow adequate time for activities; instruct in gradual position changes.
   f. Safety education.
      - Identify risks.
      - Provide instructions in writing.
      - Communicate with family and caregivers.
   g. Modify environment to reduce falls and instability: use environmental checklist.
      - Ensure adequate lighting.
      - Use contrasting colors to delineate hazardous areas, stairs.
      - Simplify environment, reduce clutter.
      - Remove throw rugs
      - Install toilet and bath/shower handrails and benches.
   h. In facilities, be sure physical therapy is part of the falls prevention team.
      - In facilities, be sure call light and bedside table are easily accessible and establish schedule for regular bathroom checks.

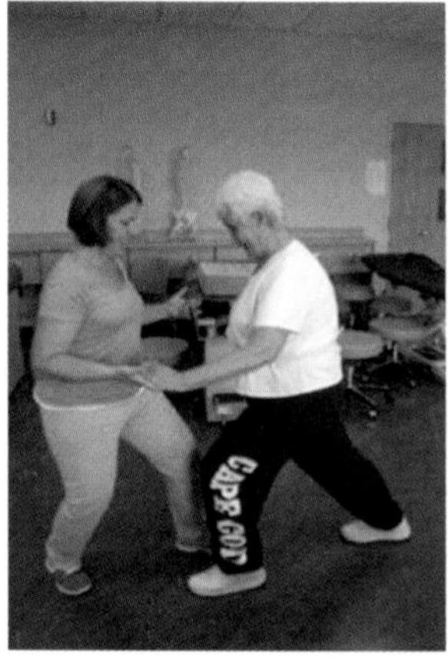

Lunge

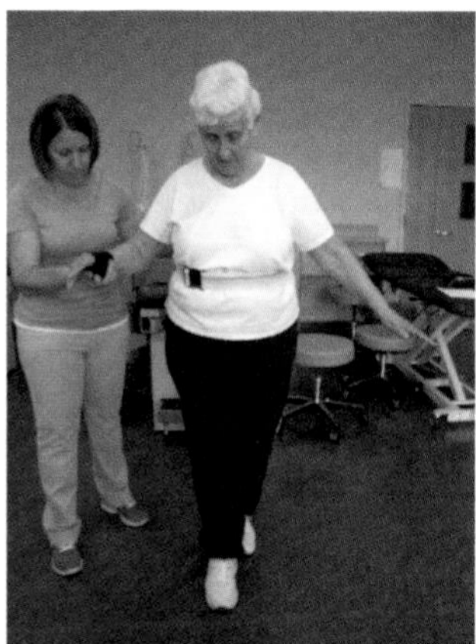

Semi-Tandem Stance

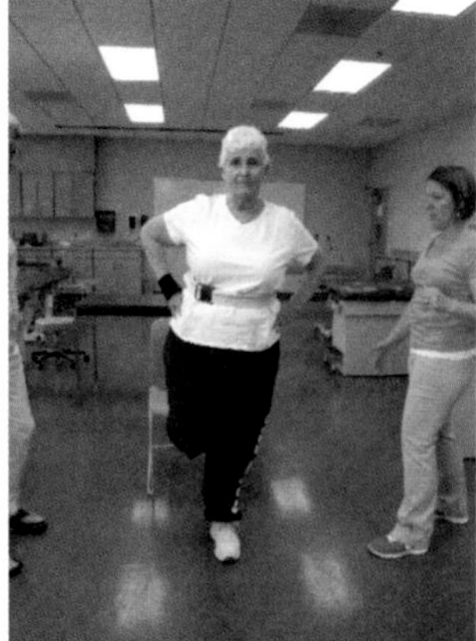

Single-Leg Stance

Figure 10-5 Balance progression examination and exercises–static balance.

4. When the patient falls.
   a. Check for fall injury.
      - Hip fracture: complaints of pain in hip, especially on palpation; external rotation of leg; inability to bear weight on leg; changes in gait, weight-bearing.
      - Head injury: loss of consciousness, mental confusion.
      - Stroke, spinal cord injury: loss of sensation or voluntary movement.
      - Cuts, bruises, painful swelling.
   b. Check for dizziness that may have preceded the fall.
   c. Provide reassurance.
   d. Do not attempt to lift patient by yourself; get help, provide first aid, and call emergency services if necessary.
   e. Solicit witnesses of fall event.
5. See additional discussion in Chapter 13 Safety and Protection.
6. Falls References
   a. The CDC's *Preventing Falls: A Guide to Implementing Effective Community-Based Fall Prevention Programs,* available at: https://www.cdc.gov/homeandrecreationalsafety/falls/community_preventfalls.html.
   b. The CDC's *Compendium of Effective Fall Interventions: What Works for Community-Dwelling Older Adults,* available at: www.cdc.gov/STEADI.
   c. Avin K.G., Hanke T.A., Kirk-Sanchez N., McDonough C.M., Shubert T.E., Hardage J., Hartley G. Management of falls in community dwelling older adults, Clinical Guidance Statement for the Academy of Geriatric Physical Therapy of APTA, *Phys Ther.* 2015; 95(6): 815–834.
   d. Gillespie LD, Robertson MC, Gillespie WJ, et al., Interventions for preventing falls in older people living in the community. *Cochrane Database of Sys Rev.*, 2012.
   e. Sherrington C, Fairhall N, Wallbank G, et al. Exercise for preventing falls in older people living in the community: an abridged Cochrane systematic review. *British Journal of Sports Medicine* 2020; 54: 885–891.
   f. Vlaeyen E, Coussement J, Leysens G et al. Characteristics and effectiveness of fall prevention programs in nursing homes: A systematic review and meta-analysis of randomized controlled trials. *J Am Geriatr Soc.* 2015; 63: 211–221.

Medication Errors

Scope of the Problem

1. Most older adults (60%–85%) utilize prescription drugs to address a chronic medical problem.
2. One-third have three or more medical problems requiring multiple medications and complex dosage schedules.
3. Average older person takes between four and seven prescription drugs each day; takes an additional three over-the-counter drugs.
4. Adverse drug reactions.
   a. Accounts for 4%–10% of hospital admissions in older adults.
      - Affects approximately 25% of all hospitalized patients over the age of 80.
      - Adverse effects are potentially disabling or life-threatening.
   b. High incidence of falls/hip fractures; e.g., psychotropic agents.
   c. Motor vehicle accidents.

Older Adults Are at Increased Risk for Drug Toxicity

1. Factors include age-related changes in pharmacokinetics.
   a. Alterations in drug absorption, distribution to tissues, oxidative metabolism.
   b. Alterations in excretion associated with a decline in hepatic and renal function: decreased clearance in certain drugs; e.g., digoxin, lithium.
   c. Altered sensitivity to the effects of drugs.
      - Increased with certain drugs; e.g., narcotic analgesics, benzodiazepines.
      - Decreased with certain drugs; e.g., drugs mediated by beta-adrenergic receptors, isoproterenol, propranolol.
   d. Drugs may interfere with brain function, cause confusion; e.g., psychoactive drugs: sedatives, hypnotics, antidepressants, anticonvulsants, antiparkinsonism agents.
   e. Older adults have less homeostatic reserve; e.g., are more susceptible to orthostatic hypotension with vasodilating drugs due to dampened compensatory baroreceptor response.
   f. Drug processing effects: multiple drugs compete for binding sites.
      - Drug-to-drug interactions; e.g., levodopa and monamine oxidase inhibitors (MAOIs) may result in hypertensive response.
      - Most drugs exert more than one specific action in the body (polypharmacological effects); e.g., prednisone prescribed for anti-inflammatory action may benefit arthritic symptoms but aggravate a coexisting diabetic state (augments blood glucose levels).
2. Physicians may prescribe inappropriate medications for elderly; estimated in 17.5% of Medicare prescriptions.
3. Most patients are not knowledgeable about drug actions, drug side effects.
4. Drug-food interactions can interfere with effectiveness of medications; e.g., efficacy of levodopa is

compromised if ingested too close to a high-protein meal; potential vitamin/drug interactions.

5. Polypharmacy phenomena: multiple drug prescriptions.
   a. Exacerbated by elderly who visit multiple physicians, use different pharmacies.
   b. Lack integrated care; e.g., computerized system of drug monitoring.
6. Health status influences/socioeconomic factors.
   a. Older adults have a high rate of medication dosage errors; associated with memory impairment, visual impairments, incoordination, and low literacy.
   b. Older adults are targeted for aggressive marketing by drug companies: may result in self-administration of medications for uninvestigated symptoms.
   c. Financial issues: due to high costs, fixed incomes, elderly may skip dosages, stop taking medications.
7. Common adverse effects.
   a. Confusion/dementia; e.g., tranquilizers, barbiturates, digitalis, antihypertensives, anticholinergic drugs, analgesics, antiparkinsonians, diuretics, beta-blockers.
   b. Sedation/immobility; e.g., psychotropic drugs, narcotic analgesics.
   c. Weakness; e.g., antihypertensives, vasodilators, digitalis, diuretics, oral hypoglycemics.
   d. Postural hypotension; e.g., antihypertensives, diuretics, tricyclic antidepressants, tranquilizers, nitrates, narcotic analgesics.
   e. Depression; e.g., antihypertensives, anti-inflammatories, antimycobacterials, antiparkinsonians, diuretics, H_2 receptor antagonists, sedative-hypnotics, vasodilators.
   f. Drug-induced movement disorders.
      - Dyskinesias (involuntary, stereotypic, and repetitive movements; i.e., lip smacking, hand movements, etc.) associated with long-term use of neuroleptic drugs and anticholinergic drugs, levodopa.
      - Akathisia (motor restlessness) associated with antipsychotic drugs.
      - Essential tremor associated with tricyclic antidepressants, adrenergic drugs.
      - Parkinsonism: associated with antipsychotics, sympatholytics.
   g. Incontinence: caused or exacerbated by a variety of drugs; e.g., barbiturates, benzodiazepines, antipsychotic drugs, anticholinergic drugs.
   h. Reference: The American Geriatrics Society continually updates the Beers Criteria for Potentially Inappropriate Medication for Use in Older Adults (https://agsjournals.onlinelibrary.wiley.com/doi/abs/10.1111/jgs.15767).

Goals, Outcomes, and Interventions

1. Assist in adequate monitoring of drug therapy.
   a. Recognize drug-related side effects, adverse reactions to drugs, potential drug interactions in the elderly.
   b. Carefully document patient responses to medications, exercise, and activity.
2. Assist in patient and family drug education/compliance; e.g., understanding of purpose of drugs, dosage, potential side effects.
3. Encourage centralization of medications through one pharmacy.
4. Assist in simplification of drug regimen and instructions.
   a. Administration of drugs; e.g., daily pill box, drug calendar.
   b. Check to see if patient is taking medications on schedule.
   c. Time doses in conjunction with daily routine.
5. Coordinate physical therapy with drug schedule/optimal dose; e.g., exercise during peak dose with individual on Parkinson's disease medications (levodopa).
6. Recognize potentially harmful interaction effects: modalities that cause vasodilatation in combination with vasodilating drugs.
7. Work closely with pharmacist and doctor as needed.

Nutritional Deficiency

Many Older Adults Have Primary Nutritional Problems

1. Nutritional problems in elderly are linked to health status and poverty rather than to age itself.
   a. Chronic diseases alter the overall need for nutrients/energy demands, the ability to take in and utilize nutrients, and overall activity levels; e.g., AD, CVA, diabetes.
   b. Limited, fixed incomes severely limit food choices and availability.
2. Both undernourishment and obesity exist in the elderly and contribute to decreased levels of vitality and fitness.
3. Contributing factors to poor dietary intake.
   a. Decreased sense of taste and smell.
   b. Poor teeth or poorly fitting dentures.
   c. Reduced gastrointestinal function.
      - Decreased saliva.
      - Gastromucosal atrophy.
      - Reduced intestinal mobility; reflux.
   d. Loss of interest in foods.
   e. Lack of social support, socialization during meals.
   f. Lack of mobility.
      - Inability to get to grocery store, shop.
      - Inability to prepare foods.

4. There is an age-related slowing in basal metabolic rate and a decline in total caloric intake; most of the decline is associated with a concurrent reduction in physical activity.
5. Dehydration is common in the elderly, resulting in fluid and electrolyte disturbances.
   a. Thirst sensation is diminished.
   b. May be physically unable to acquire/maintain fluids.
   c. Environmental heat stresses may be life-threatening.
6. Diets are often deficient in nutrients, especially vitamins A, C, B_{12}, thiamine, protein, iron, calcium/vitamin D, folic acid, and zinc.
7. Increased use of taste enhancers; e.g., salt and sugar, or alcohol influences nutritional intake.
8. Drug/dietary interactions influence nutritional intake; e.g., reserpine, digoxin, antitumor agents, excessive use of antacids.

Examination

1. Dietary history: patterns of eating, types of foods.
2. Psychosocial: mental status, desire to eat/depression, social isolation.
3. Body composition.
   a. Weight/height measures.
   b. Skin fold measurements: triceps/subscapular skin fold thickness.
   c. Upper arm circumference.
4. Sensory function: taste and smell.
5. Dental and periodontal disease; fit and use of dentures.
6. Ability to feed self: mastication, swallowing, hand/mouth control, posture, physical weakness and fatigue.
7. Integumentary: skin condition, edema.
8. Compliance to special diets.
9. Functional assessment: basic activities of daily living, feeding; overall exercise/activity levels.

Goals, Outcomes, and Interventions

1. Assist in monitoring adequate nutritional intake.
2. Assist in health promotion.
   a. Maintain adequate nutritional support.
      - Nutritional consults as necessary.
      - Nutritional educational programs.
      - Assistance in grocery shopping, meal preparation; e.g., recommendations for home health aides.
      - Elderly food programs: home-delivered/Meals on Wheels; congregate meals/senior center daily meal programs; federal food stamp programs.
   b. Maintain physical function, adequate activity levels.

APPENDIX 10A

Selected Geriatrics Outcome Measures

Table 10A-1

Mobility & Balance Outcomes Measures–Older Adults

MOBILITY OUTCOME MEASURES	TEST	NORMATIVE VALUES AND CUT–OFFS
Sit-to-Stand Transfers and Lower Extremity Strength/Power	Timed sit to stand x5	12 seconds is cut off for fall risk (Community dwelling adults age 74–98 years old) **Norms:** **Age (years)** **Time (seconds)** 60–69: 11.4 70–79: 12.6 80–89: 14.8
	Sit-to-stand (number in 30 seconds)	STS x 30 seconds below average scores: **Age (years)** **Repetitions** 60–64: Men (M): <14, Women (W) <12 65–69: M<12, W<11 70–74: M<12, W<10 75–79 M<11, W<10 80–84: M<10, W<9 85–89: M<8, W<8 90–94: M<7, W<4
Gait	Comfortable Gait Speed (CGS)	**Norms:** **Age (years)** **Mean (SD) Velocity (m/s)** 50–59: M:1.22 (.20) W: 1.11 (.22) 60–69: M: 1.03 (.20) W: 1.00 (.23) 70–79: M: 0.96 (.23) W: 0.90 (.24) ≥80: M: 0.83 (.22) W: 0.78 (.22) 1.2 m/s needed to safely cross the street 0.8–1.2 m/s for safe community ambulation
Transfer/Gait/Turns/Dynamic Stability	Timed Up and Go (TUG)	**Norms:** **Age (years)** **Time (seconds)** 60–69 8.1 70–79 9.2 80–99 11.3
Mobility/Balance with multiple tasking	Cognitive TUG (cognitive task-count backward by 3's)	>14 seconds discriminated fallers

(Continued)

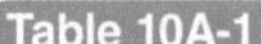
Table 10A-1

Mobility & Balance Outcomes Measures–Older Adults (Continued)

MOBILITY OUTCOME MEASURES	TEST	NORMATIVE VALUES AND CUT–OFFS
Endurance/Aerobic Capacity	6-minute walk test	**Norms:** **Age (years)** **Distance (meters)** 60–69: Men (M): 572, Women (W): 538 70–79: M: 527 W: 471 80–89: M: 417 W: 392 **Responsiveness:** Small meaningful change: 20 m Substantial meaningful change: 50 m * Measure HR at rest, post activity and 3 minutes after activity.
Static Balance	Single Leg Stance Eyes Open (SLSEO)	**Age (years)** **Time (seconds)** 60–69 27.0 70–79 17.2 80–99 8.5
CDC 4 stage balance test	Standing feet together, semi-tandem, tandem stance, SLSEO	Cut off for falls: Unable to hold tandem stance x 10 seconds (per CDC STEADI)
Functional Stability Limits	Functional Reach Test	Community-dwelling older adults 26.6 cm [95%CI: 25.14; 28.06] Non-community older adults 15.4 cm [95%CI: 13.47; 17.42]
Balance Measures–Multiple Domains	Berg Balance Scale (BBS)	**Age (years)** **Points** Norm values: 60–69 55/56 70–80 52/56 ≤50 increased fall risk
	Mini Balance Evaluation Systems Test (BEST)	**Age (years)** **Cut Point Predictive of Fall** 60–69 25/28 70–79 23/28 80–89 22/28 ≥90 17/28

References:

1. Bohannon, RW. Single Limb Stance Time. *Topics in Geriatric Rehabilitation*. 2006; 22(1): 70–77.
2. Bohannon RW. Population representative gait speed and its determinants. *J Geriatr Phys Ther*. 2008; 31(2): 49–52.
3. Hardy, S. E., S. Perera, et al. (2007). Improvement in usual gait speed predicts better survival in older adults. *J Am Geriatr Soc* 55(11): 1727–34.
4. Lusardi MM, Fritz S, Middleton A, et al. Determining risk of falls in community dwelling older adults: A systematic review and meta-analysis using posttest probability. *J Geriatr Phys Ther*. 2017 Jan/Mar; 40(1): 1–36.
5. Magnani PE, Genovez MB, Porto JM et al. Use of the BESTest and the Mini-BESTest for fall risk prediction in community dwelling older adults between 60 and 102 years of age. *J Geriatr Phys Ther*. 2020 Oct/Dec; 43(4): 179–184.
6. Middleton A, Fritz SL, Lusardi M. Walking speed: The functional vital sign. *J Aging Phys Act*. 2015 Apr; 23(2): 314–322.
7. Perera S, Mody SH, Woodman RC, Studenski SA. Meaningful change and responsiveness in common physical performance measures in older adults. *J Am Geriatr Soc*. 2006 May; 54(5): 743–749.
8. Rikli RE, Jones CJ. Development and validation of criterion-referenced clinically relevant fitness standards for maintaining physical independence in later years. *Gerontologist*. 2013 Apr; 53(2): 255–267.
9. Rosa MV, Perracini MR, Ricci NA. Usefulness, assessment and normative data of the Functional Reach Test in older adults: a systematic review and meta-analysis. *Arch Gerontol Geriatr*. 2019 Mar–Apr; 81: 149–170.
10. Shirley Ryan Agility Lab. Rehabilitation Measures Database, https://www.sralab.org/rehabilitationmeasures
11. Shumway-Cook A, Brauer S, Woollacott M. Predicting the probability for falls in community-dwelling older adults using the Timed Up & Go Test. *Phys Ther*. 2000 Sep; 80(9): 896–903.
12. Steffen TM, Hacker TA, Mollinger L. Age- and gender-related test performance in community-dwelling elderly people: Six-Minute Walk Test, Berg Balance Scale, Timed Up & Go Test, and gait speeds. *Phys Ther*. 2002 Feb; 82(2): 128–137. doi: 10.1093/ptj/82.2.128.
13. Tiedemann A, Shimada H, Sherrington C, et al. The comparative ability of eight functional mobility tests for predicting falls in community-dwelling older people. *Age Ageing*. 2008 Jul; 37(4): 430–435.

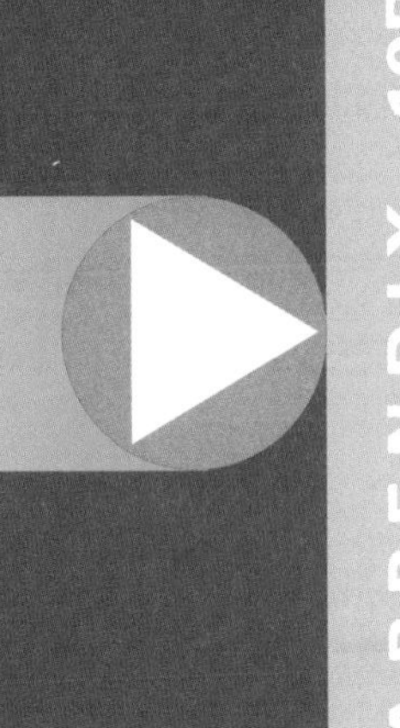

APPENDIX 10B

Review Questions and Case Study

(Answers to all Review Questions and Case Studies are found in Chapter 17)

1. What are the physiological changes that may occur in the visual system in older adults?

2. What risk factors are associated with development of osteoporosis?

3. What are the major side effects (red flags) of the use of pain medications in the geriatric population that can be a concern for physical therapists?

4. What are the most important components of the initial examination of a patient with dementia (also known as Neurocognitive Disorders)?

5. What are the major goals and interventions to minimize fall risk factors?

Case Scenario/Questions-Geriatric Physical Therapy

- **Gender:** Male
- **Age:** 76

Presenting Problem/Current Condition:

- Patient referred to outpatient physical therapy secondary to right knee pain for 3 months
- His symptoms started after falling in the grocery store. His spouse reports that he has fallen 2 times in the past year
- He rates his right knee pain as 2/10 on average and increased with stairs or squatting
- X-rays of the right knee within normal limits except mild osteoarthritis
- He denies numbness, tingling, radiating pain, or weakness in his bilateral upper or lower extremities
- The patient and his spouse report he is having difficulty with short-term memory

Past Medical/Surgical History:

- Suspected Mild Alzheimer's disease for 1 year
- Depression by 6 months
- Elevated cholesterol that is well controlled with medication
- Bilateral mild knee osteoarthritis

Other Information

- Retired history professor
- Married and lives in a one-story home

Question #1

What information from the patient or his spouse is most consistent with the diagnosis of mild Alzheimer's disease?

1. Decreased attention span and problems recognizing friends and family members
2. Increased time required to accomplish daily tasks accompanied with anxiety
3. Newly occurring sleep disorders and intermittent hallucinations
4. Difficulty with complex planning but daily life not generally affected

Question #2

The patient's spouse reports his past falls have occurred while he is multitasking or distracted (e.g., looking at his phone and walking or carrying groceries). Which of the following outcome measures would be most helpful to assess the patient's fall risk and mobility?

1. Comfortable gait speed
2. 5 times sit-to-stand
3. Timed up and go with a cognitive task
4. Single leg stance eyes open and eyes closed

Question #3

On your initial evaluation the patient's gait speed and single-leg balance are normal. He is able to complete the timed up and go with cognitive task (TUG-Cog-counting backward by 3's) in 20 seconds with 2 errors. Which of the following evidence base strategies are **BEST** for safely improving the patient's community mobility and balance?

1. Instruct the patient on use of a cane for community ambulation and conduct in clinic gait training with head turns.
2. Instruct the patient on the use of a rolling walker for community ambulation and conduct reactive postural control training in the clinic.
3. No device or patient education is needed for community ambulation, and the patient should practice the timed up and go cognitive task with his wife at home.
4. Conduct a fall risk asesessement and provide patient education and interventions to address identified fall risk factors.

11

Therapeutic Modalities

L. VINCE LEPAK III

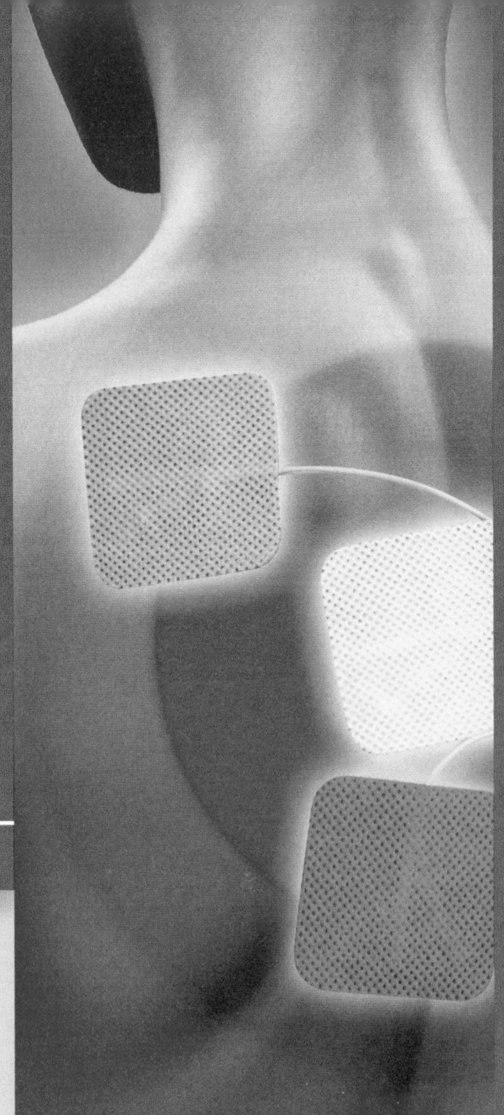

Chapter Outline

Study Tactics

Questions About Therapeutic Modalities Comprise Approximately 3.5% of the NPTE, or a Total of 6–8 Questions

Focus on:

- The selection and appropriate use of modalities, including applications, indications, precautions, contraindications, and parameters for use. Safety is a major consideration
- Electrotherapy: TENS, functional electrical stimulation (FES), high-voltage pulsed galvanic stimulation, neuromuscular electrical stimulation (NMES), interferential current, and iontophoresis
  - Parameters for use to include electrode numbers (2, 4), size and placement, duty cycle, anode/cathode, waveforms
  - Medications/polarity of substances used in iontophoresis
  - Wound healing and electrical stimulation considerations
- Ultrasound and phonophoresis: physiological effects, absorption, penetration, attenuation, frequency, precautions, and side effects
- Thermotherapy including indications, precautions, contraindications, and physiological effects
- Cervical and lumbar traction techniques including indications, precautions, contraindications, and positioning
- Intermittent compression techniques including indications, precautions, adjustments based on blood pressure, duty cycle, and frequency of treatment

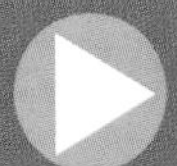

Physical Agents (See Appendix 11A for summary of Indications, Precautions, and Contraindications)

Superficial Thermotherapy

Physiological Effects of General Heat Application

1. Large areas of the body surface area are exposed to heat modality; e.g., whirlpool (hip and knee immersed) (Table 11-1).

Physiological Effects of Small Surface Area Heat Application

1. Body tissue responses to superficial heat.
   a. Skin temperature rises rapidly and exhibits greatest temperature change.
   b. Subcutaneous tissue temperature rises less rapidly and exhibits smaller change.
   c. Muscles and joints show least temperature change.
   d. Structures deeper than 3 cm require continuous ultrasound or shortwave diathermy.
2. Physiological effects on body systems and structures to small surface area heat modalities at a therapeutic level (104°F–113°F) are listed in Tables 11-2 and 11-3.

Table 11-1

Physiological Effects of General Heat Application

INCREASED	DECREASED
Cardiac output	Blood pressure
Metabolic rate	Muscle activity (sedentary effect)
Pulse rate	Blood to internal organs
Respiratory rate	Blood flow to resting muscle
Vasodilation	Stroke volume

Goals and Indications for Superficial Thermotherapy

1. Modulate pain, increase connective tissue extensibility, reduce or eliminate soft-tissue inflammation and swelling, accelerate rate of tissue healing, reduce or eliminate soft-tissue and joint restriction and muscle spasm.
2. Preparation for electrical stimulation (ES), massage, passive and active exercise.
3. Don't use passive physical agents except when necessary to facilitate participation in an active treatment program (White N, et al., *Phys Ther*. 2015).

Precautions for Use of Superficial Thermotherapy

1. Cardiac insufficiency, edema, impaired circulation, impaired thermal regulation, metal in treatment site, pregnancy, in areas where topical counterirritants have recently been applied, and open wounds.

RED FLAG CONTRAINDICATIONS: Acute and early subacute traumatic and inflammatory conditions, decreased circulation, decreased sensation, deep vein thrombophlebitis, impaired cognitive function, malignant tumors, tendency toward hemorrhage or edema, very young and very old patients. Additional contraindications are listed with each therapeutic modality.

General Treatment Preparation for Thermotherapy and Cryotherapy

1. The application of physical agents must be performed by qualified physical therapy personnel. The

Table 11-2

Increased Physiological Responses of Body Systems and Structures to Local Heat Application

SYSTEM/STRUCTURE	MECHANISM
Blood flow	Dilation of arteries and arterioles (minimal to no change in blood flow to skeletal muscle)
Capillary permeability	Increased capillary pressure
Elasticity of nonelastic tissues	Increased extensibility of collagen tissue
Cellular and metabolic rates	For every 10°C (50°F) increase in tissue temperature, the rate of cellular oxidation increases by two to three times
Vasodilation	Activation of axonal/spinal cord reflexes; Release of vasoactive agents (Kallikrein, bradykinin, histamine, prostagladins); decrease sympathetic adrenergic activity to blood vessels
Edema	Increased capillary permeability

Table 11-3

Decreased Physiological Responses of Body Systems and Structures to Local Heat Application	
SYSTEM/STRUCTURE	**MECHANISM**
Joint stiffness	Increased extensibility of collagen tissue and decreased viscosity
Strength and endurance	Decreased function of glycolytic process
Muscle spasm	Decreased firing of II afferents of muscle spindle and increased firing of Ib GTO fibers reduces alpha motor neuron activity, and thus decreases tonic extrafusal activity
Pain	Presynaptic inhibition of A delta and C fibers via activation of A beta fibers (gate theory), disruption of pain-spasm cycle

treatment and expected sensations must be explained to the patient.
2. Place patient in comfortable position.
3. Expose treatment area and drape patient properly.
4. Inspect skin and check temperature sensation prior to treatment.
5. If patient has good cognitive function, a call bell or other signaling device can be given to the patient to alert personnel of any untoward effects of treatment.
6. Check patient frequently during initial treatment.
7. Dry and inspect skin at conclusion of treatment.

Superficial Heating Physical Agents

1. Hot pack.
   a. A canvas pack filled with silica gel, heated by immersion in water between 165°F and 170°F.
   b. Method of heat transmission: conduction.
   c. Method of application.
      - Add layers of toweling between the hot pack and the patient. This can be accomplished in the following ways:
      - Place pack on patient. If patient must be placed on pack, use additional towels to minimize excessive heating of treatment area caused by weight of patient on pack and to protect bony prominences.
      - The hot pack reaches peak heat within the first 5 minutes of application; during this time, the patient is at the greatest risk for a burn. Thus, the physical therapy personnel should check the skin within the first 5 minutes of treatment and periodically thereafter, especially if the patient is lying on top of the pack.
   d. Treatment time: 20–30 minutes.
2. Paraffin bath: therapeutic application of liquid paraffin to a body part for the transmission of heat. Paraffin bath is a thermostatically controlled unit that contains a paraffin wax and mineral oil mixture in a 6:1 or 7:1 ratio. The paraffin/mineral oil mixture melts between 118°F and 130°F and is normally self-sterilizing at temperatures of 175°F and 180°F. Paraffin is primarily applied to small, irregularly shaped areas such as the wrist, hand, and foot.
   a. Method of heat transmission: conduction.
   b. Procedure.
      - Glove method (dip and wrap with plastic wrap and toweling) or immersion (part remains in the bath after final dip).
   c. Treatment time: 15–20 minutes.
   d. Indications: painful joints caused by arthritis or other inflammatory conditions in the late subacute or chronic phase, joint stiffness. Most often used on wrists and hands.

RED FLAG: Contraindications: allergic rash, open wounds, recent scars and sutures, skin infections.

   e. Unlikely to be tested on the National Physical Therapy Exam (NPTE).
3. Other superficial thermal modalities that are unlikely to appear on the NPTE are fluidotherapy and infrared lamps.
4. Hydrotherapy (whirlpool): partial or total immersion baths in which the water is agitated and mixed with air to be directed against or around the affected part. Patients can move the extremities easily because of the buoyancy and therapeutic effect of the water.
   a. Method of heat transmission: primarily convection.
   b. Treatment temperature: varies with size and status of area treated.
      - Tepid/nonthermal 79°F–92°F (26°C–33.3°C)—temperature for exercise in water.
      - Neutral 92°F–96°F (33.3°C–35.5°C)—temperature for open wounds.
      - Thermal 96°F–104°F (35.5°C–40°C)—causes stress on cardiopulmonary and nervous system—lower range increases tissue mobility—higher temperatures only used on limited body area.
   c. Treatment time: 20 minutes.
   d. Indications: subacute and chronic musculoskeletal conditions.
   e. Precautions.
      - Local immersion: decreased temperature sensation, impaired cognition, recent skin graft, confusion/disorientation, deconditioned state.

- Full-body immersion (hot water): pregnancy, multiple sclerosis, poor thermal regulation.
- Full-body immersion (tepid water): same as local immersion plus: cardiovascular medications, urinary incontinence, aquaphobia, respiratory issues.

RED FLAGS: Contraindications.
Don't use whirlpool for wound management (White N, et al., *Phys Ther.* 2015).
Local immersion: maceration, bleeding.
Full-body immersion: unstable cardiac disorder, bowel incontinence, severe epilepsy, suicidal, potential for cross-contamination.

f. Electrical safety: safety precautions must be taken with any modality that potentially exposes the patient to electrical hazards from faulty electrical connections.
   - A ground fault circuit interrupter (GFI) should be installed at the circuit breaker of the receptacle of all whirlpools. The electrical circuit is broken if current is diverted to the patient that is grounded rather than to a grounded modality.
   - All whirlpool turbines, tanks, and motors used to lift patients should be checked for current leakage (broken or frayed connections).

5. Nonimmersion irrigation device.
   a. Small, handheld electric water pump that produces a water jet to create a shearing force to loosen tissue debris. Some devices produce a pulsed lavage and include suction to remove debris.
   b. Procedure.
      - Treatment should take place in an enclosed area.
      - Face and eye protection, gloves, and waterproof gown are required.
      - Sterile, warm saline is used. Antimicrobials may be added if infection is present.
      - Select appropriate treatment pressure, usually 4–15 psi. Pressure may be increased in presence of large amounts of necrotic tissue or tough eschar. Pressure should be decreased with bleeding, near a major vessel, or if a patient complains of pain.
      - Avoid granulating tissues and use in body cavity.
      - Treatment time is usually 5–15 minutes, once a day. Wound size and amount of necrotic tissue may increase treatment parameters.

Cryotherapy

Physiological Effects of Large Surface Area Cold Application (See Table 11-4)

Table 11-4

Physiological Effects of General Cold Application

DECREASED	INCREASED
Metabolic rate	Blood flow to internal organs
Pulse rate	Cardiac output
Respiratory rate	Stroke volume
Venous blood pressure	Arterial blood pressure Shivering (occurs when core temperature drops)

Physiological Effects of Small Surface Area Cold Application

1. Effects of cold application on body tissues.
   a. Skin temperature falls rapidly and exhibits greatest temperature change.
   b. Subcutaneous temperature falls less rapidly and displays smaller temperature change.
   c. Muscles and joints show least temperature changes, requiring longer cold exposure.
2. Vasoconstriction of skin capillaries that results in blanching of skin in the center of contact area and hyperemia due to a decreased rate in oxyhemoglobin dissociation, around the edge of contact area in normal tissue.
3. Cold-induced vasodilation: cyclic vasoconstriction and vasodilation (i.e., hunting response) following prolonged cold exposure (>15 minutes and at temperatures <35°F). Occurs mostly in hands, feet, and face. The frequency of this response is inconsistent and the only clinical significance is the potential for vasodilation after 15 minutes in the distal appendages.
4. Physiological effects on body systems and structures to small surface area cold modalities (Tables 11-5 and 11-6).
5. Adverse physiological effects of cold due to hypersensitivity.
   a. Cold urticaria: erythema of the skin with wheal formation, associated with severe itching due to histamine reaction.
   b. Facial flush, puffiness of eyelids, respiratory problems, and in severe cases, anaphylaxis (decreased blood pressure, increased heart rate) with syncope are also related to histamine release.

Goals and Indications for Cryotherapy

1. Modulate pain; reduce or eliminate soft-tissue inflammation or swelling; reduce muscle spasm; reduce spasticity, cryokinetics, cryostretch; management of symptoms in multiple sclerosis.

Precautions

1. Hypertension, poor thermal regulation, impaired sensation, open wound, over superficial nerve, very old or young, cognitive changes.

Table 11-5

Decreased Physiological Responses of Body Systems and Structures to Local Cold Application

SYSTEM/STRUCTURE	MECHANISM
Blood flow	Sympathetic adrenergic activity produces vasoconstriction of arteries, arterioles, and venules Vasodilators (i.e., histamine and prostaglandins) release and production are reduced
Capillary permeability	Decreased fluids into interstitial tissue
Elasticity of nonelastic tissues	Decreased extensibility of collagen tissue
Metabolism	Decreased rate of cellular oxidation
Muscle spasm	Decreased firing of II afferents of muscle spindle, increased firing of Ib GTO fibers reduces alpha motor neuron activity and thus decreases tonic extrafusal activity
Muscle strength	Decreased blood flow, increased viscous properties of muscle (long duration: >5–10 min)
Spasticity	Decreased muscle spindle discharge (afferents: primary, secondary), decreased gamma motor neuron activity
Vasoactive agents	Decreased blood flow

Table 11-6

Increased Physiological Responses of Body Systems and Structures to Local Cold Application

SYSTEM/STRUCTURE	MECHANISM
Joint stiffness	Decreased extensibility of collagen tissue and increased tissue viscosity
Pain threshold	Inhibition of A delta and C fibers via activation of A beta fibers (gate theory), interruption of pain-spasm cycle, decreased sensory and motor conduction, synaptic transmission slowed or blocked
Increased blood viscosity	Decreased blood flow in small vessels facilitates red blood cells adhering to one another and vessel wall, impeding blood flow
Muscle strength	Facilitation of alpha motor neuron (short duration: 1–5 min)

RED FLAG: Contraindications to use of cryotherapy. Cold hypersensitivity (cold-induced uticaria manifestation), cold intolerance, cryoglobulinemia (more common with chronic liver diseases, rheumatic diseases, and multiple myeloma), peripheral vascular disease, insensate, Raynaud's disease, paroxysmal cold hemoglobinuria, over regenerating peripheral nerves.

Procedures

1. Cold packs: vinyl casing filled with silica gel or sand-slurry mixture.
   a. Method of heat transmission: conduction.
   b. Method of application.
      - Dampen a towel with warm water, wring out excess water, fold in half width-wise, and place cold pack on towel.
      - Place pack on patient and cover with dry towel to retard warming.
   c. Treatment temperature: packs are maintained in refrigerated unit at 0°F–10°F.
   d. Treatment time: 10–20 minutes.
2. Ice packs: crushed ice folded in moist towel or placed in plastic bag covered by moist towel.
   a. Method of heat transmission: conduction (abstraction).
   b. Method of application.
      - Apply the ice pack to body part.
   c. Treatment time: 10–20 minutes.
3. Ice massage: During the application of ice massage, the patient will usually experience the following sequence of physiological response stages: cold, burning, aching, and numbness.
   a. Method of heat transmission: conduction.
   b. Method of application.
      - Apply the ice massage to an area no larger than 4 × 6 inches in slow (2 inches/second) overlapping circles or overlapping longitudinal strokes, each stroke covering one-half of previous circle or stroke. If treating a large area, divide into smaller areas.
      - Do not massage over bony area or superficial nerve (e.g., peroneal/fibular).
      - Continue treatment until anesthesia is achieved.
   c. Treatment time: 5–10 minutes, or until analgesia occurs.
4. Cold hydrotherapy: See description, method of heat transmission, and method of application in superficial thermotherapy.
   a. Temperature: 32°F–79°F (0°C–26°C).
   b. Treatment time: 20 minutes.
   c. Indications: acute edema, inflammation.

RED FLAG: Precautions and contraindications: Previous risk factors for hydrotherapy and those at risk for poor thermal regulation (e.g., peripheral vascular disease, Raynaud's, elderly, and infants, etc.).

d. Advantages and disadvantages:
- Advantages: greater surface contact than any other physical modality.
- Disadvantages: Part being treated is often in a dependent position.

5. Cold compression units (e.g., Game Ready, Aircast Cryo Cuff, etc.): this combines the effects of compression and cryotherapy.
   a. Method of heat transmission: conduction and convection.
   b. Procedure:
   - Ensure no contraindication to compression
   - Inspect limb, apply hygienic sleeve to limb, and then apply compression sleeve.
   - Elevate limb.
   - Temperature 50°F–59°F (10°C–15°C).
   - Intermittent or continuous compression (5–75 mmHg).

   c. Treatment time: 15 minutes.
   d. Indications: Same as other cooling modalities.
   e. Contraindications: refer to the Red Flag Box in cyrotherapy section.

Ultrasound (US)

Biophysics Related to Ultrasound

1. Spatial characteristics of US.
   a. During continuous US, spatial characteristics of US are predominant.
   b. Continuous US is applied to achieve thermal effects.
   c. US energy (intensity) is not uniformly distributed over the surface of the transducer, because the energy is mechanically blocked by the adhesive bonding of the crystal in the transducer, and the pressure waves interfere with each other as they radiate from different areas of the crystal.
   d. Uneven intensity produces a high level of energy in the center of the US beam relative to the surrounding areas. This effect produces a "hot spot" (peak spatial intensity) in the beam. Moving the soundhead or using pulsed US tends to reduce the effect of the hot spot.
   e. Spatial average intensity. The total power (watts) divided by the area (cm^2) of the transducer head. This is typically the measurement used to document US treatments.
   f. Beam nonuniformity ratio (BNR). The ratio of spatial peak intensity to spatial average intensity. The lower the BNR, the more uniform the energy distribution, and the less risk of tissue damage. BNR should be between 2:1 and 6:1. An ideal 1:1 ratio is not technically feasible. Higher ratios result in a larger spatial peak intensity when compared to the average spatial intensity (less uniform distribution).
2. Temporal characteristics of US.
   a. During pulsed US, temporal characteristics of the US are important.
   b. Pulsed US is applied when nonthermal effects are desired (e.g., acute soft tissue injuries).
   c. Duty cycle. The fraction of time the US energy is on over one pulse period (time on + time off). For example, a 20% duty cycle could have an on-time of 2 msec and an off-time of 8 msec (2/(2+8) or 20%). A duty cycle of ≤ 50% is considered pulsed US. A duty cycle of 51%–99% produces less acoustic energy and less heat than continuous US at 100% duty cycle.
   d. Temporal peak intensity. The peak intensity of US during the on-time phase of the pulse period.
   e. Temporal average intensity. The US power averaged over one pulse period.
   f. Attenuation. The reduction of acoustical energy as it passes through soft tissue. Absorption, reflection, and refraction affect attenuation. Absorption is highest in tissues with high collagen and protein content (muscles, tendons, ligaments, capsules). The scattering of sound waves that result from reflection and refraction produces molecular friction that the sound wave must overcome to penetrate tissues.
3. Depth of penetration.
   a. At 3 MHz, greater heat production in superficial layers, caused by greater scatter (attenuation) of sound waves in superficial tissue. Used for tissues 1–2.5 cm deep.
   b. Increased heat production in deep layers at 1 MHz is caused by less scatter in superficial tissues; thus, more US energy is able to penetrate to deeper tissues. Used for tissues up to 6 cm deep.

Physiological Effects of Ultrasound

1. Thermal: produced by continuous sound energy of sufficient intensity. US intensity will vary depending on frequency, tissue type, and pathology.
   a. Intensity is based on frequency for desired thermal response in an area two times the size of the effective radiating area (ERA) in 5–10 minutes.
   - 1 MHz: 1.5–2.0 W/cm^2.
   - 3 MHz: 0.5–1 W/cm^2.

b. A significant rise in tissue temperature may take 10 minutes or more for deeper tissues with 1 MHz at 1.5 W/cm^2 in an area two times the ERA (Bellew et al., 2016, p. 96).
c. Increased tissue temperature, increased pain threshold, increased collagen tissue extensibility, alteration of nerve conduction velocity, increased enzymatic activity, and increased tissue perfusion.
d. Increased temperature at tissue interfaces due to reflection and refraction. Tissue interfaces could be bone/ligament, bone/joint capsule, and bone/muscle.
e. Excessively high temperatures may produce a sudden, strong ache caused by overheating of periosteal tissue (periosteal pain). Reduce intensity or increase surface area of treatment if periosteal pain is expressed by patient.
f. Insufficient coupling agent may produce discomfort caused by a "hot spot," which is the uneven distribution of the acoustical energy through the sound head. However, this is a greater problem if the stationary technique is used.

2. Nonthermal: generated by very low intensity or pulsed (intermittent) sound energy. Pulsed US is related to duty cycle. Typical duty cycles are 20%–50% for nonthermal intervention.
   a. Cavitation: alternating compression (condensation phase) and expansion (rarefaction phase) of small gas bubbles in tissue fluids caused by mechanical pressure waves.
      - Stable cavitation: gas bubbles resonate without tissue damage. Stable cavitation may be responsible for diffusional changes in cell membranes.
      - Unstable cavitation: severe collapse of gas bubbles during compression phase of US can result in local tissue destruction due to high temperatures.
   b. Acoustic streaming: movement of fluids along the boundaries of cell membranes resulting from mechanical pressure wave. Acoustic streaming may produce alterations in cell membrane activity, increased cell wall permeability, increased intracellular calcium, increased macrophage response, and increased protein synthesis; may accelerate tissue healing.

Goals and Indications

1. Modulate pain, increase connective tissue extensibility, reduce or eliminate soft-tissue inflammation, accelerate rate of tissue healing, reduce or eliminate muscle spasm.

Precautions

1. Acute inflammation, breast implants, open epiphyses, and US over healing fractures.

> **RED FLAG:** Contraindications.
>
> Impaired circulation; impaired cognitive function; impaired sensation; malignant tumors; over or near an area with thrombophlebitis; joint cement; directly over plastic components; over vital areas such as brain, ear, eye, heart, cervical ganglia; carotid sinuses; reproductive organs; exposed or unprotected spinal cord; over or in the area of cardiac pacemakers or in the abdomen, low back, uterus, or pelvis during pregnancy; high doses of thermal US should be avoided over open epiphyseal plates.

2. *Don't use ultrasound to reduce swelling, promote joint healing, or achieve long-term pain relief for musculoskeletal conditions* (White N, et al., *Phys Ther.* 2015).

Procedures

1. Direct contact (transducer/skin interface). Moving sound head in contact with relatively flat body surface.
   a. Apply generous amount of coupling medium (gel/cream) to skin.
   b. Select sound head size (ERA one-half the size of the treatment area). Place sound head at right angle to skin surface.
   c. Move sound head slowly (~1.5 inches/sec) in overlapping circles or longitudinal strokes, maintaining sound head to body surface angle.
   d. Each motion covers one-half of previous circle or stroke.
   e. Do not cover an area greater than two to three times the size of the effective radiating area (ERA) per 5–10 minutes of treatment. To cover an area greater than twice the ERA, apply US in two or more sections.
   f. While sound head is moving and in firm contact, turn up intensity to desired level.
   g. Treatment intensity: 0.5–2.5 w/cm^2, depending on treatment goal. Lower intensities for acute conditions or thin tissue (wrist joint); for chronic conditions or thick tissue (low back), higher intensities should be considered.
   h. Periosteal pain occurring during treatment may be caused by high intensity, momentary slowing, or cessation of moving head. If this occurs, stop treatment and readjust US intensity or add more coupling agent.
   i. Treatment time: 3–10 minutes, depending on size of area, intensity, condition, and frequency.
2. Indirect contact (water immersion). Use with irregular body parts.
   a. Fill container with water high enough to cover treatment area. A plastic container is preferred because it will reflect less acoustic energy than a metal container.

b. Place body part and sound head in water, keeping it 1 cm from skin surface and at right angle to body part.
c. Move sound head slowly, as in direct contact. If applying stationary technique, reduce intensity or use pulsed US.
d. Turn up intensity to desired level.
e. Periodically wipe off any air bubbles that may form on sound head or body part during treatment.

Phonophoresis

1. The use of US to drive medications through the skin into the deeper tissues. Local analgesics (lidocaine) and anti-inflammatory drugs (dexamethasone, salicylates) are often used.
2. Method of application is similar to direct contact technique, except that a medicinal agent is used as part of coupling medium.
   a. Mode: pulsed 20%.
   b. Treatment time: 5–10 minutes.
   c. 0.5–0.75 w/cm^2, using a medication that is prepared in a medium that will allow transmission of the US. Gel mediums or transdermal patches have good transmissivity; avoid pastes and creams.
3. Goals and indications.
   a. Pain modulation; decrease inflammation in subacute and chronic musculoskeletal conditions.
4. Evidence does not support the use of phonophoresis to treat pain and inflammation (Bellew et al., 2016, p. 128).

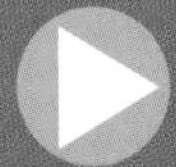

Mechanical Agents (See Appendix 11B for summary of Indications, Precautions, and Contraindications)

Mechanical Spinal Traction (Intermittent Traction)

Description

1. A distraction force applied to the spine to separate articular surfaces between vertebral bodies and elongate spinal structures. This force is applied to multiple spinal segments in the cervical and lumbar region. Many types of spinal traction are presently used, such as manual, positional, gravity-assisted, inversion, continuous, and static traction. This section will focus on mechanical traction.

Effects of Traction

1. Joint distraction: a separation of the facet joints occurs with sufficient force. This opens up the intervertebral foramen, relieves pressure on the nerve root, and decreases compressive forces on the facets. For the lumbar region, a force of 50% of the patient's body weight is required to cause separation. In the cervical region, 7% of the patient's body weight or about 20–30 lbs results in separation. In both instances, lower traction forces (lumbar: 30–40 lbs; cervical: 8–10 lbs) are recommended for initial treatment to decrease reactive muscle spasm and determine patient tolerance. In follow-up treatments, force can be gradually increased to achieve a maximal decrease in symptoms, but not to exceed 7% of body weight in the cervical region and 50% in the lumbar region.
2. Reduction of disc protrusion: separation of vertebral bodies occurs at higher forces, causing a decrease in intradiscal pressure that creates a suction-like effect on the nucleus, drawing it back in centrally. The surrounding ligamentous structures are stretched taut, which also helps to push the disc in centrally. For the lumbar region, 60–120 lbs or up to 50% of a patient's body weight, and for the cervical region, 12–15 lbs is recommended to achieve these desired effects.
3. Soft-tissue stretching: the surrounding spinal muscles, ligaments, tendons, and discs can be stretched, decreasing the pressure on the facet joints, nerve roots, vertebral bodies, and discs without achieving joint separation. Lower traction forces are sufficient to achieve this effect (lumbar region: 25% of body weight; cervical region: 12–15 lbs).
4. Muscle relaxation: both intermittent and static traction can decrease muscle tone. Traction can interrupt the pain-muscle spasm cycle by stimulating mechanoreceptors through the motion caused by interrupted traction and by inhibiting motor neuron firing with static traction. The forces recommended for soft-tissue stretching are also used for muscle relaxation.
5. Joint mobilization: at lower forces, intermittent traction stimulates the mechanoreceptors to inhibit pain and decrease spasm, while high force traction causes decreased pressure on the joints and stretches the surrounding soft tissue. Unlike manual joint mobilization, traction cannot be isolated to a particular segment and provides general mobilization in the cervical or lumbar region.

Goals and Indications

1. Decrease impairments associated with nerve root impingement.
2. Decrease chronic neck pain and improve cervical mobility.
3. Mechanical intermittent cervical traction has Grade B-Level II evidence for the treatment of chronic neck pain with mobility deficits and neck pain with radicular symptoms (see Box 2-15, Neck Pain Clinical Practice Guideline).
4. Summary evidence in systematic reviews concludes that mechanical lumbar traction has conflicting evidence (Grade D, Level IV) for the treatment of low back pain. Specifically, clinical practice guideline (see Box 2-16) suggests lumbar traction is not effective for treating acute or subacute nonspecific low back pain but may provide some benefits for some patients with signs of nerve root compression.

Precautions

1. Claustrophobia, hiatal hernia, vascular compromise, pregnancy, and impaired cognition. Any disease or condition that can compromise the structure of the spine, such as osteoporosis, tumor, infection, rheumatoid arthritis, or protracted steroid use; TMJ; problems with halter use; disc extrusion; medial disc protrusion; complete resolution of severe pain with traction.

> **RED FLAG:** Contraindications.
> Acute strains, sprains, and inflammation; spondylolisthesis, fractures, postop spinal surgery, spinal joint instability or hypermobility, and spinal cord compression; hypertension; increased peripheralization of pain, numbness or tingling, decreased myotomal strength, and decreased reflex response.

Procedure (Intermittent Traction)

1. Cervical traction.
   a. Can be seated or supine. Supine position is generally preferred.
   b. Cervical halter.
      - Head halter is placed under the occiput and the mandible.
      - Head halter is attached to the traction cord directly or to the traction unit through the spreader bar.
      - Slack is removed from the traction cord. The neck should be maintained in 20°–30° of flexion; a pillow may be used to achieve this angle.
      - Some target area specificity may be achieved by varying the neck angle approximately 0°–5° of cervical flexion to increase intervertebral space and joint separation at C1 through C5; up to 25°–30° for C5 through C7; neutral spine (approximately 20° of flexion) for disc dysfunction.
      - Traction force should be applied to the occipital region and not on the chin. If patient expresses discomfort in the temporomandibular joint area, treatment should stop and head halter should be readjusted to ensure that the force is properly applied.
   c. Cervical sliding device.
      - The head is placed on padded headrest, which positions the neck in 20°–30° of flexion.
      - Adjustable neck yoke is tightened to firmly grip just below the mastoid process.
      - Head strap is secured across the forehead.
      - Traction rope is then attached to the gliding platform of the device.
   d. Traction force is determined by treatment goals and patient tolerance.
      - Acute phase.
        - Disc protrusion, elongation of soft tissue, muscle spasm, 10–15 pounds or 7%–10% of body weight.
        - Joint distraction 20–30 pounds.
   e. Treatment time.
      - 5 to 10 minutes for acute conditions and disc protrusion, 15–30 minutes for other conditions.
   f. Duty cycle.
      - Static traction is recommended for disc protrusions or when symptoms are aggravated by motion.
      - Intermittent traction can also be used for disc protrusions and joint distraction, but a 3:1 hold/rest ratio is recommended. A 1:1 ratio is recommended when mobility is desired; i.e., joint mobilization.
2. Lumbar traction.
   a. A split table is usually used to minimize friction between the body and the table.
   b. Supine position, with pillow under the knee or small bench under lower leg, is recommended when the goal is to open up the intervertebral foramen, separate the facet joints, or elongate the muscles. The prone position may be preferable in the case of a posterior herniated lumbar disc. Some target area specificity may be achieved by varying the angle of pull (i.e., to increase intervertebral space at L5 to S1 up to 45°–60° of hip flexion, or at L3 to L4 up to 75°–90°).
   c. Apply the pelvic harness so that the top edge is above the iliac crest.
   d. Attach the thoracic harness so that the inferior margin is slightly below lower ribs.
   e. Secure the harness around the pelvis and attach it to the traction rope or spreader bar.
   f. Thoracic harness provides countertraction to the pull on the pelvis and is secured at the top of the table.
   g. Treatment force.
      - Acute phase, 30–40 pounds.
      - Disc protrusion, spasm; elongation of soft tissues, 25% of body weight.
      - Joint distraction, 50 pounds or 50% of body weight.
   h. Treatment time: 5–10 minutes for herniated disc, 10–30 minutes for other conditions.

Intermittent Mechanical Compression

Description

1. Pneumatic device that applies external pressure to an extremity through an inflatable appliance (sleeve).
2. Appliances are designed in a variety of sizes and lengths to fit either the upper or lower extremity (ankle, ankle and lower leg, or full extremity).
3. The device is attached to an inflatable pneumatic sleeve by rubber tubing.
4. The compression units and appliances are designed to inflate a single compartment to produce uniform, circumferential pressure on the extremity or multiple compartments by applying pressure in a sequential manner. Pressure is greater in the distal compartments and lesser in the proximal compartments.
5. Cold can be applied simultaneously with intermittent compression in which a coolant (50°F–77°F) is pumped through an inflatable sleeve.

Physiological Effects

1. External pressure on the extremity increases the pressure in the interstitial fluids, forcing the fluids to move into the lymphatic and venous return systems, thus reducing the fluid volume in the extremity. This reduction may stimulate increased circulation through lessening blood proximally in a limb, which results in increased peripheral blood flow (Marsico, 2016). In addition to mechanical compression, some conditions may require the daily use of compression stockings to counteract the effect of gravity on the vascular and lymph systems in the lower extremities.

Goals and Indications

1. Amputation, decrease edema, postmastectomy lymphedema, DVT prevention, stasis ulcer healing, venous insufficiency, subacute injuries such as ankle sprains with traumatic edema. Manual massage/drainage techniques have supplanted use of mechanical compression in many instances.

Precautions

1. Impaired sensation; malignancy; uncontrolled hypertension; recent skin graft; dermatologic infection.

> RED FLAG: Contraindications.
> Acute inflammation, trauma, or fracture; acute deep venous thrombosis (DVT) and thrombophlebitis; obstructed lymph or venous return; arterial disease/insufficiency; arterial revascularization; acute pulmonary edema; loss of protective sensation; cancer; edema with cardiac or renal impairment; impaired cognition; infection in treatment area; hypoproteinemia (<2 g/dL); very old or young patients.

Procedure

1. Check patient's blood pressure.
2. Set the inflation and deflation ratio to ~3:1. Generally, for edema reduction, 45–90 seconds on/15–30 seconds off. To shape residual limb, a 4:1 ratio is often used.
3. Turn the power on and slowly increase the pressure to the desired level.
   a. The patient's blood pressure determines the setting of the device. Some manufacturers recommend that the setting never exceed the patient's diastolic blood pressure. Others advise that the pressure can fall between the diastolic and systolic pressure because the pressure is on for only a short period of time.
   b. Numbness, tingling, pulse, or pain should not be felt by the patient during the treatment.
4. Treatment time.
   a. The duration may vary, depending on the patient's tolerance and condition.
      - Treatment time is usually an hour every day or BID. Some conditions may warrant shorter treatment times initially, while some will increase the times to 2 to 4 hours as tolerance and benefit progresses.

Continuous Passive Motion (CPM)

Description

1. Uninterrupted passive motion of the joint through a controlled ROM. A mechanical device provides continuous movement for extended periods of time.

Physiological Effects of CPM

1. Accelerate rate of interarticular cartilage regeneration, tendon and ligament healing.
2. Decrease edema and joint effusion.
3. Minimize contractures.
4. Decrease postoperative pain.
5. Increase synovial fluid lubrication of the joint.
6. Improve circulation.
7. Prevent adhesions.
8. Improve nutrition to articular cartilage and periarticular tissues.
9. Increase joint ROM.

Goals and Indications

1. Postimmobilization fracture, tendon or ligament repair.
2. *Don't use continuous passive motion machines for the postoperative management of patients following uncomplicated total knee replacement* (White N, et al., *Phys Ther.* 2015).

Precautions

1. Intracompartmental hematoma from anticoagulant use.

> RED FLAG: Contraindications.
> Increases in pain, edema, or inflammation following treatment.

Tilt Table

Description

1. Mechanical or electrical table designed to elevate patient from horizontal (0°) to vertical (90°) position in a controlled, incremental manner.

Physiological Effects of Tilt Table

1. Stimulate postural reflexes to counteract orthostatic hypotension.
2. Facilitate postural drainage.
3. Gradual loading of one or both lower extremities.
4. Begin active head or trunk control.
5. Provide positioning for stretch of hip flexors, knee flexors, and ankle plantar flexors.

Indications

1. Prolonged bed rest, immobilization, spinal cord injury, traumatic brain injury, orthostatic hypotension, spasticity.

Procedure

1. Patient is placed in supine position.
2. Abdominal binder, long elastic stockings, or tensor bandaging to counteract orthostatic hypotension (venous pooling) may be used.
3. Patient secured to table by straps.
4. Take baseline vitals (blood pressure, heart rate, respiratory rate).
5. Table raised gradually to given angle. Incremental rise to 30°, 45°, 60°, 80°, or 85°, or as tolerated. Position can be maintained for as long as 30–60 minutes.
6. Vital signs (blood pressure, heart rate, respiratory rate) need to be monitored to assess the patient's tolerance to treatment. Cyanotic lips or fingernail beds may indicate compromised circulation.
7. Treatment time.
   a. Initially, the duration of treatment depends on the patient's tolerance, but should not exceed 45 minutes, once or twice daily.

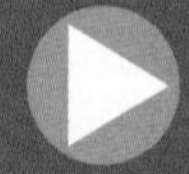

Electrical Agents (See Appendix 11C for summary of Common Applications and Parameters)

Basic Concepts of Nerve and Muscle Physiology

Properties of Electrically Excitable Cells (See Figure 11-1)

1. Resting membrane potential (RMP).
   a. The cell membrane is more permeable to potassium (K^+) compared to sodium (Na^+) and negatively charged proteins (anions).
   b. Electrical potential is generated across the cell membrane, due to the higher concentration of K^+ and anions on the inside of the cell relative to the concentration of Na^+ on the outside.
   c. A negative charge is produced within the cell, and a positive charge develops on the outside of the cell as the positively charged K^+ diffuses from the cell.
   d. RMP is –60 mV to –90 mV for excitable cells.
   e. RMP is maintained by an active sodium-potassium pump that takes in K^+ and extrudes Na^+.
2. Action potential (Figure 11-2).
   a. A stimulus (e.g., electrical) causes the cell membrane to become more permeable to Na^+ ions.
   b. An action potential (AP) is generated when the influx of Na^+ causes a reduction in RMP, which occurs slowly at first. Reduction in the RMP is called depolarization.
   c. When transmembrane potential reaches a critical threshold level (approximately –55 mV), the voltage-sensitive Na^+ and K^+ channels open widely. Permeability to Na^+ increases rapidly, whereas the permeability to K^+ increases slowly.
   d. During depolarization, transmembrane potential may rise as high as +35 mV. A positive charge is generated inside the cell, and a negative charge outside is produced, as a result of the flow of ions.
   e. The K^+ channels are fully open at about the time that the Na^+ are closed, and K^+ rushes rapidly out of the cell, making the transmembrane potential progressively more negative. This process is called repolarization.
   f. The K^+ channels remain open long enough to repolarize the membrane (10–20 mV < RMP). This is called hyperpolarization.
   g. The K^+ channels close and passive diffusion of the ions rapidly returns the RMP to its initial level.

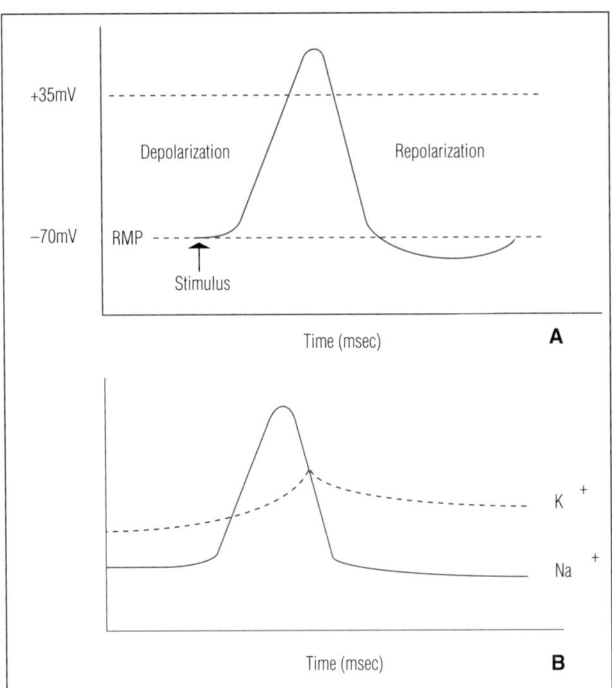

Figure 11-1 **A. Changes in transmembrane potential. B. Changes in membrane permeability of sodium and potassium during an action potential.**

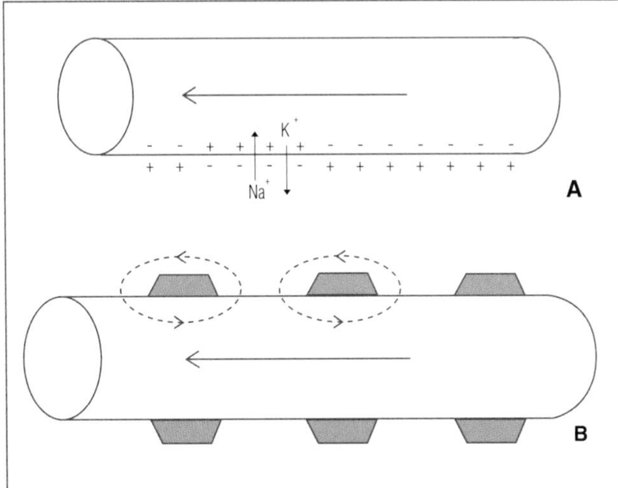

Figure 11-2 **Propagation of action potential in A. unmyelinated axon and B. myelinated axon.**

3. Propagation of the action potential. See Figure 11-2.
   a. Opening of the Na^+ and K^+ channels and voltage changes that produce an AP at one segment of the membrane triggers successive depolarization in adjacent regions of the nerve, muscle, or membranes.
   b. AP movement occurs along the surface of the nerve or muscle cell.
   c. Movement of the AP along an unmyelinated nerve is generated via sequential depolarization (eddy currents) along neighboring sites in the nerve membrane. Speed of conduction in small diameter fibers is slow due to the greater internal resistance in the small fibers.
   d. In myelinated nerve fibers, saltatory conduction occurs at discrete junctures (nodes of Ranvier) in the myelin sheath that surrounds the nerve.
   e. Na^+ and K^+ ion exchange and current flow is concentrated at these points. The impulse jumps from node to node, conducting nerve impulses at greater rates compared to smaller, unmyelinated nerve fibers.

Electrical Action of Muscle and Nerve

1. Characteristics of ES necessary to initiate excitable cell depolarization.
   a. Amplitude or intensity of the stimulus must be great enough to cause the membrane potential to be lowered sufficiently to reach threshold levels.
   b. Duration of the individual stimulus must be long enough to produce depolarization of the cell membrane. A duration of ≤1 ms is sufficient to stimulate nerve cell membrane but is too short to stimulate muscle cell membrane.
   c. Rate of rise of the current to peak intensity must be rapid enough to prevent accommodation, which is the rapid adjustment of the membrane to stimuli to prevent depolarization. Square wave delivers instantaneous rise.

Strength-Duration Curve (Figure 11-3)

1. Rheobase is the intensity of the current, with a long duration stimulus, required to produce a minimum muscle contraction.
2. Chronaxie is the pulse duration of the stimulus at twice the rheobase intensity. Chronaxie of a denervated muscle is >1 msec.
3. Very short pulse durations (<0.05 msec) with low intensities can depolarize sensory nerves. Longer

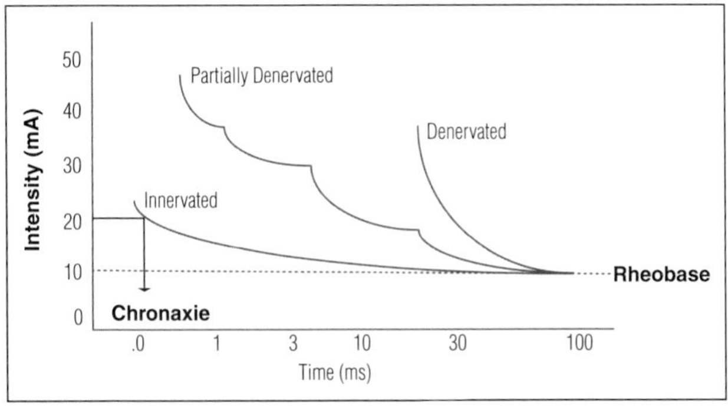

Figure 11-3 **Strength-duration curves for normally innervated, partially denervated, and completely denervated muscle.**

pulse durations (<1 msec) are required to stimulate motor nerves. Long pulse durations (>10 msec) with high intensities are needed to elicit a response from a denervated muscle.
4. Nerve conduction velocity and electromyography (EMG) have rendered strength-duration testing virtually obsolete.

Motor Point

1. An area of greatest excitability on the skin surface in which a small amount of current generates a muscle response.
2. In innervated muscle, the motor point is located at or near where the motor nerve enters the muscle, usually over the muscle belly.
3. In denervated muscle, the area of greatest excitability is located over the muscle distally toward the insertion.

Types of Muscle Contraction

1. A low-frequency pulse (1–10 pulses/sec) produces a brief muscle twitch or muscle contraction with each stimulus.
2. Increasing the number of stimuli (frequency) progressively fuses the individual muscle twitches to a point where individual twitches are not discernible. A tetanic contraction results.
3. An asynchronous or wormlike (vermicular) muscle response is noted in denervated muscle.

Basic Concepts of Electricity

1. Electrical current is the movement of electrons through a conducting medium.
2. Amperage is the rate of flow of electrons.
3. Voltage is the force that drives electrons through the conductive medium.
4. Resistance is the property of a medium that opposes the flow of electrons. A substance with a high resistance (e.g., rubber) is an insulator, and a substance with a low resistance (e.g., metal) is a conductor.
5. Ohm's law expresses the relationship between amperage, voltage, and resistance. The current is directly proportional to the voltage and inversely proportional to the resistance. The inverse of resistance is called conductance.

Electrical Stimulation (ES)

Characteristics

1. Wave forms (Figure 11-4).
   a. Monophasic: a unidirectional flow of charged particles. A current flow in one direction for a finite period of time is a phase (upward or downward deflection from and return to baseline). It has either a positive or negative charge.

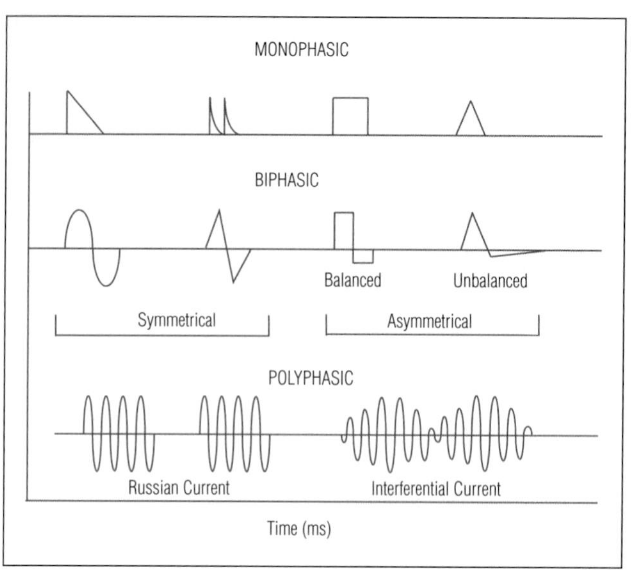

Figure 11-4 **Basic waveform characteristics.**

   b. Biphasic: a bidirectional flow of charged particles. This type of wave form is illustrated as one-half of the cycle above the baseline and the second phase below the baseline. One complete cycle (two phases) equals a single pulse. It has a zero net charge if symmetrical.
   c. Polyphasic wave: biphasic current modified to produce three or more phases in a single pulse. This waveform in medium frequency may be Russian or interferential current.

Current Modulation

1. Continuous mode: uninterrupted flow of current.
2. Interrupted mode: intermittent cessation of current flow for ≥1 second.
3. Surge mode: a gradual increase and decrease in the current intensity over a finite period of time.
4. Ramped mode: a time period with a gradual rise of the current intensity, which is maintained at a selected level for a given period of time, followed by a gradual or abrupt decline in intensity.

Goals and Indications

1. Pain modulation.
   a. Activation of gate mechanisms (gate theory).
   b. Initiation of descending inhibition mechanisms (endogenous opiate production).
2. Decrease muscle spasm.
   a. Muscle fatigue: tetanic contraction sustained for several minutes by means of continuous modulation.
   b. Muscle pump: interrupted or surge modulation producing rhythmic contraction and relaxation of the muscle to increase circulation.
   c. Pain modulation with or without muscle pumping and heat: combination of ES and US to increase

tissue temperature, produce pain modulation, and if desired, produce muscle pumping at the same time.

3. Impaired ROM (increase in or maintenance of joint mobility).
   a. Mechanical stretching of connective tissue and muscles associated with a joint. Used when muscle strength is deficient or neuromuscular dysfunction (e.g., spasticity) prevents adequate joint movement.
   b. Decrease pain to encourage joint motion.
   c. Decrease in edema if significant impediment to motion.
4. Muscle reeducation (training muscles to respond appropriately to volitional effort).
   a. Acts as an active assistive exercise.
   b. Provides proprioceptive feedback.
   c. Assists in coordinated muscle movement.
5. Disuse atrophy (muscle weakness).
   a. Used as an adjunct to volitional movement.
6. Soft-tissue repair (wound healing).
   a. Pulsed currents (monophasic, biphasic, polyphasic) with interrupted modulations. Improved circulation via the muscle pump to improve tissue nutrition and hasten metabolic waste disposal.
   b. Monophasic currents (continuous or pulsed monophasic currents).
      - Electrical potential theory. Restoration of electrical charges in wound area.
      - Bactericidal effect. Disruption of DNA, RNA synthesis, or cell transport system of microorganisms.
      - Biochemical effects. Increased adenosine triphosphate (ATP) concentration, amino acid uptake, and increased protein and DNA synthesis.
      - Cellular migration due to electrical stimulation (galvanotaxis) is influenced by more than polarity.
        - There are conflicting polarity recommendations in textbooks. In 2017, a meta-analysis conducted by Khouri et al. suggested the strength of evidence for the use of a high-volt monophasic pulsed current is strong and that switching polarities periodically is beneficial for wound healing.
   c. Both continuous and pulsed waveforms can be applied for wound healing. High-voltage pulsed monophasic current has the greatest preponderance of evidence supporting it for facilitating tissue healing.
7. Edema reduction.
   a. Muscle pump to increase lymph and venous flow.
   b. Typically a pulsed monophasic or biphasic waveform is used and set up to achieve tetany (>25–30 pps) using rhythmical muscle contractions.
8. Spasticity (ES to reduce hypertonicity).
   a. Fatigue of the agonist.
   b. Reciprocal inhibition (stimulate antagonist/inhibit agonist).
9. Denervated muscle.
   a. Controversy exists relative to the use of ES for denervated muscle. Any improvements do not persist once the stimulation ends.

Precautions

1. Precautions.
   a. Cardiac disease.
   b. Impaired mentation.
   c. In areas of impaired sensation, malignant tumors, skin irritation, or open wounds.
   d. Applying iontophoresis in the area after the application of another physical agent.
   e. In patients with hypotension or hypertension, excessive adipose tissue or edema.
   f. Bleeding disorders.
   g. Menstruating uterus.
   h. Pregnancy: during labor and delivery.

RED FLAGS: Contraindications.
- Anywhere in the body for patients with demand-type pacemakers or other electronic devices such as insulin pumps.
- Unstable arrhythmias.
- Suspected epilepsy or seizure disorder.
- Over the carotid sinus, eyes, phrenic nerve, urinary bladder stimulator, pharyngeal or laryngeal muscles, abdomen or low back during pregnancy.
- Transcerebral or transthoracic.
- Areas of uncontrolled bleeding or infection.
- Superficial metal implants.
- Areas that prohibit motion.
- Thrombosis or thrombophlebitis.

2. Procedural cautions.
   a. Do not use any electrical modality if there is evidence of broken or frayed wires or if the unit is not connected to a ground fault circuit interrupter (see Hydrotherapy section).
   b. Electrodes that are too small, have uneven contact, or are self-adhesive and no longer stick or conduct well can cause skin irritation or burns.
   c. ES should not be used while playing sports, driving, operating heavy machinery, near a diathermy device, or in conjunction with other electronic monitoring equipment.

General Guidelines for ES Procedures

1. Electrode selection.
   a. Electrode size.
      - Two electrodes (leads) are required to complete the current circuit.

- Current density (the amount of current that is dispersed under the electrode) is relative to the electrode size. A given current intensity passing through the smaller active electrode produces high current density and thus a strong stimulus, while the same current is perceived as less intense under a larger electrode because of the lesser current density.
- Electrode size should be relative to the size of the treatment site. Large electrodes in a small treatment area (i.e., forearm) could result in current overflowing to surrounding muscles and produce undesired effects.
- Conversely, small electrodes applied to a large muscle (i.e., quadriceps) could result in high current density under the electrodes that make ES uncomfortable to the patient.

b. The electrodes are placed to ensure the current path is through the desired area.

c. The space between the electrodes should be at least the diameter of the electrodes being used. The distance between the electrodes should be as great as is needed. If the electrodes are too far apart, undesired structures (i.e., other motor points) could be recruited. If that occurs, move the electrodes closer together to be more specific.

d. Inspect the patient's skin. Vigilant skin inspection and skin care are very important with long-term use of ES. This is especially important during home use of transcutaneous ES and other ES modalities. Long-term repetitive stimulation and electrode placement and removal can irritate the skin and initiate skin breakdown.

2. Muscle strengthening, muscle spasm or edema (muscle pump), ROM.
   a. Set the pulse rate to tetany (smooth muscle contraction >25–30 pps). Slowly increase intensity until a muscular response is observed.
   b. 10–25 muscle contractions may be sufficient to obtain treatment goal.
   c. Duty cycle.
      - Interrupted/ramped modulation of current allows the muscle to recover between stimulation periods.
      - On/off ratios of ≥1:3 are recommended to minimize the fatigue effects of ES.
3. Muscle spasm (fatigue).
   a. Procedure as above for innervated muscle. Current applied in continuous mode or 1:1 on/off ratio.
4. Muscle reeducation.
   a. Parameters and procedure similar to muscle strengthening techniques.
   b. Stimulation for multiple sets of singular or multiple muscle repetitions.
   c. Treatment sessions of 10–30 minutes depending on patient's mental and physical tolerance.

Iontophoresis

Description

1. The application of a continuous direct current to transport medicinal agents through the skin or mucous membranes for therapeutic purposes.

Physics

1. Like charges repel like charges.
2. Unlike charges attract unlike charges.

Electrochemical Effects Related to Iontophoresis

1. Dissolved acids, bases, salts, or alkaloids in an aqueous solution dissociate into positively or negatively charged substances (ions) when electrical current flows through a substance.
2. Polar effects.
   a. Positive ions move toward the negative pole (cathode), where a secondary alkaline reaction ($NaOH$) occurs. Current density for the anode should not exceed 1.0 mA/cm^2
   b. Negative ions move toward the positive pole (anode), where an acid is produced (HCl). Current density for the cathode should not exceed 0.5 mA/cm^2.

Ion Transfer

1. The number of ions transferred through the skin is directly related to the:
   a. Duration of treatment.
   b. Current density.
   c. Concentration of ions in the solution.

ES Characteristics of Iontophoresis

1. Direct current.
2. Maximum intensity of 4–5 mA.

Indications and Ions Commonly Used (See Table 11-7)

> **RED FLAGS:** Contraindications.
> Refer to general rules for ES.
> Impaired skin sensation.
> Allergy or sensitivity to medicinal agent or direct current.
> Denuded area or recent scars.
> Cuts, bruises, or broken skin.
> Metal in or near treatment area.

Table 11-7

Indications for the Use of Iontophoresis and Ions Commonly Used

INDICATIONS	ION	POLARITY	SOURCE
Analgesia	Lidocaine, Xylocaine Salicylate	Positive Negative	Lidocaine, Xylocaine Sodium salicylate
Calcium deposits	Acetate	Negative	Acetic acid
Dermal ulcers	Zinc	Positive	Zinc oxide
Edema reduction	Hyaluronidase	Positive	Wydase
Fungal infections	Copper	Positive	Copper sulfate
Hyperhidrosis	Water	Positive/Negative	Tap water
Muscle spasm	Calcium Magnesium	Positive Positive	Calcium chloride Magnesium sulfate
Musculoskeletal inflammatory conditions	Dexamethasone Hydrocortisone	Negative Positive	Dexamethasone phosphate Hydrocortisone sodium succinate

Transcutaneous Electrical Nerve Stimulation (TENS)

Description

1. TENS is designed to provide afferent stimulation for pain management.

Physiological Effects

1. Pain modulation through activation of central inhibition of pain transmission (gate theory).
   a. Large diameter A-beta fibers (Figure 11-5) rapidly temporally summate and activate inhibitory interneurons located in the dorsal horn of the spinal cord (substantia gelatinosa- laminae II), thus inhibiting smaller A-delta and C-fibers (pain fibers).
   b. Presynaptic inhibition of the T-cells closes the "gate" and modulates pain. The gating mechanism also includes release of enkephalins, which combine with opiate receptors to depress release of substance P from the A-delta and C-fibers.
2. Pain modulation through descending pathways generating endogenous opiates (Figure 11-6).
   a. Noxious stimuli generate endorphin production from the pituitary gland and other central nervous system (CNS) areas.
   b. Endogenous opiate-rich nuclei, periaqueductal gray matter (PAG) in the midbrain and thalamus are also activated by strong stimuli.
   c. Neurotransmitters from the PAG facilitate the cells of the nucleus raphe magnus (NRM) and reticularis gigantocellularis (RGC).
   d. Efferents from these nuclei travel through the dorsal lateral funiculus, terminating on the enkephalinergic interneurons in the spinal cord and presynaptically inhibit the release of substance P from the A-delta and C-fibers.

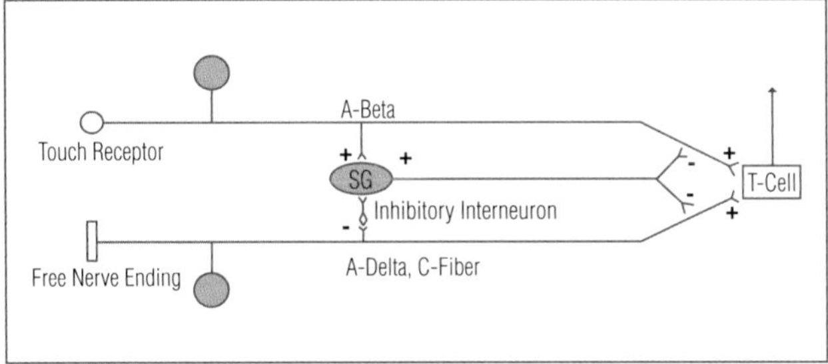

Figure 11-5 Schematic of gate control theory. (Adapted from Melzack and Wall.)

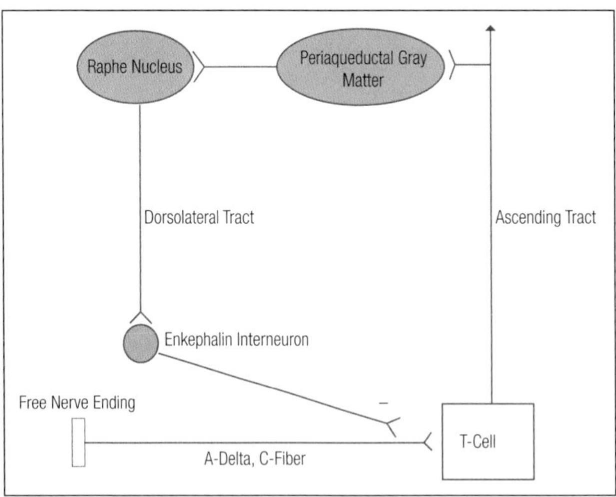

Figure 11-6 Schematic of descending inhibition mechanisms.

ES Characteristics

1. Wave form: pulsed waveforms (biphasic, monophasic, or polyphasic) have been used.
2. Current: continuous pulsatile or burst.

Procedures

1. Conventional (high rate) TENS: this most common mode of TENS can be applied during the acute or chronic phase of pain. Modulation of pain via inhibition of pain fibers by large-diameter fiber activation (gate mechanism). Onset of pain relief is relatively fast and duration of relief is relatively short.
   a. Amplitude: comfortable tingling sensation, paresthesia. No muscle response.
   b. Pulse rate: 80–110 pps.
   c. Pulse duration: 50–100 msec.
   d. Mode: continuous.
   e. Duration of treatment: 20–60 minutes.
   f. Duration of pain relief: temporary.
2. Acupuncture-like (strong low rate) TENS can be applied during the chronic phase of pain. Analgesia produced through stimulation-evoked production of endogenous opiates. Onset of pain relief may be as long as 20–40 minutes. Duration of relief may be long-lasting (≥1 hour).
   a. Amplitude: strong, but comfortable rhythmic muscle twitches.
   b. Pulse rate: 1–5 pps.
   c. Pulse duration: 150–300 msec.
   d. Mode: continuous.
   e. Duration of treatment: 30–40 minutes.
   f. Duration of pain relief: long-lasting.
3. Brief intense TENS: this mode is used to provide rapid-onset, short-term pain relief during painful procedures (wound debridement, deep friction massage, joint mobilization, or passive stretching).
   a. Amplitude: to patient's tolerance.
   b. Pulse rate: 80–150 pps.
   c. Pulse duration: 50–250 msec.
   d. Mode: continuous.
   e. Duration of treatment: 15 minutes.
   f. Duration of pain relief: temporary (30–60 minutes).
4. Burst-mode (pulse trains) TENS: combines characteristics of both high- and low-rate TENS. Stimulation of endogenous opiates, but current is more tolerable to patient than low-rate TENS. Onset of analgesia similar to low-rate TENS.
   a. Amplitude: comfortable, intermittent paresthesia.
   b. Pulse rate: 50–100 pps delivered in packets or bursts of 1–4 pps.
   c. Pulse duration: 50–200 msec.
   d. Mode: continuous.
   e. Duration of treatment: 20–30 minutes.
   f. Duration of pain relief: long-lasting (hours).
5. Hyperstimulation (point stimulation) TENS: use of a small probe to locate and noxiously stimulate acupuncture or trigger points. Multiple sites may be stimulated per treatment. Onset of pain relief is similar to acupuncture-like TENS.
   a. Amplitude: strong, to patient's tolerance.
   b. Pulse rate: 1–5 pps.
   c. Pulse duration: 150–300 msec.
   d. Duration of treatment: 15- to 30-second increments.
   e. Duration of pain relief: long-lasting.
6. Modulation mode TENS: a method of modulating the parameters of the above TENS modes to prevent neural or perceptual habituation due to constant ES. Frequencies, intensities, or pulse durations can be altered.

Electrode Placement

1. Electrode placement should have some basis in neuroanatomy and can include any of the following (or some combination of them): site of pain, peripheral nerves supplying the painful area, spinal nerve roots comprising the peripheral nerves, the segments of the spinal cord giving rise to the spinal nerve roots, related dermatomes, myotomes and sclerotomes, trigger points, motor points, nerve points or acupuncture points, or any of the aforementioned structures on the contralateral side if the area cannot be directly stimulated.

Goals and Indications

1. Acute and chronic pain modulation.

> **RED FLAGS:** Contraindications.
> Patient with demand-type pacemaker or over chest of patient with cardiac disease.
> TENS is not applied where the current path would pass through a developing fetus, over the eyes, laryngeal or pharyngeal muscles, head, carotid sinus, and neck of patient following cerebral vascular accident, or with epilepsy.

High-Voltage Pulsed Galvanic Stimulation

Description

1. High-voltage pulsed current (HVPC): typically, monophasic, twin-peaked pulses of short duration.

Physics

1. Skin offers high resistance (impedance) to the flow of low-voltage direct current.
2. Impedance is lower with HVPC than a continuous direct current. Thermal and electrochemical effects are negligible with HVPC.

ES Characteristics of HVPC

1. Wave form: paired monophasic, with an almost instantaneous rise and exponential fall of current.
2. Current: continuous, surged, or interrupted pulsatile current.

Procedure

1. Muscle stimulation protocol: refer to general application procedure.
2. Wound healing concept.
   a. Intact skin surface negative with respect to deeper epidermal layers.
   b. Injury to skin develops positive potentials initially and negative potentials during healing process.
   c. Absent or insufficient positive potentials retard tissue regeneration.
   d. Addition of positive potentials, initially through anode, may promote or accelerate healing.
3. Wound healing parameters.
   a. Amplitude: comfortable tingling sensation, paresthesia, no muscle response.
   b. Pulse rate: 50–200 pps.
   c. Pulse duration: 20–100 msec.
   d. Mode: continuous.
   e. Duration of treatment: 20–60 min.
4. Wound healing procedures.
   a. Inspect wound area.
   b. Position patient and support treatment area.
   c. Clean and débride wound site. Pack with sterile saline-soaked gauze.
   d. Both high-volt pulsed current and low-intensity continuous low-volt direct current can be used for wound healing. Although current characteristics differ, treatment parameters are similar in current intensity and treatment duration.
   e. Place active electrode over gauze.
   f. For bactericidal effect, wound electrode should be the cathode. Other microorganisms (e.g., fungi, virus) may respond better to the anode.

Goals and Indications

1. Inflammation phase: free from necrosis and exudates. Promote granulation.
2. Proliferation phase: reduce wound size, through the promotion of capillary growth and fibroblastic activity.
3. Epithelialization phase: stimulate epidermal proliferation.

Contraindications

1. See general contraindications for ES.

Concept of Medium Frequency Currents in ES

Description

1. ES frequencies in the range of 2000–5000 pps that are modulated to produce physiologically applied frequencies. This concept is utilized in the Russian (time-modulated) and the interferential (amplitude-modulated) ES techniques.

Physics Related to Medium Frequency

1. A decrease in the capacitive skin impedance of the skin is noted relative to the increase in current frequency (Figure 11-7).
2. ES frequency categories:
   a. Low frequency: 1–1000 pps.
   b. Medium frequency: 1000–10,000 pps.
   c. High frequency: >10,000 pps.

Russian Current

Description

1. A 2500-Hz sine wave (carrier frequency), which is interrupted for 10 milliseconds at 10-millisecond intervals, producing fifty 10-millisecond bursts per second. This type of time interval interruption produces time-modulated current (Figure 11-8). Also known as medium frequency, burst-alternating current.

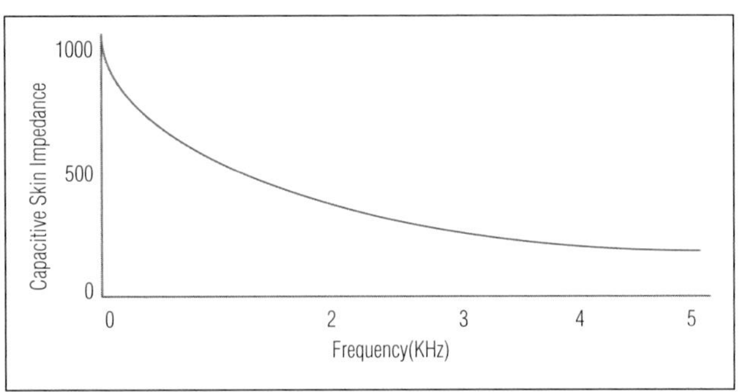

Figure 11-7 Capacitive skin resistance decreases as current frequency increases.

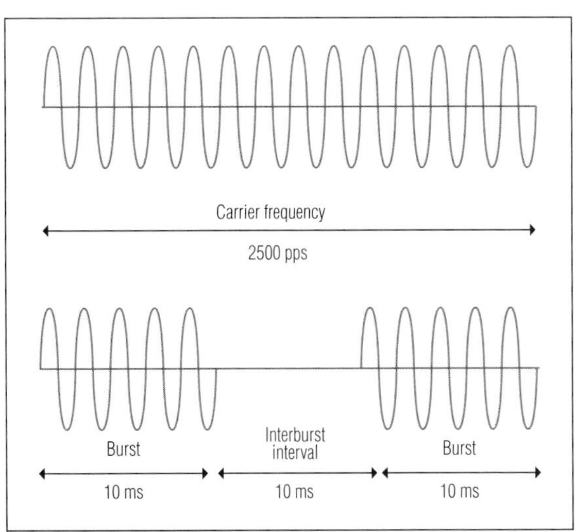

Figure 11-8 Russian current. Time-modulated polyphasic waveform.

ES Characteristics of Russian Current

1. Wave form: polyphasic sinusoidal burst.
2. Current: time modulated to create a pulsatile burst current.

Method of Application: Muscle-Strengthening Protocol

1. Amplitude: tetanic muscle contraction.
2. Pulse rate: 50–70 pps.
3. Pulse duration: 150–200 msec or 50% duty cycle.
4. Mode: interrupted.
   a. Ramp: 1–5 seconds, based on patient's tolerance.
   b. Duty cycle: 1:5.
5. Current applied to provide stimulation during the following volitional activities:
   a. Isometric exercise at several points through ROM.
   b. Slow isokinetic exercise; e.g., 5°–10°/sec.
   c. Short arc joint movement when ROM is restricted.

Muscle Spasm Protocol

1. Muscle fatigue using continuous isometric contraction for several minutes to tolerance.
2. If muscle pumping is goal, duty cycle is 1:1.
3. If ROM is goal, duty cycle is 2:5.

Contraindications

1. See general contraindications for ES.

Interferential Current (IFC)

Description

1. This current is characterized by the crossing of two sinusoidal waves with similar amplitudes, but different carrier frequencies that interfere with one another to generate an amplitude-modulated beat frequency. The consequent beat frequency is the net difference between the two superimposed frequencies.

Physics Related to IFC

1. Constructive interference: when the two waves are in phase, the sum of the superimposed wave is large (Figure 11-9A).
2. Destructive interference: the sum of the two waves is zero when the waves are 180° out of phase (Figure 11-9B).
3. Beat frequency (amplitude-modulated): resultant frequency produced by the two frequencies going into and out of phase (Figure 11-9C).
   a. Constant. Both carrier frequencies are fixed. Beat frequency is net difference between both frequencies.
   b. Variable. One carrier frequency is fixed and the other varies in frequency, generating a variable or sweep frequency. Sweep used to minimize accommodation.
4. IFC produces a cloverleaf-like pattern, since the electrical stimulating effect is at a 45° angle to the flow of current in the two circuits as interference occurs at the targeted area of the body (Figure 11-10).
   a. Static interferential fields are generated when four electrodes (two circuits) are used and the cloverleaf pattern is produced.
   b. Dynamic (scan) interferential fields occur when the interferential fields are rotated 45°, caused by the vectoring effect of rhythmically unbalancing the IFC to change the position of the stimulation areas. This effect is purported to provide a greater area of stimulation in comparison with static interferential fields.
   c. Full-field scanning produces a similar effect as dynamic interferential fields by bursting the current over the two circuits.
5. Premodulated IFC occurs when two carrier frequencies are crossed in the ES unit. The interference occurs in the unit, and the current can then be delivered through one circuit. This is ideal for small areas that would be amply covered with two electrodes.

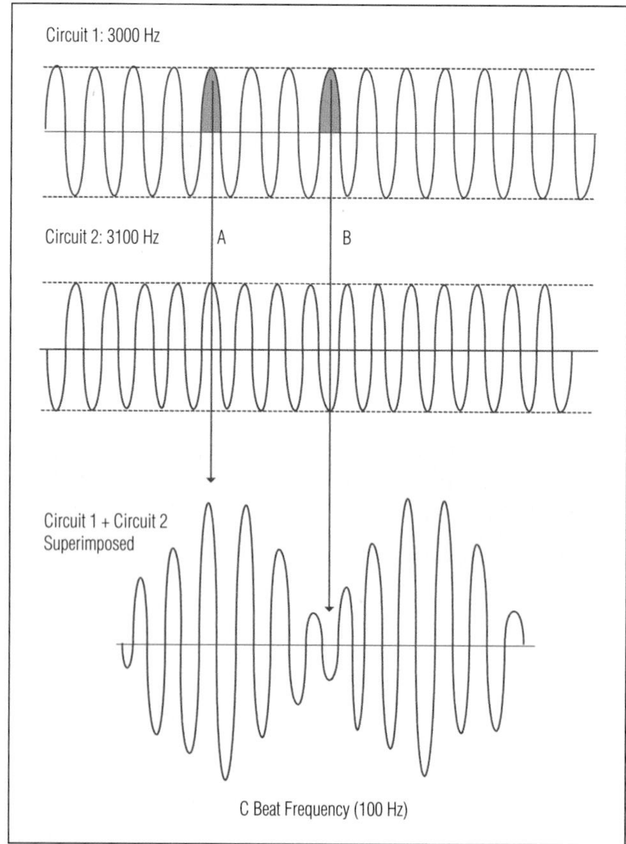

Figure 11-9 **Interferential current. Amplitude modulated polyphasic waveform.**

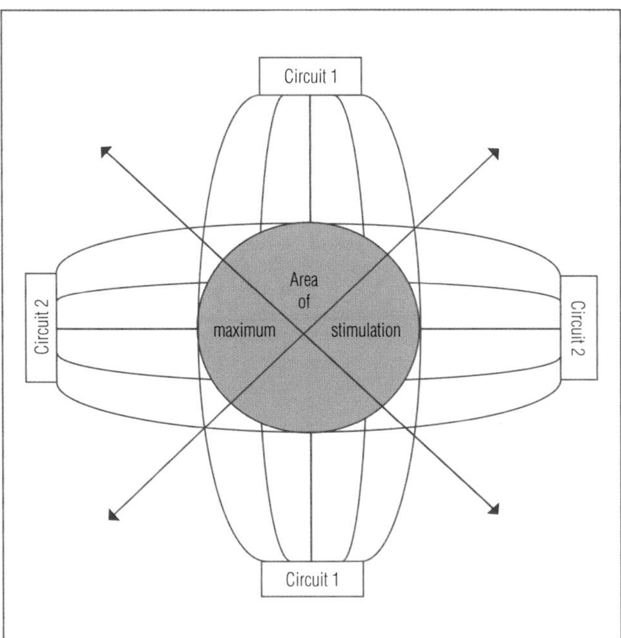

Figure 11-10 Static interference field depicting the area of maximum stimulation (circle) and the direction of maximal stimulation (arrows).

ES Characteristics

1. Wave form: polyphasic, sinusoidal (amplitude-modulated) beats.
2. Current: amplitude-modulated continuous (pain); interrupted (muscle exercise).

Procedure

1. Electrode placement (pad or suction cup electrodes).
   a. Bipolar (premodulated IFC). Two electrodes are placed to affect desired structures.
   b. Quadripolar. Two sets of electrodes placed diagonally to one another over large area (see Figure 11-10).
2. Treatment parameters.
   a. Pain protocol.
      - Similar to high- or low-rate TENS.
   b. Muscle-strengthening protocol.
      - Similar to NMES.

Goals and Indications

1. Modulate pain: increase muscle strength or ROM.

Contraindications

1. See general contraindications for ES.

Functional ES (FES)

Description

1. FES encompasses a wide range of stimulator units and techniques for disuse atrophy, impaired ROM, muscle spasm, muscle reeducation, and spasticity management.

FES is also called neuromuscular electrical stimulation (NMES) and functional neuromuscular electrical stimulation. This section will describe FES as an alternative or supplement to the use of orthotic devices.

Shoulder Subluxation

1. Patients with cerebrovascular accident (CVA) may initially exhibit weakness or flaccid paralysis of the muscles supporting the glenohumeral joint, especially the supraspinatus and posterior deltoid.
2. The force of gravity acting on the unsupported upper extremity tends to stretch the ligamentous structures surrounding the glenohumeral joint, resulting in severe pain and decreased upper extremity function.
3. ES characteristics of FES.
   a. Wave form: pulsed monophasic or biphasic waveform.
4. Procedure.
   a. Electrode placement: bipolar. Electrodes on supraspinatus and posterior deltoid.
   b. Treatment parameters.
      - Amplitude: tetanic muscle contraction to patient's tolerance.
      - Pulse rate: 25–30 pps.
      - Duration of treatment: 15–30 minutes. Three times daily, up to 6–7 hours. On/off ratio: 1:3 (2 sec: 6 sec) progressing to 12:1 (24 sec: 2 sec).

Dorsiflexion Assist in Gait Training

1. Patients with hemiplegia sometimes exhibit paralyzed dorsiflexor and evertor muscles.
2. FES controls foot drop and facilitates dorsiflexors and evertors during swing phase.
3. ES characteristics.
   a. Wave form: pulsed monophasic or biphasic waveform.
   b. Pulse duration: 20–250 μsec.
   c. Mode: interrupted by foot switch.
4. Procedure.
   a. Electrode placement: bipolar. Peroneal (fibular) nerve near head of fibula or anterior tibialis muscle.
   b. Treatment parameters.
      - Amplitude: tetanic muscle contraction sufficient to decrease plantar flexion.
      - Pulse rate: 25–30 pps. Higher rates can be used but have the potential to cause greater fatigue.
      - Treatment mode: heel switch contains pressure-sensitive contact that stops stimulation during stance phase and activates stimulation during swing phase. Hand switch also allows therapist to control stimulation during gait.

Other Gait-Assisted Protocol Considerations

1. Placement of electrodes on appropriate muscles to control muscles during push-off (plantar flexors), late

swing phase (hamstrings), quadriceps, and/or gluteals (stance phase).
2. ES characteristics: similar to dorsiflexion protocol.
3. Method of application: similar to dorsiflexion protocol, except for electrode placement.

Electromyographic (EMG) Biofeedback

Description

1. Electronic instrument used to measure motor unit action potentials (MUAP) generated by active muscles. The signals are detected, amplified, and converted into audiovisual signals that are used to reinforce voluntary control.

Principles of EMG Biofeedback

1. Motor unit: the functional unit of the neuromuscular system that consists of the anterior horn cell, its axon, the neuromuscular junction, and all the muscle fibers innervated by the axon. Motor unit potentials (MUP) are measured in microvolts (μV). The signals generated by the MUP, which contain both positive and negative phases, are also called compound action potentials (CAP) because the sensors pick up signals from multiple motor units.
2. The signal is processed through amplification, rectification (positive and negative components of the signal are made unidirectional), and integration (area under curve is computed). The integrated signal provides readings in microvolt-seconds and is displayed as the EMG biofeedback signal.
3. The EMG biofeedback signals, in conjunction with the patient's voluntary effort, are used to either increase or decrease muscle activity to achieve a functional goal.

Recording Electrodes

1. Surface electrodes.
   a. Global detection: signals from more than one muscle.
   b. Detection from mostly superficial muscles.
   c. Advantages: easy to apply, acceptable to patient/client.
   d. Disadvantages: detection from mostly superficial muscles, frequently from more than one muscle group.
2. Types of surface electrodes/sensors.
   a. Metal electrodes (silver/silver chloride): cup-shaped to accommodate conducting gel.
   b. Disposable electrodes: pregelled center with surrounding adhesive backing.
   c. Carbonized rubber electrodes (reusable): flexible to conform to body part.
3. Needle electrodes/sensors.
   a. Local detection: signals from specific muscle or muscle group.
   b. Used primarily for EMG diagnosis or research. Rarely used for EMG biofeedback.

Electrode Application

1. Electrode selection: select small electrodes (0.02 cm) for specific muscles (hand, forearm, face); large electrodes (1 cm) for large muscles or muscle groups.
2. Electrode placement.
   a. Bipolar technique: two active (positive and negative) and one reference (ground) electrode. The reference electrode may be placed between or adjacent to active electrodes. This minimizes or eliminates extraneous electrical activity (noise or cross-talk).
   b. Active electrodes are placed on or near motor point of targeted muscle or muscle group.
   c. Generally, active electrodes are placed 1–5 cm apart and parallel to muscle fibers. Reference electrode is placed near treatment site.
   d. Active electrodes are placed close together; minimizes cross-talk, yields small, more precise signals.
   e. Active electrodes are placed farther apart; yields large signals, detection from more than one muscle.

Procedure

1. Protocol for increasing muscle activity (motor recruitment or a shaping-up program).
   a. For weak muscles, begin with electrodes widely spaced and biofeedback instrument sensitivity high, to increase detection.
      • For a single weak muscle, begin with electrodes close together if a more precise signal is desired.
   b. Instruct patient to try and contract muscle (isometrically for 6–10 sec) to produce an audiovisual signal.
   c. As patient's motor recruitment ability improves, decrease the sensitivity, making it more difficult to produce an audiovisual signal.
   d. Use facilitation techniques (tapping, cross-facilitation, vibration) to encourage motor unit recruitment, if necessary.
   e. Progress from simple to more complex/functional movements as patient gains motor control.
   f. Treatment sessions may be from 5–10 minutes to ≥30 minutes, depending on patient tolerance.
2. Protocol for decreasing muscle activity (muscle relaxation or a shaping-down program).
   a. Begin with electrodes closely spaced and biofeedback instrument sensitivity low to minimize cross-talk.
   b. Instruct patient to relax, using deep breathing or visual imagery to help lower the audiovisual signal.

c. Progress from low to high sensitivity as patient gains ability to relax muscle and perform functional activities.
d. Treatment sessions may be from 5–10 minutes to ≥30 minutes, depending on patient tolerance.
e. At end of session, clean patient's skin and electrodes.

Criteria for Patient Selection for Biofeedback Training

1. Good vision, hearing, and communication abilities.
2. Good comprehension of simple commands, concentration.
3. Good motor planning skills.
4. No profound sensory or proprioceptive loss.

Acknowledgment to John Carlos, Jr, PT, PhD, and Elizabeth Oakley, PT, DHSc, MSPT, for their original contributions in formulating this chapter.

APPENDIX 11A

Thermotherapy Indications, Precautions, and Contraindications

Table 11A-1

MODALITY	INDICATIONS	PRECAUTIONS	CONTRAINDICATIONS
Cryotherapy	• Inflammation or pain • Acute edema • Muscle guarding or temporary spasticity reduction • Muscle facilitation	• Superficial nerves or open wounds • Uncontrolled hypertension • Altered sensation or mentation • Vulnerable patient populations (e.g., people with dementia, infants)	• Cold hypersensitivity or intolerance • Compromised circulation • Cryoglobulinemia • Paroxysmal cold hemoglobinuria • Raynaud's disease • Regenerating nerves
Thermotherapy	• Pain or muscle spasm • Increase soft tissue extensibility • Decrease joint stiffness • Increase circulation or metabolism	• Acute injury • Impaired circulation • Vulnerable populations (e.g., people unable to communicate) • Edema • Implants (metal conducts heat readily) • Open wounds • Over topical agents	• At risk for hemorrhaging • Deep vein thrombosis • Impaired sensation or mentation • Irradiation to eyes or reproductive organs • Pregnancy – avoid full-body heating or any heating that could potentially affect the fetus • Thrombophlebitis • Over malignant tumors
Hydrotherapy	• Superficial heating or cooling • Water exercise • Pain or edema control • Wound care (removal of necrotic tissue only)	• Local immersion: decreased temperature sensation, impaired cognition, recent skin graft • Full-body immersion (hot water): same as local immersion plus poor thermoregulation, cardiovascular medications, urinary incontinence, aquaphobia, and respiratory issues	• Local immersion: maceration, bleeding • Full-body immersion: unstable cardiac disorder, bowel incontinence, severe epilepsy, suicidal, potential for cross-contamination. Avoid full-body heating with pregnancy
Ultrasound	• Decrease pain or muscle spasm • Increase connective tissue extensibility • Reduce inflammation • Accelerate rate of tissue healing (wound healing)	• Acute inflammation (avoid continuous US) • Breast implants • Over healing fractures (high-dosage is avoided) • Directly over joint cement or plastic components (some texts list joint cement and components as contraindications)	• Impaired circulation, cognition, or sensation • High doses of thermal US should be avoided over open epiphyseal plates (nonthermal low-intensity US apply with caution) • Over malignant tumors, thrombophlebitis, or myositis ossificans • Recently irradiated tissue • Over or near cardiac pacemakers • Over the abdomen, low back, uterus, or pelvis during pregnancy • Recently irradiated tissue

Reference

1. Cameron, M. (2017). *Physical Agents in Rehabilitation: An Evidence-Based Approach to Practice.* (5th ed.). St. Louis, MO: Elsevier.

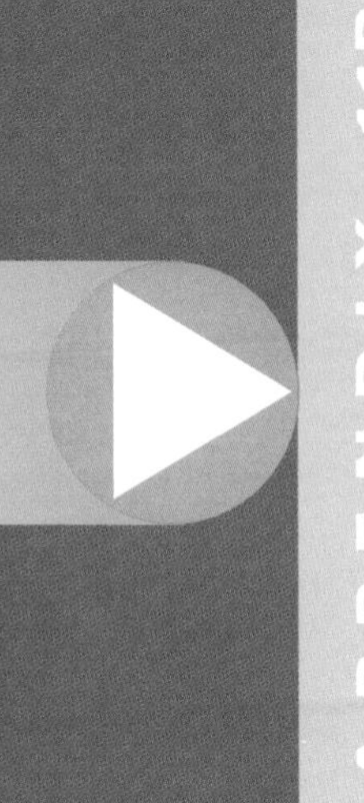

APPENDIX 11B

Mechanical Modality Indications, Precautions, and Contraindications

Table 11B-1

MODALITY	INDICATIONS	PRECAUTIONS	CONTRAINDICATIONS
Traction	• Cervical radiculopathy • Lumbar radiculopathy with radiating pain or paresthesia that does not have a directional preference (extension/ flexion) • Chronic neck pain with mobility deficits	• Significant structural disease of the spine • Pressure from belts is hazardous (pregnancy) • Disc extrusion or sequestration • Medial disc protrusion • Pain completely abolishes after treatment (check myotome, dermatome, and reflexes) • Patient is unable to tolerate prone or supine position • Claustrophobia • Altered mentation • Cervical sling traction with TMJ symptoms	• When motion is contraindicated (e.g., postop spinal surgery) • High-force tractions is avoided with joint hypermobility or instability (RA, Marfan's, high relaxin levels during pregnancy, Down syndrome) • Concerns of C1-2 stability fracture (must clear the C-spine) • Peripheralization with traction • Uncontrolled HTN (for inverse traction) • Neurologic findings worsen (check strength, sensation, and reflexes)
Compression	• Edema • DVT prevention • Venous stasis ulcers • Residual limb shaping • Hypertrophic scar management	• Neuropathy (monitor for ischemia) • Impaired mentation • Uncontrolled HTN • Potential compromise of superficial nerve • ABI between 0.5–0.8; pressures should not exceed 27 mmHg for static devices and intermittent compression devices should be avoided	• Underlying cause is unknown • Active infection or malignancy • Mechanical intermittent compressions is avoided with active DVT, PE thrombophlebitis, edema from cardiopulmonary pathology, or severe PAD • ABI less than 0.6 avoid static compression • Significant hypoproteinemia (<2 mg/ml) • Situations where limb movement is avoided
Continuous Passive Motion	• Restoration or maintenance of motion	• Significant bleeding or edema • Impaired mentation or sensation • Protection of neurovascular structures or newly repaired tissues	• Motion is contraindicated (e.g., unstable fracture) • Infection • Altered mentation

DVT = Deep Vein Thrombosis, ABI = Ankle-Brachial Index, HTN = Hypertension, RA = Rheumatoid Arthritis, PE = Pulmonary Embolus, PAD = Peripheral Arterial Disease

Reference

1. Cameron, M. (2017). *Physical Agents in Rehabilitation: An Evidence-Based Approach to Practice.* (5th ed.). St. Louis, MO: Elsevier.

APPENDIX 11C

Common Applications and Parameter Adjustments for Electrical Stimulation

Table 11C-1

Common Applications and Parameter Adjustments for Electrical Stimulation

			TIME CHARACTERISTICS			
CONDITION/ INDICATION	TYPE	DESCRIPTION OF CURRENT	PULSE FREQUENCY	PULSE DURATION	AMPLITUDE	TREATMENT VARIABLES
Weakness/ strengthen	NMES	Pulsed biphasic (most common) Pulsed monphasic Burst modulated AC (Russian stimulation)	• Tetany (smooth muscle contraction >25–30 pps)	• 300–500 μsec is common (set to patient comfort) • Russian stimulation is preset	• Goal: motor facilitation amplitude high enough for visible contraction • Goal: strengthening amplitude to maximal toleration or at least 60% maximal voluntary isometric torque	• 10 seconds on: 50 seconds off time helps minimize fatigue (shorter ratios are more practical, but introduce more fatigue) • Ramp times for comfort • 15 min treatment • 10–15 contractions • 3 treatment sessions per week
Endurance/ prevent shoulder subluxation poststroke	NMES/ FES	Pulsed current	>Tetany	See above	Submaximal	• Progress to longer ON times to shorter OFF times (1:1 or greater ratios) • Treatment times can be increased as tolerated
Muscle Reeducation (facilitation)/ Orthotic substitution	FES	Pulsed current	Tetany	See above	Intensity high enough to accomplish task	• Often hand or foot switches are used to match on/off times with task (e.g., gait or reaching activity)
Muscle Spasm	NMES	Pulsed current (most common) or Russian	>Tetany (higher frequency = greater fatigue)	See above	Maximal tolerated	• Attempting to fatigue spasm • On time = Continuous (no off time) • 10–15 minutes treatment
Pain/Acute	TENS	Pulsed current or IFC	80–110 pps	50–100 μsec	Sensory level stimulation	• Conventional TENS • Continuous for 20–60 minutes

(Continued)

Table 11C-1

Common Applications and Parameter Adjustments for Electrical Stimulation (Continued)

			TIME CHARACTERISTICS			
CONDITION/ INDICATION	**TYPE**	**DESCRIPTION OF CURRENT**	**PULSE FREQUENCY**	**PULSE DURATION**	**AMPLITUDE**	**TREATMENT VARIABLES**
Pain/Chronic	TENS	Pulsed current or IFC	1–5 pps	150–300 μsec	Motor level response that causes a comfortable rhythmical muscle contraction	• Low-rate TENS • Continuous for 30–40 minutes
Inflammation Reduction/ Medication Delivery	Ionto	DC	NA	NA	1–4 mA (clinical models) Dosage is based on mA/min: • Dose = Current (mA) x Duration (min) • Typical dose = 40–80 mA/min	• Caution: Current density [amplitude (mA)/electrode size (cm2)] should not exceed: o 0.5 mA/cm2 for cathodal electrode o 1.0 mA/cm2 for anodal electrode • See Table 11-7 for commonly used Ions
Wound Healing/ Infection	HVPC	Pulsed monophasic	30–130 pps	Depends on waveform and it could be preset	Sensory level stimulation	Pad placement over the wound: • Anode = positive pole o Reactivation of the inflammatory phase o Epithelial cell migration • Cathode = negative pole o Infection or inflammation control o Fibroplasia (granulation formation) in the proliferative phase • Same current density cautions for Iontophoresis (above) when using DC • Treatment length: 1–4 hours a day; 5–7 days a week
	DC	DC	NA	NA	• 200–1,000 microamperes = <1000 μA or <1mA	

- This appendix reflects common parameters. There are multiple combinations of parameters that might work for a condition.
- Common precautions for all electrical stimulation applications, cardiac disease, impaired mentation, in areas of impaired sensation, malignant tumors, skin irritation, or open wounds that do not require electrical stimulation for wound healing.
- Common contraindications for all electrical stimulation applications; current through or near places that might interfere with demand-type pacemakers or other electronic devices, unstable arrhythmias, untreated epilepsy or seizure disorders, over the carotid sinus, thrombosis or thrombophlebitis, eyes, or in such a manner that would allow the current to pass through the fetus during pregnancy.

APPENDIX 11D

Review Questions

(Answers to all Review Questions and Case Studies are found in Chapter 17)

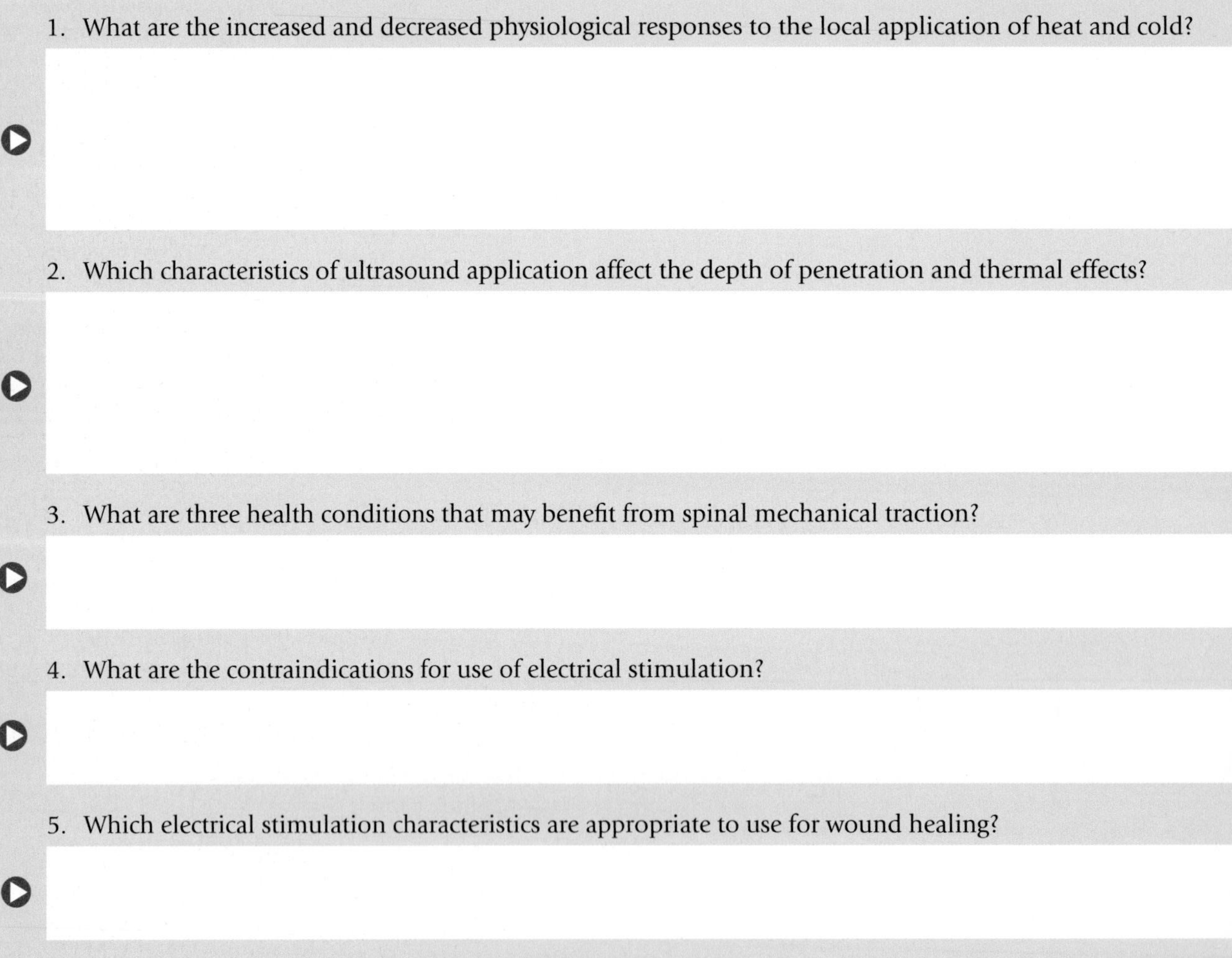

1. What are the increased and decreased physiological responses to the local application of heat and cold?

2. Which characteristics of ultrasound application affect the depth of penetration and thermal effects?

3. What are three health conditions that may benefit from spinal mechanical traction?

4. What are the contraindications for use of electrical stimulation?

5. Which electrical stimulation characteristics are appropriate to use for wound healing?

12

Functional Training, Equipment, Devices, and Technologies

JASON M. WILKEN, KELLY J. SASS, AND SUSAN B. O'SULLIVAN

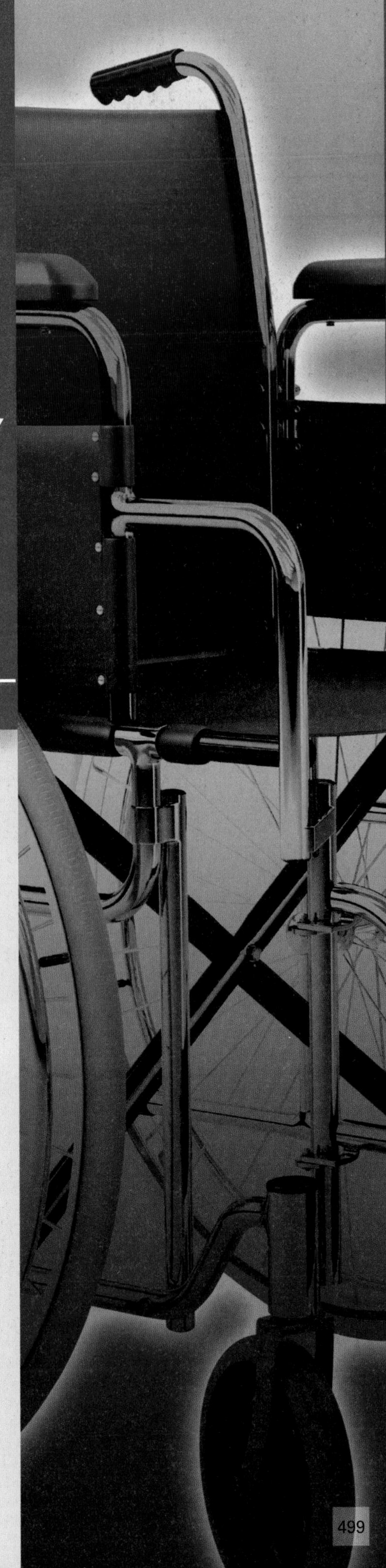

Chapter Outline

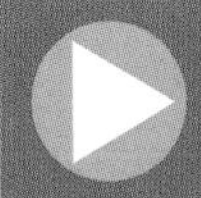

Study Tactics

Questions About Equipment, Devices, and Technologies Comprise Approximately 3% of the NPTE, or a Total of Five to Six Questions

Focus on:

- Prosthetics, orthotics, ambulation aids, wheelchairs, protective and supportive devices (slings, splints, collars, etc.), locomotor and gravity-assist devices, transfer devices, bariatric equipment, robotic exoskeletons, and more. Be judicious with the amount of time you spend preparing for the five or six questions covering this large content area!
- Different types, functions, components, characteristics, and use of a variety of prostheses, orthoses, and upper/lower extremity assistive devices
- Gait cycle. Understanding the phases of the gait cycle and common gait deviations is fundamental to establishing interventions using prosthetic devices, orthotic devices, and ambulation aids
- Prosthetics
  - Pre-prosthetic examination and management including phantom limb pain, diminished sensation, length of the residual limb, wound care, positioning and activities, types of prostheses and components (prosthetic feet, suspensions, temporary prostheses, etc.)
  - Prosthetic assessment may include alignment, gait deviations, fit, and prosthetic-related problems
- Orthotics
  - Terminology, names, functions, and components of orthotic devices
  - Orthotic assessment to address gait deviations
  - Upper or lower extremity orthoses (splints, braces) need to be reviewed as well as trunk and cervical orthoses
  - Selection of the best orthotic device to rectify or aid the situation. You might have to consider age (pediatric), occupation/athletics, prior level of function, health condition (nerve lesion, post-tendon repair), home environment, impairments (tone, joint stability), or activity limitations (transfers/gait)
  - Specific orthoses worth reviewing include ankle-foot orthoses (AFOs), reciprocating gait orthoses (RGOs), shoe inserts and modifications, spinal stabilization braces, functional wrist and finger splinting
- Wheelchairs/ambulation aids
  - Wheelchairs include modifications for specific health conditions/impairments and activity limitations. Focus on components, measurements, modifications, propulsion, and prescription. Include powered wheelchairs and bariatric dimensions.
  - Chair modifications for various adult and pediatric neuromuscular and musculoskeletal conditions
  - Crutches, canes, and walkers and their indications, particularly with regards to weight-bearing status, energy expenditure, and safety
- Supportive, protective, gravity-assisted, bariatric devices
  - Pediatric positioning devices (bolsters, pillows) and standing devices such as the parapodium or standing frame
  - Appropriate use of body-weight support devices

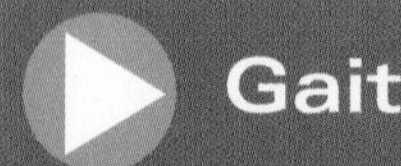

Gait

Phases of the Gait Cycle

Traditional terminology appears first and refers to points in time in the gait cycle; Rancho Los Amigos (RLA) terminology follows and refers to lengths of time in the gait cycle. Because both are in clinical use, readers should be familiar with both. These two types of terminologies do not always coincide exactly when describing the gait cycle.

Stance Phase

1. Heel Strike: the point when the heel of the lead limb contacts the ground at the beginning of stance phase.
   Initial contact (RLA): the instant the foot of the lead extremity contacts the ground.
   Muscle activation patterns (see Figure 12-1): knee extensors (quadriceps) are active at heel strike through early stance to control a small amount of knee flexion for shock absorption; ankle dorsiflexors (e.g., tibialis anterior anterior tibialis, extensor hallucis longus, extensor digitorum longus) control lowering of the foot, from heel strike to foot flat.
2. Foot Flat: the point when the sole of the foot (typically forefoot) makes contact with the ground; occurs shortly after heel strike.
   Loading response (RLA): the first period of double support from initial contact until the contralateral leg leaves the ground.

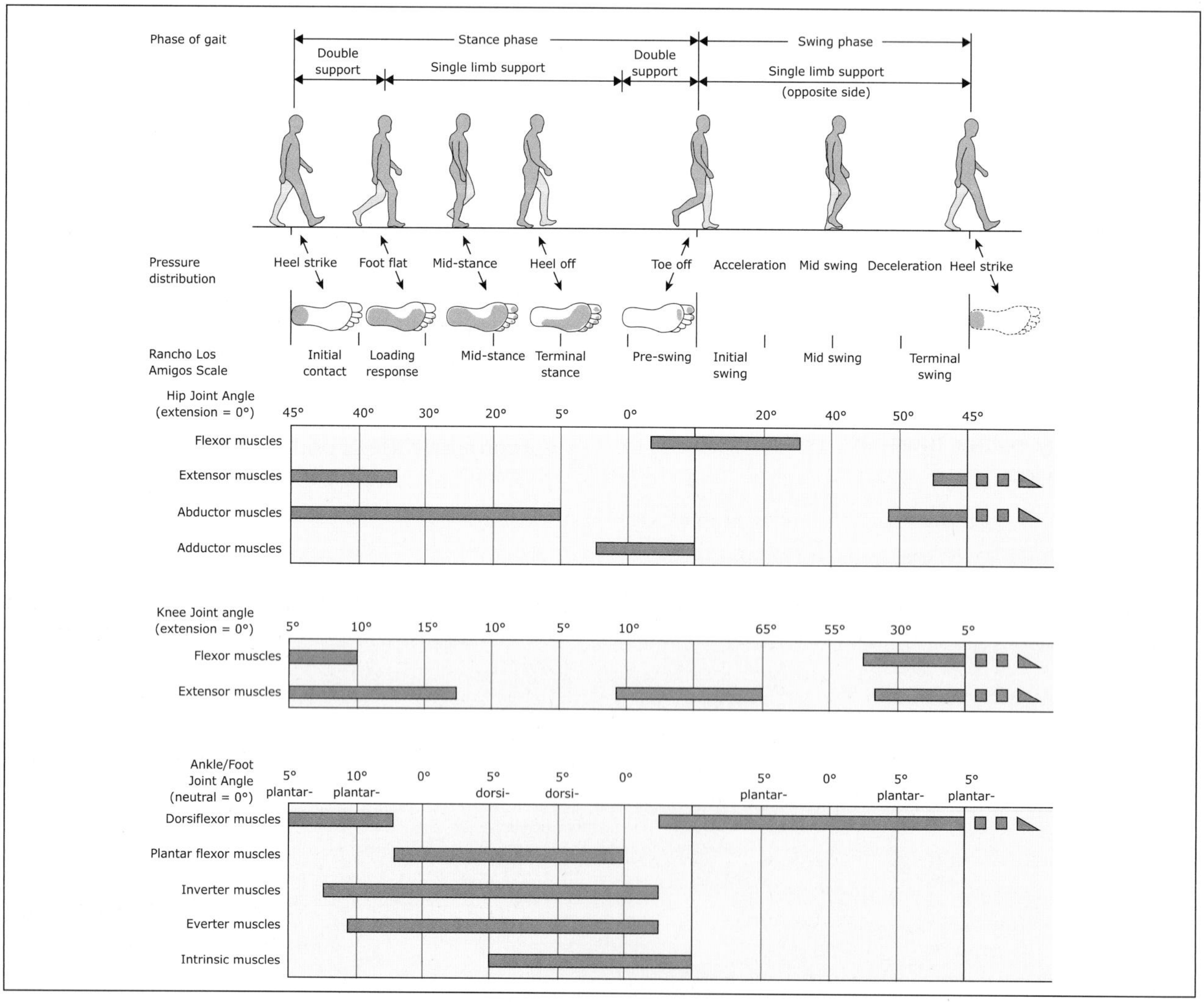

Phase of gait
Stance phase
Double support
Single limb support
Double support
Swing phase
Single limb support (opposite side)
Pressure distribution
Heel strike Foot flat Mid-stance Heel off Toe off Acceleration Mid swing Deceleration Heel strike
Rancho Los Amigos Scale
Initial contact Loading response Mid-stance Terminal stance Pre-swing Initial swing Mid swing Terminal swing
Hip Joint Angle (extension = 0°) 45° 40° 30° 20° 5° 0° 20° 40° 50° 45°
Flexor muscles
Extensor muscles
Abductor muscles
Adductor muscles
Knee Joint angle (extension = 0°) 5° 10° 15° 10° 5° 10° 65° 55° 30° 5°
Flexor muscles
Extensor muscles
Ankle/Foot Joint Angle (neutral = 0°) 5° plantar- 10° plantar- 0° 5° dorsi- 5° dorsi- 0° 5° plantar- 0° 5° plantar- 5° plantar-
Dorsiflexor muscles
Plantar flexor muscles
Inverter muscles
Everter muscles
Intrinsic muscles

Figure 12-1 **Phases of the gait cycle.**
Adapted from Susan Standring (Editor-in-Chief). Gray's Anatomy. 39th ed. 2005. P. 1533. Elsevier Churchill Livingstone.

Muscle activation patterns: gastrocnemius-soleus muscles are active from foot flat through midstance to eccentrically control forward tibial advancement.

3. Midstance: the point at which full body weight is taken by the reference or support limb.
   Midstance (RLA): the contralateral limb leaves the ground; body weight is taken and advanced over and ahead of the support limb; first period of single limb support.
   Muscle activation patterns: hip, knee, and ankle extensors are active throughout stance to oppose antigravity forces and stabilize the limb; hip extensors control forward motion of the trunk; hip abductors stabilize the pelvis during unilateral stance. Gastrocnemius-soleus muscles control forward tibial advancement, and energy is stored as Achilles tendon elongates.
4. Heel-off: occurs after midstance as the heel of the reference or support limb leaves the ground.
   Terminal stance (RLA): the last period of single limb support that begins with heel rise and continues until the contralateral leg contacts the ground (start of double limb support).
   Muscle activation patterns: peak activity of plantarflexors occurs from heel-off to toe-off and generates forward propulsion of the body and swing limb. Energy stored in Achilles tendon is released.
5. Toe-off: the last portion of stance following heel-off, when the toe of the stance limb leaves the ground.
   Preswing (RLA): the second period of double support from initial contact of the contralateral limb to lift-off of the support limb.
   Muscle activation patterns: hip and knee extensors (hamstrings and quadriceps) may contribute to forward propulsion with a brief burst of activity.

Swing Phase

1. Acceleration: the first portion of the swing phase from toe-off of the reference limb until midswing.
   Initial swing (RLA): the first portion of the swing phase from toe-off of the reference limb until maximum knee flexion of the same extremity.
   Muscle activation patterns: forward acceleration of the limb during early swing is achieved through the brief action of quadriceps; by midswing, the quadriceps is silent and pendular motion is in effect; hip flexors (iliopsoas) aid in forward limb propulsion.
2. Midswing: the midportion of the swing phase when the reference extremity moves directly below the body.
   Midswing (RLA): the portion of the swing phase from maximum knee flexion of the reference extremity to a vertical tibial position.
   Muscle activation patterns: foot clearance is achieved by contraction of the hip, knee flexors, and ankle dorsiflexors (dorsiflexors elevate the toe to improve toe clearance).
3. Deceleration: the end portion of the swing phase when the reference extremity is slowing down in preparation for heel strike.
   Terminal swing (RLA): the portion of the swing phase from a vertical tibial position of the reference extremity to just prior to initial contact.
   Muscle activation patterns: hamstrings act during late swing to decelerate the limb in preparation for heel strike; quadriceps and ankle dorsiflexors become active in late swing to prepare for heel strike.

Pelvic Motion

1. The pelvis rotates in a transverse plane (relative forward and backward motion of each side).
   a. The pelvis on the side of the swing limb moves forward to advance the limb; mean rotation is 4°.
   b. The contralateral side also rotates 4° when it is the swing limb (total of 8°).
2. The pelvis rotates in the frontal plane (lateral pelvic tilt 5°), controlled by hip abductor muscles.
   a. The side contralateral to the stance limb drops during loading response.
3. The pelvis rotates in the sagittal plane (anterior/posterior tilt). The pelvis is naturally anterior tilted 10°–15° and is pulled anterior as the hip flexors reach the end range of terminal stance.
4. The pelvis moves side to side 4 cm, moving toward the stance limb during loading response.

Cadence

1. The number of steps taken per unit of time.
2. Mean cadence is approximately 110 steps/minute.
3. Increased cadence while maintaining the same speed is the result of shorter step length.
4. Running occurs when the period of double support disappears, typically at a cadence of 180 steps/minute.

Step

1. Step length: the anterior-posterior distance between the heel at initial contact on subsequent steps (ipsi vs. contralateral, in cm or m).
2. Step time: the time (s) between initial contact on the ipsi and contralateral limb.
3. Step width: the distance between feet (e.g., base of support); measured from one heel to the same point on the opposite heel (in cm or m).
   a. Normal step width ranges between 2.54 and 12.7 cm (1 and 5 inches).
   b. Increases as stability demands rise; e.g., wide-based gait in older adults or very small children.

Stride

1. Stride length: the anterior-posterior distance between two consecutive contacts of the same limb (in cm or m).

2. Stride time: the time (s) between initial contact of the same limb on subsequent steps.

Velocity (Walking Speed)

1. The distance traveled divided by the time required (m/sec or miles/hour).
2. Average walking speed is approximately 1.3 m/s (3 miles/hour).
3. Affected by physical characteristics: height, weight, gender.
4. Decreased with age, physical disability, etc.

Acceleration/Deceleration

1. Increase/decrease in walking.
2. Measured as velocity (rate of change/time).

Energy Cost of Walking

1. Commonly measured as normalized rate of consumption (mL/kg/min) or efficiency relative to distance traveled (mL/kg/m).
2. Average oxygen rate for comfortable walking is 12 mL/kg × min.
3. Metabolic cost of walking averages 5.5 kcal/min on level surfaces; energy costs may vary widely depending on speed of walking, stride length, body weight, type of surface, gradient, and activity (e.g., stair climbing).
4. Increased energy costs can occur with age, abnormal gait (e.g., disease, muscle weakness or paralysis, physical disability), or with the use of functional devices (e.g., crutches, orthoses, prostheses).

Common Gait Deviations: Stance Phase

Trunk and Hip

1. Lateral trunk bending: the result of weak gluteus medius; will see bending to the same side as the weakness (Trendelenburg gait); also seen with pain in the hip.
2. Backward trunk lean: the result of weak gluteus maximus; will also see difficulty going up stairs or ramps.
3. Forward trunk lean: the result of weak quadriceps (decreases flexor movement at the knee), hip and knee flexion contractures.
4. Excessive hip flexion: the result of weak hip extensors or tight hip and/or knee flexors.
5. Limited hip extension: the result of tight or spastic hip flexors.
6. Limited hip flexion: the result of weak hip flexors or tight extensors.
7. Abnormal synergistic activity (e.g., stroke with lower extremity extensor synergy): excessive hip adduction combined with hip and knee extension, plantarflexion; scissoring or adducted gait pattern (e.g., spastic cerebral palsy).
8. Antalgic gait (painful gait): stance time is abbreviated on the painful limb, which results in an asymmetrical gait pattern; the uninvolved limb has a shortened step length as weight-bearing occurs sooner than normal.

Knee

1. Excessive knee flexion: the result of weak quadriceps (knee buckles) or knee flexor contracture.
   a. Will also see difficulty going down stairs or ramps.
   b. Forward trunk bending can compensate for weak quadriceps.
2. Hyperextension: the result of a weak quadriceps, plantar flexion contracture, or extensor spasticity (quadriceps and/or plantar flexion).

Ankle/Foot

1. Forefoot initial contact: Often results from weak dorsiflexors; spastic or tight plantarflexors; may also be caused by a shortened leg (leg length discrepancy).
2. Foot slap: Forefoot contacts floor with an audible slap after initial contact; the result of weak dorsiflexors or hypotonia.
3. Foot flat: Heel and forefoot contact the ground simultaneously; the result of weak dorsiflexors, limited range of motion (ROM); immature gait pattern (neonatal).
4. Calcaneus gait: Loading predominately on heel with excessive dorsiflexion and uncontrolled forward motion of the tibia: the results of weak plantarflexors.
5. Equinus gait: Heel does not touch the ground; the result of spasticity or contracture of the plantar flexors.
6. Supination: Varus calcaneus and excessive lateral loading of the foot. May occur at initial contact and correct at the foot flat with weight acceptance or remain throughout stance. Possible causes: spastic invertors, weak evertors, pes varus, genu varum.
7. Hyperpronation: excessive medial contact of foot during stance with valgus position of calcaneus. Possible causes: weak invertors, spasticity, and pes valgus.
8. Clawed toes: the result of spastic toe flexors, possibly a hyperactive plantar grasp reflex.
9. Inadequate push-off: the result of weak plantar flexors, decreased ROM into plantarflexion, or pain in the forefoot.

Common Gait Deviations: Swing Phase

Trunk and Hip

1. Insufficient forward pelvic rotation (stiff pelvis, pelvic retraction): the result of weak abdominal muscles, weak flexor muscles (e.g., stroke).

2. Insufficient hip and knee flexion: the result of weak hip and knee flexors; inability to lift the leg and move it forward.
3. Circumduction: the leg swings out to the side (abduction/external rotation followed by adduction/internal rotation); the result of weak hip and knee flexors.
4. Hip hiking (quadratus lumborum action): a compensatory response for weak hip and knee flexors, or extensor spasticity.
5. Excessive hip and knee flexion (steppage gait): a compensatory response to shorten the leg; the result of weak dorsiflexors (e.g., diabetic neuropathy, fibular neuropathy, L4-5 radiculopathy).
6. Abnormal synergistic activity (e.g., stroke with lower extremity flexor synergy): excessive hip flexion/abduction, knee flexion with ankle dorsiflexion/inversion.

Knee

1. Insufficient knee flexion: the result of extensor spasticity, pain/decreased ROM, or weak hamstrings.
2. Excessive knee flexion: the result of flexor spasticity; flexor withdrawal reflex.

Ankle/Foot

1. Foot drop (equinus): the result of weak or delayed contraction of the dorsiflexors or spastic plantarflexors.
2. Varus or inverted foot: the result of spastic invertors (anterior tibialis), weak fibularis longus/brevis, or abnormal synergistic pattern (e.g., stroke).
3. Equinovarus: the result of spasticity of the posterior tibialis and/or gastrocnemius-soleus; developmental abnormality.

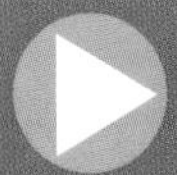

Ambulatory Aids

Canes

Indications

1. Widen base of support to improve balance; providing limited stability and unweighting (can unload forces on involved extremity by 30%); can be used to relieve pain and decrease antalgic gait pattern.

Types

1. Wood or aluminum (adjustable with pushpin lock).
2. Standard, single point cane: handle and shaft may be standard (J-shaped) or offset.
3. Quad cane: four contact points with the ground; provides increased stability but slows gait.
   a. Small-based quad cane (SBQC): useful for stairs.
   b. Wide-based or large-based quad cane (WBQC or LBQC): does not typically fit on stairs.

Cane Measurement

1. Measure a point 6 inches to the side of the toes to the ulnar styloid or wrist crease to allow for 20°–30° of elbow flexion.

Gait

1. Cane is held in the hand opposite to the involved extremity.
2. Two-point gait: cane and involved lower extremity are advanced together, followed by the uninvolved lower extremity.
3. Delayed two-point gait: cane is advanced first, followed by the involved lower extremity, and then the uninvolved lower extremity.

Crutches

Indications

1. Increase the base of support to provide a moderate degree of stability.
2. Provides a way to relieve specific weight-bearing (partial weight-bearing vs. toe-touch weight-bearing) on the lower extremities.

Types

1. Axillary crutches:
   a. Provide increased upper-extremity weight-bearing.

> **RED FLAG:** Prolonged pressure on the axillary pad can result in vascular and/or nerve damage (axillary artery/radial nerve).

2. Forearm (Lofstrand) crutches:
   a. Provide slightly less stability than axillary crutches but increased ease of movement, particularly with bilateral involvement.
   b. Frees hands for use without dropping the crutch (secured by the cuff).

Axillary Crutch Measurements

1. Crutches 6 inches in front and 2 inches lateral to the feet, axillary pads should sit two to three finger widths below the axilla.
2. Handgrip height should be at the level of the ulnar styloid or wrist crease to allow for 20°–30° of elbow flexion.

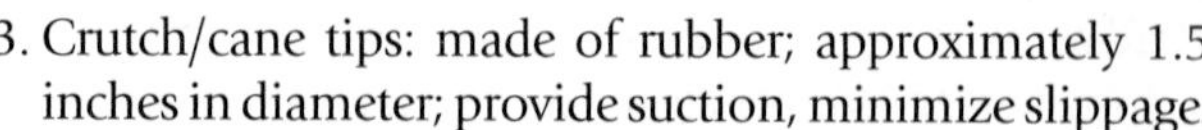

3. Crutch/cane tips: made of rubber; approximately 1.5 inches in diameter; provide suction, minimize slippage.

Gait Patterns: Use of Assistive Devices

Two-Point Gait

1. One crutch and opposite extremity move together, followed by the opposite crutch and extremity; requires use of two assistive devices (canes or crutches).
2. Allows for natural arm and leg motion during gait, good support and stability from two opposing points of contact.

Three-Point Gait

1. Crutches and involved lower extremity are advanced together, followed by the uninvolved limb.
2. Indicated for use with involvement of one extremity; e.g., lower extremity fracture.

Delayed Three-Point Gait

1. Crutches advanced first followed by the involved lower extremity; then uninvolved lower extremity.
2. Indicated when patient requires increased stability and slower movement.

Four-Point Gait

1. One crutch is advanced forward, followed by the contralateral lower extremity, then the second crutch is advanced forward, followed by that contralateral limb.
2. Used with bilateral lower extremity involvement.

Swing-to Gait

1. Crutches advanced first, and lower extremities swing forward to meet the crutches.
2. Used on non–weight-bearing status or bilateral lower extremity involvement.

Swing-Through Gait

1. Crutches advanced first, lower extremities swing forward beyond the point of crutch.
2. Used in non–weight-bearing status or bilateral lower extremity involvement.

Walkers

Indications

1. Widen base of support, providing increased lateral and anterior stability over canes or crutches.
2. Reduce weight-bearing on one or both lower extremities.
3. Frequently prescribed for patients with debilitating conditions, poor balance, or lower extremity injury when use of crutches is precluded; e.g., elderly patients, poor balance.
4. Negative features include no reciprocal arm swing, flexed posture, and encourages a step-to gait pattern.

Types of Walkers

1. Standard: four legs, typically able to fold to facilitate mobility in the community, storage in cars, etc.
2. Wheeled (rolling): available with either two or four wheels (four wheels require hand brake to provide added stability in stopping); facilitates walking as a continuous movement sequence (step-through gait pattern); allows for increased speed.
3. Hemi walker: modified for use with one hand only.

Measurement

1. Hand grip height should be at the level of the ulnar styloid or wrist crease to allow for 20°–30° of elbow flexion.

Additional Assistive Device Considerations

Weight-Bearing Status

1. Non-weight-bearing (NWB) = no weight-bearing is permitted on the affected extremity.
2. Touch or toe-touch weight-bearing (TWB) = only the toes of affected lower extremity should contact the floor to allow only minimal weight-bearing for balance purposes.
3. Partial-weight-bearing (PWB) = a percentage of the patient's weight (e.g., 50% PWB) is allowed through the affected extremity.
4. Full-weight-bearing (FWB) = there is no restriction of the amount of weight allowed through the extremity during activities.

Platforms

1. Allows weight-bearing on the forearm; used for patients who are unable to bear weight through their hands; e.g., patients with arthritis.
2. Can be added to crutches or walkers.

Crutch/Cane Tips

1. Made of rubber; must be maintained for safety to provide suction and minimize slippage.

Bariatric Equipment

1. See discussion of obesity in Chapter 8.
2. Heavy-duty equipment available for increased weight capacity and girth.
3. Heavy-duty mechanical lifts available to assist with patient transfers.

Stairs/Curbs

1. Ascent: the uninvolved lower extremity ascends the step first, followed by the assistive device and the involved lower extremity together.
2. The assistive device descends the step first, with the involved extremity or followed by the involved extremity. The univolved lower extremity then follows to the lower step.
3. Mnemonic devices to teach patient: "The good go up, the bad go down." "Up with the good, down with the bad."

Guarding

Indications

1. Protects the patient from falling.
2. Requires the use of a gait belt for initial training of most patients.

Procedure

1. Level surfaces: stand slightly behind and to one side, typically on the more involved side.
2. Stairs: therapist is always positioned below the patient.
   a. Ascent: stand behind and slightly to the involved side.
   b. Descent: stand in front and slightly to the involved side.
3. Sit-to-stand transfers.
   a. Stand to one side and slightly behind the patient.
   b. Increased levels of assistance may require therapist to stand in front of patient.

Locomotor Training

Conventional Over-Ground Training

1. Depends on an observational gait assessment.
2. Manual or verbal cues are used to provide input or guidance.
3. Often starts in parallel bars or other safe setting (e.g., body weight support).
4. Support and cues, in form of augmented and visual (mirror) feedback, are progressively decreased.

Body Weight Supported (BWS) and Treadmill Training (TT)

1. BWS: overhead harness or pressured air chamber are used to support body weight.
   a. Initially, support is high (e.g., 40% of body weight) and is progressively decreased.
   b. BWS is contraindicated if it significantly interferes with gait cycle (e.g., unable to achieve flat foot during stepping).
2. Progressive treadmill training.
   a. Progresses from treadmill walking with slow speeds (e.g., 0.6–0.8 mph) to faster, near-normal walking speeds (e.g., 2.6–2.8 mph).
   b. Progresses from level walking to slight incline walking.
   c. Progresses from treadmill walking to overground walking.
3. Manual assistance.
   a. Level of assistance decreases as training progresses (maxA, to modA, to minA, to no assistance).
   b. Assistance can include hands on pelvis (assisted pelvic motions) and hands on lower extremity (assisted stepping).

Robotic-Assisted Walking

1. An exoskeletal frame with motorized, fitted braces is used with patients with complete SCI; braces support both LEs and part of upper body.
   a. A backpack containing a computer and power supply is worn. Computer program controls hip and knee motions.
   b. Crutches or walker are required.
2. Single robotic leg brace: assists walking in individuals with single limb paralysis (e.g., chronic stroke).
3. Often paired with BWS and TT.
4. Progression is to overground walking.
5. High cost limits availability of devices.

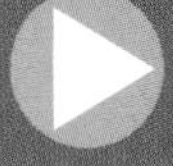

Orthotics

General Concepts

Orthosis: A Rigid or Semi-Rigid Device

1. Used to reduce functional loss due to weak, painful, diseased, or deformed joint.
2. Supports, accommodates, or protects a joint or body segment.
3. Restricts or facilitates motion.
4. Corrects alignment.

Three-Point Pressure Principle

1. Forms the mechanical basis for orthotic correction.
2. A single force is placed at the area of deformity or angulation; two additional counterforces act in the opposing direction.

Splint

1. Colloquial term to describe a temporary device that may serve the same functions.
2. Materials generally not as durable or able to withstand prolonged use.

Device Fitting and Alignment

1. Correct alignment permits effective function.
2. Limb alignment maintained or corrected to prevent further deformity.
3. Restrict or assist motion using rigid blocking or spring-like elements.
4. Transfer load to alternate structures.
5. Reduce pain and/or minimize forces by transferring them away from pressure-sensitive tissues.
6. Proper device alignment minimizes movement between limb and orthoses (e.g., pistoning) and facilitates proper device function.

Lower-Limb Orthoses: Components/Terminology

Shoes

1. The foundation for an orthosis; can substantially influence orthosis function.
2. Often used to provide support or cushioning, including reducing areas of localized high pressure.
3. Traditional leather orthopedic shoes or athletic sneakers can be worn with orthoses; attachments can be external (to the outer part of a leather shoe's sole) or internal (a molded shoe insert).
4. Components include upper, heel counter, midsole, insole, outsole, vamp, toe box.
5. Blucher opening: has vamps (the flaps contain the lace stays) that open wide apart from the anterior margin of the shoe for ease of application.
6. Bal (Balmoral) opening: has stitched down vamps, not suitable for orthotic wear.

Foot Orthosis (FO)

1. Classified as accomodative or corrective. Accomodative is used for fixed deformities and used to redistribute forces, whereas corrective is used to modify closed kinetic chain motion and loading.
2. Posting may be placed at the forefoot or hindfoot, medially or laterally, intrinsically or extrinsically, to influence motion.
3. Soft inserts (i.e., viscoelastic plastic or rubber pads or relief cut-outs) reduce areas of high loading, restrict forces, and protect painful or sensitive areas of the feet.
   a. Metatarsal pad: located posterior to metatarsal heads; moves pressure from the metatarsal heads to the metatarsal shafts; allows more push-off in weak or inflexible feet.
   b. Cushion heel: cushions and absorbs forces at heel contact; used to relieve strain on plantar fascia in plantar fasciitis.
   c. Heel-spur pad.
4. Longitudinal arch supports: prevent depression of the subtalar joint and correct for pes planus (flat foot); flat foot can be flexible or rigid.
   a. UCBL (University of California Biomechanics Laboratory) insert: a semirigid plastic molded insert to correct for flexible pes planus.
   b. Scaphoid pad: used to support the longitudinal arch.
5. Posting.
   a. Rearfoot posting: alters the position of the subtalar joint (STJ), or rearfoot, from heel strike to footflat. Must be dynamic, control but not eliminate STJ motion.
      - Varus post (medial wedge): limits or controls eversion of the calcaneus and internal rotation of the tibia after heelstrike. Reduces calcaneal eversion during running.
      - Valgus post (lateral wedge): controls calcaneus and subtalar joints that are excessively inverted and supinated at heel strike.
   b. Forefoot posting: supports the forefoot.
      - Medial wedge prescribed for forefoot varus.
      - Lateral wedge prescribed for forefoot valgus.

> **RED FLAG:** Insensitive foot—avoid modifications such as heel lifts, or rocker bars, which may increase localized forefoot pressures.

6. Heel lifts (or heel platform).
   a. Accommodates for leg length discrepancy; can be placed inside the shoe (up to 3/8 inch) or attached to the outer sole.
   b. Accommodates for limitation in ankle joint dorsiflexion.
7. Rocker bar: located proximal to metatarsal heads; improves weight shift onto metatarsals.
8. Rocker bottom: builds up the sole over the metatarsal heads and improves push-off in weak or inflexible feet.

Ankle-Foot Orthosis (AFO)

1. Typically consists of a foot plate, ankle joint or strut, and a proximal cuff or leg band below the knee.
2. Either custom-molded or off-the-shelf. Can be fabricated using many different materials including leather, thermoplastics, steel, carbon fiber, foamed plastic, or rubber.
3. Foot plate and stirrup.
   a. Foot plate: generic or custom-molded geometry. Extends to metatarsal heads or full length to tips of toes.
   b. Stirrup: a metal attachment riveted to the sole of the shoe; split stirrups allow for shoe interchange;

solid stirrups are fixed permanently to the shoe and provide for maximum stability.

4. General types:
   a. Hinged/articulating AFO (H/AAFO): single axis of rotation, allows motion in sagittal plane while controlling motion in other planes.
   b. Free motion: little or no resistance to PF or DF, helps maintain alignment and M/L stability.
      - Examples: posterior tibial tendon dysfunction (PTTD), frontal plane instabilities of subtalar, and/or talorcrural joint.
   c. Dorsiflexion assist: dynamic DF assist, primarily for weak DF, limited resistance to PF. Assist toe clearance during swing phase and help control PF at initial contact (e.g., posterior leaf spring [PLS] orthosis with narrow plastic posterior strut or lightweight carbon fiber off-the-shelf orthosis).
   d. Plantarflexion stop: blocks PF motion, allows free DF, for weak DF or tight PF, typically block PF at 90°.
   e. DF stop: blocks DF motion, allows free PF, for individuals with weak plantarflexors.
   f. Static or solid ankle AFO: provides maximum stability and control of the ankle, ankle positioned in a preferred alignment, assist swing clearance and prepositioning. Leather lacer is an example of a static AFO.
   g. Ground reaction AFO (GRAFO): controls forward progression of the tibia, primarily for PF weakness, can influence the knee by decreasing extensor moment during stance, resist DF at the ankle.
   h. Patellar tendon bearing AFO (PTBAFO): unloads the distal limb, primarily for PF weakness, anterior shell with weight-bearing capabilities, shelf transfers force to the medial tibial flare, patellar tendon bar-like prosthetic socket.
   i. Charcot restraint orthotic walker (CROW) boot: immobilizes and protects the foot and ankle; includes a rocker bottom and custom-molded insert.
      - An alternative to total contact casting in individuals with diabetes mellitus.
      - Eliminates shear forces on the plantar surface.

Knee-Ankle-Foot Orthosis (KAFO)

1. Orthosis that controls motion at the ankle, knee, and foot.
2. Can be difficult to align and adds weight to the limb.

Knee Components

1. Knee controls.
   a. Hinge joint: provides mediolateral and hyperextension control while allowing for flexion and extension.
      - Offset: the hinge is placed posterior to the weight-bearing line (trochanter-knee-ankle [TKA] line); assists extension, stabilizes knee during early stance; patients may have difficulty on ramps where knee may flex inadvertently.
   b. Locks.
      - Drop ring lock: ring drops over joint when knee is in full extension to provide maximum stability; a retention button may be added to hold the ring lock up, permitting gait training with the knee unlocked.
      - Pawl lock with bail release: the pawl is a spring-loaded posterior projection (lever or ring) that allows the patient to unlock the knee by pulling up or hooking the pawl on the back of a chair and pushing it up; adds bulk and may unlock inadvertently with posterior knee pressure.
   c. Knee stability.
      - Sagittal stability achieved by bands or straps used to provide a posteriorly directed force.
         - Anterior band or strap (knee cap): attaches by four buckles to metal uprights; may restrict sitting, increases difficulty in putting on KAFO.
         - Anterior bands: pretibial or suprapatellar or both.
      - Frontal plane controls: for control of genu varum or genu valgum.
         - Posterior plastic shell.
         - Older braces utilize valgum (medial) or varum (lateral) correction straps, which buckle around the opposite metal upright; less effective as controls than plastic shell.
2. Thigh bands.
   a. Proximal thigh band.
   b. Quadrilateral or ischial weight-bearing brim: reduces weight-bearing through the limb.
      - Patten bottom: a distal attachment added to keep the foot off the floor; provides 100% unweighting of the limb; a lift is required on the opposite leg, e.g., used with Legg-Calvé-Perthes disease.
3. Specialized KAFOs.
   a. Oregon orthotic system: a combination of plastic and metal components allows for triplanar control in three planes of motion (sagittal, frontal, and transverse).
   b. Fracture braces: a KAFO device with a calf or thigh shell that encompasses the fracture site and provides support.
   c. Functional electrical stimulation (FES) orthosis: orthotic use and functional ambulation are facilitated by the addition of electrical stimulation to specific muscles; the pattern and sequence of muscle activation by portable stimulators is controlled by an externally worn miniaturized computer pack; requires full passive range of motion (PROM); good functional endurance; in limited use with individuals with paraplegia, drop foot; also scoliosis.
4. Standing frames.
   a. Standing frames: allows for standing without crutch support; may be stationary or attached to a wheeled

mobility base (e.g., used with some patients with SCI). Provides for the benefits of weight-bearing and upright posture (e.g., reduced bone loss, supports vascular, bladder function, etc.).

Specialized Knee Orthosis (KO)

1. Articulated KO: controls knee motion and provides added stability.
   a. Postsurgery KO protects repaired ligaments from overload.
   b. Functional KO is worn long term in lieu of surgery or during selected activities (sports competitions).
   c. Examples include Lenox Hill, Pro-AM, Can-Am, Don Joy.
2. Swedish knee cage: provides mild control for excessive hyperextension of the knee.
3. Patellar stabilizing braces.
   a. Improve patellar tracking; maintain alignment.
   b. Lateral buttress (often made of felt) or strap positions patella medially.
   c. A central patellar cutout may help positioning and minimizes compression.
4. Neoprene sleeves.
   a. Nylon-coated rubber material.
   b. Provide compression, protection, and proprioceptive feedback.
   c. Provide little stabilization unless metal or plastic hinges are added.
   d. Retains body heat, which may increase local circulation.
   e. A central cutout minimizes patellar compression.
   f. Can be used in other areas of the body, such as elbow, thigh, and so on.

Hip-Knee-Ankle-Foot Orthosis (HKAFO)

1. Provides control for lower extremity joints at and above the ankle. Can consist of a hip joint and pelvic band added to a KAFO.
2. Hip joint: typically a metal hinge joint.
   a. Controls for abduction, adduction, and rotation.
   b. Controls for hip flexion when locked, typically with a drop ring lock.
3. Pelvic attachments: a leather-covered, metal pelvic band; attaches the HKAFO to the pelvis between the greater trochanter and iliac crest; adds to difficulty in donning and doffing; adds weight and increases overall energy expenditure during ambulation.

Specialized Trunk-Hip-Knee-Ankle-Foot Orthosis (THKAFO)

1. Contains a trunk band added to a HKAFO.
2. Reciprocating gait orthosis (RGO): utilizes plastic molded solid-ankle orthoses with locked knees, plastic thigh shells, a hip joint with pelvic and trunk bands; the hips are connected by steel cables, which allow for a reciprocal gait pattern (either four-point or two-point); when the patient leans on the supporting hip, it forces it into extension, while the opposite leg is pushed into flexion; allows limb advancement.

Specialized Lower Limb Devices

1. Denis Browne splint: a bar connecting two shoes that can swivel; used for correction of pes equinovarus (club foot) or developmental hip dysplasia (DDH).
2. Frejka pillow: keeps hips abducted; used for hip dysplasia or other conditions with tight adductors in young children.
3. Toronto hip abduction orthosis: abducts the hip; used in treatment of Legg-Calvé-Perthes disease.

Spinal (Trunk) Orthoses: Components/Terminology

Lumbosacral Orthosis (LSO)

1. Controls or limits lumbosacral motions.
2. Flexible LSO—corset.
   a. Uses abdominal compression to increase intra-abdominal pressure.
   b. Provides tactile reminder for postural correction.
   c. Indications: low back pain, compression of abdominal incision, respiratory assist in individual with spinal cord, sacroiliac support for pregnancy, postoperative protection, etc.
3. Rigid LSO—shell (custom or off-the-shelf).
   a. Uses three-point pressure system, intra-abdominal pressure and total contact to control flexion, extension, and lateral flexion of lumbar and sacral spinal segments.
   b. Provides tactile reminder for positioning.
   c. Trimlines/fitting:
      - Anterior: below the xiphoid process to symphysis pubis.
      - Posterior: below the inferior angle of scapula to sacro-coccygeal junction.
   d. Indications: postop protection, stenosis, low back pain, spondylolisthesis, etc.

Thoracolumbosacral Orthosis (TLSO)

1. Controls or limits thoracic and lumbosacral motions.
2. TLSO shell (custom or OTS).
   a. Uses three-point pressure system, intra-abdominal pressure, and total contact to control flexion, extension, lateral flexion, and rotation of the thoracic, lumbar, and sacral spinal segments.
   b. Trimlines/fitting:
      - Anterior: distal to the sternal notch to symphysis pubis.
      - Posterior: distal to spine of scapula to sacro-coccygeal junction.

c. Indications: postop protection, stable vertebral fracture, scoliosis (with additional thoracic pad to counter spinal curve), spinal cord injury, etc.
3. Anterior control TLSO Jewett orthosis or cruciform anterior spinal hyperextension (CASH) orthosis (both available OTS).
   a. Uses three-point pressure system and tactile reminders to control primarily flexion of thoracic and lumbar spinal segments.
   b. Fitting: sternal pad just distal to sternal notch, pubic pad just proximal to symphysis pubis, posterior pad over the thoracolumbar junction.
   c. Indications: thoracolumbar anterior vertebral compression fractures.

Cervical Orthosis (CO)

1. Soft collar.
   a. Provides minimal levels of control of cervical motion.
   b. Provides tactile reminder for postural correction.
   c. Indications: cervical pain, whiplash, cervical weakness, etc.
2. Semirigid (e.g., Miami J or Philadelphia collars):
   a. Uses three-point pressure system and tactile cues to control flexion, extension, lateral flexion, and rotation of cervical spinal segments.
   b. Trimlines/fitting:
      - Anterior: mandible to sternal notch.
      - Posterior: occiput to T1.
   c. Indications: postop protection, stable cervical vertebral injury, whiplash, etc.
3. Rigid-halo orthosis:
   a. Provides maximal control of all cervical motion with halo attachment to the skull, four uprights connect from the halo to thoracic jacket.
   b. Indications: unstable cervical vertebral fracture, spinal cord injury.
4. Minerva orthosis/cervical thoracic orthosis (CTO).
   a. Has a semi-rigid cervical collar connected to a thoracic jacket via metal uprights.
   b. Provides good control of all cervical motions.
   c. Indications: stable cervical and upper thoracic fractures and fusions.

Upper-Limb Orthoses or Splints: Components/Terminology

Goals of Upper Extremity Orthoses/Splints

1. Immobilization.
2. Protection/support.
3. Correction or prevention of deformities.
4. Substitute for weak or absent upper extremity function.
5. Serve as a base of attachment for ADL equipment.

Wrist Cock-Up Splint

1. An anterior or palmar splint that contains forearm and metacarpals. May include phalanges as well if needed for positioning.
2. Wrist can be held in neutral or in 10°–20° wrist extension.
3. For weak or absent hand strength: orthosis should support the full hand phalanges slightly flexed and with thumb in partial opposition and abduction.
4. For wrist pathologies: trim lines should be at the distal palmar crease and thenar crease to maximize hand function.
5. Used for patients with rheumatoid arthritis, fractures of carpal bones, Colles' fracture, carpal tunnel syndrome, stroke with paralysis, etc.

Thumb Spica Splint

1. A hand-based splint designed to immobilize the first carpometacarpal joint.
2. Thumb positioned in partial opposition and abduction with thumb interphalangeal joint left free for maximal function.
3. Hand-based: used for first CMC arthritis.
4. Forearm-based: used for scaphoid fracture, scaphoid-lunate instability, de Quervain's, etc.

Dorsal Wrist Splint

1. Frees the palm for feeling and grasping through use of grips that curve around over the second and fifth metacarpal heads.
2. Allows attachment of dorsal devices (i.e., rubber bands) to form a dynamic device.
3. Used for flexor tendon repairs.

Airplane Splint

1. Positions the patient's arm out to the side at 90 degrees of abduction, with elbow flexed to 90 degrees.
2. The weight of the outstretched arm is borne on a padded lateral trunk bar and iliac crest band.
3. A strap holds the device across the trunk.
4. Used to immobilize the shoulder following fracture or burn injury to prevent contracture of the axillary region.

Tenodesis Splint

1. Assists patients in use of wrist extensors to approximate the thumb and forefingers (grip) in the absence of active finger flexion.
2. Facilitates tenodesis grasp in patients with quadriplegia.

Finger Splints

1. Mallet finger: palmar DIP gutter splint to support distal phalange.
2. Boutonniere's deformity: palmar PIP gutter splint to support middle phalange.
3. Swan neck deformity: ring splints over PIP joint to prevent PIP hyperextension.

Physical Therapy Intervention

Orthotic Clinic Team

1. Physical therapist.
2. Physician.
3. Orthotist.
4. Occupational therapist.

Examination

1. Preorthotic assessment and prescription evaluate:
   a. Joint mobility.
   b. Sensation.
   c. Strength.
   d. Motor control.
   e. Functional abilities.
   f. Cognitive status.
2. Orthotic prescription considerations:
   a. Patient's abilities and needs.
      - Level of impairments, activity limitations, and participation restrictions.
      - Status: Consider whether the patient's condition is stable or progressive.
   b. Level of function, current lifestyle.
      - Consider whether the patient is going to be a community ambulator versus a household ambulator.
      - Consider recreational and work-related needs.
      - Cost vs. benefit of orthotic.
   c. Overall weight of orthotic devices vs. the strength and energy capabilities of patient. Some individuals abandon their orthoses quickly in favor of wheelchairs because of the high-energy demands of ambulating with orthoses; e.g., patients with high levels of paraplegia.
   d. Manual dexterity, mental capacity of the individual. The donning and use of devices may be too difficult or complicated for some individuals.
   e. Pressure tolerance of the skin and tissues.
   f. Use of a temporary orthosis to assess likelihood of functional independence, reduce costs; e.g., patients with high levels of paraplegia.
3. Orthotic check-out to ensure proper fit and function of the orthosis.
   a. Static assessment.
      - Ensure alignment of lower limb orthosis joints with anatomical joint axes.
      - Check skin and bony prominences for pressure intolerance; look for areas of redness that do not blanch or remain discolored after an extended time, blisters, signs of friction, etc.
   b. Dynamic assessment.
      - Assess fit of the orthosis and its effect on function during activities of daily living (ADLs) and functional mobility skills (e.g., sit-to-stand).
      - Assess fit of the orthosis and its effect on function during gait.

Orthotic Training

1. Instruct the patient in procedures for routine skin inspection and care.

> **RED FLAG:** Check for impaired sensation and areas of excessive pressure. This is important for all patients but critical for patients with impaired neurovascular status (e.g., diabetic neuropathy).

2. Ensure orthotic acceptance.
   a. Patient should clearly understand functions, limitations of an orthosis.
   b. Can use support groups to assist.
3. Teach proper application (donning/doffing) of the orthosis.
4. Teach proper use of the orthosis.
   a. Balance training.
   b. Gait training.
   c. Functional activities training.
5. Reassess fit, function, and construction of the orthosis at periodic intervals; assess habitual use of the orthosis.
6. Teach procedures for routine maintence of device.

Selected Orthotic Gait Deviations

1. Lateral trunk bending: patient leans toward the orthotic side during stance. Possible causes: KAFO medial upright too high; insufficient shoe lift; hip pain, weak or tight abductors on the orthotic side; short leg; poor balance.
2. Circumduction: during swing, leg swings out to the side in an arc. Possible causes: locked knee; excessive plantar flexion (inadequate stop, plantar flexion contractures); weak hip flexors or dorsiflexors. All of these could also cause vaulting (rising up on the sound limb to advance the orthotic limb forward).
3. Anterior trunk bending: patient leans forward during stance. Possible causes: inadequate knee lock; weak quadriceps; hip or knee flexion contracture.
4. Posterior trunk bending: patient leans backward during stance. Possible causes: inadequate hip lock; weak gluteus maximus; knee ankylosis.
5. Hyperextended knee: excessive extension during stance. Possible causes: inadequate plantar flexion stop; inadequate knee lock; poor fit of calf band (too deep); weak quadriceps; loose knee ligaments or extensor spasticity; pes equinus.
6. Knee instability: excessive knee flexion during stance. Possible causes: inadequate dorsiflexion stop; inadequate knee lock; knee and/or hip flexion contracture; weak quadriceps or insufficient knee lock; knee pain.

7. Foot slap: foot hits the ground during early stance. Possible causes: inadequate dorsiflexor assist; inadequate plantarflexor stop; weak dorsiflexors.
8. Toes first: on-toes posture during stance. Possible causes: inadequate dorsiflexor assist; inadequate plantarflexor stop; inadequate heel lift; heel pain, extensor spasticity; pes equinus; short leg.
9. Flat foot: contact with entire foot. Possible causes: inadequate longitudinal arch support; pes planus.
10. Pronation: excessive medial foot contact during stance, valgus position of calcaneus. Possible causes: transverse plane malalignment; weak invertors; pes valgus; spasticity; genu valgum.
11. Supination: excessive lateral foot contact during stance, varus position of the calcaneus. Possible causes: transverse plane malalignment; weak evertors; pes varus; genu varum.
12. Excessive stance width: patient stands or walks with a wide base of support. Possible causes: KAFO height of medial upright too high; HKAFO hip joint aligned in excessive abduction; knee is locked; abduction contracture; poor balance; sound limb is too short.

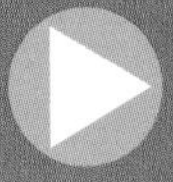

Adhesive Taping

General Concepts

Purpose
1. Limit ROM of specific joints.
2. Support injured body segment.
3. Secure protective devices such as felt, foam, gel, or plastic padding, orthoplast, or plastazote.
4. Keep dressings and bandages in place and secure.
5. Preventive support for a joint that is at risk.
6. Realign position and reduce pain; e.g., McConnell treatment for patellofemoral pain.
7. May enhance proprioception.
8. Elastic therapeutic tape (e.g., Kinesio tape) is an acrylic adhesive backed with an elastic strip. It is used with athletes and others with impairments ostensibly to alleviate pain, enhance performance, relax muscles, support muscles, and reduce inflammation. Research has shown limited evidence of benefit except for reducing pain.

Preparation
1. Part to be taped should be properly positioned and supported.
2. Select appropriate type and width of tape.
3. Body hair should be shaved, skin should be clean. Foam underwrap or stockinet may be used.
4. Lubricated pads should be placed over areas of potential blister formation from friction, e.g.; heel and lace-area pads on the foot.
5. Occlusive dressings should be applied over wounds or skin conditions to be covered by the tape.
6. Skin adherent such as benzoin should be applied to increase adhesion of the tape and to aid in toughening the skin to decrease irritation.

Application
1. If the part has not been previously injured, it should be taped in a neutral position.
2. Injured ligaments should be held in a shortened position.
   a. Lateral or inversion ankle sprains should be taped in an everted position.
   b. Tape should follow body contours and be applied primarily from medial to lateral in the case of an inversion sprain.
3. Tape should be applied with even pressure, and with overlap of previous tape strip by one-half.
4. Circular strapping should be applied very cautiously due to potential circulatory compromise.
5. Avoid creases and folds.
6. If tape is too tight, adjust by removing or modifying strips or reapply.
7. Elastic therapeutic tape is applied in a variety of configurations according to manufacturer's specifications.

Complications

RED FLAGS:
- Allergic reactions to the tape.
- Skin irritation.
- Reduced circulation.
- If tape is too tight, it might compromise the ability of the patient to perform the skill intended.
- Tape may lose its effectiveness in an hour or so, and may need to be reapplied.

Prosthetics

General Concepts

Prosthesis

1. A replacement of a body part with an artificial device; an artificial limb.

Levels of Amputation

1. Transmetatarsal amputation: partial foot amputation.
2. Ankle disarticulation (Syme's): amputation through the ankle joint; heel pad is preserved and attached to distal end of tibia for weight-bearing.
3. Transtibial amputation: below-knee (BK) amputation; ideally, 20%–50% of the tibial length is spared; short transtibial is <20% of tibial length.
4. Knee disarticulation: amputation through the knee joint; femur is intact.
5. Transfemoral amputation: above-knee (AK) amputation; ideally 35%–60% of the femoral length is spared; short transfemoral is <35% of femoral length.
6. Hip disarticulation: amputation of entire lower limb, pelvis is preserved.
7. Hemipelvectomy: amputation of entire lower limb, lower half of the pelvis is resected.
8. Hemicorporectomy: amputation of both lower limbs and pelvis below L4, L5 level.
9. Transradial amputation: below-elbow (BE) amputation.
10. Elbow disarticulation: amputation through the elbow joint.
11. Transhumeral amputation: above-elbow (AE) amputation.
12. Shoulder disarticulation: amputation through the shoulder joint.

Components

1. All prosthetic devices contain a socket and terminal device with varying components in between.
2. Sockets are custom-molded to the residual limb; total contact is desired, with the load distributed to all tissues; assists in circulation and provides maximal sensory feedback.
   a. Functions to:
      - Contain the residual tissues.
      - Provide a means to suspend the prosthetic limb.
      - Transfer forces from the prosthesis to the residual limb.

   b. Selective loading: pressure-tolerant areas are built up to increase loading, while pressure-sensitive areas are relieved to decrease loading (i.e., relief for bony prominences, nerves, and tendons).

   c. Liners.
      - Used in every suspension system except anatomical suction.
      - Comprised of silicone or gels to protect the residual limb and minimize the shear forces between the socket and the skin.

   d. Socks.
      - Socks are used to accommodate changes in volume in the residual limb.
      - Increase the number of sock plies when limb volume is decreased.
      - Decrease the number of sock plies when limb volume is increased.
      - Excessive thickness of socks (>15 ply) can alter fit and weight-bearing ability of the socket.
3. Terminal device (TD).
   a. Provides an interface between the amputee's prosthesis with the external environment.
   b. Lower-limb prosthesis: TD is a foot.
   c. Upper-limb prosthesis: TD is a hook or hand.

Lower-Limb Prosthetics (LLPs)

Partial-Foot Prosthesis

1. Plastic foot replacement: restores foot length, protects amputated stump.
2. Function may be assisted by the addition of a rocker bottom or plastic calf shell.

Transtibial (Below Knee) Prosthesis

1. Foot-ankle assembly.
   a. Functions to:
      - Absorb shock at heel strike.
      - Plantarflex in early stance to achieve foot flat.
      - Dorsiflexion during mid- and terminal stance to store energy.
      - Plantarflexion in pre-swing to push-off.
      - Provide a cosmetic replacement of the foot.

   b. Solid ankle cushion heel (SACH) foot.
      - The most commonly prescribed foot; non-articulated; contains an energy-absorbing cushion heel and internal wooden keel that limits sagittal plane motion, primarily to plantarflexion.
      - Permits a very small amount of mediolateral (frontal plane) and transverse plane motion.
      - Assists in hyperextension of knee (knee stability) during stance.
      - Used primarily in youth and more sedentary individuals.

c. Single axis foot.
- Articulated foot with the lower shank.
- Motion is controlled by anterior and posterior rubber bumpers that limit dorsiflexion and plantarflexion.
- More stable (permits only sagittal plane motion); promotes knee stability in stance phase.

d. Multi-axis foot.
- Articulated foot with the lower shank.
- Allows plantarflexion, dorsiflexion, inversion, and eversion to conform to uneven surfaces.
- Not used often due to the weight of the device.
- Indicated for medium to highly active individuals but has poor shock absorption and energy return.

e. Energy storing foot.
- Dynamic foot for active/community ambulators.
- Leaf-spring shank (with cosmetic foot cover) used with an endoskeletal prosthesis; the long band of carbon fiber originates directly from the shank; stores energy in early stance for later use during push-off.
- Decreased energy consumption due to smoother gait pattern and energy return during terminal stance and preswing and light weight.
- Some models may include shock absorption or rotational components.

f. Microprocessor foot.
- Microcomputer control of dorsiflexion and plantarflexion based on the position of the foot.
- Improves ability to ambulate on inclines, stairs, and uneven surfaces.
- Not widely used due to weight, maintenance, and cost.

2. Shank.

a. Functions to:
- Provide leg length and shape.
- Connect and transmit weight from socket to foot.

b. Exoskeletal: conventional components, usually made of wood with a plastic laminated finish; colored for cosmesis; durable.

c. Endoskeletal: contains a central metal shank (aluminum, titanium, and other high-strength alloys), may be covered by soft foam and external stocking for cosmesis; modular components allow for increased ease of prosthetic adjustment.

3. Socket.

a. PTB (patellar tendon-bearing) socket: a total contact socket that allows for moderate loading over the area of the patellar tendon.

b. Pressure-sensitive areas of the typical transtibial residual limb include:
- Anterior tibia condyle.
- Anterior tibial crest.
- Fibular head and neck.
- Fibular nerve.
- Distal cut end of tibia and fibula.

c. Pressure-tolerant areas of the typical transtibial residual limb include:
- Medial tibial plateau.
- Tibial and fibular shafts.
- Distal end (rarely, may be sensitive).
- Gastrocnemius muscles.

d. TSB (total surface bearing) socket: total contact socket with lower profile and rounder shape than PTB socket for a more intimate fit.
- Weight is borne equally throughout the socket on bones and soft tissues.
- Must use a gel-type liner for suspension and to distribute pressures.

4. Suspension.

a. Suction.
- Silicone liners rolled over the residual limb for increased suspension and proprioception.
- Uses either a pin lock or cuff to attach/seal to socket.

b. Supracondylar (SC) socket suspension: medial and lateral walls of the socket extend up and over the femoral condyles; a removable medial wedge assists in donning and removal; provides increased mediolateral stability for very short residual limbs.

c. External suspension sleeve: neoprene type sleeve that covers the proximal socket and distal thigh to suspend the limb.
- May be used alone or in conjunction with other suspension options.

Transfemoral (Above-Knee) Prosthesis

1. Knee unit (ranked by stability).

a. Manual locking knee.
- Lock is engaged for standing and walking; manually unlocked for sitting.
- Maximal stability for individuals with significant weakness in the lower extremity.
- Difficulty with clearance of the leg during swing can be controlled by shortening the total prosthetic limb length.

b. Microprocessor/Computerized knee.
- Knee stability in stance and ability to flex in swing are controlled electronically.
- Prevents knee from buckling when weighted.
- Adapts swing resistance automatically to allow variable gait speeds.
- Can be used to ascend and descend stairs step-over-step.

c. Single axis/weight activated stance control.
- Permits knee motions to occur around a fixed axis.

- Weight-activated friction braking increases friction at midstance to prevent knee flexion, but permits smooth knee motion through the rest of the gait cycle.
- Requires extension assist: internal coiled spring that assists in terminal knee extension during late swing.

d. Polycentric systems (multiple axes): changing axis of motion allows for adjustments to the center of knee rotation.
- Stable in stance phase due to knee center position.

e. Hydraulic knee units (fluid-controlled) or pneumatic knee units (air-controlled): adjusts resistance dynamically to the individual's walking speed.
- Appropriate for younger, more active individuals.

f. Single axis/constant friction.
- Continuous resistance is provided by a clamp that acts on the knee mechanism.
- Least stable knee as friction does not increase in stance phase; must have good hip extensor strength to promote knee extension in midstance.

2. Socket.
   a. Ischial containment socket.
   - Triangular-shaped socket that holds the femur in an adducted position.
   - Lateral wall of socket extends more proximally to provide lateral stability and to ensure the ischial tuberosity is seated within the socket for a more intimate fit.

   b. Quadrilateral socket.
   - Rectangular socket with a broad horizontal posterior shelf for seating of the ischial tuberosity and gluteals.
   - The medial wall is the same height as the posterior wall, while the anterior and lateral walls are 2½–3 inches higher.
   - A posterior directed force is provided by the anterior and lateral walls to ensure proper seating.
   - Reliefs are provided for the adductor longus tendon, hamstring tendons, sciatic nerve, gluteus maximus, and rectus femoris.
3. Suspension.
   a. Anatomical suction suspension.
   - Suction is employed to maximize contact and suspension; air is pumped out through a one-way air release valve located at the socket's bottom.
   - Good proprioception due to direct skin to socket total contact.

   b. Silicone suction suspension.
   - Silicone liner with either a locking pin and/or cuff is used to maintain the prosthesis on the limb.
   - Reduces shear within the socket and provides pressure relief for the residual limb to increase comfort.

   c. TES (Total Elastic Suspension).
   - Neoprene belt is applied to prosthesis and wraps around the pelvis to anchor the prosthesis on the residual limb. Can be used alone or in conjunction with other methods.
   - Adjustable and readily accommodates to volume changes.
   - May cause pistoning of the residual limb in the socket when it is the sole type of suspension.

   d. Silesian belt.
   - Strap that anchors the prosthesis by reaching around the pelvis (below iliac crest).
   - Able to control rotation in the transverse plane.
   - Used as an auxiliary suspension.
   - Poor cosmesis.

   e. Hinge suspension.
   - Hinged hip joint attached to a metal/leather pelvic band, anchored around the pelvis.
   - Adds control for medial/lateral stability of hip (rotation, abduction/adduction).
   - Reduces Trendelenburg gait deviation, but adds extra weight and bulk.

Knee Disarticulation Prosthesis

1. Functional, allows weight-bearing on the distal end of the femur.
2. Problems with cosmesis, added thigh length with the knee joint attached, especially noticeable in sitting.
3. Lower shank is shortened to balance leg length in standing.

Hip Disarticulation Prosthesis

1. Socket is molded to accommodate the pelvis; weight-bearing occurs on ischial seat, iliac crests.
2. Endoskeletal components frequently used, decreases weight of prosthesis.
3. Stability achieved with hip extension aid; posterior placement of knee joint with anterior placement of the hip joint to the weight-bearing line.

Immediate Postoperative Prosthesis

1. Temporary plastic or plaster of Paris socket with the capability to attach a foot and pylon.
2. Advantages.
   a. Allows early, limited weight-bearing ambulation within days of surgery.
   b. Limits postoperative sequelae: edema, postoperative pain.
   c. Enhances wound healing.
   d. Allows for earlier fit of permanent prosthesis.
3. Limitations.
   a. Requires skilled application and close monitoring.
   b. Does not allow for daily wound inspection; contraindicated for older patients with cardiovascular compromise and increased risk for wounds.

Upper-Limb Prosthetics (ULPs)

Below Elbow (BE) Prosthesis

1. Contains terminal device (TD), wrist joint, and forearm socket.

Above Elbow (AE) Prosthesis

1. Contains a terminal device (TD), wrist device, elbow joint, and upper arm socket.

Types of UE Prostheses

1. Conventional/body-powered system.
   a. Power for voluntary opening of the TD (hook or hand) is transmitted by a cable from a figure-of-eight shoulder harness to the TD.
   b. Rubber bands are used for closure and prehensile strength.
   c. Forearm rotation is done by manual prepositioning of the TD through the wrist joint.

Movement Control

1. BE prosthesis: bilateral scapular abduction, depression, or ipsilateral flexion of the humerus is used to pull on the cable and force opening of the hook.
2. AE prosthesis (dual control system): the same motions can be used to flex the elbow in the AE prosthesis; when the elbow is locked out, the forces are then transmitted to operate the TD.

Myoelectric System

1. Utilizes surface electrical activity of various muscles (e.g., wrist flexors/extensors, scapular, and pectoral muscles).
2. Small electric motors (battery-powered) operate the TD. The intensity of the signal from the muscle allows for different functions and graded power output to the TD.
   a. Benefits: Improves ease of function, prehensile strength, and requires no harnessing.
   b. Disadvantages: Adds weight, increased maintenance, cost.

Physical Therapy Intervention

Prosthetic Clinic Team

1. Physical therapist.
2. Physician.
3. Prosthetist.
4. Occupational therapist.

Preprosthetic Management

1. Preprescription examination.
   a. Skin: inspect incision for healing; scar tissue; other lesions.
   b. Residual limb.
      - Circumference measurements: check for edema.
      - Length: bone, soft tissue length.
      - Shape: should be cylindrical or conical; check for abnormalities (i.e., bulbous end, dog ears, adductor roll).
   c. Vascular status of sound limb, residual limb: examine pulses, color, temperature, trophic changes, pain/intermittent claudication.
   d. AROM and PROM: examine for contractures that might interfere with prosthetic prescription (e.g., hip and knee flexion contractures are most common).
   e. Sensation.
      - Assess proprioception, visual and vestibular function, and its contributions to balance.
      - Phantom limb sensation: a feeling of pressure or paresthesia as if coming from the amputated limb. Sensations are normal, not painful; may last for the lifetime of the individual.
      - Phantom pain: an intense pain felt to be emanating from the amputated limb; potentially interfering with rehabilitation and contributing to activity limitations and participation restrictions.
   f. Strength: examine strength of residual limb as tolerated; strength of the sound limb, trunk, and upper extremities needed for function. Hip extension and abduction strength are critical for gait.
   g. Functional status.
      - Functional mobility skills: bed mobility, transfers, wheelchair use.
      - Activities of daily living: basic, instrumental (use of telephone, shopping, etc.).
   h. Cardiopulmonary function, endurance.
      - The shorter the residual limb, the greater the energy demands; i.e., oxygen consumption is increased 65% over normal walking in the patient with transfemoral amputation.
      - Functional capacity further limited by concomitant diseases (e.g., cardiovascular disease, diabetes), individual fitness level, pain.
   i. Neurologic factors.
      - Cognitive function.
      - Check for neuropathy.
      - Check for neuroma: an abnormal growth of axons that occurs in the residual limb after amputation.
   j. Psychosocial factors: motivation, adjustment and acceptance, availability of support systems.
2. Preprosthetic training: goals and interventions.
   a. Ideally begins preoperatively and continues postoperatively.
   b. Facilitate psychological acceptance.
   c. Postoperative dressings: applied to the residual limb; helps to limit edema, accelerate healing,

reduce postoperative pain, and shape the residual limb.
- Elastic wraps: flexible, soft bandaging, inexpensive; requires frequent reapplication, with pressure greatest distal to proximal; if wraps are allowed to loosen, may have problems with edema control; avoid circular wrapping, which produces a tourniquet effect.
- Stump shrinkers: flexible, soft, inexpensive, readily available in different sizes.
- Semirigid dressings: Unna paste dressing (zinc oxide, gelatin, glycerin, and calamine); applied in the operating room.
- Rigid dressings: plaster of Paris dressing; applied in the operating room; a component of immediate postoperative fitting; allows for edema reduction and early ambulation with a temporary prosthesis (pylon and foot).

d. Desensitizing activities: pressure, rubbing, stroking, bandaging of the residual limb.
e. Hygiene: inspection and care of the residual limb.

> **RED FLAGS:** Positioning for prevention of contracture; positions to avoid include:
>
> Transtibial: prolonged flexion and external rotation at the hip, knee flexion; counteract with use of a posterior board to keep knee straight while in wheelchair; regularly scheduled time in prone-lying.
>
> Transfemoral: flexion, abduction, external rotation of hip; counteract with regularly scheduled time in prone-lying time.

f. Flexibility exercises.
- Full AROM and PROM, active stretching, especially in hip and knee extension on the involved extremity.
- Flexibility of sound limb and trunk.

g. Utilize a general strengthening exercise program with special emphasis on:
- Hip extensors: especially for the patient with transfemoral amputation.
- Knee extensors: the patient with transtibial amputation.
- Hip abductors: for stance phase pelvic stability.
- Dynamic exercises: utilize gravity and body weight to provide resistance during functional mat activities.

h. Functional mobility training.
- Sit-to-stand transitions, transfers, standing.
- Wheelchair independence.
- Hopping on the sound limb; mobility in the seated position; i.e., scooting for patients with bilateral transfemoral amputation.
- Early walking with crutches or walker; consider early ambulation with a temporary prosthesis.

i. Bilateral lower-extremity amputation.
- Wheelchair training important. Will be primary means of locomotion, especially early on.
- Prolonged wheelchair time increases likelihood of hip and knee flexion contractures; prone positioning program is important.
- Energy expenditure during prosthetic ambulation is increased dramatically; a trial period with temporary prostheses can be used to evaluate ambulation potential with permanent prostheses.
- Bilateral transfemoral amputation: ambulation usually requires walker; loss of lower-extremity proprioception increases balance difficulties; loss of knee extensor function will result in significant later difficulties with stair-climbing, curbs, stepping.
- Bilateral transfemoral amputation modification: patients can be fitted with shortened prostheses (stubbies) consisting of a socket and foot component (modified rocker feet) with no knee joints; increases ease of use, and function can be useful for in-home function.

Prosthetic Management

1. Prosthetic check-out.
   a. Prosthesis: delivered as ordered, proper functioning; inspect both on and off the patient.
   b. Static assessment.
   - Alignment and comfort in standing, sitting.
   - Leg length discrepancy: pelvis level.
   - Fit and suspension: pistoning when pelvis is lifted.

   c. Dynamic assessment.
   - Sit-to-stand transitions.
   - Gait: smooth, safe gait, absence of significant gait deviations; gait speeds normally decrease to reduce high levels of energy expenditure.
   - Stairs and inclines.

> **RED FLAGS:** Inspection of the residual limb with the prosthesis off.
>
> Proper loading: transient redness is to be expected in pressure-tolerant areas after prosthetic use.
>
> No redness should be seen in pressure-sensitive areas.

2. Prosthetic training: goals and interventions.
   a. Donning and doffing of the prosthesis: training specific to type of socket and type of suspension.
   b. Strengthening, flexibility exercises.
   - Emphasis on hip extension and knee extension (transtibial) with the prosthesis on.

c. Balance and coordination.
   - Symmetrical stance and weight-bearing on prosthetic limb.
   - Weight shifting to limits of stability.
   - Dynamic balance control; e.g., stepping activities.

d. Gait training.
   - Conventional training: focus on smooth weight transfer from sound limb to prosthetic limb, continuous movement sequence.
   - Feedback training: use of mirrors, tactile cues to restore typical gait pattern and facilitate weight-bearing.
   - Start training in parallel bars.
   - Initially utilize assistive devices (walker/crutches to cane) and progress to independent ambulation as the ability to shift weight to the prosthesis and safety allow.

e. Functional activities training: including transfers, stairs, curbs, ramps, down and up from floor, recreational activities, etc.

f. Regular inspection and maintenance of the prosthesis.

g. Hygiene: care of stump socks, interior of the socket.

h. Facilitate prosthetic acceptance.

Selected Prosthetic Gait Deviations

1. Transfemoral amputation.
   a. Circumduction: the prosthesis swings out to the side in an arc. Possible causes: a long prosthesis, locked knee, small or loose socket, inadequate suspension, foot plantar flexed, abduction contracture, poor knee control.
   b. Abducted gait: prosthesis is laterally displaced to the side. Possible causes: crotch or medial wall discomfort, long prosthesis, low lateral wall or malalignment, tight hip abductors.
   c. Vaulting: the patient rises up on the sound limb to swing the prosthesis through. Possible causes: prosthesis too long, inadequate suspension, socket too small, prosthetic foot set in too much plantarflexion, too little knee flexion.
   d. Lateral trunk bending during stance: the trunk bends toward the prosthetic side. Possible causes: low lateral wall, short prosthesis, high medial wall, weak abductors, abductor contracture, hip pain, short amputation limb.
   e. Forward flexion during stance: the trunk bends forward. Possible causes: unstable knee unit, short ambulatory aids, hip flexion contracture.
   f. Lumbar lordosis during stance: exaggeration of the lumbar curve. Possible causes: insufficient support from anterior or posterior walls, painful ischial weight-bearing, hip flexion contracture, weak hip extensors or abdominals.
   g. High heel rise: during early swing, the heel rises excessively. Possible causes: inadequate knee friction, too little tension in the extension aid.
   h. Terminal swing impact: the prosthesis comes to a sudden stop as the knee extends during late swing. Possible causes: insufficient knee friction or too much tension in the extension aid; patient fears that the knee will buckle; forceful hip flexion.
   i. Swing phase whips: at toe-off, the heel moves either medially or laterally. Possible causes: socket is rotated, knee bolt is rotated, foot is malaligned.
   j. Foot rotation at heel strike: as the heel contacts the ground, the foot rotates laterally, sometimes with vibratory motion. Possible causes: foot is malaligned, stiff heel cushion, or plantar flexion bumper.
   k. Foot slap: excessive plantar flexion at heel strike. Possible cause: heel cushion or plantar flexion bumper is too soft.
   l. Uneven step length: patient favors sound limb and limits weight-bearing time on the prosthetic limb. Possible causes: socket discomfort or poor alignment; hip flexion contracture or hip instability, patient habit, and need for focused gait training.

2. Transtibial amputation.
   a. Excessive knee flexion during stance. Possible causes: socket may be aligned too far forward or tilted anteriorly; plantar flexion bumper is too hard and limits plantar flexion; high heel shoes; knee flexion contracture or weak quadriceps.
   b. Inadequate knee flexion during stance. Possible causes: socket may be aligned too far back or tilted posteriorly; plantar flexion bumper or heel cushion too soft; low heel shoes; anterodistal discomfort, weak quadriceps.
   c. Lateral thrust at midstance. Possible cause: foot is inset too much.
   d. Medial thrust at midstance. Possible cause: foot is outset too much.
   e. Drop off or premature knee flexion in late stance. Possible causes: socket is set too far forward or excessively flexed; dorsiflexion bumper is too soft, resulting in excess dorsiflexion of the foot; prosthetic foot keel too short; knee flexion contracture.
   f. Delayed knee flexion during late stance: patient feels as though walking "uphill." Possible causes: socket is set too far back or lacks sufficient flexion; dorsiflexion bumper is too stiff, causing excess plantar flexion; prosthetic foot keel too long.

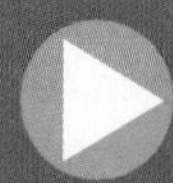

Wheelchairs

Components

Postural Support System

1. Seating.
   a. Sling seat: standard on wheelchairs. Hips tend to slide forward, thighs tend to adduct and internally rotate. Reinforces poor pelvic position (posterior pelvic tilt).
   b. Insert or contour seat creates a stable, firm sitting surface; made of wood or plastic, padded with foam.
      - Improves pelvic position (neutral pelvic position).
      - Reduces the tendency for the patient to slide forward or sit with a posterior pelvic tilt (sacral sitting).
   c. Seat cushion: distributes weight-bearing pressures. Assists in preventing decubitus ulcers in patients with decreased sensation, prolongs wheelchair sitting times.
      - Pressure-relieving, contoured foam cushion: uses dense, layered foam; accommodates moderate to severe postural deformity. Easy for caregivers to reposition patients, low maintenance. May interfere with slide transfers.
      - Pressure-relieving fluid/gel or combination cushion (fluid/gel plus foam). Can be custom-molded. Accommodates moderate to severe postural deformity. Easy for caregivers to reposition patients. Requires some maintenance, heavier, more expensive.
      - Pressure-relieving air cushion. Accommodates moderate to severe postural deformity. Lightweight, improved pressure distribution. Expensive, base may be unstable for some patients. Requires continuous maintenance.
   d. Adds to measurements to determine back height.

> **RED FLAG:** Pressure relief activities are required, typically every 15–20 minutes (e.g., for the patient with SCI). Examples include wheelchair push-ups, lateral or forward leaning; can also use tilt-in-space or reclining wheelchair to change position.

2. Back: support to the mid-scapular region is provided by most standard sling-back wheelchairs.
   a. Lower back height may increase functional mobility, i.e., sports chairs; may also increase back strain.
   b. High back height may be necessary for patients with poor trunk stability or with extensor spasms.
   c. Insert or contour backs: improve trunk extension and overall upright alignment.
   d. Lateral trunk supports: improve trunk alignment for patients with scoliosis, poor trunk stability.
3. Armrests.
   a. Full-length or desk length; desk length facilitates proximity to a desk or table but can inhibit use during sit to stand transitions.
   b. Fixed-height or adjustable height.
   c. Removable armrests: facilitate transfers.
   d. Wraparound (space saver) armrests: reduce the overall width of the chair by 1½ inches.
   e. Upper extremity support surface (trays or troughs) can be secured to the armrests; provides additional postural assistance for patients with decreased use of upper extremities, allows for ADL activities such as using utensils to feed oneself.
4. Leg rests.
   a. Fixed or swing.
   b. Swing-away, detachable: facilitates ease in transfers, front approach to wheelchair when ambulating.
   c. Elevating: indicated for LE edema control, postural support; contraindicated for patients with knee flexor (hamstring) hypertonicity or tightness.
5. Footrests.
   a. Footplates: provide a resting base for feet, feet are neutral with knees flexed to 90°; footplates can be raised or removed to facilitate transfers.
   b. Heel loops: help maintain foot position, prevent posterior sliding of the foot.
   c. Straps (ankle, calf): can be added to stabilize the feet on the foot plates.

Wheeled Mobility Base

1. Frame.
   a. Fixed or folding.
      - Folding facilitates mobility in the community, ease of storage.
      - Rigid frame facilitates stroke efficiency; increases distance per stroke.
   b. Frames available in different weights.
      - In general, the lighter the weight of the frame, the greater the ease of use.
      - Level of expected activity and environment should be considered when deciding on frame construction.

2. Wheels, hand rims.
   a. Casters: small front wheels, typically 3 to 8 inches in diameter.
   b. Drive wheels: large rear wheels used for propulsion; outer rims allow for hand grip and propulsion.
      - Projections may be attached to the rims (vertical, oblique, or horizontal) to facilitate propulsion in patients with poor handgrip, e.g., quadriplegia; horizontal or oblique projections widen the chair and may limit maneuvering in the home.
      - Friction rims/leather gloves: increase handgrip friction, ease of propulsion in patients with poor handgrip.
      - Standard spoke and mag wheels available. Mag wheels are heavier but require less maintenance.
3. Tires.
   a. Standard hard rubber tires: durable, low maintenance, indoor only.
   b. Pneumatic (air-filled) tires: provide a smoother ride, increased shock absorption; require more maintenance.
   c. Flat free insert tires: nonpneumatic, foam-filled tubes inserted in tires to decrease maintenance.
4. Brakes.
   a. Most brakes consist of a lever system with a cam.
   b. Brakes must be engaged for all transfers in and out of chair.
   c. Extensions may be added to increase ease in both locking and unlocking; e.g., for upper extremity weakness, arthritis.
5. Additional attachments.
   a. Seat belts (pelvic positioner): belt should grasp over the pelvis at a 45° angle to the seat.
   b. Seat positioners: can use lateral positioners at the hip and knee or medial thigh support (abductor pommel) to maintain neutral alignment of the hips and knees; a seat wedge or tilt-in-space chair can be used to maintain neutral hip position and control for extensor spasms or thrusting.
   c. Seat back positioners: can add lateral trunk positioners to maintain alignment, control for scoliosis.
   d. Antitipping device: a posterior extension attached to the lower horizontal supports, prevents tipping backward in the chair; also limits going up curbs or over door sills.
   e. Hill-holder device: a mechanical brake that allows the chair to go forward, but automatically brakes when the chair goes in reverse; useful for patients who are not able to ascend a long ramp or hill without a rest.

Specialized Wheelchairs

1. Reclining back: indicated for patients who are unable to independently maintain upright sitting position.
   a. Reclining wheelchairs include an extended back and typically elevating leg rests; head and trunk supports may also be added.
   b. Electric reclining back helps to redistribute weight-bearing if patient cannot do active push-ups or pressure-relief maneuvers.
2. Tilt-in-space: motorized; entire seat and back may be tipped backward (normal seat to back angle is maintained); indicated for patients with extensor spasms that may throw the patient out of the chair, or for pressure relief.
3. One-arm drive: drive mechanisms are located on one wheel, usually with two outer rims (or by push lever); patient propels the wheelchair by pushing on both rims (or lever with one hand); difficult for some patients to use, e.g., patients with left hemiplegia, cognitive/perceptual impairments.
4. Hemiplegic chair (hemi chair): designed to be low to the ground, allowing propulsion with the noninvolved upper and lower extremities.
5. Amputee chair: wheelchair is modified by placing the drive wheels posterior to the vertical back supports (2 inches backward); increases the length of the base of support and posterior stability; prescribed for patients with bilateral lower-extremity amputations, whose center of gravity is now located more posterior when seated in the wheelchair.
6. Powered wheelchair: utilizes a power source (battery) to propel the wheelchair; prescribed for patients who are not capable of self-propulsion or who have very low endurance.
   a. Microprocessors allow the control of the wheelchair to be adapted to various controls; i.e., joystick, head controls.
   b. Proportional drives: changes in pressure on the control result in directly corresponding changes in speeds.
   c. Microswitching systems: speed is preset; controls turn system on and off; i.e., sip-n-puff tubes for individuals with quadriplegia.
7. Bariatric wheelchair: heavy-duty, extra-wide wheelchair designed to assist mobility in individuals who are obese.
   a. Selection based on patient characteristics, safety, and function.
   b. The bariatric client has a center of body mass that is positioned several inches forward compared to the normal-sized person.
      - In order to ensure wheelchair stability, the rear axle is displaced forward compared to the standard wheelchair.

- This forward position allows for a more efficient arm push (full-arm stroke with less wrist extension).

c. Bariatric wheelchair can be ordered with special adaptations.
- Hard tires versus pneumatic tires for increased durability.
- Adjustable backrest to accommodate excessive posterior bulk.
- Reclining wheelchair to accommodate excessive anterior bulk, cardiorespiratory compromise (e.g., orthostatic hypotension).
- Power application attached to a heavy-duty wheelchair to accommodate excessive fatigue.

8. Sports wheelchair: variable; generally includes lightweight, solid frame, low seat, low back, seat that accommodates a tucked position, leg straps, slanted drive wheels, small push rims.

Wheelchair Measurements

General Concepts

1. Overall, the size of the wheelchair must be proportional to the size of the patient and take into account the demands of expected use and the environment in which the chair will be used.
2. Assessments should be taken with the patient on a firm surface (seated or supine).

Six Key Measurements

1. Seat width.
   a. Measurement on the patient: width of the hips at the widest part.
   b. Chair measurement: add 2 inches to the patient's measurement.
   c. Potential problems.
   - Excessive width of the wheelchair will result in added difficulties in reaching the drive wheels and propelling the chair.
   - A wheelchair that is too narrow will result in pressure/discomfort on the lateral pelvis and thighs; lateral space should allow for changes in the thickness of clothing.

   d. The bariatric client with a pear shape will have increased gluteal femoral weight distribution. Measurement should consider the widest portion of the seated position (e.g., at the forward edge of the seated position). Also consider room for weight-shifting maneuvers for pressure relief, and possible use of lift devices.
2. Seat depth.
   a. Measurement on the patient: posterior buttock to the posterior aspect of the lower leg in the popliteal fossa.
   b. Chair measurement: subtract 2–3 inches from the patient's measurement.
   c. Potential problems.
   - Seat depth that is too short fails to support the thigh and decreases surface area to distribute forces.
   - Seat depth that is too long may compromise posterior knee circulation or result in a kyphotic posture, posterior tilting of pelvis, and sacral sitting.
3. Leg length/seat to footplate length.
   a. Measurement on the patient: from the bottom of the shoe (customary footwear) to just below the thigh in the popliteal fossa; when a seat cushion is used, the height must be added from the patient's measurement.
   b. Potential problems.
   - Excessive leg length will encourage sacral sitting and sliding forward in the chair.
   - Length that is too short will create uneven weight distribution on thigh and excessive weight on the ischial seat.
4. Seat height.
   a. No patient measurement.
   b. Chair measurement: minimum clearance between the floor and the footplate is 2 inches, measured from the lowest point on the bottom of the footplate.
5. Armrest height (hanging elbow height).
   a. Measurement on the patient: from the seat platform to just below the elbow held at 90° with the shoulder in neutral position.
   b. Chair measurement: add 1 inch to the patient's hanging elbow measurement.
   c. Potential problems.
   - Armrests that are too high will cause shoulder elevation.
   - Armrests that are too low will encourage leaning forward or laterally.
6. Back height: Height will vary depending upon the amount of support the patient needs.
   a. Measurement on the patient: from the seat platform to the lower angle of the scapula, mid-scapula, top of shoulder, based on the degree of support desired.
   b. If the patient plans to use a seat cushion, the height of the cushion must be added to the patient's measurement.

Table 12-1

Standard Wheelchair Dimensions (in Inches)

CHAIR STYLE	SEAT WIDTH	SEAT DEPTH	SEAT HEIGHT
Adult	18	16	20
Narrow adult	16	16	20
Slim adult	14	16	20
Hemi/low seat			17.5
Junior	16	16	18.5
Child	14	11.5	18.75
Tiny tot	12	11.5	19.5

c. Potential problems.
- Added back height may increase difficulty in getting the chair into a car or van.
- Added back height may also prevent the patient from hooking onto the push handle for stabilization and weight relief; e.g., the patient with quadriplegia.

Standard Dimensions (See Table 12-1)

1. Custom-made wheelchairs add significantly to the cost of a wheelchair.
2. Whenever possible, patients should be matched to standardized chairs.

Wheelchair Training

Basic Instruction

1. Many first-time users require instruction in use and care of a wheelchair.
2. Instruct in good sitting posture and pressure relief.
   a. Instruct in use of wheelchair cushion: care and maintenance, schedule of use (whenever sitting); limitations of cushion.
   b. Instruct in periodic pressure reliefs: arm push-ups; weight shifts—leaning to one side, then other.

Wheelchair Propulsion

1. Instruct in manual wheelchair propulsion.
   a. Both arms on drive (push) wheels, one arm on drive wheel/one foot pulls diagonally across floor under chair (e.g., the patient with hemiplegia), or one arm (one-arm drive, both outer rims located on one side).
   b. Propulsion: forward/backward, flat surfaces, uneven surfaces.
   c. Turning: pushing harder with one hand than other; sharp turning: pull one wheel backward while pushing other wheel forward.
   d. Negotiation of obstacles.
2. Power chair training: focus on driving skill and safety; instruct in use of switches (on/off, turns), joystick; maneuverability, safe stopping.

Wheelchair Management

1. Instruct in use of wheel locks (brakes), foot supports (foot plate, leg rest), elevation of leg rests, and armrest.
2. Instruct in routine maintenance of wheelchair; normal cleaning and maintenance, power chair (battery) maintenance.

Community Mobility

1. Ramps.
   a. Ascending: forward lean of head and trunk, use shorter strokes; move hands quickly for propulsion.
   b. Descending ramps: grip hand rims loosely, control chair's descent; or descend in wheelie position (steep ramp).
2. Wheelies: instruct in how to "pop a wheelie" in order to negotiate curbs; the patient learns how to come up onto and balance on the rear wheels with the front casters off the ground (e.g., the patient with paraplegia).
   a. Practice maintaining balance point in wheelie position (therapist tips chair back into position).
   b. Practice moving into wheelie position: patient places hands well back on hand rims; then pulls (moves) them forward abruptly and forcefully. The head and trunk are moved forward to keep from going over backward. Use lightweight wheelchair to facilitate training.
   c. Balancing in wheelie position: chair tips farther back when wheels are pushed forward; chair tips toward upright when wheels are pulled back.
   d. Practice curb ascent: place the front casters up on the curb, the patient then pushes rear wheels up curb; momentum used to assist.
   e. Practice curb descent: descending backward with forward head and trunk lean; descending forward in wheelie position.
3. Practice ascending/descending stairs: in wheelchair, on buttocks.
4. Instruct in how to fall safely, return to wheelchair.
5. Instruct in how to transfer into a car, place wheelchair inside car by pulling wheelchair behind the car seat, or to use a wheelchair lift (van-equipped).

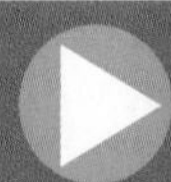

Transfer Training

Dependent Transfers

General Concepts: Minimal or No Active Participation By Patient

Dependent Lift Transfer ("Quad-Pivot" Transfer)

1. Wheelchair is positioned parallel to surface.
2. Patient is flexed forward at hips in tucked position with hips and knees flexed.
3. Therapist locks patient's tucked knees between legs; places one hand under buttocks and one hand on transfer belt.
4. Patient is rocked forward and lifted using a backward weight shift with therapist in a semisquat position.
5. Therapist then pivots using small steps and gently lowers patient to support surface.

Dependent Stand-Pivot Transfer

1. Similar to above, but patient's lower extremities are extended and in contact with floor.

Hydraulic Lift Transfer

1. Positioning and widening of base of device is critical to stability.

Assisted Transfers

General Concepts

1. Requires some participation by patient; levels of assistance include stand-by, minimal, moderate, or maximal assistance.
2. Includes verbal cueing or manual assistance for lift, support, or balance control.
3. Transfer belts, trapeze bars, overhead loops can be used to provide additional control.

Assisted Stand-Pivot Transfer

1. Used for patients who are unable to stand independently and can bear some weight on lower extremities (e.g., patients with cerebrovascular accident [CVA], incomplete SCI, hip fracture/replacement).
2. Wheelchair is placed parallel to surface (on the patient's sound or stronger side).
3. Therapist can block out one or both of the patient's knees to provide stability; support can be added by placing both hands on the patient (on both buttocks or the gait belt, both on upper back, or one on buttock/one on upper back).
4. Patient rocks forward and pushes up into standing.
5. Therapist assists patient with forward weight shift and standing, pivoting toward chair, and controlled lowering toward the support surface.
6. Variation: assisted squat-pivot transfer (partial stand-pivot) for patients who are unable to stand fully; Patient is assisted as above but does not come to a full standing position.

Assisted Transfer Using a Slide Board

1. Wheelchair is placed parallel to surface.
2. Patient moves forward in chair and board is placed well under buttocks.
3. Patient performs transfer by doing a series of push-ups and lifts along board.
4. Therapist assists in lift (hands on buttocks, on gait belt, or one on buttock/one on belt).
5. Care must be taken not to pinch fingers under board or drag/traumatize skin.
6. Feet can remain on foot pedals or be positioned on the floor.
7. Patients with complete level C6 SCI can be independent with transfer board on level surfaces.

Sit-Pivot

1. Transfer used for patients with good sitting balance who can lift buttocks clear of sitting surface; can be a progression in transfer training from using a slide board.
2. The patient utilizes the head-hips relationship to successfully complete the transfer (movement of head in one direction results in movement of hips in the opposite direction/toward the support surface being transferred to).

Training

Practice

1. In and out of bed.
2. In and out of wheelchair.
   a. Level surfaces.
   b. Unlevel surfaces: to floor.
3. On and off toilet, tub seat.
4. In and out of car.

Instructions

1. Inform patient about the transfer, as well as expectations for the patient.
2. Synchronize actions using commands and counts.
3. Reduce assistance as appropriate.

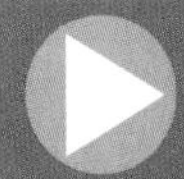

Environmental Considerations

Environmental Modification

Purpose

1. Assess degree of safety, function, and comfort of the patient in the home, community, and work environments.
2. Provide recommendations to ensure a barrier-free environment, greatest level of functional independence.

Standard Adult Wheelchair Dimensions for Environmental Access

1. Width: 24–26 inches from rim to rim.
2. Length: 42–43 inches.
3. Height (push handles to floor): 36 inches.
4. Height (armrest to floor): 29–30 inches.
5. Footrests may extend for very large people.
6. 360° turning space = 60 inches × 60 inches.
7. 90° turning space = minimum of 36 inches.
8. Minimum clear width for doorways and halls = 32 inches; ideal is 36 inches.
9. High forward reach = maximum of 48 inches from floor; low forward reach = a minimum of 15 inches from the floor.
10. Side reach = maximum of 24 inches.

Home

1. Entrance: accessible; stairs with handrail, ramp, platform to allow for ease of door opening.
2. Floors: nonskid surface, carpeting securely fastened; no throw rugs.
3. Furniture arrangement: should allow sufficient room to maneuver easily; e.g., with wheelchair or ambulation with assistive device.
4. Doors: thresholds should be flush or level (no doorsills); standard door width is 32 inches; outside door swing area requires a minimum of 18 inches for walkers and 26 inches for wheelchairs.
5. Stairs: uniform riser heights (7 inches high) with a tread depth (a minimum of 11 inches); handrails, recommended height is 32 inches, ½ to 2 inches in diameter; nonslip surface; well lighted; color code with warm colors (red, orange, yellow) if visual impairments exist.
6. Bedroom: furniture arrangement for easy maneuverability; a minimum of 3 feet on side of bed for wheelchair transfers; firm mattress, stable bed, sufficient height to facilitate sit-to-stand transfers; phone accessibility; appropriate height for wall switches is 36–48 inches; outlets a minimum of 18 inches above the floorboard.
7. Bathroom: optimal toilet seat height is 17–19 inches; tub seat, nonskid tub surface or mat; grab bars securely fastened; optimal height of horizontal grab bars is 33–36 inches.
8. Kitchen: appropriate height of countertops, for wheelchair users no higher than 31 inches; counter depth of at least 24 inches; accessible equipment and storage areas.

Community/Workplace

1. Steps: recommended height is 7–9 inches.
2. Ramps: recommended ratio of slope to rise is 1:12 (for every inch of vertical rise, 12 inches of ramp is required); minimum of 36 inches wide, with nonslip surface; handrail waist high for ambulators (34–38 inches) and should extend 12 inches beyond the top and bottom of runs; ramp should have level landing at top and bottom.
3. Parking (handicapped parking): parking space with adjacent 4-foot aisle for wheelchair maneuverability; accessible within a short distance of buildings; curb cutouts.
4. Building entrance: accessible; accessible elevator.
5. Access to public telephones, drinking fountains, bathrooms.
6. Ergonomic assessment of immediate work area: appropriate lighting, temperature, seating surface, height and size of work counter.
7. Public transportation: accessible.

Acknowledgments: Gerard Dybel

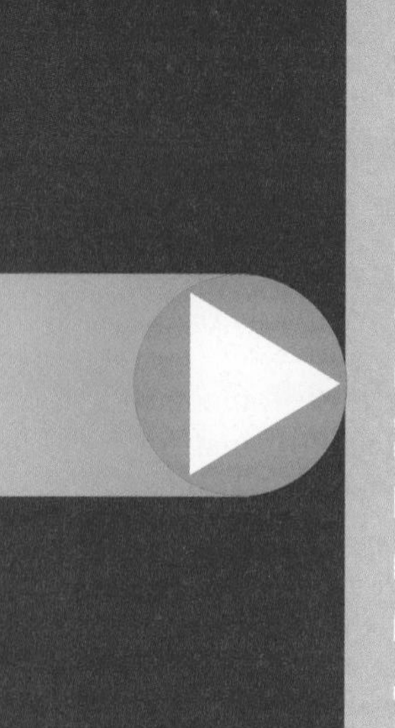

APPENDIX 12A

Review Questions

(Answers to all Review Questions and Case Studies are found in Chapter 17)

1. What are the muscle activation patterns during heel strike (initial contact) and heel-off (terminal stance) for the quadriceps, pretibial muscles, and plantar flexors?

2. What type of equipment and ambulatory aids might be needed to progress a morbidly obese patient from a sedentary bed-bound situation to independent ambulation?

3. How does rearfoot posting in a foot orthosis control for valgus or varus?

4. What are the pressure-tolerant areas in the typical transtibial residual limb that are suitable for a total contact socket?

5. What are two conditions that may warrant a therapist recommending a motorized tilt-in-space wheelchair for a patient?

13

Safety and Protection

SUSAN O'SULLIVAN AND RAYMOND SIEGELMAN

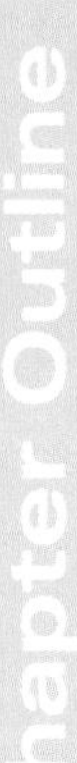

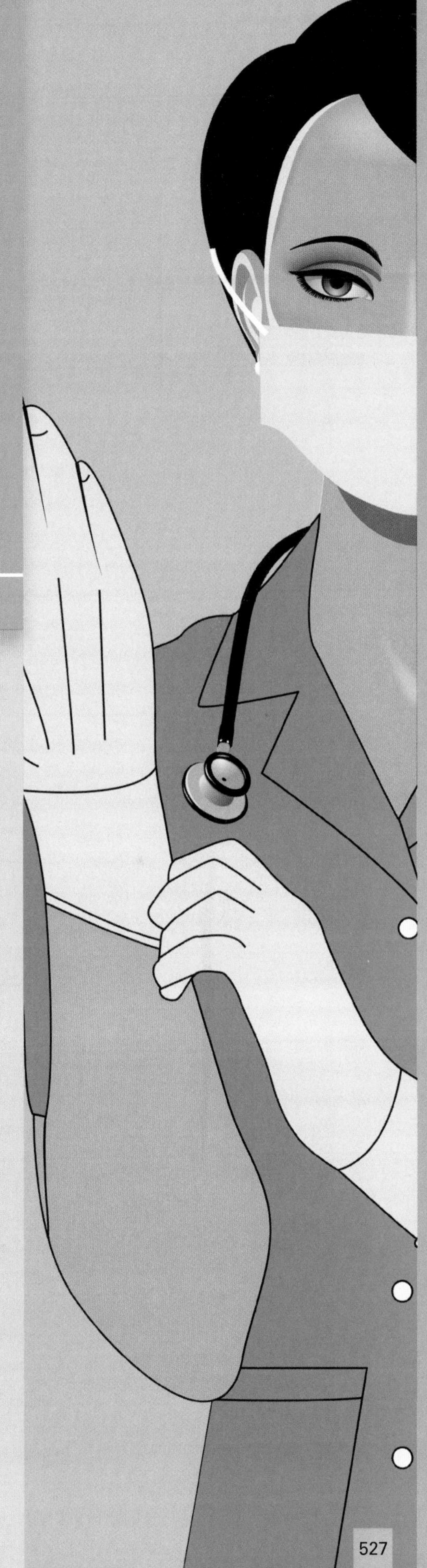

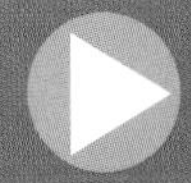

Study Tactics

Questions About Safety and Protection Comprise Approximately 3% of the NPTE, or a Total of Five to Six Questions

Focus on:

- Safety and protection throughout the NPTE. While there are only five to six questions in this section, the responsibility of the physical therapist for ensuring that the patient or client is protected and safe is emphasized throughout the exam
- Appropriate decisions for care of patients or clients that exhibit heat- or cold-related problems, diaphoresis, syncope (fainting), shock, bleeding, diabetic reactions, seizures, drug overdose, orthostatic hypotension, autonomic dysreflexia, DVT, and pulmonary embolus
- Protocols for administering CPR and basic first aid for adults or children
- Emergency preparedness for disaster situations such as a pandemic, tornado, hurricane, major fire, earthquake, domestic or foreign terrorist situation in a hospital or clinic. How can a therapist protect patients or provide care for others in these circumstances? What is the therapist's role in planning for disasters?
- Standard/universal precautions and transmission-based/isolation precautions
    - When and how to use gloves, gowns, masks, and infection control using dressings and bandages
    - Consider patients with HIV/AIDS, tuberculosis, or hepatitis
- Injury prevention, proper body mechanics, and other factors affecting PT and patient well-being:
    - Use of proper body mechanics for both the clients as well as the therapist to prevent injury. Think of proper lifting techniques and safe patient handling
    - Assessing and minimizing fall risk. Consider environmental factors such as adequate light, rugs, pets, medications and so on
    - Safe use of equipment and guarding the patient during transfers or ambulation
    - Safe use of interventions (manual therapy, exercise and modalities)
    - Equipment such as chest tubes, IVs, ventilators, dialysis precautions, shunts, arterial lines (Swan-Ganz), catheters, and monitoring devices are worth understanding relative to PT care. What to do if a line becomes dislodged? Are there any precautions regarding positioning or ambulation?
- Recognition of signs and symptoms for physical, sexual, and psychological abuse and neglect as well as reporting procedures for suspected abuse

Factors Influencing Safety and Injury Prevention

Falls

1. About one in three adults over 65 living in the community will have at least one fall a year, and about half of these have more frequent falls. The rate of fall-related injuries increases with age.
2. Falls are the leading cause of fatal and nonfatal injuries among adults 65 and older; one in five falls results in serious injury: fractures, head injury.
3. Factors that increase fall risk.
   a. 74–85 years of age.
   b. Adults with limitations in walking, ADLs, and transfers.
   c. Two or more falls in 1 year.

Clinical Assessment and Risk Factors

1. Assess the number and circumstances of previous falls.
2. Review medication history: identification of high-risk medications with possible adverse effects.
   a. Medications that affect the brain (psychotropic drugs).
      - Anxiolytics/sedative-hypnotics used for antianxiety (anxiolytic) and sedative/hypnotic properties (e.g., benzodiazepines, non-benzodiazepine prescription sedatives; anticholinergics, sedating antihistamines).
      - Antipsychotics increase fall risk due to syncope, sedation, slowed reflexes, loss of balance, and impaired psychomotor function (e.g., haloperidol [Haldol], risperidone [Risperdal], quetiapine [Seroquel], aripiprazole [Abilify]).
      - Antidepressants can cause hyponatremia/low sodium levels (except for Wellbutrin); hyponatremia is an independent risk factor for falls (e.g., sedating antidepressants—despipramine [Norpramin], imipramine [Tofranil]; mirtazapine [Remeron], trazadone); (SSRIs: sertraline [Zoloft], paroxetine [Paxil], fluoxetine [Prozac]).
      - Anticonvulsants/mood stabilizers (e.g., Depakote, Neurontin).
      - Opioid (narcotic) analgesics can increase fall risk (e.g., codeine, hydrocodone, oxycodone, morphine, fentanyl, methadone).

   b. Medications that affect blood pressure/antihypertensives can cause or worsen a drop in blood pressure (BP)/postural hypotension (e.g., Flomax, alpha-blockers [doxazosin, prazosin, terazosin]).
   c. Medications that lower blood sugar in older adults with diabetes resulting in hypoglycemia.
      - Oral or injectable medications.

   d. Diuretics can cause orthostatic hypotension; risk is increased with dehydration (e.g., Thiazide diuretics).
   e. Referral to primary medical provider is indicated for adjustment of medications as necessary.
3. Examine/evaluate personal risk factors.
   a. Visual impairments: visual screening for decreased visual acuity, depth perception, contrast sensitivity. Refer for corrective actions for refractive error, cataracts.
   b. Changes in postural blood pressure: orthostatic hypotension.
   c. Impairments in balance.
   d. Impairments in gait.
   e. Foot pain or poor footwear.
   f. Sensory changes: decreased proprioception.
   g. Impairments in cognition: confusion, memory loss.
   h. Impairments in muscle strength.
   i. Impairments in flexibility and range of motion (ROM), especially lower extremities, feet.
   j. Impairments in cardiovascular function: syncope, arrhythmias.
   k. Chronic health conditions (e.g., arthritis, stroke, Parkinson's disease).
   l. See additional discussion in Chapter 10, Geriatric Physical Therapy.
4. Examine/evaluate behavioral risk factors.
   a. History of inactivity.
   b. History of risky behaviors (e.g., standing on chair or ladder).
   c. Alcohol or recreational drug use.
5. Most falls are caused by a combination of risk factors. The more risk factors a person exhibits, the greater the fall risk.
6. Fear of falling (kinesiophobia) results in further limitations in activity and increases fall risk.
7. For individuals with limited English proficiency (LEP), eliminate language barriers by using interpreters (family, professional interpreters).

Intervention of Underlying Causes of Falls

1. Exercise.
   a. Strengthening exercises and stretching.
   b. Balance training: static/dynamic balance work.
   c. Gait training.
   d. Fitness training: low-impact cardiovascular fitness program.
2. Encourage appropriate footwear.
3. Functional training.
   a. Teach safe strategies for transitions (supine-to-sit, sit-to-stand, floor-to-standing).
   b. Teach safe strategies, protective reactions during a fall, getting up from a fall.
   c. Provide protective equipment (e.g., hip pads) for individuals at high risk for falls and hip fracture.

4. Evaluate, instruct in avoiding high-risk activities.
5. Educate in need for adequate hydration, nutritional counseling.
6. Use compensatory strategies as needed to ensure safety.
   a. Elevating head of the bed for supine-to-sit transitions.
   b. Elevated seating for sit-to-stand transitions.
   c. Assistive devices, as necessary such as walking sticks, cane, or walker.
   d. Use safe handling and guarding techniques: gait belts, assisted walking strategies, as needed.
   e. Hip protectors for preventing hip fractures in older adults.

Reduction of Environmental Fall Risk Factors

1. In-hospital: evaluate/reduce hazards in the hospital.
   a. Keep equipment (e.g., walking aids) within clear reach for easy access.
   b. Inspect all equipment for safety (e.g., canes, walkers, wheelchairs).
   c. Remove unused equipment.
   d. Keep room paths clear.
   e. Keep electric cords/tubes out of path.
   f. Keep bed in locked position.
2. Home: evaluate/reduce hazards in the home.
   a. Remove throw rugs or clutter that can be tripped over.
   b. Ensure adequate lighting without glare and use of nightlights in bedroom, hallways, and bathroom.
   c. Use/install nonslip bathmats, bath bars inside and outside tub or shower and next to toilet.
   d. Correct broken or uneven steps; add stair rails on both sides of stairs; use contrasting colors as needed to enhance depth perception.
   e. Instruct the person to avoid use of multifocal glasses while walking and stair climbing.
   f. Instruct the person to avoid walking hazards, including pets.
3. Community environmental hazards.
   a. Poorly designed public spaces.
   b. Lack of accessible public transport.
4. Community interventions.
   a. Increase public awareness, provide education about fall prevention.
   b. Institute fall-prevention programs using trained instructors (see resources).

Resources: Fall Prevention

1. Centers for Disease Control and Prevention (cdc.gov).
   a. *Preventing Falls: A Guide to Implementing Effective Community-Based Fall Prevention Program* (http://www.cdc/homeandrecreationalsafety/pdf/falls/fallpreventionguide-2015-a.pdf).
   b. *CDC Compendium of Effective Fall Interventions: What Works for Community-Dwelling Older Adults* (www.cdc.gov/STEADI/compendium.html).
2. National Council on Aging, Falls Prevention (www.ncoa.org).
3. APTA (apta.org).
   a. Balance and Falls webpage.
   b. *Safety Aspects of Mobilizing Acutely Ill Patients* (July 2008).
4. Cochrane Library (cochranelibrary.com).
   a. *Preventing Falls and Fall-Related Injuries in Older People* (Oct. 2018).
   b. *Interventions for Preventing Falls in Older People in Care Facilities and Hospitals* (Sept. 2018).
   c. *Interventions Based on Individual Assessment of Falls Risk and Multiple Component Interventions for Preventing Falls in Older People in the Community* (July 2018).

Equipment Maintenance

1. Therapeutic modalities and technologies: electrical safety.
   a. Precautions must be in place that potentially exposes any patient, therapist, or other person from electrical hazards from faulty electrical connections.
   b. A ground fault circuit interrupter (GFI) must be installed for devices used in wet or moist environments. It is a fast-acting circuit breaker that activates if there is a fault in grounding the electricity. It can prevent a dangerous shock or even electrocution to a patient or anyone else in contact with the modality.
   c. Any electrical modality or device, including those using a motor or turbine to lift patients, should be checked for current leakage as a result of broken or frayed wires. It is best if any electrical device is connected to a GFI.
2. Wheelchair maintenance.
   a. Therapist and patient should pay attention to routine cleaning and maintenance of wheelchairs. This includes tires, brakes, arm rests, leg rests, and foot plates.
   b. Power chairs require battery checks.
3. Ambulatory aids.
   a. Crutches, canes, and walkers require inspection and correction, if needed, of tips, hand grips, screws/nuts, and any other accessories.

Accountability

1. Policies and procedures manual.
   a. Safety procedures regarding risk management are specified for all personnel.
   b. Guidelines include equipment management, cleaning, maintenance, training requirements, and safety inspections.
   c. Hazardous waste and disposal of syringes ("sharps") might be considerations.
   d. Disciplinary procedures and consequences for noncompliance are established.

Function, Implications, and Related Precautions of Lines, Tubes, Catheters, and Monitors

Urinary Catheters

1. A Foley® or indwelling catheter is a flexible tube inserted into the bladder. It is held in place by a balloon that is filled with sterile water (Figure 13-1).
2. The catheter might be needed for retention of urine or incontinence, urinary output monitoring, spinal cord trauma, imaging, or surgery.
3. In a hospital situation, the urinary collecting bag is often hung on a railing below the level of the bladder to prevent reflux. Do not lift the bag above that level during transfers or ambulation.
4. In a nonemergent situation where intake and output (I&O) are being monitored, do not empty the collecting bag, as the contents need to be measured.

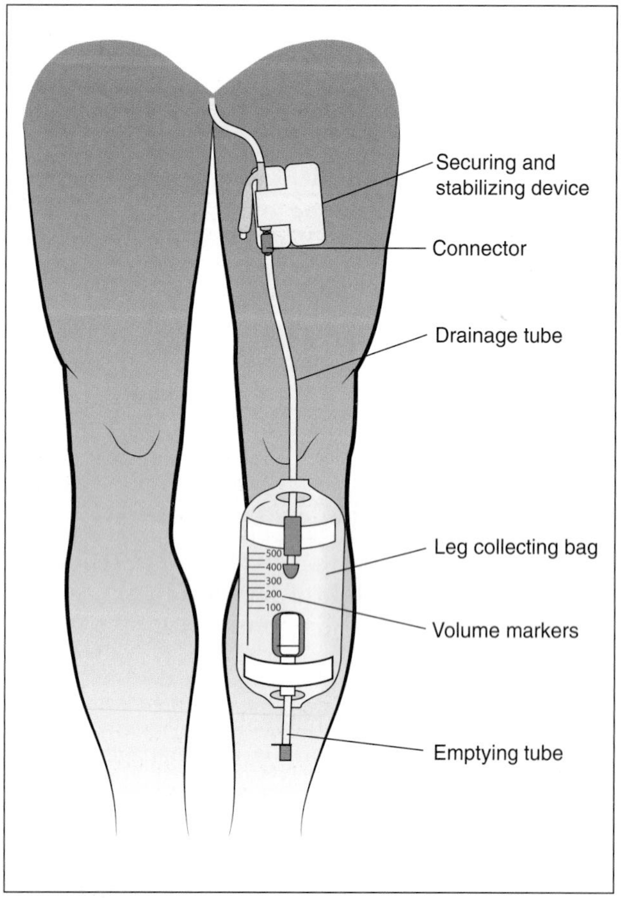

Figure 13-1 Foley® catheter.
Courtesy of Memorial Sloan Kettering Cancer Center. New York City, NY.

> **RED FLAG:** Autonomic dysreflexia is an emergency situation that can occur with spinal cord lesions usually above T6. A common cause is bladder distension from an overfull collecting bag; a blocked, twisted, or kinked collecting tube; UTI; and other causes. Sit the patient upright and empty the collecting bag or correct the tube blockage after signaling the emergency or calling 911. See Chapter 3, Neuromuscular Physical Therapy for more information.

5. A patient discharged or at home with an indwelling catheter will use a leg bag to get around. This collecting bag is secured by Velcro or tape below the knee. At bedtime, a night collecting bag is used, which is hung at the side of the bed below the level of the bladder, often, into a lined wastepaper basket.
6. Be on the alert for signs of infection such as pain, fever, foul-smelling urine, and hematuria.

Chest Tubes

1. A tube that is surgically inserted into the chest wall and sutured in place. It is attached to a vacuum line, and a water seal prevents any air from entering the tube (Figure 13-2).

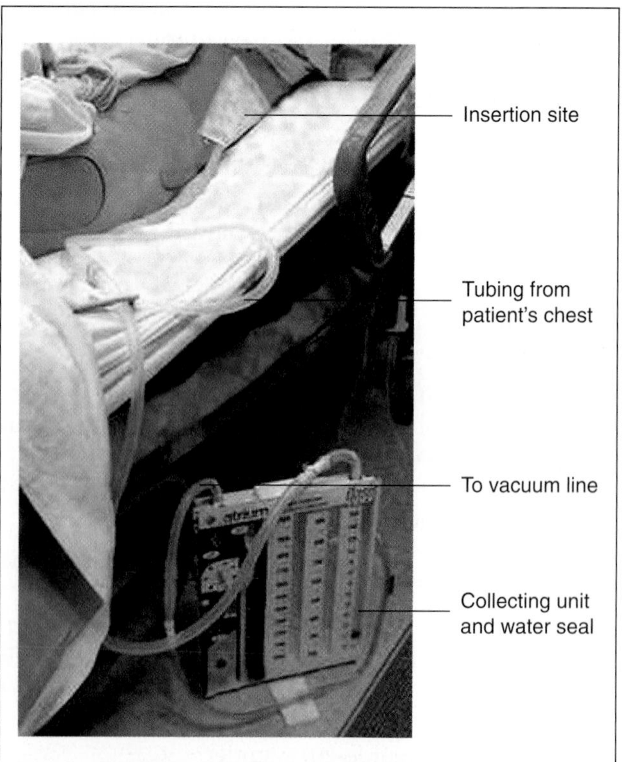

Figure 13-2 Chest tube.
Courtesy of Saddleback College. Mission Viejo, CA.

2. It is placed in the intrapleural space to evacuate air, blood, fluid, or other material following pneumothorax, cardiothoracic surgery, pleural effusion, and other conditions.
3. The tube must remain below the level of the patient's chest as the drain with the water seal is often on the floor. The patient can stand at bedside if the tube length is sufficient. A portable suction device on a moveable platform or trolley allows for ambulation.
4. Breathing maneuvers, postural drainage positioning, shaking, percussion, vibration, relaxation, and ROM exercises are permissible to the patient's tolerance. Positive pressure devices are contraindicated.

> RED FLAG: If a tube ever becomes disconnected from the patient; ask the patient to exhale fully, and place a gauze or gloved hand over the defect at the end of the exhalation. Call for medical assistance ASAP.

Intravenous Catheters

1. Peripheral IV.
   a. Short-term infusion of fluids into a peripheral vein usually in the upper extremity.
   b. The fluids might be electrolytes, blood or blood products, and other medications.
   c. Complications the therapist should be aware of include:
      - Phlebitis.
      - Infiltration of fluid to surrounding tissue with no tissue damage (nonvesicant).
      - Extravasation is infiltration of a medical fluid that can cause tissue damage (vesicant) with burning, stinging, redness, blistering, and possible necrosis.

   d. There are no contraindications to physical therapy treatment of patients with IV lines.

> RED FLAG: The upper extremity should not be raised above the level of the IV medication for any length of time or backflow of blood may occur.

   e. Rolling IV poles allow for mobility. If an infusion pump is being used, a battery backup system also allows mobility.
   f. Therapists should be aware if the IV solution is dangerously low or close to empty as air embolism is a danger.
2. Central venous catheter (CVC), also called a central line.
   a. Allows venous access for 6 days duration or longer based on patient's condition and needs.
   b. Access is to the superior vena cava, jugular, subclavian, or femoral vein.
   c. A peripherally inserted central catheter (PICC or PICC line) accesses an upper arm vein with direct access to the superior vena cava. It is used primarily for outpatient care. Activity is not limited.
   d. In the ICU, patients with central lines can undergo bed mobility activities, sitting at bedside, transfer to a bedside chair, standing, and walking short distances. Catheter dislodgement is unlikely.

> RED FLAG: When a femoral line is in place, repetitive hip flexion is contraindicated (e.g., cycling) and, in some cases, hip flexion is limited to less than 45 degrees.

Central Arterial Catheters

1. Lines that afford direct access to the arterial vessels.
   a. Access is via the radial, brachial, or femoral artery.
   b. The purpose is primarily to monitor intra-arterial blood pressure and get repeated blood gas sampling. Not used to administer medications.
   c. Early mobilization is generally safe in the ICU. This includes progressive mobility activities to tolerance such as sitting at bedside, standing at bedside, transferring to a chair or stretcher, and taking steps with a walker away from the bed. Hip flexion activity may be limited.
   d. Activities are excluded if the patient has a femoral sheath catheter.
   e. Policies differ from institution to institution.
   f. A Swan-Ganz catheter or pulmonary artery catheter is used to monitor pulmonary artery pressure, cardiac output, and oxyhemoglobin saturation.
   g. The physical therapist should inspect the catheter site before and after treatment for any sign of bleeding.

> RED FLAG: If an arterial line becomes dislodged, immediate, firm pressure must be applied to or above the arterial insertion site to try and control bleeding. Then seek immediate medical assistance.

Cardiac Monitors

1. There are a variety of reasons for continuous cardiac monitoring. Assessment can be made of heart rate (HR), rhythm, conduction, variability, or any arrhythmias.
2. Types of monitors.
   a. Mobile cardiac telemetry can monitor a patient's ECG for an extended period of time.
   b. A Holter® monitor, (a type of mobile telemetry) can be used for up to 14 days. The device is attached by leads and cannot get wet. It records to a chip which is later analyzed (Figure 13-3).

c. The mobile cardiac telemetry device (MCT) can store information in the cloud or be read in real time on a monitor. The MCT is often used at the onset of cardiac rehabilitation (a week or so) to assess how the patient accommodates to exercise or activity from a cardiac standpoint.
d. Insertable or implantable cardiac monitoring can be done for a year or more. These devices are placed under the skin and used as a long-term Holter monitor without the bulk and lack of compliance associated with the Holter. They are not pacemakers and only record information. They will be detected by airport scanning.
e. A Zio® patch is a small, self-contained device that attaches directly to the skin on the upper left chest. It is used for about 2 weeks and stores data that is analyzed upon return. There are no exercise restrictions (Figure 13-4).
f. Exercise cardiac monitors. The field is rapidly evolving. Data can be detected and seen in real time and/or downloaded to a computer, tablet, smartphone, or smartwatch for analysis and correlated with exercise parameters.
   - An ear clip, chest strap, finger sensor, or wrist strap can be sites for data collection.
   - HR, workout intensity, calories used, workout time, laps, target, and maximum HR are just some of the areas that can be monitored.
g. A pulse oximeter is a device that measures the degree of oxygen saturation of hemoglobin in the arterial blood (SaO_2). A finger clip or telemetry can be used. HR is usually monitored by this device as well. Normal SaO_2 values are usually 95%–100% oxygen saturation. (See Chapter 4, Cardiovascular and Lymphatic Physical Therapy for more information.)

3. Precautions with monitored patients/clients.
   a. Stop exercise or activity if there is irregular heartbeat, if patient/client feels weak, dizzy, light-headed, short of breath, has blurry vision, or SaO_2 drops to unacceptable levels.
   b. See additional discussion in Chapter 4.

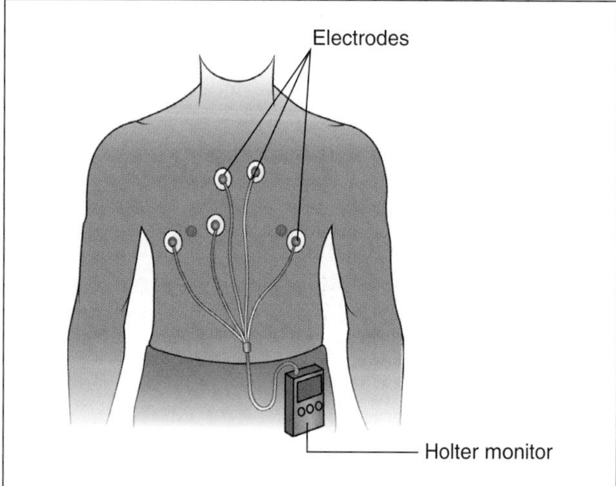

Figure 13-3 Holter monitor.
Adapted from Johns Hopkins Medicine.org. 2019.

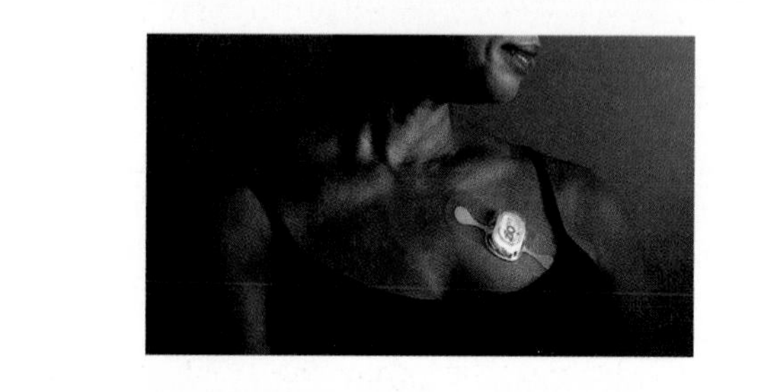

Figure 13-4 Zio patch.
Science and Enterprise-Technology News and Literature. March 2018.

Mechanical Ventilation

1. Mechanical ventilation is the use of artificial means to support or replace spontaneous ventilation (Figure 13-5).
2. Patients receiving mechanical ventilation require intubation with an endotracheal (oral), nasotracheal (nasal), or tracheal (through a tracheostomy) tube.
   a. Endotracheal and nasotracheal tubes are taped in place.
   b. Tracheal tubes are sutured in place.

RED FLAG: When a patient is intubated, avoid placing extensive tension on or movement of the tube. This could reduce optimal ventilation.

3. Monitor patient performance on the ventilator monitor for vital and other pulmonary function signs.

RED FLAG: Alarms: Red = apnea or a disconnected circuit. Yellow = low tidal volume, high respiratory rate or high pressure (PIP).

   a. A peak inspired pressure (PIP) of >30 cm H_2O might indicate a kinked tube, a need for patient suctioning, or perhaps bronchospasm (Figure 13-6).
   b. The head of the bed should be elevated between 30°–45° at all times if the patient condition allows.
4. There are no absolute contraindications for bedside physical therapy with patients undergoing mechanical ventilation. Stationary devices such as peddlers can be used bedside as well as light weights, elastic bands (TheraBand®), and so on.

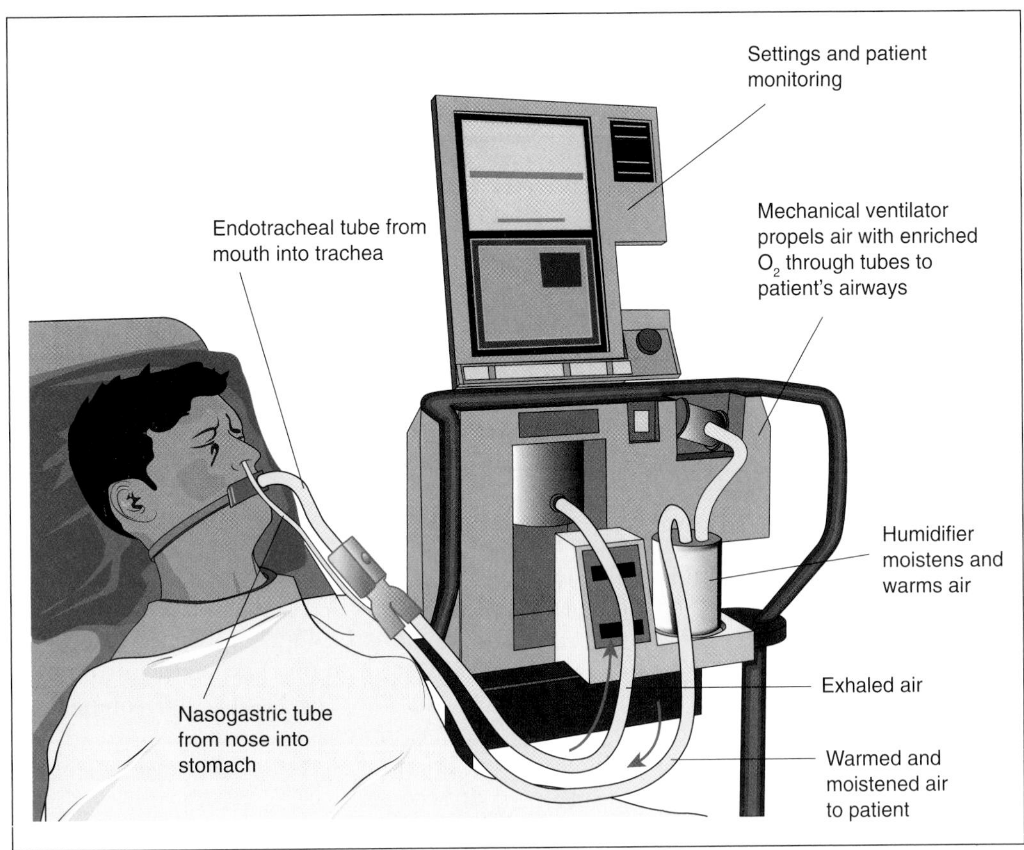

Figure 13-5 **Mechanical ventilation.**
Adapted from Nursing Standard. October 2018.

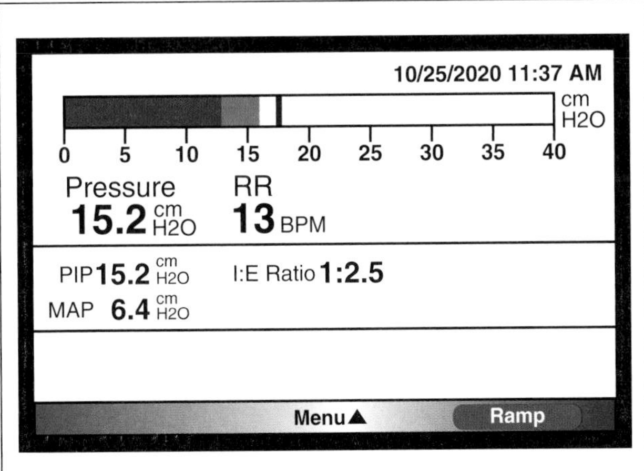

Figure 13-6 **Example of a peak-inspired screen on a mechanical ventilator.**
MAP = mean airway pressure.

5. Patient weaning from mechanical ventilation.
   a. Important to monitor exercise tolerance.
   b. If respiratory rate increases, tidal volume decreases, or there is an increase in accessory muscle use, the patient needs to rest.

Oxygen Delivery Systems

1. May be needed by patients with COPD, pneumonia, asthma, cystic fibrosis, or cardiac issues for hypoxemia.
2. Indicated if SaO_2 is <88% or PaO_2 is <55 mmHg regardless of activity level. Recall that oxygen saturation may drop to these levels with activity and the therapist should monitor O_2 saturation to ensure adequate oxygenation.
3. A portable oxygen cylinder or concentrator is attached to a delivery device such as a nasal cannula, mask, or manual resuscitator bag during exercise or mobility training.
   a. If using an oxygen cylinder, ensure that the tubing is long enough if working on stair climbing.
4. Ensure that the order for physical therapy stipulates the SaO_2. For example, "Maintain the SaO_2 >90%" or any other value.
   a. The PT may titrate the oxygen flow to maintain that saturation level while monitoring the values carefully during an activity or exercise session.
   b. The PT should also assess vital signs, heart rhythm, and other signs of distress.

c. At the end of the session return the flow rate to the original setting if it had been altered during the therapy session.

d. An appropriate exercise prescription including breathing exercises, other activities, and rest intervals should be stipulated and modified as needed.

5. See additional discussion in Chapter 5, Pulmonary Physical Therapy.

Emergency Preparedness

Guidelines for Cardiopulmonary Resuscitation (CPR) and Conversion (ECC)

Adapted from *Highlights of the American Heart Association, Guidelines for CPR and ECC*, updated 2015 and 2018. Retrieved February 2, 2019 from http://eccguidelines.heart.org.

1. Basic Life Support and CPR: adult, child, infants. (See Table 13-1.)
2. CPR and ECC.
   a. If victim is found to be unresponsive, call for help/activate the emergency response system, get an automated external defibrillator (AED), and start CPR.
   b. Check for breathing and pulse. If no breathing or only gasping and no pulse within 10 seconds, begin compressions.
   c. Deliver high-quality chest compressions: position on a hard service, use adequate rate and depth ("push hard and fast"). Minimize interruptions in compressions and allow for full chest recoil.
   d. Untrained rescuers should provide compressions only (hands-only).
   e. A trained rescuer or a second rescuer can perform rescue breaths. Apply 2 breaths after 30 compressions with each breath delivered over 1 second; observe for chest rise.
   f. AED available: a trained rescuer (health care professional) can attach the AED as soon as possible. Determine rhythm.
      - If rhythm is shockable (e.g., ventricular fibrillation or rapid ventricular tachycardia), give 1 shock and resume CPR for about 2 minutes. AED will prompt rhythm recheck. Continue until medical emergency team (MET) arrives or victim starts to move.
      - If rhythm is NOT shockable (e.g., asystole or slow, wide QRS complexes without palpable pulses [PEA]), resume CPR for 2 minutes until AED prompts for rhythm recheck. Continue compressions until MET arrives or victim starts to move.
   g. For patients with normal breathing and pulse, continue to monitor until MET arrives.
   h. For patients with no normal breathing and have pulses, provide rescue breathing: 1 breath every 5–6 seconds or about 10–12 breaths per minute. Check pulse every 2 minutes. For patients with possible opioid overdose, trained rescuers can administer intramuscular or intranasal naloxone if available, per protocol.

RED FLAG: Do not compress at a rate slower than 100/min or faster than 120/min. Do not compress greater than 2.4 inches (6 cm).

Do not lean on chest between compressions: need to allow for the heart to fill completely before the next compression.

Do not interrupt compressions for greater than 10 seconds.

Do not provide excessive ventilation.

Disaster Preparedness and Response

1. Types of disasters.
   a. Internal source.
      - Power, utility, communication, or equipment failures.
      - Fire, gas leak, hazardous material, explosion.
      - Workplace violence—active shooter, bomb scare.
   b. External source.
      - Terrorism, extremism, hate crimes.
      - Civil disturbances.
      - Mass casualty incidents.
      - Floods, hurricanes, tornados, earthquakes, tsunamis, wildfires, blizzards.
2. Risk factors.
   a. Geographic area more prone to certain types of natural disasters.
   b. Demographic area more prone to violence, extremism, civil disturbances, or mass casualties.
   c. Facilities more at risk for violent behavior are inpatient and acute psychiatric services, geriatric long-term care settings, high-volume urban emergency departments.
3. Emergency Action Plan (EAP).
   a. Methods for reporting emergencies within a facility and to external sources including contact information under the EAP.

Table 13-1

Summary of Key Basic Life Support (BLS) Components for Adults, Children, and Infants

	RECOMMENDATIONS		
COMPONENT	**ADULTS**	**CHILDREN**	**INFANTS**
Recognition	Unresponsive (all ages) No breathing, not breathing normally (e.g., only gasping)	Same as for adults	Same as for adults
CPR Sequence	CAB	CAB	CAB (ABC for neonates)
Compression Rate	100–120/min, adults	Same as for adults	Same as for adults
Compression Depth	At least 2 inches (5 cm)	At least 1/3 AP depth, about 2 inches (5 cm)	At least 1/3 AP depth, about 1½ inches (4 cm)
Hand placement	2 hands on lower half of sternum	2 hands or 1 hand on lower half of sternum	2 fingers in center of chest
Chest Wall Recoil	Allow complete recoil between compressions, HCPs rotate compressors every 2 minutes	Same as for adults	Same as for adults
Compression Interruption	30:2 (1 or 2 rescuers)	30:2 single rescuer, 15:2 2 HCP rescuers	30:2 single rescuer, 15:2 2 HCP rescuers
Airway	Head tilt-chin lift (HCP suspected trauma: jaw thrust)	Same as for adults	Same as for adults
Compression to Ventilation Ratio (until advanced airway placed)	30:2 (1 or 2 rescuers)	30:2 single rescuer or 15:2 2 HCP rescuers	30:2 single rescuer or 15:2 2 HCP rescuers
Ventilations: when rescuer untrained or trained and not proficient	Compressions only	Compressions only	Compressions only
Ventilations with Advanced Airway (HCP)	1 breath every 6–8 seconds (8–10 breaths/min) Asynchronous with chest compressions About 1 second per breath Visible chest rise	Same as for adults	Same as for adults
Defibrillation	Attach and use AED as soon as available. Minimize interruptions in chest compressions before and after shock, resume CPR, beginning with compressions immediately after each shock	Same as for adults	Same as for adults

Key: CAB: compressions, airway, breathing; HCP: health care provider; CPR: cardiopulmonary resuscitation; AED: automatic electronic defibrillator
From 2010 American Heart Association Guidelines for CPR and ECG. Downloaded from http://circ.ahajournals.org on July 5, 2011.

b. Evacuation policy and procedures including route assignments and escape procedures.
c. Protecting and evacuating patients/clients.
d. Practice of the EAP frequently using a variety of scenarios (e.g., "I hear gunshots!" "I smell gas," and so on).

4. Workplace violence, including active shooter or terrorism.
   a. RUN first.
      - Evacuate and help others, especially patients, to escape if possible.
      - Consider best escape route.
   b. HIDE (shelter in place) if escape not possible.
      - Block entrance. In physical therapy clinics use weights or other heavy apparatus.
      - Silence cell phone, call 911 with exact location and leave line open.
   c. FIGHT.
      - If unable to run or hide and life is in imminent danger.
      - Improvise weapons, yell, act aggressively, throw things, and attack if all else fails.
5. Physical therapist role in constructing an EAP.
   a. Liaison with local first responders as well as other agencies such as OSHA or Homeland Security, especially if in a smaller practice or clinic.
   b. Help develop the communication responsibilities needed during a disaster.
   c. Formulate plans for assisting patients/clients, especially those with limited mobility, during a disaster.
   d. Implement fairly frequent disaster drills of various scenarios.

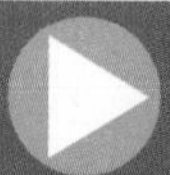

First Aid

1. First aid involves recognizing, assessing, and prioritizing the need for assistance given to any person suffering a serious injury or illness.
2. Initial care is provided within the scope of the knowledge and skills of the health care provider (HCP).
3. The HCP needs to know when to refer for additional help (activate EMS/call 911) and seek advanced medical care. For many conditions, timeliness is critical (e.g., stroke, concussion with hemorrhage).
4. Adapted from *2015 American Heart Association and American Red Cross Guidelines Update for First Aid.* Retrieved 6/14/2020 from https://www.ahajournals.org/doi/10.1161/CIR.0000000000000269.

Musculoskeletal

1. Positioning of an ill or injured person with suspected spine, hip, or pelvis injury.
   a. If spinal injury is suspected, have the injured person remain as still as possible while awaiting the arrival of EMS.
   b. HPCs should apply spinal motion restriction while waiting for EMS to arrive. Manual restriction of spinal motion should be provided as necessary.
   c. HPCs trained in advanced spinal motion restriction techniques, such as spine boarding and application of cervical collars, may attempt these procedures when appropriate support is available on-site. Lay providers or untrained HCPs should not attempt these procedures.
2. Sprains, strains, and muscle contusions.
   a. Cold application decreases hemorrhage, edema, pain, and disability.
   b. Cooling is best applied using a plastic bag or damp cloth filled with a mixture of ice and water (not ice alone). Refreezeable gel packs can be used but do not cool as effectively as an ice-water mixture.
   c. Limit application of cold to 20 minutes or less to prevent cold injury. Use a barrier cloth between the cold and skin.
   d. Heat application is contraindicated.
   e. Compression bandage may be considered for some areas.
3. Long bone fractures.
   a. A suspected long bone fracture should be splinted in a way that limits pain, reduces the chance for further injury, and facilitates safe and prompt transport. Activate EMS and facilitate transport to a medical facility as needed.
   b. HCPs should not move or try to straighten an injured extremity with angulated fractures. However, if an injured extremity is blue or extremely pale, the HCP may try to gently straighten the limb to reduce neurovascular compromise. EMS should be activated immediately.

RED FLAG: Significant trauma, to include fractures to the long bones and pelvis, may result in fat embolus syndrome (FES). HCPs must recognize that symptoms of respiratory distress may indicate the cascade of FES is beginning and activate EMS as soon as possible.

Neuromuscular

1. Stroke assessment: use of a stroke assessment system is recommended (see Box 13-1). If stroke symptoms are present, activate EMS, seek medical assistance immediately.
2. Concussion: adapted from *HEADS UP to Brain Injury Awareness*, CDC Injury Center. Retrieved February 6, 2019, from https://www.CDC.gov/headsup/index.html.
   a. HCPs should evaluate persons with concussion for signs and symptoms. See Box 13-2.
   b. Persons with mild concussion have no loss of consciousness and symptoms that last for less than 15 minutes.

BOX 13-1 Stroke Early Warning Signs: F.A.S.T.

- **F – Face Drooping**: Does one side of face droop or is it numb? Ask the person to smile.
- **A – Arm Weakness**: Is one arm weak or numb? Ask the person to raise both arms. Does one arm drift downward?
- **S – Speech Difficulty**: Is speech slurred, are they unable to speak, or are they hard to understand? Ask the person to repeat a simple sentence, such as, "The sky is blue." Is the sentence repeated correctly?
- **T – Time** to call 911: If the person shows any of these symptoms, even if the symptoms go away, call 911 and get the person to the hospital immediately for emergency stroke treatment.
- Beyond F.A.S.T.: other possible symptoms: sudden numbness or weakness of the leg; sudden confusion or trouble understanding; sudden trouble seeing with both eyes; sudden trouble walking, dizziness, loss of balance or coordination; sudden severe headache with no known cause.

Retrieved February 6, 2019, from https://www.stroke.org/understand-stroke/recognizing-stroke/act-fast/.

BOX 13-2 ▷ Concussion Signs and Symptoms

Signs of Concussion
- Change in the level of consciousness, appears dazed or stunned
- Can't recall events prior to or after a hit or fall (retrograde or anterograde amnesia)
- Forgets an instruction, appears confused
- Moves clumsily
- Answers questions slowly
- Loses consciousness, even briefly
- Shows mood, behavior, or personality changes

Symptoms of Concussion
- Headache or pressure in head
- Nausea or vomiting
- Balance problems, dizziness, blurry vision
- Sensitivity to light or noise
- Feeling sluggish, hazy, foggy, or groggy
- Confusion, concentration, or memory problems
- Just not "feeling right" or "feeling "down"

Severe Concussion: Activate EMS

Seek immediate medical care if the person experiences any of the following:
- Drowsiness or inability to wake up; loss of consciousness for longer than 30 seconds
- One pupil larger than the other pupil
- Repeat vomiting or nausea, convulsions, or seizures
- Headache that gets worse with time
- Slurred speech, numbness, or decreased coordination
- Changes in behavior: irritability, restlessness, agitation
- Confusion, disorientation, or amnesia

c. Persons with moderate concussion have no loss of consciousness and symptoms that last longer than 15 minutes.
d. Both groups should be monitored closely. Return to normal activity and sports participation is contraindicated. Medical clearance is required for resumption of activity. Recovery with absence of symptoms can take hours, days, or weeks.
e. Persons with severe concussion demonstrate loss of consciousness and more severe symptoms. (See Box 13-2.)
f. Symptoms of an expanding brain lesion (hematoma or hemorrhage) can indicate a life threatening situation. Activate EMS and seek immediate medical care. (See Box 13-1.)
g. See Chapter 3, Neuromuscular Physical Therapy for additional discussion.

BOX 13-3 ▷ Signs and Symptoms of Seizures

- Altered consciousness
- Altered motor activity: convulsions, involuntary contractions, rhythmic jerking of extremities
- Sensory phenomena: somatosensory, visual, auditory, olfactory, gustatory, and vertiginous sensations
- Autonomic phenomena: sudden anxiety, tachycardia, sweating, piloerection, loss of bladder control
- Cognitive phenomena: sudden failure to communicate, comprehend, hallucinations, intense feelings

3. Seizures.
   a. Evaluate for signs and symptoms of seizure. See Box 13-3.
   b. If the person is lying down, ensure an open airway: position the patient in lateral sidelying with their mouth pointing to the ground to establish airway and prevent aspiration. Protect the person's head by preventing it from hitting the floor. Some individuals can be helped to sit down in a safe place.
   c. Protect patient from injury: loosen restrictive clothing, remove potentially harmful nearby objects.
   d. Do not restrain the victim during a seizure as this can lead to injury and make the person more confused, agitated, or aggressive.
   e. Do not try to open the victim's mouth or place any object between the victim's teeth or in the mouth.
   f. Do not give water, pills, or food by mouth unless the person is fully alert.
   g. Always stay with the person until the seizure is over. Time the length of the seizure and how long it takes for a person to recover and return to usual activity. It is not unusual for the victim to be unresponsive or confused for a short time after a seizure.
   h. Activate EMS, seek medical assistance if:
      - A seizure lasts 5 minutes or longer.
      - Status epilepticus occurs: a seizure lasts longer than 5 minutes or when seizures occur close together without regaining consciousness. Can be life-threatening.
      - Breathing is difficult or the person is choking.
      - Injury may have occurred.
      - The person asks for medical help.

Cardiopulmonary

1. Chest pain.
   a. Chest pain can result from multiple causes: minor chest wall strains, pneumonia, rib fracture, angina, or myocardial infarction (MI).
   b. The HCP needs to be able to recognize signs and symptoms of MI.

- Classic signs: chest pain, chest discomfort or pressure, pain in other parts of the body (shoulders, one arm, back, neck or jaw), shortness of breath (SOB), and other symptoms (nausea, sweating, light-headedness, or dizziness).
- Women may present with vague or silent symptoms including uncomfortable pressure in the chest; stomach pain; sudden sweating or shortness of breath (SOB), nausea, or light-headedness without exertion; sweating that feels as if stress-related when there is no real cause.

c. Activate EMS, seek medical assistance immediately for anyone with chest pain and signs of heart attack.

d. While waiting for EMS:
- The HCP may encourage a person with chest pain to chew 1 adult or 2 low-dose aspirin if signs and symptoms suggest a heart attack and the person has no allergy or contraindication to aspirin, such as recent bleeding.
- If the person's pain does not suggest a cardiac origin, aspirin should not be encouraged; the decision to administer can be left to the EMS provider.
- The person can be given a nitroglycerin tab sublingually if available and prescribed for that person.

2. Asthma.

a. Persons may experience shortness of breath and wheezing from asthma (reactive airway disease) as well as with bronchitis and chronic obstructive pulmonary disease (COPD).

b. Asthma attacks are triggered primarily by allergic reactions.

c. Signs and symptoms include short, shallow, fast breaths; wheezing or whistling sound with breathing; frequent cough; trouble talking; and panicky feelings.

d. Typically these individuals may carry prescribed short-acting inhaled medications; treatment should be started immediately; patients should not use a long-acting medication for acute exacerbations.

e. HCPs can assist as needed with the administration of prescribed bronchodilators when a person with asthma is having trouble breathing.

f. Depending on the severity of the symptoms and treatment effectiveness of inhaler, EMS may need to be activated.

3. Shock.

a. Shock is the failure of the circulatory system to perfuse vital organs (hypoperfusion). Blood is shunted from the periphery to maintain vital organs and core temperature.

b. Types and causes of shock.
- Cardiogenic: may occur with hypotension, MI, or cardiac arrest.
- Hemorrhagic: severe internal or external bleeding.
- Metabolic: loss of body fluids from heat (dehydration) or severe vomiting and diarrhea.
- Anaphylactic: severe allergic reaction from drugs, food, or insect stings.
- Respiratory: respiratory illness or arrest.
- Septic: severe infections cause blood vessels to dilate.
- Neurogenic: significant trauma (e.g., TBI, SCI) or other neural trauma causing disruption of the ANS. The victim may lose consciousness as the brain is affected.
- If HR and rhythm are affected, can ultimately progress to cardiac arrest and death.

c. Signs and symptoms.
- Pale, gray or blue, cool skin.
- Increased and weak pulse.
- Increased respiratory rate.
- Decreased blood pressure.
- Drowsiness, diminishing level of consciousness, irritability, or restlessness.
- Nausea or vomiting.

d. Management of shock.
- Examine victim for airway, breathing, circulation (ABCs), and bleeding.
- Assess level of consciousness.
- Determine skin characteristics and perform capillary refill test.
  - Capillary refill test: squeeze fingernail for 2 seconds.
  - In healthy individuals, the nail will blanch and turn pink when pressure is released.
  - If nail bed does not refill and turn pink within 2 seconds, the cause could be that blood is being shunted away from the periphery.
- Position a victim who is in shock, responsive, and breathing normally in the supine position. If there is no evidence of trauma or injury, passive leg raising 6–12 inches (30°–60°) can be used to improve vital signs. Do not raise the feet if the movement or position cause pain.
- Cover the person with a blanket.
- Treat any specific condition identified, if possible: bleeding, anaphylaxis, and so on.
- Activate EMS ASAP. Reassure the victim and continue to monitor ABCs.
- Do not give any food or drink.

4. Vasovagal syncope: fainting with sudden drop in HR and BP. This is usually harmless but may result in injury during the episode.

a. Symptoms can include pale skin; light-headedness; tunnel vision; nausea; feeling warm; cold, clammy sweat; and blurred vision.

b. May see slow, weak pulse; dilated pupils; and jerky, abnormal movements.

c. Person should lie down with legs lifted. Alternately, the person can sit down with head between knees. The person should remain in this position until symptoms resolve, typically within 15–30 minutes. Standing up too soon puts the person at risk of fainting again.

Bleeding and Superficial Wounds

1. Minor bleeding.
   a. Usually clots within 10 minutes.
   b. If the person is taking aspirin or nonsteroidal anti-inflammatory drugs (NSAIDS), clotting may be prolonged.
2. Severe bleeding.
   a. Arterial bleed: blood spurts from the wound under high pressure; bright red blood.
   b. Venous bleed: low pressure bleed, steady flow, dark red or maroon blood.
   c. Capillary bleed: low pressure, oozing, dark red blood.
3. Blood that fails to clot even after measures to control bleeding have been taken may indicate hemophilia or other blood clotting disorders.
4. Management of bleeding.
   a. Use standard precautions: wash hands well, wear gloves if available.
   b. To control open bleeding, apply direct pressure using sterile gauze to the bleeding site until it stops. If gauze is unavailable, use a clean cloth, towel, or gloved hand. If blood soaks through, do not remove the gauze; add additional layers.
   c. Do not attempt to wash out a major wound.
   d. Once bleeding has stopped, apply a pressure bandage, such as roller gauze over the gauze pads.
   e. An ice pack can be applied over the bandage or dressing. Use with caution with children because of the risk of hypothermia.
   f. Elevate the body part above the level of the heart until bleeding stops.
   g. Brachial and femoral artery pressure points should not be utilized to stop arterial bleeding.
   h. A tourniquet should be used when standard first aid hemorrhage control does not control severe external limb bleeding. Note the time the tourniquet is first applied and communicate this information to EMS providers.
   i. Continue to monitor ABCs and overall status of patient.
   j. Activate EMS as necessary.
5. Superficial wounds: lacerations and abrasions.
   a. If there are no foreign objects, cover with a clean occlusive dressing and apply pressure to stop bleeding.
   b. Thoroughly irrigate the wound with a large volume of lukewarm water with or without soap until there is no foreign matter in the wound. Do not remove any imbedded objects (e.g., glass); seek medical advice.
   c. Cover the wound with a bandage or gauze pad.
   d. Seek medical help if the wound is bleeding heavily, does not stop after 5–10 minutes, is close to the eye, caused by a puncture wound from a dirty or rusty object, has ragged or separated edges, is caused by an animal or human bite, or shows signs of infection.
6. Impaled objects and puncture wounds.
   a. Usually do not present with significant external bleeding.
   b. May present with internal bleeding.
   c. Never remove an impaled object.
   d. Apply a dressing that stops bleeding and secures the impaled object for removal in a location where significant arterial bleeding can be most appropriately managed (e.g., emergency room).

Internal Bleeding

1. Often the result of blunt force trauma rupturing a blood vessel or an organ or injury from a fall.
2. Severe internal bleeding may be life-threatening. Signs and symptoms include:
   a. Ecchymosis (black and blue skin areas) in the injured area.
   b. Body part, especially the abdomen, may be swollen, tender, and firm; patient may exhibit rebound tenderness.
   c. Skin may appear pale or gray and cool or moist (e.g., shock).
   d. Respiratory rate is increased.
   e. Pulse rate is increased and weak.
   f. Blood pressure is decreased.
   g. Person may be nauseated or vomit.
   h. Person may exhibit anxiety or restlessness.
   i. Level of consciousness may decline.
3. Management of internal bleeding.
   a. Activate EMS immediately.
   b. Monitor closely: ABCs and vital signs.
   c. Keep person comfortable and quiet; avoid having them get overheated or chilled.

Integumentary

1. Thermal burns.
   a. Burns can result from a variety of causes including fire and scalds from hot water.
   b. Cool thermal burns with cool water ASAP and for at least 10 minutes. If cool water is not available, a cool compress can be applied.

   c. Do not apply ice directly to a burn as it can produce tissue ischemia.
   d. Monitor for hypothermia when cooling large burns. This is especially important in children who have a larger body surface area for their weight.
   e. After cooling, the burn can be loosely covered with a sterile, dry dressing.
   f. Avoid all natural remedies, such as honey.
   g. Activate EMS, seek advanced medical care with burns involving blistering or broken skin; difficulty breathing; burns on the face, neck, hands, or genitals; and burns involving a large surface area, such as the trunk and extremities.
2. Electric injury.
   a. Severity of electric injuries can vary widely including unpleasant tingling sensations as a result of thermal burns, cardiopulmonary arrest, and death.
   b. Thermal burns are typically present at the entrance and exit points of the electric current and along its internal pathway.
   c. Cardiac arrhythmias can include ventricular tachycardia progressing to ventricular fibrillation and ventricular asystole.
   d. Respiratory arrest can result from electric injury to the respiratory center in the brain or from tetanic contractions or paralysis of respiratory muscles.
   e. Do not touch an electrocuted victim while the power is on. Turn the power off at its source.
   f. Assess the victim, administer CPR, defibrillation, and treatment for shock and thermal burns as needed.
   g. Activate EMS, seek advanced medical care ASAP.

Hypoglycemia

1. Signs and symptoms:
   a. Rapid heartbeat, heart palpitations.
   b. Anxious feeling, panic attacks.
   c. Excessive sweating (diaphoresis) unrelated to exercise or activity or environment that comes on suddenly.
   d. Feelings of queasiness or hunger and food cravings.
   e. Dizziness, light-headedness, and headache.
   f. Blurred vision.
   g. Trouble sleeping.
   h. Inability to concentrate, confusion.
   i. Lack of coordination.
   j. Altered behavior or mood problems (e.g., angry outbursts).
2. Management.
   a. If a person with diabetes reports low blood sugar or exhibits signs and symptoms of mild hypoglycemia and is able to follow simple commands and swallow, oral glucose tablets (often carried by the victim) or dietary sugars (sucrose candy, orange juice, fructose/fruit leather, or whole milk) should be given.
   b. Symptoms may not resolve for 10–15 minutes; HCPs should therefore wait at least 10–15 minutes before calling EMS or retreating the person with additional oral sugars.
   c. If a person's status deteriorates during that time or does not improve, activate EMS immediately.
   d. If the person with diabetes demonstrates severe hypoglycemia and is unconscious, exhibits seizures, or is unable to follow simple commands or swallow safely, activate EMS immediately.

Anaphylaxis

1. Persons with severe allergic reactions may progress to anaphylaxis.
2. Symptoms may include respiratory difficulty (e.g., wheezing), cutaneous manifestations (e.g., hives or swelling of the lips or eyes), cardiovascular manifestations (e.g., hypotension, cardiovascular collapse, shock), or gastrointestinal cramping and diarrhea.
3. Epinephrine should be administered. Persons at risk are typically prescribed and carry an epinephrine autoinjector (EpiPen®). Dosage is administered intramuscularly.
4. The HCP can administer the EpiPen® using an intramuscular injection typically in the thigh if the person is unable to do so.
5. Activate EMS immediately. If the person with anaphylaxis does not respond to the initial dose in 5–10 minutes, a repeat dose may be considered.

Environmental Emergencies

1. Exertional dehydration.
   a. HCPs my assist at "hydration stations" at sporting events. Vigorous exercise particularly in hot and humid environments can lead to significant dehydration.
   b. In the absence of shock, confusion, or inability to swallow, the individual with exertional dehydration should be given oral rehydration fluids, preferably carbohydrate-electrolyte (CE) fluids. If these beverages are not available, potable water may be used.
2. Individuals with severe dehydration with shock, confusion, or symptoms of heat stroke require advanced medical care. Activate EMS immediately.
3. Heat-induced symptoms precipitated by vigorous exercise include heat cramps, heat exhaustion, and heat stroke.
   a. Heat cramps are painful involuntary muscle spasms often affecting the calves, arms, abdominal muscles, or back.
      - First aid includes rest, cooling off, and drinking a CE solution if available. Stretching, icing, and massage may relieve painful muscles.
      - Exercise should not be resumed until all symptoms are resolved.

b. Heat exhaustion is caused by exercise-induced heat and fluid/electrolyte loss as sweat.
   - Signs and symptoms can start suddenly and include nausea, dizziness, muscle cramps, feeling faint, headache, fatigue, and heavy sweating.
   - This is a serious situation that can rapidly advance to heat stroke.
   - Treatment involves having the victim lie down in a cool place, removing as many clothes as possible, and cooling the victim with a cool water spray. The victim should also be encouraged to drink cool fluids, preferably CE fluids.

c. Heat stroke includes all of the symptoms of heat exhaustion plus additional central nervous system (CNS) signs (e.g., dizziness, syncope, confusion, or seizures).
   - Immediate cooling is necessary, preferably by immersing the victim up to the chin in cool water.
   - Activate EMS immediately.
   - Emergency treatment is needed with intravenous fluids. Do NOT try to force the victim to drink fluids.

4. Hypothermia.
   a. Hypothermia is caused by prolonged exposure to cold. Length of exposure and the victim's body temperature determine the urgency of treatment.
   b. Begin rewarming of the victim: move the person to a warm environment, remove wet clothing, and wrap the exposed body surfaces with blankets or dry clothing.
   c. Active rewarming can include placing the victim near a heat source and placing containers or warm, but NOT hot, water in contact with the skin.
   d. If frostbite of an exposed part (typically the extremities and nose) is present, remove wet clothing, dry and cover the victim to prevent hypothermia.
   e. Activate EMS immediately, or transport to a medical facility immediately. Protect frostbitten parts from refreezing.

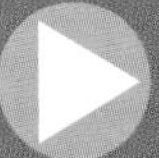

Infection Control Procedures

1. Adapted from *Centers for Disease Control and Prevention (CDC) Guidelines for Standard Precautions and Transmission-Based Precautions* (last updated February 28, 2017), retrieved February 20, 2019, from https://www.cdc.gov/infectioncontrol/guidelines/.

Standard/Universal Precautions

1. Based on a risk assessment and the use of practices and protective equipment to protect HCPs from infection and prevent the spread of infection from patient to patient.
2. Standard precautions include:
   a. Perform hand hygiene.
      - Hand washing with antimicrobial soap and water; hand antisepsis with an alcohol-based hand rub or antiseptic hand wash.
      - Decontaminate hands before direct contact with patients, or after contact with the patient's skin, body fluids or excretions, nonintact skin, and wound dressings.
      - Decontaminate hands before and after donning sterile gloves.

   b. Use personal protection equipment (PPE) whenever there is an expectation of possible exposure to infectious material.
      - Gloves and gowns.
      - Mouth, nose, and eye protection (e.g., face shield) during patient-care activities that are likely to generates splashes or sprays of blood, body fluids, secretions, or during aerosol-generating procedures.

   c. Follow respiratory hygiene/cough etiquette principles.
   d. Ensure appropriate patient placement. High-risk patients are placed in an isolation/single-patient room. Triage and isolation of patients with COVID-19 are essential to minimize risk of infection among patients and health care workers.
   e. Clean and disinfect the environment appropriately.
      - Clean and disinfect surfaces in direct contact with the patient (e.g., treatment areas, frequently touched surfaces, waiting room).
      - Use EPA-registered disinfectants with known microbiocidal activity.
      - Clean and disinfect multiuse equipment and devices used during delivery of patient care including mobile devices moved in and out of patient rooms.
      - Multiple patients receiving therapy at the same time and place using shared equipment are at increased risk of infection and cross-contamination.
      - Plastic, single patient, disposable liners should be used for hydrotherapy tanks.
      - Hydrocollator tanks should be emptied and cleaned every 2 weeks.
      - Paraffin baths should be cleaned monthly.
      - Toys used with young pediatric patients that may put them in their mouths should be cleaned with diluted alcohol or bleach solutions and rinsed prior to and after use.

   f. Handle textiles and laundry carefully.
   g. Follow safe injection practices. Handle with care needles and other sharp instruments.

Transmission-Based/Isolation Precautions

1. Are used in addition to standard precautions previously discussed for patients with known or suspected infections.
2. Contact precautions.
   a. Indicated for patients with known or suspected infections that represent an increased risk for contact transmission.
   b. The patient is placed in a single patient room (acute care hospital) to limit the potential transmission of infectious agents. In ambulatory settings, place patients requiring contact precautions in a private exam room or cubicle ASAP.
   c. PPE including gloves and gown is used for all interactions that involve contact with the patient or the patient's environment.
   d. PPE is donned upon room entry and properly discarded before room exit.
   e. Transport and movement of the patient outside the room is limited to medically necessary purposes.
   f. Disposable or dedicated patient-care equipment (e.g., blood pressure cuffs) is used. Common use equipment is cleaned and disinfected before use on another patient.
   g. Cleaning and disinfecting the room is prioritized (e.g., at least daily).
3. Droplet precautions.
   a. Used for patients known or suspected to be infected with pathogens transmitted by respiratory droplets that are generated by the patient who is coughing, sneezing, or talking. COVID-19 is primarily spread by respiratory droplets.
   b. The patient is instructed to wear a mask during triage or transport.
   c. Same as for contact precautions:
      - Ensure appropriate single room placement.
      - Use PPE appropriately; HCP should don mask upon entry into the patient room or patient space.
      - Limit transport and movement of patients.
4. Airborne precautions.
   a. Used for a patient with known or suspected infections with pathogens transmitted by the airborne route (e.g., tuberculosis, measles, chickenpox, disseminated herpes zoster, COVID-19).
   b. The patient is placed in an airborne infection isolation room (AIIR) if available.
   c. The patient is instructed to wear a mask if transported outside the AIIR.
   d. Entry of susceptible HCPs is restricted (e.g., unvaccinated HCPs).
   e. Essential HCPs wear PPE, including a high-level respirator (NIOSH-approved N95 or higher).
   f. Transport and movement of the patient outside the room is limited to medically necessary purposes. The patient is instructed to wear a surgical mask when transported outside the AIIR room.
   g. Susceptible persons are immunized ASAP following unprotected contact with vaccine-preventable infections (e.g., measles, varicella, or smallpox).
5. Respiratory hygiene/cough etiquette principles.
   a. Recommended for all persons with signs and symptoms of respiratory infection.
   b. The person with a respiratory infection is instructed to:
      - Cover their mouth and nose with a tissue when coughing or sneezing.
      - Use the nearest no-touch waste receptacle to dispose of tissue after use.
      - Perform hand hygiene.
      - HCPs should offer masks to persons with symptoms who are coughing. If at an outpatient facility, masks should be offered at entry into the facility.
      - Observe droplet precautions.

Disinfection and Sterilization

1. Disinfection is the process of reducing or eliminating the microorganisms on hands, surfaces, or equipment.
2. Chemical disinfectants are most commonly used. They must be approved by the Environmental Protection Agency (EPA).
3. These agents are microbicidal and can eliminate most bacteria and viruses. Spores must be eliminated by sterilization.
4. Proper dilutions, usage, and safety issues associated with each type are stipulated.
5. Types.
   a. Isopropyl or ethyl alcohol sometimes combined with quaternary ammonium compounds or phenolics in the form of pads or towelettes. Examples are Gym Wipes, ShockWave, or Microban.
   b. Chlorine and chlorine compounds. Bleach such as Clorox is most common.
   c. Hydrogen peroxide (H_2O_2).
   d. Formaldehyde. Examples are Microban and Metri-Cide.
   e. Glutaraldehydes. Examples are CaviWipes and McKesson.
   f. Quaternary ammonium compounds. Examples are types of Lysol and Zephiran (benzalkonium chloride).
6. Sterilization is an absolute method for killing all microorganisms.
   a. In physical therapy, certain instruments or devices may need to be sterilized such as scissors or forceps used in wound debridement or certain respiratory interventions that use tubing.
   b. Steam (autoclave) is the most common method.
   c. Other methods may use dry heat at high temperatures, chemical vapors, or ionizing radiation.

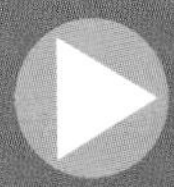

Abuse, Neglect, and Sexual Harassment

Child Abuse and Neglect

1. Can originate from parent, family member, caregiver, or family friend. Signs and symptoms include the following.
2. Physical abuse.
   a. Bruises, burns, welts, injury marks from a hand or belt.
   b. Medical or dental issues that have gone untreated.
   c. Child avoids touch or contact; seems fearful or on high alert.
3. Sexual abuse.
   a. Child demonstrates highly sexualized behavior, e.g., inappropriate language or touching.
   b. Child avoids certain people or caregiver.
   c. Bruising, bleeding, or pain around genitals, anus, or breasts.
   d. Pregnancy or STDs for those less than 14 years of age.
4. Emotional abuse.
   a. Depression or low self-esteem.
   b. Constant worrying about wrongdoing.
   c. Behavioral extremes. Child is either excessively demanding or obedient.
   d. Disinterested in others.
5. Child neglect.
   a. Diminished weight or stunted growth.
   b. Unkempt, dirty-looking, poor hygiene.
   c. Actual or fear of abandonment, being left alone, or unsupervised.
   d. Improper medical care such as untreated illnesses or injuries.
   e. Frequently absent from school or has unattributable learning problems.

Elder Abuse and Neglect

1. Can originate from caregiver, family member, or neighbor. Signs and symptoms include the following.
2. Physical abuse.
   a. Hitting, kicking, burns.
   b. Locking the individual in a room. Inappropriate use of restraints.
   c. Administering incorrect or dangerous medications.
   d. Individual exhibits repeated injuries, broken bones, contusions, lacerations.
3. Sexual abuse.
   a. Inappropriate touching.
   b. Genital contusions.
   c. Forced to view pornography.
4. Psychological abuse.
   a. Depressed or withdrawn.
   b. Frightened or agitated.
   c. Confused or incoherent.
   d. Caregivers don't meet individual's needs in terms of food, water, bathing.
5. Elder neglect.
   a. Individual appears unclean or unkempt.
   b. Evidence of weight loss.
   c. Individual might be missing hearing aids, glasses, walker, and other functional necessities.
   d. Individual not taking medications as prescribed.

Disabled Abuse and Neglect

1. Can originate from caregiver, family member, or other residents if in a skilled nursing facility. Signs and symptoms:
   a. Very similar to signs and symptoms of elder/abuse neglect.
   b. Physical, emotional, sexual neglect or abandonment.
   c. Caretaker or family member may exploit the disabled individual by concealing or misusing funds targeted for the disabled person.
   d. Be aware of unexplained pressure sores or bruises.

Abuse/Neglect Management and Reporting

1. Perform an examination and evaluation to establish a diagnosis and prognosis.
   a. Document thoroughly.
2. Reporting.
   a. Physical therapists are mandated reporters of child, elder, and disabled abuse/neglect in all 50 states and territories.
   b. All states have abuse/neglect "hot lines."
   c. Triggers and reporting thresholds may vary from state to state.
   d. Person reporting suspected abuse/neglect is immune from criminal or civil liability.

> RED FLAG: *Failure* to report suspected abuse/neglect by a health professional is considered a crime in most jurisdictions. Loss of license and other penalties may accrue.

   e. Facilities may have specific reporting protocols.

Sexual Misconduct and Sexual Harassment

1. Sexual misconduct.
   a. Physical therapists shall not engage in any sexual relationship or act with patients/clients, students, or supervisees.
   b. Integrity in relationships should also extend to colleagues and members of the health care team.
   c. Therapists should discourage sexual misconduct by others.
      - Communication with the individuals involved is the first step.
      - If the behaviors continue, the therapist is obligated to report misconduct, which may be illegal or unethical to the proper authority.
2. Romantic/sexual relationships with former patients/clients.
   a. There is no hard or fast rule.
   b. In some cases such relationships would "not offend." In other cases it might never be considered appropriate (e.g., a post-therapy relationship, which is solely used by the therapist as a means of exploiting the former patient financially or in other ways).
3. Sexual harassment.
   a. Sexual harassment includes unwelcome sexual advances, inappropriate sexual remarks or requests for sexual favors, or other verbal or physical advances in the workplace or other professional/social situations.
   b. The harasser can be a supervisor, co-worker, client, or any other person doing business with the facility.
   c. Included are a range of actions from inappropriate touching, rude comments, graphic art of a sexual nature, whistling, and leering to sexual abuse and assault.
   d. Adverse effects of sexual harassment can include stress, social withdrawal, sleep disorders, eating difficulties, or other health impairments.
   e. This conduct can affect an individual's employment, unreasonably interfere with work, or create a hostile or offensive environment.
   f. The victim may be of any gender and, not necessarily, of the opposite sex.
   g. The victim does not have to be the person harassed but is affected by the offensive conduct.
   h. The offended individual should inform the harasser that the conduct is unwelcome and must stop immediately.
   i. If the behavior continues, the victim or offended individual should report the behavior to a supervisor and file a report using an available employee complaint mechanism.
   j. If an HCP witnesses sexual harassment, bystander intervention can include intervening to give the person being harassed a chance to leave the situation.
      - Create a distraction.
      - Talk with the person being harassed and offer to accompany them during interactions with the harasser.
      - Enlist others for help and talk with a supervisor.
   k. Title VII of the Civil Rights Act of 1964 prohibits employment sexual harassment.
   l. Principle 4 of the Code of Ethics states, "Physical therapists shall not harass anyone verbally, physically, emotionally or sexually."
4. Inappropriate sexual behaviors by a patient/client.
   a. Patients with a traumatic brain injury or dementia with damage to the area controlling sexual function may demonstrate inappropriate sexual behaviors. Secondary factors that can intensify the behaviors include stress, depression, and anxiety.
   b. Signs and symptoms include:
      - Disinhibition.
      - Hypersexuality and arousal.
      - Exhibitionism and genital touching.
      - Coercive sexual assault.
      - Inappropriate and sexually charged comments.
   c. Management of inappropriate sexual behavior.
      - Talking with the health care team to develop management strategies.
      - Consistent behavioral techniques utilized by the whole team.
      - Set professional boundaries in relationships with patients/clients.
      - Provide verbal feedback and set limits as to what interactions are acceptable and what are not.

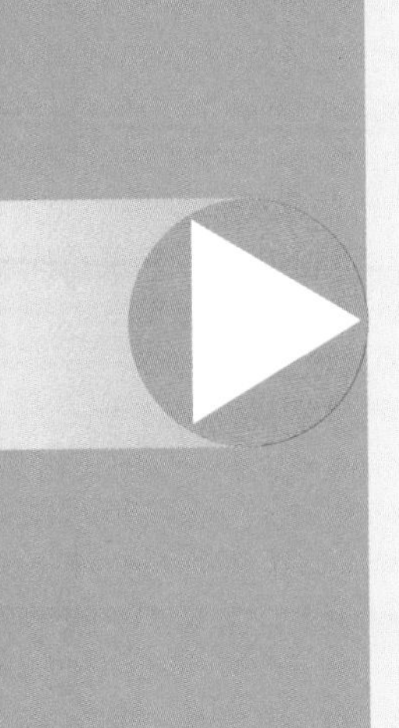

APPENDIX 13A

Review Questions

(Answers to all Review Questions and Case Studies are found in Chapter 17)

1. Identify three risk factors in each of the following categories that increase the likelihood of falls in older adults: medications, personal risk factors, and chronic diseases.

2. Differentiate between key basic life support (CPR) components for adults, children, and infants in terms of compression rate and depth.

3. A physical therapist should be on the alert for which possible signs and symptoms of physical, emotional, and sexual child abuse?

4. As a physical therapist practicing in a health care facility, what are possible internal and external sources of disasters that might trigger the initiation of an Emergency Action Plan (EAP)?

14

Professional Responsibilities

STEPHEN L. GOFFAR, CHAD W. JACKSON, AND
JENNIFER C. KISH

Chapter Outline

Study Tactics

Questions About Professional Responsibilities Comprise Approximately 2% of the NPTE, or a Total of Four to Five Questions

Focus on:

- Patient/client rights and legal/ethical obligations
  - Current major federal acts that impact patients' access to health care, licensure, and confidentiality. This includes Medicare/Medicaid, Health Insurance Portability and Accountability Act (HIPAA), Americans with Disabilities Act (ADA), and Individuals with Disabilities Education Act (IDEA). Review the role of Occupational Safety and Health Administration (OSHA), Joint Commission, and Commission on Accreditation of Rehabilitation Facilities (CARF).
  - Workplace transgressions such as sexual harassment, negligence/liability, and malpractice
  - Cultural and socioeconomic factors such as language, disability, ethnicity, religion, and sexual preference which might affect patient management
- Documentation and risk guidelines
  - Documentation guidelines. This might include SOAP notes and informed consent
  - Risk management and quality assurance (informed consent, incident/occurrence report, peer review, etc.)
  - Health information technology (electronic medical records, telemedicine)
- Roles and responsibilities of other health care workers
  - Definitions of various health professionals, support staff, students, and volunteers. You may be asked when it is appropriate to refer patients to other professionals or to delegate responsibilities to support staff. Be thoroughly familiar with the role and responsibilities of the PTA
  - Health care ethical principles (autonomy, justice, beneficence, nonmaleficence) and APTA Code of Ethics/Principles
  - Billing, coding, or reimbursement

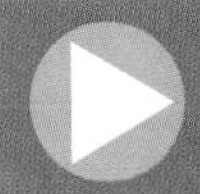

Institutional Types

Practice Environments

Acute Care (Short-Term Hospital)

1. Treatment for a short-term illness or health problem.
2. Average patient length of stay is 4–5 days.
3. Provider may be physician, physician assistant (PA), nurse, physical therapist (PT), etc.
4. Rapid discharge for next level of care makes the PT's role in patient and family education and in discharge planning increasingly important.

Primary Care

1. Basic or first-level health care.
2. Includes health services that cover a range of prevention, wellness, and treatment for common patient concerns. Primary care providers (PCPs) include doctors, nurses, nurse practitioners, and physician assistants. They often maintain long-term relationships with patients.
3. Provided on an outpatient basis.
4. PTs support primary care teams through examination, evaluation, diagnosis, prognosis, and prevention of musculoskeletal and neuromuscular disorders.
5. Often the PCP is the "gatekeeper" to other subspecialists, including physical therapy.

Secondary Care (Specialized Care)

1. Second-level medical services.
2. Provided by medical specialists, such as cardiologists, urologists, and dermatologists, who do not have first contact with patients.
3. This care often requires inpatient hospitalization or ambulatory same-day surgery such as hernia repair.
4. Physical, occupational, respiratory, and speech-language pathologists often work in secondary care settings.

Tertiary Care (Tertiary Health Care)

1. Highly specialized, technologically based medical services; e.g., heart, liver, or lung transplants, and other major surgical procedures.
2. Provided by highly specialized physicians in a hospital setting.
3. PTs respond to requests for consultation made by other health care practitioners.

Subacute Care

1. An intermediate level of health care for medically fragile patients too ill to be cared for at home.
2. Provided by medical and nursing services as well as rehabilitative services; e.g., PT, occupational therapy (OT), and speech-language pathology (SLP) at a higher level than is offered in a skilled nursing facility (SNF) on a regular basis.
3. Provided within the hospital or SNF setting.

Long-Term Acute Care Hospital (LTACH)

1. Patients require complex medical intervention from specialized staff including 24-hour physician, nursing care, and therapy.
2. Diagnoses treated include respiratory failure, ventilator dependency and weaning (e.g., COVID-19 respiratory disease), septicemia with major complications, skin ulcers with major complications.
3. Patient stays must be an average of 25 days or more.

Ambulatory Care (Outpatient Care)

1. Includes outpatient preventative, diagnostic, and treatment services.
2. Provided at medical offices, surgery centers, or outpatient clinics.
3. Providers may be physicians, PAs, nurse practitioners, PTs, or others.
4. Less costly than inpatient care. Favored by managed-care plans.
5. Outpatient rehabilitation centers, PT clinics, outpatient satellites of institutions, or privately owned outpatient clinics.

Skilled Nursing Facility

1. Free-standing or part of a hospital transitional care unit.
2. Care provided by continuous nursing, rehabilitation, and other health care services on a daily basis.
3. Skilled nursing services or skilled rehabilitation services (or a combination of these services) must be needed and provided on a "daily basis," i.e., on essentially a 7-days-a-week basis. A patient whose inpatient stay is based solely on the need for skilled rehabilitation services would meet the "daily basis" requirement when they need and receive those services on at least 5 days a week. (If therapy services are provided less than 5 days a week, the "daily" requirement would not be met.)
4. Patients are not in an acute phase of illness, but require skilled care on an inpatient basis.
5. SNFs must be certified by Medicare and meet qualifications, including 24-hour nursing coverage, availability of PT, OT, and SLP.

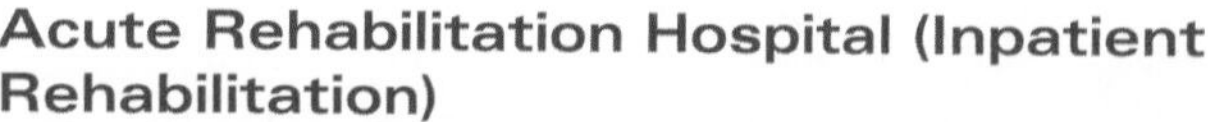

Acute Rehabilitation Hospital (Inpatient Rehabilitation)

1. Facility that provides coordinated rehabilitation, social, and vocational services to disabled individuals to facilitate their return to maximal functional capacity.
2. Patients must be able to participate in a minimum of 3 hours of daily therapy. Most common diagnoses treated are stroke, brain injury, other neurologic conditions (Parkinson's disease, multiple sclerosis), multiple trauma, general rehabilitation (spinal injury, amputation).
3. Average length of stay is 13 days.

Nursing Home (Long-Term Care Facility)

1. Long-term care facility provides services to patients for 60 days or more.
2. Medical services provided to patients with permanent or residual disability caused by a nonreversible pathological health condition.
3. May require specialized care/rehabilitation.

Custodial Care Facility

1. Patient care that is not medically required but necessary for the patient that is unable to care for him-/herself.
2. Custodial care may involve medical or nonmedical services that do not seek a cure.
3. This type of care is usually not covered under most health care plans.
4. Daily care is delivered by nonmedical support staff.

Hospice Care

1. Care available for terminally ill patients having 6 months or less to live as well as their families at home or the inpatient setting.
2. Hospice team includes: nurses, social workers, chaplains, volunteers, and physicians. PT and OT services are optional.
3. Eligibility for reimbursement.
   a. Medicare eligibility.
   b. Certification by physician of terminal illness (≤6 months of life).
   c. Authorized for two 90-day benefit periods and unlimited 60-day extension periods.

Home Health Care

1. Health care provided to individuals and their families in their homes.
2. Provided by a home health agency (HHA), which may be governmental, voluntary, or private; nonprofit or for-profit.
3. Eligible patients.
   a. Are homebound or have great difficulty leaving the home without assistance or an assistive device.
   b. Would experience a health risk leaving the home.
   c. Require intermittent skilled care from one of the following services: nursing, PT, OT, or SLP.
   d. Have physician certification.
   e. Either show potential for progress, need skilled therapy to develop, or safely and effectively perform maintenance therapy for their condition.
   f. Have more than housekeeping deficits.
4. Environmental safety is consideration of PT or OT; e.g., proper lighting; securing of scatter rugs, handrails, wheelchair ramps.
5. Supplemental equipment may be necessary; e.g., raised toilet seats, grab bars, long-handled utensils, if delivered by a licensed durable medical equipment vendor to the home at the time of hospital discharge. It may be reimbursable.
6. Adaptive equipment ordered in the home is not reimbursable, except for items such as wheelchairs, commodes, and hospital beds.
7. Indications of substance abuse recognized by the PT should be reported immediately to the physician.
8. Suspected physical abuse or neglect should be communicated immediately and directly to the proper authorities; e.g., Department of Social Services or equivalent should be notified if child abuse is suspected.
9. The laws that mandate reporting of abuse of an elder, disabled individual, or minor may vary from state to state.

School System

1. Goal of PT treatment is to promote student access to school environments and benefit from the educational program.
2. Major goal of PT treatment is the child's functioning in the school setting.
3. Recommendations are made for adaptive equipment to facilitate improved posture, head control, and function; e.g., using a computer, viewing a blackboard, improving mobility from class to class.

Private Practice

1. Entrepreneurial PTs who work for or own a freestanding, independent PT practice.
2. May accept all insurances with provider numbers or be a cash-based practice which does not accept insurance.
3. Settings may include any general outpatient or any speciality practice area.
4. May occupy a physical space or have a mobile clinician model.
5. Must document every visit and complete reevaluations at least every 30 days for reimbursement purposes.

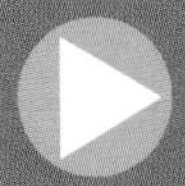

The United States Health Care System

Organization

Overview

1. A group of decentralized subsystems that serve different populations.
2. Most Americans have private health insurance via managed-care plans (health maintenance organizations, preferred provider organizations), traditional fee-for-service plans, or participate in public programs, such as Medicare or Medicaid.
3. Decentralization results in overlap in some areas and competition in others; therefore, health care is primarily a business that is market-driven, especially for patients covered by managed-care insurance.
   a. Patients are viewed as consumers because of this economic focus.
   b. Cost containment while maintaining quality of service is a delicate balancing act that is not always achieved.
4. PCPs have increased significance as the first line for evaluation and intervention, and as the referral source for specialized and/or ancillary services.

Health Care Regulations

1. Health care is a highly regulated industry, with most regulations mandated by law at both the state and federal levels.
2. Legally mandated regulations are set forth by the Center for Medicare and Medicaid Services (CMS), a division of U.S. Department of Health and Human Services.
   a. CMS is the federal agency that develops rules and regulations pertaining to federal laws, specifically the Medicare and Medicaid programs.
   b. Facilities that participate in Medicare and/or Medicaid programs are monitored regularly for compliance with CMS guidelines by federal and state surveyors.
   c. Often, state departments of public health monitor Medicare/Medicaid compliance of inpatient institutions, and "fiscal intermediaries" are contracted to monitor compliance of Medicare Part B regulations.
   d. Facilities that repeatedly fail to meet CMS guidelines may lose their Medicare and/or Medicaid certification (e.g., "provider status").
3. Standards related to safety are set forth and enforced by the Occupational Safety and Health Administration (OSHA), a division of the U.S. Department of Labor.
   a. Structural standards and building codes are established and enforced by OSHA to ensure the safety of structures.
   b. The safety of employees and consumers is regulated by OSHA standards for handling infectious materials and blood products, controlling blood-borne pathogens, operating machinery, and handling hazardous substances.
   c. Material Safety Data Sheets are mandated by OSHA. These documents give employees information about potentially hazardous materials in the workplace and how to protect themselves.
   d. The blood-borne pathogen and needlestick prevention standard requires institutions to have processes in place to reduce the risk of exposure to blood-borne pathogens. This includes a written safety plan, employee training, and proper disposal practices.
   e. Other OSHA standards cover x-ray safety, electrical and fire safety, and provide for the provision of personal protective equipment (PPE). Additionally, an emergency action plan (EAP) is a written document required by particular OSHA standards. The purpose of the EAP is to facilitate and organize employer and employee actions during workplace emergencies.
4. Individual states develop their own requirements with state agencies to enforce these regulations. State accreditation to obtain licensure for a health care facility is mandatory.
5. Local or county entities also develop regulations pertaining to health care institutions (i.e., physical plant safety features such as fire, elevator, and boiler regulations).

Voluntary Accreditation

1. Voluntary accreditation and self-imposed compliance with established standards is sought by most health care organizations.
2. Accreditation is a status awarded for compliance with standards and regulations, promulgated by the specific accrediting agency.
3. Accreditation ensures the public that a health care facility is adequately equipped, meets high standards for patient care, and has qualified professionals and competent staff.
4. Accreditation affirms the competence of practitioners and the quality of health care facilities and organizations.
5. Although national accreditation through an accrediting agency is voluntary, it is mandatory for most third-party reimbursement and to meet eligibility requirements for federal government grants and contracts.

6. CMS and many states accept certain national accreditations as meeting their respective requirements for participation in the Medicare and Medicaid programs and for a license to operate.

Voluntary Accrediting Agencies

1. The Joint Commission (TJC).
   a. A not-for-profit organization that accredits/certifies health care organizations and programs according to TJC standards.
   b. Health care organizations and facilities volunteer to be evaluated for accreditation or certification.
   c. TJC accredits hospitals, SNFs, home health agencies, preferred provider organizations (PPOs), rehabilitation facilities, health maintenance organizations (HMOs), behavioral health (including mental health and chemical dependency facilities, ambulatory clinics, physician's networks, hospice care, long-term care facilities, and others).
2. Commission on Accreditation of Rehabilitation Facilities (CARF): a nonprofit organization that provides accreditation at the request of free-standing rehabilitation facilities and the rehabilitative programs of larger hospital systems in the areas of behavioral health, employment (work hardening) and community support services, and medical rehabilitation (spinal cord injury, chronic pain).
3. Some accreditation bodies may perform unannounced or unscheduled site surveys to ensure ongoing compliance.

Reimbursement/Third-Party Payers for Health Care Services

Medicare

1. Administered by federal government CMS, through the extension of Title XVIII of the Social Security Act, 1965.
2. Provides medical coverage and health care services to individuals:
   a. ≥65 years.
   b. Disabled.
   c. End-stage renal disease (ESRD).
3. Social Security Amendment of 1983.
   a. Established Medicare's prospective payment system.
      - Based on diagnostic-related groups (DRGs).
        - Classification system that places patients into disease categories or groups.
        - Basis for Medicare's prospective payment system.
      - Hospital paid a specific amount per diagnosis, regardless of the length of stay, number of services provided, or tests performed.
4. Medicare Part A benefits.
   a. Hospital insurance that covers:
      - Inpatient hospital care.
        - Limits number of hospital days.
      - Skilled nursing facilities—first 100 days.
      - Home Health Agencies.
      - Hospice care.
   b. Provides basic protection against the cost of health care.
   c. Does not cover all medical expenses or the cost of long-term or custodial care.
   d. Provides coverage for patients that have been on Social Security disability for 24 months.
   e. Annual deductible fees paid by the patient.
   f. Services provided by a student physical therapist may be reimbursible under appropriate supervision.
   g. Services may be provided by a physical therapy aide if allowed by the jurisdiction.
5. Medicare Part B.
   a. Medical insurance that covers:
      - Physician visits.
      - Outpatient laboratory tests and x-rays.
      - Ambulance transportation.
      - Outpatient physical and occupational therapy services (hospital and private practice).
      - Home health care provided by a PT in independent practice (PTIP).
      - Durable medical equipment (e.g., wheelchairs, canes, walkers) determined to be "medically necessary."
      - Medical supplies not covered by hospital insurance.
      - Residents of long-term care facilities.
   b. Each patient must pay a monthly premium.
   c. PT treatment does not need to be given on a daily basis.
   d. The physician responsible for the care of the patient referred for PT must "certify" the plan of care.
   e. Only PT care that is considered to be "skilled," "necessary," and "certified" by the referring physician will be reimbursed by Medicare.
   f. Reimbursement mandates successfully reporting data using quality outcome measures.
   g. Student physical therapist services provided may be reimbursable under direct "in-room" supervision.
   h. Care provided by a physical therapy aide is not reimbursable regardless of supervision.
   i. Time-based billing requires documentation of:
      - Time-in and time-out or total time.
      - Services described by timed codes, untimed codes, and unattended activities.
      - Total number of units billed is limited by the total minutes of the one-on-one encounter.

Medicaid

1. A joint state and federal program mandated by Title XIX of the Social Security Act.
2. Provides health services to the poor, elderly, and disabled who do not receive Medicare, regardless of age.
3. Benefits vary from state to state.
4. Preauthorization is needed by a physician before treatment can begin.
5. Individual states can determine the scope, duration, and amount of services provided.

Workers' Compensation

1. Regulated by state statutes and administered by private insurers, self-insured employers, or other agencies in some states.
2. Provides health care for individuals injured on the job.
3. Some states limit the number of visits per diagnosis and/or require a preapproval process for reimbursement.
4. Other states require that the total number of visits, total number of weeks (duration), and number of treatments per week (frequency) to be usual, customary, and reasonable.
5. Employers only contribute to the fund.
   a. All large employers (≥10 employees) or high-risk employers must contribute to workers' compensation.

Private Health Insurance

1. Includes commercial insurance, fee-for-service or traditional indemnity plans, or employers who are self-insured.
2. Patient has freedom to choose his/her providers.
3. Preauthorization may not be needed.
4. The number of PT visits should be usual, customary, and reasonable, which are often defined contractually in the insurance policy.

Managed Health Care Systems

1. Third-party payers direct patients to certain providers and monitor services in order to avoid excessive and inappropriate treatment and limit access.
   a. Third-party payers frequently use gatekeepers (usually the PCP) to manage access to certain providers, including PT.
   b. Use techniques such as preadmission certification, concurrent reviews, financial incentives, or penalties.
   c. Goal is to contain costs and ensure favorable patient outcomes.
2. Health Maintenance Organization (HMO).
   a. A form of managed care that provides a broad spectrum of health services to individuals and families for a preset amount of money.
   b. Employers contract for these services as a benefit to their employees.
   c. Employees may pay a fee per visit (copay).
   d. Patients are locked into use of the system of member health care providers and affiliating facilities.
   e. Some HMOs allow patients to seek care "out of network," but at a higher or additional cost to the patient.
   f. PCPs chosen by individuals act as gatekeepers for medical care beyond their scope of practice.
      - Must authorize PT services before they can be provided.
   g. Total number of visits per diagnosis is limited.
   h. Types of HMOs.
      - Individual Practice Associations (IPAs).
        - Physician groups contract independently with the HMO.
        - Physicians work out of their own offices instead of a central facility.
      - Prepaid Group Plan (PGP).
        - Physicians practice out of a central location.
3. Preferred provider organization (PPO).
   a. A group of providers, usually physicians or hospitals, that offer health care services as an entity to employers.
   b. Providers discount their fees to attract patients.
   c. Patients are not locked into PPO providers but receive financial incentives to use services through the PPO network.
   d. An employer can offer its employees a traditional health plan, HMO, or PPO.
   e. Preauthorization is needed before services can be provided.
4. Both HMOs and PPOs employ one or more of the following payment mechanisms for care sought.
   a. Fee for service: model in which providers are paid retrospectively for each service performed.
   b. Case-based rate: a flat bundled reimbursement rate is established prospectively based on the diagnosis.
      - Per diem: flat rate per day.
      - Per visit: flat rate per visit.
      - Per episode of service.
      - Made at the time of the service.
      - Predetermined dollar amount.
   c. Coinsurance: insured's share of the cost of covered service.
      - Expressed as a percentage of the net charges; e.g., 80% paid by insurance and 20% paid by insured.
   d. Each payment model balances risk and incentives for utilization of services.

Health Savings Accounts

1. Tax-free savings account that can be used to pay for health-related expenses and retiree health expenses.
2. Must have a high-deductible health plan, which is an insurance product that covers catastrophic health occurrences.

Personal Payment and Free Care

1. Individuals without health insurance must personally pay for all medical care.
2. Individuals who cannot pay for health care can receive pro bono, or free, care through philanthropic donations and services.
3. Many states have programs that offset some of the expense of providing free care by relying on other not-for-profit organizations.

Restructuring the Health Care System

1. Cost containment created incentives for health care providers and hospitals to control both cost and utilization of inpatient services by:
   a. Reducing average length of hospital stay.
   b. Reducing routine and/or unnecessary diagnostic testing and treatment.
   c. Increasing use of outpatient diagnostic testing and treatment.
   d. Increasing utilization of home care and skilled long-term care.

Affordable Care Act

1. Because many Americans were uninsured due to finances and/or preexisting conditions, the Patient Protection and Affordable Care Act (March 23, 2010) was enacted at the federal level. The overall goal is to provide quality affordable health care for all Americans. Some features include:
   a. Patient bill of rights.
   b. Increased cost-free preventive services.
   c. Closing the gap in Medicare Part D prescription drug plan coverage or Medicare Advantage plan coverage where the Medicare plan member was 100% responsible for the cost of their prescription drugs (donut hole).
   d. Mandatory and regulated affordable insurance options for small businesses and individuals through a marketplace exchange.
   e. Young adult coverage.
   f. Prohibiting denial of coverage for preexisting conditions in children.
   g. Establishment of Accountable Care Organizations.

Accountable Care Organizations (ACOs)

1. On October 20, 2011, the Centers for Medicare & Medicaid Services (CMS), an agency within the Department of Health and Human Services (HHS), finalized new rules under the Affordable Care Act to help physicians, hospitals, and other health care providers better coordinate care for Medicare patients through ACOs.
2. Under the final rule, an ACO refers to a group of providers and suppliers of services (e.g., hospitals, physicians, and others involved in patient care) that will work together to coordinate care for the Medicare fee-for-service patients they serve. The goal of an ACO is to deliver seamless, high-quality care for Medicare beneficiaries, instead of the fragmented care that often results from a fee-for-service payment system in which different providers receive different, disconnected payments. The ACO will be a patient-centered organization where the patient and providers are partners in care decisions.
3. An ACO can be based in physician practices, hospitals, or via networks comprised of partnerships or joint venture arrangements between hospitals and ACO professionals.

Defensible Documentation

The International Classification of Functioning, Disability, and Health Resources (ICF) Model (See Box 14-1)

1. Developed by the World Health Organization (WHO) and endorsed by the American Physical Therapy Association (APTA), the World Confederation for Physical Therapy, and other international organizations.
2. The ICF Model.
   a. Identifies dimensions of function (body functions and body structures, activities, participation) and disability (participation restrictions).
   b. Serves as a platform for communication among medical personnel, patients, and their family/caregivers.
   c. Serves as a platform for selecting and comparing examination techniques, outcomes, and interventions.
   d. Uses a unified, standard language and framework and permits documentation of functioning and disability as a multidimensional phenomena experienced at the level of the body, the person, and society.

Outcome Measures Organized by the ICF Categories

1. Physical therapists select tests and measures as a means to:
   a. Identify and characterize signs and symptoms of pathology/pathophysiology, impairments, functioning, and disability.
   b. Establish a diagnosis and prognosis, select interventions, and document changes in patient/client status.
   c. Monitor outcomes, document end points of care, and ensure appropriate and timely discharge.
2. Documentation is enhanced by using measurements with demonstrated reliability and validity.

Medical Records

1. Complete, timely, and accurate documentation is essential for:
   a. Patient safety.
   b. Accurate communication between health care providers.

BOX 14-1 Terminology: Functioning, Disability, and Health

Health Condition is an umbrella term for disease, disorder, injury, or trauma, and may also include other circumstances, such as aging, stress, congenital anomaly, or genetic predisposition. It may also include information about pathogeneses and/or etiology.

Body Functions are physiological functions of body systems (including psychological functions).

Body Structures are anatomical parts of the body such as organs, limbs, and their components.

Impairments are the problems in body function or structure, such as a significant deviation or loss.

Activity is the execution of a task or action by an individual.

Participation is involvement in a life situation.

Activity Limitations are difficulties an individual may have in executing activities.

Participation Restrictions are problems an individual may experience in involvement in life situations.

Contextual Factors represent the entire background of an individual's life and living situation.

- **Environmental Factors** make up the physical, social, and attitudinal environment in which people live and conduct their lives, including social attitudes, architectural characteristics, and legal and social structures.
- **Personal Factors** are the particular background of an individual's life, including gender, age, coping styles, social background, education, profession, past and current experience, overall behavior pattern, character, and other factors that influence how disability is experienced by an individual.

Performance describes what an individual does in his or her current environment.

Capacity describes an individual's ability to execute a task or an action (highest probable level of functioning in a given domain at a given moment).

From The World Health Organization. International Classification of Functioning, Disability, and Health Resources (ICF). World Health Organization, Geneva, 2002. http://www.who.int/classifications/en/

c. Compliance with federal and state regulations.
d. Appropriate utilization for third-party payers.
e. Historical record for potential legal situations.

2. General guidelines for documentation.
   a. All documentation must comply with all applicable state, federal, and regulatory agency laws and regulations.
   b. All documentation must comply with Medicare guidelines and any other guidelines required by the local insurance carrier to ensure reimbursement.
   c. Patient's right to privacy must always be respected and protected.
   d. Release of any medical information must be authorized by the patient.
   e. Records must be kept in a safe and secure place for a certain number of years (varies from state to state; usually 7 years).
3. Basic principles of documentation (see Guide to Physical Therapist Practice, APTA).
   a. Documentation should be consistent with Guidelines for Physical Therapy Documentation, APTA.
   b. All documents must be legible.
   c. Only medically approved abbreviations or symbols can be used.
   d. Mistakes should be crossed out with a single line through the error, and then initialed and dated by the therapist.
   e. White-out material should never be used to correct text in a medical record.
   f. Informed consent for treatment must be given only by a competent adult.
   g. Noncompetent adults or minors must have a parent or legal guardian give written consent/proxy.
   h. Document each episode of treatment.
   i. Patient name and some other unique identifier should be on each page.
   j. Date each entry (some payers require length of time per visit, particularly Medicare and Medicaid).
   k. Sign each entry with first and last names and professional designation.
   l. Record significant events; e.g., phone conversations with the physician or nurse.
   m. Document treatment rendered in objective, measurable, and functional terms.
   n. Document patient's response to treatment.
   o. When goals and outcomes are reached, complete a discharge plan.
   p. Electronic documentation systems must have both security and confidentiality provisions in place. These electronic medical record systems are usually cloud-based and encrypted, especially if being used on mobile devices.
   q. A computer signature is acceptable on a secured computer documentation system.
   r. When correcting a charting error on an electronic medical record, it must be clearly indicated that a change was made without deletion of the original medical record.

4. Initial visit note.
   a. Referral mechanism by which services are initiated.
   b. Patient reported health status.
   c. Systems review.
   d. Tests and measures.
   e. Evaluation.
   f. Diagnosis/PT diagnosis.
   g. Prognosis.
   h. Plan of care.
   i. Authentication.
5. Progress notes.
   a. Document specific treatment, equipment provided; include signature of therapist who provides care.
   b. Document patient response to treatment, functional progress, goals achieved, revision of goals, and treatment plan modifications.
   c. Interim progress notes can be written by:
      - PT.
      - Physical therapist assistant (PTA).
      - Student (PT or PTA) notes must be cosigned by supervising therapist.
6. Reevaluation/summary progress report.
   a. Completed minimally every 30 days for all Medicare patients; includes:
      - Restatement of initial problem.
      - Length of time patient has been treated.
      - Progress or regression since last summary or initial evaluation.
      - Rationale for continued care.
      - Revision of goals and outcomes.
      - Revision of plan of care.
      - Changes documented are stated in behavioral, objective, measurable, and functional terms; e.g., range of motion, strength, sitting tolerance.
   b. Must be written by a PT.
      - PT students can complete if cosigned by supervising therapist.
7. Discharge/Conclusion of the episode of care summary includes:
   a. Restatement of initial problem.
   b. Length of time the patient has been treated.
   c. Progress since initial evaluation.
   d. Patient progress toward goal and outcome achievement.
   e. Reason for discharge.
   f. Must be written by a PT.
      - PT students can complete if cosigned by supervising therapist.
8. Conclusion of care plan.
   a. Referrals, written or verbal, related to patient's continued care.
      - Additional services.
      - Type of supervision the patient will require.
      - Home care.
      - Family intervention.
      - Patient and family education requirements.
      - Written home exercise program (HEP).
      - List of equipment ordered, vendor's name, and delivery date.
      - Social and community needs of the patient.
      - Date of discharge.
      - A PT should discharge a patient from PT treatment when maximum benefit is reached.
      - Identifies needs of patient after discharge from a facility.
         - Preferable setting for discharge.
   b. Must be written by a PT.
      - PT students can complete if cosigned by supervising therapist.
9. Advance directives.
   a. A legal document that delineates a patient's wishes for future medical care or no medical care.
   b. Are implemented if the patient is cognitively impaired.
   c. Can include living wills and durable power of attorney.

Common Reasons for Payment Denials

1. Incomplete/insufficient documentation. Documentation that is submitted without required documentation elements may result in a denial of payment.
2. Medically unnecessary. Poor documentation that does not fully explain the reasons for therapeutic interventions may result in denial of payment.
3. Incorrect coding.
   a. Failure to document using proper ICD codes. Failure to document the proper CPT (Current Procedural Terminology), World Health Organization's International Classification of Diseases, 9th Revision, Clinical Modification (ICD-9-CM 2001) or other diagnosis or treatment codes can result in denial of payment.
4. Pay for performance.
   a. As pay for performance programs (payment based on improved functional outcomes) grow, poor documentation may result in reduced payments for services.

Elements of Patient/Client Management

Initial Examination/Evaluation/Diagnosis/Prognosis

1. The PT performs an initial examination and evaluation to establish a diagnosis and prognosis prior to intervention.
2. The PT examination.
   a. Identifies the PT needs of the patient or client.
   b. Incorporates appropriate tests and measures to facilitate outcome measurement.

c. Produces data that are sufficient to allow evaluation, diagnosis, prognosis, and the establishment of a plan of care.
d. May result in recommendations for additional services to meet the needs of the patient or client.
e. Used to determine proper diagnosis and treatment coding.

Examination

1. History.
   a. Patient's name, age, race, education, gender, and primary language.
   b. Chief complaint and risk factors, relevance for PT intervention, if applicable.
   c. Referral source.
   d. Pertinent diagnosis and medical history.
   e. Demographic characteristics, including pertinent psychological, social, cultural, and environmental factors.
   f. Concurrent medical services provided.
   g. Pertinent problems.
   h. Statement describing patient's understanding of problem.
   i. Review of systems.
      - All major systems to establish need for further evaluation.
      - Cardiovascular, pulmonary, EENT, GI, GU, lymph, integument, neuromusculoskeletal.
2. Systems review.
   a. Physiologic and anatomic status.
      - Cognitive status, alertness, judgment, communication.
      - Neurological status: pain, sensation, reflexes, balance, motor function, etc.
      - Musculoskeletal: joint range of motion, strength, posture, etc.
      - Cardiovascular: vital signs, endurance, etc.
      - Integumentary.
   b. Functional status: mobility, transfers, activities of daily living (ADLs), work, school, or athletic performance, etc.
   c. Communication ability, affect, cognition, language, and learning style.

Evaluation

1. Analysis of current impairments and effect on function.
2. Analysis of prolonged impairment, functional limitation, and disability.
3. Analysis of living environment, potential discharge destination, and social supports.

Diagnosis

1. Diagnostic label consistent within the legal boundaries governing PT practice.
2. Encompasses a cluster of signs, symptoms, syndromes, or categories.
3. Guides therapist in determining appropriate interventions strategy.
4. Guides therapist in referring patient/client to an appropriate practitioner for services outside the scope of PT.

Prognosis

1. Includes predicted optimal level of improvement in function and amount of time needed to reach that level.
2. Can also predict levels of improvement at various intervals during the course of therapy.

Plan of Care

1. The PT establishes a plan of care for the individual patient/client based on the examination, evaluation, diagnosis, prognosis, anticipated goals, and expected outcomes of the planned interventions for identified impairments, functional limitations, and disabilities.
2. The PT, in consultation with appropriate disciplines, plans for conclusion of care/discharge of the patient/client, taking into consideration achievement of anticipated goals and expected outcomes, and provides for appropriate follow-up or referral.
3. The PT also addresses risk reduction, prevention, impact on societal resources, and patient/client satisfaction.
4. Identifies realistic long-term and short-term goals and expected functional outcomes.
   a. Goals establish the intended impact on function, structures, activity, and participation of the implementation of the plan of care.
   b. Goals should be measurable, functional, and time-specific.
      - Who will participate in the activity?
      - A detailed description of the activity.
      - The connection of the activity to a specific function.
      - A specific measure for success.
      - A time measure.

Intervention

1. The PT provides, or directs, and supervises the PT intervention consistent with the results of the examination, evaluation, diagnosis, prognosis, and plan of care.
2. The intervention is:
   a. Provided under the ongoing direct care or supervision of the PT.
   b. Provided in such a way that delegated responsibilities are commensurate with the qualifications and the legal limitations of the PT support and professional personnel involved in the intervention.
   c. Altered in accordance with changes in response or status.
   d. Provided at a level that is consistent with current PT practice.
   e. Interdisciplinary when necessary to meet the needs of the patient or client.

3. Documentation of the intervention is:
   a. Dated and appropriately authenticated by the PT or, when permissible by law, by the PTA, or both.

Reexamination

1. The PT reexamines the patient/client as necessary during an episode of care to evaluate progress or change in patient/client status, and modifies the plan of care accordingly or discontinues PT services.
2. The PT reexamination:
   a. Identifies ongoing patient/client needs.
   b. May result in recommendations for additional services, discharge, or discontinuation of PT needs.

Discharge/Discontinuation of Intervention

1. Discharge.
   a. The PT discharges the patient/client from PT services when the anticipated goals or expected outcomes for the patient/client have been achieved.
   b. Occurs at the end of an episode of care and is the end of PT services provided during that episode.
2. Discontinuation.
   a. The PT discontinues intervention when the patient/client is unable to continue to progress toward goals or when the PT determines that the patient/client will no longer benefit from PT.
   b. Discontinuation also occurs when the patient/client, caregiver, or legal guardian declines to continue intervention.

Successful Documentation Practices

1. Incorporate evidence-based practice principles. Use standard tests and measures that are valid and reliable, and select interventions based on research and practice.
2. Demonstrate progress in specific and functional terms.
3. Document medical necessity and reasons for skilled care.
4. Document to stand up in a court of law. Document fully, and limit the use of jargon and obscure abbreviations. Sign and date all entries. Be factual and objective.

Telehealth/Telerehabilitation

1. Telehealth requires review and integration of regulatory issues, interstate licensure laws, risk management, privacy (HIPAA), and reimbursement concerns prior to implementation of services.
2. Please see the American Physical Therapy Association Telehealth website for updates and additional resources (https://www.apta.org/telehealth/).

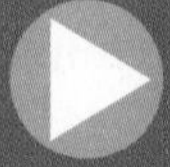

Management and Legal Issues

Human Resources

Interview

1. Performed by supervisor, director, and also possibly a member of the human resources department.
2. Purpose is to meet with prospective employee.
   a. Exchange questions and answers to obtain enough information to make an informed decision.
   b. Questions asked are informational to encourage discussion rather than questions that require "yes or no" answers.
   c. The Equal Employment Opportunity Commission (EEOC) clearly states that "an employer may not base hiring decisions on stereotypes and assumptions about a person's race, color, religion, sex (including gender identity, sexual orientation, and pregnancy), national origin, age (40 or older), disability or genetic information" (EEOC, https://www.eeoc.gov/laws/practices/, 2018).
   d. Information regarding academic record, educational program, or references cannot be obtained without consent.
   e. Many employers will require a criminal background check (criminal offender record information referred to as CORI) that requires the consent of the applicant to pursue.
   f. Interviewer provides information about:
      - Advantages and disadvantages of the organization.
      - Benefits available.
      - Work hours.
      - Vacation, sick, and personal time.
      - Salary range.
      - Job description.
3. Employers look for the following information in an interview.
   a. Decision-making style.
   b. Communications skills.
   c. Interpersonal skills: poise, tact, ability to work in groups.
   d. Leadership.
   e. Achievement record and relevant employment experience.
   f. Sense of personal direction.
4. Documents reviewed for employment.
   a. Job application: completeness, attention to detail.
   b. Previous employment experience.
   c. Transcript from educational institution (especially for new graduates): grade point average and

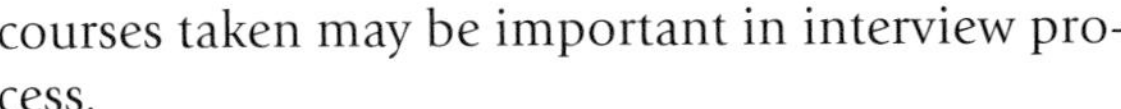

courses taken may be important in interview process.

d. Résumé: a brief written summary that highlights personal, educational, and professional qualifications and experience.

e. References.
   - Professional: former employers, clinical supervisors, faculty.
   - Character: family, friend, clergy.

Job Descriptions

1. General summary of responsibilities.
   a. Provides overview of position including supervisor relationships.
2. Specific job responsibilities.
   a. Identifies the specific responsibilities of the position.
   b. Establishes performance standards.
   c. Establishes skilled and nonskilled requirements of job.
   d. Formalizes basic performance expectations by describing duties in detail.
   e. Establishes degree of decision-making authority and autonomy.
   f. Organizational and supervisory relationships of position.
      - Position title.
      - Department division.
      - Title of position's supervisor.
3. Job specifications.
   a. Educational requirements; e.g., graduate from accredited PT program.
   b. State licensure.
   c. Previous experience requirements.
   d. Essential job functions or specific physical and mental demands of position.
      - Lifting requirements.
      - Transferring requirements.
      - Ambulatory or positioning requirements.
      - Proficiency in reading/writing/comprehension.
      - Maintaining static postures: performing therapeutic procedures for several minutes.
   e. Ability to plan and organize time and other work habits.
   f. Problem-solving skills.

Performance Appraisal

1. Assesses an employee's performance in relation to performance expectations established with objective criteria.
2. Written report and discussed verbally.
3. Frequency can be 3–6 months or annually.
4. Correlates to job description and goals of the organization.
5. Improves communication between the employee and employer.
6. Feedback should be immediate, specific, and communicated directly.
7. Outcomes of performance appraisals can be motivational and used as a reward system; e.g., raises, bonuses, promotions. May also identify performance issues and areas for improvement.
8. Examples of methods of review:
   a. Essay appraisal: short paragraph on strengths and weaknesses.
   b. Performance criteria-based method: based on functional job description using a weighted rating scale (most important task gets highest rating); e.g., patient evaluation, weighted average of 5, and personal appearance 2.
9. Objective performance goals should be established for the next review.

Unions

1. Organized group of workers with the same goals and objectives.
2. Provides collective bargaining when negotiating work contracts.
   a. Salaries.
   b. Fringe benefits.
   c. Hours of work.
   d. Conditions of work site.
3. Mediates grievances due to labor disputes, disciplinary problems, etc.

Policy and Procedure Manual

1. Provides extensive information on what shall be done and how it shall be done in a PT department.
2. Required by JCAHO, CARF, and other accrediting agencies. Often required by other state regulatory bodies, such as state boards of public health.
3. Policies are broad statements that guide in decision-making. They may include:
   a. Scope of service.
      - Mission and philosophy statement.
      - Identifies the types of services provided, hours available, referral requirements (if applicable), staffing, and other general information about the service.
   b. Operational policies.
      - Billing policies.
      - Referral policies (if appropriate).
      - Medical record management.
      - Quality assurance and improvement activities.
      - Other applicable clinical policies.
   c. Human resources policies.
      - Vacation: paid time off; varies according to length of employment, seniority, or other criteria.
      - Introductory period (also called probationary period).
      - Job descriptions and performance appraisal policies.
      - Time off, leave of absence, sabbaticals.
         - Military service.
         - Maternity/paternity leave.

        ○ Medical leave.
        ○ Jury duty.
    - Dress code.
4. Procedures: specific guides to job behaviors for all departmental personnel, visitors, and patients that standardize activities with a high level of risk.
    a. Safety and emergency procedures.
    b. Equipment management, cleaning, maintaining, training requirements, safety inspections.
    c. Hazardous waste management.
    d. Disciplinary procedures.
        - Manager presents problem in clear and concise terms, and specifically references the problem to the job description and expectations.
        - Discussion is on performance discrepancy.
        - Employee is given chance to respond.
        - Manager presents action to be taken and why.
        - Follow-up date for reevaluation is set.
        - Consequences of noncompliance are established.
        - Documentation of meeting is objective.

Employee Engagement/Staff Motivation

1. Sustains individual behavior toward attainment of an objective or goal by providing:
    a. Challenging work, varied treatment assignments with opportunity to receive feedback regarding performance.
    b. Good working conditions.
        - Essential equipment should be available for proper patient care.
    c. Recognition of performance (praise or positive feedback, salary, bonuses, raises, and/or promotions).
    d. Enhanced opportunity to achieve job-related goals.
        - Outline of policies.
        - Development of a clear job description.
        - Outline job responsibilities.
    e. Concern as a supervisor in resolving work-related problems.
    f. Acknowledgment of the contributions of the staff toward realization of the mission, and scope of the service and/or institution.
    g. Fair compensation based on market factors and required qualifications, while ensuring equity among the staff of the department/service.
    h. Consultation with supervisor and involved staff member regarding problems that affect his or her employment.
    i. Realistic job expectations.
        - Supervisor should avoid promising more than can be delivered; e.g., promising a promotion to a senior position when no budget has been approved.

Continuing Education

1. Ongoing educational activities to foster lifelong learning.
    a. Enhances clinical knowledge.
    b. Exposes, instructs, and teaches therapists/assistants new techniques and technologies.
2. Educational programs can be delivered a variety of ways.
    a. On-site programs.
        - In-services.
        - Journal clubs.
        - Case presentations.
    b. Off-site programs.
        - Continuing education programs.
        - National and state physical therapy meetings.
        - Special interest group–sponsored courses.
        - Online course offerings.
3. Frequency can vary according to time and resources.
4. Employers should support and may subsidize staff member's attendance. Should promote professionalism, educational development, and continued competence.
5. Each state has its own requirements and expectations for licensee continuing education.

Non-Discrimination Laws

1. Prevent a facility from discrimination against employees regarding race, color, religion, gender, or national origin.
2. Title VII of the Civil Rights Act of 1964 prohibits employment discrimination based on:
    a. Race.
    b. Color.
    c. Gender.
    d. Religion.
    e. National origin.
    f. Sexual harassment.
3. The Age Discrimination and Employment Act of 1967.
    a. Prohibits employers from discriminating against persons from 40–70 years of age in any area of employment.
4. 1973 Rehabilitation Act.
    a. Prohibits employment discrimination based on disability in:
        - Federal executive agencies.
        - All institutions receiving Medicare, Medicaid, and other federal support.
5. The Americans with Disabilities Act (ADA), 1990.
    a. Prevents discrimination against people with disabilities.
    b. Ensures their integration into mainstream American life.
    c. The definition of "disabilities" encompasses a wide range of physical and mental conditions.

d. Requires businesses of ≥15 employees to accommodate needs of people with disabilities to facilitate their economic independence in both the public and private sectors.
e. Equal Employment Opportunity Commission (EEOC) oversees issues and interprets regulations.
f. Requires reasonable accommodation to the workplace by removing barriers unless this would cause "undue hardship" (an action requiring significant difficulty or expense).
   - Installing an elevator so the individual could access upper floors might be considered an undue hardship.
g. PTs serve as consultants to:
   - Employers helping them meet their responsibilities.
   - Disabled, helping them achieve their rehabilitation potential and rights under law.

Departmental Operations Management

Meetings

1. Staff meeting.
   a. Regularly held departmental meetings with a specific agenda set in advance.
   b. Purpose is to discuss department or hospital/management business, state or national PT issues, and to educate staff members.
   c. Agendas are predetermined to ensure that the objectives and purpose of the meeting are clear.
2. Supervisory meeting.
   a. Supervisor and staff meet regularly.
      - To discuss patient-care issues.
   b. One-on-one meeting designed to meet the needs of the staff member.
3. Team meeting.
   a. Usually scheduled at least weekly.
   b. Interdisciplinary (physicians, nurses, PTs, OTs, social services, etc.) to improve communication between all staff.
   c. Purpose is to:
      - Discuss and coordinate patient care services.
      - Set goals and outcomes for individual patients.
      - Discuss goal/outcome achievement necessary for discharge.
      - Discuss discharge plans including destination, equipment needs, home-care services, etc.

Strategic Planning

1. Organizational planning process for goal achievement and future goals.
   a. Based on the organization's mission and philosophy statement.
   b. Used for developing plans for implementation to achieve identified goals.
2. Results of strategic planning process summarized in strategic plan.
   a. Provides focused direction so goals of organization are achieved.
   b. Identifies individuals responsible to develop and carry out the plan; e.g., staff members, department director sets the timeline, and the expected outcomes.
   c. Informs external parties about organization.
   d. Goals are time related; e.g., 1-year, 3-year, or 5-year plans.
   e. Methodology for evaluating the progress of the plan should be developed as part of the plan.
   f. Analysis of progress toward goals should be done by the director/manager at least quarterly.
3. Strategic plans are always driven by and consistent with the organization's mission and philosophy.

Incident/Occurrence and Sentinel Event Reporting

1. Incident/occurrence report is used to document incidents that involve patients and/or staff and that result in harm and/or the potential for harm to the patient and/or staff.
   a. Incident reports are not part of the medical record, nor are they referenced in the medical record.
   b. Used to document additional information, circumstances, contributing factors that would not be appropriate to include in the medical record.
   c. Used to evaluate systems and processes that hold the potential or have contributed to a negative patient outcome.
   d. Are part of an internal quality improvement program.
   e. Can be used as a component of individual employee performance appraisal and improvement.
2. Sentinel event: a patient safety event that reaches the patient and results in any of the following: death, permanent harm, severe temporary harm with intervention required to sustain life.
   a. Monitoring of sentinel events is a critical part of a comprehensive quality assurance and improvement program.
   b. When a sentinel event occurs, a "root cause" analysis is done to identify underlying problems with processes, systems, or performance that can be improved to reduce the likelihood of recurrence.
   c. Many regulatory and accrediting agencies require sentinel event reporting and analysis, particularly on specific types of incidents.

Health Care Marketing

1. Begins with an assessment of the true needs and wants of the patient/client and key stakeholders.

2. Analyze the strengths, weaknesses, opportunities, and threats (SWOT Analysis) of the organization to meet the needs of the customer.
3. A needs assessment should be conducted, before providing a service or planning a new facility to determine:
   a. Where is the market (consumer)?
   b. Does a need for the service exist (environment)?
   c. Who is the competition?
   d. In-depth analysis of the marketplace, including demographical and epidemiological data.
   e. Review of the literature.
   f. Survey of colleagues and referral sources.
4. Marketing methods:
   a. Website and social media.
   b. Brochures, newsletters, education, and pamphlets.
   c. Guest appearances on television, radio, and at local organizations.
   d. Professional referral.
   e. Word of mouth.
   f. Direct marketing to managed-care groups; e.g., sport injuries, low back pain, and referral sources.
   g. Community sponsorship.
   h. Advertising.

Service Management

1. Management principles, functions, and strategies.
   a. Management with a positive attitude about change and innovation fosters best practice.
   b. Successful management supports open communication, team building, decentralization of resources, and the sharing of power.
   c. Management that utilizes strategic thinking in a systems model can respond proactively to market demands and changes.
   d. The use of different management styles (i.e., the manager's characteristic way of performing management tasks) has a significant impact on productivity, change, and growth.
   e. Management's understanding and application of theories of motivation and behavior facilitates appropriate and effective responses to situations, fosters program efficacy, and promotes employee satisfaction.
   f. Administrative functions of management include program development, fiscal and personnel management, and program evaluation.
   g. Management by objective (MBO): a complete system of management based on a set of core goals to be accomplished by a program.
      - Mission and goals are established.
      - Measurable objectives are quantified.
      - Specific time frames for accomplishment of objectives are established.
      - Staff training needs and deterrents to progress are identified.
      - Program evaluation is instituted.
2. Program development.
   a. Purposes of developing specific programs.
      - To directly meet the needs of a specific population(s) or group(s).
      - To clearly focus evaluation and intervention efforts and activities.
      - To increase visibility and use of available services (e.g., offering an outpatient cardiac rehabilitation program is more visible than individual referrals, resulting in increased recognition and utilization of this service).
      - To convert an idea into a practice reality.
   b. Basic steps of program development.
      - Needs assessment.
         - Describe the community, its physical, social, cultural, and economic factors, and populations at risk.
         - Describe the target population's demographics, disorder(s), functional level, and presenting problems.
         - Identify specific needs of target population.
            - Perceived needs of the population as reported by others (e.g., family, physicians, and other professionals).
            - Perceived needs as stated by the individual members of the target population.
            - Real needs, which are the actual disabilities and functional limitations of the target population.
      - Determine discrepancy between real and perceived needs.
      - Determine unmet needs according to priority.
      - Identify resources available for program implementation.
         - Formal or institutional resources such as staff, supplies, money, space.
         - Informal resources such as family, friends, cultural or religious figures, self-help/consumer groups.
      - Needs assessment methods.
         - Survey, interview, or self-report of target population. A representative sample is required.
         - Key informant involves the surveying of specific individuals who are knowledgeable about the target population's needs.
         - Community forums to obtain information through public meetings or panels.
         - Service utilization review of records and reports.
         - Analysis of social indicators to identify social, cultural, environmental, and/or economic factors that can predict problems.
   c. Program planning.
      - Define a focus for the program based on needs assessment results.
         - Problem areas, functional/activity limitations, and unmet needs that are relevant to the majority of the target population are the priority focus.

- Program level of difficulty as determined by the range of population's functional levels and the level required by the current and expected environment.
- Adopt a frame of reference that is most likely to successfully address and meet the needs that are the program's focus.
- Establish objectives and goals of the program specifically related to primary focus.
  - Set individual goals to be met by the program.
  - Determine programmatic goals to establish standards for program evaluation.
- Describe integration of program into existing system of care.
  - Establish realistic timetable for program implementation.
  - Define staff roles, responsibilities, and assignments.
  - Identify methods for professional collaboration.
  - Determine the physical setting and space requirements.
  - Consider potential barriers to program implementation.
  - Develop methods to deal effectively with identified obstacles before program implementation.
- Develop a referral system for entry into, completion of, and discharge from the program.
  - Evaluation protocols standardize information to be obtained from each person referred to the program and assess the type of program services needed.
  - Criteria for acceptance into the program and for movement through program levels are set.
  - Discharge criteria determine when an individual has achieved maximum gain from the program, usually defined as the achievement of program goals.
- Describe the fiscal implications of the program plan.
  - Determine projected volume or service demand to estimate revenue.
  - Identify resource utilization and projected expenses to estimate costs.
  - Directly compare estimated revenue and estimated expenses to determine financial viability of program.

d. Program implementation.
- Initiate program according to timetable and steps set forth in the program plan.
- Document program activities, procedures, and use.
- Communicate and coordinate with other programs within the system.
- Promote program to ensure it reaches target population.

e. Program evaluation.
- Determine whether program should continue, change, or be discontinued.
- Establish and analyze metrics and benchmarks for success.

Fiscal Management

Budget

1. A financial plan, for a specific time period, of the amount of funds allotted to cover specific expenses of operating a PT department or private practice.
2. An integral part of the planning process.
3. Provides a mechanism of assessing the financial success of the practice, programs, or projects.
4. Expresses anticipated income and expenditures over specific time periods.
5. Operating budgets are usually planned for a one-year duration (e.g., the organization's fiscal year), and can be "flexible," changing according to volume and other factors.
6. A budget is planned for capital expenses, including all major renovation expenses or the purchase of equipment that is reusable and will last a minimum of 3 years. Capital budgeting should be part of the strategic plan.

Expense Budgets

1. Represent the amount of money spent by an organization to provide goods and services within a specific period of time.
2. Two types of expense budgets:
   a. Operating expense budgets.
   - Related to the day-to-day operation of the organization.
   - Include categories relating to salaries, benefits (sick, vacation, etc.), supplies, utilities (telephone and electric), linen, housekeeping, maintenance, continuing education, etc.

   b. Capital budgets.
   - Deal with the purchase of larger items that will be utilized for >3 years, such as new equipment or new buildings.
   - Capital expense is equipment that is depreciable, and usually costs >$1,000.

Costs

1. There are direct and indirect, fixed and variable, and discretionary costs associated with providing a PT service.
   a. Direct costs are directly associated with the production of a service.
   - The cost of salaries for professional staff.
   - Treatment supplies (ultrasound gel, massage lotion).

- Treatment equipment.
- Continuing education.

b. Indirect costs are necessary to produce a service but are indirectly associated with that service.
- Utilities (telephone and electric).
- Housekeeping, laundry.
- Marketing services, etc.

c. Fixed costs remain unchanged, even with changes in volume.
- Air conditioning.
- Rent.

d. Variable costs increase and decrease in direct proportion to the volume of activity.
- Linen and labor costs increase as volume increases.

e. Discretionary expenses are those costs that are not essential for providing PT services. They may include budgeting for continuing education or recognition activities.

Accounts Payable

1. Money owed to a creditor (individual who provides a service or equipment) for services rendered.
2. A part of the budget where debts are listed.

Accounts Receivable

1. Money owed to a company (hospital, PT practice) for providing a service; e.g., PT treatment on credit.
2. An asset expected to benefit future operations.

Quality Assurance and Quality Improvement

Quality Assurance (QA)

1. Monitor quality.
2. Monitor appropriateness of care.
3. Resolve identified problems.

Continuous Quality Improvement

1. A systematic process that involves ongoing, deliberate, and continuous monitoring of the systems and processes that affect patient care to ensure the highest quality outcomes possible.

Utilization Review (UR)

1. Written plan to determine:
   a. Appropriate use of resources.
   b. Medical necessity of services provided.
   c. Cost efficiency.
2. Methods for UR.
   a. Prospective review.
   - Evaluation of proposed treatment plan that specifies how care will be provided.
   - Used by third-party payers to approve proposed PT treatment program.

   b. Concurrent review.
   - Evaluation of ongoing treatment program during hospitalization or treatment.
   - Method to ensure that appropriate care is being delivered.

   c. Retrospective review.
   - Audits of medical records after treatment was rendered.
   - Method to ensure appropriate care was given.
   - Time-consuming, expensive method for third-party payers.

   d. Statistical utilization review health informatics/ "Big Data."
   - Review of network, regional, or national claims data, such as pricing and utilization, are analyzed.
   - Determines which providers offer the most efficient and cost-effective care.
   - Establishes norms for application in predictive analytics to reduce fraud, waste, and abuse.

   e. Peer review.
   - Performed by peer groups of health professionals.
   - Retrospective and concurrent review of clients' records to determine whether services provided are necessary, appropriate, and comprehensive in relation to the patient's needs.
     - Educational, not punitive.
     - Aim is improvement of quality of care.
     - Focuses on how well services are performed in the delivery of care under review.
     - Determines whether the patient's needs have been met.
   - May also be performed by peer review organization (PRO).
     - Reviews services provided to Medicare and Medicaid beneficiaries and some managed care plans.
     - Determines appropriateness of services delivered to patients.

   f. Audit or program evaluation.
   - Assessment of the management of patients with a specific diagnosis.
     - Objectives are established for patients; e.g., total hip replacements.
     - Outcomes are evaluated in terms of range of motion, strength, pain, function, gait level, ability to climb stairs, etc.
     - Comparisons made between treating therapists, other facilities, etc.
     - Programs can be modified or improved when indicated.
   - Payment audits.
     - May be performed by third-party payers.
     - Medicare Fee-for-Service Recovery Audit Program identifies and corrects past Medicare improper payments.

Professional Standards

1. Standards are developed by professional associations and are binding only to association members.
2. Code of Ethics helps PTs and PTAs understand how to act morally and professionally.
   a. Code of Ethics (APTA) has been codified as law in many state practice/licensure law and regulations. It is often adopted by many institutions as the standard of behavior for PTs.
   b. Download and review the APTA Code of Ethics for Physical Therapist at https://www.apta.org/apta-and-you/leadership-and-governance/policies/code-of-ethics-for-the-physical-therapist.
   c. APTA Standards of Ethical Conduct for the Physical Therapist Assistant (PTA) provides a foundation for PTA conduct.
3. The APTA Guide for Professional Conduct assists in the interpretation of the Code of Ethics (see https://www.apta.org/your-practice/ethics-and-professionalism/apta-guide-for-professional-conduct).
4. The APTA Standards of Practice for Physical Therapy defines performance expectations. (See https://www.apta.org/apta-and-you/leadership-and-governance/policies/standards-of-practice-pt for additional information).

Caregiver Definitions and Roles

Physical Therapist (PT)

1. A skilled health professional with a minimum of a baccalaureate degree; current accreditation standards mandate a postbaccalaureate degree (doctorate).
2. Licensed by each state or jurisdiction following successful performance on National Physical Therapy Examination.
3. Examines patient; evaluates data; establishes diagnosis, prognosis, and plan of care; administers or supervises treatment.
4. May delegate portions of plan of care to supportive personnel; e.g., PTA.
5. Supervises and directs supportive staff (PTA, PT aide) in designated tasks.
6. Reevaluates and adjusts plan of care as appropriate.
7. Performs and documents final evaluation and establishes discharge and follow-up plans.
8. Consultation by giving professional opinions to others to identify problems, recommend solutions, or produce a specific outcome.
   a. May be patient-related consultation to evaluate the quality of PT services.
   b. May be client-related consultation to a business, school, organization, or government agency.
      - Expert witness.
      - ADA compliance.
      - Work-related injury prevention.
      - Request for a second opinion.

Physical Therapy Director

1. Oversees function, responsibilities, and relationships of all personnel.
2. Establishes, revises, and ensures that policies and procedures are carried out according to established policy and procedures.
3. Acts as liaison with facility administration.
4. Sets department goals and strategic plan.

Physical Therapy Supervisor

1. Qualified experienced PT with a variety of skills:
   a. Motivates subordinates.
   b. Evaluates staff and gives oral and written feedback.
   c. Interviews new staff and helps develop their skills.
   d. Delegates tasks to appropriate staff.
2. Patient care may or may not be primary responsibility of the supervisor.

Physical Therapist Assistant (PTA)

1. Licensed or certified skilled physical therapy clinicians, usually with a 2-year associate degree.
2. Must work under the direction and supervision of a PT in all practice settings in accordance with jurisdictional requirements.
   a. When the PT and PTA are not within the same physical setting, delegated functions by the PTA must be safe and legal physical therapy practice based on:
      - Complexity and acuity of the patient's needs.
      - Proximity and accessibility to the PT.
      - Supervision available in the event of emergencies.
      - Type of setting in which the service is provided.
   b. In home health, regularly scheduled and documented supervisory meetings are established between the PT and PTA; the frequency is determined by the needs of the patient and the needs of the PTA, and include:
      - On-site reassessment of the patient.
      - On-site review of the plan of care with appropriate revision or termination.
      - Assessment and recommendation for utilization of outside resources.
3. Able to adjust treatment procedure in accordance with changes in patient status within the scope of the established plan of care.
4. May not evaluate, develop, or change plan of care, or write discharge plan or summary.
5. May carry out routine operational functions, including supervision of the physical therapy aide and documentation of patient progress.

Physical Therapy Aide

1. A nonlicensed worker, specifically trained under the direction of a PT or PTA.

2. Functions only with continuous on-site supervision by a PT or, where allowable by law or regulation, the PTA.
3. Performs designated routine tasks related to the operation of a physical therapy service.
4. Supervised job responsibilities may include:
   a. Functional and ambulation activities.
   b. Application of specific heat, cold, and whirlpool treatments.
   c. Equipment maintenance.
   d. Patient transportation.
   e. Secretarial or housekeeping duties.
5. Aides are not licensed by the state, and some state laws limit or prohibit treatment procedures by aides.

Physical Therapy and Physical Therapist Assistant Student

1. Performs duties commensurate with level of education.
2. PT clinical instructor (CI) is responsible for all actions and duties of affiliating student.
3. PT may supervise both PT and PTA students.
4. PTA may supervise only a PTA student.

Physical Therapy Volunteer

1. Member of the community.
   a. Interested in assisting PTs with departmental activities.
   b. Takes phone messages, does filing and other basic secretarial tasks.
   c. May not provide or set up patient treatment, transfer patients, clean whirlpools, or maintain equipment.

Home Health Aide

1. A nonlicensed worker (e.g., nursing/rehabilitation assistant) specifically trained to:
   a. Provide personal care and home-management services.
   b. Assist patients to remain in the home environment.
2. Supervised by a nurse.
3. Responsibilities include:
   a. Bathing, grooming, light housework, shopping, or cooking in some circumstances.
   b. Supervision of home exercise program (HEP) as directed by the PT; e.g., ambulation.

Occupational Therapist (OT)

1. A skilled health professional that holds a minimum of a baccalaureate degree (most have master's degrees and some clinical doctorates) and has passed a national certification examination (NBCOT exam). OTs are licensed by some, but not all, states. The OT provides:
   a. Education and training in ADLs.
   b. Fabrication of orthoses (splints).
   c. Guidance in selection and use of adaptive equipment.
   d. Therapeutic activities to enhance functional performance, and cognitive/perceptual function.
   e. Consultation concerning the adaptation of physical environments for the handicapped.
   f. Creative activities in treatment of physically and emotionally disabled patients.
2. Services are provided on an inpatient basis, outpatient basis, and in industrial environments.

Certified Occupational Therapist Assistant (COTA)

1. Skilled technician who holds an associate degree and has passed a national certification examination.
2. Works under the direction of an OT to carry out established treatment.
   a. Cannot evaluate, establish, or revise a plan of care.
3. Performs duties in a rehabilitation or home setting.
   a. Concerned with functional deficits in ADLs, including dressing, grooming, hygiene, housekeeping, etc.

Speech-Language Pathologist (SLP)

1. A skilled health professional that holds a master's degree in communication disorders, has completed 1 year of field experience, and has passed a national examination to obtain the Certificate of Clinical Competence authorized by the American Speech and Hearing Association.
2. Conducts remedial programs to restore or improve communication of patients with language and speech impairments.
   a. May arise from physiological or neurological disturbances and defective articulation.
3. Works with OT to correct swallowing problems and cognitive processing deficits; and with PT in the area of positioning and mobility.

Certified Orthotist (CO)

1. Designs, fabricates, and fits orthoses (braces, splints, collars, corsets) prescribed by physicians.
2. Successfully completed the examination by the American Orthotic and Prosthetic Association.
3. Provides these devices to patients with disabling conditions of limbs and spine.
4. Works directly with physicians and physical and occupational therapists.

Certified Prosthetist (CP)

1. Designs, fabricates, and fits prostheses for patients with partial or total absence of a limb (amputation).
2. Successfully completed the examination by the American Orthotic and Prosthetic Association.
3. Works directly with physicians, PTs, and OTs.
4. Individuals may be certified in both orthotics and prosthetics (CPO).

Certified Respiratory Therapist (CRT)

1. A skilled technician holding an associate degree from a 2-year training program accredited by the Committee in Allied Health Education and Accreditation.
   a. Passes a national exam to become registered.
2. Administers respiratory therapy as prescribed and supervised by a physician.
   a. Performs pulmonary function tests.
   b. Treatments consist of oxygen delivery, aerosols, and nebulizers.
   c. Maintains all respiratory equipment and assists patients in their use; i.e., ventilators, oxygen, pressure machines, etc.
   d. Coordinates care with pulmonary PT treatments.

Primary Care Physician (PCP)

1. A practitioner, usually an internist, general practitioner, or family medicine physician, who provides primary care services and manages routine health care needs.
2. Acts as the gatekeeper for patients covered by managed health care.
3. May be an MD or DO (Doctor of Osteopathic Medicine).
   a. Authorizes referrals to other specialty physicians or services, including PT.

Physician Assistant (PA-C) and Nurse Practitioner (NP)

1. Skilled health care professional, graduate of an accredited program at the graduate level.
   a. Required to pass national certification examination.
   b. Direct patient contact required during training in a variety of settings or specialty area.
2. Under the supervision of a physician, performs routine diagnostic, therapeutic, preventative, and health maintenance services in any setting in which the physician renders care.
   a. Specialties include family medicine, obstetrics, pediatrics, orthopedics, emergency medicine, and others.
3. Able to write PT orders, order medical tests, and prescribe most medications.
4. Often referred to as Physician Extenders.
5. An NP must also be a registered nurse (RN).

Physiatrist

1. A physician specializing in physical medicine and rehabilitation.
   a. Certified by the American Board of Physical Medicine and Rehabilitation.
   b. Diagnoses and treats patients with disabilities involving musculoskeletal, neurological, cardiovascular, or other body systems.
2. Primary focus on maximal restoration of physical, psychological, social, and vocational function, and alleviation of pain.
3. May lead the rehabilitation team in coordination of patient care.
   a. Works directly with PTs, OTs, and speech-language pathologists (SLP).

Chiropractor (DC)

1. An alternative medical practitioner, usually licensed by a state board.
   a. Deals with relationship of the nervous system and the spinal column in the restoration and maintenance of health.
2. Services are covered for individuals in most group health plans.
3. Patients may see a chiropractor and PT at the same time.
   a. PT, with patient's permission, should contact chiropractor to coordinate care.

Registered Nurse (RN)

1. A skilled health professional that is a graduate of an accredited nursing program, and licensed by the state board following successful performance on licensure exam.
2. Primary liaison between the patient and the physician.
   a. Communicates to physician changes in patient's medical or social condition.
   b. Educates the patient and family to facilitate recovery.
   c. Makes referrals to other services under physician's direction.
   d. Supervises other levels of nursing care (licensed practical nurse [LPN], home health aide).
   e. Administers medication but cannot change drug dosages.
   f. Carries out range of motion, bed exercises, transfers, and ambulation as instructed by the PT.

Rehabilitation Counselor (Vocational Rehabilitation Counselor)

1. Counsels physically and mentally handicapped individuals.
   a. Helps patients improve their ability to function optimally in society.
   b. Administers vocational tests, procures vocational training, and provides occupational information for job placement.

Audiologist

1. A health professional with a graduate degree in audiology.
2. A specialist in hearing disorders and evaluation who works to rehabilitate individuals with hearing loss.
   a. Uses audiometric tests to assess sensitivity of sense of hearing.
   b. Uses speech audiometric tests to assess ability to understand selected words.
   c. Audiometrist is a technician trained to administer audiometric tests selected and evaluated by the audiologist.

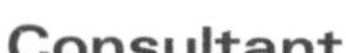

Consultant

1. A person that, by training and experience, has acquired a special knowledge in a subject area that has been recognized by a peer group.
2. A person that analyzes situations, offers advice and solutions to problems.
   a. For example: physician referral for consultation or advice regarding diagnosis or treatment of a patient.
   b. Consultant reviews history, examines patient, and writes opinion.
   c. Responsibility of patient care not delegated to consultant.

Athletic Trainer Certified (ATC)

1. A health professional with a minimum of a baccalaureate degree who is an integral part of the health care system associated with sports.
   a. Usually works under supervision of a physician.
   b. Provides injury prevention, recognition, treatment, and rehabilitation after athletic trauma.
2. Settings for delivery of care:
   a. Secondary schools, colleges and universities, professional athletic organizations, and private or hospital-based clinics.

Social Worker (MSW)

1. Usually completed a master's degree from a school of social work accredited by the Council on Social Work Education. After 1 year of practical field work, they are licensed or registered by the state.
2. Acts as a resource director assisting patients and families with necessary applications for financial resources, appropriate discharge destinations (e.g., skilled nursing facility, custodial care facility), rental and loaner equipment, and support groups, etc.
3. Acts as a personal or family counselor.
4. Educates the patient and family about their medical problems. Also educates home health staff, helping them understand patient and family interaction, and crisis management.
5. Acts as an advocate for the patient in dealing with outside agencies and procuring support services.
6. Mediates between the patient and family by alleviating fears, developing realistic expectations of the patient to the family, and interpreting the patient and families' situation to outside relatives and the home health care team.

Alternative Support Staff: (e.g., Massage Therapists, Exercise Therapists, Acupuncturists)

1. May work within the supervision of a PT.
2. Employed under their appropriate titles.
3. Involvement in patient care activities should be within the limits of their education and in accordance with applicable laws and regulations and the discretion of the PT.

Team Roles and Principles of Collaboration

1. Overview.
   a. A team is a group of equally important individuals with common interests who collaborate to develop shared goals and build trusting relationships to achieve these shared goals.
   b. Members of the team include the patient/client/consumer; his/her family, significant others, and/or caregivers, health care professionals; and the reimburser's gatekeepers.
   c. Professional members on the team will vary according to practice setting.
   d. The consumer, family, significant other, and/or caregiver role on the team has become increasing important. Collaboration with these individuals is even mandated by law (e.g., Omnibus Budget Reconciliation Act of 1990 [OBRA '90], Individuals with Disabilities Education Act [IDEA]).
2. Principles of collaboration.
   a. Factors that influence effective team functioning.
      - Member skill and knowledge.
      - Membership stability.
      - Commitment to team goals.
      - Good communication.
      - Membership composition.
      - Common language and goals.
      - Effective leadership.
3. Types of teams.
   a. Multidisciplinary.
      - A number of professionals from different disciplines conduct assessments and interventions independent from one another.
      - Member's primary allegiance is to his/her discipline. Some formal communications occur between team members.
      - Limited communications may result in lack of understanding of different perspectives.
      - Resources and responsibilities are individually allocated between disciplines; therefore, competition among team members may develop.
   b. Interdisciplinary.
      - All disciplines relevant to the case agree to collaborate for decision-making.
      - Evaluation and intervention are still conducted independently within defined areas of each profession's expertise. However, there is a greater understanding of each discipline's perspective.
      - Outcomes and goals are team-directed and not bound to discipline specific roles and functions.
      - Members tend to use group process skills effectively (e.g., during team planning meetings).
      - The exchange of information, prioritization of needs, allocation of resources, and responsibilities are based on members' expertise and skills, not on "turf" issues.

- Ongoing training, support, supervision, cooperation, and consultation among disciplines are important to this model to ensure that professional integrity and quality of care are maintained.

c. Intradisciplinary.
- One or more members of one discipline evaluate, plan, and implement treatment of the individual; e.g., PT, PTA, PT consultant.
- Other disciplines are not involved; communication is limited, thereby limiting perspectives on the case.
- This "team" is at risk due to potential narrowness of perspective.
- Comprehensive, holistic care can be questionable.

d. Team efficacy.
- Interdisciplinary teams are the most common and considered to be the most effective in today's health care system.

Statutory Laws

Health Insurance Portability and Accountability Act (HIPAA)

1. Elements of the act include standards and safeguards to ensure:
   a. An individual's right to continuity in health care.
   b. Privacy and security of health care records.
   c. Portability of health insurance.
2. HIPAA privacy rule.
   a. Elements:
   - Standards address the use and disclosure of "protected health information" (PHI).
   - Standards address an individual's privacy rights to understand and control use of PHI.

   b. Applies to (Covered Entities) health plans, health care clearing houses, and any health care provider who transmits PHI electronically and their business associates.
   c. Protected health information.
   - Past, present, or future physical/mental health conditions.
   - Care provided to an individual.
   - Past, present, or future payment for care provided.
   - Individually identifiable health information (e.g., name, address, birth date, SSN, phone number, email address, or any information that could reasonable lead to the identity of an individual).

   d. Disclosures.
   - Covered entities may not disclose PHI except when the privacy rule permits or written authorization by the individual or their appointed representative.
   - Covered entities must disclose PHI to individuals when requested and to HHS when conducting an investigation.

   e. General information.
   - Patient confidentiality is maintained in all oral, written, and electronic forms.
   - Technical, administrative, and physical safeguards must protect PHI.
   - All individuals must be informed of a facility's privacy policies.
   - Written consent must be obtained before any personal health information is disclosed or used for other purposes.
     - Exemptions to written consent may be made in emergencies or if delay will prevent timely care.
     - If language barriers preclude signed consent in emergent or crucial situations, treatment may commence if the physician believes that consent is implied.
   - Prior to discussion of a person's status with a family member or other providers, the person may grant permission or object.
     - Providers can use clinical judgment to decide whether to discuss a case if the person cannot give permission, or even if there is an objection.
     - Documentation for this decision is essential.

   f. All information disclosed must be the minimum needed for the immediate purpose.
3. Practice implications.
   a. Physical identifiability of patients must be reduced.
   b. Charts and other documentation must be stored out of public view and secured.
   c. Any information stored or transmitted by computers must be safeguarded.
   d. Faxes must be sent with cover sheets on dedicated lines to secure locations.
   e. All e-mails should be password-protected.
   f. All conversations regarding a person's health status must occur in private areas with minimal disclosure.
   g. Cover sheets should be used on clipboards that contain patient paperwork.
   h. Treatment may be provided in groups or open clinics. Discussions about these treatments should be done quietly and in a private space.
   i. There is no guarantee of 100% confidentiality. Reasonable and vigilant safeguards are required.
   j. HIPAA does not override state laws with more restrictive privacy policies and defers to state laws regarding minors.
4. Individual Rights.
   a. An individual can request to see and obtain copies of all information in their medical or health records.
   - Providers have up to 30 days to respond.
   - A reasonable charge can be imposed for copying.

   b. An individual has the right to request that information in their record be amended.
   - The provider may refuse, but must provide a rationale.
   - The provider may comply and provide a reason for amending the record. Original documentation is not removed.

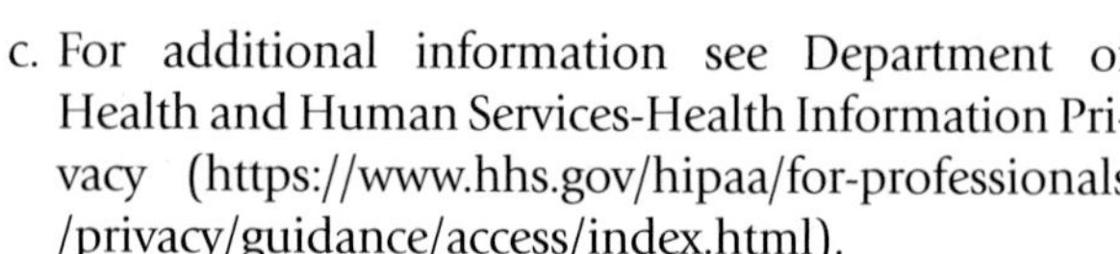

c. For additional information see Department of Health and Human Services-Health Information Privacy (https://www.hhs.gov/hipaa/for-professionals/privacy/guidance/access/index.html).

Professional Licensing Laws Are Enacted by All States

1. Protect the consumer against professional incompetence and exploitation by opportunists.
2. Determine the minimal standards of education.
   a. Graduation from an accredited program or its equivalent in PT.
   b. Successful completion of a national licensing examination.
   c. Ethical and legal standards relating to continuing practice of PT.
   d. All PTs must have a license to practice.
   e. Each state determines criteria to practice and issue a license.
   f. Licensure examination and related activities are the responsibility of the Federation of State Boards of Physical Therapy.
      - All states belong to this association.

Individuals with Disabilities Education Act (IDEA)

1. Enacted in 1975 with the most recent revision in December 2015. Ensures that children with disabilities receive appropriate, free public education.
2. IDEA provides statutes and guidelines for states and school districts regarding the provision of special education and related services to eligible infants, toddlers, children, and youth with disabilities.
3. Establishes Early Intervention Programs (EIP) including PT, OT, SLP, and other services as needed.
   a. Services are provided to children with developmental delays (physical, emotional, cognitive, or communicative).
   b. Services provided to infants or toddlers "at risk" for developing delays.
   c. Provision for necessary adaptive equipment.
4. Requires creation of individualized education plans (IEPs).
   a. Guides the team; however, child has the option of not attending planning meetings for the IEP.
   b. Considers evaluation results and child's concerns.
      - Functional needs, strength, ROM.
      - Factors such as English proficiency, behavioral issues, vision, hearing, and communication needs.
      - Need for assistive devices.

Safety

Assuring Patient Safety

1. Risk management programs.
   a. Identify, evaluate, and take corrective action against risk.
      - Potential patient, employee, and/or visitor injury.
      - Property loss or damage with resulting financial loss or legal liability.
   b. Efforts taken to decrease risk in PT.
      - Equipment maintenance: e.g., documented maintenance and calibration of electrical equipment.
      - Staff education; e.g., safety training for staff in use of equipment.
        - Regular check of essential safety equipment.
      - Policies to clean equipment and reduce the potential for spreading infection.
      - Use of incidence reports to quantify safety events.
   c. Patient and staff safety.
      - PTs must follow strict federal standards when using any form of patient restraint.
        - Restraint must be used for a specific reason, i.e., patient safety.
        - Restraints are considered temporary and may not be used for an indefinite amount of time.
        - A patient in restraints must be checked on every 30 minutes.
        - Restraints are not for punishment or to substitute proper staff supervision.
        - Use proper patient identifiers, such as wrist bands, with patient date of birth, first and last names, or other unique patient identifiers.
   d. Identify risk factors in patient care or patient and therapist safety; e.g., more than three incidents of patient falls on the rehabilitation floor may require an in-service in transfer training.
   e. Proper and timely reporting of adverse patient occurrence or reactions as required by federal or state statute. These may include:
      - Adverse reactions to regulated medicines.
      - Incidents involving abuse or neglect of patient.
      - Outbreaks of disease that may affect public safety (i.e., influenza).
      - "Reportable" occurrences such as violence against patients where significant harm is caused to the patient (i.e., nursing home patient with a fall resulting in severe fracture or death).
   f. Annual certification/recertification of staff in cardiopulmonary resuscitation (CPR).

Malpractice/Negligence

Malpractice

1. PTs are personally responsible for negligence and other acts that result in harm to a patient through professional/patient relationships.

Negligence

1. An act or omission by a medical professional that deviates from the accepted standard of care expected from a reasonable competent practitioner.
2. To find a practitioner negligent, harm must have occurred to the patient.

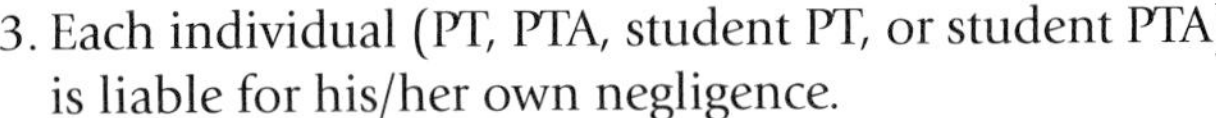

3. Each individual (PT, PTA, student PT, or student PTA) is liable for his/her own negligence.
4. Both administrative and clinical supervisors may also be found negligent due to the actions of their workers if they provided faulty supervision or inappropriate delegation of responsibilities.
5. Ethical principles are violated in caring for patients; e.g., acting without consent, breaking of confidentiality, lack of respect for patients.
6. Patients may also contribute to negligence if they do not follow directions of the therapist.
7. The institution is usually found negligent if a patient was harmed as a result of an environmental problem.
   a. Slippery floor.
   b. Fall in a poorly lit hall.
8. The institution is also liable if an employee was incompetent or not properly licensed.
9. Examples of negligence in physical therapy practice include but are not limited to:
   a. Adverse reaction to treatment, such as pain, burns, falls, injuries from therapeutic exercise, or harm from defective equipment.
   b. Failure to follow referral orders.
   c. Failure to obtain informed consent.
   d. Any action or inaction that is inconsistent with the Code of Ethics or the Standards of Practice that results in harm to a patient.

Acknowledgment to Judith D. Hershberg, PT, DPT, MS; Catherine S. Lane, PT, DPT, MS; Linda Arslanian, PT, DPT, MS; Rita P. Fleming-Castaldy, PhD, OTL, FAOTA; William Farina, PT, DPT, MBA, FACHE; and Lois Siegelman, MS, FACHE, for their original contributions in formulating this chapter.

APPENDIX 14A

Review Questions

(Answers to all Review Questions and Case Studies are found in Chapter 17)

1. What is defined as protected health information and what actions must be taken to secure it?

2. Compare and contrast the requirements for supervision of the PTA and PT aide in the provision of care.

3. What are the documentation requirements for time-based billing for Medicare beneficiaries?

4. Compare and contrast payment mechanisms used in managed care.

15

Teaching and Learning

SUSAN B. O'SULLIVAN

Chapter Outline

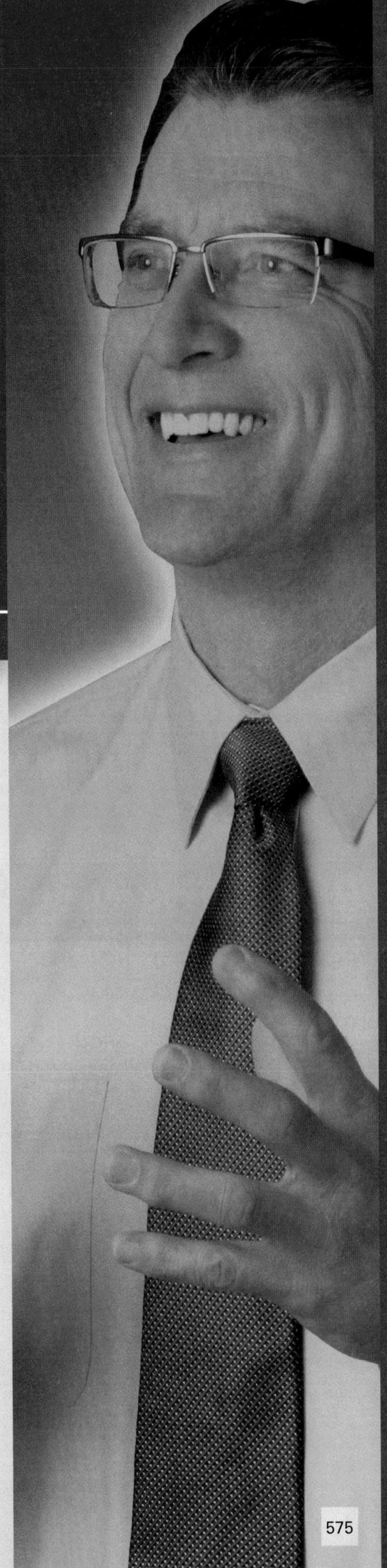

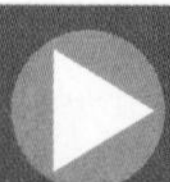

Physical Therapist Roles and Responsibilities

Patient/Client-Related Instruction

Basic Concepts

1. The process of informing, educating, or training patients/clients, families, significant others, and caregivers in order to promote and optimize physical therapy services.
2. Provided across all settings for all patients/clients.
3. Components include:
   a. Current condition, impairments, activity limitations and participation restrictions.
   b. Anticipated goals and expected outcomes, plan of care, specific intervention elements, and self-management strategies.
   c. Elements necessary for the smooth transition to home or an alternative setting, work, and community.
   d. Individualized family service plans (IFSPs) or individualized education plans (IEPs).
   e. Safety awareness, and risk factor reduction and prevention.
   f. Health promotion, wellness, and fitness.

Educational Programs

Instruction and Educational Programs Are Provided for the Following

1. Other therapists, health care providers, staff and/or students in academic and/or clinical settings. Programs can be formal or informal.
2. Instruction and educational programs are provided for local, state, and federal agencies.
3. The general public to increase awareness of health issues and roles of the physical therapist.

Clinical Education of Students

Instruction and Supervision of Physical Therapy or Physical Therapist Assistant Students

1. Provided by clinical instructors during scheduled clinical education experiences.
2. Close communication and collaboration with the school and the academic coordinator of clinical education are necessary.

Educational Concepts

Learning Styles

Characteristic Mode

1. Of gaining, processing, and storing information. Learning styles differ across dimensions.

Analytical versus Intuitive Learners

1. Analytical/objective learner.
   a. Processes information in a step-by-step order.
   b. Perceives information in an objective manner; is able to use facts and easily understand relationships between them.
   c. Perceives information in an abstract, conceptual manner; information does not need to be related to personal experience.
   d. Learns best with structure, step-by-step learning; may have difficulty comprehending the big picture.
2. Intuitive/global learner.
   a. Processes information all at once, in a simultaneous manner, not in an ordered sequence.
   b. Perceives information in a subjective manner: reflects on personal experiences.
   c. Perceives information in a concrete manner: information assimilated about practical, real-life experiences.
   d. Learns best if information is connected to personal experiences and presented in a practical, real-life context. If not, knowledge may be disregarded. May have difficulty ordering steps and comprehending details.

Reasoning: Inductive versus Deductive

1. Inductive reasoner (assimilator): observes similarities, can develop theoretical models to explain relationships.
2. Deductive reasoner (converger): analyzes problems in depth; applies information, theoretical models to practical situations.

Initiative: Active versus Passive Learner

1. Active/aggressive learner: exhibits initiative, actively seeks information; may reach conclusions quickly before all information is gathered.
2. Passive learner: often exhibits little initiative; responds best to directed learning.

Learning Theories

Behaviorist (Stimulus-Response Theory)

1. Basic premises.
   a. Behavior is modified in response to a given stimulus.
   b. Behavior is determined by its consequences; the response of one behavior becomes the stimulus for the next response (chaining).
   c. Learning occurs because the behavior is reinforced (learned association).
2. Behavior can be controlled or shaped by operant conditioning (behavior modification techniques).
   a. Desired or correct behaviors are identified.
   b. Frequent and scheduled reinforcements are given to reinforce the desired behaviors; e.g., praise, encouragement, candy.
      - Accuracy of reinforcement is critical; e.g., use of rewards that are meaningful to the individual.
      - Timing of reinforcement is critical: immediate versus distant or delayed; e.g., use of a reinforcement schedule.
   c. Negative behaviors are ignored; unreinforced behaviors are weakened and eventually extinguished.
   d. Behavior that has aversive consequences (punishment) is less likely to occur again; aversive conditioning is less powerful as a tool for learning than positive reinforcements.
   e. The environment is altered to promote correct responses; e.g., a closed environment with reduction of distractors.
   f. Repetition is a necessary prerequisite for learning.
   g. Clinical uses: limited; e.g., may be used when working with adults with impaired or limited cognitive abilities (traumatic brain injury, stroke) or young children.
3. Prominent theorists: B.F. Skinner, G. Watson.

Cognitive Theory

1. Basic premises.
   a. Focus is on cognitive development of intellectual abilities and skills, from:
      - Symbolic function (ages 2–8).
      - Concrete mental operations (ages 8–12).
      - Conceptual thought (ages 12 and up).
   b. Thinking emerges with language development.
   c. Perceptual features are important conditions of learning; e.g., figure-ground, directional signs, sequence.
2. Cognitive strategies are used; e.g., repeated challenges to thinking.
   a. Knowledge is organized by the teacher; the teacher is the expert; a pedagogical approach (the art and science of teaching children).
   b. Learning is culturally relative.
   c. Cognitive feedback is used to confirm and correct knowledge.
   d. Goal-setting by learner is important for motivation.
   e. Both divergent and convergent theory is nurtured.
3. Prominent theorists: J. Piaget, J.S. Bruner.

Humanist

1. Basic premises.
   a. Personal freedom and dignity of the individual is emphasized in the learning process.
   b. Understanding of the learner's needs and feelings is sought.
   c. The learner experiences unconditional positive regard, acceptance, and understanding.
2. Teaching is student-centered; e.g., self-discovery, self-appropriated learning, experiential learning.
   a. Promotes active learning (self-initiated) rather than passive; e.g., knowledge is organized by the learner, not for the learner.
   b. Learning addresses relevant problems and issues.
   c. A positive learning climate is facilitated.
   d. The teacher is a facilitator and resource-finder.
   e. Learning is evaluated by the learner; e.g., self-assessment.
3. Prominent theorists: Carl Rogers, A.H. Maslow.

Adult Learning (Andragogy)

1. Basic characteristics of adult learners.
   a. The learner is self-directed: goal-oriented, seeks knowledge for own sake.
   b. Has a rich core of experience that serves as a broad base for learning.
   c. Demonstrates a readiness to learn.
   d. Demonstrates a problem-centered orientation to learning.
2. Teaching is learner-centered.
   a. The teacher interacts with the learner: helps to clarify the learning problem, structure the learning environment to enhance learning, provide resources.
   b. Learners share the responsibility for planning the learning experience; actively participate in the learning process.
   c. The learning process makes use of the experiences of the learner.
3. Prominent theorists: M. Knowles, J.R. Kidd.

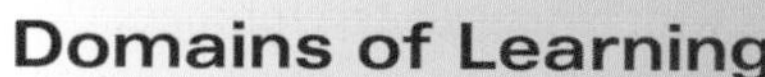

Domains of Learning

Cognitive

1. Objectives concern mental and intellectual processes.
2. Include recall of knowledge, comprehension, application, analysis, synthesis, and evaluation.

Affective

1. Objectives concern feelings and emotions.
2. Include receiving (attending to phenomena and stimuli); awareness of environment (people and situations); responding (compliance, acceptance of responsibility, satisfaction); valuing (accepting and internalizing worth or value), organization of a value system; and characterization by a value or value complex (persistent and consistent behaviors influenced by a value system).

Psychomotor

1. Objectives concern motor skills.
2. Include writing, speaking, performing motor skills safely, correctly, and independently.

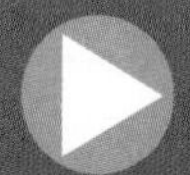

Instruction

Instructional Process

Needs Assessment

1. During the needs assessment, the therapeutic relationship is established, including active listening and positive verbal and nonverbal interactions.
2. Includes the identification of relevant characteristics and needs of the learner prior to the educational experience; establish therapeutic relationship including active listening and positive verbal and nonverbal interactions.
   a. Determine what the learner needs to know.
      - Current level of knowledge.
      - Plans/needs for the future.
   b. Determine what the learner brings to the learning experience.
      - Educational background, previous knowledge and experiences, health beliefs, valued activities, and potential treatment barriers.
      - All instruction should take into account the influences of age, culture, race, gender, gender roles, sexual orientation, and socioeconomic status.
   c. Determine the learner's readiness to learn.
      - Learning style.
      - Capabilities, attentiveness, energy level.
   d. Identify impairments that may have impact on learning: e.g., perceptual deficits, visual impairments, communication impairments, confusion, memory loss, emotional dysregulation.
   e. Identify available resources; e.g., information about facilities, materials, time available for the instructional process.

Analysis of Data, Formulation of Objectives of Instruction

1. Specify what the learner should learn (goals and behavioral objectives).
   a. Identify what the learner will do; e.g., describe, discuss, explain.
   b. Identify what the criteria of performance are; e.g., given a list of risk factors that the learner will correctly identify.
   c. Specify the conditions of the performance; e.g., 75% of the time.
   d. Set goals that are attainable, mutually agreed upon by learner and instructor.
   e. Use clear, unambiguous, and measurable terms; e.g., family/caregiver will demonstrate understanding of safety measures to prevent falls by correctly describing proper use of brakes and transfer sequence 100% of the time within 2 weeks.
2. Set priorities.
   a. Determine which educational goals are most important, what sequence is needed.
   b. Ensure maximum utilization of available teaching time.
   c. Avoid bombardment; e.g., too much, too soon.
   d. Repetition is important for learning; build in experiences that reinforce instruction.

Analysis of Instruction/Planning: What, How, Where, When

1. Select what materials to use; options include print, audiovisual media, computer-assisted instruction, models.
2. Select what methods of teaching are appropriate; options include individual instruction, group discussion, organized classes/lecture, demonstration and modeling, tutorials. Also includes written or pictorial instruction; e.g., home exercise program.
   a. Choice of method is dependent on:
      - The individual learner/unique characteristics; e.g., preferences for rate and style of learning, motivation.
      - Objectives of instruction.
   b. A variety of teaching methods is typically helpful to reinforce the learning.

3. Select what activities are likely to help the learner achieve the stated objectives.

Implementation: Strategies to Affect Mastery of Learning

1. Individuals learn best when:
   a. They are actively involved in goal-setting and the learning process; learning is not dictated by the instructor.
   b. Learners need to feel free to express their own ideas, beliefs, and concerns.
   c. There is respect and trust between learner and instructor.
   d. The instructor is supportive and nonjudgmental.
2. Therapist/teacher should recognize that:
   a. Individuals learn at different rates.
   b. Trial and error and introspection are an essential part of the learning process.
   c. Experiential learning is more effective than didactic learning.
   d. Reinforcement is necessary to ensure a sense of competence and success.
3. Therapist/teacher roles and responsibilities.
   a. Gain the learner's attention, motivation, and active participation.
   b. Provide an overview of the learning process: objectives, purposes, nature of the task, and procedures to follow.
   c. Stimulate recall of previous learning; relate present learning to past and future learning.
   d. Monitor and control the learning.
      - Organize learning units over a period of time.
      - Break down learning into a series of steps or units.
      - Determine the best sequence(s) of learning units and experiences; e.g., sequence from familiar to unfamiliar, simple to complex, concrete to abstract.
      - Provide ample opportunity for practice and repetition.
      - Progress at a comfortable pace for the learner.
      - Give timely feedback, provide accurate knowledge of results.
      - Reward successful behaviors.
   e. Monitor and control the environment.
   f. Reduce conditions that have a negative impact on learning; e.g., pain or discomfort, anxiety, fear, frustration, feelings of failure, humiliation or embarrassment, boredom, time pressures.

Evaluation

1. Initial evaluation.
   a. Determine relevant previous achievement, learning skills.
   b. Utilize diagnostic tests.
   c. Determine aptitude/choice of learning approaches.
2. Formative evaluation (diagnostic-progress assessment).
   a. Analyze what learning has occurred, what must still be learned.
   b. Institute appropriate changes/modifications in the teaching plan.
3. Summative evaluation (outcome assessment).
   a. Assess attainment of learning objectives and content/skills.
   b. Determine effectiveness of teaching materials/methods.
4. Sources: direct observation of behaviors, written and verbal feedback, formal checklists, questionnaires, pre- and post-tests.

Documentation

1. Provide a complete record of activities and outcomes to ensure accountability, continuity of care. Include
   a. Educational plan: objectives and activities.
   b. Progression and modification of the educational plan; document the need for change.
   c. Outcomes: document the learner's progress and attainment of the learning objectives.

APPENDIX 15A

Review Questions

(Answers to all Review Questions and Case Studies are found in Chapter 17)

1. Differentiate between deductive and inductive reasoning.

2. How might operant conditioning be used to shape behavior in a noncompliant patient with TBI?

16

Research and Evidence-Based Practice

MARK E. LESTER AND SUSAN B. O'SULLIVAN

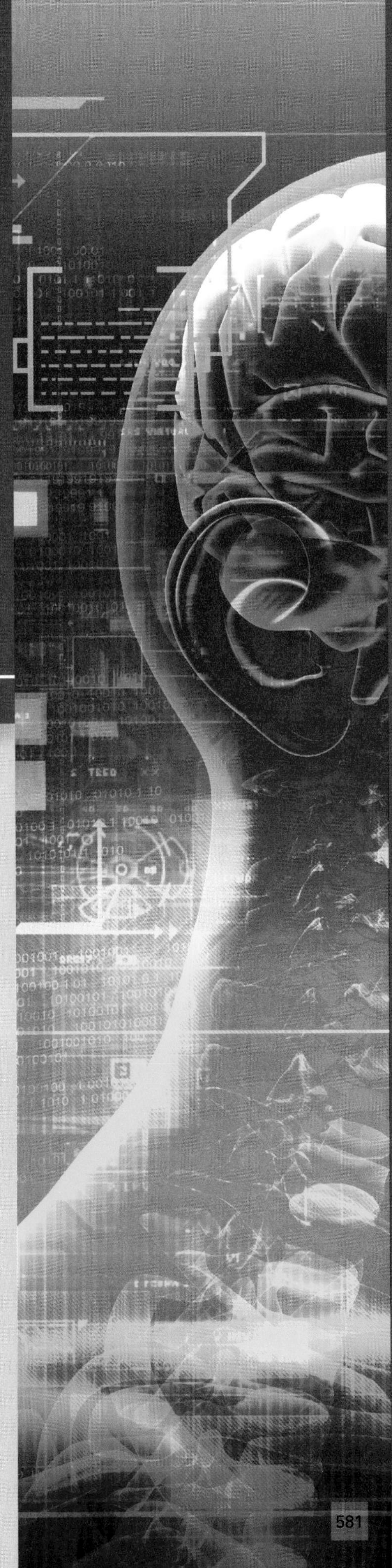

Chapter Outline

Study Tactics

Approximately 2% of the NPTE, or a Total of 3–5 Questions, Will Focus on Research and Evidence-Based Practice

Stick to Reviewing the 11 Concise Pages in This Chapter. Focus Specifically on the Following Terms and Concepts and Understand How to Interpret Their Values:

- Evidence-based practice principles
- Types of research such as descriptive, experimental, correlational, and epidemiological
- Choosing or assessing an experimental design with consideration of controls and hypotheses.
- Hierarchy of evidence (scientific rigor of research studies)
- Normal distribution curve, mean, median, and mode
- Standard deviation from the mean and other measures of variance
- Reliability (interrater, intrarater)
- Validity—internal, content, construct
- Types of research errors
- Correlation coefficients
- Analysis of variance, t-test, and chi-square
- Measures of statistical significance (p-values)
- Measures of Diagnostic Accuracy (sensitivity, specificity, and likelihood ratios)
- Confidence intervals
- Effect size

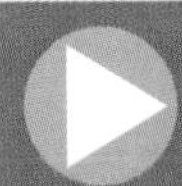

Physical Therapist Roles and Responsibilities

Physical Therapists Use Evidence-Based Practice (EBP)

Definition of EBP

"The conscientious, explicit, and judicious use of current best evidence in making decisions about the care of individual patients" (Sackett et al., 2000).

Clinical Decisions Are Based On

1. The highest level of external clinical evidence available. For example, systematic reviews with meta-analysis of multiple large, rigorously conducted, randomized controlled trials.
2. Clinical expertise of the therapist; proficiency and judgment acquired through clinical practice, acquisition of clinical skills, and continued educational development. For example, the clinician accurately identifies the patient's health status and needs, and the risks and benefits of potential interventions.
3. Patient values: values and unique qualities (preferences, concerns, expectations) are identified and integrated into clinical decisions.

EBP Is a Four-Step Process (See Table 16-1)

Electronic Medical Databases Can Be Used to Search for Current Best Evidence (See Table 16-2)

APTA Clinical Research Agenda

1. Support, explain, and enhance physical therapy clinical practice by facilitating research that is primarily useful to clinicians.

Clinical Practice Guidelines (CPGs)

1. Systematically developed statements to assist clinicians and patients in decisions about appropriate courses of action.
2. CPGs are developed through a combination of current best scientific evidence (e.g., systematic research and meta-analysis), expert judgment, and analysis of patient preferences combined with outcome-based guidelines.
3. Guidelines issued by professional groups and governmental agencies are developed by expert consensus.
   a. APTA currently has a program to assist CPG development, resources, and a submission/acceptance process.

Clinical Prediction Rule (CPR)

1. A combination of clinical findings that have statistically demonstrated meaningful predictability in guiding clinical decision-making.
2. A mathematical, evidence-based tool that can be used to assist clinicians in determining a diagnosis (diagnostic CPRs), prognosis (prognostic CPRs), or intervention (prescriptive CPRs).
3. Combined with clinical expertise and patient preference to improve overall quality of care.

Table 16-1

Steps in Evidence-Based Practice

Step 1	A clinical problem is identified, and an answerable research question is formulated. • The question is clearly defined and related to a clinical decision (e.g., what tests and measures have the best diagnostic utility, what therapeutic interventions have the most success with particular patient classifications). • The question is focused to clarify the target of the literature search.
Step 2	A systematic literature review is conducted and the best evidence is collected. • Sources of evidence may include books, journals, clinical protocols, or colleagues. • Stronger sources of evidence include a systematic review using an electronic search of the medical literature; see Electronic Medical Databases and Resources (Table 16-2). • Articles are selected that are most likely to provide valid results (e.g., randomized controlled trials [RCTs]).
Step 3	The research evidence is summarized and critically analyzed. • The type (design) of the study is identified. • Study methods are identified (e.g., Were appropriate samples of patients used? What are the inclusion and exclusion criteria? Were all patients who entered the trial properly accounted for and attributed at the conclusion of the study?). • Statistical methods and analysis are identified (e.g., Are results presented clearly? Are they statistically significant? Are they clinically meaningful?).
Step 4	The research evidence is synthesized and applied to clinical practice. • Best evidence is available and applied to clinical practice using clinical decision analysis.

Table 16-2

Electronic Medical Databases and Resources
PubMed • US National Library of Medicine's search service to Medline and Pre-Medline (database of medical and biomedical research) http://www.ncbi.nlm.nih.gov/pubmed/
Cochrane Database of Systemic Reviews (Cochrane Reviews) • Database of systematic reviews of RCTs; primary source for clinical effectiveness information http://www.cochrane.org/reviews
Physiotherapy Evidence Database (PEDro) • Database of physical therapy RCTs, systematic reviews, and evidence-based clinical practice guidelines http://www.pedro.fhs.usyd.edu.au/index.html
ERIC • Database of education research https://eric.ed.gov/
CINAHL • Database of nursing and allied health research http://www.cinahl.com
Ovid • Database of health and life science research http://www.ovid.com
APTA Evidence-Based Practice Resources • Provides APTA members easy access to journals and other resources relevant to clinical practice https://www.apta.org/patient-care/evidence-based-practice-resources

Physical Therapy Outcomes Registry (APTA)

1. An organized system for collecting data to evaluate patient function.
2. Includes clinically relevant measures for the population of patients receiving physical therapy services.
3. Use of standardized outcome measures improves practice (patient outcomes, patient satisfaction, PT clinical decision-making), informs payment for physical therapy services, and promotes research.

Research Is Conducted in Academic and Clinical Settings

1. The research question/proposal is developed and submitted for ethical approval (Institutional Review Board) and funding (Grants through Private, Public, or Government Agencies).
2. The research study is conducted.
3. The research data is analyzed and reported (i.e., presentation and written publication).

Research Evidence Is Incorporated into Clinical Practice

1. Steps: see Table 16-1.
2. Sources: evidence is presented in publications, websites (Table 16-2), discussion groups, presentations.
3. Changes in clinical practice are based on consultation with the patient, to arrive at a determination of which option best suits the patient (a client-centered approach).
4. Physical therapists must exercise good clinical judgment in determining applicability of the research results to the specific patient (i.e., similarity to the research group).

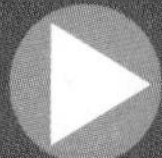

Research Design

Methods

Common steps in research design include development of a problem statement, formation of a research question, collection and analysis of data, interpretation of results, and discussion of the relationship of findings to existing body of evidence.

Variables

General Concepts

1. Independent variable: a variable that stands alone and isn't changed by any other variables being measured (e.g., age and time) in an experiment, the variable that is being manipulated.

2. Dependent variable: the variable that is being studied and measured; in an experiment, it changes when the independent variable is manipulated (e.g., how tall you are at different ages).

Levels of Measurement Data Types (See Table 16-3)

1. Variables may be categorical or continuous.
   a. Categorical variables are categorized according to a trait or characteristic that does not have inherent numerical value. Categorical data include nominal and ordinal scales.
      - Nominal scale: classifies variables or scores into two or more mutually exclusive categories based on a common set of characteristics; the lowest level of measurement (e.g., subjects are classified by sex, race, or ethnicity).
      - Ordinal scale: classifies and ranks variables or scores in terms of the degree to which they possess a common characteristic.
        - Intervals between ranks are NOT equal (e.g., visual analog pain scale; manual muscle test grades of normal, good, fair, poor, trace, zero).

   b. Continuous variables measure a characteristic with inherent numerical value. Continuous data include interval and ratio scales.
      - Interval scale: classifies and ranks variables or scores based on predetermined equal intervals.
        - Does not have a true zero point (e.g. temperature scales (Fahrenheit or Celsius), IQ test with scores ranging from 0–200).
      - Ratio scale: classifies and ranks variables or scores based on equal intervals and a true zero point.
        - The highest, most precise level of measurement; equal intervals and true zero point (e.g, range of motion, scales for weight, force production using a dynamometer).

Types of Research

1. Biomedical research can be described by the timeframe used to collect data (cross-sectional, retrospective, or prospective) and/or by the goal of the research design (to describe, associate, predict, or compare phenomena).

Research Type by Time Frame

1. Cross-sectional Research
   a. Data are collected on an individual or groups of individuals at a single point in time.

Table 16-3

Examples of Statistical Analyses According to the Study's Purpose and the Data's Level of Measurement

PURPOSE	LEVEL OF MEASUREMENT	STATISTICS
Describe*	Nominal	Frequency, Percentage
	Ordinal	Median, Mode, Range
	Interval/Ratio	Mean, Variance, Standard Deviation, Skew and Kurtosis of the Distribution
Associate**	Nominal	Chi Square, Phi coefficient, point biserial, rank biserial
	Ordinal	Spearman's Rank Order or Kendall's Tau Correlations
	Interval/Ratio	Pearson's Product Moment Correlation
Predict	Nominal/Ordinal	Logistic Regression, Discriminant Analysis
	Interval/Ratio	Simple Regression, Multiple Regression
Compare	Nominal	One group: Chi Square Two groups: Independent: Chi Square; Paired: McNemar Test More than two groups: Independent: Chi Square; Paired: Cochran's Q
	Ordinal	Two groups: Independent: Mann-Whitney U; Paired: Wilcoxon Signed Rank More than two groups: Independent: Kruskal-Wallis; Paired: Friedman ANOVA
	Interval/Ratio	Two groups: Independent: t-test; Paired: Paired t-test; Statistical Control: ANCOVA More than two groups: Independent: ANOVA; Repeated Measures: Repeated Measures ANOVA; Statistical Control: ANCOVA

Nominal: characteristics into categories
Ordinal: rank ordering, no specific intervals between ranks
Interval: values rank ordered on a scale that has equal distances (intervals) between points on that scale
Ratio: values rank ordered on a scale that has equal intervals and a true zero point
*Descriptive statistics used for lower levels of measurement can also be used at higher levels of measurement
**Choosing the correct correlation statistic to use depends on the level of measurement of both variables of interest
Adapted from table prepared by Nina Coppens, PhD, RN, University of Massachusetts, Lowell.

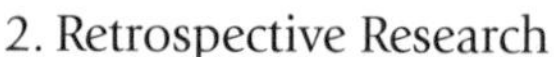

2. Retrospective Research
   a. Individuals or groups of individuals are enrolled in the study at a particular timepoint or following the occurrence of a target event and historical data are collected; the study proceeds backwards in time. Data are typically collected from subject interview or review of records.
3. Prospective Research
   a. Individuals or groups of individuals are enrolled in the study at a particular timepoint and followed forward in time to determine if a particular outcome occurs.

Research Type by Research Goal

1. Descriptive Research
   a. Involves collecting data about conditions, attitudes, or characteristics of subjects or groups of subjects.
   b. Determines and reports existing phenomena.
   c. Data collection: typically done through questionnaire survey, interview, or observation.
      - Permits classification, identification.
      - Data can be used for prediction, decision-making.
   d. Examples of descriptive research.
      - Case studies or clinical reports: in-depth investigation of an individual, group, or institution.
      - Developmental research: studies of behaviors that differentiate individuals at different levels of age, growth, or maturation.
      - Longitudinal studies: differentiate changes in an individual or group of individuals over time (e.g., disease progression).
      - Normative research: investigates standards of behavior, standard values for given characteristics of a sample (e.g., gait characteristics).
      - Qualitative research: seeks to understand concepts, opinions, or experiences related to social phenomena and complex human behavior.
        - Utilizes people's own written or spoken words, behaviors through interview or observation.
        - Develops concepts, insights, and understanding from patterns in the data; uses inductive reasoning.
        - Emphasis is on understanding of human experience (e.g., holistic view of people and settings).
2. Correlational Research
   a. Attempts to determine the presence and magnitude of relationships or associations between two or more variables.
   b. Describes or predicts relationships among variables without active manipulation of the variables.
   c. Limitations.
      - Measures degree of association, not level of agreement between variables.
      - Cannot establish cause-and-effect relationships.
      - May fail to consider all variables that contribute to a relationship.
   d. When a study is attempting to find the presence and magnitude of a relationship between variables, the statistic of interest is the correlation coefficient. Correlation coefficients range from -1 to $+1$.
      - If the correlation is >0, the variables are positively correlated.
      - If the correlation is 0, the variables are not related.
      - If the correlation is <0, the variables are inversely related.
      - The closer the correlation is to $+1$ or -1, the stronger the association between the variables.
   e. When a study is attempting to predict the occurrence of one variable from another variable, the statistics of interest are the regression equation and the coefficient of determination.
      - The regression equation predicts how much the dependent variable will change given a specific change in the independent variable.
      - The coefficient of determination is the square of the correlation coefficient. It describes how strong the linear relationship between the variables is (e.g., how accurately changes in the independent variable predict changes in the dependent variable).
   f. Examples of correlational research.
      - Retrospective: investigation of data collected in the past. Prospective: recording and investigation of present data.
      - Descriptive: investigation of several variables at once; determines existing relationships among variables.
      - Predictive: useful to develop predictive models.
3. Experimental Research
   a. Attempts to define a cause-and-effect relationship through group comparisons.
   b. Alleged cause or treatment (the independent variable) is manipulated.
   c. Effect or difference (the dependent variable) is determined.
   d. Designs.
      - True experimental design: includes random assignment into experimental group (receives treatment) or control group (no treatment). All other experiences are held similar.
      - Cohort design: quasi-experimental design, subjects are identified and followed over time for changes/outcomes following exposure to an intervention; lacks randomization, may or may not have a control group.
      - Within-subject design (repeated measures): subjects serve as their own controls; randomly assigned to treatment or no treatment blocks.

- Between-subject design: comparisons made between groups of subjects.
- Single-subject experimental design: involves a sample of one with repeated measurements and design phases. Single-subject designs include:
  - A-B design: involves two phases, a pretreatment or baseline phase followed by an intervention or treatment phase.
  - A-B-A design (multiple baseline design): involves three phases—a baseline phase and a treatment phase, followed by a second baseline phase.
  - A-B-A-B (multiple baseline, multiple treatment): includes baseline, treatment, and additional baseline and treatment phases.
- Factorial design: refers to the number of independent variables utilized (e.g., single factor, multifactor).

4. Causal-Comparative Research
   a. Attempts to define a cause-and-effect relationship through group comparisons.
   b. Ex post facto research: the cause or independent variable has already occurred; cannot be manipulated (e.g., gender) or should not be manipulated (e.g., type of brain injury).
   c. Groups are compared based on the dependent variable.
5. Epidemiology
   a. The study of disease frequency and distribution in a community.
   b. The science concerned with examining and determining the specific causes of health problems and interrelationships of factors.

Hypothesis

General Concepts

1. A hypothesis is a tentative and testable explanation of the relationship between variables; the results of an experiment determine whether the hypothesis is accepted or rejected.
2. Null hypothesis: states that no relationship exists between variables, a statistical hypothesis; any relationship found is the result of chance or sampling error.
   a. The null hypothesis is rejected; meaning that a significant difference was observed between groups or treatments.
   b. The null hypothesis is accepted; meaning that no significant difference was observed between groups or treatments.
3. Research hypothesis: states that a relationship between variables exists and manipulating the independent variable will bring about a change in the dependent variable.
   a. May be nondirectional or directional. Nondirectional hypotheses predict that the dependent variable will change when the independent variable changes, but do not specify if the change will be an increase or a decrease in magnitude. Directional hypotheses predict that the change will occur in a specified direction (increase or decrease).

Sampling

Selection of Sample

1. The selection of individuals for a study from a population. The sample represents the larger group from which they were selected.
2. Random: all individuals in a population have an equal chance of being chosen for a study.
3. Systematic: individuals are selected from a population list by taking individuals at specified intervals (e.g., every tenth name).
4. Stratified: individuals are selected from a population from identified subgroups based on some predetermined characteristic (e.g., by height, weight, or gender).
5. Double-blind study: an experiment in which the subject and the investigator are not aware of group assignment.
6. Effect size: the size (quantity, magnitude) of the differences between sample means; allows a statistical test to find a difference when one really does exist.
7. Generalizability: the degree to which a study's findings based on a sample apply to an entire population.

Instrumentation

Selection

1. Instruments are chosen with established validity and reliability.
2. Gold standard: an instrument with established validity can be used as a standard for assessing other instruments.

Informed Consent

General Concepts

1. A document that includes consent of an individual prior to participation in a study with full disclosure of risks and benefits; ethical disclosure.
2. Components.
   a. Information about the general nature of what is to take place.
   b. Any risks to the individual and what will be done to minimize the risks.
   c. Possible benefits.
   d. An ethical disclosure.

Determining the Quality of Research

Control

1. The researcher attempts to remove the influence of any variable other than the independent variable in order to evaluate its effect on the dependent variable.
   a. Control group: the group in a research study that resembles the experimental group, but which does not receive the new or different treatment (e.g., treated as usual); provides a baseline for interpretation of results.
   b. Experimental group: the group in a research study that receives a new or novel treatment that is under investigation.
   c. Intervening variable: a variable that alters the relationship (intervenes) between the independent and dependent variable; may not be directly observable or easy to control (e.g., anxiety).
      - If the presence of the intervening variable is known, its presence and magnitude can be recorded, making it a control variable.
      - If the presence of the intervening variable is not known or its presence and magnitude are not recorded, it may become a confounding variable and make the true nature of the relationship between the independent and dependent variables difficult to identify or understand.

Validity

1. The degree to which a test, instrument, or procedure accurately measures what it is supposed to or intended to measure.
2. Types.
   a. Face validity: the assumption of validity based on the appearance of an instrument as a reasonable measure of a variable; may be used for initial screening of a test instrument but psychometrically unsound. Poorest form of validity.
   b. Internal validity: the degree to which the observed differences on the dependent variable are the direct result of manipulation of the independent variable and not some other variable.
   c. External validity: the degree to which the results are generalizable to individuals (general population) or environmental settings outside of the experimental study.
   d. Content validity: the degree to which an instrument measures an intended content area.
      - Determined by expert judgment.
      - Requires both item validity and sampling validity.
   e. Concurrent validity: the degree to which the scores on one test are related to the scores on another criterion test with both tests being given at relatively similar times; usually involves comparison to the gold standard.
   f. Predictive validity: the degree to which a test is able to predict future performance.
   g. Construct validity: the degree to which a test measures an intended hypothetical abstract concept (non-observable behaviors or ideas).

Threats to Validity

1. Sampling bias (selection bias): the researcher introduces systematic sampling error (e.g., a sample of convenience) (the use of volunteers or available groups) instead of random selection of subjects.
2. Failure to exert rigid control over subjects and conditions: intervening variables interact with the dependent variable (e.g., in a longitudinal pediatric study, the outcome is due to the maturation of the child rather than the treatment intervention).
3. The administration of the pretest influences scores on the post-test (e.g., a learning effect occurs as a result of taking a test).
4. The measurement instrument is not accurate, the test does not measure the characteristic it purports to measure (e.g., muscle strength, not motor control).
5. Pretest-treatment interaction: subjects respond differently to the treatment because of the pretest.
6. Multiple treatment interference: more than one treatment is being given to the subjects at the same time; or carry-over effects from an earlier treatment influence the results of a later treatment (e.g., effects of ultrasound following application of a hot pack).
7. Experimenter bias: expectations of the researcher about the expected outcomes of the study influence the results of a study.
8. Hawthorne effect: the subject's knowledge of participation in an experiment influences the results of a study.
9. Placebo effect: subjects respond to a sham treatment with positive effects (e.g., taking a sugar pill instead of an experimental drug results in a change).

Reliability

1. The degree to which an instrument measures a phenomenon accurately, dependably, time after time, and without variation.
   a. Interrater (intertester) reliability: the degree to which two or more independent raters can obtain the same rating for a given variable; the consistency of multiple raters.
   b. Intrarater (intratester) reliability: the degree to which one rater can obtain the same rating for a given variable on multiple measurement trials; an individual's consistency of rating.
   c. Test-retest reliability: the degree to which the scores on a test are stable or consistent over time; a measure of instrument stability.
   d. Split-half reliability: the degree of agreement when a test is split in half and the reliability of the first half is compared to the second half; a measure of internal consistency of an instrument.

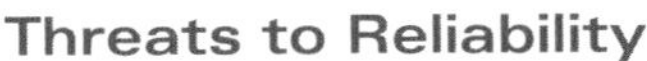

Threats to Reliability

1. Errors of measurement: random errors or systematic errors (e.g., repeat measurements of blood pressure may vary as a result of physiological changes) (fear, anxiety).

Objectivity

1. Agreement among expert judges on what is observed or what is done (e.g., scoring of a perceptible sign or symptom is the same) regardless of who is observing the phenomena (e.g., licensure exam).

Subjectivity

1. Refers to a testing format that may differ depending upon the person grading the test (e.g., figure skating judging).

Testing Diagnostic Accuracy

1. Sensitivity: a test's ability to correctly identify the proportion of individuals who truly have a disease or condition (a true positive).
2. Specificity: a test's ability to correctly identify the proportion of individuals who do not have a disease or condition (a true negative).
3. Predictive value: a test's ability to estimate the likelihood that a person will test positive (or negative) for a target condition.
4. True positive: individuals are correctly identified as having the target condition.
5. True negative: individuals are correctly identified as not having the target condition.
6. False positive: individuals are identified as having the target condition when they do not.
7. False negative: individuals are identified as not having the target condition when they do.
8. Both sensitivity and specificity are expressed as values between 0 and 1. Values very close to 1 are ideal.
9. Sensitivity and specificity values may be combined to obtain a likelihood ratio, used to determine how much the test influences identification of a condition or limitation in function.
10. Sensitive tests help to rule out a condition when the test is negative and the condition is not present—this can be remembered by the acronym SnNOut (Sensitive Negative Rule Out).
11. Specific tests help to rule a condition in when the test is positive and the condition is present—this can be remembered by the acronym SpPIn (Specific Positive Rule In).

Responsiveness

1. Used to determine if a measure is able to reflect meaningful change in status.
2. Minimal detectable change (MDC): the smallest amount of change in a measurement that exceeds the measurement error of the instrument; reflects a true change in status.
3. Minimally important clinical difference (MCID): is the smallest difference in a measured variable that signifies a clinically important change in status.

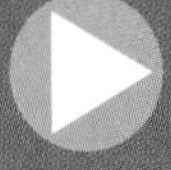

Data Analysis and Interpretation

Descriptive Statistics

Purpose: Summarize and Describe Data

Measures of Central Tendency: A Determination of Average or Typical Scores

1. Mean: the arithmetic average of all scores (X).
   a. Add all scores together and divide by the number of subjects (N).
   b. The most frequently used measure of central tendency; appropriate for interval or ratio data.
2. Median: the midpoint, 50% of scores are above the median and 50% of scores are below; appropriate for ordinal data.
3. Mode: the most frequently occurring score; appropriate for nominal data.

Measures of Variability: A Determination of the Spread of a Group of Scores

1. Range: the difference between the highest score and the lowest score.
2. Standard deviation (SD): a determination of variability of scores (difference) from the mean.
   a. Subtract each score from the mean, square each difference, add up all the squares, and divide by the number of scores.
   b. The most frequently used measure of variability.
   c. Appropriate with interval or ratio data.
3. Normal distribution: a symmetrical bell-shaped curve indicating the distribution of scores; the mean, median, and mode will be similar.
   a. Half the scores are above the mean and half the scores are below the mean.

b. Most scores are near the mean, within one standard deviation; approximately 68% of scores fall within −1 or +1 SD of the mean.
c. Frequency of scores decreases farther from the mean.
   - Approximately 95% of scores fall within −2 or +2 SD of the mean.
   - Approximately 99% of scores fall within −3 or +3 SD of the mean.
d. Distribution may be skewed (not symmetrical) rather than normal: scores are extreme, clustered at one end or the other; the mean, median, and mode are different.

4. Percentiles and quartiles: describe a score's position within the distribution, relative to all other scores.
   a. Percentiles: data are divided in 100 equal parts; position of score is determined.
   b. Quartiles: data are divided into four equal parts and position of score is placed accordingly.

Inferential Statistics

Purpose

1. Help determine how likely the results of a study of a sample can be generalized to the whole population.

Concepts

1. Standard error of measurement: an estimate of expected errors in an individual's score; a measure of response stability or reliability.
2. Tests of significance: an estimation of true differences, not due to chance; a rejection of the null hypothesis.
   a. Probability levels are associated with inferential analyses. Alpha level: preselected level of statistical significance.
      - Most commonly set at 0.05 or 0.01; indicates that the expected difference is due to chance (e.g., at 0.05, only 5 times out of every 100 or a 5% chance) often expressed as a value of P.
      - Allows rejection of the null hypothesis: there are true differences on the measured dependent variable.
   b. Degrees of freedom: based on number of subjects and number of groups; allows determination of level of significance based on consulting appropriate tables for each statistical test.
   c. Errors.
      - Standard error: expected chance variation among the means, the result of sampling error.
      - Type I error: the null hypothesis is rejected by the researcher when it is true (e.g., the observed difference in the means of scores is concluded to be truly different when the difference is due to chance).
      - Type II error: the null hypothesis is not rejected by the researcher when it is false (e.g., the observed difference in the means of scores is concluded to be due to chance when the difference is real).
      - Statistical Power is the ability to observe a difference in the tested sample when a real difference exists in the population.
         - Increasing sample size, increasing the effect size, increasing the alpha level, and decreasing observed variance will increase statistical power and decrease the occurrence of Type I and Type II errors.

Correlational Statistics

1. Used to determine the relative strength of a relationship between two variables (e.g., compare progression of radiologically observed joint destruction in rheumatoid arthritis and its relationship to demographic variables [gender, age], disease severity, and exercise frequency).
2. Pearson product-moment coefficient (r): used to correlate continuous data with underlying normal distribution on interval or ratio scales (e.g., the relationship between proximal and distal development in infants is examined).
3. Spearman's rank correlation coefficient (r_s or Spearman's rho): a nonparametric test used to correlate ordinal data (e.g., the relationship of verbal and reading comprehension scores is examined).
4. Point biserial correlation: one variable is dichotomous (nominal) and the other is ratio or interval (e.g., the relationship between elbow flexor spasticity and side of stroke [left or right] in stroke patients is examined).
5. Rank biserial correlation: one variable is dichotomous (nominal) and the other is ordinal (e.g., the relationship between gender and functional ability is examined).
6. Phi coefficient: both variables are dichotomous (nominal) (e.g., the relationship between sex and eye color is examined).
7. Intraclass correlation coefficient (ICC): a reliability coefficient based on an analysis of variance.
8. Strength of relationships.
   a. Positive correlations range from 0 to +1: indicates that as variable X increases, so does variable Y.
      - Good reliability >0.75
      - Moderate reliability = 0.50 to 0.75
      - Poor reliability <0.50
   b. Negative correlations range from −1 to 0: indicates that as variable X increases, variable Y decreases; an inverse relationship.
9. Coefficient of Determination: a representation of the degree that variation in one variable is attributable to another variable.

a. Determined by squaring the correlation coefficient (e.g., a correlation coefficient of 0.70 means that the coefficient of determination is 49%), i.e., a linear relationship between the variables can be determined with 49% accuracy.

Linear Regression

1. Used to determine the relationship between two variables as a basis for prediction.
2. An examination of two continuous variables that are linearly correlated. The variable designated X is the independent or predictor variable. The variable designated Y is the dependent or criterion variable.
3. The purpose is to generate an equation that relates X to Y, such that if given values of X, Y can be predicted (e.g., blood pressure [Y] is examined by age [X]) answers the question: Can systolic blood pressure be predicted from age?
4. See Figure 16-1 for determining appropriate statistical tests.

Parametric Statistics

1. Testing is based on population parameters; includes tests of significance based on interval or ratio data.
2. Assumptions.
   a. A normal distribution exists in the population studied of the variable measured, or distribution is known. In a large, representative sample, the assumption of normal distribution is probably met.
   b. Random sampling is performed.
   c. Variance in the groups is equal.

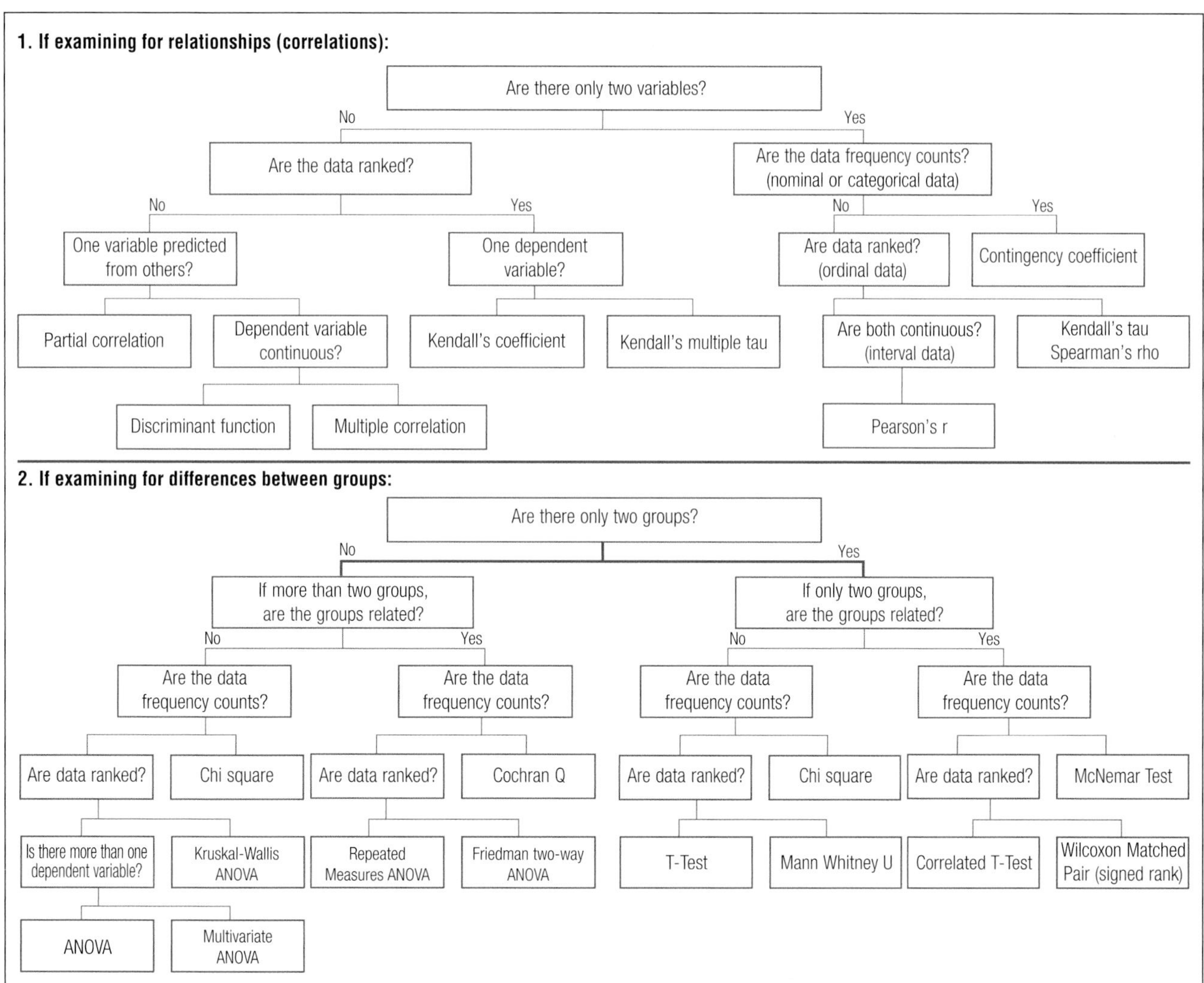

Figure 16-1 **Flow diagram for determining appropriate statistical tests.**

Key: follow flow diagram to the right with yes answers; follow flow diagram to the left with no answers
Adapted from materials prepared by Dr. L Zaichkowsky, Boston University

3. T-test: a parametric test of significance used to compare two independent groups created by random assignment and identify a difference at a selected probability level (e.g., 0.05).
   a. T-test for independent samples: compares the difference between two independent groups (e.g., a test to determine whether an intervention [a new hand splint] improves the function of patients with rheumatoid arthritis).
   b. T-test for paired samples: compares the difference between two matched samples (e.g., Does therapy improve function in siblings with autism?).
      - One-tailed t-test: based on a directional hypothesis; evaluates differences in data on only one end of a distribution, either negative or positive (e.g., patients who receive a certain treatment exhibit better rehabilitation outcomes than those who do not).
      - Two-tailed t-test: based on a nondirectional hypothesis; evaluates differences in data on both positive and negative ends of a distribution; tests of significance are almost always two-tailed (e.g., either group of patients [treatment or control] may exhibit better rehabilitation outcomes).
   c. Inappropriate use of t-tests: use of a t-test to compare more than two means within a single sample (e.g., three modes of exercise are compared within a single sample).
4. Analysis of variance (ANOVA): a parametric test used to compare three or more independent treatment groups or conditions at a selected probability level.
   a. Simple (one-way) ANOVA: compares multiple groups on a single independent variable; e.g., three sets of post-test scores (balance scores from a Balance Master) are compared from three different categories of elderly: young elderly (65–74); old elderly (75–84); and old and frail elderly (>85).
   b. Factorial ANOVA (multifactorial) compares multiple groups on two or more independent variables (e.g., two groups of injured patients [those with severe ankle sprain and moderate ankle sprain] and a control group are compared for muscle activation patterns and sensory perception in each limb).
5. Analysis of covariance (ANCOVA): a parametric test used to compare two or more treatment groups or conditions while also controlling for the effects of intervening variables (covariates) (e.g., two groups of subjects are compared on the basis of gait parameters using two different types of assistive devices), subjects in one group are taller than subjects in the second group; height then becomes the covariate that must be controlled during statistical analysis.

Nonparametric Statistics

1. Testing is not based on population parameters; includes tests of significance based on ordinal or nominal data.
2. Used when above parametric assumptions cannot be met.
3. Less powerful than parametric tests, more difficult to reject the null hypothesis (e.g., can be used with small sample and with ordinal or nominal level data).
4. Chi-square test: a nonparametric test of significance used to compare data in the form of frequency counts occurring in two or more mutually exclusive categories (e.g., subjects are asked to rate treatment preferences).

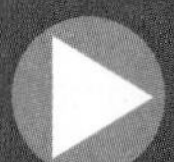

Evaluating the Evidence: Levels of Evidence and Grades of Recommendation

Definitions

Systematic Review (SR)

1. SR is a type of literature review in which the primary studies are summarized, critically appraised, and statistically combined.
2. Usually quantitative in nature (RCTs) with specific inclusion/exclusion criteria.
3. Meta-analysis is a statistical analysis that combines the results of multiple conceptually similar scientific studies; results in a higher statistical power and more robust findings.

Randomized Controlled Trial (RCT)

1. RCT is an experimental study in which participants are randomly assigned to either an experimental or control group to receive different interventions or a placebo.

Cohort Study

1. A cohort study is a prospective (forward-in-time) study; a group of participants (cohort) with a similar condition is followed for a defined period of time.
2. Comparison is made to a matched group that does not have the condition.

Homogeneity/Heterogeneity

1. Homogeneity: an SR free of variations in the directions and degree of results between individual studies.
2. Heterogeneity: an SR with variations.

Case-Control Study

1. A retrospective (backward-in-time) study.
2. A group of individuals with a similar condition (disease) is compared with a group that does not have the condition to determine factors that may have played a role in the condition.

Case Report Study

1. A type of descriptive research in which only one individual is studied in depth, often retrospectively.

Levels of Evidence

Grades (See Table 16-4)

1. Includes criteria to determine the level of evidence and the accompanying grade of recommendation.
2. Level I is based on the highest level of evidence and Level V is the lowest level of evidence.
3. Grades are used when evaluating interventions and supporting action statements for best practice (CPGs).
4. Synopses of CPGs are presented in individual chapters.

Table 16-4

Levels of Evidence and Grades of Recommendation

LEVEL	DESCRIPTION
I	Evidence is based on SR of high-quality RCTs (or meta-analyses) with adequate size to ensure low risk of bias, substantial agreement of size and direction of treatment effects; or individual RCT with narrow confidence level, treatment effects precisely defined, and low risk of bias; prospective studies.
II	Evidence is based on SR lesser-quality RCT (e.g., too small to provide Level I evidence) weaker diagnostic criteria and reference standards, improper randomization; <than 80% follow-up of subjects enrolled in study or SR of cohort studies with homogeneity; prospective studies.
III	Evidence is based on SR of nonrandomized, controlled cohort studies or individual case-control study; retrospective studies.
IV	Evidence is based on case series studies and poor-quality cohort or case-control studies (comparison groups not adequately defined, exposures and outcomes not measured objectively, lack of control for confounders, insufficient follow-up—cohort studies only).
V	Evidence is based on expert opinion without critical appraisal, or based on physiology, bench research.
GRADES OF RECOMMENDATION BASED ON	**STRENGTH OF EVIDENCE**
A—Strong evidence	A preponderance of Level I and/or Level II studies support the recommendation. This must include at least one Level I study.
B—Moderate evidence	A single, high-quality RCT or a preponderance of Level II studies support the recommendation.
C—Weak evidence	A single Level II study or a preponderance of Levels III and IV studies, including statements of consensus by content experts, support the recommendation.
D—Conflicting evidence	Higher-quality studies conducted on this topic that disagree on conclusions. The recommendation is based on these conflicting studies.
E—Theoretical/ foundational evidence	A preponderance of evidence from animal or cadaver studies, from conceptual models/principles, or from basic sciences/bench research support this conclusion.
F—Expert opinion	Best practice based on the clinical experience of the guideline's development team.

RCT = randomized controlled trials; SR = systematic review

Grades of recommendation adapted from Knee Pain and Mobility Impairments: Meniscal and Articular Cartilage Lesions. Clinical Practice Guidelines linked to the International Classification of Functioning, Disability, and Health from the Orthopedic Section of the American Physical Therapy Association, Summary of Recommendations. *JOSPT*; 6(40): A30, 2010.

APPENDIX 16A

Review Questions

(Answers to all Review Questions and Case Studies are found in Chapter 17)

1. What is the difference between independent and dependent variables?

2. What is the significance of validity and reliability regarding a clinical test? What are the possible threats to each?

3. What is the significance of sensitivity and specificity regarding a clinical test?

4. From highest to lowest level of rigor, what is the hierarchy of evaluating and grading levels of evidence? Give an example of each.

17

Answers to Chapter Review Questions and Case Studies

Chapter Outline

Chapter 2, Appendix 2C
Review Questions and Case Studies

Musculoskeletal Physical Therapy

1. Which motion at the glenohumeral joint has the greatest limitation if the diagnosis is adhesive capsulitis?

External rotation (capsular pattern).

2. When considering the concave-convex rule, to which joints in the spine does the concave rule apply?

Every joint below the second cervical vertebra. Only the atlanto-occipital joint is convex.

3. Which special test when applied to the ankle/foot is BEST used to identify ligamentous instability of the calcaneofibular ligament?

Talar tilt.

4. What are the major differences in diagnostic characteristics and pattern of joint dysfunction between osteoarthritis and rheumatoid arthritis?

Osteoarthritis is first manifested by changes in joint cartilage with eventual erosion to subchondral bone. All joints are not equally affected. The DIPs, PIPs, the CMC of the thumb, cervical and lumbar spine, hips, knees, and MTPs are the primary sites.

Rheumatoid arthritis is an autoimmune disease that primarily affects the synovium. The synovium proliferates, dissolves collagen, and extends over the joint cartilage. There is persistent inflammation and systemic complaints such as morning stiffness, fever, and loss of appetite. Joints are affected in a bilateral symmetrical pattern. All joints including the spine and TMJ can be involved.

5. Based on Clinical Practice Guidelines for Knee Ligament Sprain, which intervention has the strongest overall evidence for effectiveness?

Therapeutic exercise, including NWB open-chain and WB closed-chain activities, is the most effective based on evidence when dealing with patients with knee instability and movement coordination impairments.

Other interventions, such as bracing, CPM, early intervention, etc., demonstrate moderate to weak evidence based on available studies.

6. Following a total hip replacement, in the acute phase, which positions should be avoided in bed positioning and activities involving bed mobility?

A wedge should be used in positioning to prevent hip adduction. Hip flexion should not exceed 90°. Adduction and internal rotation should be limited when moving in bed.

7. For an anteriorly displaced articular disc at the TMJ, what is the primary joint mobilization technique?

If TMJ restriction is present, primary glide is inferior, which gaps the joint, stretches the capsule, and allows relocation of the disc.

Case Study #1

Patient Profile

- Gender: Female
- Age: 49

Presenting Problem/Current Condition

- Patient referred to outpatient physical therapy with a chief complaint of right-sided neck pain
- Insidious onset upon waking up 3 days ago
- Pain and numbness extending to right posterior forearm and dorsum of hand, occasionally extending to the 3rd digit
- Arm weakness

Past Medical History

- History of hypertension
- Occasional headaches associated with neck pain

Other Information

- School teacher
- Obese, BMI=34
- Occasional consumption of alcohol

1. What elements from the patient interview make a diagnosis of cervical radiculopathy most likely?

Dermatomal paresthesia or numbness and myotomal muscle weakness is correct. Neck pain outlined in a narrow band that follows a dermatomal pattern is most suggestive of radiculopathy. History of myotomal weakness is a common finding associated with cervical radiculopathy.

2. What are the most common findings in the clinical examination for patients with cervical radiculopathy?

(+) ULTT, (+) Spurling's test, (+) cervical distraction test, painful ROM is correct. These findings are part of a clinical prediction rule test cluster for diagnosing a cervical radiculopathy.

3. What intervention is the **BEST** choice for reducing pain and improving function in acute cervical radiculopathy?

Mobilizing and stabilizing exercise is correct. There is consistent albeit weak evidence that mobilizing and stabilizing exercises are effective in reducing pain and improving function in patients with acute radiating (radicular) neck pain. Cervical collar and laser therapy are also recommended for acute radiating (radicular) neck pain based on current best evidence.

4. During the patient interview, the therapist learns that the patient has rheumatoid arthritis. What special test is most appropriate to determine if the patient has upper cervical spine instability?

Sharp Purser test is correct. The Sharp Purser test assesses the integrity of the transverse ligament, which holds the dens (odontoid process) of the axis against the anterior arch of the atlas. The transverse ligament is also damaged in patients with rheumatoid arthritis.

Case Study #2

Patient Profile

- Gender: Female
- Age: 68

Presenting Problem/Current Condition

- Referred to physical therapy with a chief complaint of right posterior thigh/knee pain for the past 6 weeks
- Onset after a long period of sitting during a train ride
- Knee stiffness on waking in the morning that lasts for less than 30 minutes
- Pain worsens with inactivity and improves with staying active

Past Medical History

- History of left knee replacement 2 years ago

Other Information

- DVT ruled out with Doppler ultrasound
- Denies any neurologic symptoms or low back pain

1. What elements from the patient interview make a diagnosis of knee osteoarthritis (OA) more likely?

Knee stiffness upon first waking that lasts less than 30 minutes is correct. Pain associated with knee OA typically occurs after waking up in the morning or a period of rest and lasts less than 30 minutes.

2. What are most common findings in the clinical examination and diagnostic imaging for patients with knee osteoarthritis?

Hypomobile, painful joint; decreased joint space and osteophytes on radiographs is correct. Patients with knee osteoarthritis typically present with bony enlargement, crepitus, joint effusion, and decreased range of motion. Classic radiographic findings in OA include osteophyte formation, joint space narrowing, subchondral sclerosis, and bone cysts.

3. What interventions offer strong evidence for reducing pain and improving function in osteoarthritis?

Therapeutic exercise (neuromuscular and functional exercises) is correct. There is strong and consistent evidence that neuromuscular and functional training exercise are effective in reducing pain and improving function in patients with osteoarthritis. Effective interventions include isometric, isotonic, functional, and proprioception/balance exercises. Evidence supports both supervised and home exercise interventions.

Chapter 3, Appendix 3B
Review Questions and Case Studies

Neuromuscular Physical Therapy

1. Which cranial nerves may play any role in vision? What findings are normal or abnormal?

CN II (Optic)	Optic-visual acuity or visual fields, pupillary constriction
CN III (Oculomotor)	Pupillary size, extraocular movement
CN IV (Trochlear)	Extraocular movement
CN V (Trigeminal)	Corneal reflex
CN VI (Abducens)	Extraocular movement
CN VII (Facial)	Ability to close eyes tightly (may be absent in Bell's palsy)
CN VIII (Vestibulocochlear)	Nystagmus (secondary to brain dysfunction)

2. Following a CVA, what are the major considerations when examining the patient for perceptual deficits?

Testing for visual field deficits such as homonymous or bitemporal hemianopsia.

Examine for body scheme or image such as unilateral neglect or somatognosia.

Examine for spatial relations such as figure-ground, depth perception, vertical disorientation, etc.

Examine for agnosia such as the inability to recognize familiar objects with an impaired sensory modality.

Examine for apraxias such as dressing apraxias, agraphia, etc.

3. When examining deep tendon reflexes, what is the score reported for an obligatory and sustained response?

0 = absent reflex

1+ = tone change but no movement

2+ = visible movement of extremity

3+ = exaggerated full movement of extremity

4+ = obligatory and sustained movement lasting >30 seconds

4. What are the characteristics in terms of communication, gait, tone, balance, and respiratory function in a patient with late Parkinson's disease (Stage IV Hoehn and Yahr)?

Communication: dysarthria, hypophonia (low volume), masklike face, small writing.

Gait: poverty of movement, festinating gait possible.

Tone: cogwheel rigidity.

Balance: impaired postural reactions including trunk rigidity and lack of rotation.

Respiratory function: decreased chest expansion, decreased vital capacity.

5. What are the initial physical therapy goals and interventions upon receiving a referral for a patient recently diagnosed with a unilateral vestibular disorder?

Implement safety measures first. Teach sensory substitution (visual, tactile) and compensatory strategies and provide an ambulatory aid as indicated. Later on, habituation training, eye and head exercises, and postural stability activities can be implemented.

6. Following an MVA, a patient with a complete SCI at the C7 level has been admitted to a rehab facility after a lengthy stay at an acute care hospital. What are the components of the physical therapist's initial examination?

Vital signs, respiratory function, skin condition, muscle tone, DTRs, sensation, muscle strength, functional status, wheelchair skills, and administration of a standardized test such as the FIM.

7. What is the common pattern of fatigue in many patients with multiple sclerosis?

High energy in early morning, followed by early afternoon fatigue and exhaustion, and then some recovery by early evening. Thus, schedule these patients for morning intervention or consider this pattern for job or other ADL tasks.

Case Study #1

Patient Profile

- Gender: Male
- Age: 63

Presenting Problem/Current Condition

- Patient is referred to inpatient physical therapy secondary to a right ischemic stroke with left hemiparesis.
- Patient was admitted to the hospital 3 days ago with an intense headache and left upper greater than lower extremity weakness.
- Patient also exhibits neglect of the left side of their body.

Past Medical/Surgical History

- History of hypertension by 10 years
- Bilateral knee osteoarthritis
- Right knee arthroscopy with meniscal debridement

Other Information

- College basketball coach
- Married and lives in a 2-story home

1. Which of the following arteries is occluded and most closely associated with the patient's presenting symptoms?

Middle cerebral artery (MCA) is correct. Middle cerebral artery strokes are characterized by upper greater than lower extremity involvement. Non-dominant (typically right side) hemisphere MCA strokes also have a higher likelihood of neglect or perceptual deficits.

2. What impairments and/or activity limitations are most consistent with the patient's presenting symptoms and an acute right (nondominant hemisphere) MCA stroke?

Inability to roll to the left side is correct. Secondary to the patient's left-sided neglect, they will not orientate or turn their head to the left. The patient will also have a flaccid left upper extremity and low tone in the left lower extremity, making it difficult to initiate and complete rolling to the left. Rolling to the left side must be done with caution and assistance.

3. When completing your initial evaluation on this patient you determine they have significant neglect of the left side with complete paresis/sensory loss of the left upper extremity and moderate hypotonia/weakness of the left lower extremity. What initial intervention is the **BEST** choice for improving this patient's function?

Midline orientation and approximation of the left upper extremity in sitting are safe and appropriate initial treatments to treat neglect and hypotonia/sensory deficits of the left upper extremity.

4. The patient is making progress with midline orientation in sitting, but once you transition them from sit to stand you notice they forcefully shift weight from the right to the left side. You are concerned about Pusher's syndrome. Which of the following interventions would be **BEST** to maintain a midline posture?

Visual feedback with a mirror provides patients with a reference of their orientation and can be combined with verbal and tactile cueing to improve alignment to gravity and a neutral posture.

Case Study #2

Patient Profile

- Gender: Female
- Age: 55

Presenting Problem/Current Condition

- Patient is referred to outpatient physical therapy secondary to an ataxic gait and three falls in the past 6 months.
- Patient also reports consistent burning pain, numbness/tingling, and weakness in the bilateral fingers/thumbs, ankles, feet, and toes for the past year.
- She denies specific aggravating factors and reports that her numbness and tingling are constant.
- She reports her falls typically happen when she is walking in the dark or on an unlevel surface.

Past Medical/Surgical History

- History of hypertension and diabetes by 15 years. Hypothyroidism by 7 years.
- Obesity (>36 BMI)
- Lumbar and bilateral knee osteoarthritis
- Past surgeries: bilateral carpal tunnel releases 8 years ago

Other Information

- Occupation: information technology manager
- Lives alone

1. Which of the following health conditions is the most likely cause of the patient's presenting symptoms?

Polyneuropathy is correct. The patient has several risk factors for polyneuropathy and presents with a classic glove and stocking pattern of sensory loss.

2. Which of the following examination findings would reinforce both small and large myelinated neural fiber impairments and increased risk for foot ulceration?

Monofilaments test discriminate touch and large myelinated pathways. Pinprick tests can detect painful stimuli and small neural pathway pathology. This combination places patients at increased risk for foot ulcerations. If these tests are positive, the patient is at increased risk for foot ulcerations.

3. When completing your initial evaluation on this patient you determine they have significant sensory impairments at the ankles, feet, and toes. They also have atrophy of their intrinsic muscles of the feet/toes, but normal strength at and above the ankles. Which of the following impairments in balance/mobility are most consistent with polyneuropathy, the patient's history and sensory/strength findings?

Tandem stance creates a narrow base of support and with elimination of vision the patient is not able to compensate and requires a steppage strategy to maintain safety.

4. Which of the following compensatory strategies is BEST to enhance this patient's safety when ambulating in the community?

A cane or walking stick will provide sensory feedback and allow for correction of posture using feedforward (visual cues) and feedback from the cane/walking stick.

Chapter 4, Appendix 4B
Review Questions and Case Study

Cardiovascular and Lymphatic Physical Therapy

1. What risk factors contribute to the development of coronary artery disease?

   Risk factors include age, gender, family history, cigarette smoking, sedentary lifestyle, obesity (BMI >30 kg/m or waist girth >40 inches), hypertension, dyslipidemia, prediabetes, increased plasma glucose, diabetes.

2. What are the expected ST segment changes following an acute myocardial infarction and with impaired coronary perfusion?

   Following an acute MI the ST segment will be elevated.

   In case of impaired perfusion as in coronary artery disease, the ST segment becomes depressed and can be upsloping, horizontal, or downsloping.

3. How would you instruct your patient regarding possible circumstances that could elicit angina pectoris?

   Increased demands on the heart could elicit angina pectoris. These can include physical exertion, emotional stress, smoking, temperature extremes (especially cold), and overeating.

4. When exercising a patient with diabetes and coronary artery disease who is taking beta blockers, what is the best measure to monitor exercise performance?

   Borg's Ratings of Perceived Exertion scale (RPE scale or Modified RPE scale) can be used. RPE increases linearly with increasing exercise intensity and correlates closely with HR and work rate.

   Beta blockers blunt heart rate response to increasing exercise intensity. Thus, HR is not a reliable sign to monitor under these circumstances.

5. What are the goals of inpatient cardiac rehabilitation in the acute stage or Phase 1?

   The acute stage, lasting perhaps 3–5 days (sometimes longer), should focus on early return to independence in ADL, counteract effects of bed rest by reducing risk of thrombi, maintain muscle tone, reduce orthostatic hypotension, maintain joint mobility, help allay anxiety, provide patient and family education, and promote risk factor reduction.

6. When managing edema secondary to lymphatic dysfunction, use of manual lymph drainage (MLD) emphasizes which directional principles?

   Emphasis is on decongesting proximal segments first, then extremities. The flow within segments is distal to proximal.

Case Study

Patient Profile

- Gender: Male
- Age: 84

Presenting Problem/Current Condition

- Seen in emergency room for primary complaint of chest tightness
- Cardiac enzymes were positive for myocardial infarction
- Had surgery for three-vessel coronary artery bypass graft
- Physical therapy consulted to initiate phase 1 cardiac rehabilitation

Past Medical History

- Hypertension
- Hyperlipidemia
- Smokes 1 pack per day × 60 years

Other Information

- Patient is postoperative day 3 with usual postoperative course.
- Patient lives alone and uses a cane to ambulate.
- Patient has fallen three times in the last month.

1. What would the therapist expect on the initial physical therapy examination?

Patients are given several liters of fluid during surgery to combat the effects of volume depletion. This results in peripheral edema, which can negatively impact a patient's balance and ability to ambulate.

A patient with a coronary artery bypass graft will have had a sternotomy, which causes pain with breathing. The pain leads to symmetrical decreases in breathing pattern, an ineffective cough, and abnormal breath sounds (either decreased due to lack of air movement or crackles from atelectasis or pulmonary edema).

2. The first time the patient mobilizes from supine to standing, he demonstrates a drop in blood pressure (supine: 128/72, standing: 106/68). What is the MOST likely explanation for this response?

Due to effects of medications and increased IV fluids, often in the extravascular space, a patient will have decreased intravascular volume postoperatively. This can lead to orthostatic hypotension.

A minimal drop in blood pressure does occur with position changes, but the body accommodates quickly, so a decrease of 22 mmHg is too much. Similarly, activity should not be necessary to increase the blood pressure. Moving from supine to standing is minimal activity and would not cause the blood pressure to drop due to excessive myocardial demand.

3. The physical therapist designs a phase 1 walking program for the patient. What is the MOST appropriate program?

Interval walking allows the patient to work harder for short periods with equal rest periods to allow recovery. The intensity of activity must be less than 70% of HRmax, which is necessary for a patient within 4–6 weeks of a myocardial infarction.

Chapter 5, Appendix 5A
Review Questions and Case Study

Pulmonary Physical Therapy

1. What are the PaO_2 and FiO_2 normal values in room air?

The partial pressure of oxygen in the arterial blood (PaO_2) is 95–100mm Hg in young healthy individuals. It decreases with age.

The fraction of oxygen in inspired room air (FiO_2) is the percentage of oxygen in the air, which is 21% or written out as 0.21. Use of supplemental oxygen will increase FiO_2.

2. When auscultating the lungs, what are the main characteristics of crackles, wheezes, vesicular, and bronchial breath sounds?

Crackles (rales, crepitations) are crackling sounds heard during inspiration that indicate pathology such as pulmonary edema, fibrosis, or atelectasis.

Wheezes are musical sounds heard during expiration, especially with COPD.

Vesicular sounds (normal breath sounds) are soft, rustling sounds heard throughout inspiration and the beginning of expiration.

Bronchial sounds are hollow, echoing sounds usually heard over the right main stem bronchus during inspiration and expiration. They are normal sounds.

3. What are the expected physical, imaging, PFT, and laboratory findings associated with moderate to severe asthma?

Physical findings: productive cough, dyspnea, decreased breath sounds, wheezes, crackles, tachypnea, tachycardia, increased accessory muscle use, anxiety.

Imaging findings: hyperlucency and flattened diaphragms.

PFT findings: decreased FEV_1/FVC ratio, decreased FEV_1, lower flow rates.

Laboratory findings: ABG hypoxemia and hypercapnea with severe disease.

4. What are the precautions when using postural drainage in the Trendelenburg position?

Care should be exercised and use of the Trendelenburg (head down) position possibly limited or eliminated in situations involving congestive heart failure, significant hypertension, pulmonary edema, increased intracranial pressure, aneurysm, severe SOB, obesity, ascites, pregnancy, and hiatal hernia.

Case Study

Patient Profile

- Gender: Female
- Age: 72

Presenting Problem/Current Condition

- Recent 3-day admission to the hospital with increased shortness of breath and productive cough with yellowish-green sputum
- Treated with high-dose steroids and antibiotics, along with bronchodilators for a chronic obstructive pulmonary disease exacerbation
- Referred to outpatient pulmonary rehabilitation 2 weeks after her hospital discharge

Past Medical History

- Hypertension
- Hyperlipidemia
- Type II diabetes
- Obstructive sleep apnea
- Obesity
- Smoking 1–2 packs per day × 45 years

Other Information

- Patient uses CPAP at night for obstructive sleep apnea.
- She receives assistance from a local agency for house cleaning and grocery shopping.
- She lives alone and uses a rollator for community ambulation.

1. What is the most likely sequelae of the patient's medical treatment in the hospital that the physical therapy should consider during their examination?

   Patients given high-dose steroids are at risk for proximal muscle weakness after just 1–2 doses. It is important to screen for muscle weakness and address it with strengthening exercises in order to maximize the patient's function.

   A patient admitted to the hospital could have delirium and it is important to consider, but there is no evidence in the case that this patient was delirious. Antibiotics do not cause incontinence. There is not any evidence that the patient was immobile in the case that would warrant concern for their integument.

2. What is one of the primary benefits of pulmonary rehabilitation for patients with chronic obstructive pulmonary disease after an exacerbation of their disease?

   Patients consistently report improvements on quality of life measures, including the St. George's Respiratory Questionnaire. Patients often improve on the impact and the activities sections of the questionnaire, even without a significant change in the patient's symptoms. While some patients may experience the changes described in the other choices, these benefits are inconsistent across a heterogeneous population.

3. Which intensity of walking program would be the **BEST** option for the patient to start in pulmonary rehabilitation?

   The patient should start an exercise program at a light or moderate intensity. Working at 50% of the patient's maximum is in that range. Since the intensity is lower, working at 5 days per week is manageable and will help to increase the patient's endurance. Current guidelines recommend at least 20 minutes per day for this patient population. Neither 20% nor 30% are sufficient intensity to affect a change to the cardiovascular system. And 85% is too high for the patient to work at initially, especially following a recent hospitalization.

Chapter 6, Appendix 6A
Review Questions and Case Study

Therapeutic Interventions

1. During strength training, what is the influence of the Valsalva maneuver regarding intrathoracic pressure, heart rate, venous pressure, and cardiac work?

   The Valsalva maneuver (forced exhalation with a closed glottis) results in increased intrathoracic pressure, venous pressure, cardiac work, and decreased heart rate.

2. What are the implications of the FITT equation in terms of strategies to develop cardiovascular endurance?

   The FITT equation includes the factors of frequency, intensity, time, and type of exercise. Intensity (overload) is the primary way to increase cardiovascular endurance. At least 2 days (frequency) of exercise a week or more is needed to increase endurance. Duration (time) of exercise depends on initial fitness level. The goal would be 20–30 minutes, 3–5 days a week for conditioned people. Initial time would be significantly curtailed for deconditioned or obese individuals. The type of exercise should involve large muscle groups.

3. When exercising a patient in an aquatic environment, what are the factors that can make the activity easier to perform? More difficult to perform?

   Easier: movement horizontal to or upward toward the water surface, use of a flotation device, a paddle turned to slice through the water, decreased speed of movement, exercising in deeper water increases buoyancy.

   More difficult: increased speed of movement, use of fins, paddles, and boots to increase resistance, exercise in shallower water, movement downward in the water, increased speed of movement.

4. What is the main principle being employed when using the PNF-facilitated stretching technique of contract-relax?

   The muscle to be stretched relaxes as a result of autogenic inhibition possibly from Golgi tendon organ firing. The muscle can be further relaxed through the effects of reciprocal inhibition if active contraction is performed.

5. What are the most common errors associated with training a patient to improve postural stability?

   Inadequate stretching of tight pelvic and hip musculature prior to training; inadequate core muscle control; starting at too high a functional level or progressing too rapidly; exercising past the point of fatigue.

Case Study

Patient Profile

- Gender: Male
- Age: 35

Presenting Problem/Current Condition

- Referred to physical therapy with a diagnosis of right biceps brachii Grade II muscle strain
- Sustained injury playing recreational softball 3 weeks ago
- Initially placed in sling for a suspected rotator cuff tear
- Now has full range of motion of RUE but weakness of biceps brachii muscle due to inactivity (MMT = 3+/5 or Fair+)
- No current pain with ADLs

Past Medical History

- No prior medical history or prior surgical history involving the RUE

Other Information

- Denies neck pain
- Denies any neurologic symptoms of the RUE

1. What is the typical healing timeline for a Grade II muscle injury?

Grade II muscle strains can take from 3–12 weeks to completely heal. See the Stages of Soft Tissue Healing section on pg. 130 for a review of healing timelines of specific tissues and injuries.

The typical healing time for a Grade 1 muscle injury is 0–4 weeks. Four weeks to 6 months is more consistent with the range of healing time for a Grade III muscle strain, which may require surgery and months of rehabilitation. Six to 12 months may be required for healing of significant cartilage and ligamentous injuries.

2. Which set of exercise parameters should be used to initiate a resistance training program for this patient?

Three days per week, 12–15 repetitions of 3 sets at 50% of the 1-RM weight is the correct answer. These parameters are based on the ACSM Guidelines (2018) for evidence-based resistance exercise (see Table 6-3). These recommendations state that individuals beginning a resistance program to improve strength should exercise 2–3 days per week, at 40–50% of the 1-RM weight, and 2–4 sets of 8–12 repetitions per set.

3. Which adjustment should be made to progress the rehabilitation program and increase strength of the affected muscle?

Intensity (resistance) is the correct parameter to increase in order to improve muscle strength. The ACSM Guidelines state that while 40–50% of the 1-RM is beneficial for individuals *beginning* an exercise program like the patient in this scenario, 60–70% of the 1-RM (moderate-to-vigorous intensity) should be prescribed to increase strength.

Chapter 7, Appendix 7B
Review Questions and Case Study

Integumentary Physical Therapy

1. Differentiate between the viral infections herpes simplex and herpes zoster in terms of expected symptoms.

   Herpes simplex is preceded by itching and soreness followed by vesicular eruptions. A good example is a cold sore.

   Herpes zoster (shingles) is the result of reactivation of the varicella-zoster virus (chickenpox). Often results in pain, tingling, and vesicle formation along dermatomes of spinal or cranial nerves. May last a long time. Superficial or deep heat contraindicated.

2. When performing a physical examination of pressure injury (ulcer), what elements should be part of the physical therapist's examination?

   Determine the location of the wound; assess the length, width, girth, and depth of the wound; examine for tunneling; determine type, amount, color, and odor of exudates if any; determine presence of necrotic or granulation tissue; determine wound temperature using thermistor probe.

3. Differentiate between a superficial partial-thickness burn and a full-thickness burn.

   Superficial partial-thickness: epidermis and upper dermis damage, bright pink or red, blisters, moderate edema, painful.

   Full-thickness: complete destruction of epidermis, dermis, and subcutaneous tissues; white, gray, or charred appearance; poor circulation; dry, leathery surface; little pain as nerve endings destroyed.

4. Differentiate between venous and arterial ulcers in terms of expected clinical presentation.

   Venous ulcers: irregular shape and dark appearance; shallow, often at medial malleolus; pulses present; little pain; fair amount of exudate.

   Arterial ulcers: smooth edges; deep, often on toes, lateral malleoli and shin; pulses often absent; painful; no drainage.

5. Which categories of wound dressings can be used for exudative wounds?

   Many modern dressings can be used for exudative wounds. Some are more suited for heavy exudation. Some are better if the exudate is moderate or mild.

   Categories include hydrocolloids, hydrogels, foams, alginates, and gauze. The dressing category not used with exudates is transparent films.

6. What are the important clinical changes affecting the prognosis for a patient with diffuse systemic sclerosis?

   Diffuse systemic sclerosis/scleroderma has a poorer prognosis than limited systemic sclerosis/scleroderma (LSS). The integumentary changes are more rapid and widespread, there is earlier involvement of visceral organs (e.g., kidneys, heart, and lungs), and mortality occurs sooner than someone with LSS and no organ involvement. Monitoring vital signs and blood pressure for acute hypertension is essential.

Case Study

Patient Profile

- Gender: Male
- Age: 75

Presenting Problem/Current Condition

- Patient referred to physical therapy for management of wound at amputated site.
- Digits 1–3 on the right foot were amputated 2 months ago due to gangrene.
- The amputation site has not healed. The patient has been using a silver-based wound gel with a gauze dressing cover changed twice a day.
- The wound bed is pale and dry. The skin below the knees is dry, hairless, atrophied, and shiny.
- Patient is experiencing numbness in the legs, feet, and toes.

Past Medical History

- 15-year history of diabetes (most recent A1C = 7.3%); takes Metformin once a day with meals
- 20-year history of hypertension and peripheral vascular disease
- Smoked one-half a pack of cigarettes for 60 years (30 pack-years), stopped smoking last year
- Raynaud's disease

Other Information

- Retired respiratory therapist
- Regular consumption of alcohol (2–3 drinks a day)
- BMI = 20

1. What is the most likely reason the wound is not healing?

Inadequate blood flow to allow for healing is the correct answer. The cause of the blood flow restriction is multifactorial (hypertension, peripheral vascular disease, smoking history, Raynaud's disease). Additionally, his prior history of gangrene (often related to ischemia) and description of the skin and wound (i.e., shiny, atrophied, hairless, pale, dry) are consistent with decreased blood flow. Although his BMI is on the low side of ideal and proper wound healing requires increased caloric and protein intake, there is nothing presented that would indicate a significant nutritional deficit. This patient's A1C is also only slightly elevated and does not indicate gross mismanagement of their condition. Finally, there are no overt signs of infection (e.g., purulent exudate, fever, erythema, red streak, increasing pain, swelling, or odor).

2. Which of the following diagnostic tests is **BEST** to establish the ideal level for future amputation of this limb?

The correct answer is Transcutaneous oximetry (TcPOS). $TcPO_2$ reflects the amount of local oxygen available, which closely resembles the PaO_2. The $TcPO_2$ is often used to determine which tissues have the highest probability of healing. Multiple factors affect $TcPO_2$ measurements and include: room/skin temperature, smoking, coffee consumption, pain, and anxiety. Although the ABI helps the clinician understand the severity of arterial disease and if a distal wound will heal (must be greater than 0.5), it does not specifically establish where there is adequate blood flow to support healing. Similar to the ABI, capillary refill is used to screen for peripheral arterial disease, but it is inadequate to discern healthy from compromised circulation. The SWM is used to assess tactile sensation (5.07 monofilament exerts 10 g of force, which assesses protective sensation of the feet) but does not examine circulation.

3. Which of the following interventions are important to implement in a person with a gangrenous toe due to ischemia?

The correct answer is to keep the limb in a dependent position. Maintaining the limb in a dependent position promotes blood flow and helps to prevent additional circulatory compromise. It might seem simple, but it is often overlooked. A gangrenous toe due to ischemia typically mummifies (shrinks, becomes dry, turns black) and results in dry-gangrene. Wet-gangrene occurs when bacteria invades the tissue and it becomes soft, malodorous, edematous, and dark. Wet-gangrene can quickly lead to sepsis and potentially death. Dry-gangrene can become wet or infected if the affected area is moistened or kept moistened; therefore, hydrotherapy and dressings that promote moisture are contraindicated for dry (ischemic) gangrene. Sharp debridement is also contraindicated for this wound as it may introduce bacteria. The appropriate treatment for this wound is to keep it clean and dry until self (the toe may detach due to mummification) or surgical amputation occurs.

Chapter 8, Appendix 8A Review Questions and Case Study

Other Systems

1. What are the adverse side effects of cancer treatment that can impact physical therapy intervention?

Chemotherapy may cause fatigue, gastrointestinal symptoms (i.e., anorexia, nausea, vomiting, diarrhea, ulcers, hemorrhage), bone marrow suppression (i.e., anemia, leukopenia, thrombocytopenia), skin rashes, neuropathies, or phlebitis. Leukopenia can result in increased susceptibility to infection. Thrombocytopenia can result in increased bleeding. Anemia can decrease aerobic capacity.

Long-term use of corticosteroids causes immunosuppression and associated symptoms. It also increases the risk of diabetes, hypertension, obesity, osteoporosis, and easily bruised skin.

Immunosuppression can result in fatigue, weight loss, flu-like symptoms (fever, chills), nausea, vomiting, anorexia, or fluid retention (edema).

Radiation can result in pain, fatigue, fibrosis, burns, delayed wound healing, edema, and nervous system effects (radiation encephalopathy, peripheral neuropathy with unique feature of rapid motor weakness that can occur acutely or several years after radiation).

2. What are the typical medications that may be prescribed for a patient diagnosed with GERD?

Proton pump inhibitors (PPIs) such as Prilosec; H_2 blockers such as cimetidine (Tagamet) and antacids such as Tums.

3. What are three possible interventions a physical therapist might use in the management of stress incontinence?

Use of Kegel's (pelvic floor) strengthening exercises, functional electrical stimulation, and biofeedback.

4. What are some of the long-term complications of diabetes that a physical therapist needs to consider during examination and treatment?

There are many complications. A partial list includes retinopathy, renal disease, polyneuropathy, atherosclerosis, CVA, MI, peripheral arterial disease, joint stiffness, osteoporosis, gastroparesis, GERD, liver disease, skin ulcers, and amputations.

5. Differentiate between hypothyroidism and hyperthyroidism in terms of expected symptoms.

Hypothyroidism: weight gain, lethargy, low blood pressure, constipation, intolerance to cold, dry skin, appearance of goiter (thyroid gland enlargement).

Hyperthyroidism: nervousness, hyperreflexia, tremor, hunger, weight loss, fatigue, heat intolerance, tachycardia, diarrhea.

Case Study

- Gender: Male
- Age: 64

Presenting Problem/Current Condition

- Patient referred to outpatient physical therapy with low back pain × 5 years with increased symptoms over the past year.
- No known mechanism of injury.
- Rates pain as a constant 4/10 with no consistent aggravating or easing factors
- Denies numbness, tingling, or weakness in either lower extremity
- Denies bowel or bladder incontinence but reports frequent urination, nocturia, and difficulty starting urination

Past Medical/Surgical History

- Well-controlled hypertension for 7 years
- Well-controlled high cholesterol for 8 years

Other Information

- Mechanic
- Married
- Does not smoke and has 1–2 drinks a week

1. Which of the following questions is BEST for determining if prostate dysfunction is contributing to the patient's low back pain?

Genital and sacral pain is the correct answer. These regions are identified as common pain referral areas from prostate dysfunction. Pain in the suprapubic area is most commonly the result of bladder dysfunction. "Having foul smelling urine" is associated with urinary tract infections which may be the result of multiple causes, to include prostate dysfunction. Blood in the stool is the result of problems with the colon or rectum.

2. The patient shares that he has noticed periodic blood in his urine, increased pain at night, and erectile dysfunction over the past 6 months. These symptoms are most consistent with which medical diagnosis?

Prostrate cancer is the correct answer. Prostate cancer, unlike prostatitis and benign prostratic hyperplasia, may include blood in the urine/semen, bone and night pain, weight loss without trying, and erectile dysfunction. Bladder cancer typically results in consistent and large amounts of blood in the urine, but not erectile dysfunction.

3. The patient is diagnosised with prostrate cancer and undergoes surgery and radiation. The patient is referred for evaluation and treatment secondary to significant pelvic floor dysfunction. What is the BEST option for initially starting pelvic floor exercises?

The correct answer is to instruct the patient to lay supine with knees bent and complete Kegel exercises. Performing Kegel exercises while voiding is contraindicated and may impair urinary reflexes and potentially contribute to urinary tract infections. Performing these exercises in sitting or when transitioning from sit to stand involves more advanced positions that require a higher degree of pelvic floor motor control and strength.

Chapter 9, Appendix 9A
Review Questions and Case Study

Pediatric Physical Therapy

1. In the developing infant, what are the differences in terms of age of onset and response between the asymmetrical tonic neck reflex (ATNR) and the symmetrical tonic neck reflex (STNR)?

   ATNR is normally present at birth. Rotation of the head to one side results in flexion of the skull-side limbs and extension of face-side limbs.

   STNR usually appears between 4 and 6 months of age. Cervical flexion results in flexion of the arms and extension of the legs. Cervical extension results in extension of the arms and flexion of the legs.

2. When performing an examination of the skeletal system in a full-term neonate, what possible abnormal bony conditions should be part of the screening process?

   Fractured clavicle, hip dysplasia, spinal curvature including kyphosis and scoliosis, spina bifida occulta (dimple or tuft of hair), and talipes equinovarus.

3. What are the typical lower extremity contractures seen with the child with spastic cerebral palsy?

   Hip flexors, adductors, and internal rotators. Knee flexors and ankle plantar flexors.

4. What is a realistic expectation for functional mobility in the community and in the household for a patient with myelodysplasia affecting the midlumbar levels (about L3)?

   Wheelchair for community mobility. Orthoses with walker or crutches for household ambulation.

Case Study

Patient Profile

- Gender: Male
- Age: 12 months

Presenting Problem/Current Condition

- The infant has been referred to physical therapy for part of early intervention services
- Diagnosis is Down Syndrome (Trisomy 21)

Past Medical/Surgical History

- Born at full term via Cesarean section
- Ventricular septal defect that the pediatric cardiologist hopes will close as he gets older
- Receiving speech therapy due to delays in expressive communication skills

Other Information

- Child is currently in foster care due to neglect and is awaiting adoption.
- Foster care provider is unfamiliar with Down Syndrome and has many questions about the condition and prognosis.
- Child is pleasant and smiles at everyone.
- Fine motor skills are age-appropriate.
- Child can belly crawl, sit independently, get into the quadruped position, and is starting to pull to stand
- Prefers to sit in a W-sitting position and sleep in prone with hips in abduction, ER, and flexion
- Transitions into sitting from prone by pushing up on hands and maximally abducting hips
- Very little interest in toys

1. Which of the following would be the **GREATEST** priority in your role as the PT when planning education with the foster care provider?

Children cannot be tested for AA instability until they are 3 years old. Until that time, it should be assumed that they have instability. Families need to be educated on the precautions and contraindications since forceful neck flexion and rotation could result in a significant injury to the spinal cord. The child will have low muscle tone and a potential for joint laxity, and education about this should occur; however, it is a greater priority to prevent an injury to the spinal cord with education about AA instability. PTs should also provide education about the prognosis of gross motor skills and a timeline for ambulation, but it is not the greatest priority in this case. Although the potential causes of the septal defect can be discussed, if this defect is already present it is the physician's role to discuss the intervention options for this congenital heart condition, which may require surgical closure.

2. Which of the following is potentially **MOST** problematic with his preferred W-sitting posture?

W-sitting can cause an increase in hip internal rotation and typically a decrease in external rotation. This type of sitting can also result in femoral anteversion. Both the anteversion and excessive internal rotation of the hip can cause "toeing-in." W-sitting does not cause kyphosis. The child may possibly develop an excessive lordosis in the lumbar spine. W-sitting causes laxity of the medial collateral ligaments, not the lateral. Femoral retroversion is rare and results in "toeing-out" but is not associated with W-sitting.

3. What is the prognosis for children with Down Syndrome in terms of independent ambulation?

Most children with Down Syndrome will have gross motor delays and will not walk on time (normally 9–15 months). But all children with Down Syndrome will walk and most by the age of 2 years. A small portion will not walk until they are 5 years old. Although this can be variable and all children develop on slightly different timetables, all children with Down Syndrome will be able to ambulate.

Chapter 10, Appendix 10A Review Questions and Case Study

Geriatric Physical Therapy

1. What are the physiological changes that may occur in the visual system in older adults?

   May include general decline in visual acuity; presbyopia; decreased ability to adapt to light and dark; diminished oculomotor responses; cataracts; glaucoma.

2. What risk factors are associated with development of osteoporosis?

   Hormonal deficiency associated with menopause; nutritional deficiency of calcium, excessive alcohol and caffeine consumption; decreased physical activity; hyperthyroidism; diabetes; celiac disease; corticosteroids, thyroid hormone; family history, Caucasian and Asian races.

3. What are the major side effects (red flags) of the use of pain medications in the geriatric population that can be a concern for physical therapists?

   Increased fall risk, disorientation, and sedation.

4. What are the most important components of the initial examination of a patient with dementia?

   History including onset and progression of symptoms; cognitive function (e.g., Mini-Mental State Examination); impairments of communication and perception; behavior changes; self-care; motor function including gait, balance, and dyspraxia; environmental safety.

5. What are the major goals and interventions to minimize fall risk factors?

   Based on examination findings, identify fall risk. Eliminate or minimize fall risk factors with consideration of disease and medications. Increase strength and flexibility. Implement balance and gait training. Compensate for sensory deficiencies. Functional training including sit-to-stand, stairs, walking, turning. Provide assistive devices as needed. Allow adequate time for activities. Safety education. Modify environment.

Case Study

- Gender: Male
- Age: 76

Presenting Problem/Current Condition

- Patient referred to outpatient physical therapy secondary to right knee pain for 3 months.
- His symptoms started after falling in the grocery store. His spouse reports that he has fallen 2 times in the past year.
- He rates his right knee pain as 2/10 on average and increased with stairs or squatting.
- X-rays of the right knee within normal limits except mild osteoarthritis.
- He denies numbness, tingling, radiating pain, or weakness in his bilateral upper or lower extremities.
- The patient and his spouse report he is having difficulty with short-term memory.

Past Medical/Surgical History

- Suspected Mild Alzheimer's disease for 1 year
- Depression by 6 months
- Elevated cholesterol that is well controlled with medication
- Bilateral mild knee osteoarthritis

Other Information

- Retired history professor
- Married and lives in a one-storey home

1. What information from the patient or his spouse is most consistent with the diagnosis of mild Alzheimer's disease?

Increased time required to accomplish daily tasks and anxiety are common in patients with mild Alzheimer's disease. Decreased attention span and problems recognizing friends and family members are findings that are more consistent with moderate Alzheimer's disease. Sleep disorders (sundowner's syndrome) and intermittent hallucinations are also seen in moderate Alzheimer's disease or in patients with Diffuse Lewy Body disease. Difficulty with complex planning but daily life not generally affected are more consistent with mild cognitive impairment.

2. The patient's spouse reports his past falls have occurred while he is multitasking or distracted (e.g., looking at his phone and walking or carrying groceries). Which of the following outcome measures would be most helpful to assess the patient's fall risk and mobility?

Timed up and go with a cognitive task is the correct answer. This real-world task examines various components of community mobility and balance and includes cognition and multitasking. Patients who can complete this task in less than 14 seconds have decreased fall risk. Comfortable gait speed, 5 times sit-to-stand, and single leg stance eyes open/closed are helpful for specific components of balance but do not challenge multiple components of balance and do not require multitasking.

3. On your initial evaluation, the patient's gait speed and single-leg balance are normal. He is able to complete the timed up and go with cognitive task (TUG-Cog-counting backward by 3's) in 20 seconds with 2 errors. Which of the following evidence base strategies are **BEST** for safely improving the patient's community mobility and balance?

The patient's performance on the TUG-Cog is abnormal (>14 seconds-Appendix 10A) and emphasizes the need for further fall risk assessment, to include screening for intrinsic/extrinsic fall risk factors (Tables 10-5 and 10-6). The patient should also attend clinic and have interventions and education based on identified risk factors (Table 10-7).

Chapter 11, Appendix 11A Review Questions

Therapeutic Modalities

1. What are the increased and decreased physiological responses to the local application of heat and cold?

   Increased with heat: blood flow, capillary permeability, elasticity, metabolism, edema.

   Increased with cold: joint stiffness, pain threshold, blood viscosity.

   Decreased with heat: joint stiffness, muscle strength, muscle spasm, pain.

   Decreased with cold: blood flow, capillary permeability, elasticity, metabolism, muscle spasm, muscle strength, spasticity.

2. Which characteristics of ultrasound application affect the depth of penetration and thermal effects?

   Frequency in MHz determines depth of penetration. Three MHz produces greater heat in superficial tissues. One MHz increases heat production in deep layers. Temporal characteristics are a major factor in determining thermal characteristics. Pulsed US (duty cycle <50%) produces less acoustic energy and less heat and is considered nonthermal. Continuous US produces thermal effects and increases tissue temperature.

3. What are three health conditions that may benefit from spinal mechanical traction?

   Cervical radiculopathy; chronic neck pain with mobility deficits; lumbar radiculopathy that does not have a directional preference (extension/flexion). See Chapter 11, and Neck and Low Back Pain Clinical Practice Guidelines in Chapter 2 for additional information.

4. What are the contraindications for use of electrical stimulation?

   Near demand-type pacemakers; unstable arrhythmias; epilepsy; seizure disorder; active bleeding; near thrombophlebitis; superficial metal implants; over or near the carotid sinus, thoracic region, phrenic nerve, urinary bladder stimulators, low back during pregnancy, pharyngeal region.

5. Which electrical stimulation characteristics are appropriate to use for wound healing?

   High-volt pulsed galvanic current and low-intensity, low-volt continuous direct current can be used for wound healing.

Chapter 12, Appendix 12A Review Questions

Functional Training, Equipment, Devices, and Technologies

1. What are the muscle activation patterns during heel strike (initial contact) and heel-off (terminal stance) for the quadriceps, pretibial muscles, and plantar flexors?

   Initial contact: Quadriceps is active for shock absorption and to control for knee flexion; pretibial muscles (anterior tibialis, extensor hallucis longus, and extensor digitorum longus) control plantar flexion by decelerating the foot.

   Terminal stance: peak activity of the plantar flexors to generate forward propulsion.

2. What type of equipment and ambulatory aids might be needed to progress a morbidly obese patient from a sedentary bed-bound situation to independent ambulation?

   Heavy-duty mechanical lift (e.g., Hoyer lift) to help transfer a patient from sit-to-stand.

   Body weight support system (BWS) with an overhead harness to unload some body weight in a progressive manner.

   Heavy-duty, extra-wide walker.

3. How does rearfoot posting in a foot orthosis control for valgus or varus?

   Rearfoot posting acts primarily on the subtalar joint from initial contact to loading response.

   A medial wedge (varus post) limits or controls calcaneal eversion and internal rotation of the tibia.

   A lateral wedge (valgus post) controls an excessively inverted and supinated calcaneus and subtalar joint.

4. What are the pressure-tolerant areas in the typical transtibial residual limb that are suitable for a total contact socket?

   The areas that can tolerate pressure are the patellar tendon, medial tibial plateau, tibial and fibular shafts, and the distal end of the residual limb. The distal end can be problematic if there are open wounds or sensitivity issues.

5. What are two conditions that may warrant a therapist recommending a motorized tilt-in-space wheelchair for a patient?

   A tilt-in-space chair allows the seat and back to be tipped backward as a unit. It is indicated for patients with significant extensor spasms that could eject the patient from the chair.

   Another indication would be for pressure relief. This situation is one in which the impairment prevents or limits the patient from changing positions and redistributing weight independently.

Chapter 13, Appendix 13A Review Questions

Safety and Protection

1. Identify three risk factors in each of the following categories that increase the likelihood of falls in older adults: medications, personal risk factors, and chronic diseases.

Medications that increase the likelihood of falls include:

- Medications that affect the brain (psychotropic drugs)
  - o Anxiolytics/sedative-hypnotics used for antianxiety (anxiolytic) and sedative/hypnotic properties (e.g., benzodiazepines, non-benzodiazepine prescription sedatives; anticholinergics, sedating antihistamines)
  - o Antipsychotics increase fall risk due to syncope, sedation, slowed reflexes, loss of balance, and impaired psychomotor function (e.g., haloperidol [Haldol], risperidone [Risperdal], quetiapine [Seroquel], aripiprazole [Abilify])
  - o Antidepressants can cause hyponatremia/low sodium levels (except for Wellbutrin); hyponatremia is an independent risk factor for falls (e.g., sedating antidepressants—despipramine [Norpramin], imipramine [Tofranil]; mirtazapine [Remeron], trazadone); SSRIs (e.g., sertraline [Zoloft], paroxetine [Paxil], fluoxetine [Prozac])
  - o Anti-convulsants/mood stabilizers (e.g., Depakote, Neurontin)
  - o Opioid (narcotic) analgesics can increase fall risk (e.g., codeine, hydrocodone, oxycodone, morphine, fentanyl, methadone)
- Medications that affect blood pressure/antihypertensives can cause or worsen a drop in BP/postural hypotension (e.g., Flomax, alpha-blockers [doxazosin, prazosin, terazosin])
- Medications that lower blood sugar in older adults with diabetes resulting in hypoglycemia.
  - o Oral or injectable medications
- Diuretics can cause orthostatic hypotension; risk is increased with dehydration (e.g., Thiazide diuretics)

Personal risk factors that increase the likelihood of falls:

- Vision problems: decreased visual acuity, depth perception, contrast sensitivity; cataracts
- Changes in postural blood pressure: orthostatic hypotension
- Impairments in balance
- Impairments in gait
- Foot pain or poor footwear
- Sensory changes: decreased proprioception
- Impaired cognition
- Decreased muscle strength
- Decreased flexibility and ROM, especially lower extremities, feet

Chronic diseases that increase the likelihood of falls:

- Cardiovascular disease: syncope, arrhythmias, blood pressure changes
- Arthritis
- Stroke
- Parkinson's disease

2. Differentiate between key basic life support (CPR) components for adults, children, and infants in terms of compression rate and depth.

The compression rate is the same for all three groups, 100–120/minute. The compression depth varies among the groups: for adults—at least 2 inches (5 cm); for children—at least 1/3 AP depth, about 2 inches (5 cm); and for infants—at least 1/3 AP depth, about 1½ inches (4 cm).

3. A physical therapist should be on the alert for which possible signs and symptoms of physical, emotional, and sexual child abuse?

Some possible signs and symptoms of child abuse can include the following:

- Physical abuse
  - o Bruises, burns, welts, injury marks from a hand or belt
  - o Medical or dental issues that have gone untreated
  - o Child avoids touch or contact; seems fearful or on high alert
- Sexual abuse
  - o Child demonstrates highly sexualized behavior (e.g., inappropriate language or touching)
  - o Child avoids certain people or caregiver
  - o Bruising, bleeding, or pain around genitals, anus, or breasts
  - o Pregnancy or STDs for those less than 14 years of age
- Emotional abuse
  - o Depression or low self-esteem
  - o Constant worrying about wrongdoing
  - o Behavioral extremes; child is either excessively demanding or obedient
  - o Disinterested in others

4. As a physical therapist practicing in a health care facility, what are possible internal and external sources of disasters that might trigger the initiation of an Emergency Action Plan (EAP)?

- Internal sources
  - o Power, utility, communication or equipment failures
  - o Fire, gas leak, hazardous material, explosion
  - o Workplace violence—active shooter, bomb scare
- External sources
  - o Terrorism, extremism, hate crimes
  - o Civil disturbances
  - o Mass casualty incidents
  - o Floods, hurricanes, tornados, earthquakes, tsunamis, wildfires, blizzards

Chapter 14, Appendix 14D Review Questions

Professional Responsibilities

1. What is defined as protected health information, and what actions must be taken to secure it?

Public Health Information (PHI) as **individually identifiable health information**, held or maintained by a covered entity or its business associates acting for the covered entity, that is transmitted or maintained in any form or medium (including the **individually identifiable health information** of non–U.S. citizens).

A variety of actions to provide physical security for information must be taken, such as locking cabinets and doors that contain personal information, FAX cover sheets, maintaining password protection on computers, and considering who is in the area when discussing patient information.

2. Compare and contrast the requirements for supervision of the PTA and PT aide in the provision of care.

- A physical therapist assistant operates under the direction of the physical therapist who must be available at least by telecommunications
- A physical therapist aide operates under the **direct, on-site** supervision of the physical therapist or physical therapist assistant

3. What are the documentation requirements for time-based billing for Medicare beneficiaries?

- Time-in and time-out or total time
- Services described by timed codes, untimed codes, and unattended activities
- Total number of units billed is limited by the total minutes of the one-on-one encounter

4. Compare and contrast payment mechanisms used in managed care.

- Capitation: Payment to primary care provider is based solely on the number of enrolled beneficiaries. Their care is managed using these funds. If enrollees remain healthy, provider profits are greater.
- Fee for service: Providers are paid after services are provided to the patient
- Case-based rate: Payment to providers is made based on the diagnosis. Often payment is bundled by the day, the visit, or the episode of care.

Chapter 15, Appendix 15A Review Questions

Teaching and Learning

1. Differentiate between deductive and inductive reasoning.

   Deductive reasoning is the process whereby conclusions are drawn based on information, theoretical models, laws, rules, or accepted principles.

   Inductive reasoning is the process whereby conclusions are drawn by extrapolating specific situations to larger circumstances. It does not guarantee the conclusion in every case.

2. How might operant conditioning be used to shape behavior in a noncompliant patient with TBI?

   Behavior modification uses operant conditioning techniques by identifying the desired behavior and reinforcing the desired behavior immediately in a meaningful way. Negative behaviors are ignored, aversive behavior (punishment) is minimized, and a closed environment with few distractions is preferred.

Chapter 16, Appendix 16A Review Questions

Research and Evidence-Based Practice

1. What is the difference between independent and dependent variables?

   The independent variable is the treatment or cause believed to bring about a change. The dependent variable is the change, outcome, or difference in behavior resulting from the independent variable.

2. What is the significance of validity and reliability regarding a clinical test? What are the possible threats to each?

   Validity is the degree to which an instrument or procedure accurately measures what it purports to measure. Threats to validity include sampling bias, lack of controls over the subjects, inaccurate measuring instrument, experimenter bias, variables in treatment administration, placebo effect, and Hawthorne effect (subject's knowledge of participation in an experiment).

   Reliability is the consistency with which a test measures what it purports to measure. Threats to reliability may deal with intrarater or interrater factors, errors of measurement, and systemic or environmental factors.

3. What is the significance of sensitivity and specificity regarding a clinical test?

   Sensitivity is a test's ability to correctly identify the proportion of those that truly have the condition, impairment, or disease. It is the true positive rate.

   Specificity is a test's ability to correctly identify the proportion of those who do NOT have the condition, impairment, or disease. It is the true negative rate.

4. From highest to lowest level of rigor, what is the hierarchy of evaluating and grading levels of evidence? Give an example of each.

   Level 1 (Grade A): systematic reviews including meta-analysis, individual randomized control trials

   Level 2 (Grade B): cohort studies

   Level 3 (Grade B): case-control studies, retrospective studies

   Level 4 (Grade C): case-series or poor quality cohort and case-control studies; descriptive studies

   Level 5 (Grade D): expert opinion or observations

18

Online Simulated Examination Answers and Teaching Points

STEP 1 Follow the instructions found in the front inside cover of this book to access the TherapyEd Online Learning Portal and take an examination.
STEP 2 After completing the exam, review your performance analysis.
STEP 3 As needed, review exam questions and answers plus TEACHING POINTS which contain explanations of correct answer, incorrect choices, and reasoning subtype for that examination.
There are a total of three examinations.

Domains of Knowledge

- Cardiovascular/Pulmonary
- Musculoskeletal
- Neuromuscular
- Integumentary
- Metabolic and Endocrine
- Gastrointestinal
- Genitourinary
- Lymphatic
- System Interactions
- Nonsystem

Categories

- Examination
- Evaluation, Diagnosis
- Interventions
- Equipment, Devices, and Technologies
- Therapeutic Modalities
- Safety and Protection
- Professional Responsibilities
- Research and Evidence-Based Practice

Critical Reasoning Strategies

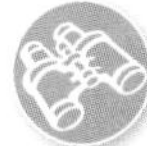 Inductive Reasoning

 Analytical Reasoning

 Evaluative Reasoning

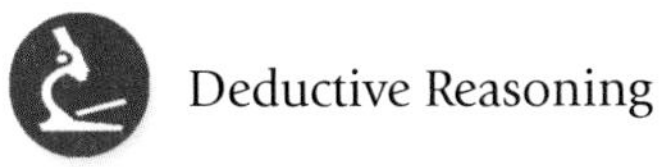
Deductive Reasoning

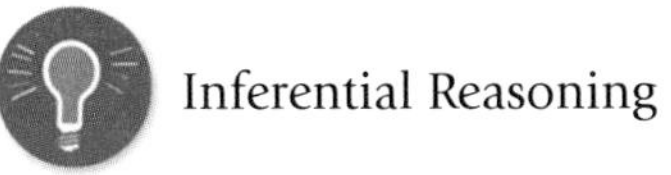
Inferential Reasoning

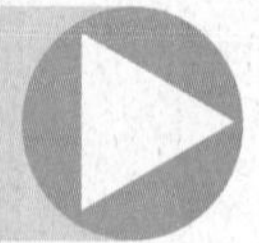

Examination A

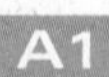

A1

Metabolic and Endocrine | Evaluation, Diagnosis

An elderly patient with hypothyroidism is recovering from a fall and is referred to physical therapy to increase exercise tolerance and safety. The patient denies numbness but reports significant muscle pain in both lower extremities. What additional musculoskeletal effects should the therapist examine for?

Choices:

1. Distal muscle weakness.
2. Proximal muscle weakness.
3. Joint laxity.
4. Increased deep tendon reflexes.

Teaching Points

Correct Answer: 2

Hypothyroidism can have numerous musculoskeletal effects, including myalgia (muscle pain) and proximal muscle weakness.

Incorrect Choices:

Additional musculoskeletal effects include stiffness (not joint laxity) and delayed relaxation (decreased) deep tendon reflexes.

Type of Reasoning: Inferential

For this question, the test-taker must determine what is most likely to be true based on knowledge of hypothyroidism. Questions of this nature, where one must infer information, require inferential reasoning skill. In this case, one should infer that proximal muscle weakness is most likely to be present. If answered incorrectly, review information on hypothyroidism.

A2

Genitourinary | Examination

A patient is referred to a woman's health clinic with moderate to severe uterine prolapse. What symptoms should the therapist examine for?

Choices:

1. Absent perineal sensation.
2. Bowel leakage.
3. Low back pain and perineal discomfort aggravated by prolonged standing.
4. Low back pain and perineal discomfort aggravated by lying down.

Teaching Points

Correct Answer: 3

Low back pain and perineal discomfort aggravated by prolonged standing are common with uterine prolapse.

Incorrect Choices:

Perineal sensation is not decreased; patients typically experience a sensation of heaviness or pulling in the pelvis. Pain is often relieved by lying down (not aggravated). Constipation and painful bowel movement are common.

Type of Reasoning: Inferential

This question requires one to determine what is most likely to be true based on knowledge of uterine prolapse. Questions of this nature often require inferential reasoning skill. In this case, one should infer that back and perineal pain aggravated by prolonged standing are often associated with uterine prolapse. If answered incorrectly, review signs and symptoms of uterine prolapse.

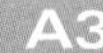
A3 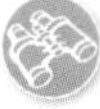

Integumentary | Evaluation, Diagnosis

A child experienced a superficial partial-thickness burn from a scalding pot of water affecting 26% of the thorax and neck. On what should the therapist's **INITIAL** plan of care focus?

Choices:

1. Return to preburn function and activities of daily living.
2. Pain management.
3. Infection management.
4. Chest wall mobility and prevention of scar contracture.

Teaching Points

Correct Answer: 4

Prevention of scar contracture and preservation of chest wall mobility and normal neck range of motion (ROM) are the initial major goals to focus on with this patient.

Incorrect Choices:

Return to preburn function and ADLs is an important treatment goal but is not the initial focus. Pain and infection management are important goals of the medical team and are typically managed by the medical team.

Type of Reasoning: Inductive

For this question, the test-taker must use clinical judgment to determine a best course of action, which necessitates inductive reasoning skill. Knowledge of effective treatment approaches for burns is paramount to arriving at a correct conclusion. In this case, chest wall mobility and prevention of scar contracture should be the initial focus of the therapist. Review treatment approaches for burns, especially in children, if answered incorrectly.

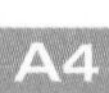

A4

Cardiovascular/Pulmonary | Evaluation, Diagnosis

A patient with coronary artery disease has been doing regular aerobic exercise on a treadmill. If the patient fails to comply in taking prescribed beta-blocker medication and continues to exercise, what potential rebound effects could result?

Choices:

1. Increase in blood pressure and decrease in heart rate during exercise.
2. Decrease in blood pressure and heart rate during exercise.
3. Increase in blood pressure and heart rate during exercise.
4. Decrease in blood pressure and increase in heart rate during exercise.

Teaching Points

Correct Answer: 3

Beta-blockers affect the beta-1 adrenergic receptors. Blocking these inhibits the sympathetic response. However, when abruptly terminated, they cause a reflexive opposite response. This patient will demonstrate increased contractility, blood pressure (BP), and heart rate (HR) as a result.

Incorrect Choices:

This patient's BP will increase, but the patient's HR will not decrease with exercise. The HR and BP will increase, not decrease with exercise on a beta-blocker or when it is quickly removed. The BP will increase, not decrease with activity due to the abrupt stopping of the medication.

Type of Reasoning: Inferential

This question requires one to determine the likely effects of exercise and not taking beta-blocker medication. Questions of this nature, where one must infer what is most likely to be true of a situation, require inferential reasoning skill. For this scenario, one should infer that the patient would have an increase in blood pressure and heart rate with exercise. If answered incorrectly, review information on effects of beta-blockers and exercise.

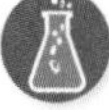

A5

Musculoskeletal | Examination

A patient has persistent midfoot pain with weight bearing. The injury occurred during a soccer match when an opposing player stepped on the patient's right foot when it was planted and cutting to the left. Patient locates the pain where laces are tied. Upon examination there is splaying of the first metatarsal and increased pain when passively stressing the foot with plantarflexion and rotation. What injury should the therapist suspect the patient has sustained?

Choices:

1. Lisfranc injury.
2. Turf toe.
3. Calcaneocuboid joint subluxation.
4. Hallux rigidus.

Exam A

Teaching Points

Correct Answer: 1

The Lisfranc injury (also known as the Lisfranc fracture, tarsometatarsal injury, or simply midfoot injury) is an injury of the foot in which one or all of the metatarsal bones are displaced from the tarsus. Direct Lisfranc injuries are usually caused by a crush injury, such as when a heavy object falls onto the midfoot, or when landing on the foot after a fall from a significant height. The injury often occurs when an athlete has his or her foot plantar flexed and another player lands on his or her midfoot.

Incorrect Choices:

Turf toe is a sprain of the MTP joint of the first toe due to hyperextension, such as when pushing off into a sprint and having the toe get stuck flat on the ground. Calcaneocuboid joint subluxation (also known as cuboid syndrome) is defined as a minor disruption or subluxation of the structural congruity of the calcaneocuboid portion of the midtarsal joint. The disruption of the cuboid's position irritates the surrounding joint capsule, ligaments, and fibularis longus tendon. Hallux rigidus (stiff big toe) is a degenerative arthritis and stiffness due to bone spurs that affects the MTP joint at the base of the hallux. Symptoms include pain and stiffness in the joint at the base of the big toe during use (walking, standing, bending, etc.).

Type of Reasoning: Analytical

This question requires one to determine a type of injury sustained based on a description of mechanism of injury and symptoms. Questions that necessitate analyzing information to determine a reasonable conclusion often utilize analytical reasoning skill. For this situation, the symptoms are consistent with Lisfranc injury. Review signs and symptoms of Lisfranc injury if answered incorrectly.

A6 

System Interactions | Evaluation, Diagnosis

A patient is referred to physical therapy with a 10-year history of rheumatoid arthritis (RA). What are possible extra-articular complications?

Choices:

1. Disc degeneration.
2. Psoriatic skin and nail changes.
3. Vasculitis.
4. Conjunctivitis and iritis.

Teaching Points

Correct Answer: 3

Rheumatoid arthritis is a progressive autoimmune disease affecting primarily joints and synovial tissue. Extra-articular complications of the disease can include vasculitis.

Incorrect Choices:

The other choices are not expected extra-articular complications in patients with RA. Disc degeneration is seen in degenerative disc disease. Psoriatic skin and nail changes and conjunctivitis and iritis can be seen in psoriatic arthritis.

Type of Reasoning: Inferential

For this question, the test-taker must infer or determine what is most likely to be true for a patient with rheumatoid arthritis. This requires inferential reasoning skill. In this case, possible extra-articular complications include vasculitis. Review information on rheumatoid arthritis if answered incorrectly.

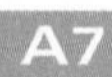

Integumentary | Evaluation, Diagnosis

A physical therapist is instructing an elderly patient how to perform bed mobility following a total hip replacement. The therapist should carefully consider the effects of aging that relate to skin. What is one such effect?

Choices:

1. Increased perception of pain.
2. Impaired sensory integrity.
3. Increased skin elasticity.
4. Increased acute inflammatory response.

Teaching Points

Correct Answer: 2

Changes in skin composition associated with aging include decreased sensitivity to touch, decreased perception of pain and temperature, and increased risk of injury.

Incorrect Choices:

Perception of pain is decreased (not increased). The dermis thins, and elasticity is decreased (not increased). The elderly often exhibit low-grade inflammation; acute inflammatory responses are commonly caused by tissue injury or infections.

Type of Reasoning: Inferential

For this question, the test-taker must recall the effects of aging and then determine the most likely effect that relates to the skin. This requires inferential reasoning skill. For this situation, the most likely skin effect is impaired sensory integrity. Review effects of the aging process, especially those that affect the skin, if answered incorrectly.

A8 

Cardiovascular/Pulmonary | Examination

What would a therapist who is examining the breathing pattern of a patient with a complete (ASIA A) C5 spinal cord injury expect to observe?

Choices:

1. Asymmetric lateral costal expansion due to ASIA A injury.
2. An increased subcostal angle due to air trapping from muscle weakness.
3. No diaphragmatic motion since the diaphragm is below the level of the lesion.
4. Rising of the abdomen due to no abdominal muscle tone on the abdominal viscera.

Teaching Points

Correct Answer: 4

The abdominal musculature provides external stability to the abdominal viscera. Without this, the viscera are displaced with respiration.

Incorrect Choices:

With an ASIA A injury, the muscle weakness would be symmetric. The diaphragm is innervated by C3–5 nerve roots, so it will be functioning in this patient. Muscle weakness will cause a restrictive disorder (inability to generate negative pressure), not an obstructive disorder (air trapping).

Type of Reasoning: Inferential

One must determine what is most likely to be true for patients with cervical spinal cord injury in order to arrive at a correct conclusion. Questions that ask one to predict possible outcomes often necessitate inferential reasoning skill. For this case, the therapist should anticipate rising of the abdomen due to no abdominal muscle tone on the abdominal viscera. Review cervical spinal cord injury effects on respiration if answered incorrectly.

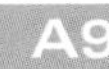

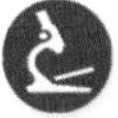

Metabolic and Endocrine | Evaluation, Diagnosis

Men are at risk for development of metabolic syndrome if they exhibit which of the following symptoms?

Choices:

1. An HDL level lower than 45 mg/dL.
2. A waist size greater than 40 inches.
3. Triglyceride levels greater than 100 mg/dL.
4. Fasting blood glucose less than 100 mg/dL.

Teaching Points

Correct Answer: 2

Criteria for diagnosis of metabolic syndrome include abdominal obesity (waist circumference >40 inches in men or >35 inches in women).

Incorrect Choices:

Other criteria include elevated triglycerides (150 mg/dL or higher); low HDL levels (<40 mg/dL in men or <50 mg/dL in women); and a fasting plasma glucose level >110 mg/dL.

Type of Reasoning: Deductive

This question requires the test-taker to recall the guidelines for risk of developing metabolic syndrome. This is factual information, which is a deductive reasoning skill. For this situation, a waist size greater than 40 inches would be a risk factor. Review metabolic syndrome guidelines if answered incorrectly.

A10 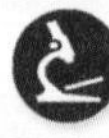

Musculoskeletal | Examination

During an examination, the limitations of ultrasound imaging include which of the following?

Choices:

1. Inability to clearly see cartilage in infants.
2. Disruption of cardiac pacemakers.
3. Difficulty penetrating bone and therefore visualizing internal structure of bones.
4. Inability to give a clear picture of tendons and therefore diagnose tendon tears.

Teaching Points

Correct Answer: 3

Ultrasound has difficulty penetrating bone. Ultrasound images are typically used to help diagnose tendon tears, such as tears of the rotator cuff in the shoulder or Achilles tendon in the ankle; abnormalities of the muscles, such as tears; bleeding or other fluid collections within the muscles, bursae, and joints; benign and malignant soft tissue tumors; early changes of rheumatoid arthritis; fluid in a painful hip joint in children; lumps in the neck muscles of infants; and soft tissue masses (lumps/bumps) in children.

Incorrect Choices:

The other choices are not limitations of diagnostic ultrasound.

Type of Reasoning: Deductive

One must recall the limitations of ultrasound in order to arrive at a correct conclusion. This necessitates factual recall of guidelines, which is a deductive reasoning skill. For this scenario, difficulty penetrating bone and visualizing internal structure of bones is a limitation of ultrasound. Review ultrasound guidelines and limitations if answered incorrectly.

A11 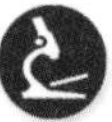

Metabolic and Endocrine | Evaluation, Diagnosis

A patient with a body mass index (BMI) of 37 is referred to physical therapy for exercise conditioning. What are additional clinical manifestations associated with the BMI that this patient might exhibit?

Choices:

1. Hyperpnea and hyperpituitarism.
2. Hypertension and hyperinsulinemia.
3. Hormone-related cancer.
4. Hypolipoproteinemia and hypotension.

Teaching Points

Correct Answer: 2

Obesity is associated with hypertension, dyslipidemia, hyperinsulinemia (type 2 diabetes), and hyperglycemia. The presence of these comorbidities increases risk, resulting in the need for additional medical screening before exercise testing.

Incorrect Choices:

Hyperpituitarism, hormone-related cancer, and hypotension are not associated with obesity.

Type of Reasoning: Deductive

For this question, the test-taker must recall the clinical manifestations associated with a high BMI (obesity). This is factual information, which necessitates deductive reasoning skill. In this case, the clinical manifestations include hypertension and hyperinsulinism. Review obesity guidelines if answered incorrectly.

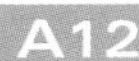

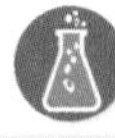

Musculoskeletal I Evaluation, Diagnosis

An 8-year-old boy is referred to physical therapy with chronic pain in the hip, thigh, and knee without any precipitating trauma or other known cause. The symptoms initially began as soreness and progressively worsened. The physical therapist notes that the patient walks with exaggerated trunk and pelvic movements, and there is significantly limited range of motion with hip abduction and extension. Examination of the knee region is normal. What is the **MOST LIKELY** diagnosis?

Choices:

1. Hip dysplasia.
2. Legg-Calvé-Perthes disease.
3. Growing pains.
4. Slipped capital femoral epiphysis.

Teaching Points

Correct Answer: 2

Legg-Calvé-Perthes disease is an idiopathic childhood hip disorder initiated by disruption of blood flow to the femoral head, leading to avascular necrosis. Age of onset is between 2–13 years and is four times more likely in boys than girls. Characteristic clinical examination findings are gradual onset and limited range of motion in abduction and extension (due to collapse of subchondral bone at the femoral neck/head). The gait deviation is called a psoatic limp due to weakness of the psoas major muscle. The patient moves in hip external rotation, flexion, and adduction along with exaggerated trunk and pelvic movements.

Incorrect Choices:

Slipped capital femoral epiphysis (SCFE) is also a common hip disorder observed in adolescents. However, the age of onset in males is usually 10–17 years (average 13 years). Patients with SCFE demonstrate a Trendelenburg gait and limited range of motion in abduction, flexion, and internal rotation. Hip dysplasia is an abnormality in the size, shape, orientation, or organization of the femoral head and/or acetabulum that can result in hip subluxation or dislocation. Hip dysplasia is more common in females than males. Legg-Calvé-Perthes disease is often misdiagnosed as growing pains in early stages. However, children experiencing growing pains typically present with increased pain at night and do not commonly exhibit loss of range of motion or a dysfunctional gait.

Type of Reasoning: Analytical

This question requires the test-taker to analyze pieces of information in order to draw a reasonable conclusion. This type of reasoning process is analytical, where the test-taker weighs the individual symptoms to determine a likely diagnosis. The symptoms presented in this situation are most likely consistent with Legg-Calvé-Perthes disease. Review information on Legg-Calvé-Perthes disease if answered incorrectly.

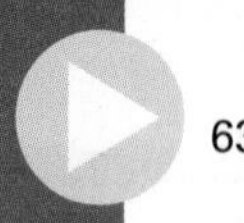

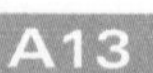

A13 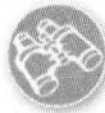

Neuromuscular | Interventions

To prepare a patient with a cauda equina lesion for ambulation with crutches, what upper quarter muscles would be the most important to strengthen?

Choices:

1. Upper trapezius, rhomboids, and levator scapulae.
2. Deltoid, coracobrachialis, and brachialis.
3. Middle trapezius, serratus anterior, and triceps.
4. Lower trapezius, latissimus dorsi, and pectoralis major.

Teaching Points

Correct Answer: 4

The muscles needed for crutch use include the shoulder depressors and extensors along with elbow extensors.

Incorrect Choices:

All other choices include muscles that enhance shoulder elevation or abduction.

Type of Reasoning: Inductive

For this question, one must utilize clinical judgment to determine the most important muscles to strengthen for crutch use. This requires inductive reasoning skill. For this scenario, the therapist should focus on strengthening the lower trapezius, latissimus dorsi, and pectoralis major. Review muscles needed for crutch use if answered incorrectly.

A14 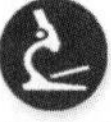

Cardiovascular/Pulmonary | Examination

What will a patient with a significant right thoracic structural scoliosis demonstrate on examination?

Choices:

1. Decreased breath sounds on the right.
2. Decreased thoracic rib elevation on the right.
3. Increased lateral costal expansion on the right.
4. Shortened internal and external intercostals on the right.

Teaching Points

Correct Answer: 3

With a right thoracic scoliosis, the convex side is on the right. This would allow for increased aeration and mobility on that side.

Incorrect Choices:

The ribs would elevate normally or more on the right side. The remaining choices would be true on the contralateral or shortened side of the scoliosis. The left side would have shortened muscle length and decreased aeration.

Type of Reasoning: Deductive

This question requires the test-taker to recall the structural changes that occur with thoracic scoliosis. This necessitates the recall of facts, which is a deductive reasoning skill. For this case, the therapist should anticipate that the patient will demonstrate an increased lateral costal expansion on the right. Review scoliosis information, especially thoracic scoliosis and structural changes, if answered incorrectly.

A15 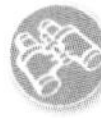

Musculoskeletal | Interventions

A therapist has been treating a patient for several weeks for decreased shoulder elevation and a loss of external rotation. Recovery has been good; however, the patient still complains of being unable to reach the upper shelves of kitchen cabinets and closets. To help the patient achieve this goal, what should be the focus of manual therapy?

Choices:

1. Superior glide.
2. Inferior glide.
3. Anterior glide.
4. Grade II oscillations.

Teaching Points

Correct Answer: 3

Anterior glide would help increase external rotation (ER), which is a component of full elevation. Performing anterior glides to improve ER and late flexion will help increase overhead reach since ER of humerus occurs with flexion.

Incorrect Choices:

Superior glide is not a joint mobilization for any pathology of the shoulder. Inferior glide would help increase shoulder abduction. Grade II mobilization would not improve motion.

Type of Reasoning: Inductive

One must utilize knowledge of joint mobilization techniques and benefits of specific mobilization approaches in order to arrive at a correct conclusion. This necessitates clinical judgment, which is an inductive reasoning skill. For this situation, the therapist should focus on anterior glides to improve ER and late flexion. Review joint mobilization techniques if answered incorrectly.

A16 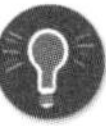

Neuromuscular | Interventions

Which activity would help break up obligatory lower extremity synergy patterns in a patient with hemiplegia?

Choices:

1. High kneeling position, ball throwing.
2. Standing, alternate marching in place with hip and knee flexion and hip abduction.
3. Sitting, alternate toe tapping.
4. Sitting, foot slides under the seat.

Teaching Points

Correct Answer: 1

Kneeling positions with the hip in extension and knee flexed to 90° is an out-of-synergy position. Additionally, kneeling provides an opportunity to work on balance (e.g., reaching, ball throwing) and postural control in a safe position that reduces fall risk.

Incorrect Choices:

Marching with hip and knee flexion and hip abduction, toe tapping in sitting, and foot slides using knee flexors in sitting all utilize movement in synergy or a synergy-supported position (see Table 3-8 for abnormal synergy patterns). Marching is also a higher-level activity and introducing this exercise too soon puts the patient at increased risk of falling.

Type of Reasoning: Inferential

For this question, the test-taker must recall out-of-synergy positions and then use that knowledge to determine which described position would be most beneficial for breaking up lower limb synergy. This requires inferential reasoning skill. In this case, having the patient in a high kneeling position with ball throwing will accomplish this. Review out-of-synergy positions if answered incorrectly.

A17 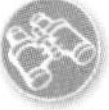

Neuromuscular | Examination

A patient recovering from a partial spinal cord injury reports lack of feeling in the more-affected hand. Monofilament testing reveals lack of ability to tell when the stimulus is being applied (only 1 correct response out of 5 tests). What additional sensory tests should the therapist perform?

Choices:

1. Test for sharp sensation.
2. Test for two-point discrimination.
3. Test for vibration.
4. Test for joint proprioception (thumb up/thumb down).

Teaching Points

Correct Answer: 1

Testing for perception of sharp sensation can be performed as pain and temperature are carried in a different pathway (anterolateral spinothalamic pathways) from other answer options; monofilament, vibration, and joint proprioception are carried in the dorsal column-lemniscal pathways.

Incorrect Choices:

All other choices test for discriminative sensations (two-point discrimination, vibration, and joint proprioception) and require intact dorsal column–medial lemniscal pathways projecting to the somatic sensory cortex.

Type of Reasoning: Inductive

For this question, one must utilize knowledge of sensory testing and sensory pathways in order to determine the test that is best to perform next. This reasoning process requires inductive reasoning skill, where clinical judgment is paramount to arriving at a correct conclusion. For this case, the therapist should test for pain to assist in localized/involvement of the lesion. Review the sensory pathways if answered incorrectly.

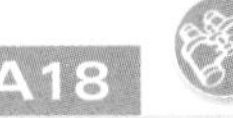

A18

Musculoskeletal I Interventions

A basketball player is referred to a physical therapist with a diagnosis of a quadriceps muscle contusion. The injury occurred 24 hours earlier when the player was struck in the thigh by an opponent's knee. Which intervention is contraindicated at this time?

Choices:

1. Isometric quadriceps femoris exercises.
2. Knee and hip range of motion in a pain-free range.
3. Aggressive quadriceps femoris stretching.
4. Ice baths.

Teaching Points

Correct Answer: 3

Aggressively stretching a muscle following direct trauma that results in formation of a hematoma may induce myositis ossificans, which is a painful condition of abnormal calcification within a muscle belly. The quadriceps, brachialis, and biceps brachii muscles are the most frequent locations for myositis ossificans. While flexibility exercises in a pain-free range are appropriate, aggressive stretching exercises into the painful range should be avoided.

Incorrect Choices:

Quadriceps setting exercises, gentle knee and hip range of motion exercises, and ice baths are all appropriate choices of interventions after a muscle contusion that do not increase the risk of developing myositis ossificans.

Type of Reasoning: Inductive

For this question, the test-taker must recall intervention approaches that should be avoided after muscle contusion. This requires inductive reasoning skill, where one utilizes clinical judgment and knowledge of intervention guidelines to arrive at a correct conclusion. For this case, the therapist should avoid aggressive quadriceps femoris stretching in order to avoid inducing myositis ossificans. If answered incorrectly, review intervention guidelines for patients with muscle contusions.

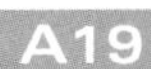

A19

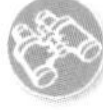

Musculoskeletal I Interventions

A patient is referred to physical therapy with a diagnosis of carpal tunnel syndrome (CTS) that has been confirmed by electrodiagnostic studies. The patient's chief complaint is intermittent hand paresthesias, which affects their quality of sleep. What is the **BEST** choice of initial intervention for this patient?

Choices:

1. Iontophoresis to the carpal tunnel region.
2. Neutral-positioned wrist orthosis worn at night.
3. Neutral-positioned wrist orthosis worn during the day.
4. Thermal ultrasound to the carpal tunnel region.

Teaching Points

Correct Answer: 2

According to the 2019 CTS Clinical Practice Guideline (see Box 2-3), there is moderate evidence to support the use a neutral-positioned wrist orthosis worn at night for short-term symptomatic relief and functional improvement in patients with CTS.

Incorrect Choices:

According to the clinical practice guideline, there is weak evidence to support the use of a splint during the day. Iontophoresis and thermal ultrasound are not recommended as interventions for CTS.

Type of Reasoning: Inductive

For this question, one must utilize knowledge of carpal tunnel intervention approaches in order to arrive at a correct conclusion. This requires inductive reasoning where clinical judgment and knowledge of intervention approaches guides critical thinking. In this case, the BEST choice of initial intervention is a neutral-position-ing wrist orthosis worn at night. If answered incorrectly, review intervention approaches for carpal tunnel syndrome.

A20 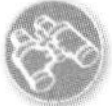

Cardiovascular/Pulmonary | Evaluation, Diagnosis

A patient with a long history of cigarette smoking has been admitted to the hospital and presents with tachy-cardia, signs of lung infection, abnormal breath sounds in both lower lobes, and dullness to percussion. What should the therapist's **INITIAL** intervention focus on with this patient?

Choices:

1. Getting the patient to quit smoking.
2. Breathing reeducation to increase efficiency of ventilation.
3. Airway clearance and secretion removal.
4. Graded inspiratory muscle training.

Teaching Points

Correct Answer: 3

The patient has signs and symptoms consistent with pneumonia. It is most important to assist with secre-tions clearance to assist with recovery from the infection and to improve gas exchange.

Incorrect Choices:

Quitting smoking is an appropriate goal for this patient but would be best timed after the acute period has passed. It isn't stated that the patient's breathing pattern is impaired and therefore it is not imperative to address it at this time. If there is an increased work of breathing, it will be rectified by clearing the secretions. Patients with a history of chronic obstructive pulmonary disease (COPD), which is presumed in this case due to the long history of tobacco use, do benefit from inspiratory muscle training (IMT). However, this is best timed after the acute infection has resolved.

Type of Reasoning: Inductive

This question requires one to utilize clinical judgment to consider a best course of action for a patient with pneumonia. Knowledge of effective intervention approaches for pneumonia is paramount to arriving at a cor-rect conclusion and requires inductive reasoning skill. For this case, the therapist should focus on airway clear-ance and secretion removal initially. Review intervention approaches for pneumonia if answered incorrectly.

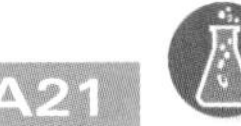

A21 Musculoskeletal I Evaluation, Diagnosis

A patient presents to a physical therapy clinic after a traumatic anterior glenohumeral joint dislocation. The patient complains of numbness in the lateral part of the upper arm. During the physical examination, the therapist confirms that there is numbness in the deltoid region, in addition to painful limited range of motion and weakness with shoulder abduction and external rotation. Which neurological diagnosis is consistent with the findings in this patient?

Choices:
1. Thoracic outlet syndrome.
2. Axillary nerve injury.
3. C7–C8 radiculopathy.
4. Radial tunnel syndrome.

Teaching Points

Correct Answer: 2

Injury to the axillary nerve is a well-documented complication of glenohumeral dislocation, reported in as many as 40% of cases. The incidence of concomitant axillary nerve injuries increases with age. Patients with this injury typically present with numbness or paresthesias in the lateral shoulder region and weakness with shoulder abduction.

Incorrect Choices:

Thoracic outlet syndrome occurs with compression of neurovascular structures in the region of the scalene triangle, between the clavicle and 1st rib, or between the pectoralis minor and thoracic wall. Pain and paresthesias may be present and are typically reported in the medial forearm and hand. A radiculopathy that involves the C7 and C8 nerve roots would primarily affect forearm and intrinsic hand muscles and the patient would present with pain and paresthesias along the C7 and C8 dermatomes. Radial tunnel syndrome is an entrapment neuropathy of the lateral elbow region causing pain and paresthesia in the posterolateral forearm and dorsum of the hand.

Type of Reasoning: Analytical

This question requires the test-taker to analyze the presenting symptoms and determine the likely diagnosis that is consistent with the findings. This requires analytical reasoning skill where pieces of information are weighed for their significance and flowing from that, a reasonable conclusion of what the information means. In this case, the findings are consistent with axillary nerve injury. Review information on axillary nerve injury if answered incorrectly.

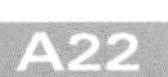
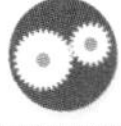

A22 Nonsystem I Professional Responsibilities

While performing an evaluation for a 17-year-old patient for neck pain, the patient expresses the need for housing assistance after being laid off recently due to budget cuts. As a result, the therapist helps the patient coordinate an appointment with a social worker. According to the Health Insurance Portability and Accountability Act (HIPAA), which of the following pieces of information is **MOST** likely inappropriate to share with the social worker?

Choices:
1. The patient was laid off.
2. The patient has neck pain.
3. The patient needs housing assistance.
4. The patient is 17 years old.

Teaching Points

Correct Answer: 2

Health care providers can communicate information relevant to mutual patients, but not communicate information that is irrelevant to another provider's care. In this example, the patient's neck pain is most likely to be irrelevant information to the social worker relative to the other items.

Incorrect Choices:

The information regarding being laid off, need for housing assistance, and the patient's age are valuable background information for the social worker. This information is sensitive but must be shared to allow the social worker to have a basic understanding of why assistance is needed.

Type of Reasoning: Evaluative

For this question, the test-taker must weigh the information presented and then apply knowledge of the HIPAA to arrive at a correct conclusion. This requires weighing the information for its merits, which is an evaluative reasoning skill. For this case, it would be most likely inappropriate to share that the patient has neck pain. If answered incorrectly, review HIPAA guidelines.

A23 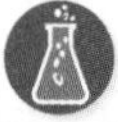

Nonsystem | Safety and Protection

A patient in the ICU is two days post-CABG. What is the primary purpose of the tubing inserted into this patient?

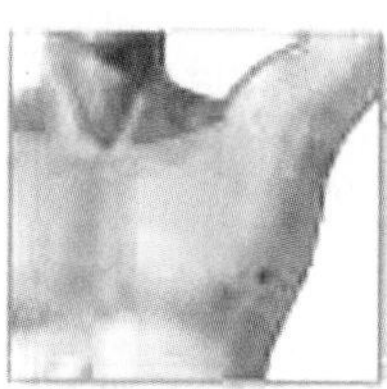

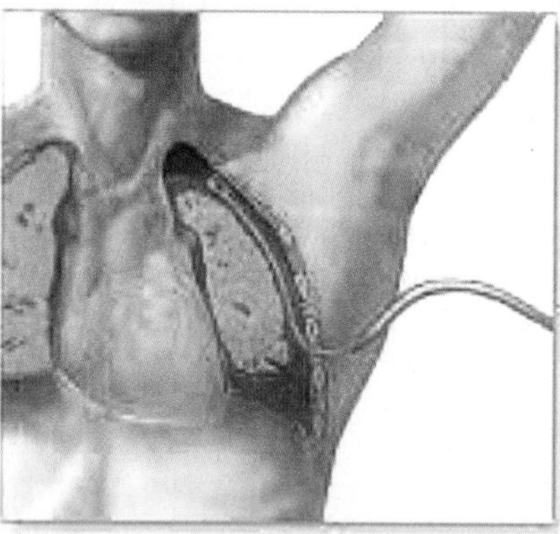

Choices:

1. To provide moistened room air directly to the patient.
2. To provide heated and moistened pure O_2 directly to the patient.
3. To measure pulmonary artery pressure and cardiac output via a Swan-Ganz catheter.
4. To evacuate air and/or blood from the intrapleural space.

Teaching Points

Correct Answer: 4

A chest tube has been inserted into the intrapleural space. It would be attached to a vacuum line with a water seal interspersed. Air, blood, or other fluid is evacuated from the pleural space following a pneumothorax, cardiothoracic surgery, pleural effusion, or other condition to allow the lung to fully expand. The water seal prevents any air from back-flowing into the thoracic cavity. Chest physical therapy is permitted in this area.

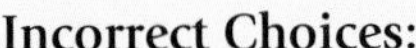

Incorrect Choices:

Supplemental O_2 is provided by use of a nasal cannula, mask, or manual resuscitator bag. Mechanical ventilation is a means to replace spontaneous breathing. Moistened and heated O_2 is administered via endotracheal, nasotracheal, or tracheal means. A chest tube is not applicable for these purposes.

A Swan-Ganz catheter, also known as a pulmonary catheter, is a thin tube inserted directly into the pulmonary artery. It can measure pulmonary artery pressure, cardiac output, and oxyhemoglobin saturation.

Type of Reasoning: Analytical

For this question, the test-taker must analyze the information in the picture in order to make a determination of the primary purpose of the tubing inserted into the patient. This requires analytical reasoning skill, where determining a correct answer through the review of pictures, charts, and graphs is utilized. For this case, the tubing is placed to evacuate air and/or blood from the intrapleural space. Review ICU guidelines, especially types of drainage tubes, if answered incorrectly.

A24 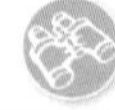

Cardiovascular/Pulmonary I Interventions

Following a motor vehicle accident, a patient with chest trauma developed atelectasis. Which intervention is ineffective in the immediate management of atelectasis?

Choices:

1. Pain reduction techniques.
2. Segmental breathing.
3. Incentive spirometry.
4. Paced breathing.

Teaching Points

Correct Answer: 4

In order to reverse atelectasis, the patient needs a technique to facilitate deep breathing. Paced breathing controls the rate of breathing, not the depth of breathing, and will therefore be ineffective.

Incorrect Choices:

Reducing the patient's pain associated with the trauma will allow the patient to take deeper breaths, which will decrease atelectasis. Segmental breathing will allow for prolonged inspiration with a breath hold. The long inspiration will facilitate deeper breathing, which can reverse the atelectasis. A breath hold will allow collateral ventilation via the pores of Kohn, which will result in increased pressures to inflate alveoli and therefore reverse atelectasis. Incentive spirometry will cause increased deep breathing with visual feedback, which can reverse atelectasis.

Type of Reasoning: Inductive

This question requires clinical judgment and knowledge of atelectasis in order to determine a best course of action. This necessitates inductive reasoning skill where clinical judgment is used to reach a sound conclusion. In this case, the least effective treatment would be paced breathing. Review atelectasis and treatment approaches if answered incorrectly.

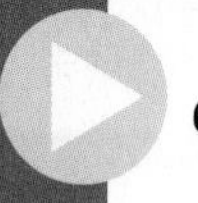

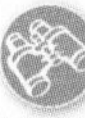

A25

Musculoskeletal | Evaluation, Diagnosis

Following a reattachment of the flexor tendons of the fingers, the patient is in a splint. One physical therapy goal is to minimize adhesion formation. What should the physical therapist teach the patient to perform after 72 hours postsurgery?

Choices:

1. Passive extension and active flexion of the interphalangeal joints.
2. Active extension and flexion of the interphalangeal joints.
3. Active extension and passive flexion of the interphalangeal joints.
4. Gentle passive extension and flexion of the interphalangeal joints.

Teaching Points

Correct Answer: 3

Severe edema increases tendon drag and likelihood of rupture. Therefore, wait until 48–72 hours postop prior to initiating range of motion (ROM) therapy. This patient is a few days postop and can begin passive finger flexion with caution so as not to disrupt the repair. Begin by blocking the metacarpophalangeal (MCP) in full flexion and actively extend interphalangeal (IP) joints, followed by passive proximal interphalangeal (PIP) flexion and active extension.

Incorrect Choices:

Generally for weeks 1 through 3 there should be no active flexion of the involved digits, as this could damage and/or tear the repair. Passive extension of the fingers should not be done until there is adequate strength of the repair.

Type of Reasoning: Inductive

One must utilize clinical judgment coupled with knowledge of flexor tendon repairs in order to arrive at a correct conclusion. This requires inductive reasoning skill. For this scenario, the therapist should teach the patient to perform active extension and passive flexion of the interphalangeal joints. If answered incorrectly, review treatment approaches for flexor tendon repairs.

A26

Musculoskeletal | Evaluation, Diagnosis

A patient complains of pain and paresthesias affecting the right foot. The right patellar tendon reflex is diminished and there is decreased sensation to light touch on the medial aspect of the foot and heel. Based on these findings, manual muscle testing results might also demonstrate weakness in which muscle?

Choices:

1. Tibialis anterior.
2. Adductor longus.
3. Biceps femoris.
4. Gastrocnemius.

Teaching Points

Correct Answer: 1

This question describes a patient with a suspected L4 nerve root problem. The patellar tendon reflex is mediated at the L4 spinal cord level, and the sensory deficit is in the L4 dermatome. The only L4-innervated muscle among the answer choices is the tibialis anterior (L4-5).

Incorrect Choices:

The nerve root innervation levels for the other answer choices are adductor longus (L2-3), biceps femoris (L5-S1), and gastrocnemius (S1-2).

Type of Reasoning: Inferential

One must determine which muscle is likely to show weakness based on presenting patient symptoms. This requires one to determine what is likely to be true of a situation, which often necessitates inferential reasoning skill. For this case, the patient is likely to demonstrate weakness of the tibialis anterior muscle. Review L4 nerve root innervation and dysfunction if answered incorrectly.

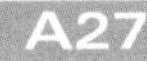
A27
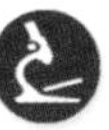

Nonsystem I Therapeutic Modalities

A patient's plan of care includes use of iontophoresis for the management of calcific bursitis of the shoulder. To administer this treatment using the acetate ion, what current characteristics and polarity should be used?

Choices:

1. Monophasic twin-peaked pulses using the positive pole.
2. Monophasic twin-peaked pulses using the negative pole.
3. Direct current using the positive pole.
4. Direct current using the negative pole.

Teaching Points

Correct Answer: 4

The acetate ion has a negative charge, and thus a negative pole will be needed to repel the drug into the tissue. Direct current will continuously drive the acetate into the tissue during the treatment time.

Incorrect Choices:

While monophasic, twin-peaked current has polarity, it is a pulsed current and will not be able to continuously drive the acetate into the tissue, resulting in less medication being delivered to the site. The positive pole will not repel the acetate ion.

Type of Reasoning: Deductive

For this question, one must recall the guidelines for application of iontophoresis and treatment using the acetate ion. This necessitates factual recall of information, which is a deductive reasoning skill. In this case, the therapist should use direct current using the negative pole. Review iontophoresis guidelines if answered incorrectly.

A28

Musculoskeletal I Evaluation, Diagnosis

A patient is seen in a physical therapy clinic for a traumatic knee injury. The patient sustained the injury by falling "up the stairs" in their house and striking the proximal tibia directly against the edge of a step. During the examination of the patient, the therapist notes diffuse bruising around the tibial tuberosity. What structure was **MOST LIKELY** injured?

Exam A

Choices:
1. Anterior cruciate ligament.
2. Posterior cruciate ligament.
3. Medial patellofemoral ligament.
4. Popliteal artery.

Teaching Points

Correct Answer: 2

The PCL is the primary restraint to posterior displacement of the tibia on the femur. The scenario describes one of the three most common mechanisms of injury of the PCL. This occurs when the knee is flexed, and an object forcefully strikes the proximal anterior tibia and displaces it posteriorly. The most common causes of PCL injury are motor vehicle accidents (dashboard injury) and athletics.

Incorrect Choices:

The usual mechanism of injury for the ACL is noncontact deceleration that produces a valgus twisting injury (e.g., athlete quickly pivoting in the opposite direction). Other mechanisms of injury of the ACL include hyperextension and severe medial tibial rotation.

The medial patellofemoral ligament is typically injured during a lateral patellar dislocation. The most common mechanism for a patellar dislocation is a powerful contraction of the quadriceps in combination with sudden flexion and external rotation of the tibia on the femur. This question describes trauma to the tibia, not the patella.

Injuries of the popliteal artery are rare and typically result from severe trauma resulting in (1) a dislocation of the tibia on the femur or (2) a fracture of the distal femur with posterior displacement of the short distal fragment.

Type of Reasoning: Inferential

For this question, the test-taker must draw from knowledge of anatomy, coupled with an understanding of the mechanism of injury in order to determine which structure was most likely injured. This requires inferential reasoning skill, where one must determine what is likely to be true of a situation. For this case, the posterior cruciate ligament was likely injured. Review mechanisms of injury of the PCL if answered incorrectly.

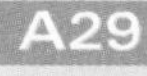
A29
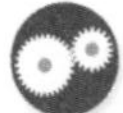

Musculoskeletal | Evaluation, Diagnosis

A physical therapist examines a tall, thin adult patient whose chief complaint is intense mid-back pain that is described as a dull ache and throbbing. The patient is unable to identify any aggravating or easing factors, and the therapist is unable to change the patient's symptoms with any type of position changes or functional tests. The therapist notices that the patient has an indented sternum (pectus excavatum). In this situation, what action should the therapist take?

Choices:
1. Treat the patient with grades III and IV mobilizations of the thoracic spine and costovertebral joints.
2. Begin the patient on a strengthening program targeting the chest, back, and core muscles.
3. Recommend an x-ray to rule out a fracture of the thoracic spine and sternum.
4. Refuse to treat the patient and immediately consult with the patient's primary care provider for further evaluation.

Teaching Points

Correct Answer: 4

This question describes a patient with a possible thoracic aortic aneurysm (TAA). Although less prevalent than abdominal aortic aneurysms, a TAA should still be treated as an emergency situation. Patients often describe the pain of an aneurysm as throbbing or pulsating, and the pain location of a TAA is typically between the shoulder blades or substernal. Risk factors for aortic aneurysms include connective tissue disorders such as Marfan's syndrome. Patients with Marfan's syndrome are tall and thin and often have deformities of the sternum.

Incorrect Choices:

There are no indications in this scenario that the patient's back pain is musculoskeletal in nature. Each of the incorrect choices describe intervention options for a musculoskeletal problem and ignore the fact that what is described is a potential emergency situation. If there had been a fracture of a thoracic vertebra, changes in positions and activities certainly would have provoked the patient's symptoms.

Type of Reasoning: Evaluative

One must determine a best course of action based on presenting signs and symptoms in order to arrive at a correct conclusion. This requires evaluative reasoning skill where one must weigh the merits of a course of action to make sound decisions. For this situation, the therapist should refuse to treat the patient and immediately consult with the patient's primary care provider for further evaluation. Review symptoms of thoracic aortic aneurysm if answered incorrectly.

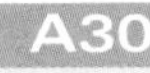
A30
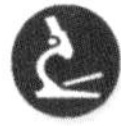

Lymphatics | Interventions

A patient with right upper extremity lymphedema is receiving care in a physical therapy clinic. The therapist decides to perform manual lymphatic drainage and provide 24-hour compression. What is the **BEST** way to apply compression to sustain the gains made during manual lymphatic drainage?

Choices:

1. Elastic bandages with multilayered foam padding applied distal to proximal.
2. Elastic bandages with multilayered foam padding applied proximal to distal.
3. Short stretch bandages with multilayered foam padding applied distal to proximal.
4. Short stretch bandages with multilayered foam padding applied proximal to distal.

Teaching Points

Correct Answer: 3

The best choice for compression treatment following manual lymphatic drainage utilizes short stretch bandages with multilayered foam padding applied distal to proximal. Short stretch bandages have low resting and high working pressures and do not create a barrier to lymph flow at rest. However, when exercising, compression against the bandage increases to provide a more effective and consistent change in pressure during the contraction cycle, enhancing lymph flow. Bandages should be applied from distal to proximal, with higher pressure distally to avoid constricting lymph flow to the torso.

Incorrect Answers:

Elastic bandages are not appropriate for this treatment because of the excessive pressures placed on the lymphatic and vascular systems.

Type of Reasoning: Deductive

For this question, the test-taker must recall how to correctly apply compression bandaging for lymphedema in order to draw a correct conclusion. This requires the recall of factual guidelines, which is a deductive reasoning skill. For this scenario, the best method of application is using short stretch bandages with multilayered foam padding applied distal to proximal. If answered incorrectly, review lymphedema treatment guidelines, especially bandaging.

A31 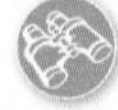

Musculoskeletal | Interventions

A patient presents with a chronic restriction of the temporomandibular joint (TMJ). The physical therapist observes the situation seen in the picture during mouth-opening range of motion (ROM) assessment. What is the **BEST** intervention if the patient has a classic TMJ unilateral capsular restriction?

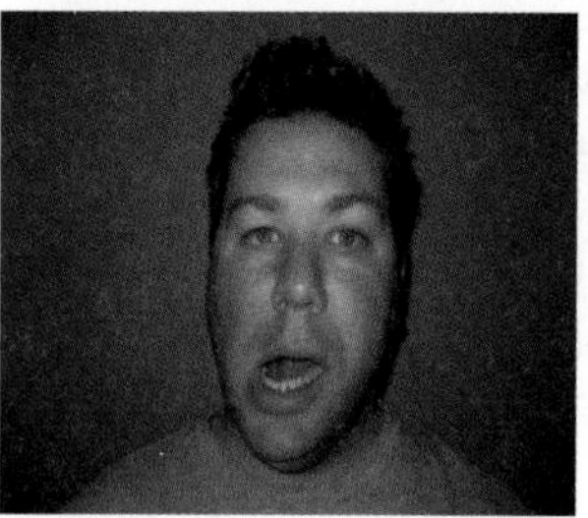

Choices:

1. Left TMJ, superior glide manipulation.
2. Left TMJ, inferior glide manipulation.
3. Right TMJ, superior glide manipulation.
4. Right TMJ, inferior glide manipulation.

Teaching Points

Correct Answer: 4

Right TMJ, inferior glide. In the photo, the chin has deviated to the right at terminal opening. The active range of motion (AROM) will be limited with ipsilateral opening and a lateral deviation to the side of restriction for patients with a TMJ capsular pattern of restriction.

Incorrect Choices:

The left TMJ incorrectly states the capsular pattern. Additionally, superior glide manipulation on the right would compress the joint, not affording a stretch to the capsule tightness.

Type of Reasoning: Inductive

This question requires clinical judgment in order to determine a best intervention approach for a patient with TMJ dysfunction. Knowledge of effective intervention approaches for the TMJ is paramount to arriving at a correct conclusion, necessitating inductive reasoning skill. For this case, the **BEST** intervention approach is right TMJ, inferior glide manipulation. Review intervention approaches for the TMJ if answered incorrectly.

A32 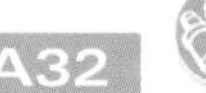

Neuromuscular | Examination

A patient in Hoehn and Yahr Stage 3 Parkinson's disease exhibits episodes of akinesia while walking. What should the therapist examine?

Choices:

1. Primary involvement of the head and trunk.
2. Associated dyskinesias.
3. Primary involvement of the hips and knees.
4. Triggers that precipitate the freezing episodes.

Teaching Points

Correct Answer: 4

Freezing of gait (episodes of akinesia) is typically associated with a trigger (e.g., turning, changing direction or speed, doorways). Identification of triggers is helpful in developing the plan of care.

Incorrect Choices:

Freezing is most often evident during gait and typically involves the entire body, not individual segments of the body. Associated dyskinesias may be present but do not typically influence freezing episodes.

Type of Reasoning: Inductive

For this question, one must utilize clinical judgment and knowledge of Parkinson's disease in order to arrive at a correct conclusion. This requires inductive reasoning skill. For this situation, the therapist should examine triggers that precipitate the freezing episodes. Review Parkinson's disease, especially examination of akinesia, if answered incorrectly.

A33 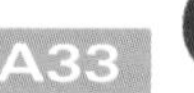

Metabolic and Endocrine | Evaluation, Diagnosis

A patient is referred to physical therapy for balance and gait training following two falls in the home in the past month. The therapist notes in the medical record that the patient has adrenal insufficiency. What are the metabolic abnormalities associated with adrenal insufficiency?

Choices:

1. Hypokalemia.
2. Hyponatremia.
3. Hyperglycemia.
4. Alkalosis.

Teaching Points

Correct Answer: 2

Metabolic abnormalities seen in adrenal insufficiency include hyponatremia (decreased sodium concentration in the blood) secondary to renal loss of sodium ions. A decrease in cortisol results in an inability to regulate potassium and sodium. Symptoms include general fatigue and anorexia.

Incorrect Choices:

Patients with adrenal insufficiency will be hyperkalemic, hypoglycemic, and may have acidosis.

Type of Reasoning: Deductive

For this question, the test-taker must recall the metabolic abnormalities that are often associated with adrenal insufficiency in order to arrive at a correct conclusion. This necessitates the recall of factual information, which is a deductive reasoning skill. For this case, hyponatremia is often associated with adrenal insufficiency. Review signs and symptoms of adrenal insufficiency if answered incorrectly.

A34 

Nonsystem I Safety and Protection

A physical therapist is treating a patient with active infectious hepatitis B. In addition to wearing a protective gown when in the patient's room, what precautions should be taken to avoid transmission of the disease?

Choices:

1. Avoid direct contact with the patient's blood or blood-contaminated equipment by wearing gloves.
2. Avoid direct contact with any part of the patient.
3. Have the patient wear a mask to minimize droplet spread of the organisms from coughing.
4. Provide tissues and no-touch receptacles for disposal of tissues.

Teaching Points

Correct Answer: 1

Hepatitis B is transmitted in blood, body fluids, or body tissues. Precautions should include avoiding direct contact with blood or blood-contaminated equipment.

Incorrect Choices:

This is not an airborne infectious disease. The patient does not need to wear a mask or have specific no-touch tissue receptacles. Contact with body surfaces with no blood droplets or open wounds should also not be an issue.

Type of Reasoning: Deductive

For this question, one must recall the guidelines for standard precautions. This is factual information, which is a deductive reasoning skill. For this case, in addition to wearing a protective gown, the therapist should avoid direct contact with the patient's blood or blood-contaminated equipment by wearing gloves. Review standard precautions, especially for hepatitis B, if answered incorrectly.

A35 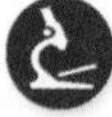

Musculoskeletal I Examination

Idiopathic scoliosis is suspected in a 12-year-old girl. During the physical examination, what is the standard screening test for this condition?

Choices:

1. Longsitting, forward bend test.
2. Standing, forward bend test.
3. Sitting, rotation test to the right and left.
4. Standing, backward extension test.

Teaching Points

Correct Answer: 2

Screening is most commonly done on adolescents. Females achieve adolescence about 2 years before males and are afflicted with scoliosis requiring treatment three to four times more frequently than males. The forward bend test is the standard screening test for scoliosis. During the test, the child will bend forward with feet together, knees straight, and arms hanging free. The therapist observes child from the back, looking for a difference in the shape of the ribs on each side. A spinal deformity is most noticeable in this position.

Incorrect Choices:

All other choices are not appropriate for examining for scoliosis (e.g., backward extension, trunk rotation, forward bending in longsitting).

Type of Reasoning: Deductive

For this question, the test-taker must recall the guidelines for conducting a scoliosis screening test in order to arrive at a correct conclusion. This necessitates factual recall of testing guidelines, which is a deductive reasoning skill. For this situation, the standard screening test is standing, forward bend test. Review scoliosis screening guidelines if answered incorrectly.

A36 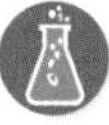

System Interactions | Evaluation, Diagnosis

A college student is seen by a physical therapist 3 weeks after having an open reduction and internal fixation (ORIF) for a talus fracture. There was no known nerve damage associated with the original injury or surgery. After several treatment sessions the therapist notices that the patient's pain is out of proportion to what is expected at this stage of recovery. The therapist observes that the patient's ankle and foot are still markedly swollen, and the skin appears mottled (red and white). The injured foot feels sweaty compared to the unaffected side. What condition should the therapist suspect?

Choices:

1. Infection in the ankle joint.
2. Complex regional pain syndrome (Type I).
3. Complex regional pain syndrome (Type II).
4. Post-traumatic arthritis.

Teaching Points

Correct Answer: 2

Complex regional pain syndrome (CRPS) Type I was formerly known as Reflexive Sympathetic Dystrophy. This question describes classic symptoms of CRPS, which include unexplained and hypersensitive pain, temperature changes, skin changes, and swelling of the affected area. In CRPS Type I, there is no known nerve damage, whereas in CRPS Type II (formerly causalgia) there is a known nerve injury, such as a crush injury to a peripheral nerve.

Incorrect Choices:

An infection of the ankle joint would have presented differently than what is described in the question stem. Signs of infection include fever and chills, palpable warmth in the infected area, and pain, redness, and possible purulent drainage at the surgical incision site. Post-traumatic arthritis may develop in the ankle or subtalar joints following a surgical repair of the talus, but it would typically take months to develop. Additionally, the clinical presentation described in this scenario is not consistent with the pain and stiffness patients describe in an arthritic joint.

Type of Reasoning: Analytical

For this question, the test-taker must analyze the presenting symptoms of the patient and determine the likely diagnosis. This requires analytical reasoning skill where pieces of information are analyzed to draw reasonable conclusions. For this situation, the symptoms are consistent with CRPS (Type I). If answered incorrectly, review information on CRPS, especially Type I symptoms.

A37 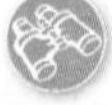

Genitourinary I Interventions

A woman is referred to physical therapy with a diagnosis of pelvic floor weakness after delivering a baby. Proper instructions for pelvic floor exercises would **NOT** include which of the following?

Choices:

1. Stop and start the flow of urine every time you go to the toilet.
2. Squeeze the muscles around the vagina, imagining you are stopping the flow of urine, hold for 5–10 seconds, then relax.
3. Repeat the exercises 10 times, three times a day.
4. Start in supine position and progress to sitting and standing practice.

Teaching Points

Correct Answer: 1

Kegel exercises (pelvic floor exercises) should not include stopping and starting the flow of urine every time one goes to the toilet. This can be used once as a test to find if the correct muscles are contracting. Continued use can result in bladder complications (e.g., infection, overuse).

Incorrect Choices:

Proper instructions for Kegel exercises include: lie down, sit, or stand with your legs slightly apart and relax your thighs, buttocks, and abdomen muscles. Tighten the ring of muscle around your front and back passages, drawing the pelvic floor muscles up inside. Hold for 5–10 seconds and relax. Repeating the exercise 10 times, three times a day is the recommended intensity and frequency.

Type of Reasoning: Inductive

This question requires one to recall Kegel exercise guidelines in order to determine an approach that is **NOT** appropriate to provide as part of instruction for exercise. This requires inductive reasoning skill, where clinical judgment is paramount to arriving at a correct conclusion. For this case, it is NOT appropriate to stop and start the flow of urine every time when going to the toilet. Review Kegel exercise guidelines if answered incorrectly.

A38 

Musculoskeletal I Examination

During observation of bilateral active straight leg raising in a supine position, the patient demonstrates progressively increasing lumbar lordosis during lowering of the limbs with each successive lift. What is the **MOST LIKELY** cause of the observed excessive lordosis during the bilateral straight leg activity?

Choices:

1. Muscle imbalance between the rectus femoris and the sartorius muscles.
2. Weakness of both quadratus lumborum muscles.
3. Weakness of the rectus abdominis and oblique muscle groups.
4. Excessive elastic shortening of the ipsilateral hamstring muscle group.

Teaching Points

Correct Answer: 3

During a dynamic activity such as the performance of a bilateral active straight leg raise, the weight of the limbs lifted produces an anterior torque on the pelvis. During this dynamic activity, excessive lordosis typically is associated with excessive anterior pelvic rotation. Normally muscles that control anterior pelvic rotation (posterior pelvic rotators) act to counter the anterior torques produced by the mass of the lower limbs lifted off the table, helping to prevent unwanted sagittal plane movements of the lumbar spine. Contractile activities of the anterior trunk muscles (rectus and obliques) provide a posterior rotation moment on the pelvis, helping to stabilize the pelvis. Fatigue weakness of the anterior trunk muscles in this patient could result in poor control of sagittal plane rotation of the pelvis, leading to the observed increasing lumbar lordosis.

Incorrect Choices:

The quadratus lumborum acts as a stabilizer and an extensor of the lumbar spine in the sagittal plane, and one would not suspect weakness as the cause of the observed excessive lordosis. Lack of hamstring lengthening could not directly produce the observed increasing lordosis. While the rectus femoris and sartorius are capable of anterior pelvic rotation when the lower limbs are fixed, they offer no direct force to produce unwanted anterior pelvic rotation and subsequent lordosis in this case in which the limbs have been lifted off the table.

Type of Reasoning: Inferential

For this question, one must infer, or draw a reasonable conclusion, for an increasing lumbar lordosis during bilateral straight leg raising. Questions that require one to determine what is most likely to be true often necessitate inferential reasoning skill. For this case, the cause is most likely fatigue weakness of the rectus abdominis and oblique muscle groups. Review causes of lumbar lordosis if answered incorrectly.

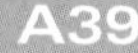

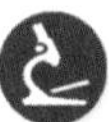

System Interactions | Evaluation, Diagnosis

The therapist is treating a patient with chronic Lyme disease of more than 1 year's duration. What joints are likely to demonstrate more arthritic changes and therefore should be the focus of physical therapy interventions?

Choices:

1. Small joints of the hands and feet.
2. Large joints of the body, especially the knee.
3. Axial joints, especially the lumbrosacral spine.
4. Axial joints, especially the cervical and thoracic spine.

Teaching Points

Correct Answer: 2

Stage 3 Lyme disease (late or chronic Lyme disease) is characterized by intermittent arthritis with marked pain and swelling, especially in the large joints. Permanent joint damage can occur.

Incorrect Choices:

Other joints may be affected, though not with the same frequency as the large joints.

Type of Reasoning: Deductive

This question requires the test-taker to recall the stages of Lyme disease and presenting symptoms in order to arrive at a correct conclusion. This necessitates the recall of facts and guidelines, which is a deductive reasoning skill. For this situation, the patient is likely to show arthritic changes of the large joints of the body, especially the knee. Review Lyme disease stages and symptoms if answered incorrectly.

A40 

Cardiovascular/Pulmonary | Examination

A physical therapist is preparing to treat a patient in an inpatient setting. The therapist observes the following readout for the patient's cardiac rhythm on a telemetry unit. What is the patient's heart rate?

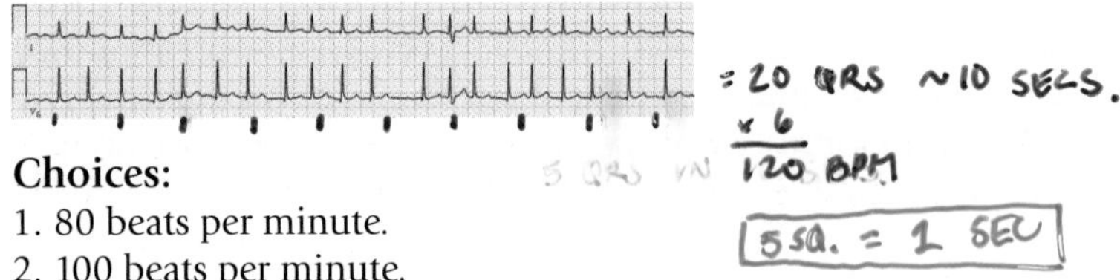

Choices:

1. 80 beats per minute.
2. 100 beats per minute.
3. 120 beats per minute.
4. 140 beats per minute.

Teaching Points

Correct Answer: 3

Each square on the electrocardiogram (ECG) paper is 5 mm long, which represents 0.2 seconds. Five squares are equal to 1 second. There is a total of 50 squares on this strip, which equals a total 10 seconds. The number of QRS peaks on the strip is 20. Therefore, there is a total of 20 QRS peaks on this 10-second ECG strip, which translates to a heart rate of 120 beats per minute.

Incorrect Answers:

All of the other answers are incorrect because they do not consider the entire strip to account for all the available beats, which is necessary if the rhythm is irregular.

Type of Reasoning: Deductive

For this question, the test-taker must recall the guidelines of how to read the heart rate on an electrocardiogram (ECG) in order to arrive at a correct conclusion. This requires deductive reasoning skill, where factual recall of information guides critical thinking. For this case, the patient's heart rate according to the ECG is 120 beats per minute. If answered incorrectly, review guidelines for reading electrocardiograms.

A41 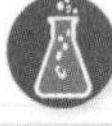

Neuromuscular | Examination

A physical therapist observes a full-term infant in the neonatal intensive care unit (NICU) just after birth. In the supine position, the shoulders are abducted and externally rotated, elbows and fingers are flexed, hips are abducted and externally rotated, and knees are flexed. What would this posturing be an indication of?

Choices:

1. Upper extremity tone is abnormal.
2. Lower extremity tone is abnormal.
3. Tone is abnormal in both upper and lower extremities.
4. Tone is normal in both upper and lower extremities.

Teaching Points

Correct Answer: 4

A full-term infant in the NICU can have low Apgar scores, respiratory distress, or any one of a number of specific diagnoses (none listed in this case). Initial tone and posturing involve some flexion of the limbs. At 1 month, decreased flexion can be expected.

Incorrect Choices:

All other choices indicate that the flexor tone and posturing noted in a newborn's upper and lower limbs are abnormal.

Type of Reasoning: Analytical

For this question, one must analyze the description of posture in an infant and make a determination of what the posturing indicates. This requires analytical reasoning skill. For this case, the posturing indicates that tone is normal in both upper and lower extremities. Review posturing in infants if answered incorrectly.

A42 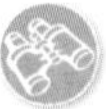

Metabolic and Endocrine | Interventions

A patient with type 1 diabetes mellitus has generalized osteoporosis. What is the **BEST** exercise to include in this patient's plan of care?

Choices:

1. Bilateral quadriceps presses against resistance in sitting.
2. Aquatic exercises.
3. Running on a treadmill.
4. Partial squats in standing.

Teaching Points

Correct Answer: 4

Extensor stabilization exercises in weight-bearing postures provide the best stimulus to bone (e.g., standing, holding against resistance, standing partial squats).

Incorrect Choices:

High-load, short-duration activities (jumping, running, weights) provide less stimulus to bone while posing increased risk of muscle strain and injury. The buoyancy of water limits the load on bone during aquatic exercises.

Type of Reasoning: Inductive

This question requires the test-taker to utilize clinical judgment in order to determine a best course of action. Questions of this nature often require inductive reasoning skill. For this case, the best exercise to include for osteoporosis is partial squats in standing. Review exercise guidelines for osteoporosis if answered incorrectly.

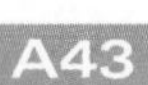

A43

Nonsystem | Safety and Protection

Patients may sustain injuries that cause external or internal bleeding. Which finding is **MOST LIKELY** to be present in patients with internal bleeding?

Choices:

1. Decreased level of consciousness.
2. Cool, moist skin with a pale or gray appearance.
3. Restlessness or anxiety.
4. Referred pain.

Teaching Points

Correct Answer: 4

Referred pain is present when visceral structures are impacted by injury, tumors, or abnormal pressure. Patients who suffer blunt trauma may sustain bleeding that creates abnormal pressure on visceral structures that refer to a predictable body region (e.g., liver referred to the right shoulder). Patients with a history of blunt trauma, who present with referred pain, should be emergently referred to a physician for assessment.

Incorrect Choices:

Restlessness and anxiety, decreased levels of consciousness, and skin changes (cool, moist, pale/gray) are symptoms related to shock. Patients may experience any of these symptoms due to hypovolemia or psychogenic reasons. Patients with both external or internal bleeding may experience symptoms of shock. Symptoms of shock are very concerning, and in response, health care providers should place patients in supine, elevate the legs if appropriate, and activate EMS if symptoms are not quickly resolved.

Type of Reasoning: Inferential

For this question, the test-taker must infer what is likely to be true of a situation, based on clinical symptoms. Questions of this nature often require inferential reasoning skill. For this situation, referred pain is most likely to be present with internal bleeding. If answered incorrectly, review information on internal bleeding and common findings.

A44

Neuromuscular | Evaluation, Diagnosis

While gait training a patient following a stroke, the therapist observes the knee on the hemiparetic side going into recurvatum during stance phase. What is the **MOST LIKELY** cause of this deviation?

Choices:

1. Severe spasticity of the hamstrings or weakness of the gastrocnemius-soleus.
2. Weakness or severe spasticity of the quadriceps.
3. Weakness of the gastrocnemius-soleus or spasticity of the pretibial muscles.
4. Weakness of both the gastrocnemius-soleus and pretibial muscles.

Teaching Points

Correct Answer: 2

Weakness or severe spasticity of the quadriceps is the most likely cause of genu recurvatum.

Incorrect Choices:

Spasticity of the hamstrings or pretibial muscles is unlikely and would cause the knee to buckle. Weakness of the gastrocnemius-soleus would cause lack of push-off, while weakness of the pretibial muscles would cause a drop foot.

Type of Reasoning: Inferential

For this question, one must determine the most likely cause of genu recurvatum and use this knowledge to arrive at a correct conclusion. Questions of this nature often require inferential reasoning skill. For this case, the cause is most likely due to weakness or severe spasticity of the quadriceps. Review gait patterns, especially genu recurvatum, if answered incorrectly.

A45 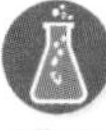

Lymphatic I Examination

This picture depicts a clinician assessing for Stemmer's sign. The clinician is examining for what condition?

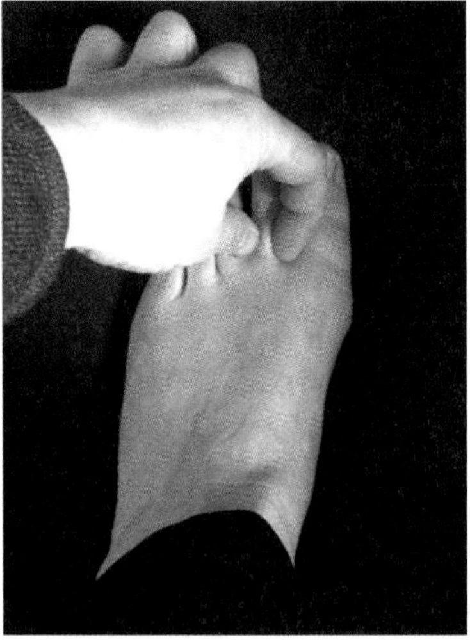

Choices:

1. Metatarsalgia.
2. Hammer toe.
3. Lymphedema.
4. Fracture of the second toe.

Teaching Points

Correct Answer: 3

Stemmer's sign is assessed by pulling up on the skin at the base of the second toe or finger, which the clinician is doing in this picture. If the skin is unable to be pulled up, then it is a sign of lymphedema, usually primary but also advanced secondary.

Incorrect Choices:

A bunion is diagnosed by the metacarpophalangeal (MCP) joint angle. A fracture is diagnosed by radiology. A hammer toe is usually diagnosed by visual inspection of the foot.

Type of Reasoning: Analytical

For this question, one must utilize knowledge of Stemmer's sign and analyze the information present in the picture in order to arrive at a correct conclusion. Questions that accompany pictures often necessitate analytical reasoning skill. For this situation, the picture depicts an examination for the presence of lymphedema. Review Stemmer's sign if answered incorrectly.

A46 

Neuromuscular | Evaluation, Diagnosis

An infant has been diagnosed with a complete rupture of C8 and T1 resulting in Klumpke's paralysis. Which movement can be expected to be impaired?

Choices:

1. Shoulder elevation.
2. Wrist and finger flexion.
3. Elbow extension.
4. Elbow supination.

Teaching Points

Correct Answer: 2

Klumpke's paralysis involves muscles innervated by the lower roots of the brachial plexus (C8–T1 nerves). Paralysis affects the intrinsic hand muscles (interossei, thenar, and hypothenar muscles), flexors of the wrist and fingers (flexor carpi ulnaris and ulnar half of flexor digitorum profundus), and forearm pronators. Typical presentation is an intrinsic minus or claw hand. Horner's syndrome can also be present with involvement of T1 affecting the dilators of eye and eyelid elevation.

Incorrect Choices:

Shoulder and elbow movements are not impaired with Klumpke's paralysis.

Type of Reasoning: Inferential

This question requires one to determine the expected motion impaired by Klumpke's paralysis. This necessitates understanding of the diagnosis and muscles innervated by the lower roots of the brachial plexus in order to arrive at a correct conclusion. For this scenario, one would expect wrist flexion to be impaired. Review Klumpke's paralysis and movements impaired by the injury if answered incorrectly.

A47 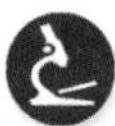

Gastrointestinal | Evaluation, Diagnosis

What is pain and tenderness with palpation over McBurney's point associated with?

Choices:

1. Acute appendicitis.
2. Hiatal hernia.
3. Acute cholecystitis.
4. GERD.

Teaching Points

Correct Answer: 1

Pain and tenderness with palpation over McBurney's point are associated with acute appendicitis. McBurney's point is located half the distance between the anterior superior iliac spine (ASIS) and the umbilicus in the right lower abdominal quadrant.

Incorrect Choices:

A positive Murphy's sign (pain and tenderness over the costovertebral angle) is associated with acute cholecystitis or acute pyelonephritis. Hiatal hernia pain is usually sharp and localizes to the lower esophagus/upper stomach area. Gastroesophageal reflux disease (GERD) produces persistent burning pain in the esophagus, throat, or chest.

Type of Reasoning: Deductive

This question requires factual recall of information in order to arrive at a correct conclusion. This is a deductive reasoning skill. One must recall what pain and tenderness of McBurney's point indicates. In this case, it is indicative of acute appendicitis. Review testing guidelines for acute appendicitis if answered incorrectly.

A48 

Cardiovascular/Pulmonary I Examination

What is the expected hemodynamic response for a patient on a beta-adrenergic blocking agent during exercise?

Choices:

1. Heart rate to be low at rest and rise minimally with exercise.
2. Heart rate to be low at rest and rise continuously to expected levels as exercise intensity increases.
3. Systolic blood pressure to be low at rest and not rise with exercise.
4. Systolic blood pressure to be within normal limits at rest and progressively fall as exercise intensity increases.

Teaching Points

Correct Answer: 1

A beta-blocker will decrease the sympathetic response to activity. This will decrease the heart rate at rest and will blunt the heart rate response to activity.

Incorrect Choices:

The heart rate response to exercise will be blunted. The blood pressure will rise with exercise, just not to the expected levels. The systolic blood pressure will be lowered at rest and will increase with activity, but not to normal levels.

Type of Reasoning: Inferential

For this question, one must determine what is most likely to be true of a situation, which is an inferential reasoning skill. One must utilize knowledge of beta-blockers and exercise with beta-blocker use in order to arrive at a correct conclusion. For this situation, one would expect heart rate to be low at rest and rise minimally with exercise. If answered incorrectly, review beta-blocker effects during exercise.

A49 

Neuromuscular I Evaluation, Diagnosis

A new child is moving into a school district and entering 2nd grade. A physical therapy request has been made. In reviewing the chart from the previous school, the therapist notes that the child has cerebral palsy. Using the Gross Motor Classification System (GMFCS) for Cerebral Palsy, the child is reported at a Level V. The reason for the referral is MOST LIKELY for which of the following goals?

Choices:

1. Independent in advanced gross motor skills such as jumping, climbing, and riding a bike.
2. Independent and safe in gait and stair climbing using an assistive device.
3. Independent in use of manual wheelchair for primary mobility.
4. Maintain range of motion and skin integrity with use of positioning devices.

Teaching Points

Correct Answer: 4

A Level V indicates that the child is severely limited even with the use of assistive technology. So the referral is most likely to prevent further impairments and maintain educational goals.

Incorrect Choices:

Jumping, climbing describe a Level I; stair training describes a Level III; manual wheelchair use describes a level III or IV.

Type of Reasoning: Inferential

One must infer or determine what is most likely to be true of a situation in order to reach a reasonable conclusion. This requires inferential reasoning skill, where the test-taker is tasked with determining the most likely reasoning for the child's referral to PT. In this case, the referral was MOST LIKELY for maintaining range of motion and skin integrity with use of positioning devices. If answered incorrectly, review the Gross Motor Function Classification System.

A50 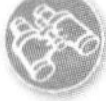

Neuromuscular | Examination

A patient sustained a right middle cerebral artery stroke 2 weeks ago with the primary impairments of contralateral upper greater than lower extremity hemiparesis and hemisensory loss. What examination item is **BEST** to assess the patient's primary impairments?

Choices:

1. Functional Independence Measure (FIM).
2. Berg Balance Scale.
3. Fugl-Meyer Assessment of Motor Performance.
4. NIH Stroke Scale.

Teaching Points

Correct Answer: 3

The Fugl-Meyer assessment of motor performance is the best option and contains specific tests to assess upper and lower extremity function, strength, coordination, sensation, and range of motion.

Incorrect Choices:

The Berg Balance Scale, FIM, and the NIH Stroke Scales assess function across multiple areas and domains but are not specific to sensory and motor impairments. Please see Box 3-1 and Table 3-13 for additional information.

Type of Reasoning: Inductive

For this question, the test-taker must utilize clinical judgment to determine a best course of action. This necessitates inductive reasoning skill. In this case, one must be familiar with the examinations presented in order to choose the examination that will best assess the patient's primary impairments. For this scenario, the Fugl-Meyer Assessment of Motor Performance is best. If answered incorrectly, review information on CVA assessment, especially the Fugl-Meyer Assessment of Motor Performance.

A51 

Neuromuscular | Evaluation, Diagnosis

A young adult who is comatose (Glasgow Coma Scale score of 3) is transferred to a long-term care facility for custodial care. On initial examination, the therapist determines the patient is demonstrating decerebrate posturing. Which limb or body position is indicative of this?

Choices:

1. The upper extremities in flexion and the lower extremities in extension.
2. Extreme hyperextension of the neck and spine with both lower extremities flexed and the heels touching the buttocks.
3. All four limbs in extension.
4. All four limbs in flexion.

Teaching Points

Correct Answer: 3

With decerebrate posturing (decerebrate rigidity), the upper and lower extremities are held rigidly in extension.

Incorrect Choices:

In decorticate posture, the upper extremities are held rigidly in flexion while the lower extremities are extended. With opisthotonos, extreme hyperextension of the neck and spine is evident, with both lower extremities flexed and the heels touching the buttocks. All limbs flexed is not typically found in the comatose patient.

Type of Reasoning: Deductive

This question requires the test-taker to recall factual guidelines related to posturing with individuals who are comatose. Recall of facts and guidelines often necessitates deductive reasoning skill. For this case, decerebrate posturing would present as all four limbs in extension. Review various types of posturing with coma if answered incorrectly.

A52 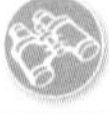

Gastrointestinal | Interventions

A patient is recovering from a mild stroke with trunk weakness and postural instability. The patient complains of severe heartburn. What is the **BEST** choice to maximize stroke recovery and improve trunk stabilization while minimizing heartburn?

Choices:
1. Perform trunk stabilization exercises with the patient in the semi-Fowler position.
2. Begin with bridging exercises progressing to sitting holding.
3. Perform resisted holding in sitting using rhythmic stabilization.
4. Instruct the patient to take antacids right before physical therapy.

Teaching Points

Correct Answer: 3

Heartburn is a common symptom of gastroesophageal reflux disease (GERD) and can be aggravated by positioning in supine, prone, or bridging. Modifying the patient's position to upright can alleviate the symptoms and demonstrate to the patient the therapist's concern.

Incorrect Choices:

Semi-Fowler position (supine, head and torso elevated 30°) is not an effective position to work on trunk stabilization. Bridging will aggravate heartburn. Prophylactic use of antacids before therapy is not indicated. With severe heartburn, the patient will likely be on a proton pump inhibitor (PPI) such as Prilosec, Nexium, or Prevacid.

Type of Reasoning: Inductive

For this question, the test-taker must utilize clinical judgment in order to arrive at a correct conclusion. This necessitates inductive reasoning skill. In this situation, the best choice for a patient with severe heartburn is to perform resisted holding in sitting using rhythmic stabilization. Review information regarding GERD and exercise approaches if answered incorrectly.

A53

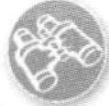

Integumentary | Interventions

A physical therapist is educating a patient with diabetic polyneuropathy. What is the BEST foot care precaution information to share with this patient?

Choices:
1. Apply moisturizing cream daily in between the toes and on the heels.
2. It is best to shop for new shoes at the beginning of day.
3. Keep your feet warm at night with a heating pad or hot water bottle.
4. Use a pumice stone to gently remove calluses.

Teaching Points

Correct Answer: 4

Foot care precaution for patients with diabetic polyneuropathy should include the use of a pumice stone to gently file calluses. Other advice includes examining footwear for proper fit to prevent callus and corn development. Additionally, patients should never use anything sharp or chemicals to debride corns or calluses.

Incorrect Choices:

It is important to moisturize but not between the toes as it contributes to skin maceration. It is best to buy shoes at the end of the day when the feet are larger. Buying shoes at the beginning of the day could result in an improper fit. Finally, heating pads and hot water bottles are contraindicated in someone with polyneuropathy. If the patient's feet are cold, it is recommended they wear socks.

Type of Reasoning: Inductive

For this question, the test-taker must utilize knowledge of diabetic foot care in order to determine the best foot care precaution information to share with the patient. This necessitates clinical judgment, which is an inductive reasoning skill. For this case, the therapist should share with the patient use of a pumice stone to gently remove calluses. If answered incorrectly, review diabetic foot care information.

A54 

Neuromuscular I Examination

A therapist wishes to examine the balance of an elderly patient with a history of falls. The Berg Balance Test is selected. Which area is **NOT** examined using this test?

Choices:

1. Sit-to-stand transitions.
2. Functional reach in standing.
3. Turning head while walking.
4. Tandem standing.

Teaching Points

Correct Answer: 3

The Berg Balance Test (BBT) is a test of static and dynamic balance in sitting and standing. It includes transitional items of sit-to-stand and stand-to-sit. It does not include items on gait. Turning while walking is an item on both the Tinetti Performance-Oriented Mobility Assessment and the Dynamic Gait Index.

Incorrect Choices:

All other choices are items on the BBT.

Type of Reasoning: Deductive

For this question, the test-taker must recall the features of the BBT in order to arrive at a correct conclusion. This is factual recall of information, which is a deductive reasoning skill. In this case, the BBT does not examine turning while walking. Review the BBT if answered incorrectly.

A55 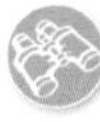

Musculoskeletal I Interventions

The physical therapist is instructing a new mother to perform range of motion and stretching for her newborn who has a clubfoot. In what directions should the therapist advise her to carefully stretch?

Choices:

1. Plantarflexion and inversion.
2. Plantarflexion and eversion.
3. Dorsiflexion and inversion.
4. Dorsiflexion and eversion.

Teaching Points

Correct Answer: 4

The term "clubfoot" (talipes equinovarus) refers to the way the foot is positioned at a sharp angle to the ankle, like the head of a golf club. It describes a range of foot abnormalities usually present at birth in which the infant's foot is twisted into an equinovarus deformity. Stretching should be opposite the direction of the deforming position; therefore, stretch is into dorsiflexion and eversion.

Incorrect Choices:

All other choices would not be beneficial when stretching a clubfoot.

Type of Reasoning: Inductive

This question requires one to determine a best course of action using clinical judgment, based on knowledge of clubfoot. Questions of this nature, where clinical judgment is utilized to reach a sound conclusion, often necessitate inductive reasoning skill. In this case, the therapist should recommend stretching in the opposite direction of the deforming position, which is dorsiflexion and eversion. Review clubfoot and treatment guidelines if answered incorrectly.

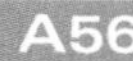

Cardiovascular/Pulmonary I Interventions

Pursed lip breathing as part of the treatment regimen would be **MOST** appropriate for a patient with which condition?

Choices:

1. Circumferential thoracic burns.
2. Asbestosis.
3. Rib fracture.
4. Emphysema.

Teaching Points

Correct Answer: 4

Pursed lip breathing gives increased resistance to the airways on exhalation. The resistance causes increased pressure, which helps to prevent airway collapse (likely sequelae given the pathophysiology of emphysema). This occurs via collateral ventilation through pores of Kohn and canals of Lambert.

Incorrect Choices:

Circumferential thoracic burn is a restrictive disorder, and pursed lip breathing will not have any effect on this. Asbestosis is an interstitial lung disease where there are fibrotic changes within the lung tissue. Pursed lip breathing will have no effect on this patient's breathing pattern. Rib fractures are also a restrictive disorder. In order to improve the breathing pattern, it would be most beneficial to control pain. Pursed lip breathing will have little effect.

Type of Reasoning: Inferential

This question requires one to utilize knowledge of pursed lip breathing in order to determine a best course of action in choosing this approach for a specific diagnosis. This requires clinical judgment, which is an inductive reasoning skill. For this situation, pursed lip breathing is most appropriate for emphysema. If answered incorrectly, review pursed lip breathing guidelines and intervention approaches for emphysema.

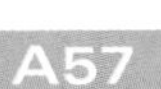

A57

Musculoskeletal | Examination

A patient has normal quadriceps strength but unilateral weakness (3/5) of the hamstring muscles on the right. What might the therapist observe during swing phase of gait?

Choices:

1. Excessive compensatory hip extension on the sound side.
2. Decreased hip flexion followed by increased knee flexion on the weak side.
3. Excessive hip extension followed by abrupt knee extension on the weak side.
4. Excessive hip flexion followed by abrupt knee extension on the weak side.

Teaching Points

Correct Answer: 4

The hamstring muscles primarily control the forward swing of the leg during terminal swing. Loss of function may result in abrupt knee extension and increased hip flexion.

Incorrect Choices:

Excessive compensatory hip extension on the sound side would help in pulling the weak side into flexion due to weak hip flexors. This is not the case. Decreased hip flexion followed by increased knee flexion on the weak side would be the result of weak hip flexors and knee extensors during terminal swing. There would be abrupt knee extension as the hamstrings need to decelerate the tibia at terminal swing; however, one would not have excessive hip extension.

Type of Reasoning: Inferential

This question asks one to determine what is likely to be true for a patient with unilateral weakness of the hamstring muscles during gait. This requires one to infer information and recall the effects of muscle weakness on gait, necessitating inferential reasoning skill. For this case, the therapist is likely to see excessive hip flexion followed by abrupt knee extension on the side with hamstring weakness. Review gait abnormalities associated with muscle weakness if answered incorrectly.

A58

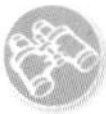

Musculoskeletal | Interventions

An adult patient sustained an elbow dislocation while completing a military obstacle course eight weeks ago and continues to have limited elbow flexion. Which joint mobilization technique is **BEST** to improve elbow flexion?

Choices:

1. Posterior glide of the radial head on the humerus.
2. Anterior glide of the radial head on the humerus.
3. Lateral glide of the radial head on the humerus.
4. Medial glide of the radial head on the humerus.

Teaching Points

Correct Answer: 2

An anterior glide of the radius on the humerus would be used to increase elbow flexion. In this case, and according to the concave-convex rule, a concave surface is moving on a convex surface, so the anterior glide will occur in the same direction as the osteokinematic motion of flexion. See Table 2-1 for a review of the concave-convex rule application to peripheral joints.

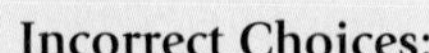

Incorrect Choices:

Medial and lateral glides may be used to augment overall mobility but are not the best choice to improve elbow joint flexion. Posterior glide of the radial head would be used to increase elbow extension.

Type of Reasoning: Inductive

This question requires the test-taker to recall joint mobilization information and then apply them to a patient who sustained an elbow dislocation with resultant decreased elbow flexion. This requires inductive reasoning skill, where clinical knowledge is applied to therapeutic situations. For this situation, the therapist should select an anterior glide of the radial head on the humerus. If answered incorrectly, review joint mobilization guidelines, especially for the elbow.

A59 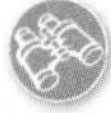

Neuromuscular | Interventions

A patient with a complete tetraplegia (ASIA A) at the C6 level is initially instructed to transfer using a transfer board. With shoulders externally rotated, how should the remaining upper extremity (UE) joints be positioned?

Choices:

1. Forearms pronated with wrists and fingers extended.
2. Forearms supinated with wrists extended and fingers flexed.
3. Forearms pronated with wrists and fingers flexed.
4. Forearms supinated with wrists and fingers extended.

Teaching Points

Correct Answer: 2

The patient with tetraplegia at the C6 level does not have triceps to assist in transfers. Independent transfers can be achieved using muscle substitution and positioning to lock the elbow. The hands are positioned anterior to the hips; the shoulders are externally rotated with the elbows and wrists extended, forearms supinated, and fingers flexed. Strong contraction of the anterior deltoid, shoulder external rotators, and clavicular portion of the pectoralis major flexes and adducts the humerus, causing the elbow to extend.

Incorrect Choices:

Fingers are always flexed (not extended) to preserve tenodesis grasp. Forearms are supinated (not pronated) and the wrist is extended (not flexed).

Type of Reasoning: Inductive

This question requires one to determine, through clinical judgment, what would be the best UE joint positioning for a patient with C6 tetraplegia in order to perform a transfer using a transfer board. This necessitates clinical judgment and use of knowledge of transfers with tetraplegia, which is an inductive reasoning skill. For this case, the therapist should ensure the forearms are supinated with wrists extended and fingers flexed. Review transfer guidelines for patients with tetraplegia if answered incorrectly.

A60 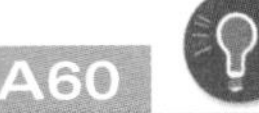

Integumentaryl Evaluation, Diagnosis, Prognosis

Which of the following is the **MOST** valid prognostic indicator of early wound healing of a diabetic foot ulceration?

Choices:

1. Increase in the granulation formation within the first month.
2. A reduction of the wound surface area in the first month.
3. A reduction in the exudate production in the first few weeks.
4. Epithelialization is present within the first month of care being initiated.

Teaching Points

Correct Answer: 2

A significant decrease in wound area during the first month is the most significant prognostic indicator of full wound closure for diabetic foot ulcerations. Significant reduction of wound area in the first few weeks is also a predictor of complete wound healing in venous and pressure ulcerations.

Incorrect Choices:

Although the other options are important for wound healing and contribute to a reduction in wound surface area, individually they represent an earlier stage of wound healing and are not as predictive of complete wound healing.

Type of Reasoning: Inferential

For this question, the test-taker must infer what is most likely to be true for the healing of a diabetic foot ulceration. Specifically, the test-taker must review the information presented and determine which is the most reliable prognostic indicator for future healing. This necessitates inferential reasoning skill. For this scenario, a reduction of the wound surface area in the first month is the most reliable indicator for future healing. Review wound healing guidelines, especially diabetic foot ulcers, if answered incorrectly.

A61 

Musculoskeletal I Examination

A patient is seen in the physical therapy clinic with a complaint of shoulder and neck pain following an injury sustained during a lacrosse game. The patient complains of local pain and denies any associated paresthesia or numbness. The therapist suspects a suprascapular nerve injury. Which resisted motion test results would support this diagnosis?

Choices:

1. Weakness with shoulder extension.
2. Weakness with shoulder abduction and lateral rotation.
3. Weakness with shoulder medial rotation.
4. Weakness with shoulder adduction and medial rotation.

Exam A

Teaching Points

Correct Answer: 2

The suprascapular nerve innervates the supraspinatus and infraspinatus, which are tested with the actions of shoulder abduction and lateral rotation, respectively. There is no cutaneous nerve field for the suprascapular nerve.

Incorrect Choices:

The long head of the triceps brachii (radial nerve) and posterior deltoid (axillary nerve) muscles are tested with shoulder extension. The subscapularis muscle produces medial rotation and is innervated by the upper and lower subscapular nerve. Combined shoulder adduction and medial rotation are produced by the pectoralis major (medial and lateral pectoral nerves), latissimus dorsi (thoracodorsal nerve), and teres major (upper and lower subscapular nerve) muscles. See Table 2-4 for a review of upper extremity muscles and their innervation.

Type of Reasoning: Inferential

For this question, the test-taker must infer what is likely to be true of a clinical situation in order to arrive at a correct conclusion. This requires inferential reasoning skill. For this case, weakness with shoulder abduction and lateral rotation would support a diagnosis of suprascapular nerve injury. If answered incorrectly, review information on suprascapular nerve injury.

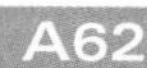
A62 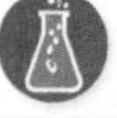

Musculoskeletal | Evaluation, Diagnosis

A competitive gymnast is examined by the physical therapist. The chief complaint is nagging, localized pain in the anterior left lower leg that is consistently present at night and increases during activity with swelling. What are these complaints **MOST** characteristic of?

Choices:

1. Bone tumor.
2. Anterior compartment syndrome.
3. Shin splints.
4. Stress fracture.

Teaching Points

Correct Answer: 4

Symptoms of a stress fracture may include pain and swelling, particularly with weight bearing on the injured bone. Stress fractures should be considered in patients who present with tenderness or edema after a recent increase in activity or repeated activity with limited rest. The differential diagnosis varies based on location but commonly includes tendinopathy, compartment syndrome, and nerve or artery entrapment syndrome.

Incorrect Choices:

Bone tumor is a possibility but not the most characteristic in this scenario. Pain may be increased at night. In this case there was pain at night but not increased. Activity may also increase the amount of pain. There may also be swelling with a bone tumor. Imaging is required.

Compartment syndrome is a painful condition that occurs when pressure within the muscles builds to dangerous levels. This pressure can decrease blood flow, which prevents nourishment and oxygen from reaching nerve and muscle cells. Compartment syndrome can be either acute or chronic. Acute compartment syndrome is a medical emergency. It is usually caused by a severe injury. There may be pain, decreased pulses, paresthesias, pallor, and paralysis. Chronic compartment syndrome, also known as exertional compartment syndrome, is usually not a medical emergency. It is most often caused by athletic exertion. However, the patient usually complains of a bursting type of pressure and pain, and that was not the case here.

Shin splints (medial tibial stress syndrome) is a common condition that can be distinguished from tibial stress fractures by nonfocal tenderness (diffuse along the mid-distal, posteromedial tibia) and a lack of edema.

Type of Reasoning: Analytical

This question requires one to determine the most likely diagnosis based on a description of symptoms. Questions of this nature often necessitate analytical reasoning skill, where information is analyzed in order to draw reasonable conclusions. For this scenario, the symptoms are most consistent with a stress fracture. Review signs and symptoms of stress fractures if answered incorrectly.

A63 

Gastrointestinal | Evaluation, Diagnosis

A patient is referred to physical therapy with a chief complaint of pain involving their hips, low back, and shoulders. The patient is unable to identify any precipitating event or trauma that led to their symptoms. During the physical examination of these regions, the therapist is unable to reproduce the patient's symptoms. The patient also reports experiencing recent bouts of diarrhea, abdominal pain, and skin rashes. The therapist suspects that a systemic disorder may account for all of the patient's complaints. Which disease is the most likely explanation for this patient's clinical presentation?

Choices:

1. Colorectal cancer.
2. Inflammatory bowel disease.
3. Diverticulitis.
4. Pancreatitis.

Teaching Points

Correct Answer: 2

Inflammatory bowel disease (IBD) refers to two inflammatory conditions: Crohn's disease and ulcerative colitis. The etiology of these two disorders is unknown but thought to be due to genetic or immunologic influences on the gastrointestinal (GI) tract. Both diseases cause inflammation inside the intestine as well as significant problems in other parts of the body including polyarthritis and migratory arthralgias. Diarrhea, constipation, abdominal pain, fever, rectal bleeding, night sweats, skin rashes and uveitis are other clinical signs and symptoms of IBD. IBD is a different clinical entity than IBS–irritable bowel syndrome.

Incorrect Choices:

Common signs and symptoms of colorectal cancer include rectal bleeding; hemorrhoids; abdominal, pelvic, back, and sacral pain; diarrhea, nausea and vomiting; constipation; and unexplained weight loss. Diverticulitis involves inflamed pouches of intestine that can also lead to abdominal pain and nausea. Left lower quadrant pain is another common symptom of diverticulitis, along with flatulence, bloody stools, and constipation. Patients with pancreatitis typically complain of epigastric pain that radiates to the mid back; nausea, vomiting and diarrhea; abdominal distention; and malaise. They may also exhibit jaundice and in severe cases may exhibit a bluish discoloration of the abdomen (Cullen's sign) or discoloration of the flanks (Grey Turner's sign) due to hemorrhage.

Type of Reasoning: Inferential

For this question, one must weigh the patient's symptoms and then infer which disease is most likely to be present. This requires inferential reasoning skill, where the test-taker predicts what is true of a situation. In this case, the symptoms are most likely to be due to IBD. If answered incorrectly, review IBD symptoms.

A64 

Nonsystem I Research

A research team compares the effects of exercise mode (concentric and eccentric strengthening) on patients with chronic Achilles' tendinopathy. Measurements of disability and performance are collected at baseline, after 12 weeks of treatment, and at 1 year post-treatment. Which is the best statistical test to use to determine which exercise mode is best at decreasing disability over time?

Choices:

1. One-way analysis of variance (ANOVA).
2. Repeated measures ANOVA.
3. Two-way ANOVA with repeated measures on one factor.
4. Two-way ANOVA with repeated measures on both factors.

Teaching Points

Correct Answer: 3

The study has two independent variables (exercise mode and time). Exercise mode is a between-subjects (nonrepeated) factor with two levels (concentric and eccentric). Time is a within-subjects (repeated) factor with three levels (baseline, 12 weeks, and 1 year). The two-way ANOVA with repeated measures on one factor (also called a two-way mixed model ANOVA) is used to compare each factor independently (main effects) as well as the effect of one factor on the other (interaction effect).

Incorrect Choices:

The one-way ANOVA is used to compare a single independent variable (between subjects factor) with at least three levels. A repeated measures ANOVA is used to compare a single independent variable (within-subjects factor) with at least three levels. A two-way ANOVA with repeated measures on both factors is used to compare two independent variables that are both within-subjects factors (all participants are exposed to all levels of each independent variable). Each independent variable would have to have at least two levels in this case.

Type of Reasoning: Deductive

For this question, the test-taker must recall research guidelines in order to arrive at a correct conclusion. This necessitates deductive reasoning skill, where factual recall of information guides conclusions. For this case, the best statistical test is the two-way ANOVA with repeated measures on one factor. If answered incorrectly, review statistical tests information.

A65 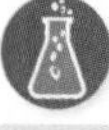

Cardiovascular/Pulmonary I Evaluation, Diagnosis

A patient presents with hemosiderin changes and increased lower extremity edema. What diagnosis are these changes consistent with?

Choices:

1. Chronic venous insufficiency.
2. Acute venous insufficiency.

3. Acute arterial insufficiency.
4. Chronic arterial insufficiency.

Teaching Points

Correct Answer: 1

Lower extremity edema is usually due to incompetent valves, which causes the edema. Long-standing edema causes staining of the legs because of increased iron from pooling blood.

Incorrect Choices:

While lower extremity edema would be present in acute venous insufficiency, there is not any time for leg staining. Acute arterial insufficiency would cause significant pain, pale or cyanotic skin, and decreased or absent pulses. Chronic arterial insufficiency would cause pain, decreased or absent pulses, and dependent rubor along with trophic changes (nail changes, loss of hair, and pale, shiny skin).

Type of Reasoning: Analytical

For this question, one must analyze the symptoms presented and make a determination of the most likely diagnosis. This necessitates analytical reasoning skill, where symptoms are assessed to determine a sound conclusion. For this situation, the symptoms are consistent with chronic venous insufficiency. If answered incorrectly, review venous insufficiency information.

A66 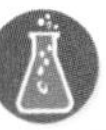

Neuromuscular | Evaluation, Diagnosis

A patient experienced a cerebrovascular accident (right CVA) 2 weeks ago. The patient has motor and sensory impairments primarily in the left lower extremity; the left upper extremity shows only mild impairment. The patient exhibits some confusion and perseveration. Based on these findings, what type of stroke syndrome does this patient present with?

Choices:

1. Posterior cerebral artery stroke.
2. Internal carotid syndrome.
3. Anterior cerebral artery syndrome.
4. Middle cerebral artery syndrome.

Teaching Points

Correct Answer: 3

These signs and symptoms are characteristic of anterior cerebral artery (ACA) syndrome, with contralateral hemiplegia and lower extremities more affected than upper extremities.

Incorrect Choices:

Posterior cerebral artery (PCA) syndrome typically presents with visual impairments, pain, and involuntary movements. Contralateral hemiplegia may also be present, but lacks specific findings with regards to greater impact on the upper or lower extremities. Middle cerebral artery (MCA) syndrome results in contralateral hemiplegia with greater involvement of the upper extremities than lower. Internal carotid lesions typically involve a massive infarction in the areas of the brain supplied by the MCA and ACA, producing significant edema with possible uncal herniation, coma, and death.

Type of Reasoning: Analytical

For this question, the test-taker must analyze the symptoms presented and determine the specific type of stroke syndrome. Questions that require one to determine a diagnosis based on symptoms often necessitate analytical reasoning skill. In this case, the symptoms are consistent with anterior cerebral artery syndrome. Review types of stroke if answered incorrectly.

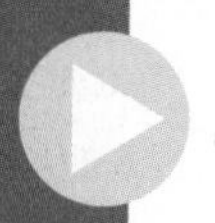

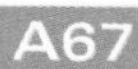

A67

Cardiovascular/Pulmonary | Examination

A patient with Guillain-Barré syndrome was just weaned from a ventilator. The patient has a maximal inspiratory pressure (MIP) of $-35cmH_2O$ and maximal expiratory pressure (MEP) of $40cmH_2O$. Which of the following is an expected finding on examination?

Choices:

1. Asymmetrical decreased costal expansion.
2. Increased inspiration: expiration (I:E) ratio.
3. Increased subcostal angle.
4. Ineffective cough for secretion clearance.

Teaching Points

Correct Answer: 4

Both the MIP and MEP findings indicate significant ventilator muscle weakness. The patient will have difficulty drawing air in and forcefully expelling it, which are two phases of an effective cough. Therefore, the patient will have difficulty clearing their secretions. See Tables 5-1 and 5-2 for normal values of MIP and MEP.

Incorrect Choices:

A patient with Guillain-Barré syndrome will present as if they have a restrictive lung disease. The patient will have decreased costal expansion, but it will be symmetrical. Both increased I:E ratio and subcostal angle are findings consistent with someone with obstructive lung disease and lung hyperinflation, not restrictive lung disease.

Type of Reasoning: Analytical

This question provides pulmonary findings and the test-taker must determine the expected finding on examination. One must weigh the information presented to draw a reasonable conclusion, necessitating analytical reasoning skill. For this case, the MIP and MEP findings indicate ineffective cough for secretion clearance. If answered incorrectly, review pulmonary guidelines, especially MIP and MEP.

A68

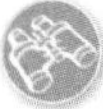

Cardiovascular/Pulmonary | Evaluation, Diagnosis

A therapist is planning to use percussion and shaking for assisting airway clearance with a patient diagnosed with chronic obstructive pulmonary disease (COPD). What major precaution might curtail selection of this form of intervention?

Choices:

1. A platelet count of 20,000.
2. Dyspnea when in the Trendelenburg position.
3. SaO_2 range of 88%–94% on room air.
4. Diagnosis of multilobe pneumonia.

Teaching Points

Correct Answer: 1

A patient with a platelet count of 20,000 is at increased risk for bleeding. Percussion may cause microtraumas and increased bleeding risk.

Incorrect Choices:

While dyspnea in Trendelenburg is uncomfortable, the position could be modified so that percussion and vibration can be completed. While an SaO2 range of 88%–94% on room air is a consideration, it would not preclude this intervention. This should be monitored closely while considered positions maximize ventilation and perfusion. While this patient will require assistance for positioning, it doesn't eliminate this treatment intervention. Pneumonia is an indication for manual airway clearance techniques. The therapist will need to complete the techniques in multiple postural drainage positions to optimize efficiency.

Type of Reasoning: Inductive

This question requires the test-taker to utilize clinical judgment in order to determine a best course of action. This requires inductive reasoning skill. In this case, a platelet count of 20,000 would curtail selection of the specific intervention approach. Review indications and contraindications for airway clearance techniques if answered incorrectly.

A69 

Musculoskeletal | Examination

A patient with degenerative joint disease of the right hip complains of pain in the anterior hip and groin, which is aggravated by weight bearing. There is decreased range of motion and capsular restrictions. Right gluteus medius weakness is evident during ambulation, and there is decreased tolerance of functional activities including transfers and lower extremity dressing. In this case, a capsular pattern of joint motion should be evident by which of the following?

Choices:

1. Hip flexion, abduction, and internal rotation.
2. Hip flexion, adduction, and internal rotation.
3. Hip extension, abduction, and external rotation.
4. Hip flexion, abduction, and external rotation.

Teaching Points

Correct Answer: 1

The capsular pattern of the hip is limitation of flexion/internal rotation with some limitation of abduction. Additionally, according to the Hip Pain/Hip Osteoarthritis Clinical Practice Guideline (see Box 2-1), hip IR or flexion that is 15° less than the nonpainful side is strongly associated with hip OA.

Incorrect Choices:

The other patterns are not representative capsular patterns of the hip.

Type of Reasoning: Inferential

One must recall the capsular patterns of the hip in order to determine what is likely to be true for the patient in this question. This requires inferential reasoning skill, where one utilizes knowledge to determine likely symptoms or presentation of problems. In this case, the patient would likely show limitations in hip flexion, abduction, and internal rotation. Review capsular patterns of the hip if answered incorrectly.

Exam A

A70 

Musculoskeletal | Examination

Confirmation of a diagnosis of spondylolisthesis can be made when viewing an oblique radiograph of the spine. What is the relevant diagnostic finding?

Choices:
1. Posterior displacement of L5 over S1.
2. Bamboo appearance of the spine.
3. Compression of the vertebral bodies of L5 and S1.
4. Bilateral pars interarticularis defects.

Teaching Points

Correct Answer: 4

Spondylolisthesis is defined as forward translation of a vertebral body with respect to the vertebra below. Spondylolysis, a break in the vertebra typically in the region of the pars interarticularis, may or may not be associated with a spondylolisthesis. If the pars defect is bilateral, it may allow slippage of the vertebra, typically L5 on S1, resulting in spondylolisthesis. Most cases are thought to result from minor overuse trauma, particularly repetitive hyperextension of the lumbar spine.

Incorrect Choices:

Posterior displacement of L5 over S1 is the wrong direction. Bamboo appearance of the spine would be found with ankylosing spondylitis. Compression of the vertebral bodies of L5 and S1 would be classified as compression fractures and generally would not result in forward slippage of a vertebra.

Type of Reasoning: Inferential

One must recall the typical diagnostic finding of spondylolisthesis in order to arrive at a correct conclusion. This requires the test-taker to infer the likely symptoms based on knowledge of the diagnosis, which is an inferential reasoning skill. For this situation, one would expect to see bilateral pars interarticularis defects. If answered incorrectly, review radiograph findings of spondylolisthesis.

A71 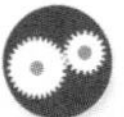

Nonsystem | Professional Responsibilities

A physical therapist and physical therapist assistant are conducting a cardiac rehabilitation session for 20 patients. The therapist is suddenly called out of the room. The physical therapist assistant should do which of the following?

Choices:
1. Terminate the exercises and have the patients monitor their pulses until the therapist returns.
2. Have the patients continue with the same exercise until the therapist returns.
3. Have the patients switch to a less intense exercise until the therapist returns.
4. Continue with the outlined exercise progression for that session.

Teaching Points

Correct Answer: 4

The physical therapist provided an exercise program, and it is appropriate for the PTA to continue to follow it.

Incorrect Choices:

There is no need to terminate exercise since the patients have an established exercise program. It is within a PTA's scope of practice to progress a program, so there is no need to maintain the same intensity of exercise. There is no need to reduce the intensity of the program, as the PTA can monitor and progress a program.

Type of Reasoning: Evaluative

This question requires one to determine a best course of action based on knowledge of supervisory guidelines and scope of practice information. This requires evaluative reasoning skill, where one weighs the options presented and determines a best course of action. For this scenario, the PTA should continue with the outlined exercise progression for that session. Review scope of practice guidelines if answered incorrectly.

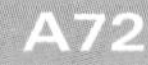

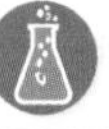

Neuromuscular | Evaluation, Diagnosis

A patient reports progressive fatigue, muscle weakness, and soreness in the bilateral shoulder and pelvic girdle muscles for the past 4 months. The patient's past medical history is unremarkable with the exception of a 10-year history of high cholesterol and hypertension. Neuromuscular screening of the bilateral upper and lower extremities revealed weakness (4-/5 manual muscle testing) of various shoulder/scapular and pelvic muscles bilaterally. Cranial nerve, sensory, and reflex (to include Babinski/Clonus) testing are normal. Which of the following health conditions is most consistent with the patient's signs and symptoms?

Choices:

1. Guillain-Barré syndrome.
2. Myopathy.
3. Myasthenia gravis.
4. Amyotrophic lateral sclerosis.

Teaching Points

Correct Answer: 2

Myopathy typically impacts proximal muscles to a greater extent than distal muscles. Cholesterol lowering drugs (statins) are a risk factor for the development of myopathy.

Incorrect Choices:

Guillain-Barré syndrome (GBS) typically follows a respiratory illness or vaccination and causes rapid demyelination of multiple peripheral nerves resulting in rapid and acute proximal to distal weakness. Although myasthenia gravis causes fatigue and ultimately weakness in multiple muscles in the bilateral upper and lower extremities, it also presents with mild ptosis and involvement of ocular and/or oropharyngeal muscles. Amyotrophic lateral sclerosis may also cause fatigue/weakness, but it typically presents with asymmetric weakness and is defined by both lower and upper motor neuron involvement.

Type of Reasoning: Analytical

This question provides a group of symptoms and the test-taker must determine the most likely condition. This necessitates analytical reasoning skill, where information is analyzed to determine its meaning and significance, then draw a reasonable conclusion. For this case, the symptoms are consistent with myopathy. If answered incorrectly, review information on myopathy, especially signs and symptoms.

A73 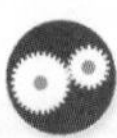

Nonsystem I Professional Responsibilities

Initially, a patient was seen by a physical therapist (PT) in an outpatient clinic for 2 weeks. As it was difficult for the patient to arrange transportation, the therapist has decided to follow this patient by using telerehabilitation. After 6 weeks, the therapist decides that the patient's exercise regime needs to be progressed. How should these exercise progressions **BEST** be implemented?

Choices:

1. Send the patient an app showing the exercise progressions and then watch the patient's performance using electronic means.
2. Have the patient make a trip back to the clinic to be taught the new exercise variations.
3. Describe the exercise progressions over the phone to the patient, while simultaneously viewing their performance electronically.
4. Demonstrate the exercises to the patient electronically and then view the patient's performance.

Teaching Points

Correct Answer: 4

Telehealth/telerehabilitation involves two-way, visual communication between the parties involved, in this case, between the PT and the patient at home. Often, tablets are used and visual insets of the participants are seen on both devices. In this case, the exercises are to be progressed. It would be **BEST** and quite efficient for the PT to demonstrate to this patient what needs to be done differently and then view how the patient performs. Recall that the PT and patient have been conducting electronic rehabilitation for some time. The process is interactive. There is no implication that the plan of care is to be radically changed.

Incorrect Choices:

While sending an app may be a supplementary way for reinforcing the exercise progressions, it is not the best means to ensure correct compliance. Comprehension of written English, difficulty with interpreting what needs to be done or pictorial instruction, and other factors may be deterrents to correct performance.

Describing the exercises on the phone to the patient is unnecessary as two-way visual communication is available and well established.

Having the patient return to the clinic is unnecessary at this time. If there was a significant change to the plan of care, if a reexamination of the patient was necessary, or perhaps a discharge visit was required, then a trip to the clinic would be in order. That's not the case here.

Type of Reasoning: Evaluative

For this question, the test-taker must weigh the potential approaches and determine which approach is best for the patient. Evaluative reasoning skills are utilized whenever one must weigh the benefits and potential drawbacks of a potential course of action. For this scenario, the therapist should demonstrate the exercises to the patient electronically and then view the patient's performance. Review telerehabilitation guidelines if answered incorrectly.

A74 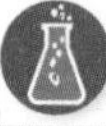

Musculoskeletal I Evaluation, Diagnosis

A patient is seen in physical therapy with a complaint of ring finger pain and weakness after an injury sustained while playing football. The patient describes grabbing an opponent's uniform and feeling a painful pop in the finger during an attempted tackle. During the physical examination, the therapist observes swelling of the distal and middle phalanges of the ring finger, tenderness to palpation of the distal interphalangeal (DIP) joint region, and inability to produce flexion at the DIP joint. What is the **MOST LIKELY** diagnosis?

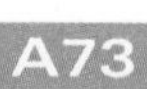

Choices:

1. Boutonniere deformity.
2. Mallet finger.
3. Swan neck deformity.
4. Jersey finger.

Teaching Points

Correct Answer: 4

Jersey finger is the eponym for a rupture or avulsion fracture of the flexor digitorum profundus (FDP) tendon at its insertion on the distal phalanx. The ring finger is involved in 75% of cases of jersey finger because it is more prominent than the other digits during grip. The mechanism of injury is forceful extension of the DIP joint during maximal contraction of the FDP. The key physical examination finding is an inability to actively flex the DIP joint in isolation.

Incorrect Choices:

A boutonniere deformity results from rupture of the central tendinous slip of the extensor tendon mechanism. With boutonniere deformities, the PIP is in a position of flexion and between the two lateral bands of the extensor mechanism. A swan neck deformity results from injury to the volar plate or transverse retinacular ligament, producing a deformity of flexion of the MCP and DIP joints with relative hyperextension of the PIP. Boutonniere and swan neck deformities may result from trauma but are often seen in patients with rheumatoid arthritis. A mallet finger results from rupture or avulsion of the terminal tendon of the extensor mechanism at the insertion on the distal phalanx. The mechanism of injury is usually traumatic forced flexion of the DIP joint and results in a deformity of flexion of the DIP with an inability to produce active extension.

Type of Reasoning: Analytical

This question requires one to analyze the symptoms presented and determine the likely diagnosis. This requires analytical reasoning skill, where pieces of information are evaluated in order to conclude what they mean as a whole. In this case, the presenting symptoms are most likely associated with jersey finger. Review information on jersey finger, especially symptoms and mechanism of injury, if answered incorrectly.

A75 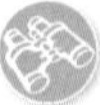

Cardiovascular/Pulmonary | Evaluation, Diagnosis

A patient with chronic asthma has been admitted to the hospital for an acute exacerbation. What is the **MOST** important information the therapist needs in order to determine the patient's prognosis with physical therapy?

Choices:

1. A current medication list.
2. A previous history of the disease.
3. The most recent chest x-ray results.
4. The most recent pulmonary function test results.

Teaching Points

Correct Answer: 4

Recent pulmonary function test results will give the therapist information regarding the severity of the lung disease. This information will assist in determining how much the patient will progress.

Incorrect Choices:

While the current medication list will help determine how the patient is currently being managed, it doesn't give any information about his or her function. The previous history of the disease will not translate well into what the patient's function has been. It is possible that he or she has been quite functional despite terrible disease such that an acute exacerbation with little reserve will leave him or her quite limited. An acute asthma exacerbation will likely not appear on a chest x-ray, nor would chronic disease.

Type of Reasoning: Inductive

One must utilize clinical judgment in order to determine the most important information about a patient with asthma. Questions of this nature, where clinical judgment and knowledge are applied to patient cases, often necessitate inductive reasoning skill. For this situation, the most important information is the most recent pulmonary function test results. If answered incorrectly, review pulmonary rehab, including pulmonary testing information.

A76 

Nonsystem I Equipment, Devices

A therapist is examining the gait of a patient with a transfemoral prosthesis. The patient circumducts the prosthetic limb during swing. The therapist needs to identify the cause of the gait deviation. What is the **MOST** likely prosthetic cause?

Choices:

1. Unstable knee unit.
2. Inadequate socket flexion.
3. High medial wall or abducted hip joint.
4. Increased knee flexion resistance.

Teaching Points

Correct Answer: 4

Prosthetic causes of circumduction include a long prosthesis, locked knee unit, inadequate knee flexion, inadequate suspension, small or loose socket, and plantar flexed foot.

Incorrect Choices:

An unstable knee unit will cause forward flexion during stance. Inadequate socket flexion will result in lordosis during stance. A high medial wall or abducted hip joint will result in an abducted gait.

Type of Reasoning: Inferential

For this question, one must determine the reason for a specific gait deviation in order to arrive at a correct conclusion. One must apply knowledge of prosthetics in order to infer the most likely reason, which necessitates inferential reasoning skill. For this situation, the most likely cause is increased knee flexion resistance, which will not allow adequate knee flexion during swing phase. Review lower extremity prosthetics information if answered incorrectly.

A77 Neuromuscular | Examination

A middle-aged adult experienced a mild traumatic brain injury 1 month ago and has been undergoing rehabilitation. The patient initially had intermittent headaches, dizziness, and difficulty with dynamic balance, but now reports resolution of all symptoms. The dizziness handicap inventory score on the last visit was 1/100 at baseline and 3/100 after walking 10 minutes. The Mini-Balance Evaluation System Test (Mini-BEST) on the last visit was 26/28. The patient would like to go back to their previous active lifestyle, to include running. Which of the following examination items would provide the most complete assessment for safe return to work and recreation?

Choices:

1. Functional Gait Assessment (FGA).
2. Four Square Step Test (FSST).
3. Functional Independence Measure (FIM).
4. Community Balance and Mobility Scale (CBMT).

Teaching Points

Correct Answer: 4

The patient's performance on the dizziness handicap inventory and Mini-BEST reinforce their symptoms (both at rest and exertion) have improved and fall risk is very low. The CBMT is the correct answer as it includes higher level balance and mobility items, to include running short distances. It is also a reliable and valid tool for patients who have experienced a TBI (see Table 3-16).

Incorrect Choices:

The FGA and FIM do not assess higher level balance and mobility items. The FSST requires dynamic mobility and balance in multiple planes but does not specifically address running or other higher level community tasks.

Type of Reasoning: Inductive

This question requires one to use clinical judgment to determine the best examination item to assess for safe return to work and recreation. This requires inductive reasoning skill. For this situation, the best examination item is the CBMT. If answered incorrectly, review information on brain injury assessment, especially the CBMT.

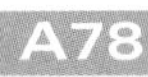

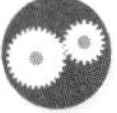

A78 System Interactions | Evaluation, Diagnosis

An elderly patient with degenerative joint disease is seen by a physical therapist 3 days following a total knee replacement. Which of these findings would be an indication for the therapist to contact the surgeon?

Choices:

1. Patient is noncompliant when learning to transfer properly.
2. Patient cannot ambulate at least 50 feet with a standard walker.
3. Patient fails to recognize the therapist on the third consecutive postoperative visit.
4. Patient complains of soreness at the incision site.

Teaching Points

Correct Answer: 3

Postoperative adverse effects on the cardiac, pulmonary, and neuromuscular systems and on cognitive function are the main concerns for elderly surgical patients who are at high risk. Postoperative delirium is characterized by incoherent thought and speech, disorientation, impaired memory, and attention. Elderly patients usually manifest delirium following a lucid interval of 1 postoperative day or more, a condition known as interval delirium. Symptoms are often worse at night. Alternatively, the condition can be silent and unnoticed, or misdiagnosed as depression. However, the effects of elderly postoperative delirium are evident in increased morbidity, delayed functional recovery, and prolonged hospital stay. Fortunately, the postoperative cognitive dysfunction is a reversible condition in the majority of elderly surgical patients. Preoperative risk factors of bilateral total knee arthroplasty are associated with a significantly higher incidence of acute delirium than unilateral total knee arthroplasty in patients over 80 years.

Failing to recognize the therapist after three visits is an indication of a declining mental condition. This would definitely be a safety consideration as the patient may not be able to follow all the precautions and may also put himself or herself in danger by walking without an ambulatory aid, etc. Wound infection is also a consideration. Contacting the surgeon is necessary.

Incorrect Choices:

Soreness at the incision site would be an expected common complaint. The patient being noncompliant could potentially be a safety issue; however, the therapist should first attempt behavior modification. If that failed, they could get advice from a co-worker and possibly counseling for the patient if deemed necessary. Not being able to ambulate 50 feet could be due to many problems, including pain, weakness, and balance issues. None of these factors require consultation with the surgeon at this time.

Type of Reasoning: Evaluative

For this question, one must determine a best course of action based on presenting signs. Questions of this nature, where information is weighed to determine its significance, often necessitate evaluative reasoning skill. For this scenario, the patient failing to recognize the therapist on the third consecutive postoperative visit would be an indication to contact the surgeon. Review adverse postoperative effects, especially in older adults, if answered incorrectly.

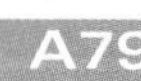

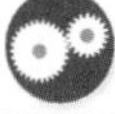

Nonsystem | Safety and Protection

The Emergency Activation Plan (EAP) has been activated at a large rehabilitation hospital. A disgruntled former employee is roaming the corridors making threats and promising violence. At this time, the therapeutic gymnasium is busy with patients with a variety of serious disabilities undergoing treatment. In this situation, which action should the therapists take **FIRST**?

Choices:

1. Rapidly return all patients to their rooms in order to shelter-in-place.
2. Evacuate the gym via the designated fire stairs to get outside the building.
3. Create a barrier to the main entrance to the gym using available heavy equipment or weights.
4. Shelter all patients in a corner of the gym and surround and protect them with all available equipment and devices.

Teaching Points

Correct Answer: 3

Blockading the entrance is the FIRST thing to do. There is no mention of an active shooter. May have a knife or other weapon, even a gun; however, up to this point it is verbal threats only. In this scenario, locking and/or blocking the gym entrance would be the most prudent thing to do first considering the patient population in the gym at the time. Disaster protocols may vary among clinical facilities and each employee must be aware of that protocol.

Incorrect Choices:

Using fire stairs impractical with wheelchairs and patients with serious disabilities. Evacuation would not be the first action to take based on the situation. Returning patients to their rooms may put therapists and patients in harm's way as a confrontation with the perpetrator is more likely.

Placing all patients together in one dead-end space could make them all an easy target even if trying to protect them. Barring the perpetrator from the gymnasium would be a more logical action.

Type of Reasoning: Evaluative

For this question, one must make a value judgment of a best course of action, based on the presenting information. This requires the test-taker to weigh the merits of the potential courses of action in order to determine which option should be utilized first. In this scenario, the therapists should create a barrier to the main gym entrance using available heavy equipment or weights first. Review emergency procedures, especially disaster protocols and guidelines.

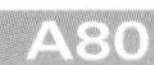

Cardiovascular/Pulmonary I Examination

Following a hard tackle, a football player exhibits signs of fractured ribs and a pneumothorax. When auscultating during inhalation over the injured area, what would the physical therapist expect to hear?

Choices:

1. Soft, rustling sounds on inhalation.
2. Decreased or no breath sounds.
3. Crackles.
4. Wheezes.

Teaching Points

Correct Answer: 2

The fractured ribs will cause the patient to have pain and therefore not take deep breaths. More importantly, the pneumothorax will cause an increasing positive pressure on the lung, not allowing it to inflate. The result will be minimal air movement and decreased or absent breath sounds.

Incorrect Choices:

Soft, rustling sounds are normal, vesicular breath sounds. These would not be present with these injuries. Crackles would indicate atelectasis or secretions, but it would not be possible to hear these sounds with these injuries because there is minimal air movement. Likewise, wheezes wouldn't be possible to hear.

Type of Reasoning: Deductive

One must recall the auscultation sounds with a pneumothorax in order to arrive at a correct conclusion. This necessitates the recall of factual information, which is a deductive reasoning skill. For this case, one would expect to hear decreased or no breath sounds. Review auscultation guidelines, especially with pneumothorax, if answered incorrectly.

A81 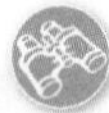

Cardiovascular/Pulmonary I Interventions

Which common musculoskeletal complication of cystic fibrosis is important to combat with a resistance training program?

Choices:

1. Carpal tunnel syndrome.
2. Polyarthralgia.
3. Decreased bone density.
4. Joint contractures.

Teaching Points

Correct Answer: 3

In addition to production of a thick and sticky mucus that blocks the airways, patients with CF also produce a thick mucus that can block the common bile duct leading to malabsorption of nutrients and resulting in decreased bone density. A resisted exercise program can assist with reversing the effects of the disease process.

Incorrect Choices:

CF primarily affects the respiratory and digestive systems. There is no evidence that carpal tunnel syndrome or other peripheral neuropathies are a common complication of cystic fibrosis. Patients with cystic fibrosis may present with polyarthralgias (joint swelling and stiffness) and joint contractures, but a strength training program would not be the best intervention to address these impairments.

Type of Reasoning: Inductive

For this question, the test-taker must recall the complications of cystic fibrosis and then prioritize which complication is most important to combat with a resistance training program. This necessitates clinical judgment and knowledge, which is an inductive reasoning skill. For this case, decreased bone density is most important. Review information on cystic fibrosis, especially musculoskeletal complications, if answered incorrectly.

A82 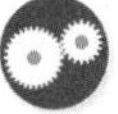

Nonsystem I Safety and Protection

While ambulating a patient in the clinic, the patient trips and falls, hitting his head on the corner of a treatment table. The patient lies motionless on the floor, exhibiting a loss of consciousness lasting 2 minutes and then a drowsiness or inability to fully wake up. What is the first thing the therapist should do?

Choices:

1. Determine the patient's heart rate and blood pressure.
2. Check the head for signs of an external wound.
3. Call emergency medical services.
4. Perform a brief cognitive assessment once the patient is awake.

Teaching Points

Correct Answer: 3

The patient is exhibiting signs of a severe concussion with loss of consciousness for longer than 30 seconds. The therapist should call for emergency medical services immediately.

Incorrect Choices:

Once EMS is activated, the head can be checked for wounds, and resting vital signs (HR and BP) can be taken. A brief cognitive assessment is not appropriate at this time. Other signs of severe concussion the patient may exhibit include one pupil larger than the other, nausea or vomiting, seizures, headache that gets worse with time, slurred speech, decreased coordination, and changes in behavior (irritability, restlessness, agitation).

Type of Reasoning: Evaluative

For this question, the test-taker must weigh the significance of the information presented and make a decision on a best course of action. This necessitates evaluative reasoning skill, where decisions are often made based on the relevance of the information presented. In this case, the information presented is of high importance, necessitating a call for emergency medical services. If answered incorrectly, be sure to review emergency procedures for patient injuries.

A83 

Integumentary | Examination

A therapist is examining a patient with an ulcer in the lower leg/ankle and suspects it is an arterial rather than a venous ulcer. One of the factors the therapist uses to determine this is based on the location of the ulcer. What is the typical location of an arterial ulcer?

Choices:

1. Medial malleolus.
2. Posterior tibial area.
3. Lateral malleolus.
4. Medial distal tibia.

Teaching Points

Correct Answer: 3

The typical location of an arterial ulcer is the distal lower leg (toes, foot), the lateral malleolus, or the anterior tibial area.

Incorrect Choices:

The typical location of a venous ulcer is the distal lower leg and the medial malleolus.

Type of Reasoning: Inferential

One must determine what is likely to be true of a situation in order to arrive at a correct conclusion for this question. This necessitates inferential reasoning skill. The test-taker must utilize knowledge of arterial ulcers to determine what is likely to be true. In this case, the typical location of an arterial ulcer is on the lateral malleolus. Review information on arterial ulcers if answered incorrectly.

A84 

Genitourinary | Evaluation, Diagnosis

During pregnancy, the presence of the hormone relaxin can lead to abnormal movement and pain. Which joints are typically affected?

Choices:

1. Glenohumeral joints.
2. Hip joints.
3. Lumbrosacral joints.
4. Sacroiliac joints.

Teaching Points

Correct Answer: 4

The sacroiliac (SI) joints are most often affected in pregnancy, resulting in pain.

Incorrect Choices:

The other joints are not typically affected. Low back pain is common in pregnancy, largely resulting from the physical changes (added weight, poor muscle tone, increased lordosis, loose pelvic ligaments).

Type of Reasoning: Deductive

For this question, the test-taker must recall the typical joints that are affected by pregnancy and may result in pain in order to arrive at a correct conclusion. This necessitates the recall of factual information, which is a deductive reasoning skill. For this scenario, the sacroiliac joints are typically affected by pregnancy. Review pregnancy and common physical changes if answered incorrectly.

A85 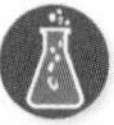

Lymphatic | Interventions

A client with Stage I lymphedema of the right lower extremity is referred for physical therapy. The therapist considers a program of complete decongestive therapy (CDT). An important component of CDT is manual lymphatic drainage. How should the therapist **BEST** perform this procedure?

1. Starting at the distal portion of the limb and working proximally to move the lymph toward the right lymphatic duct.
2. Starting at the proximal portion of the limb and working distally to move the lymph toward the thoracic duct.
3. Following application of intermittent pneumatic compression to the right lower extremity.
4. By performing deep tissue friction massage for several minutes on fibrotic areas prior to CDT.

Teaching Points

Correct Answer: 2

Manual lymphatic drainage is a component of a CDT plan for patients with lymphedema. Because of the very low forces present in the lymph system, lymph load in proximal areas must be relieved prior to progressing to areas where lymphedema is present. This proximal to distal approach maximizes any benefits that may occur from this treatment technique. Additionally, the anatomy of the lymph system requires movement of lower extremity lymph toward the thoracic duct. Only right upper quarter lymph would be directed toward the right lymphatic duct.

Incorrect Choices:

Intermittent pneumatic compression may be a treatment alternative when care is utilized to avoid damaging the lymph system by using low pressure, sequential compression. Additionally, the practice is limited to use in the upper extremity due to the unacceptable risk of causing genital lymphedema if performed in the lower extremity. Deep tissue friction massage is not indicated in patients with lymphedema. Aggressive manipulation of the integument may cause damage to lymphatic structures.

Type of Reasoning: Analytical

For this question, the test-taker must analyze the symptoms presented in order to determine the most likely diagnosis. This requires analytical reasoning skill, where pieces of information are analyzed in order to draw a logical conclusion. In this situation, the symptoms are indicative of secondary lymphedema. Review secondary lymphedema if answered incorrectly.

A86 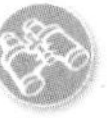

Nonsystem I Equipment, Devices

A patient has a body mass index (BMI) of 32 kg/m^2 with excessive tissue mass in the hip area. What accommodations are needed to the wheelchair prescription for this patient?

Choices:

1. Move the small front casters closer to the drive wheels to increase stability.
2. Add friction rims to increase handgrip function.
3. Add an antitipping device to prevent falls going up curbs.
4. Displace the rear axle forward for more efficient arm push.

Teaching Points

Correct Answer: 4

This patient is obese. A bariatric wheelchair with heavy-duty, extra-wide wheels is necessary. The rear axle is displaced forward compared to the standard wheelchair to allow for more efficient arm push.

Incorrect Choices:

Moving the front casters closer to the drive wheels would decrease stability (not increase). Friction rims and antitipping devices are adjustments that may be necessary for the patient with a spinal cord injury.

Type of Reasoning: Inductive

For this question, one must utilize knowledge of wheelchair prescription for patients with obesity in order to arrive at a correct conclusion. Clinical judgment coupled with knowledge of wheelchair prescription guidelines are required, which necessitates inductive reasoning skill. For this case, the therapist should recommend a wheelchair in which the rear axle is displaced forward for more efficient arm push. Review wheelchair prescription guidelines, especially for patient with obesity, if answered incorrectly.

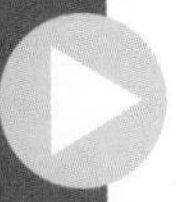

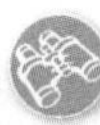

A87

Neuromuscular | Interventions

A patient is diagnosed with benign paroxysmal positional vertigo (BPPV). What intervention should the plan of care for this patient emphasize?

Choices:

1. Gaze stability exercises using horizontal head rotation (X1 viewing).
2. Canalith repositioning treatment.
3. Postural stability exercises in sitting using a therapy ball.
4. Habituation exercises using provocative positions and movements.

Teaching Points

Correct Answer: 2

The goal of treatment is to remove the otoconia that have become dislodged and are free-floating in the semicircular canal (SCC), or canalithiasis. The patient's head is guided through a series of movements to move the debris out of the involved SCC and into the vestibule. Once moved, the symptoms should resolve. Canalith repositioning maneuver (modified Epley) is used for canalithiasis.

Incorrect Choices:

Gaze stability exercises and postural stability exercises (sitting on a ball) are treatments used for unilateral and bilateral vestibular hypofunction (UVH, BVH). Habituation training (motion sensitivity training) is used when a patient with UVH presents with continual complaints of dizziness. Patients with central vestibular lesions may also benefit from habituation exercises.

Type of Reasoning: Inductive

For this question, the test-taker must recall intervention approaches for BPPV in order to arrive at a correct conclusion. Based on knowledge of effective approaches, one will utilize inductive reasoning skill to determine the intervention approach that is most effective. In this case, canalith repositioning treatment is the best approach. Review intervention approaches for BPPV if answered incorrectly.

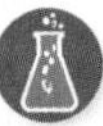

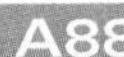

A88

Lymphatic | Evaluation, Diagnosis

An athlete sees a physical therapist with a complaint of "right groin strain." Examination of the musculoskeletal system in the groin is inconclusive; however, the therapist does detect swollen inguinal lymph nodes on the right side only. What should the therapist do next?

Choices:

1. Refer the athlete to a primary care physician to rule out systemic disease.
2. Examine lymph nodes of the neck which may be swollen if mononucleosis is suspected.
3. Ask the patient questions relating to possible STD as many symptoms are mistaken for other conditions.
4. Examine the right foot, leg, and hip for injury or infection.

Teaching Points

Correct Answer: 4

The most common cause of unilateral inguinal lymph node swelling is injury or infection involving the distal foot, leg, thigh, or hip. Abrasions in these areas, fairly routine for many athletes, are potential sources. Insect bites are another possible cause. The therapist should perform a thorough examination and treat any injuries or wounds appropriately.

Incorrect Choices:

Although mononucleosis (Epstein-Barr virus) is prevalent in young athletes, there were no complaints of sore throat or fatigue. The only swollen lymph nodes detected were in the right inguinal area. It is unlikely that mononucleosis is the source. Asking the patient about STDs at this point in the examination is also premature. STDs can result in swollen lymph nodes (chlamydia, gonorrhea, etc.) and not necessarily present with other symptoms, but is this the next step in the PT examination? If the swollen lymph nodes were more extensive and had remained so for 2 or 3 weeks, then referral to a physician would be in order.

Type of Reasoning: Analytical

For this question, the test-taker must utilize knowledge of symptoms that indicate injury or infection to the distal extremity in order to determine a best course of action. This necessitates analytical reasoning skill, where the presenting symptoms are analyzed in order to determine the likely cause and ultimately, the next course of action. For this situation, the symptoms are indicative of potential injury or infection of the distal extremity, and examination of the foot, leg, and hip is the next course of action. Review signs and symptoms of injury and infection in the lower extremity, especially in athletes, if answered incorrectly.

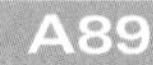

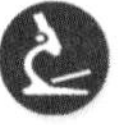

Cardiovascular/Pulmonary I Interventions

What is an acceptable modified position to drain the posterior basal segment of the left lower lobe in a patient with pulmonary infiltrate?

Choices:

1. Side-lying on the right, with a pillow under the right hip and the bed flat.
2. Prone, with a pillow under the hips and the bed flat.
3. Side-lying on the right, with a pillow between the legs and the foot of the bed elevated 18 inches.
4. Prone, with a pillow under the hips and the head of the bed elevated 18 inches.

Teaching Points

Correct Answer: 2

Prone, with a pillow under the hips and the bed flat, will raise the posterior basal segments up to facilitate drainage. This is an acceptable modified position for drainage of the posterior basal segment of the left lower lobe.

Incorrect Choices:

The side-lying position with the bed flat will drain the lingula more than the posterior basal segments. With the bed elevated in side-lying, the pillow position is just for comfort but will not facilitate drainage. Raising the bed up will cause drainage to go toward the base of the lungs, which would not be effective. If the head of the bed is elevated up in prone, drainage will also be more difficult.

Type of Reasoning: Deductive

One must recall the proper positions for posterior basal segment drainage of the left lower lobe in order to arrive at a correct conclusion. This requires recall of facts and guidelines, which is a deductive reasoning skill. In this case, the therapist should position the patient in prone, with a pillow under the hips and the bed flat. Review postural drainage techniques if answered incorrectly.

A90 

Musculoskeletal | Evaluation, Diagnosis

An adult patient is seen in a physical therapy clinic one day after sustaining an ankle inversion injury. The lateral aspect of the ankle is swollen. The patient is having difficulty bearing weight on the involved lower extremity. The therapist is concerned about the possibility of a fracture. What other physical exam finding would indicate a need for ankle radiographs?

Choices:

1. Palpation tenderness at the distal lateral malleolus.
2. Inability to fully dorsiflex the ankle.
3. Positive anterior drawer test.
4. Weak and painful resisted eversion.

Teaching Points

Correct Answer: 1

The Ottawa Ankle Rules (see Box 2-10) were developed to provide clinicians with guidelines for determining when to order an x-ray following an acute ankle injury. Palpation tenderness of either malleoli is one of the criteria. The Ottawa Ankle Rules are highly sensitive and accurately rule out a fracture following an acute ankle injury.

Incorrect Choices:

The other choices are each common and important examination findings in patients after ankle sprain, but none of them is a component of the Ottawa Ankle Rules.

Type of Reasoning: Deductive

For this question, the test-taker must draw from factual recall of the Ottawa Ankle Rules to guide clinical decision-making about when to order ankle radiographs. This requires deductive reasoning skill, where factual information is used to guide clinical reasoning. For this situation, weak and painful resisted inversion would indicate a need for radiographs. Refer to the Ottawa Ankle Rules if answered incorrectly.

A91 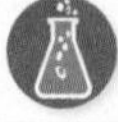

System Interactions | Evaluation, Diagnosis

A patient complains of excessive upper and lower extremity muscle aching, cramping, and right upper quadrant pain when exercising. The patient has a history of chronic alcoholism and was placed on atorvastatin (a statin drug) 2 months ago. The therapist should refer the patient to the primary care physician for which reason?

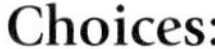

Choices:

1. For an exercise test to determine the right intensity for exercise.
2. To rule out cirrhosis of the liver.
3. To rule out liver and muscle dysfunction from statin.
4. To rule out gallstones that may be obstructing the bile duct.

Teaching Points

Correct Answer: 3

A small percentage of patients (<5%) who take statins (atorvastatin such as Lipitor, or others) can experience myalgia, cramps, stiffness, spasm, or weakness affecting exercise tolerance. The patient needs to see the primary care physician to have the dose or medication changed.

Incorrect Choices:

Determining the appropriate exercise intensity is within the scope of a physical therapist's practice. A physical therapist (PT) is the appropriate professional in this case, so no referral is needed. These signs and symptoms are not consistent with cirrhosis or gallbladder disorders. Exercise would not worsen this condition.

Type of Reasoning: Analytical

For this question, the test-taker must analyze the symptoms presented and determine the likely reason for the symptoms. This necessitates analytical reasoning skill. In this case, the symptoms and current use of a statin drug should prompt the therapist to refer the patient to the physician to rule out liver and muscle dysfunction from statin use. Review side effects of statin use if answered incorrectly.

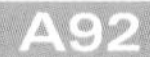

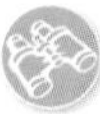

A92

Neuromuscular | Interventions

A patient recovering from traumatic brain injury (TBI) is unable to bring the right foot up on the step during stair climbing training. What is the **BEST** choice to promote independent stair climbing for this patient?

Choices:

1. Practice marching in place.
2. Strengthen the hip flexors using an isokinetic training device before attempting stair climbing.
3. Passively bring the foot up and place it on the 7-inch step.
4. Practice stair climbing inside the parallel bars using a 3-inch step.

Teaching Points

Correct Answer: 4

The most appropriate lead-up activity to promote the skill of stair climbing is practice using a 3-inch step in the parallel bars.

Incorrect Choices:

Passive movements do not promote active learning. Marching in place and isokinetic training may improve the strength of the hip flexors but do not promote the same synergistic patterns of muscle activity as the desired skill.

Type of Reasoning: Inductive

One must determine through clinical judgment the **BEST** approach for promoting the skill of stair climbing. This question requires inductive reasoning skill, in which the test-taker must first determine the problem and then judge which intervention approach leads up to improving stair climbing ability. If this question was answered incorrectly, review information on exercises to promote stair negotiation.

A93 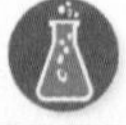

Integumentary | Evaluation, Diagnosis

A physical therapist is performing an examination of an elderly patient who is confined to bed in a custodial care facility. A large ulcer is observed on the right heel as shown in the picture. Based on the staging of pressure ulcers, how would this ulcer be classified?

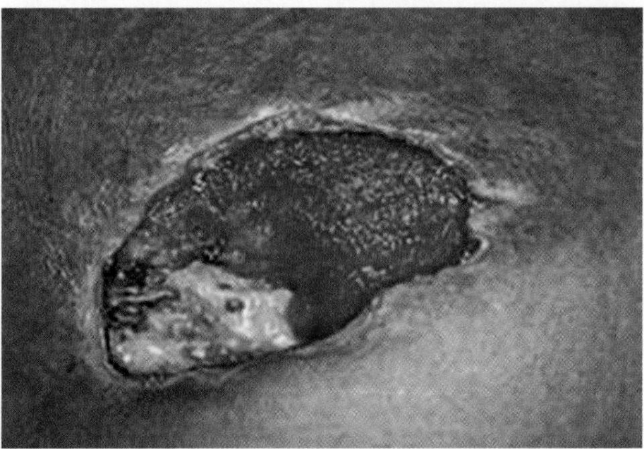

From: Perry, Potter, and Elkin, 2012/Courtesy Laurel Wiersma, RN, MSN, CNS, Barnes-Jewish Hospital.

Choices:

1. Stage I ulcer.
2. Stage II ulcer.
3. Stage III ulcer.
4. Stage IV ulcer.

Teaching Points

Correct Answer: 3

A stage III ulcer is characterized by full-thickness skin loss with damage to or necrosis of subcutaneous tissue. It presents clinically as a crater.

Incorrect Choices:

A stage I ulcer is characterized by nonblanchable erythema of intact skin. A stage II ulcer is characterized by partial-thickness skin loss involving the epidermis or dermis. The ulcer is superficial and presents clinically as an abrasion, blister, or shallow crater. A stage IV ulcer is characterized by full-thickness skin loss with extensive destruction, tissue necrosis, and damage to muscle, bone, or supporting structures. Undermining or sinus tracts may be present.

Type of Reasoning: Analytical

For this question, the test-taker must examine the picture provided and determine the most likely stage of ulceration based on the picture. This requires analysis of information, which is an analytical reasoning skill. For this case, the picture represents a stage III ulcer. Review stages of ulcers if answered incorrectly.

A94 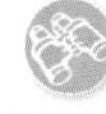

Musculoskeletal | Evaluation, Diagnosis

A patient was referred to a physical therapist with chief complaints of neck and posterior arm pain and paresthesias in the thumb and index finger. A C6 radiculopathy is suspected. The therapist decides to treat the patient with mobilizations of the lower cervical spine. Which statement indicates a favorable response to the treatment?

Choices:

1. Neck pain improves, and distal symptoms increase.
2. Neck pain improves with no change in distal symptoms.
3. No change in neck pain, and distal symptoms increase.
4. No change in neck pain, and distal symptoms decrease.

Teaching Points

Correct Answer: 4

The theme of this question is the centralization phenomenon. McKenzie reported that centralization occurred when a patient's symptoms moved from a distal or peripheral area to a location closer to the spine. Numerous studies have reported that patients with spinal pain who describe a centralization of their symptoms exhibit greater reductions in pain and disability and a better prognosis compared with those who were unable to centralize symptoms. See Box 2-15 for the Neck Pain Clinical Practice Guideline.

Incorrect Choices:

An increase in distal symptoms is a sign that the C6 nerve root is being irritated, which may lead to a deterioration in the patient's neurologic status. An improvement in neck pain with no change in distal symptoms is an acceptable response, but not preferred.

Type of Reasoning: Inductive

For this question, the test-taker must utilize clinical judgment in order to determine which response to treatment indicates a favorable response. This requires inductive reasoning skills. For this scenario, no change in neck pain and distal symptoms decreasing would indicate a favorable response to treatment. Review treatment guidelines for the lower cervical spine, especially mobilizations, if answered incorrectly.

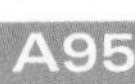
A95
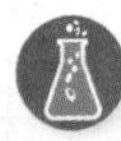

Musculoskeletal | Examination

The physical therapist is examining the muscle length of the patient's left hip and knee. How should the therapist interpret the muscle length test shown in the picture?

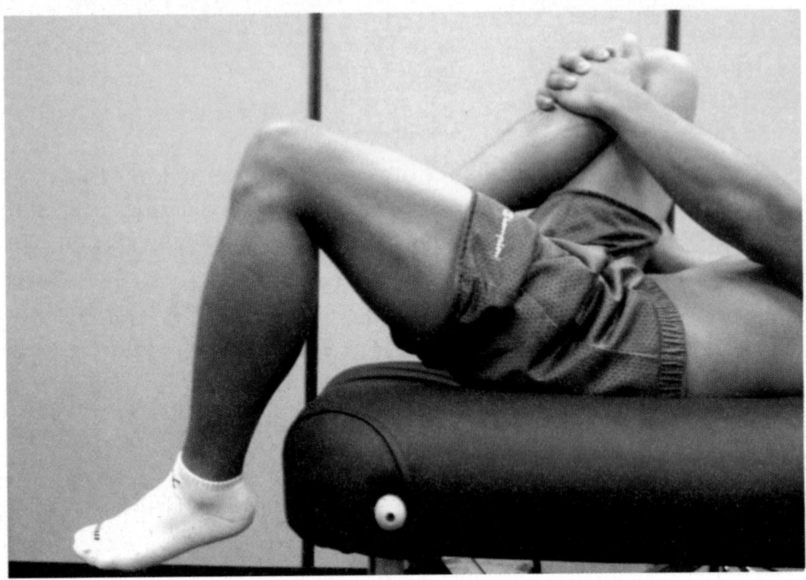

Choices:

1. Shortness of one joint and two joint hip flexors.
2. Shortness of one joint hip flexor with normal two joint hip flexors.
3. Normal one joint hip flexors with tightness of two joint hip flexors.
4. Normal one joint and two joint hip flexors.

Teaching Points

Correct Answer: 2

The posterior thigh does not touch the table, and the knee can be flexed as many degrees beyond 80° as the hip is flexed. The Thomas test is utilized to test for hip flexor length and to distinguish between one joint and two joint hip flexor tightness. With low back and sacrum flat on the table, a normal one joint hip flexor length would be with thigh flat on the table. Normal two joint hip flexor length would be 80° of knee flexion.

Incorrect Choices:

The other choices do not correctly interpret the test results.

Type of Reasoning: Analytical

For this question, one must analyze the information presented in the picture and make a determination of the likely outcome of the test conducted. This necessitates analytical reasoning skill, which is often used when analyzing information presented in pictures. For this situation, the therapist should interpret shortness of one joint hip flexor with normal two joint hip flexors. If answered incorrectly, review the Thomas test.

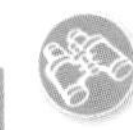

A96

Musculoskeletal | Interventions

A therapist is instructing the family of a 9-year-old boy with Duchenne's muscular dystrophy (MD). What should be the main focus of the plan of care for maintaining function in the lower extremities?

Choices:

1. Strengthening the knee extensors and plantar flexors.
2. Strengthening the plantar flexors and stretching the hip extensors.
3. Stretching the hip flexors and plantar flexors.
4. Strengthening the hip flexors and knee extensors.

Teaching Points

Correct Answer: 3

Duchenne's MD is a rapidly progressive disorder characterized by muscle wasting and atrophy. Contractures of the hips, knees, plantar flexors, and iliotibial band are common. Scoliosis occurs at around age 11 or 12. The main focus is preventing contractures, maintaining activities of daily living (ADL), energy conservation, family education, and positioning.

Incorrect Choices:

Strenuous exercise and strengthening may cause breakdown of muscle fibers. Low repetition active range of motion (AROM) is safe but not strengthening.

Type of Reasoning: Inductive

This question requires the test-taker to draw from knowledge of Duchenne's MD in order to determine a best course of action. This necessitates clinical judgment, which is an inductive reasoning skill. For this scenario, the therapist should focus on stretching the hip flexors and plantar flexors. Review Duchenne's MD if answered incorrectly.

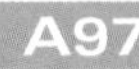

A97

Nonsystem | Equipment, Devices

A soccer player with a Q angle in excess of 30° exhibits abnormal patellofemoral tracking. While playing soccer, what is the **MOST** often used orthotic device to address this problem?

Choices:

1. Patellar stabilizing brace with a lateral buttress.
2. Patellar stabilizing brace with a medial buttress.
3. Neoprene sleeve with a patellar cutout.
4. Derotation brace.

Teaching Points

Correct Answer: 1

An increased valgus deformity can result in a greater lateral displacement force on the patella, which can disrupt patella tracking and could even lead to subluxation. The theory behind the lateral buttress brace is that it provides support to help prevent subluxation and tries to maintain the normal patella tracking.

Incorrect Choices:

A medial buttress would be on the wrong side. A neoprene sleeve provides some increased warmth and could be beneficial to a painful arthritic knee but would be of no benefit in patella alignment problems. A derotation brace is designed for rotary instabilities secondary to cruciate injuries.

Type of Reasoning: Inferential

For this question, the test-taker must utilize knowledge of abnormal patellofemoral tracking and devices used in order to arrive at a correct conclusion. One must infer what is most often used for the problem, which necessitates inferential reasoning skill. In this case, a patellar stabilizing brace with a lateral buttress is most often used. Review devices used in abnormal patellofemoral tracking if answered incorrectly.

A98 

Nonsystem I Therapeutic Modalities

A patient with diabetes mellitus has had a stage III pressure ulcer over the right ischial tuberosity for the past 5 months. The ulcer is infected with *Staphylococcus aureus*, and necrotic tissue covers much of the wound. What therapeutic modality is **CONTRAINDICATED** in this situation?

Choices:

1. Low-voltage, constant microamperage direct current.
2. High-voltage monophasic pulsed current.
3. Pulsed monophasic current.
4. Moist hot packs.

Teaching Points

Correct Answer: 4

Both a moist environment and heat can accelerate bacterial growth. Hot packs would be contraindicated in this case.

Incorrect Choices:

None of the other options are contraindicated for the treatment of this wound. They might aid in wound healing.

Type of Reasoning: Deductive

This question requires one to recall knowledge of wound treatment contraindications in order to arrive at a sound conclusion. This necessitates the recall of facts, which is a deductive reasoning skill. For this situation, moist hot packs are contraindicated. Review wound treatment guidelines and contraindications if answered incorrectly.

A99 

Neuromuscular I Interventions

A therapist is treating a child with spastic diplegia. What intervention can be used to promote relaxation?

Choices:

1. Rhythmic stabilization.
2. Slow rocking on a therapy ball.
3. Spinning in a hammock.
4. Rolling and spinning on a scooter board.

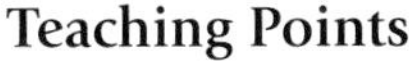

Teaching Points

Correct Answer: 2

Relaxation can be achieved using slow rocking (slow vestibular stimulation).

Incorrect Choices:

Rhythmic stabilization is a proprioceptive neuromuscular facilitation (PNF) technique used to improve postural stability. Spinning and rolling on a scooter board are interventions used to increase mobility based on fast vestibular stimulation.

Type of Reasoning: Deductive

For this question, the test-taker must recall intervention approaches that promote relaxation for spastic musculature in order to arrive at a correct conclusion. This requires the recall of factual information, which is a deductive reasoning skill. For this case, slow rocking is an intervention approach that promotes relaxation. Review intervention approaches for relaxation of spastic muscles if answered incorrectly.

A100 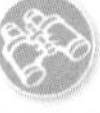

Musculoskeletal | Interventions

A patient presents to physical therapy with a complaint of anterior knee pain. There was no history of trauma associated with the onset of the pain. The patient interview and physical examination are consistent with patellofemoral pain syndrome (PFPS). Which of the following is the **BEST** intervention for most patients with PFPS?

Choices:

1. Running gait retraining.
2. Patellar taping.
3. Patellofemoral knee orthoses.
4. Exercises targeting hip and knee muscles.

Teaching Points

Correct Answer: 4

According to the Patellofemoral Pain Clinical Practice Guidelines (CPG; see Box 2-9), there is *strong* evidence to support the prescription of therapeutic exercises that target both the hip and knee musculature. Hip exercises should focus on the gluteal muscles. Knee exercises may include both weight-bearing and non-weight-bearing exercises targeting the quadriceps and hamstring muscles.

Incorrect Choices:

According to the Patellofemoral Pain CPG, there is only *moderate* evidence for the use of the other three answer choices. Running gait retraining, patellar taping, and patellofemoral knee orthoses are all interventions that physical therapists may consider in patients with patellofemoral pain. Running gait retraining may include multiple sessions of cuing to adopt a non-rearfoot strike pattern, cuing to increase cadence, and cuing to reduce peak hip adduction.

Type of Reasoning: Inductive

For this question, one must draw upon knowledge of effective intervention approaches for PFPS to arrive at a correct conclusion. This requires inductive reasoning skill, where clinical judgment is paramount to making a best intervention decision. In this situation, the best intervention is exercises targeting hip and knee muscles. If answered incorrectly, review intervention approaches for PFPS and the Patellofemoral Pain Clinical Practice Guidelines.

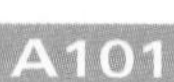
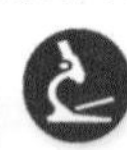

A101

Nonsystem | Research

A research team is interested in determining if video taken on a smartphone is as accurate as a three-dimensional motion capture system at estimating step length, step width, and gait velocity. Which type of validity is the research team trying to establish?

Choices:
1. Face validity.
2. Content validity.
3. Predictive validity.
4. Concurrent validity.

Teaching Points

Correct Answer: 4

Concurrent validity is a type of criterion validity. It is used when comparing two measures at the same time to determine if the experimental measure (in this case the smartphone video) can be used as a substitute for the reference measure/gold standard (three-dimensional motion capture).

Incorrect Choices:

Face validity indicates that a measure appears to measure what it is intended to measure. It is the weakest form of validity. Content validity is used to determine if the items that make up an instrument represent all possible content that defines the variable of interest. Predictive validity is a type of criterion validity and is used to determine if an experimental measure can predict a future outcome.

Type of Reasoning: Deductive

The test-taker must draw from knowledge of research guidelines in order to arrive at a correct conclusion for this question. This requires deductive reasoning skill, where factual information is used to determine which type of validity is being established. For this situation, the research team is establishing concurrent validity. Review research guidelines and types of validity if answered incorrectly.

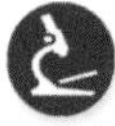

A102

Musculoskeletal | Examination

A physical therapist examines a patient who sustained a noncontact injury of the knee. During the examination, the therapist performs the pivot shift test. What is the pivot shift test used to examine?

Choices:
1. Patellar tendon rupture.
2. Anterolateral rotary instability or ALRI.
3. Posterior instability.
4. Anteromedial instability or AMRI.

Teaching Points

Correct Answer: 2

The pivot shift test is used to determine the presence of a rotary component to anterior knee instability. The Lachman's test and anterior drawer test measure straight plane anterior instability. The pivot shift test provides additional information about the lateral stabilizers of the knee, such as the capsule and anterolateral ligament. The Slocum test is also used to identify ALRI. There is a modified pivot shift test used for the examination of suspected meniscal tears. See Box 2-6 for the Knee Ligament Sprains Clinical Practice Guideline.

Incorrect Choices:

A patellar tendon rupture is determined by observation and palpation of a defect in the tendon between the patella and tibial tuberosity. The mechanism of injury is a sudden eccentric loading contraction of the quadriceps femoris muscle, such as when landing from a jump or fall. Special tests used to assess the PCL or posterior instability of the knee include the posterior drawer and quad active test. Hyperextension or a dashboard injury are common mechanisms of injury for the PCL.

Type of Reasoning: Deductive

This question requires the test-taker to recall the utility of the pivot shift test. This necessitates the recall of factual guidelines, which is a deductive reasoning skill. For this case, the test is used to determine the presence of anterolateral rotary instability or ALRI. If answered incorrectly, review the pivot shift test.

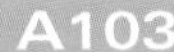

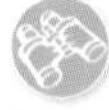

Nonsystem I Therapeutic Modalities

When using continuous ultrasound in treating the hip of an obese patient, the **GREATEST** benefit might occur if the ultrasound frequency and dosage (intensity) are set at which parameters?

Choices:

1. 1 MHz and 1.5 watts/cm^2.
2. 1 MHz and 0.5 watts/cm^2.
3. 3 MHz and 1.5 watts/cm^2.
4. 3 MHz and 0.5 watts/cm^2.

Teaching Points

Correct Answer: 1

1 MHz frequency is recommended for target tissue deeper than 2 cm, and 1.5 watts/cm^2 would increase the rate of heating, allowing it to be treated in a reasonable time frame.

Incorrect Choices:

The frequency 3 MHz does not penetrate past 2 cm and would not be effective at the hip. A rate of heating of 0.5 watts/cm^2 intensity is very slow and would result in a prolonged treatment time.

Type of Reasoning: Inductive

For this question, one must utilize knowledge of ultrasound guidelines in order to determine which frequency and rate of heating would provide the greatest benefit. This requires clinical judgment, which is an inductive reasoning skill. For this scenario, 1 MHz and 1.5 watts/cm^2 would provide the greatest benefit. Review ultrasound guidelines, especially for the hip, if answered incorrectly.

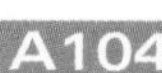

A104

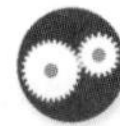

Integumentary | Interventions

A patient presents with a stage III pressure ulcer with a moist, necrotic wound. A hydrocolloidal dressing is being used. During the dressing change, the therapist detects a strong odor, and the wound drainage has a yellow color. What is the therapist's **BEST** course of action?

Choices:

1. Reapply a new gauze dressing instead of hydrocolloid and report the findings to the physician.
2. Speak to the nurse about changing to a hydrogel dressing.
3. Leave the dressing off the wound and report the findings immediately to the physician.
4. Reapply a new hydrocolloid dressing and record the findings in the chart.

Teaching Points

Correct Answer: 4

Hydrocolloidal dressings are typically changed every 3 to 5 days or when drainage leaks out. An odor and yellowish color are to be expected as the dressing material melts.

Incorrect Choices:

The decision about what type of dressing to apply to a wound is the physician's in collaboration with the wound care team. This is not an emergency situation.

Type of Reasoning: Evaluative

For this question, the test-taker must weigh the potential courses of action and determine which one will have the most beneficial outcome. This necessitates evaluative reasoning skill, where the value of information is weighed to make decisions on next steps. For this situation, the therapist should reapply a new hydrocolloid dressing and record the findings in the chart. Review wound care guidelines, especially the use of hydrocolloidal dressings, if answered incorrectly.

A105

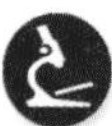

Musculoskeletal | Examination

During examination of a patient with degenerative osteoarthritic changes in the carpometacarpal (CMC) joint of the right thumb, the physical therapist notes a 20-degree loss of thumb palmar abduction. What translatory joint play motion (based on the traditional concave/convex rules of motion) is associated with thumb palmar abduction and should be examined?

Choices:

1. Dorsal translation of the metacarpal on the trapezium.
2. Palmar translation of the metacarpal on the trapezium.
3. Ulnar translation of the metacarpal on the trapezium.
4. Radial translation of the metacarpal on the trapezium.

Exam A

Teaching Points

Correct Answer: 1

The carpometacarpal joint of the thumb is considered a saddle joint in which the articular surface geometry is generally concave in one plane and convex in a plane perpendicular to the other. The proximal joint surface of the first metacarpal is generally convex in the palmar to dorsal direction and concave in the medial to lateral direction. The articular surface of the base of the first metacarpal typically presents as the convex member of this joint when movement occurs in palmar abduction. Thumb palmar abduction thus involves a convex metacarpal surface moving on the concave surface of the trapezium. Following the traditional concave/convex rules of motion, one would expect a combination of palmar roll and dorsal translatory motion of the metacarpal on the trapezium during palmar abduction. In this case, a therapist would be sure to evaluate dorsal glide of the metacarpal on the trapezium.

Incorrect Choices:

The other examples of joint play motion are not congruent with palmar abduction of the thumb.

Type of Reasoning: Deductive

For this question, one must recall the translatory joint play motion of the CMC joint of the thumb in order to arrive at a correct conclusion. This necessitates the recall of facts, which is a deductive reasoning skill. For this case, the expected motion is dorsal translation of the metacarpal on the trapezium. Review joint play of the CMC joint of the thumb if answered incorrectly.

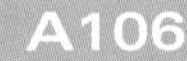
A106 

Neuromuscular | Evaluation, Diagnosis

Following a cerebrovascular accident involving the right hemisphere, a patient is exhibiting unilateral neglect. What might the patient do as a result?

Choices:

1. Eat food only from the left side of a plate.
2. Bump his wheelchair into things on the right side.
3. Ignore or deny the existence of the right upper extremity.
4. Shave only on the right side of the face.

Teaching Points

Correct Answer: 4

A patient with a right hemisphere lesion (left hemiplegia) will tend to ignore items or body parts on the left side while favoring items or body parts on the right side.

Incorrect Choices:

All other choices do not match the above description and favor items or body parts on the left side.

Type of Reasoning: Inferential

One must infer, or determine what is likely to be true of a situation, in order to reach a sound conclusion. This necessitates inferential reasoning skill, where behavior in patients is predicted. In this case, one might expect the patient to shave only on the right side of the face. Review information on unilateral neglect if answered incorrectly.

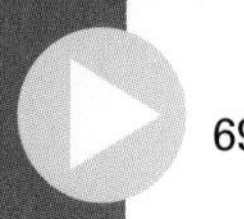

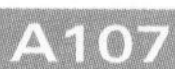

A107

Musculoskeletal | Evaluation, Diagnosis

Damage as a result of a Salter-Harris type IV supracondylar humeral epiphyseal fracture will **MOST LIKELY** result in what consequence?

Choices:

1. Refracture at a future time.
2. Nonunion.
3. Arrested growth.
4. Severing of the radial nerve.

Teaching Points

Correct Answer: 3

Supracondylar fractures are the most common pediatric elbow fracture, occurring most commonly between 3 and 10 years of age. Extension fractures account for about 95% of supracondylar fractures. The mechanism of injury is a fall on an outstretched hand with elbow hyperextended.

Type IV is a fracture through all three elements of the bone: the growth plate, metaphysis, and epiphysis (10% incidence). Type IV growth plate fractures start above the growth plate, cross the growth plate, and exit through the joint cartilage. These injuries can affect the joint cartilage and may impair normal growth. See Table 2-31 for a review of Salter-Harris fracture classifications.

Incorrect Choices:

Nonunion of pediatric fractures is a rare complication. However, in one study of nonunion fractures, 47% were above the elbow, with most of the nonunions at the lateral condyle. Refractures of the forearm have an incidence of about 5%. Overall, the incidence of supracondylar-associated neurovascular injury is 12% and increases with displacement to between 19% and 49%. Excessive swelling and ecchymosis are a significant risk factor for compartment syndrome, and a thorough neurovascular exam should be performed and should focus on the brachial artery as well as the median and radial nerves.

Type of Reasoning: Inferential

This question requires the test-taker to determine the most likely consequence of a Salter-Harris type IV supracondylar humeral epiphyseal fracture. This requires knowledge of the Salter-Harris classification system in order to determine the most likely outcome. For this scenario, the most likely outcome is arrested growth. Review Salter-Harris fractures if answered incorrectly.

A108

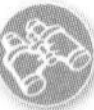

Cardiovascular/Pulmonary | Examination

What is the **BEST** way to monitor the intensity of exercise for a patient limited mostly by claudication?

Choices:

1. Assessing ankle-brachial index (ABI) during exercise.
2. Maintaining heart rate (HR) between 60% and 70% of age-predicted HR_{max} during exercise.
3. Sustaining pain levels of at least 2 out of 4 on the claudication scale during exercise.
4. Upholding rate of perceived exertion (RPE) levels of 11 to 13 out of 20 during exercise.

Exam A

Teaching Points

Correct Answer: 3

It has been established that in order to generate collateral circulation in patients with ischemia (i.e., claudication), patients need to exercise with at least moderate claudication pain. This level of blood and oxygen deprivation over time initiates the generation of collateral circulation. This correlates to 2 out of 4 on the claudication scale.

Incorrect Choices:

The ABI is not practical to assess during exercise because the patient cannot be moving during this test. While the RPE and HR_{max} are at moderate levels, this may not be at an intensity that elicits claudication symptoms.

Type of Reasoning: Inductive

For this question, one must utilize clinical judgment in order to determine the best way to monitor the intensity of exercise for a patient with claudication. This requires knowledge of the effects of exercise on claudication, which is an inductive reasoning skill. For this case, the best way to monitor exercise is to sustain pain levels of at least 2 out of 4 on the claudication scale during exercise. Review information on claudication and exercise if answered incorrectly.

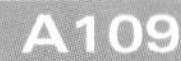

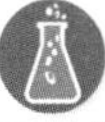

Musculoskeletal I Evaluation, Diagnosis

A weightlifter with hypertrophy of the scalene muscles complains of pain and paresthesia in the right upper extremity when lifting weight overhead. What is the **MOST LIKELY** cause?

Choices:

1. Thoracic outlet syndrome.
2. Vertebral artery obstruction.
3. Cervical radiculopathy.
4. Complex regional pain syndrome type 1.

Teaching Points

Correct Answer: 1

Hypertrophied scalene muscles can result in thoracic outlet syndrome due to their close anatomical relationship to the neurovascular structures. The neurovascular bundle passes between the anterior and middle scalene muscles and could be under pressure from hypertrophied scalenes. The anterior and middle scalenes attach to the first rib, and tightness in these muscles could result in elevation of the first rib, thereby compressing the neurovascular bundle. Neurogenic (neurological) thoracic outlet syndrome is characterized by compression of the brachial plexus. In the majority of thoracic outlet syndrome cases, the symptoms are neurogenic. Signs and symptoms of neurological thoracic outlet syndrome often include wasting in the thenar area, numbness or tingling in the fingers, pain in the shoulder and neck, ache in the arm or hand, and weakening grip.

Incorrect Choices:

The clinical presentation of vertebral artery occlusion varies with the area of ischemia and cause of occlusion. Vertigo, dizziness, nausea, vomiting, and head or neck pain are the most common initial symptoms reported. Other common signs and symptoms include weakness, hemiparesis, ataxia, diplopia, pupillary abnormalities, speech difficulties, and altered mental status.

Cervical radiculopathy pain travels down the arm in the area of the involved nerve. Pain is usually described as sharp. There can also be a "pins and needles" sensation or even complete numbness. In addition, there may be a feeling of weakness with certain activities. Symptoms can be worsened with certain movements, like extending or straining the neck or turning the head.

Complex regional pain syndrome (CRPS) is a chronic pain condition that is believed to be the result of dysfunction in the central or peripheral nervous systems. Typical features include dramatic changes in the color and temperature of the skin over the affected limb or body part, accompanied by intense burning pain, skin sensitivity, sweating, and swelling. The key symptom of CRPS is continuous, intense pain out of proportion to the severity of the injury (if an injury has occurred), which gets worse rather than better over time. None of these are normally associated with hypertrophy of the scalene muscles.

Type of Reasoning: Analytical

This question provides a group of symptoms, and the test-taker must determine the most likely cause. Questions that require one to determine a diagnosis based on a description of symptoms often necessitate analytical reasoning skill. For this situation, the symptoms are indicative of thoracic outlet syndrome. Review thoracic outlet syndrome if answered incorrectly.

A110

Cardiovascular/Pulmonary | Evaluation, Diagnosis

A patient is immersed up to the neck in a therapeutic pool. While exercising this patient, the therapist should take into consideration the physiological effects of immersion. Which significant result might occur?

Choices:

1. Increased forced vital capacity.
2. Increased expiratory reserve volume.
3. Increased work of breathing.
4. Decreased pulmonary blood flow.

Teaching Points

Correct Answer: 3

Full chest immersion in a pool can result in increased work of breathing as a result of increased hydrostatic pressure.

Incorrect Choices:

The other choices are not consistent with the physiological effects resulting from full chest immersion in a pool.

Type of Reasoning: Inferential

This question requires one to determine what is most likely to be true for a patient who is immersed up to the neck in a therapeutic pool. Questions that require one to make a determination of what is true of a situation often necessitate inferential reasoning skill. For this scenario, full chest immersion would likely result in increased work of breathing. Review effects of immersion if answered incorrectly.

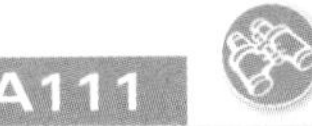

A111

Neuromuscular | Interventions

What intervention **BEST** illustrates selective stretching when working with a patient with a spinal cord injury (C6 complete)?

Choices:

1. Long finger flexors are fully ranged into extension with wrist extension.
2. Hamstrings are fully ranged to 110° in supine.
3. Low back extensors are fully ranged in longsitting.
4. Hamstrings are fully ranged in longsitting.

Teaching Points

Correct Answer: 2

Hamstrings need to be fully ranged to 110° in the supine position. This allows for function in the longsitting position (e.g., dressing, leg management during transfers).

Incorrect Choices:

Ranging the hamstrings or low back extensors in long sitting will result in overstretched low back extensors (needed for stability in sitting). The long finger flexors are ranged into full extension with wrist flexion (not wrist extension). This allows the hand to be used functionally for tenodesis grasp.

Type of Reasoning: Inductive

One must utilize knowledge of spinal cord injury and selective stretching techniques in order to arrive at a correct conclusion. This necessitates clinical judgment, which is an inductive reasoning skill. In this case, the intervention that best demonstrates this is when the hamstrings are fully ranged to 110° in supine. Review stretching techniques for spinal cord injury if answered incorrectly.

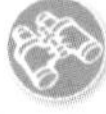

A112

Musculoskeletal | Interventions

Strengthening of the lateral pterygoid, anterior head of the digastric muscle, and suprahyoid muscles would be the **MOST BENEFICIAL** intervention to improve which of the following?

Choices:

1. Mouth closing.
2. Mouth opening.
3. Mouth protrusion.
4. Mouth retrusion.

Teaching Points

Correct Answer: 2

The muscles involved in opening include the lateral pterygoid, anterior head of the digastric muscle, and suprahyoid muscles.

Incorrect Choices:

The muscles that assist with mouth closing are the masseter, temporalis, medial pterygoid, and lateral pterygoid. The muscles that assist with protrusion are the temporalis, medial pterygoid, and lateral pterygoid. The muscles that assist with retrusion are the temporalis and suprahyoid muscles.

Type of Reasoning: Inductive

For this question, one must utilize knowledge of musculoskeletal anatomy and muscle strengthening in order to determine the most beneficial intervention approach. This is an inductive reasoning skill. In this case, the approach improves mouth opening. If answered incorrectly, review lateral pterygoid and suprahyoid muscles.

A113 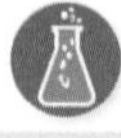

Neuromuscular | Evaluation, Diagnosis

A patient with suspected right cubital tunnel syndrome presents with sensory loss (light touch and sharp/dull) and radiating pain in the medial arm, medial forearm, medial hand, and little and ring fingers. The patient also has 4/5 muscle testing in all C8-T1 muscles in the right upper extremity with the exception of C8 muscles innervated by the right radial nerve. The patient has no neck pain and Spurling's and cervical quadrant testing are negative. Past medical history includes breast cancer (treated with surgery/radiation and chemotherapy) that has been in remission for 2 years. Past social history includes a 35-year history of smoking. Which of the following health conditions is most consistent with the patient's signs and symptoms?

Choices:

1. Cubital tunnel syndrome.
2. Ulnar/median neuropathy at the axilla.
3. Medial cord brachial plexopathy.
4. C8-T1 radiculopathy.

Teaching Points

Correct Answer: 3

The patient's history and physical examination findings are most consistent with medial cord brachial plexopathy. This can occur secondary to a Pancoast tumor (tumor of the upper lobe of the lung). Smoking and a past history of cancer are risk factors for this type of tumor.

Incorrect Choices:

Isolated ulnar nerve involvement does not explain the patient's weakness in other C8-T1 muscles that are not innervated by the ulnar nerves. It also does not explain the patient's more proximal medial arm and forearm sensory loss. Medial and ulnar compression at the axilla are also not consistent with the patient's symptoms, and specifically the involvement of the median nerve would result in weakness in forearm flexors and pronator teres (non C8-T1 muscles), as well as sensory loss of the right palmar hand, thumb, index, long and ring fingers. C8-T1 radiculopathy would explain the majority of the patient's findings, but if these nerve roots were involved the patient would also have weakness of radial-C8 innervated muscles.

Type of Reasoning: Analytical

This question provides a group of symptoms and the test-taker must determine the most likely health condition based on those symptoms. This necessitates analytical reasoning skill, where one must draw a reasonable conclusion about a situation based on pieces of information. For this situation, the symptoms are consistent with medial cord brachial plexopathy. Review the brachial plexus and associated conditions, especially medial cord plexopathy, if answered incorrectly.

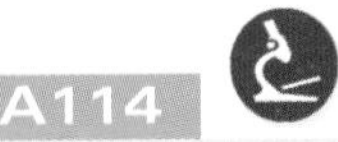

Nonsystem I Research

What is the **BEST** evidence to determine orthotic intervention to prevent inversion ankle sprains?

Choices:

1. Systematic review and meta-analysis of cohort studies.
2. Systematic review and meta-analysis of randomized controlled trials.
3. Meta-analyses of multiple case studies.
4. Randomized double-blind controlled trials.

Teaching Points

Correct Answer: 2

Systematic review including meta-analysis of randomized controlled trials (RCTs) provides the best research evidence of effectiveness of an intervention.

Incorrect Choices:

Meta-analysis is not applied to cohort studies or multiple case studies. While an RCT can provide strong evidence of the effectiveness of an intervention, evidence derived from a meta-analysis that combines multiple RCTs is stronger.

Type of Reasoning: Deductive

In order to arrive at a sound conclusion, the test-taker must recall research designs, specifically which designs provide the strongest research evidence. This necessitates the recall of facts, which is a deductive reasoning skill. For this scenario, systematic reviews of randomized controlled trials provide the best evidence. Review research designs if answered incorrectly.

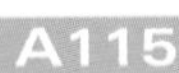
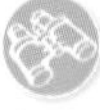

Musculoskeletal I Interventions

A patient presents with insidious onset of low back pain that started 10 days ago. Examination reveals an Oswestry Disability Index score of 40%, a Fear Avoidance Belief Questionnaire for Physical Activity score of 16, hypomobility at L4–5 with posteroanterior (PA) glide, and pain that radiates into the right buttock. Lumbar active range of motion (AROM) is painful at 50% of expected range in all directions. Hip passive range of motion (PROM) is within normal limits. Abdominal strength is fair. Based on this data, what is the **BEST** intervention for this patient?

Choices:

1. Abdominal stabilization.
2. Manipulation.
3. Positional distraction.
4. Transcutaneous electrical nerve stimulation (TENS) and ice.

Teaching Points

Correct Answer: 2

If a patient presents with four out of five criteria listed in the examination findings, the patient has a 95% chance of benefiting from manipulation using the lumbopelvic regional thrust manipulation technique.

This percentage for treatment success is based on the clinical prediction rule validated by Childs et al., 2004, *Ann Intern Med*. Additionally, see Box 2-16 for the Low Back Pain Clinical Practice Guideline.

Incorrect Choices:

Abdominal stabilization is a good secondary intervention. Since the patient does not fit the clinical practice rules for abdominal stabilization, it should not be the first choice for intervention. Positional distraction would be appropriate for radicular pain; however, that is not the case here.

Type of Reasoning: Inductive

One must utilize clinical judgment in order to determine the best intervention approach for this patient. This requires one to have knowledge of the various intervention approaches and examination results, which necessitates inductive reasoning skill. For this situation, the best intervention approach is manipulation. Review intervention approaches for low back pain if answered incorrectly.

A116 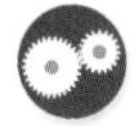

Gastrointestinal | Evaluation, Diagnosis

A patient who is well known to the physical therapy clinic for treatment of chronic neck pain now presents with a new complaint of acute mid-back pain. Current symptoms also include abdominal pain and distension, which, along with the mid-back pain, intensify soon after meals. The patient also reports having a recent episode of chronic neck pain that resolved after taking 5,000 mg of acetaminophen daily for 2 weeks. What action should the therapist take?

Choices:

1. Refer the patient to their primary care physician with possible nephrolithiasis.
2. Treat the patient with cryotherapy for pain relief and instruct the patient in a core strengthening program.
3. Refer the patient to their primary care physician with possible pancreatitis.
4. Instruct the patient to rest and continue to take acetaminophen as needed for their pain.

Teaching Points

Correct Answer: 3

This question describes a patient with acute pancreatitis, likely due to taking excessive amounts of acetaminophen. The maximum daily dosage of acetaminophen is 4,000 mg. Drug toxicity can bring on an acute attack of pancreatitis. In addition to those described in the question stem, common clinical findings include epigastric pain radiating to the back; nausea, vomiting, and diarrhea; fever and sweating; tachycardia; malaise; bluish discoloration of the abdomen or flanks (called Cullen's sign); and jaundice.

Incorrect Choices:

Nephrolithiasis, or kidney stones, have a different clinical presentation than what is described here. Pain typically occurs in the low back or under the lower ribs and radiates into the abdomen and groin. Painful urination, a persistent need to urinate, and cloudy or foul-smelling urine are all common symptoms of a kidney stone. Cryotherapy is an intervention that would be appropriate if the patient had back pain due to some type of musculoskeletal injury or dysfunction. Choice 4 fails to consider the patient's gastrointestinal symptoms and the possibility that the excessive dosage of acetaminophen might have contributed to the current complaints.

Type of Reasoning: Evaluative

For this question, one must determine a best course of action based on presenting patient symptoms. This necessitates evaluative reasoning skill, where information is weighed to determine the significance. For this situation, the therapist should refer the patient to their primary care physician for possible pancreatitis. If answered incorrectly, review signs and symptoms of pancreatitis.

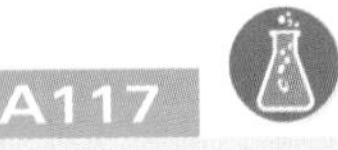

A117

Lymphatic I Evaluation

A client is seen in physical therapy with a chief complaint of aching in the left lower extremity along with a feeling of tightness and heaviness. The onset of symptoms occurred soon after the client returned from a vacation to a tropical country. Upon examination, the physical therapist observes pitting edema and notes that the skin of the involved leg feels thick and dry compared with the uninvolved side. Which pathology is **MOST LIKELY** to result in the client's signs and symptoms?

Choices:

1. Chronic venous insufficiency (CVI).
2. Lipedema.
3. Congestive heart failure (CHF).
4. Secondary lymphedema.

Teaching Points

Correct Answer: 4

Aching, tightness, and a sensation of heaviness in the involved limb are common complaints from a patient with lymphedema. A known risk factor for secondary lymphedema is filariasis, a mosquito-borne illness that is prevalent in tropical and subtropical climates.

Incorrect Choices:

While lower extremity swelling is frequently seen in patients with CVI, CHF, and lipedema, the swelling is typically bilateral and symmetrical. A patient with CVI may also present with varicose veins and would describe any pain or achiness they experience along the course of superficial veins. A patient with CHF would experience a number of other cardiovascular symptoms, including shortness of breath, heart palpitations, and fatigue.

Lipedema is a disorder characterized by excessive subcutaneous fat deposition. The appearance may be similar to lymphedema, but the patient does not experience the skin changes (thickening) associated with lymphedema. Pain and bruising are prominent features of lipedema, and swelling is absent in the feet and hands.

Type of Reasoning: Analytical

For this question, the test-taker must analyze the symptoms presented in order to determine the most likely diagnosis. This requires analytical reasoning skill, where pieces of information are analyzed in order to draw a logical conclusion. In this situation, the symptoms are indicative of secondary lymphedema. Review secondary lymphedema if answered incorrectly.

A118 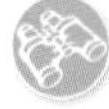

Neuromuscular I Evaluation, Diagnosis

A patient with a 7-year history of Parkinson's disease is hospitalized. The patient is ambulatory but requires close supervision to prevent falls. What should be the focus of the physical therapist's plan of care?

Choices:

1. Manual balance perturbation training.
2. Transfer and wheelchair training.
3. Caregiver training for contact guarding during level walking and stairs.
4. Locomotor training using a rolling walker.

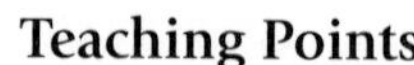

Exam A

Teaching Points

Correct Answer: 3

Caregiver training with safety instruction in contact guarding during level walking and stairs is the best choice to keep this patient functional in the home environment.

Incorrect Choices:

Manual balance perturbation training will likely result in a rigid response, decreasing use of normal synergistic movements. This patient should be kept safe and ambulatory for as long as possible and not be relegated to a wheelchair. A rolling walker is contraindicated for patients with a forward, flexed posture (typical in patients with Parkinson's disease).

Type of Reasoning: Inductive

This question requires clinical judgment in order to determine a best course of action. Utilizing knowledge of Parkinson's disease and the current level of function, inductive reasoning skills are utilized to determine the focus for the plan of care. In this case, the focus should be on caregiver training for contact guarding during level walking and stairs. Review Parkinson's disease if answered incorrectly.

A119 

Integumentary | Examination

A patient is referred to physical therapy with a diagnosis of congestive heart failure. During the initial session, the physical therapist examines the skin for suspected changes. What appearance can be expected?

Choices:

1. Pale, washed-out color.
2. Yellowish discoloration.
3. Slightly bluish, slate-colored discoloration.
4. Cherry-red discoloration.

Teaching Points

Correct Answer: 3

Slightly bluish, grayish, slate-colored discoloration of the skin along with clubbing of the nails is characteristic of chronic hypoxia.

Incorrect Choices:

Pallor (lack of skin color, paleness) is indicative of anemia, internal hemorrhage, or lack of sunlight exposure. Yellowish discoloration of the skin is indicative of jaundice (liver disease). Cherry-red discoloration of the skin is indicative of carbon monoxide poisoning.

Type of Reasoning: Inferential

This question requires one to infer what is likely to be true of a situation in order to reach a sound conclusion. This necessitates inferential reasoning skill. For this situation, the patient with congestive heart failure is expected to show slightly bluish, slate-colored discoloration. Review congestive heart failure information if answered incorrectly.

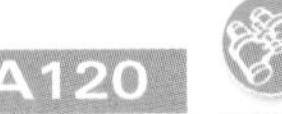

A120

Integumentary I Interventions

A patient with a 10-year history of discoid lupus erythematosus presents with multiple discoid skin lesions that are raised and red and contain scaling plaques with central atrophy on the lower extremities. Topical corticosteroid creams are being used. What should be the focus of the therapist's initial plan of care?

Choices:

1. Range of motion (ROM) exercises and prevention of deformity.
2. Lightweight splints to provide joint protection.
3. Aerobic training using a treadmill.
4. Resistive training using weights at 60%–80%, one repetition maximum.

Teaching Points

Correct Answer: 1

Range of motion (ROM) exercises and prevention of deformity are important elements of the plan of care.

Incorrect Choices:

Lightweight splints are not an initial priority and can contribute to contracture development if worn too long. Furthermore, there are no reports of arthralgia in this case. Regular exercise is important but should not be aggressive (resistive training). Also, long-term use of corticosteroids puts this patient at risk for osteoporosis. Aerobic (treadmill) training might be indicated but is not an initial priority. Splints to provide joint protection are also not an initial priority.

Type of Reasoning: Inductive

This question requires one to determine a best course of action based on knowledge of discoid lupus erythematosus. This necessitates clinical judgment, which is an inductive reasoning skill. For this scenario, range of motion (ROM) exercises and prevention of deformity should be the initial focus. If answered incorrectly, review information on discoid lupus erythematosus.

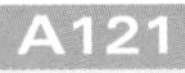

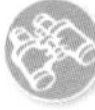

A121

Genitourinary I Evaluation, Diagnosis

On the third day following a cesarean delivery, what should a physical therapist's interventions include?

Choices:

1. Gentle partial sit-ups and head lifts.
2. Breathing, coughing, and pelvic floor exercises.
3. Low-intensity aerobic conditioning.
4. Pelvic tilts on all fours.

Teaching Points

Correct Answer: 2

Initial postpartum interventions (days 1 to 3) should include breathing, coughing, and pelvic floor exercises.

Incorrect Choices:

All other choices can be part of the postpartum exercise program during later recovery.

Type of Reasoning: Inductive

This question requires one to utilize knowledge of postpartum intervention approaches in order to arrive at a correct conclusion. This necessitates clinical judgment, which is an inductive reasoning skill. For this case, the therapist should include breathing, coughing, and pelvic floor exercises. Review postpartum intervention approaches if answered incorrectly.

A122

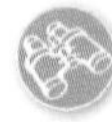

Cardiovascular/Pulmonary I Interventions

A patient with post–traumatic brain injury (Rancho Los Amigos Levels of Cognitive Functioning Scale level III) has evidence of retained secretions on auscultation and chest films. What is the **BEST** mode of airway clearance for this patient?

Choices:

1. Active cycle of breathing.
2. Autogenic drainage.
3. Use of the FLUTTER device.
4. Use of high-frequency chest wall oscillation.

Teaching Points

Correct Answer: 4

High-frequency chest wall oscillations (HFCWO) via a device such as the Vest Airway Clearance System allow for control of inspiratory and expiratory flow rates. The device can be used in any position regardless of the patient's cognitive status.

Incorrect Choices:

The first two choices require a patient to consistently follow commands and potentially complete the activity alone, which would be difficult for a patient in this cognitive stage of recovery. Oscillatory positive expiratory pressure (PEP) using a FLUTTER device requires a patient to breathe through a mouthpiece with inspiration unimpeded and long exhalation against a back pressure, also impossible for this patient.

Type of Reasoning: Inductive

For this question, one must determine a best course of action for airway clearance, based on knowledge of effective airway clearance approaches. This necessitates inductive reasoning skill, where clinical judgment is paramount to arriving at a correct conclusion. For this situation, the best mode of airway clearance is high-frequency chest wall oscillation. Review airway clearance approaches if answered incorrectly.

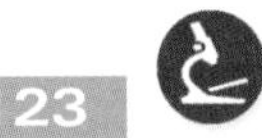

Neuromuscular | Examination

A physical therapist is performing sensory tests on a patient diagnosed with C6 nerve root impingement. Where should the testing concentrate?

Choices:
1. Second, third, and fourth fingers, palmar surface.
2. Ulnar border of the hand (fifth finger).
3. Palmar surface of the thumb and distal, radial forearm.
4. Medial (ulnar) forearm.

Teaching Points

Correct Answer: 3
The C6 nerve root supplies both sides of the thumb and the radial aspect of the forearm.

Incorrect Choices:
The C7 root supplies the middle of the hand (second, third, and fourth fingers, palmar surface). The C8 root supplies the ulnar border of the hand (fifth finger). The T1 root supplies the medial surface of the forearm.

Type of Reasoning: Deductive
One must recall sensory testing guidelines in order to arrive at a correct conclusion for this question. This requires the recall of facts, which is a deductive reasoning skill. For this situation, the therapist should focus on the palmar surface of the thumb and distal, radial forearm. Review sensory testing for the upper extremity, especially the C6 distribution, if answered incorrectly.

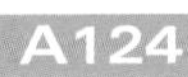

Neuromuscular | Evaluation, Diagnosis

A patient is experiencing left foot weakness and toe drag when walking greater than 10 minutes for the past 3 months. Muscle spasms and weakness in the right hand are also present for the past 3 weeks. Neuromuscular screening examination reveals 4/5 MMT and fasciculations in the left extensor hallicus longus, left tibialis anterior, and right first dorsal interossei. Reflex testing reveals a 3+ in the right triceps and biceps and a positive right Hoffman's sign. Sensory testing for light touch and vibration of the upper and lower extremities is normal. Which of the following health conditions is most consistent with the patient's signs and symptoms?

Choices:
1. Polyneuropathy.
2. Cervical myelopathy.
3. Myasthenia gravis.
4. Amyotrophic lateral sclerosis.

Teaching Points

Correct Answer: 4
The presence of upper and lower motor neuron (UMN and LMN) involvement without sensory loss is most consistent with amyotrophic lateral sclerosis (ALS). In early or Stage 1 of ALS, patients will often display mild focal weakness with asymmetrical distribution to include symptoms of hand cramping and fasciculations.

Incorrect Choices:

Polyneuropathy involves bilateral distal extremity motor, sensory, and autonomic impairments without UMN involvement. Cervical myelopathy may involve both LMN (at the level of compression) and UMN involvement (distal to compressed cervical level) but typically results in bilateral lower extremity involvement and both motor and sensory impairments (ataxia). Myasthenia gravis results in fatigue and ultimately weakness in multiple muscles in the bilateral upper and lower extremities but does not result in UMN involvement.

Type of Reasoning: Analytical

For this question, the test-taker must analyze the symptoms presented and determine the likely diagnosis. This requires analytical reasoning skill, where pieces of information are analyzed for their significance in order to draw a reasonable conclusion. For this case, the symptoms are consistent with ALS. If answered incorrectly, be sure to review information on ALS, including early/stage 1 symptoms.

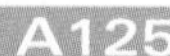
A125

Musculoskeletal | Evaluation, Diagnosis

A physical therapist examines an elderly patient whose chief complaint is deep, boring pain in the pelvis and thighs. The patient also complains of weakness, fatigue, and headaches. Paget's disease is suspected. Which clinical examination finding may corroborate the diagnosis of Paget's disease?

Choices:

1. Pain, redness, and swelling of the 1st metatarsal joint.
2. Increased skin temperature over long bones.
3. Tachycardia, hyperreflexia, and decreased muscle strength.
4. Kyphosis and easy bruising.

Teaching Points

Correct Answer: 2

Increased skin temperature over affected long bones is a common finding in individuals with Paget's disease, a focal inflammatory condition that produces disordered bone remodeling. There is increased vascularity associated with the bone remodeling, leading to the increased skin temperature in affected areas. The bones that are most commonly involved are the pelvis, skull, femur, tibia, spine, shoulders, and ribs.

Incorrect Choices:

Pain, redness, and swelling of the 1st metatarsal joint is a hallmark finding of gout. The combination of tachycardia, hyperreflexia, and decreased muscle strength is characteristic of Graves' disease or hyperthyroidism. Kyphosis and easy bruising are common findings in Cushing's syndrome, along with the telltale "moon face" and buffalo hump appearance of individuals with the disorder.

Type of Reasoning: Inferential

For this question, a diagnosis is provided and the test-taker must determine the likely symptoms consistent with this diagnosis. This requires inferential reasoning skill, where one infers or determines what is likely to be true of a situation. For this case, symptoms of increased skin temperature over long bones would corroborate a diagnosis of Paget's disease. If answered incorrectly, review symptoms of Paget's disease.

A126 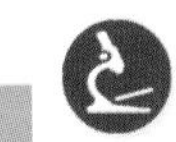

Neuromuscular | Evaluation, Diagnosis

A physical therapist is working with a patient who exhibits fluent aphasia. What is a typical characteristic of this form of aphasia?

Choices:
1. Impaired auditory comprehension.
2. Slow, hesitant speech.
3. Good comprehension.
4. Impaired articulation.

Teaching Points

Correct Answer: 1
Fluent aphasia is characterized by impaired auditory comprehension and fluent speech that is of normal rate and melody (e.g., Wernicke's aphasia).

Incorrect Choices:
Nonfluent aphasia is characterized by speech that is slow, hesitant, awkward, interrupted, and produced with effort (e.g., Broca's aphasia). Patients tend to have good awareness of their deficit and comprehension. Impaired articulation characterizes the patient with dysarthria (a motor speech disorder).

Type of Reasoning: Deductive
One must recall the characteristics of fluent aphasia in order to arrive at a correct conclusion. This necessitates the recall of facts, which is a deductive reasoning skill. For this case, fluent aphasia is characterized by impaired auditory comprehension. Review types of aphasia, especially fluent aphasia, if answered incorrectly.

A127 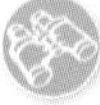

Neuromuscular | Interventions

Three months following a left cerebrovascular stroke and a 4-week stay of inpatient rehabilitation, a patient is receiving home care physical therapy. The patient's movements in the right extremities show good recovery (out-of-synergy). Functional level is a 6 on the Functional Independence Measure (FIM) for self-care items. At this juncture, what should be the focus of motor learning strategies?

Choices:
1. Use of mental practice to improve performance.
2. Breaking down complex tasks into component parts.
3. Use of serial practice order of related skills.
4. Consistency of performance in variable environments.

Teaching Points

Correct Answer: 4
This patient demonstrates good functional recovery. Motor learning for the autonomous stage of motor learning should utilize variable practice in variable environments.

Incorrect Choices:

Mental practice and breaking down tasks into components can be helpful in the early cognitive stage of motor learning. Serial practice order is indicated for the middle, associative stage of motor learning.

Type of Reasoning: Inductive

One must utilize clinical judgment in order to determine a best intervention approach for a patient with CVA. Having knowledge of the stages of recovery, coupled with sound inductive reasoning skills, one should conclude that consistency of performance in variable environments is the best focus for intervention. Review motor learning strategies for CVA if answered incorrectly.

A128 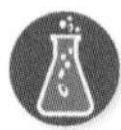

Musculoskeletal | Examination

A physical therapist evaluates a patient with low back pain and radiating pain and paresthesias into the right buttock, posterior thigh, lateral leg, and lateral foot. An S1 radiculopathy is suspected. Which special test is **BEST** for ruling **IN** a lumbosacral radiculopathy?

Choices:

1. Straight leg raise.
2. Crossed straight leg raise.
3. Prone instability test.
4. Femoral nerve traction test.

Teaching Points

Correct Answer: 2

This question requires knowledge of lumbar spine musculoskeletal special tests along with the application of their established sensitivity and specificity values. The crossed straight leg raise (SLR) is considered to be a highly specific test, which when positive helps to rule in the diagnosis of a herniated nucleus pulposus or lumbosacral radiculopathy. See Table 2-21 for a summary of the diagnostic accuracy of lumbar spine and pelvis special tests.

Incorrect Choices:

The SLR (Lasegue's) test is a highly sensitive test and is therefore helpful in ruling out a lumbosacral radiculopathy when negative. The SLR test is an integral part of a comprehensive physical examination of a patient with LBP, but given its poor specificity, it is not helpful for ruling in a lumbar radiculopathy. The prone instability test is clinically useful for assessing lumbar spine instability. The femoral nerve traction test is helpful for assessing neurological dysfunction involving the femoral nerve and/or lumbar nerve roots L2–L4.

Type of Reasoning: Analytical

For this case, the test-taker must evaluate the symptoms presented and determine the special test that will rule in a diagnosis. This necessitates analytical reasoning skill, where symptoms are analyzed to draw reasonable conclusions. For this scenario, the therapist should conduct a crossed straight leg raise to rule in lumbosacral radiculopathy. If answered incorrectly, review information on special testing for lumbosacral radiculopathy.

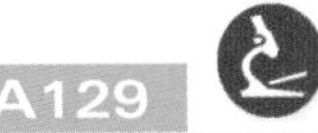

Neuromuscular | Examination

What is the most effective form of diagnostic imaging for patients with multiple sclerosis (MS) to help determine level of disease activity?

Choices:

1. Positron emission tomography (PET).
2. Magnetic resonance imaging (MRI).
3. Computed tomography (CT).
4. Transcranial sonography.

Teaching Points

Correct Answer: 2

MRI is highly sensitive for detecting MS plaques in the white matter of the brain and spinal cord. Lesions are seen as areas of increased signal intensity (bright spots). Contrast-enhanced scans are used for more long-term disease activity.

Incorrect Choices:

All other choices of diagnostic imaging techniques do not offer the same sensitivity and specificity for detecting plaques.

Type of Reasoning: Deductive

One must recall the most effective diagnostic tool for MS in order to arrive at a correct conclusion. This requires the recall of factual information, which is a deductive reasoning skill. For this scenario, the most effective test is magnetic resonance imaging (MRI). Review diagnostic imaging techniques, especially for MS, if answered incorrectly.

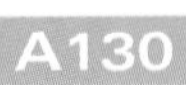
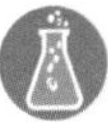

Genitourinary | Evaluation, Diagnosis

An elderly male patient is not able to participate in rehabilitation. He is lethargic, complains of nausea and painful urination, and seems to be feverish. The therapist should inform his primary care physician if which of the following is suspected?

Choices:

1. Bladder cancer.
2. Benign prostatic hyperplasia.
3. Urinary tract infection.
4. Renal calculi (kidney stones).

Teaching Points

Correct Answer: 3

These are signs and symptoms of urinary tract infection. Evidence of fever is especially significant. The physician should be informed.

Incorrect Choices:

The other choices do present with these same signs and symptoms. Fever is uncommon.

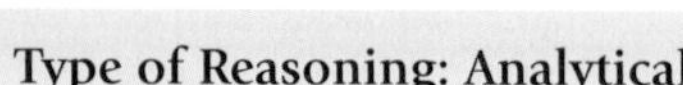

Type of Reasoning: Analytical

For this question, one must analyze the symptoms presented in order to determine the most likely diagnosis. Questions of this nature often necessitate analytical reasoning skill. For this situation, the symptoms are consistent with a urinary tract infection. Review signs and symptoms of urinary tract infection if answered incorrectly.

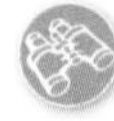

A131

Musculoskeletal | Evaluation, Diagnosis

The left phrenic nerve of a patient was accidentally severed during thoracic surgery. Which muscles should the physical therapist strengthen in order to provide substitute function?

Choices:

1. Tranversus abdominis.
2. Scalenes.
3. Internal obliques.
4. External obliques.

Teaching Points

Correct Answer: 2

The phrenic nerve arises from the neck (C3–5) and innervates the diaphragm. The diaphragm is responsible for 45% of the air that enters the lungs during quiet breathing. During quiet breathing, the predominant muscle of respiration is the diaphragm. As it contracts, pleural pressure drops, which lowers the alveolar pressure and draws in air down the pressure gradient from mouth to alveoli. Expiration during quiet breathing is predominantly a passive phenomenon; as the respiratory muscles relax, the elastic lung and chest wall return passively to their resting volume. With paralysis of the diaphragm, the accessory muscles of respiration should be strengthened. These include the scalenes and sternocleidomastoid.

Incorrect Choices:

During active expiration, the most important muscles are those of the abdominal wall (including the rectus abdominis, internal and external obliques, and transversus abdominis), which drive intra-abdominal pressure up when they contract and thus push up the diaphragm, raising pleural pressure, which raises alveolar pressure, which in turn drives air out. These muscles do not substitute for diaphragmatic function.

Type of Reasoning: Inductive

One must utilize knowledge of accessory muscles of respiration in order to arrive at a correct conclusion. Based on this knowledge, one can determine the best muscles to focus on for intervention, which is an inductive reasoning skill. In this case, the scalenes should be the focus. Review accessory muscles for respiration if answered incorrectly.

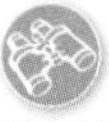

A132

Neuromuscular | Interventions

A patient recovering from surgery to remove a cerebellar tumor presents with pronounced ataxia and problems with standing balance and postural stability. To help improve this situation, what would be the **BEST** approach to incorporate in the intervention?

Exam A

Choices:

1. Lower extremity splinting and light touch-down hand support.
2. Rhythmic stabilization during holding in kneeling.
3. Perturbed balance activities while standing on carpet.
4. Stabilizing reversals during holding in side-lying.

Teaching Points

Correct Answer: 2

Rhythmic stabilization is a proprioceptive neuromuscular facilitation (PNF) technique designed to improve stability. The high kneeling position is a good choice to begin with for the patient with pronounced ataxia. The posture is upright; while the center of mass (COM) is lowered, the degrees of freedom are reduced by kneeling (foot and ankle control not required), and the base of support (BOS) is increased over standing.

Incorrect Choices:

Splinting and touch-down support are compensatory interventions not likely to improve recovery. Perturbed balance activities are contraindicated for the patient with poor postural stability and pronounced ataxia. Stabilizing reversals in side-lying are also not indicated, as the side-lying position does not require upright control.

Type of Reasoning: Inductive

One must utilize clinical judgment in order to determine the best intervention approach for this client. This necessitates inductive reasoning skill. For this scenario, the therapist should choose rhythmic stabilization during holding in kneeling to improve stability. Review intervention approaches for stability, especially rhythmic stabilization, if answered incorrectly.

A133 

Musculoskeletal I Examination

What would be a typical finding during the physical therapist's examination of a patient diagnosed with myofascial pain syndrome (MPS)?

Choices:

1. Few localized trigger points with referred patterns of pain during palpation.
2. Multiple generalized local tender points in muscle without referred patterns of pain.
3. Chronic fatigue, decreased exercise tolerance, and headaches.
4. Irritable bowel syndrome and sleep disturbance.

Teaching Points

Correct Answer: 1

MFP is a chronic pain disorder characterized by localized trigger points and referred patterns of pain. Pressure on sensitive points in muscle (trigger points) causes referred pain in seemingly unrelated parts of the body.

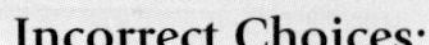

Incorrect Choices:

Chronic fatigue, sleep disturbances, generalized tender points, and irritable bowel syndrome are symptoms of fibromyalgia and not necessarily of myofascial pain syndrome.

Type of Reasoning: Inferential

One must infer or determine what is likely to be the findings of a patient with myofascial pain syndrome in order to arrive at a correct conclusion. Questions that provide a diagnosis and require the test-taker to identify likely symptoms or findings often necessitate inferential reasoning skill. For this case, one should expect to see few localized trigger points with referred pattern of pain during palpation. If answered incorrectly, review information on myofascial pain syndrome.

A134 

Musculoskeletal | Examination

Which special test of the knee region may assist in the classification of patellofemoral pain syndrome (PFPS)?

Choices:

1. Patellar apprehension test.
2. Thessaly test.
3. Patellar tilt test.
4. Noble compression test.

Teaching Points

Correct Answer: 3

The patellar tilt test is a nonprovocative test used to identify reduced patellar mobility (positive test), which prompts a moderate change in the likelihood of patellofemoral pain being present. Specifically, the test is used to determine the structural tightness of the lateral patellar retinaculum. The test also assists in classifying patients into the category of patellofemoral pain with mobility impairments. See Box 2-9 for the Patellofemoral Pain Clinical Practice Guidelines.

Incorrect Choices:

The Thessaly test is a pain provocation test for meniscal injuries. The patellar apprehension test is utilized to determine if patellar instability is present. The Noble compression test is a provocative test for iliotibial band friction syndrome.

Type of Reasoning: Inferential

This question requires the test-taker to infer which special test will be best in assisting in the classification of PFPS. This requires inferential reasoning skill where one uses judgment to determine what is likely to be a best course of action in a situation. For this case, the patellar tilt test may assist in the classification of PFPS. Review the Patellofemoral Pain Clinical Practice Guidelines if answered incorrectly.

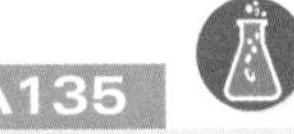

A135

Musculoskeletal | Examination

Six weeks following the conclusion of the football season, a therapist examines a player whose chief complaint is right thigh pain and decreased knee range of motion. Radiographic imaging of the area is shown in the picture. Intervention for this individual should be based on which diagnosis?

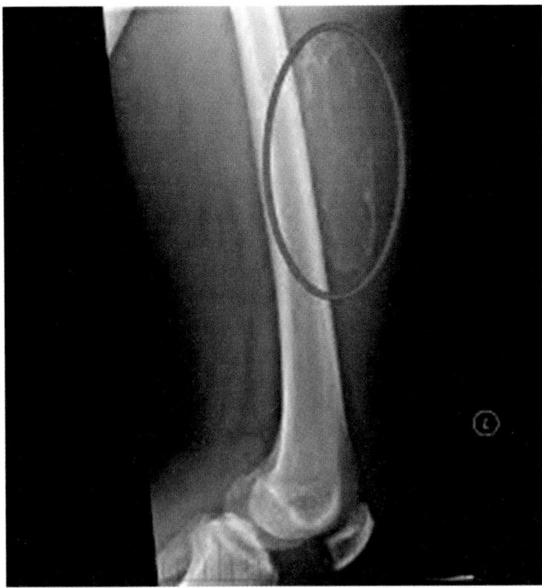

Choices:

1. Femoral stress fracture.
2. Neoplasm.
3. Quadriceps hematoma.
4. Myositis ossificans.

Teaching Points

Correct Answer: 4

Soft tissues that were injured in a traumatic event initially develop a hematoma and subsequently can develop into myositis ossificans. Myositis ossificans is a benign, ossifying soft-tissue lesion typically occurring within skeletal muscle, usually in adolescents and young adults. The most frequent symptoms and signs are pain and tenderness with a soft tissue mass. Approximately 80% of cases arise in the large muscles of the proximal extremities.

Incorrect Choices:

A stress fracture is an overuse injury. Bone is constantly attempting to remodel and repair itself, especially when extraordinary stress is applied. When enough stress is placed on the bone, it causes an imbalance between osteoclastic and osteoblastic activity, and a stress fracture may appear. Insidious onset of pain and swelling over the affected region is the most important complaint, initially during the activity. Neoplasms, or cancer of bone, change the appearance of bone on an x-ray. Bone may look ragged or may appear to have a hole in it. Hematomas look very different from tumors or bones on an x-ray because they are mostly fluid, and tumors and bones are solid.

Type of Reasoning: Analytical

For this question one must analyze the symptoms and information presented in the picture in order to determine the most likely diagnosis. This requires analytical reasoning skill, where assessing information from pictures is often used to reach sound conclusions. In this case, the symptoms presented and the picture depict myositis ossificans. Review signs and symptoms of myositis ossificans if answered incorrectly.

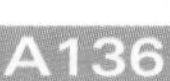
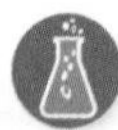

A136

Neuromuscular I Examination

During a finger-to-nose test, a patient demonstrates hesitancy in getting started and is then unable to control the movement. The finger slams into the side of the face, missing the nose completely. How should the therapist document this finding?

Choices:

1. Dysmetria.
2. Dysdiadochokinesia.
3. Dyssynergia.
4. Intention tremor.

Teaching Points

Correct Answer: 1

Dysmetria is an inability to judge the distance or range of movement. It includes both overestimation (hypermetria) and underestimation (hypometria) of the required range needed to reach the goal.

Incorrect Choices:

Dysdiadochokinesia is an impaired ability to perform rapid alternating movements (RAM). Dyssynergia is an impairment in movement composition. Movements are typically performed in component parts rather than as a single, smooth activity. Intention (kinetic) tremor is an involuntary oscillatory movement that occurs during voluntary movement.

Type of Reasoning: Analytical

For this question, one must analyze the symptoms presented in order to determine the most likely cause. This requires analytical reasoning skill. For this situation, the symptoms are consistent with dysmetria. Review signs of dysmetria if answered incorrectly.

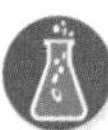

A137

Gastrointestinal I Evaluation

A physical therapist has been treating a 40-year-old female patient who is 5′3″ and 185 lbs. She is receiving therapy for low back pain. The patient recently returned from a vacation where she reports she was "not really watching her diet." She now complains of new pain in the right upper quadrant (RUQ), some mild nausea, as well as pain near her right scapula. These pains become worse with meals. Based on her symptoms, which is the **MOST LIKELY** source of these new complaints?

Choices:

1. Cirrhosis.
2. Acute pancreatitis.
3. Renal stones.
4. Gallstones.

Teaching Points

Correct Answer: 4

Classic symptoms of gallstones include nausea and RUQ pain, which can radiate to the right scapula. Gallstones are found more commonly in patients who are overweight or obese, female, and around the fourth decade of life. Gallstones occur more commonly in patients eating meals high in fat/cholesterol.

Incorrect Choices:

Cirrhosis does not typically cause any pain as the primary complaint. Ascites, which is not seen in all cases of cirrhosis, can cause abdominal distension, which is described as "discomfort" more than pain. Patients with acute pancreatitis will present very ill and not often ambulatory. The pain is severe and usually in the epigastrium radiating to the mid back. Patients often experience nausea and vomiting. Although alcohol consumption can lead to pancreatitis, this patient did not mention heavy alcohol use. Renal stones will often present with flank pain, and in some cases the pain can radiate to the groin depending on the location of the stone. This pain is also very severe and can cause vomiting.

Type of Reasoning: Analytical

This question requires one to analyze the symptoms presented in order to draw a logical conclusion about the most likely cause for them. When pieces of information are analyzed in order to draw a conclusion, analytical reasoning skills are utilized. For this situation, the most likely source of the symptoms is gallstones. Review signs and symptoms of gallstones if answered incorrectly.

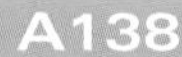
A138
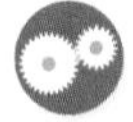

Nonsystem I Therapeutic Modalities

A physician requests that a physical therapist perform interferential current for pain management over the left shoulder of a patient with adhesive capsulitis. The therapist discovers that the patient has a pacemaker. In this case, what should the therapist do?

Choices:

1. Perform the treatment since there is no contraindication.
2. Refer the patient to another physical therapist who has greater expertise in using electrical modalities for patients with pacemakers.
3. Do not perform the treatment since it is contraindicated.
4. Administer the treatment with a waveform that does not penetrate as deep as interferential current.

Teaching Points

Correct Answer: 3

All applications of electrical stimulation are contraindicated in the presence of a pacemaker. Consultation with the referring physician is necessary.

Incorrect Choices:

All other options resulting in the administration of electrical stimulation near or through a pacemaker are contraindicated.

Type of Reasoning: Evaluative

This question requires the test-taker to weigh the potential courses of action and determine which response will have the most beneficial outcome. This necessitates evaluative reasoning skill. For this scenario, the therapist should not perform the electrical stimulation and should instead consult with the physician about alternative forms of therapy. Review contraindications for electrical stimulation if answered incorrectly.

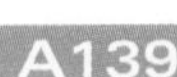

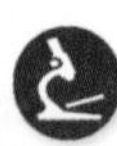

A139

Metabolic/Endocrine | Evaluation, Diagnosis

A physical therapist evaluates a patient for chronic low back pain. The patient is currently taking a diuretic (hydrochlorothiazide or hctz) to manage their hypertension. What is a potential adverse side effect of taking the diuretic?

Choices:

1. Water intoxication.
2. Metabolic acidosis.
3. Hypoglycemia.
4. Potassium depletion.

Teaching Points

Correct Answer: 4

Diuretics inhibit potassium, sodium, and water resorption by the kidneys. For patients taking diuretics, the therapist must monitor for possible symptoms consistent with potassium depletion and dehydration. Clinical signs and symptoms of potassium depletion include muscle weakness, fatigue, cardiac arrhythmia, abdominal distention, and nausea.

Incorrect Choices:

Water intoxication results from intake of large amounts of water without balanced solute ingestion. This may occur in individuals who drink only water after having the flu or in athletes who have lost a large amount of body fluid during strenuous exercise that has been replaced by water only. Symptoms include sleepiness, confusion, decreased alertness, poor motor coordination, and hyperventilation. Common causes of metabolic acidosis include drug or chemical toxicity, renal failure, severe diarrhea, and diabetic ketoacidosis. Symptoms of metabolic acidosis are headache, fatigue, drowsiness, nausea, hyperventilation, and convulsions. Hypoglycemia is often seen in patients with diabetes mellitus and is usually the result of a decrease in food intake or an increase in physical activity soon after insulin administration. Symptoms of hypoglycemia include shakiness, perspiration, irritability, pallor, weakness, blurred vision, headache, slurred speech, and hunger.

Type of Reasoning: Deductive

For this question, the test-taker must recall the adverse side effects of a diuretic in order to arrive at a correct conclusion. This requires deductive reasoning skill, where factual information is recalled in order to determine a correct answer. For this situation, a potential adverse side effect is potassium depletion. Review information on diuretics, especially adverse side effects, if answered incorrectly.

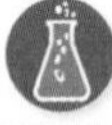

A140

Musculoskeletal | Evaluation, Diagnosis

During gait analysis, a therapist notes that a patient is lurching backward during stance phase. What is the cause of this compensatory motion?

Choices:

1. Gluteus medius weakness.
2. Hip and knee flexion contractures.
3. Quadriceps weakness.
4. Gluteus maximus weakness.

Teaching Points

Correct Answer: 4

Lurching backward during stance is a compensation for weak hip extensors, commonly called a gluteus maximus gait. Leaning backward during loading response inclines the ground reaction force vector posteriorly from its point of application at the hindfoot. Because the vector passes closer to the hip joint's lateral axis, its moment arm is shorter, and it produces a smaller hip flexor moment. If it falls behind the axis it can produce a hip extensor moment.

Incorrect Choices:

Gluteus medius weakness produces a Trendelenburg gait, or leaning to the side opposite the weakness.

When the quadriceps are weak, the person must compensate to preserve knee stability. Two of the common compensations will be hyperextension of the knee and forward trunk lean to put the center of gravity in front of the knee.

Hip and knee flexion contracture would produce a "short limb" during stance. This would result in the opposite extremity having to circumduct, hip hike, and steppage gait to get the lower extremity (LE) through swing. It will also lead to a shorter stride. Lumbar spine extension can effectively compensate for hip flexion contractures up to about 15°. When hip flexion contractures exceed 15° (a common occurrence) or there is limited lumbar spine extension range available (also common), the patient is forced to adopt a forward trunk tilt in terminal stance in order to complete the step. With a knee flexion contracture, it is more difficult to advance the ground reaction force vector anterior to the knee, its normal midstance position. This will force an increase in the muscular demands placed on the quadriceps muscle to maintain weight-bearing through a flexed knee.

Type of Reasoning: Analytical

One must analyze the gait abnormality in order to determine the most likely cause for it. This requires analysis of specific deficits, which necessitates analytical reasoning skill. For this case, the lurching backward during gait is caused by gluteus maximus weakness. Review gait analysis guidelines and effects of gluteus maximus weakness if answered incorrectly.

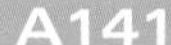
A141
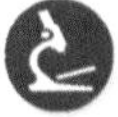

Cardiovascular/Pulmonary | Evaluation, Diagnosis

What are some common adverse effects that patients taking nitrates, diuretics, beta-blockers, or calcium antagonists might experience?

Choices:

1. Hypotension and dizziness.
2. Arrhythmia and unstable blood pressure.
3. Extreme fatigue and arrhythmias.
4. Hypotension and decreased electrolytes.

Teaching Points

Correct Answer: 1

All of these medications lower blood pressure. If the dosage is too great for patients, they will be hypotensive and likely feel dizzy.

Incorrect Choices:

Beta-blockers and calcium antagonists control arrhythmias. All medications stabilize blood pressure. If the dose of all these medications is too great, then the patient might experience extreme fatigue.

Type of Reasoning: Deductive

One must recall the adverse effects of various medications in order to arrive at a correct conclusion. This necessitates the recall of facts, which is a deductive reasoning skill. For this case, all of the medications may cause hypotension and dizziness. Review adverse effects of cardiac medications if answered incorrectly.

A142 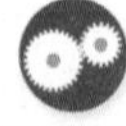

Neuromuscular | Evaluation, Diagnosis

A 3-year-old child with Arnold-Chiari malformation has a ventriculoperitoneal shunt in place. During physical therapy treatment, the child becomes agitated and irritable, then drowsy and listless. What should the therapist do in this situation?

Choices:

1. Immediately place firm pressure over the fontanel.
2. Administer emergency oxygen.
3. Place the child in a head-down position.
4. Call for emergency medical services.

Teaching Points

Correct Answer: 4

These are all signs of shunt blockage. Emergency medical services are indicated.

Incorrect Choices:

All other choices are inappropriate given the emergency nature of this problem and they may also be harmful, exacerbating the developing pressure in the brain (especially the head-down position).

Type of Reasoning: Evaluative

For this question, the test-taker must weigh the options presented and determine which option will most effectively address the problem at hand. This requires evaluative reasoning skill in order to reach a sound conclusion. For this situation, the therapist should call for emergency medical services. Review emergency procedures for shunt blockage if answered incorrectly.

A143 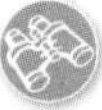

Neuromuscular | Interventions

A patient with a 6-year history of Parkinson's disease (PD) has experienced two recent bouts of pneumonia and limited functional mobility in the home. The therapist's plan of care focuses on improving respiratory function and postural control. What is the **BEST** choice for intervention to address these issues at this time?

Choices:

1. Supine, UE PNF lift and reverse lift patterns using rhythmic initiation.
2. Quadruped, alternate arm and leg raises.
3. Sitting, bilateral symmetrical UE PNF D2 flexion patterns using rhythmic initiation.
4. Standing, bilateral symmetrical UE PNF D2 flexion patterns using dynamic reversals.

Teaching Points

Correct Answer: 3

Sitting, bilateral symmetrical UE PNF D2 flexion patterns using rhythmic initiation are the best choices to open up the chest and enhance lung function (restrictive lung function is common in patients with PD). The sitting posture is a good starting position for a patient with postural instability since the base of support (BOS) is wide and the center of mass (COM) is lowered compared to standing.

Incorrect Choices:

Progression can occur from sitting to standing postures, but beginning in standing is not a good choice. Supine, UE PNF lift, and reverse lift patterns using rhythmic initiation can be used to improve rolling in patients with PD. Quadruped, arm and leg raises do not address the problem of restrictive lung disease.

Type of Reasoning: Inductive

This question requires one to utilize clinical judgment coupled with knowledge of PNF approaches to determine a best course of action for a patient with PD. This necessitates inductive reasoning skill. For this situation, sitting, bilateral symmetrical UE PNF D2 flexion patterns using rhythmic initiation is best. Review PNF approaches and intervention approaches for PD if answered incorrectly.

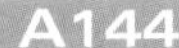
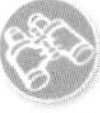

A144

System Interactions | Evaluation, Diagnosis, Prognosis

An elderly patient with diabetic peripheral neuropathy and retinopathy is having difficulty with balance when ambulating at home. The patient has fallen three times in the last month. What is the first priority of the home physical therapist's plan of care?

Choices:

1. Gait training with a cane to ensure safety.
2. Color-coding raised surfaces, such as steps, with a sharp color contrast.
3. Ambulation practice on changing floor to carpet surfaces in the home.
4. Installing nightlights in strategic areas throughout the house and keeping them lit continuously.

Teaching Points

Correct Answer: 1

The first priority of the home physical therapist should be gait training with a cane to ensure safety. This compensatory strategy is necessary as this patient is demonstrating complications of diabetes, which are chronic and progressive.

Incorrect Choices:

Color-coding steps and installing nightlights may also be necessary compensatory strategies to modify the home environment. However, they are not the first priority. Ambulation practice without a cane will not ensure the safety of this patient.

Type of Reasoning: Inductive

This question requires clinical judgment in order to determine a best course of action for an elderly patient with a history of falls. This necessitates inductive reasoning skill coupled with knowledge of effective approaches for home safety and fall prevention. For this scenario, the therapist should focus on gait training with a cane to ensure safety. Review fall prevention and home safety guidelines if answered incorrectly.

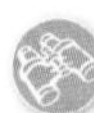

A145

Cardiovascular/Pulmonary I Interventions

A patient with deconditioning and a BMI of 52 presents to physical therapy for aerobic conditioning to assist with weight loss. To help increase the patient's functional capacity, the therapist initiates inspiratory muscle training. The patient's baseline maximal inspiratory pressure (MIP) is −65 ccH_2O. What is the most appropriate training program to increase the patient's MIP?

Choices:

1. Resistance = 65 ccH_2O, 15 minutes continuously.
2. Resistance = 26 ccH_2O, 15 minutes continuously.
3. Resistance = 59 ccH_2O, 30 minutes continuously.
4. Resistance = 13 ccH_2O, 30 minutes continuously.

Teaching Points

Correct Answer: 2

This represents 40% of the patient's MIP, which is within the optimal training range for increasing ventilatory muscle strength (30%–75% of MIP).

Incorrect Choices:

65 and 59 ccH_2O are at 100% and 90% of the patient's maximum, which is too hard of a training protocol. 13 ccH_2O is only 20% of the patient's maximum, which is too easy to cause changes in strength or endurance.

Type of Reasoning: Inductive

For this question, one must utilize knowledge of inspiratory muscle training guidelines and MIP values to determine a correct course of action. This requires clinical judgment, which is an inductive reasoning skill. For this case, the therapist should choose resistance = 26 ccH_2O, 15 minutes continuously to increase the patient's functional capacity. If answered incorrectly, review inspiratory muscle training guidelines and MIP values.

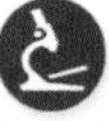

A146

Cardiovascular/Pulmonary I Examination

A therapist is monitoring the blood pressure of a healthy athlete exercising on a treadmill. The speed and incline steadily increase during the exercise period. The therapist would expect the blood pressure response to demonstrate which of the following?

Choices:

1. Blunted rise in systolic pressure and a slight decrease in diastolic pressure.
2. Slight drop in systolic pressure and either a slight increase or decrease in diastolic pressure.
3. Steady increase in systolic pressure accompanied by a steady increase in diastolic pressure.
4. Steady increase in systolic pressure and either a slight increase or decrease in diastolic pressure.

Teaching Points

Correct Answer: 4

A steady increase in systolic pressure and either a slight increase or decrease in diastolic pressure is a normal response to ramp exercise protocol. With a continual, steady increase in exercise, the systolic blood pressure will continue to rise because the patient is not permitted to reach steady state.

Incorrect Choices:

In a healthy individual, there should not be a blunted systolic blood pressure response. This occurs most frequently in patients on a beta-blocker. In a normal patient who is not on medications, it is not a normal response to have a drop in blood pressure. A drop in blood pressure would indicate an inability to maintain cardiac output at that intensity of exercise. Diastolic blood pressure does not increase steadily with activity. The normal increase or decrease of diastolic blood pressure is 10 mmHg.

Type of Reasoning: Deductive

One must recall the expected changes in blood pressure during treadmill exercise in order to reach a sound conclusion. This necessitates the recall of facts, which is a deductive reasoning skill. For this case, the therapist should expect a steady increase in systolic pressure and either a slight increase or decrease in diastolic pressure. Review responses to treadmill exercise if answered incorrectly.

A147 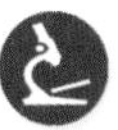

Musculoskeletal | Evaluation, Diagnosis

A physical therapist examines an elderly patient whose chief complaint is a sudden onset of muscle pain around the neck, shoulders, and hips. The patient also complains of fatigue, temporal headaches, and vision changes. The referring physician suspects polymyalgia rheumatica. Which laboratory test would help establish the diagnosis of this disease?

Choices:

1. Myelin basic protein.
2. Serum uric acid.
3. Creatine kinase.
4. Erythrocyte sedimentation rate.

Teaching Points

Correct Answer: 4

Polymyalgia rheumatica is a systemic inflammatory disorder that primarily affects proximal muscles in the shoulder and pelvic girdles, and muscular arteries such as the temporal artery. The erythrocyte sedimentation rate (ESR) and C-reactive protein (CRP) blood tests are general markers of inflammation and are markedly elevated in patients with the disorder. In addition to those described in the question stem, common clinical findings include weakness, malaise, low grade fever, sweats, weight loss, and depression.

Incorrect Choices:

Myelin basic protein levels are determined following a lumbar puncture with aspiration of cerebrospinal fluid. Elevated myelin basic protein levels are suggestive of demyelinating diseases such as multiple sclerosis. Elevated serum acid levels are seen in patients with gout and may be seen in patients with other conditions such as diabetes, hypothyroidism, and obesity. Creatine kinase levels are used to help diagnose conditions associated with muscle damage such as rhabdomyolysis and myocardial infarction.

Type of Reasoning: Deductive

For this question, the test-taker must recall laboratory testing guidelines related to polymyalgia rheumatica in order to reach a correct conclusion. This is factual information, which is a deductive reasoning skill. For this case, an erythrocyte sedimentation rate test would best establish the diagnosis of this disease. Review laboratory testing guidelines for polymyalgia rheumatica and other forms of arthritis if answered incorrectly.

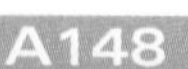
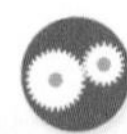

A148

System Interactions I Evaluation, Diagnosis

A patient recovering from a total hip arthroplasty is seen by the physical therapist for early mobilization out of bed. While sitting on the edge of the bed, the patient experiences rapid onset of dyspnea, sudden chest pain, and cyanosis. What action should the therapist take?

Choices:

1. Return the patient to supine and monitor vital signs for the next 5 minutes.
2. Stabilize the patient and contact medical services immediately.
3. Allow the patient to rest for a few minutes and continue with the therapy session.
4. Return the patient to supine and reschedule the therapy session for later in the afternoon.

Teaching Points

Correct Answer: 2

This patient is exhibiting signs and symptoms of pulmonary embolism. This is an emergency medical situation and a cause of death in a substantial number of patients.

Incorrect Choices:

All other choices do not address the life-threatening and emergency nature of this situation.

Type of Reasoning: Evaluative

For this question, one must determine the best course of action by weighing the options presented. This requires analysis of the symptoms in order to determine the severity of the situation to reach a sound conclusion, which is an evaluative reasoning skill. In this case, the therapist should stabilize the patient and contact medical services immediately. Review emergency procedures for pulmonary embolism if answered incorrectly.

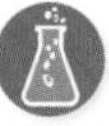

A149

Neuromuscular I Examination

A physical therapist is examining a patient recently admitted to inpatient rehabilitation following a severe traumatic brain injury (TBI). Which of the following examination items provides the most complete assessment of consciousness, including formalized examination of brain stem reflexes?

Choices:

1. Glasgow Coma Scale.
2. Rancho Los Amigos Levels of Cognitive Functioning.
3. Coma Recovery Scale-Revised.
4. Glasgow Outcome Scale-Extended.

Teaching Points

Correct Answer: 3

The Coma Recovery Scale-Revised examines multiple domains (auditory, visual, motor, verbal, communication, and arousal) of consciousness and function to include brain stem reflexes (pupillary light reflex, corneal reflex, spontaneous eye movements, oculocephalic reflex, and postural responses). It is recommended for use in multiple settings (acute care, inpatient/outpatient rehabilitation, long-term acute care/skilled nursing) and patients with various health conditions (TBI, stroke, brain tumor) that result in altered levels of consciousness.

Incorrect Choices:

The Glasgow Coma Scale (GCS) is typically used to assess acute concussions/TBIs, but is limited to assessing eye, verbal, and motor responses (see Table 3-15). The Rancho Los Amigos Levels of Cognitive Functioning (LOCF) is recommended for various settings and is used to delineate eight levels of cognitive and behavioral function in patients recovering from moderate to severe TBI (See Table 3-17). Although commonly used, the GCS and Rancho Los Amigos LOCF do not specifically include assessment of brain stem reflexes. The Glasgow Outcome Scale-Extended is a structured interview that does not include physical examination items. It is most often used in research studies to classify global functional outcome states (death, vegetative, moderate/severe disability) for patients who have experienced a TBI.

Type of Reasoning: Analytical

For this question, the test-taker must analyze the examination requirements presented and determine which formalized examination best meets these parameters. This requires analytical reasoning skill. For this case, the Coma Recovery Scale-Revised provides the needed measures of consciousness and formalized examination of brainstem reflexes. Review assessments for TBI, especially coma recovery and the Coma Recovery Scale-Revised, if answered incorrectly.

A150 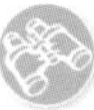

Neuromuscular | Interventions

When working with a child with Down syndrome and severe hypotonicity, how would it be best to activate the postural extensor muscles during early intervention?

Choices:

1. Slow, repetitive rocking movements with the child seated on a large gymnastic ball.
2. Prone positioning on a large gymnastic ball with the child looking up.
3. Quadruped, opposite arm and leg lifts.
4. Standing, weight shifts in modified plantigrade.

Teaching Points

Correct Answer: 2

The child with Down syndrome typically demonstrates hypotonia, developmental delay in postural stability, and poor use of proprioception for postural control. Prone positioning on a large gymnastic ball and having the child look up (neck extension) and/or reach up is a good early intervention to activate the postural extensors.

Incorrect Choices:

Slow, repetitive rocking on a large ball is relaxing and not indicated for patients with hypotonia. Quadruped opposite arm and leg lifts and standing, weight shifts in modified plantigrade are dynamic stability (controlled mobility) activities and are too advanced for this child, who lacks basic stability.

Type of Reasoning: Inductive

One must utilize knowledge of effective intervention approaches to activate postural extensor muscles in order to arrive at a correct conclusion. This necessitates clinical judgment, which is an inductive reasoning skill. For this scenario, the therapist should place the child in prone on a large ball with the child looking up. Review intervention approaches for promoting extensor muscle activation if answered incorrectly.

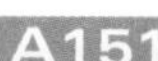

A151 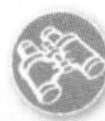

Neuromuscular | Interventions

A patient recovering from stroke demonstrates dyspraxia. Which of the following physical therapy interventions is the **BEST** option for treatment of dyspraxia?

Choices:

1. Reeducation of weak muscles using isokinetics before activity practice.
2. Compensatory training strategies with maximum use of environmental cues.
3. Task-specific practice of familiar activities progressing from parts to whole.
4. Maximum use of manual facilitation of movements and new tasks.

Teaching Points

Correct Answer: 3

Dyspraxia is an impairment of skilled learned movement (a disconnect between the idea for movement and its motor execution). Task-specific practice using familiar activities and progression from parts to whole is the best choice to enhance learning.

Incorrect Choices:

Reeducation of weak muscles in isolated movements will not carry over to improved functional task performance. Compensatory techniques may be necessary if the dyspraxia is severe and the patient fails to benefit from a remedial intervention program (not evident in this case). Manual facilitation may benefit the patient during task practice, but both maximum use and practice of new tasks are not likely to benefit the patient.

Type of Reasoning: Inductive

For this question, the test-taker must draw from knowledge of dyspraxia and effective intervention approaches to arrive at a correct conclusion. This necessitates clinical judgment, which is an inductive reasoning skill. In this case, the focus of intervention should be task-specific practice of familiar activities progressing from parts to whole. If answered incorrectly, review intervention approaches for dyspraxia.

A152 

Musculoskeletal | Interventions

A patient presents with a limitation of wrist flexion. The joint mobilization technique that would **BEST** improve the patient's range of motion is which of the following Grade IV descriptions?

Choices:

1. Posterior to anterior glide of the proximal carpal row on distal radius and ulna.
2. Posterior to anterior glide of the lunate on capitates.
3. Anterior to posterior glide of the proximal carpal row on distal radius and ulna.
4. Anterior to posterior glide of lunate on capitates.

Teaching Points

Correct Answer: 3

A Grade IV anterior to posterior glide of proximal carpal row on distal radius and ulna is the correct choice because during wrist flexion, the proximal row moves dorsally on the distal radius and ulna.

Incorrect Choices:

Posterior to anterior glide of the proximal carpal row on distal radius and ulna is a component motion for wrist extension. Posterior to anterior glide of the lunate on capitates would likely improve wrist extension. Anterior to posterior glide of lunate on capitates may assist with flexion but does not address the primary area of motion during wrist flexion.

Type of Reasoning: Inferential

This question requires one to determine which intervention approach will have the optimal outcome in improving a wrist flexion limitation. This requires one to determine what is most likely to be true, which is an inferential reasoning skill. For this case, the best technique would be a Grade IV anterior to posterior glide of the proximal carpal row on distal radius and ulna. Review joint manipulation techniques, especially for the wrist, if answered incorrectly.

A153 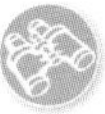

Neuromuscular | Examination

An older adult with a 3-year history of Parkinson's disease is referred secondary to initial and mild difficulties with balance. The patient has had two near falls in the past 3 months with both occurring after he was accidently bumped in the community. Which of the following examination items is **BEST** to assess the patient's current balance and fall risk?

Choices:

1. Berg Balance Scale (BBS).
2. The Mini-BEST (Balance Evaluation System Test).
3. Functional Gait Assessment (FGA).
4. Timed Up & Go with Cognitive Task (TUG-Cog).

Teaching Points

Correct Answer: 2

The patient's past falls are a result of delayed reactive postural control (the ability to recover balance after an external perturbation). The Mini-BEST has strong psychometric properties and measures various domains of balance to include reactive postural control (see Table 3-9). The Mini-Best is also recommended by the APTA Neurology Section Parkinson's Disease EDGE Task Force (see Table 3-19).

Incorrect Choices:

The BBS, FGA, and TUG-Cog do not directly assess reactive postural control.

Type of Reasoning: Inductive

For this question, the test-taker must utilize knowledge of examination approaches for patients with Parkinson's disease in order to arrive at a correct conclusion. This requires clinical judgment, which is an inductive reasoning skill. For this case, the Mini-BEST would best assess the patient's current balance and fall risk. If answered incorrectly, review balance and fall risk assessments, especially the Mini-BEST.

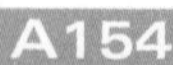
A154 

Metabolic and Endocrine | Interventions

A patient with insulin-dependent diabetes is participating in an aerobic exercise class. The therapist recognizes that important dietary recommendations to prevent delayed-onset hypoglycemia after exercise include intake of which of the following?

Choices:

1. Fruit juice or candy.
2. Crackers or bread.
3. Beef jerky and string cheese.
4. Carrot sticks and cherry tomatoes.

Teaching Points

Correct Answer: 2

Slowly absorbed carbohydrates (crackers, bread, or pasta) can help prevent delayed-onset hypoglycemia.

Incorrect Choices:

Rapidly absorbed carbohydrates (e.g., fruit juice, candy, honey) are given during exercise to help prevent hypoglycemia. Foods with saturated fats (beef jerky, string cheese) should be limited. Carrot sticks and cherry tomatoes do not have major effects in preventing hypoglycemia.

Type of Reasoning: Inferential

This question requires one to recall slowly absorbed carbohydrates in order to arrive at a correct conclusion. This necessitates the recall of factual information, which is a deductive reasoning skill. For this situation, crackers or bread should be chosen to prevent delayed-onset hypoglycemia after exercise. Review dietary recommendations to prevent hypoglycemia if answered incorrectly.

A155 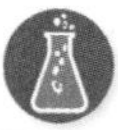

Musculoskeletal | Examination

A physical therapist is examining a patient who is complaining of pain in the left shoulder region. The examination of the shoulder elicits pain in the last 30° of shoulder abduction range of motion. This finding is most congruent with which of the following diagnoses?

Choices:

1. Calcific supraspinatus tendinitis.
2. Subacromial bursitis.
3. Acromioclavicular (AC) sprain.
4. Thoracic outlet syndrome.

Teaching Points

Correct Answer: 3

Typically, AC sprains will have pain at extremes of active range of motion (AROM), especially horizontal adduction and full elevation and pain on passive horizontal adduction and elevation. There are special tests for AC joint disorders:

- Acromioclavicular shear test: positive if abnormal movement of AC joint or pain at joint
- Passive cross-chest adduction

Incorrect Choices:

Calcific tendinitis may be asymptomatic and an incidental finding on an imaging study. If it is symptomatic, it can behave similarly to impingement syndrome. Supraspinatus tendinitis and subacromial bursitis will typically have a painful arc of motion from 60° to 120° of elevation and not at end range. TOS will usually manifest itself with proximal (supraclavicular and shoulder) pain and distal neurovascular symptoms of the upper extremity.

Type of Reasoning: Analytical

For this question, the test-taker must analyze the symptoms presented in order to draw a sound conclusion about the likely diagnosis. This necessitates analytical reasoning skill, where pieces of information are analyzed to determine their relevance. In this case, the symptoms are consistent with acromioclavicular (AC) sprain. Review symptoms of AC sprain if answered incorrectly.

A156 

Neuromuscular I Examination

A patient is recovering from a stroke (left cerebrovascular accident) and demonstrates difficulty with articulation. The therapist decides to test for function of the hypoglossal nerve (CN XII). Which of the following is the **BEST** test for hypoglossal function?

Choices:

1. Stimulate the back of the throat on each side and observe for gag reflex.
2. Instruct the patient to clench the teeth and hold against resistance.
3. Instruct the patient to show the teeth and puff out the cheeks.
4. Instruct the patient to protrude the tongue, observe for unilateral deviation.

Teaching Points

Correct Answer: 4

The hypoglossal nerve innervates the tongue. It is best tested by having the patient protrude the tongue. The therapist observes for deviation to the affected side. The tongue should also be inspected for muscle wasting and fasciculations. Articulation problems (dysarthria) occur with lesions of CN XII.

Incorrect Choices:

The gag reflex is impaired with lesions of CN IX Glossopharyngeal and CN X Vagus. Clenching the teeth and holding against resistance are tests for CN V Trigeminal. Showing the teeth and puffing out the cheeks are tests for CN VII Facial.

Type of Reasoning: Deductive

For this question, the test-taker must recall the guidelines for testing hypoglossal nerve (CN XII) function. This is factual information, which requires deductive reasoning skill. In this case, the therapist should instruct the patient to protrude the tongue and observe for unilateral deviation. If answered incorrectly, review testing guidelines for the hypoglossal nerve.

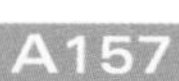

A157

Musculoskeletal | Examination

A patient presents with an acquired flatfoot deformity. The therapist recognizes that this can result from injury to a foot tendon. Which structure should be examined?

Choices:

1. Anterior tibialis tendon.
2. Posterior tibialis tendon.
3. Fibularis longus tendon.
4. Achilles tendon.

Teaching Points

Correct Answer: 2

The posterior tibial tendon helps hold the arch up and provides support when stepping off on the toes when walking. If this tendon becomes inflamed, overstretched, or torn, one may experience pain on the inner ankle and gradually lose the inner arch on the bottom of the foot, leading to flatfoot (posterior tibial tendon dysfunction [PTTD]).

Incorrect Choices:

The other choices are not associated with acquired flatfoot.

Type of Reasoning: Deductive

For this question, one must recall the tendon that is associated with flatfoot deformity. This necessitates the recall of factual information, which is a deductive reasoning skill. For this scenario, the tendon to be examined is the posterior tibialis tendon. Review flatfoot deformity if answered incorrectly.

A158

Musculoskeletal | Evaluation, Diagnosis

A physical therapist examines an elderly patient with chronic neck stiffness and shoulder pain. The patient exhibits significant kyphosis of the thoracic spine and a forward head posture. After completing the clinical examination, the therapist suspects a cervical spine myelopathy. Which physical examination finding would help corroborate the diagnosis of cervical myelopathy?

Choices:

1. Diminished patellar tendon and Achilles tendon reflexes.
2. Loss of sensation in the L5 dermatome.
3. Positive Hoffman's test.
4. Muscle weakness in the S1 distribution.

Teaching Points

Correct Answer: 3

Due to compression of the spinal cord, patients with a cervical myelopathy typically exhibit upper motor neuron signs, such as the presence of pathological signs (Hoffman's, Babinski, clonus), hyperreflexia, and ataxia. Additional clinical findings include loss of strength in the upper extremities, clumsiness, and bilateral upper extremity paresthesias.

Incorrect Choices:
Each of the incorrect choices is characteristic of the presentation of a patient who might have a lumbo-sacral radiculopathy. These findings include signs of lower motor neuron disease in a myotomal pattern or sensory deficits in a dermatomal distribution.

Type of Reasoning: Inferential
This question requires the test-taker to infer what is likely to be true of a situation after weighing the information provided. Inferential reasoning skill is often used to draw conclusions about likely findings or symptoms based on a provided diagnosis. In this case, a positive Hoffman's test would corroborate the diagnosis of cervical myelopathy. If answered incorrectly, review information on cervical myelopathy and Hoffman's sign.

A159 

Neuromuscular | Interventions

A patient with complete C7 spinal cord injury is receiving physical therapy to maintain joint mobility in an inpatient rehabilitation setting. What intervention is likely to produce the **GREATEST** risk of heterotopic ossification (HO)?

Choices:
1. Prolonged positioning with resting splints.
2. Forceful passive range of motion (PROM), especially if spasticity is present.
3. Prolonged stretching using tilt table standing.
4. Joint mobilization with PROM.

Teaching Points

Correct Answer: 2
Forceful PROM in the presence of spasticity increases the risk of developing HO (osteogenesis typically occurring in the soft tissues adjacent to large joints).

Incorrect Choices:
Joint mobility can usually be successfully maintained with all other choices.

Type of Reasoning: Inferential
For this question, the test-taker is provided with a condition and must determine the greatest risk factor associated with the condition. This requires one to determine what is likely to be true of a situation, which necessitates inferential reasoning skill. For this scenario, forceful passive range of motion (PROM), especially with spasticity present, presents the greatest risk for developing HO. Review risk factors for development of HO if answered incorrectly.

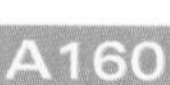

A160 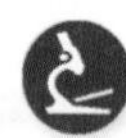

Integumentary I Examination

A patient complains of vascular changes in the hands usually experienced whenever it is cold. The therapist suspects Raynaud's disease. Which finding is consistent with this diagnosis?

Choices:

1. Hypersensitivity to tactile stimuli.
2. Loss of proprioception of the affected fingers.
3. Loss of two-point discrimination in the affected hands.
4. Temporary pallor and cyanosis of the digits.

Teaching Points

Correct Answer: 4

Raynaud's disease is a vasospastic disorder characterized by intermittent episodes of small artery constriction of the digits of the fingers (rarely the toes), causing temporary pallor and cyanosis.

Incorrect Choices:

The condition is most likely caused by hypersensitivity of the digital arteries to cold (not tactile stimulation). The condition is temporary and not associated with loss of proprioception or tactile discrimination.

Type of Reasoning: Deductive

This question provides a diagnosis, and the test-taker must infer the most likely examination findings. Questions of this nature often require inferential reasoning skill. For this situation, one would expect to see temporary pallor and cyanosis of the digits. Review signs and symptoms of Raynaud's disease if answered incorrectly.

A161 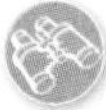

Nonsystem I Equipment, Devices

A patient sustained a trimalleolar ankle fracture on the right and a fracture of the left distal radius. For partial weight-bearing, it is **BEST** if the therapist has the patient use which device?

Choices:

1. Axillary crutches.
2. Forearm crutches.
3. Platform crutches.
4. Lofstrand crutches.

Teaching Points

Correct Answer: 3

Platform crutches allow weight-bearing on the forearms and are used for patients who are unable to bear weight through their hands, as in this case.

Incorrect Choices:

All other choices allow weight-bearing through the hands, placing stress on the distal radius.

Type of Reasoning: Inductive

For this question, one must determine the best assistive device for a patient with a trimalleolar ankle fracture on the right and a fracture of the left distal radius. This necessitates clinical judgment, which is an inductive reasoning skill. Based on the patient's injuries, platform crutches are the best choice. Review indications for platform crutches if answered incorrectly.

A162 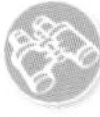

Musculoskeletal I Interventions

In a 6-month-old child demonstrating muscle contracture consistent with left torticollis, what is the **BEST** stretching technique to normalize muscle length of the sternocleidomastoid?

Choices:

1. Stabilize the left shoulder and stretch the neck into right side-bending.
2. Stabilize the left shoulder and stretch the neck into right side-bending and left rotation.
3. Stabilize the left shoulder and stretch the neck into left side-bending.
4. Stabilize the left shoulder and stretch the neck into left side-bending and right rotation.

Teaching Points

Correct Answer: 2

A left-sided torticollis is present with contracture of the left sternocleidomastoid. The muscle action of the left sternocleidomastoid is left side-bending and right rotation. To most effectively stretch the left sternocleidomastoid, stabilize the left shoulder and place the cervical spine into a combination of right side-bending and left rotation.

Incorrect Choices:

While right side-bending would still stretch the left sternocleidomastoid, the muscle is most effectively stretched with a combination of side-bending and rotation. Placing the cervical spine in left side-bending and right rotation would be an effective stretch for the right sternocleidomastoid.

Type of Reasoning: Inductive

This question requires the test-taker to recall the best treatment approaches for torticollis, specifically, stretching techniques to normalize the muscle length of the sternocleidomastoid. This requires clinical judgment, which is an inductive reasoning skill. For this case, the therapist should stabilize the left shoulder and stretch the neck into right side-bending and left rotation to stretch the sternocleidomastoid. Review stretching guidelines for torticollis if answered incorrectly.

A163 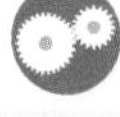

Neuromuscular I Interventions

A teenager is admitted to a skilled nursing facility with a severe traumatic brain injury and marked spasticity. Cognitive function is documented at Rancho Los Amigos Levels of Cognitive Functioning Scale level IV. Family members visit on a daily basis. In this situation, it would be BEST if passive range of motion (PROM) exercises are implemented in which way?

Choices:

1. Taught to family members in order for them to participate in the care of the patient.
2. Performed only by the physical therapist since the patient is unable to follow verbal commands.
3. Performed only by the physical therapist (PT) or physical therapist assistant (PTA) to minimize the possibility of pathological fractures.
4. Taught to all registered nurses (RNs) who might participate in the care of the patient.

Teaching Points

Correct Answer: 1

Passive range of motion (PROM) exercises can be taught to family members in order for them to participate in the care of the patient.

Incorrect Choices:

Other rehab staff, not only PTs or PTAs (e.g., rehabilitation aides, nursing assistants), can also be taught PROM techniques to maintain the joint mobility of the patient with marked spasticity. The RN is not typically engaged in this type of care of the patient.

Type of Reasoning: Evaluative

This question requires one to weigh the potential courses of action in order to determine which action will have the best therapeutic outcomes. This requires evaluative reasoning skill. For this situation, the therapist should teach family members PROM exercises so they can participate in the care of the patient. Review traumatic brain injury information and participation of family in the plan of care.

A164 

Nonsystem I Equipment, Devices

After gait training a patient with a transtibial prosthesis, a therapist notices redness along the patellar tendon and medial tibial flare. What would this finding indicate?

Choices:

1. The socket is too small and the residual limb is not seated properly.
2. The socket is too large and pistoning is occurring.
3. There is improper weight distribution during stance.
4. Pressure-tolerant weight-bearing is occurring.

Teaching Points

Correct Answer: 4

Pressure-tolerant areas of the typical transtibial residual limb include the patellar tendon, the medial tibial plateau, the tibial and fibular shafts, and the distal end.

Incorrect Choices:

These are expected areas of redness. All other choices would not result in that pattern of redness.

Type of Reasoning: Inferential

For this question, one must infer what is likely to be true for a patient who is gait training with a transtibial prosthesis. This requires inferential reasoning skill. Using knowledge of prosthetics, one should conclude that pressure-tolerant weight-bearing is occurring during stance. Review gait training guidelines with transtibial prosthetics if answered incorrectly.

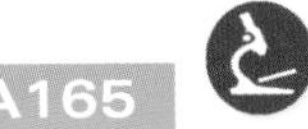

A165

Neuromuscular | Examination

During the examination of a 2-year-old child with mild cerebral palsy, the therapist is encouraged because the normal developmental milestones for a child of this age have been achieved. This was demonstrated by the child's ability to perform which activity?

Choices:

1. Hop on one foot.
2. Stand on tiptoes.
3. Go up stairs foot-over-foot.
4. Jump with two feet.

Teaching Points

Correct Answer: 3

Going up stairs foot-over-foot (reciprocal stair climbing) is a developmental skill normally achieved by 2 years.

Incorrect Choices:

The ability to hop on one foot and stand on tiptoes is normally achieved by 4 years. The ability to jump with two feet is normally achieved by 3 years.

Type of Reasoning: Deductive

One must recall motor skill development in toddlers in order to arrive at a sound conclusion for this question. This necessitates the recall of factual information, which is a deductive reasoning skill. For this situation, going up stairs foot-over-foot is a normal developmental milestone for a 2-year-old child. Review motor skill milestones, especially stair negotiation, if answered incorrectly.

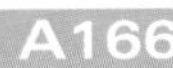
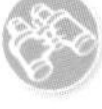

A166

Cardiovascular/Pulmonary | Interventions

A therapist sees a patient in the intensive care unit with multiple trauma and severe traumatic brain injury. A chest tube is in place and it exits from the right thorax. The patient is in need of airway clearance. What action should be taken in this case?

Choices:

1. Percussion and shaking are contraindicated due to the traumatic brain injury.
2. Percussion and shaking can be done only in the right side-lying position.
3. Percussion and shaking can be done in the area surrounding the chest tube.
4. Percussion and shaking can be done only when the chest tube is removed.

Teaching Points

Correct Answer: 3

It is possible to complete manual techniques in the area of the chest tube. It is often the area in most need of airway clearance. It is important to consider pain management when doing this intervention.

Incorrect Choices:

Percussion and shaking are not contraindicated, but it is important to consider that this may be agitating to patients with a severe brain injury. Also, placing the patient in Trendelenburg should be avoided in the acute period to eliminate increases in intracranial pressure. Percussion and shaking can be completed bilaterally and with the chest tube in place. It is important to attend to patient comfort and chest tube positioning when in right side-lying.

Type of Reasoning: Inductive

This question requires one to determine a best course of action based on knowledge of airway clearance guidelines. This requires clinical judgment, which is an inductive reasoning skill. For this scenario, it is possible to perform percussion and shaking in the area surrounding the chest tube. Review airway clearance techniques, especially around chest tube sites, if answered incorrectly.

A167 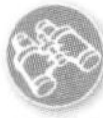

Musculoskeletal | Interventions

A patient is seen in an outpatient physical therapy clinic 3 days after a medial meniscus repair. What type of exercise should be avoided for the first 6–8 postoperative weeks to protect the repair?

Choices:

1. Ankle pumps.
2. Isometric quadriceps contractions.
3. Open chain resisted knee extension.
4. Open chain resisted knee flexion.

Teaching Points

Correct Answer: 4

The attachments of the medial meniscus include the semimembranosus tendon, MCL and fibrous capsule, and medial meniscopatellar ligament. During open chain resisted knee flexion, the semimembranosus tendon will pull on the posterior aspect of the medial meniscus and in doing so may tear the surgical repair. Resisted knee flexion should be avoided for several weeks postoperatively until the repair site is stable.

Incorrect Choices:

Ankle pumps do not produce any adverse forces on the healing meniscus and are beneficial development postsurgically and during periods of immobilization for prevention of DVT. Isometric quad sets produce little tibiofemoral joint motion. Resisted knee extension produces some anterior meniscal motion via the medial meniscopatellar ligament, but the amount of translation is minimal and not harmful to the repair.

Type of Reasoning: Inductive

One must determine the type of exercise to avoid interruption of a medial meniscus repair in order to arrive at a correct conclusion. Drawing from knowledge of kinesiology, the test-taker must utilize clinical judgment to draw a correct conclusion, which is an inductive reasoning skill. For this case, open chain resisted knee flexion should be avoided. If answered incorrectly, review exercise guidelines for medial meniscus repair.

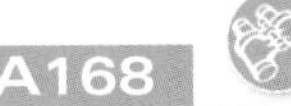

A168

Nonsystem I Equipment, Devices

To promote upright posture and higher walking speeds in a child with spastic diplegia, which ambulatory aid is **MOST** beneficial?

Choices:

1. A reciprocating gait orthosis.
2. An anterior rolling walker.
3. A posterior rolling walker.
4. Loftstrand (forearm) crutches.

Teaching Points

Correct Answer: 3

A posterior rolling walker is used to promote an upright posture (eliminates the forward lean seen in use of the standard anterior walker). The addition of wheels improves walking speed and reduces energy expenditure.

Incorrect Choices:

All other choices do not achieve these same goals.

Type of Reasoning: Inductive

One must utilize knowledge of mobility devices in order to arrive at a sound conclusion for this question. This necessitates clinical knowledge and judgment, which is an inductive reasoning skill. For this scenario, the therapist should choose a posterior rollator walker to promote an upright posture and higher walking speeds. Review mobility devices, especially rolling walkers, if answered incorrectly.

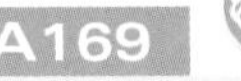
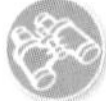

A169

Cardiovascular/Pulmonary I Interventions

Which high-intensity interval training program would be best for a patient with compensated New York Heart Association Class III heart failure?

Choices:

1. Time: 5–10 minutes; Intensity: 40%–50% of peak VO_2; Frequency: 2–3 times/week; Duration: 4–6 weeks
2. Time: 5–10 minutes; Intensity: 90%–95% of peak VO_2; Frequency: 5–7 times/week; Duration: 4–6 weeks.
3. Time: >35 minutes; Intensity: 90%–95% of peak VO_2; Frequency: 2–3 times/week; Duration: 8–12 weeks.
4. Time: >35 minutes; Intensity: 40%–50% of peak VO_2; Frequency: 5–7 times/week; Duration: 8–12 weeks.

Teaching Points

Correct Answer: 3

Choice 3 incorporates all parameters suggested by the Clinical Practice Guideline for the Management of the Patient with Heart Failure (see Table 4-18).

Incorrect Choices:

A training period of 5–10 minutes is too short and 40%–50% of peak VO_2 is not a sufficient intensity. A frequency of 5–7 times/week is too often and increases risk for injury. A duration of 4–6 weeks is too short to improve aerobic fitness.

Exam A

Type of Reasoning: Inductive

This question requires one to determine through clinical judgment the best high-intensity interval training program for a patient with compensated Class III heart failure. This requires knowledge of cardiac rehabilitation guidelines, which is an inductive reasoning skill. For this situation, the best program would be >35 minutes; intensity: 90%–95% of peak VO_2 with a frequency 2–3 times/week and a duration of 8–12 weeks. If answered incorrectly, review high-intensity interval training programs, especially for compensated Class III heart failure.

A170 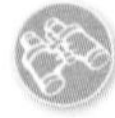

Neuromuscular I Examination

An independent community dwelling adult with multiple sclerosis is referred to physical therapy secondary to a recent exacerbation that has resulted in a significant increase in fatigue with activities of daily living and their work as an accountant. Which of the following examination items are **BEST** to serve as initial outcome measures for this patient?

Choices:

1. 12-item Multiple Sclerosis Walking Scale and Dynamic Gait Index.
2. Multiple Sclerosis Quality of Life Measure and Timed Up & Go.
3. Visual Analog Scale (Fatigue) and 2-minute walk test.
4. Fatigue Scale of Motor/Cognitive Function and 6-minute walk test.

Teaching Points

Correct Answer: 3

The visual analog scale (Fatigue) measures self-report of fatigue for daily life, grooming, and household/ occupational activities. Normative values for the 2-minute walk test have also been established for patients with multiple sclerosis.

Incorrect Choices:

None of the other options, except for the Fatigue Scale of Motor/Cognitive Function, directly measure the patient's primary impairment of fatigue. Additionally, secondary to the recent exacerbation it is important that the patient is not overexerted with more demanding (e.g., running) and increased duration activities (e.g., 6-minute walk test). Please see Table 3-18 for the APTA Neurology Section Multiple Sclerosis EDGE Task Force recommended examination items.

Type of Reasoning: Inductive

For this question, the test-taker must utilize clinical judgment to determine the best examination item for a patient with multiple sclerosis. This necessitates inductive reasoning skill. In this case, one must be familiar with the examinations presented in order to choose the examination that will best assess the patient's symptoms. For this scenario, the Visual Analog Scale (Fatigue) and 2-minute walk test are best. If answered incorrectly, review information on assessments for multiple sclerosis, especially the Visual Analog Scale (Fatigue) and the 2-minute walk test.

Neuromuscular I Intervention

A therapist is working with a patient with early myasthenia gravis with a focus on improving endurance, strength, and community participation. Which of the following signs are most consistent with exacerbation of myasthenia gravis and a need to stop or modify an exercise session?

Choices:

1. Double or blurred vision, decreased voice projection, and difficulty with repetitive sit-to-stand.
2. Dyspnea, syncope, and cold hands and feet.
3. Hyperreflexia, muscle spasms, and an inability to stand on one foot with eyes open.
4. Increased muscle and joint pain, inability to sleep, and irritability.

Teaching Points

Correct Answer: 1

Patients with myasthenia gravis (MG) typically have involvement of bulbar (extraocular, facial, and muscles of mastication) and proximal limb-girdle muscles. If overworked, patients will exhibit visual changes and difficulty with prolonged speaking, eating, or reading. They will also have weakness with repetitive testing of exercise of proximal limb muscles.

Incorrect Choices:

Shortness of breath, syncope, and cold distal extremities are more consistent with cardiovascular and respiratory conditions and not typically associated with MG unless it is severe (e.g., myasthenic crisis). Hyperreflexia and muscle spasm are more closely associated with upper motor neuron lesions and CNS involvement. Joint and muscle pain, inability to sleep, and irritability are more consistent with an active arthritic process or fibromyalgia.

Type of Reasoning: Inferential

This question requires the test-taker to infer or determine what is likely to be true for symptoms that are consistent with exacerbation of myasthenia gravis. This necessitates inferential reasoning skill. For this situation, double or blurred vision, decreased voice projection, and difficulty with repetitive sit-to-stand would indicate an exacerbation of myasthenia gravis. Review information on myasthenia gravis, especially response to exercise, if answered incorrectly.

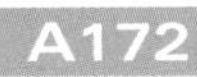 

Musculoskeletal I Intervention

An adult patient is referred to physical therapy with a diagnosis of central spinal stenosis. The patient's chief complaint is low back pain that radiates into the posterior aspect of both legs. Prolonged walking is an aggravating factor. The therapist identifies several hypomobile lumbar segments and plans to treat the patient with graded posterior-to-anterior mobilizations. How should the therapist position the patient in order to avoid exacerbating the lower extremity symptoms?

Choices:

1. Prone with the patient propped up on elbows.
2. Prone with a pillow placed under the patient's hips and lumbar spine.
3. Prone with the foot of the bed slightly elevated.
4. Prone with the head of the bed slightly elevated.

Teaching Points

Correct Answer: 2

Patients with central spinal stenosis have a position preference of flexion of the lumbar spine. Flexion of the low back opens the vertebral canal and lumbar foramina, thereby relieving pressure on lumbosacral nerve roots. The "shopping cart sign" is an illustration of how leaning forward in flexion can help alleviate symptoms in patients with spinal stenosis. Placing a pillow under the hips and low back of the prone patient puts the lumbar spine into some flexion and is more comfortable than prone lying in neutral.

Incorrect Choices:

Each of the other options places the patient into lumbar spine extension and will exacerbate the patient's symptoms.

Type of Reasoning: Inductive

For this question, the test-taker must determine a best course of action, based on knowledge of the diagnosis and positions that alleviate symptoms of the condition. This requires clinical judgment, which is an inductive reasoning skill. For this case, the therapist should place the patient in prone with a pillow placed under the patient's hips and lumbar spine. Review positioning techniques for central spinal stenosis if answered incorrectly.

A173 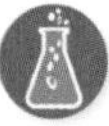

Musculoskeletal | Examination

After sustaining direct trauma to his anterior leg, a construction worker complains of severe leg pain and numbness and tingling on the dorsum of the foot. On examination, the physical therapist notes a tensely swollen leg, weak ankle dorsiflexors, and an absent dorsalis pedis pulse. What is the **MOST LIKELY** diagnosis?

Choices:

1. Syndesmosis injury.
2. Chronic exertional compartment syndrome.
3. Acute anterior compartment syndrome.
4. Medial tibial stress syndrome.

Teaching Points

Correct Answer: 3

Acute compartment syndromes are usually the result of direct trauma or a tibial fracture, resulting in swelling and increased compartmental pressure that results in local muscle ischemia. The six Ps of a compartment syndrome are pain, palpable tenderness, paresthesia, paresis, pallor, and pulselessness. Four of the Ps were described in the question stem: severe pain, paresthesias, paresis (weak ankle dorsiflexors), and pulselessness.

Incorrect Choices:

While a syndesmosis injury is possible, that type of injury does not typically present with any type of neurovascular deficit. Chronic exertional compartment syndrome and medial tibial stress syndrome are both overuse disorders, whereas an acute traumatic injury was described in this question.

Type of Reasoning: Analytical

For this question, the test-taker must analyze the symptoms presented in order to make an accurate determination of the diagnosis. This requires analytical reasoning skill, where pieces of information are weighed to draw correct conclusions. For this scenario, the symptoms most likely indicate acute anterior compartment syndrome. If answered incorrectly, review information on acute anterior compartment syndrome.

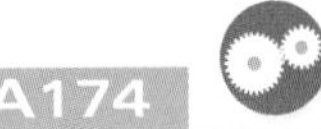

A174

System Interactions | Evaluation, Diagnosis

A physical therapist is treating a terminally ill patient with AIDS at home. What would be a major psychological focus or consideration when managing this patient?

Choices:

1. Discontinue treatment if the patient/therapist relationship becomes overly dependent.
2. Encourage expression of feelings and memories.
3. Keep the patient's friends and relatives up to date on the patient's treatment and state of mind.
4. Discontinue any activities that may cause the patient discomfort in order to keep anxiety levels low.

Teaching Points

Correct Answer: 2

When treating the patient with a terminal illness, the therapist should provide support and understanding of the grief process, encourage expression of feelings and memories, and respect privacy, cultural, or religious customs.

Incorrect Choices:

The therapist needs to maintain the boundaries of treatment and not discharge the patient. Keeping friends and relatives updated would violate the patient's privacy unless specific permission is given by the patient. The patient should be kept involved in the decision planning in order to reduce anxiety.

Type of Reasoning: Evaluative

One must weigh the options presented in order to determine the best course of action for a patient with AIDS. This necessitates evaluative reasoning skill, where one weighs the benefits of potential courses of action. For this scenario, the therapist should encourage expression of feelings and memories. Review the grief process for patients with terminal illness if answered incorrectly.

A175

Neuromuscular | Evaluation, Diagnosis

A patient with a transverse spinal cord injury has total lack of hip flexion, abduction, and knee extension. This functional loss is consistent with a designation of a complete spinal cord lesion at which level?

Choices:

1. L1.
2. L3.
3. L4.
4. L5.

Teaching Points

Correct Answer: 1

Hip flexors are innervated and functional at the L2 spinal cord level (key muscle). Therefore, an L1 lesion would produce complete loss of this muscle function.

Incorrect Choices:

Key muscles innervated and therefore functional at the remaining lumbar segments include knee extensors at L3, ankle dorsiflexors at L4, and long toe extensors at L5.

Type of Reasoning: Deductive

For this question, the test-taker must recall the innervation levels of the lumbar spine in order to arrive at a correct conclusion. This necessitates the recall of facts, which is a deductive reasoning skill. For this case, the lack of hip flexion, abduction, and knee extension are consistent with an L1 spinal cord lesion. Review innervation of the lumbar spine, especially L1, if answered incorrectly.

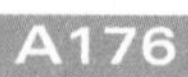
A176
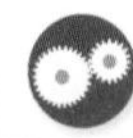

Nonsystem I Professional Responsibilities

A physical therapist (PT) is substituting for an ill colleague and is unable to access the previous PT's notes in the medical record. In this case, what should the therapist do?

Choices:

1. Ask the patient what treatment had been administered in the last session.
2. Attempt to reach the ill therapist by phone before commencing the session.
3. See if other coworkers can figure out how to access the information in the medical record.
4. Briefly examine the patient and intervene appropriately.

Teaching Points

Correct Answer: 4

If a PT accepts an individual for physical therapy services, the PT will be responsible for the examination, evaluation, and intervention of a patient. At the least, a systems review and brief plan of care should be formulated before intervening. Electronic medical records help to minimize difficulties in handwriting interpretation; however, systems aren't perfect.

Incorrect Choices:

Asking the patient for information can be unreliable. Trying to reach the ill therapist by phone is inappropriate and may also be unreliable since the ill therapist may not have access to the medical record at home. It is not the co-worker's responsibility to interpret others' notes; no one should have access to patient information if not involved in the care of that patient.

Type of Reasoning: Evaluative

This question requires one to weigh the potential courses of action and determine which action will resolve the problem at hand. This necessitates evaluative reasoning skill, where potential courses of action are weighed to draw sound conclusions. For this situation, the therapist should briefly examine the patient and intervene appropriately. Review professional roles and responsibilities if answered incorrectly.

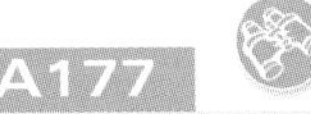

Systems Interaction | Evaluation, Diagnosis

A patient undergoing radiation therapy for breast cancer is referred for physical therapy. The radiation is limited to the involved breast. Which side effect of radiation therapy is the most important consideration for the physical therapist when developing a treatment plan?

Choices:

1. Increased possibility of hemorrhage resulting from heavy resistance exercise.
2. Gastrointestinal dysfunction.
3. Development of lymphedema in the ipsilateral upper extremity.
4. Painful upper extremity motion as a result of skin irritation and soft tissue fibrosis.

Teaching Points

Correct Answer: 4

Patients undergoing radiation therapy often experience skin irritation, swelling, and fibrosis of connective tissue at the treatment site. Ipsilateral trunk and upper extremity mobility may be painful and limited if the target of radiation therapy is the breast or in the axilla.

Incorrect Choices:

Hemorrhage following heavy resistance exercise is a possibility if the patient's platelet count drops too low, but this is a side effect of chemotherapy, not radiation therapy. Chemotherapy attacks the rapidly dividing cancer cells, but it also affects all rapidly dividing cells in the body, including all blood cell types. Chemotherapy can also be toxic to the cells that line the gastrointestinal tract and can result in nausea and vomiting, which may lead to poor nutritional intake and dehydration. Lymphedema is a complication that can occur after treatment of breast cancer as a result of the removal of lymph nodes, typically in the axillary and pectoral regions. Radiation to the axillary lymph nodes may cause lymphedema, but the treatment site in this case was the breast.

Type of Reasoning: Inductive

For this question, the test-taker must determine a best course of action in developing a treatment plan based on possible side effects associated with radiation therapy. This requires clinical judgment, which is an inductive reasoning skill. For this case, it is MOST IMPORTANT to consider the presence of painful upper extremity motion as a result of skin irritation and soft tissue fibrosis. If answered incorrectly, review side effects of radiation therapy.

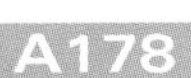

Musculoskeletal | Examination

The physical therapist receives a referral to evaluate and treat a 6-month-old infant with right congenital muscular torticollis. On initial examination, the therapist would expect the head to be in which position?

Choices:

1. Tilted toward the noninvolved side, with the chin rotated toward the same side.
2. Tilted toward the involved side, with the chin rotated toward the opposite side.
3. Limited in ROM in lateral flexion toward the involved side.
4. Limited in ROM in neck flexion and extension.

Teaching Points

Correct Answer: 2

Congenital muscular torticollis involves a shortened sternocleidomastoid (SCM) muscle with a weakened contralateral SCM muscle, with a resulting posture of lateral flexion of the head to the involved (right) side, tight SCM muscle side and rotation of the head to the noninvolved (left) side.

Incorrect Choices:

The other choices do not correctly identify the impairments in head position and ROM seen with muscular torticollis.

Type of Reasoning: Inferential

For this question, the test-taker must determine what is likely to be the clinical presentation for a child with torticollis. This requires one to recall the symptoms of congenital muscular torticollis in order to determine the likely clinical presentation, necessitating inferential reasoning skill. For this case, one would expect the head to be tilted toward the involved side with the chin rotated toward the opposite side. Review symptoms of congenital muscular torticollis if answered incorrectly.

A179 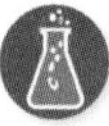

System Interactions | Evaluation, Diagnosis

An elderly female patient is being evaluated for recurrent thoracic back pain. During the history, the patient reveals a smoking habit, and she drinks four to six cups of coffee a day. Activity level is low, consisting of daily trips to the local coffee shop to socialize with friends. Body weight and height are below normal. Medical history includes Graves' disease. The therapist decides to consult the primary physician for further workup. What is the suspected problem?

Choices:

1. Osteoporosis.
2. Osteoarthritis.
3. Gout.
4. Spinal stenosis.

Teaching Points

Correct Answer: 1

This patient is exhibiting several risk factors for osteoporosis: postmenopausal age, low body weight, loss of height, sedentary lifestyle, tobacco use, and hyperthyroidism (Graves' disease). Signs and symptoms include severe and localized thoracic-lumbar pain, increased pain with prolonged upright posture, decreased pain in hook-lying, loss of height, and kyphosis (dowager's hump). Her pain is most likely due to compression fractures, which can be confirmed on x-ray. Osteoporosis can be confirmed with a bone density scan.

Incorrect Choices:

Osteoarthritis produces asymmetrical pain with typical involvement of large weight-bearing joints. Gout pain is limited to only a few joints, typically affecting the first metatarsal, the knee, or the wrist. Spinal stenosis typically occurs in the lumbar spine and is accompanied by pain when standing and walking, extending into the buttocks and proximal thigh, nocturnal pain, and lower motor neuron (LMN) signs.

Type of Reasoning: Analytical

This question provides a group of symptoms, and the test-taker must determine the most likely diagnosis based on a risk factor assessment. This requires analytical reasoning skill where symptoms are analyzed to reach sound conclusions. For this scenario, one would suspect the problem to be osteoporosis. Review risk factors for the development of osteoporosis if answered incorrectly.

A180 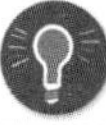

Musculoskeletal | Examination

A patient ambulates with excessive foot pronation. What will the therapist's examination **MOST LIKELY** reveal?

Choices:

1. Varus position of the heel.
2. Forefoot valgus.
3. Plantar fasciitis.
4. Valgus position of the heel.

Teaching Points

Correct Answer: 4

Excessive foot pronation is known as pes planus or pes valgus—a "flat foot deformity." The foot remains in pronation at the subtalar joint during weight-bearing. The slight pronation of both the subtalar and transverse tarsal joints seen in normal stance is exaggerated.

Incorrect Choices:

The question asks what this observation during gait would reveal. Many patients have pronated feet without plantar fasciitis. Overpronation can cause stress or chronic inflammation on the plantar fascia ligament (plantar fasciitis) and lead to numerous related foot and ankle injury conditions. Over time, the force of the impact is absorbed into the tissues, which can lead to conditions such as Achilles tendinitis, bunions, heel spurs, metatarsalgia, Morton's neuroma, plantar fasciitis (heel and arch pain), posttibial tendinitis, shin splints, and tarsal tunnel syndrome, as well as knee pain (chondromalacia, iliotibial band syndrome), hip pain, and lower back discomfort. Related conditions include corns, calluses, and hammertoes. Forefoot valgus and varus position of the heel are not congruent with foot pronation.

Type of Reasoning: Inferential

For this question, one must determine the likely clinical presentation based on the provided clinical observation. This necessitates inferential reasoning skill, where one determines what is likely to be true of a situation. In this case, one would expect valgus position of the heel to be present. If answered incorrectly, review flat foot deformity and clinical findings.

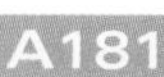
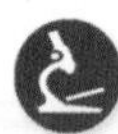

A181

Musculoskeletal | Interventions

A human bite injury resulted in laceration of the extensor tendons over the metacarpophalangeal (MCP) joints. Following surgical repair, the patient was placed in a dorsal dynamic extension splint (as pictured). Therapy is initiated in the first 24-hours, with the therapist instructing the patient to move in which way?

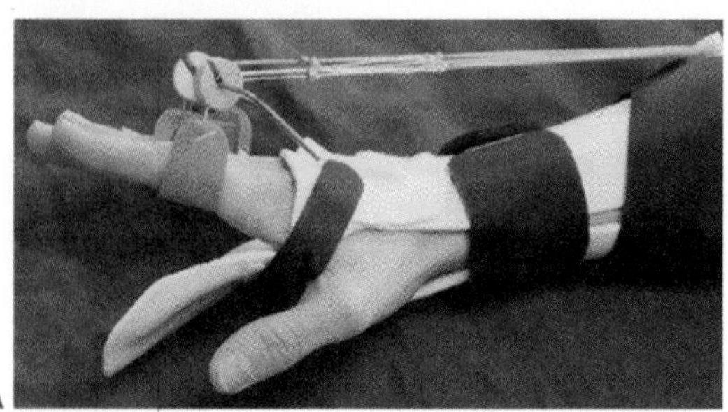
A

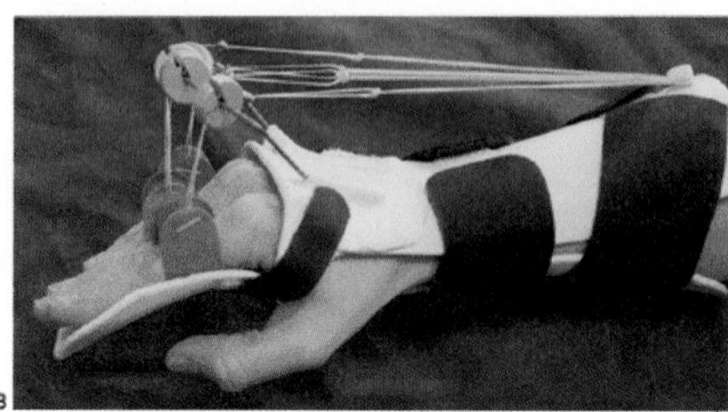
B

Choices:

1. Actively extend the wrist and passively flex the MCP joints.
2. Actively extend the wrist and MCP joints.
3. Passively extend the wrist and MCP joints.
4. Passively extend the wrist and actively flex the MCP joints.

Teaching Points

Correct Answer: 4

Goals during the first few weeks include preventing tendon rupture and promoting tendon healing as well as edema and pain control. For scar management, perform active range of motion (AROM) flexion, isolated joint and tendon gliding (hook and straight fist). Perform passive extension via elastic recoil of the dynamic splint, 10-reps hourly. Begin active MP flexion to 30°–40° (via flexion block on dynamic splint). Progress MP flexion as tolerated. Perform wrist and digit passive range of motion (PROM) in extension and tenodesis out of splint 10 repetitions hourly. Avoid making a full fist as this may place too much stress on the repair. The wrist is splinted in 40°–45° extension with 0°–20° of MP flexion and 0° of IP flexion.

Incorrect Choices:

One would not want any active extension as this could disrupt the repair. There are many different protocols, but many avoid any active extension until 4 weeks postop. Passively extending the wrist and MCP joints would be safe but would not help with preventing contractures of the repaired extensor tendons.

Type of Reasoning: Deductive

For this question, one must recall the protocol for range of motion after extensor tendon repair. This requires the recall of protocol guidelines, which is factual information and necessitates a deductive reasoning skill. For this scenario, the therapist should instruct the patient to passively extend the wrist and actively flex the MCP joints. Review extensor tendon repair range of motion guidelines if answered incorrectly.

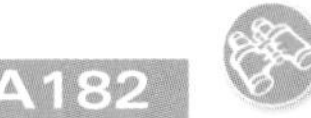

A182

Lymphatic | Interventions

The patient has phase II lymphedema in the right lower extremity resulting in fluid accumulation at the ankle. Which intervention would be most effective at reducing the edema?

Choices:

1. Crushed ice pack.
2. Intermittent compression pump.
3. Pulsed ultrasound.
4. Contrast bath.

Teaching Points

Correct Answer: 2

An intermittent compression pump provides external pressure, increasing the external hydrostatic pressure, which encourages reabsorption of the edema and minimizes fluid outflow from vessels. Pressures greater than 45 mmHg are contraindicated.

Incorrect Choices:

The other physical agents are not effective for this type of edema. In addition, the target area is too large for ultrasound (US) to cover reasonably, and a contrast bath would require the patient to be treated in a dependent position, which would further contribute to edema formation.

Type of Reasoning: Inductive

For this question, one must utilize clinical judgment in order to determine the best intervention approach for a patient with phase II lymphedema venous insufficiency. This requires inductive reasoning skill. Having knowledge of effective edema reduction techniques for this diagnosis, the therapist should choose the intermittent compression pump to reduce edema. Review edema reduction techniques for venous insufficiency if answered incorrectly.

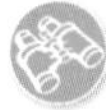

A183

Musculoskeletal | Interventions

To prevent bone density loss, which exercise activity should the physical therapist **FIRST RECOMMEND** to a previously untrained postmenopausal patient with a diagnosis of osteoporosis?

Choices:

1. High-impact aerobics for 45 minutes two to three times per week.
2. Jogging 30 minutes four times weekly.
3. Walking 30 minutes three times weekly.
4. Strengthening exercises to the upper and lower extremity muscles beginning at 75% of one rep maximum one time per week.

Teaching Points

Correct Answer: 3

Walking 30 minutes three times weekly. Weight-bearing, non-jarring exercises have been proven to reduce or slow bone loss without causing vertebral compression.

Incorrect Choices:

Individuals with osteoporosis should initially avoid high-impact exercises to limit excessive vertebral loading, which is the case with aerobics and jogging.

Initially, exercise intensity should be lower at first (50% of the one rep max and more frequently than one time per week).

Type of Reasoning: Inductive

For the question, the test-taker must utilize clinical judgment in order to determine the best recommendation for exercise for a patient with osteoporosis. This requires inductive reasoning skill, where application of clinical knowledge is paramount to arriving at a correct conclusion. For this scenario, the therapist should first recommend walking 30 minutes three times weekly. If answered incorrectly, review exercise programs for individuals with osteoporosis.

A184 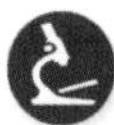

Cardiovascular/Pulmonary | Evaluation, Diagnosis

What is one of the most common early signs of right ventricular failure?

Choices:

1. Paroxysmal nocturnal dyspnea.
2. Exertional dyspnea.
3. Pulmonary edema.
4. Dependent edema.

Teaching Points

Correct Answer: 4

If the right ventricle fails, the increased fluid will back up. Traveling backward from the right ventricle, the edema goes into the right atrium and then the periphery. This causes dependent edema.

Incorrect Choices:

An inability to lie flat occurs when there is edema in the lungs (paroxysmal noctural dyspnea). This doesn't occur in isolated right ventricular failure. Exertional dyspnea occurs in right ventricular failure as a result of deconditioning after a period of time. It is not an early indication. Pulmonary edema results from increased intravascular pulmonary pressures. This doesn't occur in right ventricular failure because there is a reduction in forward flow, and therefore there are lower pulmonary arterial pressures.

Type of Reasoning: Deductive

For this question, one must recall the early signs of right ventricular failure in order to arrive at a correct conclusion. This requires the recall of factual information, which is a deductive reasoning skill. In this case, an early sign is dependent edema. Review signs and symptoms of right ventricular failure if answered incorrectly.

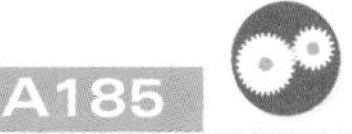

Nonsystem | Therapeutic Modalities

A physical therapist is considering the use of intermittent pneumatic compression for the presence of symmetrical bilateral lower extremity edema. Which of the following questions is **MOST IMPORTANT** to ask a patient prior to applying intermittent compression?

Choices:

1. Do you have difficulty breathing?
2. Did you recently have a "bull's-eye" rash anywhere on your body?
3. Did you recently fall and sprain your ankle?
4. Has your weight gradually changed in the past the 12 months?

Teaching Points

Correct Answer: 1

Symmetrical bilateral edema can signify congestive heart failure (CHF). Moderate to severe CHF can lead to pulmonary edema and subsequent shortness of breath. Intermittent compression may shift a significant amount of fluid from the periphery to the core circulation, thus increasing the load on the heart and immediate risk for a cardiac event. It is important to screen patients for shortness of breath as heart failure with pulmonary edema are contraindications to intermittent pneumatic compression.

Incorrect Choices:

A bull's-eye rash is associated with Lyme's disease and may cause joint pain and myalgia but would not result in bilateral lower extremity edema. Asking a patient if they experienced a fall and ankle sprain would explain unilateral localized pain and swelling but not bilateral edema. A gradual weight change over 1 year is less concerning than a rapid fluctuation in weight over days to weeks. Specifically, rapid weight changes are associated with high-risk health conditions (e.g., CHF, cancer, liver, or renal disease) that are recognized as contraindications to intermittent compression.

Type of Reasoning: Evaluative

For this question, the test-taker must weigh the questions presented and determine which question is most important to ask prior to use of intermittent compression. Evaluative reasoning skill is often used when weighing the merits of potential courses of action. For this scenario, it is most important to ask if the patient has difficulty breathing, as this can signify CHF. Review contraindications for intermittent compression, if answered incorrectly.

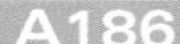 

Musculoskeletal | Examination

An ectomorphic adolescent patient presents at a physical therapy practice with a 6-month history of pain in both hands. Subjective complaints consist of pain that is worse in the morning but gradually improves throughout the day and overall fatigue. The only significant objective data from examination was mild edema and pain at end ranges of motion. What should the physical therapist do next in order to try to establish a diagnosis?

Choices:

1. Administer the Functional Independence Measure (FIM).
2. Examine for clubbing at the distal interphalangeal joints.
3. Examine for Dupuytren's contracture.
4. Refer the patient to a physician.

Teaching Points

Correct Answer: 4

This case represents the typical presentation for juvenile rheumatoid arthritis (JRA). The following are common symptoms of JRA: swollen, stiff, painful joints usually worse in the morning; fatigue; fever; swollen lymph nodes; and poor weight gain/slow growth. Additionally, the physical therapist was unable to identify specific impairments that would be potentially contributing to the patient's complaints, warranting referral to physician for additional testing.

Incorrect Choices:

The other choices do not address the findings of swollen, painful joints. The FIM evaluates functional performance (eating, dressing, grooming). Clubbing is seen with hypertrophic osteoarthropathy. Dupuytren's contracture involves flexion contractures of the fourth and fifth digits of the hand, MP, and proximal interphalangeal (PIP) joints.

Type of Reasoning: Evaluative

For this question, one must weigh the potential courses of action and determine which decision will best aid in establishing a diagnosis. This necessitates evaluative reasoning skill where one weighs the merits of each potential course of action to seek resolution. For this situation, the therapist should refer the patient to a physician. Review diagnostic approaches for JRA if answered incorrectly.

A187 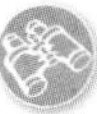

Nonsystem | Therapeutic Modalities

A therapist has decided to use mechanical lumbar traction on a patient with posterior herniated nucleus pulposus at L4-5 and signs of nerve root compression. If tolerated by the patient, what is the **BEST** positioning for this treatment?

Choices:

1. Prone, with no pillow under the hips or abdomen.
2. Prone, with a pillow under the hips and abdomen.
3. Supine, with the hips and knees flexed to 45°.
4. Supine, with hips and knees flexed to 90°.

Teaching Points

Correct Answer: 1

Neutral or extended position of the spine allows for separation of the vertebral bodies while preventing excessive stress on the posterior structures.

Incorrect Choices:

All of the other choices place the person in a flexed position, which places greater stress on the posterior structures of the disc. In the early stages of treatment, a flexed position is inadvisable with a posterior herniation.

Type of Reasoning: Inductive

For this question, one must utilize clinical judgment to determine the best positioning for lumbar traction. This requires inductive reasoning skill. For this case, the therapist should position the patient in prone, with no pillow under the hips or abdomen. Review lumbar traction techniques, especially for a posterior herniation, if answered incorrectly.

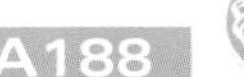

A188

Musculoskeletal I Interventions

A patient seen in a physical therapy clinic exhibits a forward head posture, excessive thoracic kyphosis, and rounded shoulders. Which muscles, in addition to the pectoralis minor, should be the focus of a therapeutic stretching plan for this patient?

Choices:

1. Rectus capitis posterior major, lower trapezius.
2. Upper trapezius, lower trapezius.
3. Rectus capitis posterior major, upper trapezius.
4. Rectus capitis posterior minor, lower trapezius.

Teaching Points

Correct Answer: 3

Muscles that will adaptively shorten in an individual with this posture also include the cervical paraspinal muscles, scalenes, levator scapulae, and suboccipital muscle group.

Incorrect Choices:

Due to the excessive kyphosis, the muscle fibers of the lower trapezius will be in a lengthened position and should be the target of strengthening exercises, not a stretching program.

Type of Reasoning: Inductive

For this question, the test-taker must draw from knowledge of treatment techniques for forward head posture, thoracic kyphosis, and rounded shoulders in order to arrive at a correct conclusion. This necessitates clinical judgment, which is an inductive reasoning skill. For this case, the therapist should focus on strengthening the pectoralis minor, rectus capitis posterior major, and upper trapezius. Review treatment techniques for postural dysfunction if answered incorrectly.

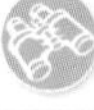

A189

Cardiovascular/Pulmonary I Interventions

A patient with restrictive lung disease secondary to circumferential thoracic burns demonstrates decreased ability to expand the lower rib cage and push the abdominal wall anteriorly. The therapist should consider the use of facilitation techniques to enhance the function of which of the following?

Choices:

1. Rectus abdominis.
2. Anterior scalenes.
3. Internal intercostals.
4. Diaphragm.

Teaching Points

Correct Answer: 4

Contraction of the diaphragm causes the ribs to move outward, which is the desired motion in this case.

Incorrect Choices:
Facilitating the rectus abdominis will cause trunk flexion, which will not increase lower rib expansion. Anterior scalenes facilitation will assist with increasing the negative pressure on inspiration; however, it will not assist with expanding the lower rib cage. Facilitation of the internal intercostals will cause the opposite motion than the desired lower rib expansion.

Type of Reasoning: Inductive
One must determine, based on the deficits presented, which muscle to facilitate in order to improve function. This requires inductive reasoning skill, where clinical judgment is paramount to arriving at a correct conclusion. For this situation, the therapist should focus on facilitating the diaphragm. If answered incorrectly, review facilitation techniques of the rib cage.

A190 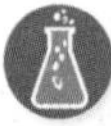

Musculoskeletal | Examination

A young, athletic patient complains of deep hip and groin pain along with a clicking sensation. The patient's symptoms are aggravated by deep squats and sports activities. Hip internal rotation is limited and the FABER and FADDIR tests are both positive. What is the **MOST LIKELY** diagnosis?

Choices:
1. Femoroacetabular impingement.
2. Trochanteric bursitis.
3. Piriformis syndrome.
4. Iliotibial band friction syndrome.

Teaching Points

Correct Answer: 1
Femoroacetabular impingement (see Box 2-4) results from a deformity of the femoral head or neck and the acetabular rim. Patients typically complain of anterior groin or hip pain reproduced by FADDIR and/or FABER tests, hip internal rotation less than 20° (with the hip at 90° of flexion), mechanical symptoms such as snapping or clicking, and radiographic findings of a cam (femoral neck/head) or pincer (acetabular rim) deformity.

Incorrect Choices:
Trochanteric bursitis is an inflammation of the deep trochanteric bursa, and the associated pain is palpable at the lateral aspect of the hip. Piriformis syndrome occurs when tightness or spasm of the piriformis muscle causes compression of the sciatic nerve. Symptoms are typically located in the buttock region, not the groin. Iliotibial band friction syndrome results from tightness of the IT band and results in pain at the distal lateral knee.

Type of Reasoning: Analytical
This question provides a group of signs and symptoms, and the test-taker must determine the most likely diagnosis. This necessitates analytical reasoning skill, where information is weighed or analyzed to draw a correct conclusion. In this case, the diagnosis is most likely femoroacetabular impingement. Review symptoms of femoroacetabular impingement if answered incorrectly.

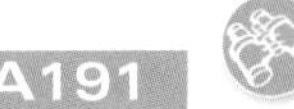

A191

Neuromuscular I Interventions

A patient with postpolio syndrome (PPS) is referred to physical therapy for exercise training. The patient reports recent general fatigue and weakness along with muscle and joint pain. What is the **BEST** initial intervention?

Choices:

1. Treadmill training at 2 mph and a 10 degree slope, 3 days/week for 30 minutes.
2. Cycle ergometry at peak heart rate, 3 days/week for 40 minutes.
3. Therapeutic aquatics, 3 days/week for 20 minutes.
4. Strength training at 70% 1 RM, 2 days/week.

Teaching Points

Correct Answer: 3

A good choice for an initial intervention is therapeutic aquatics. The warmth of the water can ease muscle and joint pain, and the buoyancy can assist fatigued limbs. An initial exercise duration of up to 20 minutes per session in 2- to 4-minute intervals is recommended.

Incorrect Choices:

All other choices are too vigorous for this patient at this time. If weakness or symptoms are recent, exercise duration should be no more than 15 minutes per session.

Type of Reasoning: Inductive

For this question, the test-taker must determine the best initial intervention approach for a patient with PPS. This necessitates clinical judgment, which is an inductive reasoning skill. For this case, the therapist should initiate intervention with therapeutic aquatics, 3 days/week for 20 minutes. Review intervention approaches for PPS if answered incorrectly.

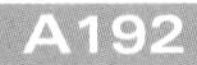
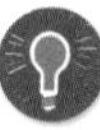

A192

Neuromuscular I Examination

A patient recovering from stroke walks with limited tibial advancement during stance on the more affected lower extremity. The therapist next examines the patient for a compensatory gait deviation. What is the **MOST LIKELY** deviation?

Choices:

1. Trendelenburg.
2. Circumduction.
3. Exaggerated flexion synergy.
4. Exaggerated extension synergy.

Teaching Points

Correct Answer: 2

Circumduction is the most likely compensatory gait deviation when tibial advancement is limited (e.g., spasticity of plantar flexors).

Incorrect Choices:

Trendelenburg gait is a lateral trunk lean that results from a weak or paralyzed gluteus medius on the stance side. An exaggerated flexion synergy results in flexion, abduction, and external rotation at the hip when the leg is lifted. An exaggerated extension synergy results in extension, adduction, and internal rotation (a scissoring pattern).

Type of Reasoning: Inferential

This question requires one to determine what is most likely to be true for a patient with a gait deviation. This requires inferential reasoning skill. Based on the description of symptoms, one should infer that circumduction would be the most likely gait deviation. Review gait deviations associated with limited tibial advancement.

A193 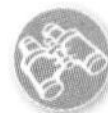

Neuromuscular | Interventions

An elderly patient with a 5-year history of Parkinson's disease (PD) demonstrates frequent freezing of gait (FOG) episodes while ambulating. What is the **BEST** choice of intervention to improve gait and reduce FOG?

Choices:

1. Part-to-whole training in sequencing of required gait elements.
2. Walking using lightly resisted progression with elastic bands to facilitate forward progression.
3. Body weight support and treadmill training (BWSTT), 40% unweighting, 3% incline, at 2.7 mph.
4. Locomotor training using a personal listening device with 80 to 100 beats/min music.

Teaching Points

Correct Answer: 4

Locomotor training using a personal listening device and 80 to 100 beats/min music has been shown to improve rhythmicity and decrease FOG episodes in patients with PD.

Incorrect Choices:

Part-to-whole training is not effective for motor skills with highly integrated elements (gait). Light resistance will likely increase the patient's stiffness during gait (already a problem with PD). BWSTT might be helpful to improve the rhythmicity of gait, but 40% unweighting is too high and 2.7 mph is too fast for this patient.

Type of Reasoning: Inductive

For this question, one must utilize knowledge of Parkinson's disease and effective gait training approaches in order to arrive at a correct conclusion. This necessitates inductive reasoning skill, where clinical judgment is paramount to choosing sound conclusions. For this situation, the best intervention approach is locomotor training using a personal listening device with 80 to 100 beats/min music. Review gait training approaches for PD if answered incorrectly.

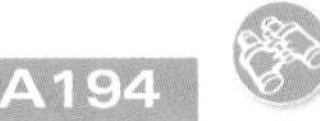

A194 Musculoskeletal | Interventions

A high school student sprained their great toe in gym class several weeks ago and continues to complain of pain and stiffness. On examination, the physical therapist notes limited first metatarsophalangeal joint extension. Which mobilization technique is **BEST** to improve extension of this joint?

Choices:

1. Medial glide of the proximal phalanx on the metatarsal.
2. Lateral glide of the proximal phalanx on the metatarsal.
3. Dorsal (anterior) glide of the proximal phalanx on the metatarsal.
4. Plantar (posterior) glide of the proximal phalanx on the metatarsal.

Teaching Points

Correct Answer: 3

An anterior or dorsal glide of the phalanx on the metatarsal would be used to increase first metatarsophalangeal extension. In this plane, a concave surface is moving on a convex surface, so the anterior glide will occur in the same direction as the osteokinematic or physiologic motion of extension.

Incorrect Choices:

Medial and lateral glides may be used to improve abduction/adduction or overall mobility of the joint. A plantar or posterior glide of the first phalanx would be used to improve metatarsophalangeal joint flexion. In this plane, a concave surface is moving on a convex surface, so the plantar glide will occur in the same direction as the physiologic motion of plantarflexion. See Table 2-1 for a review of the concave-convex rule application to peripheral joints.

Type of Reasoning: Inductive

For this question, one must recall joint mobilization guidelines and then apply them to a patient who has limited metatarsophalangeal extension with pain and stiffness. This requires inductive reasoning skill, where clinical knowledge is applied to therapeutic situations. For this case, the therapist should choose dorsal (anterior) glide of the proximal phalanx on the metatarsal. If answered incorrectly, review joint mobilization information, especially for the foot.

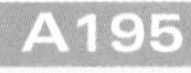

A195 Cardiovascular/Pulmonary | Evaluation, Diagnosis

A patient presents to outpatient cardiac rehabilitation. Their intake form states they had new onset atrial fibrillation 3 months ago, and their physician started a beta-blocker and placed a permanent pacemaker (dual sensing, demand pacemaker). Which statement BEST describes the anticipated patient findings or response to exercise?

Choices:

1. The pacemaker placement will have eliminated the atrial fibrillation, and the patient will have a regular heart rate.
2. The pacemaker will sense a lack of depolarization and initiate a contraction if the heart rate drops too low.
3. The patient could experience sudden cardiac death if they exercise.
4. The patient's hemodynamic response will be an unreliable measure of exercise tolerance and should not be measured.

Teaching Points

Correct Answer: 2

A dual sensing pacemaker is implanted to assess depolarization of the atrium or the ventricle. If the depolarization does not occur within the set time limits of the device, the pacemaker will initiate depolarization, which results in a ventricular contraction.

Incorrect Choices

The pacemaker has no effect on the heart rhythm in this case. The beta-blocker may lead to the patient converting to normal sinus rhythm, or more likely, the patient will remain in atrial fibrillation and the medication works to maintain the heart rate within a normal range (60–100 beats per minute). There is not any increased risk associated with exercise and a pacemaker. The hemodynamic response should be the same as any patient on a beta-blocker.

Type of Reasoning: Inferential

For this question, one must determine what is likely to be true for a patient with atrial fibrillation and a permanent pacemaker in place. This requires inferential reasoning skill, where one must predict outcomes based on information presented. For this situation, the patient's pacemaker will sense a lack of depolarization and initiate a contraction if the heart rate drops too low. Review pacemaker guidelines if answered incorrectly.

A196 

Neuromuscular I Evaluation, Diagnosis

A patient with a crush injury to the foot appears to be developing early signs of complex regional pain syndrome (CRPS). What are some early signs of this clinical condition the therapist would expect?

Choices:

1. Worsening pain with edema and atrophic skin and nail changes.
2. Cool, dry, and cyanotic skin with thickened fascia and developing contracture.
3. Hyperalgesia, allodynia, and hyperpathia.
4. Muscle atrophy, osteoporosis, and developing ankylosis.

Teaching Points

Correct Answer: 3

CRPS includes symptoms of pain, vascular changes, and atrophy. Early signs (stage 1) include hyperalgesia (increased sensitivity to pain), allodynia (all stimuli are perceived as painful), and hyperpathia (increased intensity) with edema, increased sweating, and thin, shiny skin.

Incorrect Choices:

Later signs and symptoms (stage 2) include increased pain with edema and atrophic skin and nail changes. Late stage changes (stage 3) include spreading pain; hardening of edema; cool, dry, and cyanotic skin; developing osteoporosis; and ankylosis.

Type of Reasoning: Inferential

One must infer what is likely to be true of a patient with early stage CRPS in order to arrive at a sound conclusion. This necessitates inferential reasoning skill, where one determines what is likely to be true of therapeutic situations. In this case, the early stage presentation is likely to be hyperalgesia, allodynia, and hyperpathia with edema, increased sweating, and thin, shiny skin. Review signs and symptoms of CRPS if answered incorrectly.

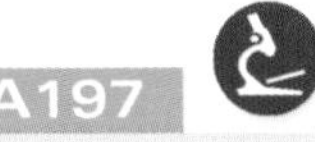

A197

Neuromuscular | Examination

A patient with long-standing diabetes mellitus is showing early signs of polyneuropathy. What is the **MOST** useful test to determine whether demyelination has taken place?

Choices:

1. Nerve conduction velocity (NCV) testing.
2. Electromyography (EMG).
3. Transcutaneous electrical nerve stimulation (TENS).
4. Motor point stimulation.

Teaching Points

Correct Answer: 1

NCV provides the most useful measurement of demyelinization in polyneuropathy. Conduction time is measured by recording the evoked potential from either a motor or sensory nerve. Speed of nerve transmission is directly related to level of myelination.

Incorrect Choices:

EMG is used to document (1) the different types of peripheral axonal injury (axonotmesis, neurotmesis) and (2) impairment of muscle recruitment. TENS is an electrical modality designed to provide afferent stimulation for pain management. Motor point stimulation is the area on the skin of greatest excitability to stimulate a muscle.

Type of Reasoning: Deductive

This question requires one to recall the benefits of each of the potential tests provided in order to choose the one that will be most useful in determining whether demyelination has taken place. This necessitates the recall of factual information, which is a deductive reasoning skill. For this situation, nerve conduction velocity (NCV) testing would be most useful. Review testing for demyelinization if answered incorrectly.

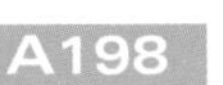

A198

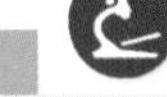

Musculoskeletal | Evaluation, Diagnosis

A physical therapist examines a young adult with a primary complaint of back and sacroiliac pain and stiffness that is worse in the morning. The patient demonstrates a kyphotic posture and extension is limited throughout the spine. Ankylosing spondylitis is suspected. Which laboratory test would help establish the diagnosis of this disease?

Choices:

1. Myelin basic protein.
2. A1c.
3. Creatine kinase.
4. HLA-B27 genetic marker test.

Teaching Points

Correct Answer: 4

The HLA-B27 test is primarily ordered to help strengthen or confirm a suspected diagnosis of ankylosing spondylitis (AS), reactive arthritis (formerly Reiter's syndrome), and juvenile rheumatoid arthritis. The test alone is not diagnostic of AS. It is ordered as part of a group of tests to help diagnose inflammatory arthritic conditions. This group of tests typically includes a rheumatoid factor, erythrocyte sedimentation rate, and a C-reactive protein.

Incorrect Choices:

Myelin basic protein levels are determined following a lumbar puncture with aspiration of cerebrospinal fluid. Elevated myelin basic protein levels are suggestive of demyelinating diseases such as multiple sclerosis. A1c, also called hemoglobin A1c or glycated hemoglobin, is hemoglobin with glucose attached. The A1c test evaluates the average amount of glucose in the blood over the last 2–3 months and is ordered to measure blood sugar levels in patients with diabetes or suspected diabetes/prediabetes. Creatine kinase levels are used to help diagnose conditions associated with muscle damage such as rhabdomyolysis and myocardial infarction.

Type of Reasoning: Deductive

This question requires the test-taker to recall laboratory testing guidelines for AS. This necessitates the recall of factual information, which is a deductive reasoning skill. For this case, an HLA-B27 test would help establish the diagnosis. Review information on AS and laboratory testing if answered incorrectly.

A199 

Cardiovascular/Pulmonary | Evaluation, Diagnosis

An adult female patient is being seen in an outpatient physical therapy clinic for hip pain. During the current visit to the clinic, the patient reports significant shortness of breath with minimal activity and no other symptoms. Past medical history is generally unremarkable to include no history of smoking or recent trauma. The patient's current medications include NSAIDS and a hormonal contraceptive medication. After walking from the waiting room to the treatment room, the patient's respiratory rate is 28, heart rate is 184, and SpO_2 = 92% on room air. What is the MOST likely cause of the patient's symptoms?

Choices:

1. Anxiety due to stress at work and home.
2. Pleural effusion due to lung cancer.
3. Pulmonary embolism due to use of birth control.
4. Tension pneumothorax due to increased exercise.

Teaching Points

Correct answer: 3

Patients taking hormonal birth control are at increased risk for pulmonary embolism or deep venous thrombosis. If a patient taking hormonal contraceptives experiences a marked increase in their respiratory and heart rates, they should be referred for emergency medical treatment. Normal adult respiratory rates are 12–20 breaths per minute and the normal adult heart rate is 60–100 beats per minute.

Incorrect Choices:

It is highly unlikely that anxiety would cause a drop in SpO_2. Pleural effusion due to lung cancer is very unlikely in a premenopausal woman with no history of smoking. A tension pneumothorax typically occurs as a result of trauma and does not usually result from exercise.

Type of reasoning: Inferential

This question requires the test-taker to analyze the presenting patient symptoms and then determine what is mostly likely to be the cause for such symptoms. This requires inferential reasoning skill, where one infers or determines what is likely to be true of a clinical situation. In this case, the symptoms are consistent with a pulmonary embolism. If answered incorrectly, review symptoms of pulmonary embolism.

A200 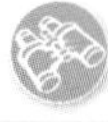

Neuromuscular I Interventions

A physical therapist is examining a patient who presents with brief episodes of vertigo when getting out of bed, bending forward, and when looking up to reach overhead. The patient has normal smooth pursuit and does not have resting or positional nystagmus during the ocular examination. When performing a Dix-Hallpike test to the right, the therapist observes a right torsional, up-beating nystagmus that lasts for 30 seconds and reproduces the patient's symptoms. What would be the most appropriate treatment for this patient?

Choices:

1. Perform a log roll maneuver.
2. Perform gaze stabilization VOR x 1 exercises in sitting.
3. Perform a canalith repositioning maneuver.
4. Perform Cawthorne-Cooksey exercises.

Teaching Points

Correct Answer: 3

The patient's presentation is consistent with right posterior canal benign paroxysmal positional vertigo (BPPV), which is treated with the canalith repositioning maneuver.

Incorrect Choices:

The log roll maneuver is used to treat horizontal canal BPPV. Gaze stabilization exercises and Cawthorne-Cooksey exercises are used to address impairments associated with vestibular hypofunction. BPPV results in overactivity of vestibular receptors due to the presence of otoconia in the semicircular canal, rather than diminished vestibular function.

Type of Reasoning: Inductive

For this question, one must recall effective treatment approaches for BPPV in order to arrive at a correct conclusion. This requires inductive reasoning skill, where clinical judgment and knowledge of treatment guidelines guide clinical reasoning. For this scenario, the most appropriate treatment is performing a canalith repositioning maneuver. Review treatment guidelines for BPPV if answered incorrectly.

Examination B

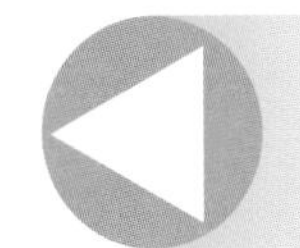

B1 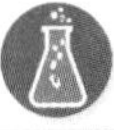

Neuromuscular | Evaluation, Diagnosis

A physical therapist is treating a child with spastic cerebral palsy who is 3 years old cognitively but at a 6-month-old gross developmental level. What is an appropriate treatment activity for this child?

Choices:

1. Reaching for a multicolored object while in an unsupported standing position.
2. Reaching for a multicolored object while in an unsupported, guarded sitting position.
3. Visually tracking a black and white object held 9 inches from his/her face.
4. Reaching for a black and white object while in the supine position.

Teaching Points

Correct Answer: 2

The appropriate task would include the 6-month-old gross developmental level activity of working on unsupported sitting. A multicolored object is appropriate for a 3-year-old cognitive level.

Incorrect Choices:

Standing and supine are not appropriate choices (too advanced or not advanced enough). The use of a multicolored object is more appropriate than a black and white object for a 3-year-old cognitive level.

Type of Reasoning: Analytical

In this question, the test-taker must take into consideration the chronological, cognitive, and gross developmental levels of the child in order to arrive at the correct conclusion. In this scenario, the test-taker must provide the appropriate physical challenge for a child developmentally functioning at 6 months in gross development, while providing activities that are appropriate for the 3-year-old cognitive level. If this question was answered incorrectly, review motor and cognitive developmental milestones.

B2 

Musculoskeletal | Interventions

A patient is receiving mobilizations to regain normal mid thoracic extension. After three sessions, the patient complains of localized pain that persists for greater than 24 hours. What is the therapist's **BEST** option?

Choices:

1. Change mobilizations to gentle, low-amplitude oscillations to reduce the joint and soft tissue irritation.
2. Continue with current mobilizations, followed by a cold pack to the thoracic spine.
3. Place the physical therapy on hold and resume in 1 week.
4. Change to self-stretching activities, because the patient does not tolerate mobilization.

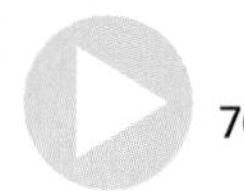

Teaching Points

Correct Answer: 1

Changing to low-amplitude oscillations will promote a decrease in the pain and tissue irritation. If pain persists for more than 24 hours, the soft tissue and joint irritation may progress.

Incorrect Choices:

Pain beyond 24 hours indicates possible tissue damage, so modification would be indicated. Placing the patient on hold would not be indicated or appropriate based on the patient's response. Self-stretching will improve the osteokinematic motion, but not the arthrokinematic motion, so this would not be an appropriate modification. It is not specific to the joint and may increase the irritation. It certainly would not decrease the pain and irritation.

Type of Reasoning: Inferential

This question requires one to understand joint mobilization techniques, coupled with recognition of possible results that may occur when utilizing the techniques. In this scenario, the patient's symptoms indicate that the joint mobilization techniques resulted in soft tissue and joint irritation. Therefore, the therapist should consider less irritating mobilization for improved tolerance. If this question was answered incorrectly, refer to joint mobilization information.

B3
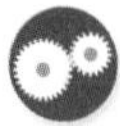

Neuromuscular | Interventions

A therapist wishes to use behavior modification techniques as part of a plan of care to help shape the behavioral responses of a patient recovering from traumatic brain injury (TBI). What intervention is the **BEST** to use?

Choices:

1. Use frequent reinforcements for all desired behaviors.
2. Encourage the staff to tell the patient which behaviors are correct and which are not.
3. Reprimand the patient every time an undesirable behavior occurs.
4. Allow the patient enough time for self-correction of the behavior.

Teaching Points

Correct Answer: 1

Behavioral modification is best achieved through use of positive reinforcements for all desired behaviors.

Incorrect Choices:

Negative behaviors should be ignored, not reprimanded. Self-correction is not a form of behavior modification.

Type of Reasoning: Evaluative

The test-taker utilizes knowledge of behavioral modification techniques to choose the correct answer in this scenario. Using evaluative skills, one determines the value of each of the four choices and which choice is most aligned with behavioral modification guidelines to promote positive behaviors via positive reinforcement techniques.

B4 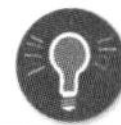

Neuromuscular | Interventions

A patient with multiple sclerosis (MS) presents with dysmetria in both upper extremities. Which of the following interventions is the **BEST** choice to deal with this problem?

Choices:

1. 3-lb weight cuffs to wrists during activities of daily living (ADL) training.
2. Isokinetic training using low resistance and fast movement speeds.
3. Pool exercises using water temperatures greater than 85 °F.
4. Proprioceptive neuromuscular facilitation (PNF) patterns using dynamic reversals with carefully graded resistance.

Teaching Points

Correct Answer: 4

Dysmetria is a coordination problem in which the patient is unable to judge the distance or range of movement (overshoots or undershoots a target). Adding manual resistance with PNF can assist the patient in slowing down the movement and achieving better control.

Incorrect Choices:

The patient lacks speed control. Low-resistance, fast-speed isokinetic training is contraindicated. The resistance of water (pool therapy) could help control the speed of movements, but the temperature is too warm (patients with MS demonstrate heat intolerance). Weight cuffs could also help slow the movements down but would unnecessarily fatigue the patient (patients with MS demonstrate problems with excessive fatigue).

Type of Reasoning: Inferential

One must understand the deficit of dysmetria in order to arrive at the correct conclusion. Using skills of inference, the test-taker uses the knowledge of dysmetria to determine what course of action is useful to promote improved coordination and motor control. If this question was answered incorrectly, review information on dysmetria.

B5 

Musculoskeletal | Interventions

A patient is seen in a physical therapy clinic several months after a total knee arthroplasty. The patient exhibits limited knee flexion with an empty end-feel detected by the therapist. There is no visible or palpable joint swelling. The therapist determines that manual therapy intervention is appropriate. Which tibiofemoral mobilization technique is the BEST initial choice to address these examination findings?

Choices:

1. Grade I/II posterior-to-anterior.
2. Grade I/II anterior-to-posterior.
3. Grade III/IV anterior-to-posterior.
4. Grade III/IV posterior-to-anterior.

Teaching Points

Correct Answer: 2

The therapist notes an empty end-feel during knee flexion suggesting that pain or muscle guarding is limiting the motion. No tissue resistance is encountered by the therapist during the passive range of motion assessment of the patient's knee. Grade I and II mobilization techniques are used to decrease pain and muscle guarding. This finding must be addressed first before considering the use of end-range mobilization techniques (grade III and IV) to improve motion. Based on the concave-convex rule, a posterior glide (anterior-to-posterior) would best facilitate knee flexion. See Table 2-1 for a review of the concave-convex rule application to peripheral joints.

Incorrect Choices:

Mobilizing the tibia in a posterior-to-anterior direction would be appropriate to improve limited knee joint extension. Grade III and IV joint mobilizations are used to improve motion by stretching tight joint capsules, ligaments, and other soft tissue structures at the end-range of motion.

Type of Reasoning: Inductive

For this question, one must recall joint mobilization guidelines and then apply them to a patient with a total knee arthroplasty with an empty end-feel during knee flexion. This requires inductive reasoning skills. For this case, the therapist should choose grade I/II anterior-to-posterior mobilization. If answered incorrectly, review joint mobilization guidelines, especially for the knee.

B6 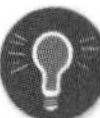

Cardiovascular/Pulmonary I Interventions

A patient recovering from cardiac transplantation for end-stage heart failure is referred for exercise training. What guidelines should the therapist follow when implementing an exercise program for this patient?

Choices:

1. Require longer periods of warm-up and cool-down.
2. Require short bouts of exercise.
3. Eliminate all resistance training.
4. Require a frequency of 2–3 times/week.

Teaching Points

Correct Answer: 1

A patient recovering from cardiac transplantation will require longer periods of warm-up and cool-down because physiological responses to exercise and recovery take longer.

Incorrect Choices:

Low- to moderate-intensity resistance training can be performed. Aerobic exercise should be performed 4–6 times/week, while progressively increasing the duration of training from 15–60 minutes per session. (Source: *ACSM Guidelines for Exercise Testing and Prescription*)

Type of Reasoning: Inferential

This question requires the test-taker to infer what may be true of a patient, given the diagnosis of cardiac transplantation. Inferential reasoning skills are utilized whenever one must predict a best course of action or determine what may be true of a person or situation. In this case, the therapist should recognize that the patient will require longer periods of warm-up and cool-down. If this question was answered incorrectly, review exercise guidelines for patients with cardiac transplantation.

B7 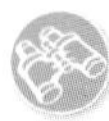

Neuromuscular | Interventions

A patient with fibromyalgia syndrome is experiencing symptoms of widespread pain, multiple tender trigger points, fatigue, sleep disturbances, and depression for the past 10 months and describes significant limitations in daily activities. The therapist wants to increase the patient's activity level with aerobic conditioning. Which of the following is the **BEST** choice for an initial exercise prescription for this patient?

Choices:

1. Treadmill walking, 20% grade, 30 minutes/session, 3–5 times/week.
2. Walking in the gym, 2–3 miles, 45–60 minutes/session, 3–5 times/week.
3. Pedaling on a cycle ergometer, 45 minutes/session, 4 times/week.
4. Pool walking, slow walking, 30 minutes/session, 2–3 times/week.

Teaching Points

Correct Answer: 4

Low-impact aerobics activities are best. Aquatic exercise (walking in a pool) has been shown to decrease pain and stiffness while increasing cardiovascular conditioning and strength. Exercise should start slow (mild intensity), 30-minute duration with rests as needed (interval training), 2–3 times per week.

Incorrect Choices:

All other choices are too aggressive (intensity, duration, frequency) and are likely to increase the patient's symptoms, resulting in increased pain. It is particularly important to start slowly. Overdoing activities can make the patient feel worse and discontinue therapy.

Type of Reasoning: Inductive

For this question, one must utilize clinical judgment to determine a best course of action. Questions where one must apply knowledge to clinical scenarios often necessitate inductive reasoning skill. For this situation, the BEST choice for an initial exercise prescription is pool walking, slow walking, 30 minutes/session, 2–3 times per week. If answered incorrectly review exercise prescription guidelines for fibromyalgia syndrome.

B8 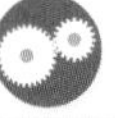

Genitourinary | Evaluation, Diagnosis

A new staff physical therapist (PT) on the oncology unit of a large medical center receives a referral for strengthening and ambulation for a woman with ovarian cancer. She is undergoing radiation therapy after a surgical hysterectomy. Her current platelet count is 17,000. What intervention is indicated for this patient at this time?

Choices:

1. Active range-of-motion (AROM) exercises and activities of daily living (ADLs) exercises.
2. Aerobic exercise 3–5 days/week at 40%–60% oxygen uptake reserve.
3. Resistance training at 60%, one repetition maximum.
4. Progressive stair climbing using a weighted waist belt.

Teaching Points

Correct Answer: 1

AROM and ADL exercises are beneficial and safe for this patient.

Incorrect Choices:

Exercise testing and training is contraindicated in patients with cancer whose platelets are <50,000, WBC <3,000, or Hemoglobin <10 g/dL. Additonal contraindications include significant bony metastases, severe cachexia, severe fatigue, or poor functional status.

Type of Reasoning: Evaluative

One must utilize knowledge of normal platelet counts and contraindications for resistive exercise in patients with cancer. In this situation, the patient's platelet count is low, which should alert the test-taker that resistive exercise should be deferred. Questions such as these require one to review the merits of a situation, which is an evaluative skill. Knowledge of normal blood counts is very useful information.

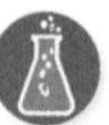

Musculoskeletal | Interventions

A patient complains of increased pain and tingling in both hands after sitting at a desk for longer than 1 hour. The diagnosis is thoracic outlet syndrome (TOS). Which treatment would be the **MOST** effective physical therapy intervention?

Choices:

1. Cardiovascular training using cycle ergometry to reduce symptoms of TOS.
2. Stretching program for the pectoralis minor and scalenes.
3. Strengthening program for the scalenes and sternocleidomastoids.
4. Desensitization by maintaining the shoulder in abduction, extension, and external rotation with the head turned toward the ipsilateral shoulder.

Teaching Points

Correct Answer: 2

TOS is described as compression to the neurovascular structures in the scalene triangle, the area defined by the anterior and middle scalenes between the clavicle and the first rib. The compression is a result of a shortened pectoralis minor and scalene muscles. Therefore, a stretching program to these muscles to gain space in the scalene triangle is appropriate.

Incorrect Choices:

Shortening of the scalenes and sternocleidomastoids may be the culprit that caused TOS to develop. Strengthening these muscles would not improve the amount of space in the scalene triangle space. Cardiovascular training, especially performed in the posture using a cycle ergometer, would not improve the disorder. The problem in TOS is too much vascular volume in too small a space. Increasing the vascular volume through that space with cardiovascular exercise will not resolve the symptoms of TOS. Desensitization by putting the shoulder and neck in this position is likely to diminish the space in the scalene triangle and further compress the neurovascular structures that run through that triangle.

Type of Reasoning: Analytical

This requires analytical reasoning. If this question was answered incorrectly, review the causes and interventions for TOS.

B10 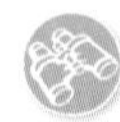

Metabolic/Endocrine | Evaluation, Diagnosis

A patient with diabetes and normal blood glucose prior to exercising reports feeling weak, dizzy, and somewhat nauseous after 1 hour of exercising in your clinic. The therapist notices that the patient is also sweating profusely and is unsteady when standing. What is the therapist's **BEST** immediate course of action?

Choices:

1. Insist that the patient sit down until the orthostatic hypotension resolves.
2. Have a nurse administer an insulin injection for hyperglycemia.
3. Have the patient sit down and administer orange juice for hypoglycemia.
4. Call for emergency services; the patient is having an insulin reaction.

Teaching Points

Correct Answer: 3

Hypoglycemia, or abnormally low blood glucose, results from too much insulin (insulin reaction). It requires accurate assessment of symptoms and prompt intervention. Have the patient sit down and give an oral sugar (e.g., orange juice).

Incorrect Choices:

Once the patient is stabilized, the physician should be notified. Emergency services are generally not needed. Profuse sweating does not usually accompany orthostatic hypotension.

Type of Reasoning: Inductive

The test-taker must first determine the cause of the patient's symptoms and then the appropriate course of action. Questions such as these utilize one's clinical judgment and diagnostic thinking, which is an inductive reasoning skill. One should recognize that these symptoms are indicative of hypoglycemia and require immediate administration of sugar to relieve symptoms.

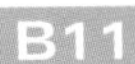 B11 

Neuromuscular | Evaluation, Diagnosis

A patient recovering from Guillain-Barré syndrome (GBS) started attending a supervised outpatient exercise program. The patient failed to show up for follow-up sessions. The patient reported increased muscle pain and being too weak to get out of bed for the past 2 days. The patient is afraid to continue with the exercise class. What is the therapist's **BEST** course of action regarding the patient's exercise program?

Choices:

1. Discharge the patient from the program because exercise is counterproductive in GBS.
2. Reschedule exercise workouts for early morning when there is less fatigue.
3. Decrease the intensity and duration, but maintain a frequency of 3 times/week.
4. Decrease the frequency to once a week for an hour session, keeping the intensity moderate.

Teaching Points

Correct Answer: 3

Clinical manifestations of GBS include myalgias, weakness, as well as excessive fatigue with minimal activity. Nonexhaustive exercise and general body conditioning are indicated. A change in the exercise prescription (intensity and duration) is warranted.

Incorrect Choices:

The patient should not exercise to the point of fatigue and exhaustion. A frequency of once a week is too little to be beneficial. Rescheduling exercise to early morning does not address the needed change in exercise prescription. Stopping exercise completely will not help this patient.

Type of Reasoning: Inferential

This question requires the test-taker first to understand the nature of GBS and then determine the appropriate exercise regimen to prevent further exacerbation of symptoms. Therefore, one must infer, or draw conclusions, from the evidence presented to arrive at the correct decision. If this question was answered incorrectly, review information on GBS.

B12 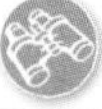

Nonsystem | Therapeutic Modalities

A physical therapist is conducting an initial examination of a client that sustained a direct blow to the knee 2 days ago. The x-ray in the emergency room was negative for a fracture. The patient is concerned about increased swelling over their "kneecap." The therapist's initial assessment is consistent with traumatic prepatellar bursitis. Which of the following would be of **MOST BENEFIT** to treat this condition?

Choices:

1. 20 minutes of cryotherapy, every 2–3 hours, for 3 continuous days.
2. 30 minutes of cryotherapy, twice a day, for 3 continuous days.
3. 1 MHz 20% pulsed ultrasound for 8 minutes three times a week.
4. 3 MHz 20% pulsed ultrasound for 8 minutes three times a week.

Teaching Points

Correct Answer: 1

This is an acute inflammatory condition. Cryotherapy is used to limit or reduce edema formation in acute situations. It should be applied as soon as possible and multiple times a day during the acute cycle. Under normal circumstances consistent vasoconstriction due to cryotherapy lasts up to about 20 minutes during the cooling cycle, which is why periods of cooling longer than 20 minutes are not recommended.

Incorrect Choices:

Thirty minutes of cryotherapy is longer than the recommended 15–20 minutes and has the potential for a hunting response. The hunting response is a phenomenon when tissue temperatures get too cold or persist too long, resulting in reflexive vasodilation. Additionally, icing two times a day is insufficient to control or prevent acute traumatic edema. Ultrasound is not recommended to limit edema formation, and three times a week of any modality is insufficient to control acute edema.

Type of Reasoning: Inductive

For this question, the test-taker must use clinical judgment and knowledge of traumatic prepatellar bursitis treatment in order to arrive at a correct conclusion. This requires inductive reasoning skill. For this case, the most beneficial treatment is 20 minutes of cryotherapy, every 2–3 hours, for 3 continuous days. If answered incorrectly, review treatment information for traumatic prepatellar bursitis.

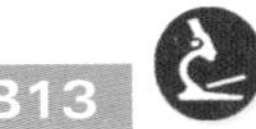

B13

Cardiovascular/Pulmonary | Interventions

A patient is recovering from open heart surgery (sternotomy and coronary artery bypass). The PT is supervising the patient's outpatient exercise program at 7 weeks postsurgery. What guidelines should be followed regarding the use of moderate to heavy weights during resistance training?

Choices:

1. Should include upper body exercises only.
2. Is contraindicated during the first 2 months.
3. Should be based on 60%–80%, one repetition maximum initially.
4. Can be included if resistance training is once a week.

Teaching Points

Correct Answer: 2

Resistive training after cardiothoracic surgery is restricted to 5 to 8 pounds for the first 5 to 7 weeks. Moderate to heavy resistance exercises are contraindicated.

Incorrect Choices:

Resistance training can begin 5 weeks postsurgery, including 4 weeks of consistent participation in a supervised cardiac rehabilitation endurance training program. Once cleared, initial loads for the upper body should be 30%–40%, one repetition max, and 50%–60% for hips and legs. (Source: *ACSM Guidelines for Exercise Testing and Prescription*)

Type of Reasoning: Deductive

One must recall the guidelines for cardiac exercise post-CABG in order to arrive at a correct conclusion. This requires recall of factual guidelines, which is a deductive reasoning skill. For this question, the key words are "7 weeks postsurgery," which should draw one to conclude that resistance training with moderate to heavy weights should be avoided during the first 3 months. If this question was answered incorrectly, review cardiac exercise guidelines, especially post-CABG.

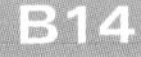

B14

Cardiovascular/Pulmonary | Evaluation, Diagnosis

A patient with asthma is taking a beta-2 agonist (sympathomimetic), albuterol (Ventolin). What is the **MOST** important effect of this medication?

Choices:

1. Increases airway resistance and decreases secretion production.
2. Reduces airway resistance by reducing bronchoconstriction.
3. Increases heart rate (HR) and BP to enhance a training effect during aerobic activity.
4. Reduces bronchial constriction and high blood pressure (BP) that accompanies exercise.

Teaching Points

Correct Answer: 2

Sympathomimetics are a class of drugs that mimic the effects of stimulation of body organs and structures by the sympathetic nervous system. Albuterol (Ventolin) has the primary action of reducing airway resistance by a decrease in bronchospasm.

Incorrect Choices:

Albuterol decreases airway resistance and has no effect on the volume or consistency of airway secretions. The primary effects of albuterol are on $\beta 2$ receptors in the bronchiole smooth muscle. It may also have an effect on $\beta 1$ receptors, producing cardiovascular adverse reactions of increased BP and tachycardia. These adverse effects can result in a patient monitoring exercise parameters at lower exercise workloads and reducing aerobic training effects.

Type of Reasoning: Inferential

This question, while requiring knowledge of the effects and side effects of medication (a deductive skill), also requires one to determine the **MOST** important effects (not adverse effects). Therefore, this question utilizes inferential reasoning, in which the test-taker must draw conclusions based on the information presented and determine what is most important, which encourages inferential deductive reasoning. If this question was answered incorrectly, refer to information on sympathomimetic medications.

B15 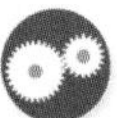

Lymphatic I Interventions

A patient who sustained a crush injury of the shoulder and upper arm has successfully completed a course of rehabilitation and is about to return to work as a painter. The patient now complains of frequent aching and pain in the axilla. The therapist is concerned that the patient is at risk for the development of lymphedema. The patient is active in team and individual sports. What is the **BEST** recreational activity for the patient to consider?

Choices:

1. Softball.
2. Cycling.
3. Bowling.
4. Jogging.

Teaching Points

Correct Answer: 2

The best choice is cycling, which does not involve the strenuous movements of the upper extremities that are required to perform the other activities.

Incorrect Choices:

Softball, bowling, and jogging are high-risk activities for patients with suspected lymphedema because of the strenuous nature and the frequent, sometimes aggressive rotational movements of the upper extremities. Softball and bowling require batting the ball and throwing from an over- or underhand position, with the potential for high centrifugal forces. Jogging is also not recommended for those at risk for developing lymphedema because of the forces placed on the upper extremity during arm carriage.

Type of Reasoning: Evaluative

For this question, one must evaluate the recreational activities presented and determine the activity that is best for a patient who is at risk for lymphedema. This requires evaluative reasoning skill, where one weighs the merits of each of the options to determine which one is best. For this case, cycling is the best activity. If answered incorrectly, review lymphedema guidelines, especially activities for patients at risk for lymphedema.

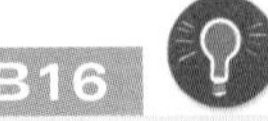

Musculoskeletal | Interventions

A therapist determines that a patient is walking with a backward trunk lean with full weight on the right leg. The patient also demonstrates great difficulty going up ramps. What is the **BEST** intervention to remediate this problem?

Choices:

1. Strengthen hip extensors through bridging.
2. Stretch hip abductors through sidelying positioning.
3. Strengthen knee extensors with weights, using 80%, one repetition maximum.
4. Stretch hip flexors through prone-lying positioning.

Teaching Points

Correct Answer: 1

Backward trunk lean (gluteus maximus gait) is the result of a weak gluteus maximus. It causes increased difficulty going up stairs or ramps. Functional training exercises such as bridging are indicated.

Incorrect Choices:

The patient is able to perform a backward trunk lean in standing, indicating adequate range in hip flexors. Ability to take full weight on the limb without knee buckling indicates adequate strength of knee extensors. Tightness in hip abductors is rare and would result in the posture (lateral lean) being maintained during all phases of gait.

Type of Reasoning: Inferential

In this question, the test-taker must determine the cause of a backward trunk lean and difficulty ascending ramps and which muscle groups require strengthening. This type of question requires one to make inferences or draw conclusions from the evidence presented in order to make a clinical decision. If this question was answered incorrectly, review knowledge of gait deviations and their causes.

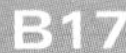

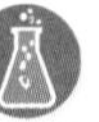

Integumentary | Examination

A patient has developed a thick eschar secondary to a full-thickness burn. What is the antibacterial agent **MOST** effective for infection control for this type of burn?

Choices:

1. Sulfamylon.
2. Nitrofurazone.
3. Panafil.
4. Silver nitrate.

Teaching Points

Correct Answer: 1

Sulfamylon penetrates through eschar and provides antibacterial control.

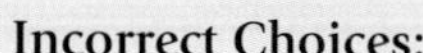

Incorrect Choices:

Silver nitrate and nitrofurazone are superficial agents that attack surface organisms. Panafil is a keratolytic enzyme used for selective debridement.

Type of Reasoning: Analytical

This question requires recall of the properties of each agent in antibacterial control and then determination of which one would **MOST** effectively promote infection control. Therefore, the test-taker must analyze each agent and rely on knowledge of these agents to arrive at the correct conclusion. If this question was answered incorrectly, review information on agents used after burns.

B18 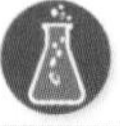

Neuromuscular | Evaluation, Diagnosis

An elderly person has lost significant functional vision over the past 4 years and complains of blurred vision and difficulty reading. The patient frequently mistakes images directly in front of them, especially in bright light. When walking across a room, the patient is able to locate items in the environment using peripheral vision when items are located to both sides. Based on these findings, what is the visual condition this patient is **MOST** likely experiencing?

Choices:

1. Glaucoma.
2. Cataracts.
3. Homonymous hemianopsia.
4. Bitemporal hemianopsia.

Teaching Points

Correct Answer: 2

Cataracts, which cause a clouding of the lens, result in a gradual loss of vision; central vision is lost first, then peripheral.

Incorrect Choices:

Glaucoma produces the reverse symptoms: loss of peripheral vision occurs first, then central vision, progressing to total blindness. Hemianopsia is a field defect in both eyes that often occurs following stroke. There was no mention of cerebrovascular accident (CVA) in the question.

Type of Reasoning: Analytical

In this question, symptoms are presented and one must make a determination of the most likely diagnosis. These types of questions require analysis of the meaning of information presented that utilizes analytical reasoning skill. If this question was answered incorrectly, refer to information on visual deficits associated with aging.

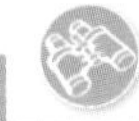

B19

Musculoskeletal | Examination

An office worker complains of intermittent numbness and tingling in the thumb, index finger, and middle finger of the right hand. Carpal tunnel syndrome is suspected. What is the **BEST** physical examination item to corroborate this diagnosis?

Choices:

1. Allen's test.
2. Finkelstein's test.
3. Semmes-Weinstein monofilament testing.
4. Watson (scaphoid shift) test.

Teaching Points

Correct Answer: 3

There is strong evidence to support the utilization of Semmes-Weinstein monofilament testing in patients with suspected CTS (see Box 2-3). Clinicians should assess the middle finger using a 2.83 or 3.22 monofilament as threshold normal for light-touch sensation and static 2-point discrimination. In patients with suspected moderate to severe CTS, clinicians should assess the thumb or index finger with a 3.22 monofilament as threshold for normal.

Incorrect Choices:

Allen's test is a measure of arterial blood flow to the palm and hand. A positive Finkelstein's test is diagnostic of de Quervain's tenosynovitis. The Watson test is used to diagnose carpal bone (scaphoid) instability.

Type of Reasoning: Inductive

For this question, the test-taker must utilize clinical judgment to determine a best course of action for a patient with suspected carpal tunnel syndrome. This requires inductive reasoning skill, where one must draw upon clinical judgment to draw correct conclusions. For this case, it is BEST to choose Semmes-Weinstein monofilament testing. If answered incorrectly, review Semmes-Weinstein monofilament testing information.

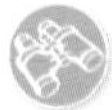

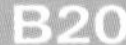

B20

Neuromuscular | Interventions

A patient incurred a right CVA 1 month ago and demonstrates moderate spasticity in the left upper extremity (predominantly increased flexor tone). The major problem at this time is a lack of voluntary movement control. There is minimal active movement, with ¼ inch subluxation of the shoulder. What initial treatment activity is the **BEST** choice for this patient?

Choices:

1. Sitting, left active shoulder protraction with extended elbow and shoulder flexed to 90°.
2. Sitting, weight-bearing on extended left upper extremity, weight shifting.
3. Quadruped, rocking from side to side.
4. PNF D2 flexion pattern, left upper extremity.

Teaching Points

Correct Answer: 2

Sitting, weight-bearing, and rocking on an extended left upper extremity will help to decrease the flexor tone. It also provides joint compression (approximation) at the shoulder, which will help maintain shoulder position and stimulate stabilizing muscles.

Incorrect Choices:

Quadruped is too strenuous for this patient at this time (maximum weight-bearing on a weak, unstable upper extremity). The other two activities demand more voluntary control than this patient currently demonstrates.

Type of Reasoning: Inductive

The test-taker must make a determination of where the patient is currently functioning and match this knowledge to what the patient could most likely tolerate and achieve success in during interventions. In this situation, the patient would benefit the most from weight-bearing activities through the affected extremity with weight shifting. Questions such as these require clinical judgment, which is an inductive reasoning skill.

B21 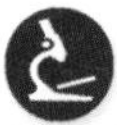

Musculoskeletal I Examination

An athlete sustains a twisting injury of the knee while playing basketball. The physical therapist suspects a meniscus injury. What is the **BEST** choice of special tests to confirm this diagnosis?

Choices:

1. Lachman and anterior drawer tests.
2. Joint line tenderness and Thessaly test.
3. Noble compression and Ely's tests.
4. Varus and valgus stress tests.

Teaching Points

Correct Answer: 2

This question describes a common mechanism of injury for a meniscus tear. The Clinical Practice Guideline for meniscus injuries recommends utilization of the Thessaly and McMurray tests (see Box 2-8). The combination of a positive Thessaly or McMurray test, along with palpable joint line tenderness, yields good diagnostic utility for ruling in a meniscal tear (high specificity and positive likelihood ratio values).

Incorrect Choices:

The Lachman and anterior drawer tests are utilized to assess the integrity of the ACL. The Noble compression test is used for the diagnosis of iliotibial band friction syndrome, and Ely's test is used to identify rectus femoris muscle tightness. Varus and valgus stress tests are used to assess the medial and lateral stability of the knee joint.

Type of Reasoning: Deductive

For this question, one must recall the tests that are conducted to confirm a meniscus injury. This is factual recall of guidelines, which is a deductive reasoning skill. For this case, the therapist should examine for joint line tenderness and administer the Thessaly test. If answered incorrectly, review joint line tenderness and the Thessaly test.

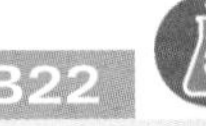

B22

Musculoskeletal | Examination

The therapist in the photograph is testing which muscle?

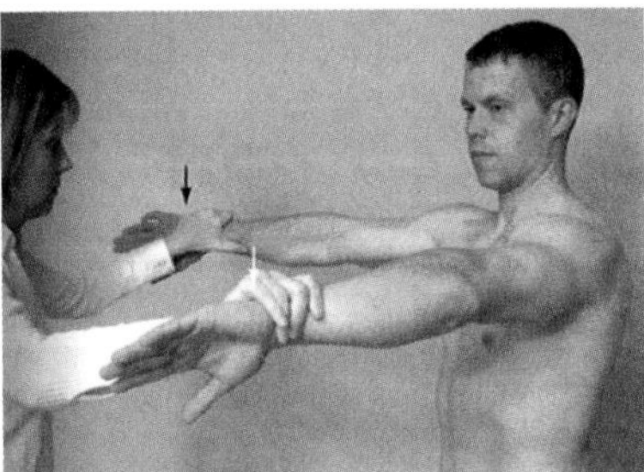

Choices:

1. Upper trapezius.
2. Middle deltoid.
3. Supraspinatus.
4. Anterior deltoid.

Teaching Points

Correct Answer: 3

The muscle being tested is the supraspinatus. The empty-can position puts the supraspinatus muscle in its most effective position for contraction. Weakness may be a result of inflammation, neuropathy of the suprascapular nerve, or a tendon tear.

Incorrect Choices:

The muscle test for the anterior deltoid would have the humerus and forearm in neutral rather than internal rotation of the humerus and pronation of the forearm shown in the picture. The muscle test for the middle deltoid would have the shoulder in abduction to 90°. The muscle test for the upper trapezius is the shoulder shrug.

Type of Reasoning: Analytical

In this situation, the test-taker must recall knowledge of muscle testing of the supraspinatus to arrive at the correct conclusion. Whereas recall of muscle testing positions and procedures can be simple recall, the picture utilizes analysis of information coupled with recall, which becomes an analytical skill. If this question was answered incorrectly, refer to information on special tests of the shoulder complex.

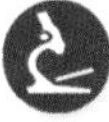

B23

Neuromuscular | Examination

A physical therapist is screening an individual who sustained a direct blow to the head while playing soccer 3 hours ago. Which of the following examination items is **BEST** for assessing the level of consciousness and severity of the potential concussion/traumatic brain injury (TBI) in this individual?

Choices:

1. Glasgow Coma Scale.
2. Rancho Los Amigos Levels of Cognitive Functioning.
3. Duration of post-traumatic amnesia.
4. Duration of the alteration of consciousness.

Teaching Points

Correct Answer: 1

The Glasgow Coma Scale (GCS) is commonly used to acutely assess patient's level of consciousness and severity of TBI (see Chapter 3 and Table 3-15). Specifically, a <13 GCS score 2 hours after injury requires immediate emergency evaluation.

Incorrect Choices:

The Rancho Los Amigos Levels of Cognitive Functioning is recommended for various inpatient and rehabilitation settings for patients recovering from moderate to severe traumatic injury (see Table 3-17) but is not indicated in acute concussion assessment. The duration of post-traumatic amnesia (1–7 days = moderate TBI; >7 days = severe TBI) and alteration of consciousness (>24 hours = moderate/severe TBI) are also helpful in determining the severity of TBI, but this patient's injury only happened 3 hours ago.

Type of Reasoning: Deductive

For this question, one must recall the features of each of the presented examination items and determine the exam that will best assess the level of consciousness and severity of a potential concussion/TBI. This necessitates the recall of factual information, which is a deductive reasoning skill. For this scenario, the GCS is best. Review examinations for concussions and TBI, especially the GCS, if answered incorrectly.

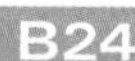

Musculoskeletal I Examination

A patient is referred to physical therapy after an antero-inferior dislocation of the right shoulder. What positive examination finding on the involved side is expected as a result of this dislocation?

Choices:

1. Weak rhomboids.
2. Positive drop arm test.
3. Positive Neer's test.
4. Weak deltoids.

Teaching Points

Correct Answer: 4

Because of the anatomical position of the axillary nerve, it can be damaged by an antero-inferior dislocation at the glenohumeral joint. This may result in weak deltoids.

Incorrect Choices:

A drop arm test evaluates the integrity of the rotator cuff. A Neer's test evaluates impingement of the shoulder. The rhomboids are innervated by the dorsal scapular nerve. Anatomically, the dorsal scapular nerve is medial and posterior to the shoulder joint.

Type of Reasoning: Analytical

This question requires one to recall musculoskeletal anatomy of the shoulder and the various tests that can be administered to determine dysfunction in the shoulder. For this case, the drop arm test and Neer's test are not administered to determine anterior shoulder dislocation, and rhomboids do not play a role in anterior shoulder stability. Through analysis of the information presented, the test-taker should conclude that weak deltoids are the most likely result of the dislocation.

B25 Nonsystem | Research

A physical therapist is analyzing data as part of a research team. The therapist finds a statistically significant interaction effect between the two independent variables. A post-hoc multiple comparison tests is then performed to investigate the interaction. If the therapist does not use a correction formula to adjust the alpha level when performing the multiple comparison tests, which statistical error may occur?

Choices:

1. Sampling error.
2. Type I error.
3. Residual error.
4. Type II error.

Teaching Points

Correct Answer: 2

A Type I error occurs when the conclusion is made that a difference between groups exists when no difference actually exists (a difference is observed in the average scores of the sample groups, when there is no difference between groups in the population). When multiple comparisons of the same data are made in a research study, the alpha level (which is the level of acceptable risk for making a Type I error) must be adjusted to account for the multiple comparisons. Several formulas exist to calculate the alpha level based on the number of comparisons being made.

Incorrect Choices:

Sampling error is the natural variation in the mean score of a sample with respect to the mean of the population. Residual error is the difference between individual scores and the predicted score of the dependent variable based on the score of the independent variable. Type II error is defined as stating there is no difference between groups when a real difference exists (no difference is observed in the average scores of the sample groups, when there is a difference between group scores in the population).

Type of reasoning: Deductive

For this question, the test-taker must recall research guidelines and statistical errors in order to determine a correct conclusion. This requires deductive reasoning skill, where factual guidelines help the test taker to draw a reasonable conclusion. For this situation, the error described is a Type 1 error. If answered incorrectly, review statistical guidelines, especially statistical errors.

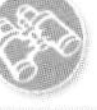

B26 Neuromuscular | Examination

An elderly individual with a history of falls in the home (four in the past 2 months with minor injury) is referred to physical therapy as a result of these falls. Which test is the **BEST** to evaluate gait, strength, and dynamic postural stability/balance?

Choices:

1. 30-Second Chair Stand.
2. Stops Walking While Talking.
3. Four Square Step Test.
4. Timed Up & Go.

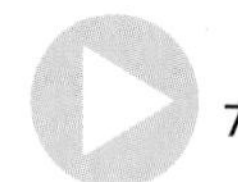

Teaching Points

Correct Answer: 4

The Timed Up & Go (TUG) test is the best choice to evaluate gait, strength, and dynamic postural stability/balance. It involves standing up and sitting down from a chair (lower extremity extensor strength), walking 3 meters, and turning.

Incorrect Choices:

All other tests can be used to assess balance but do not examine the three stated components equally well as the TUG. The 30-Second Chair Stand involves sit-to-stand-to-sit transitions (assesses lower extremity strength and endurance). The Stops Walking While Talking involves talking while walking (dual-tasking). The Four Square Step Test involves timed stepping in all directions.

Type of Reasoning: Inductive

This question requires one to utilize clinical judgment in order to determine the **BEST** test to evaluate gait, strength, and balance. Questions of this nature often necessitate inductive reasoning skill, where clinical judgment is paramount to arriving at a correct conclusion. For this scenario, the TUG test is the best choice. Review the TUG test if answered incorrectly (see Table 3-11).

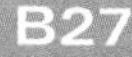
B27
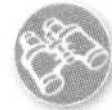

Neuromuscular | Interventions

A patient with amyotrophic lateral sclerosis is referred for physical therapy. The patient has mild to moderate weakness (2/5 to 4/5 MMT) and fasciculations in various muscles below the knees and in the right hand. Which of the following is the **BEST** choice for initial intervention strategies for this patient?

Choices:

1. Breathing exercises, full body stretching, and rolling activities to avoid overexertion.
2. Functional training activities with assistive devices as needed to support independence.
3. Daily progressive resistance exercise for all muscle groups.
4. Transfer training and wheelchair use to avoid overexertion.

Teaching Points

Correct Answer: 2

Patients with ALS who have moderate weakness in various muscles in the distal lower extremities will require assistive devices/bracing to maintain independence. Strengthening and range of motion exercises should focus on functional activities, and weak muscles (<3 out of 5 manual muscle testing) should not be overworked. Additionally, use of an assistive device and bracing can assist in maintaining independence while avoiding fatigue.

Incorrect Choices:

Breathing exercises, stretching, and rolling are for patients in the later or end stage of ALS. Daily progressive resistive exercise is not indicated for denervated and weak muscles (<3 out of 5). Transfer and wheelchair training are the focus for patients who are no longer community ambulators.

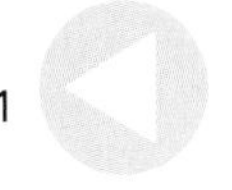

Type of Reasoning: Inductive

This question requires one to draw from clinical knowledge in order to determine a best course of action. This requires inductive reasoning skill. For this situation, the BEST initial intervention strategies would be functional training activities with assistive devices as needed to support independence. If answered incorrectly, review intervention guidelines for amyotrophic lateral sclerosis.

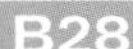

B28 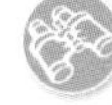

Cardiovascular/Pulmonary | Evaluation, Diagnosis

A 2-week-old infant born at 27 weeks gestation with infant respiratory distress syndrome is referred for a physical therapy consult. Nursing reports that the child "desaturates to 84% with handling" and has minimal secretions at present. What is the therapist's **BEST** course of action?

Choices:

1. Provide suggestions to nursing for positioning for optimal motor development.
2. Put the PT consult on hold because the child is too ill to tolerate exercise.
3. Delegate to a physical therapy assistant (PTA) a maintenance program of manual techniques for secretion clearance.
4. Perform manual techniques for secretion clearance, 2–4 hours daily, to maintain airway patency.

Teaching Points

Correct Answer: 1

Excessive handling of a premature infant can cause oxygen desaturation. It is in the best interests of the infant to limit the number of handlers. The PT's role should be to assist nursing in developing positioning schedules, positions for feeding, infant stimulation activities, etc.

Incorrect Choices:

At present, there is little information provided that would necessitate the PT or PTA to be a direct caregiver to this child.

Type of Reasoning: Inductive

The test-taker must utilize clinical judgment coupled with knowledge of neonatology physical therapy practice to arrive at the correct conclusion. One uses inductive reasoning skills whenever diagnostic thinking or clinical judgment is utilized. If this question was answered incorrectly, refer to information on neonatology practice.

B29 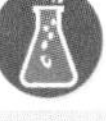

Musculoskeletal | Evaluation, Diagnosis

A patient sustained a valgus stress to the left knee while skiing. The orthopedist found a positive McMurray's test and a positive Lachman's stress test. The patient has been referred to physical therapy for conservative management of this problem. What is the **BEST** intervention for the subacute phase of rehabilitation?

Choices:

1. Open-chain exercises of the hip extensors and hamstrings to inhibit anterior translation of the femur on the tibia.
2. Closed-chain functional strengthening of the quadriceps femoris and hamstrings, emphasizing regaining terminal knee extension.
3. Closed-chain functional strengthening of the quadriceps femoris and hip abductors to promote regaining terminal knee extension.
4. Open-chain strengthening of the quadriceps femoris and hip adductors to inhibit anterior translation of the tibia on the femur.

Teaching Points

Correct Answer: 2

The evaluation is suggestive of an unhappy triad injury. Closed-chain exercises are emphasized during the **subacute phase** to enhance functional control of the muscles surrounding the knee. Terminal extension must be achieved during this stage if normal function is to occur.

Incorrect Choices:

Open-chain exercise does not promote regaining functional control for the muscle surrounding the knee. Focus on the hip abductors (rather than the hamstrings) will not promote regaining functional control of the knee joint.

Type of Reasoning: Analytical

The test-taker must have knowledge of the patient's exact deficits and appropriate interventions in order to make the correct decision in this case. This requires knowledge of McMurray's test, Lachman's test, and rehabilitation strategies after an unhappy triad injury. In this type of question, the meaning of the information presented is analyzed to make the appropriate decision.

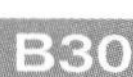

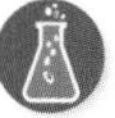

Lymphatic | Evaluation, Diagnosis

A physical therapist examines a patient with secondary lymphedema of the upper extremity following a mastectomy. The patient reports that there has been a recent increase in swelling of the upper extremity which does not resolve overnight or with elevation of the limb. No atrophic changes (skin discoloration and fibrotic skin folds) are present. Which stage of lymphedema is characterized by this clinical presentation?

Choices:

1. Stage 0.
2. Stage I.
3. Stage II.
4. Stage III.

Teaching Points

Correct Answer: 3

Stage II lymphedema is described as spontaneously irreversible and is characterized by an increase in swelling that is not reduced overnight or by elevation of the affected limb. A positive Stemmer's sign and clinical fibrosis may be present. See pg. 277 for a full description of the stages of lymphedema.

Incorrect Choices:

Stage 0 is described as a preclinical or latent stage during which the patient is at risk for development of lymphedema. The patient may complain of achiness and heaviness of the affected limb although edema is not yet evident. In Stage I pitting edema is present and is reversible with elevation. The affected area may be a normal size in the morning but swelling increases with activity, heat, and humidity. Stage III is also called elephantiasis. Severe nonpitting fibrotic edema is present along with atrophic changes (deep skin folds, discoloration, hardening of dermal tissue). These changes may limit mobility of the affected limb and the patient.

Type of Reasoning: Analytical

For this question, the test-taker must analyze the presenting symptoms and match them to a stage of lymphedema. Questions that require one to consider pieces of information to draw reasonable conclusions require analytical reasoning skill. For this case, the symptoms are consistent with Stage II lymphedema. If answered incorrectly, review stages of lymphedema, especially clinical presentation of Stage II.

B31 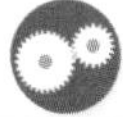

Nonsystem | Safety and Protection

During a therapy session, a patient with a past history of seizures and traumatic brain injury loses consciousness and presents with tonic-clonic movements involving all four extremities. The seizure lasts about 4 minutes before the patient slowly becomes responsive. What is the therapist's **BEST** immediate course of action?

Choices:

1. Position the patient in supine with head supported and wait out the seizure.
2. Wrap the limbs in a sheet to prevent self-harm and position in sidelying.
3. Position the patient in sidelying with the mouth pointing to the ground.
4. Initiate rescue breathing and seek emergency medical assistance.

Teaching Points

Correct Answer: 3

This is an emergency situation. To ensure an open airway and prevent aspiration, position the patient in sidelying with the mouth pointing toward the ground. The patient should be protected from injury by loosening restrictive clothing and removing potentially harmful nearby objects.

Incorrect Choices:

Supine position can be life-threatening if the tongue falls backward to restrict the airway. The patient should not be restrained as this may increase the likelihood of injury or agitation. Rescue breathing is not indicated during an active seizure. Emergency care (EMS) is required if the patient has no known history of seizures, if the seizure lasts 5 minutes or longer, or if status epilepticus occurs.

Type of Reasoning: Evaluative

This question requires one to make a value judgment of the most appropriate initial course of action in a treatment situation. In this case, the patient's symptoms constitute an emergency. The therapist should first position the patient in sidelying with the mouth pointing downward to open the airway and prevent aspiration. If this question is answered incorrectly, refer to safety and protection guidelines for patients with seizure disorders.

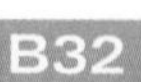
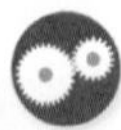

B32

Nonsystem | Safety and Protection

A cyclist has fallen and dislocated the right shoulder during a race where a physical therapist is providing medical support. While waiting for the physician to arrive at your site to determine whether it is safe to reduce the injury on-site the patient begins to become agitated, complains of nausea, and appears pale and gray. Vital signs have changed since the patient's arrival with increased pulse and respiratory rate and decreased blood pressure. What is the **BEST** action to take?

Choices:

1. Provide sips of cold fluids.
2. Place the patient in supine and elevate the legs.
3. Place the patient in sitting with the head between the knees.
4. Place the patient sidelying on his left side and protect the right shoulder.

Teaching Points

Correct Answer: 2

This patient presentation is consistent with shock. The proper positioning is in supine with the legs elevated.

Incorrect Choices:

Food and drink should never be provided to a patient experiencing symptoms of shock. If the patient vomited or lost consciousness, it would be appropriate to move them into sidelying to assist with maintaining an open airway. Patients who are experiencing vasovagal syncope may also get relief by putting their heads between their knees, but this position is not recommended for patients with shock.

Type of Reasoning: Evaluative

This question requires the test-taker to evaluate the potential courses of action and then determine which action will best remedy the symptoms, based on recognition of the symptoms that are consistent with shock. This requires evaluative reasoning skill. For this scenario, it is best to place the patient in supine and elevate the legs to remedy the symptoms. If answered incorrectly, review first aid and treatment guidelines for shock.

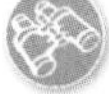

B33

Cardiovascular/Pulmonary | Interventions

A patient has a right pleural effusion postoperatively after a right lower lobe wedge resection. Which physical therapy treatment would be **MOST** effective for this patient to complete three times per day?

Choices:

1. Acapella in postural drainage positions, 10–15 breaths each session.
2. Segmental breathing while positioned in sitting and left sidelying, 10 minutes, three times per day.
3. Autogenic drainage, repeating steps as needed.
4. Percussion and shaking, 5 minutes per lobe, in prone and head of bed flat.

Teaching Points

Correct Answer: 2

Breathing will help to increase aeration to the potentially collapsed areas of the lungs. Changing positions will help to aerate different segments of the lung.

Incorrect Choices:

All other choices target airway clearance. The secretions are located between the parietal and visceral pleura, not in the airways. Therefore, these techniques will be ineffective.

Type of Reasoning: Inductive

This question requires the test-taker to recall the most effective treatment approaches for patients with pleural effusion and lobe wedge resection. This necessitates clinical judgment, which is an inductive reasoning skill. For this case, the therapist should choose segmental breathing while positioned in sitting and left sidelying, 10 minutes, three times per day. If answered incorrectly, review treatment guidelines for pleural effusion and lung aeration approaches.

B34 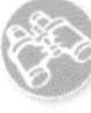

Neuromuscular | Examination

A patient is referred to physical therapy for functional gait difficulties. The patient is unable to take a normal step and drags the left foot. Examination reveals muscle weakness with fasciculations in the left lower leg. What other signs and symptoms will this patient most likely exhibit?

Choices:

1. Decreased tone and hyporeflexia.
2. Muscle spasms and positive Babinski.
3. Increased tone and hyperreflexia.
4. Dyssynergia and timing deficits.

Teaching Points

Correct Answer: 1

Muscle weakness with fasciculations is symptomatic of a lower motor neuron (LMN) lesion. Other signs and symptoms of a LMN lesion include hypotonia or flaccidity, hyporeflexia, or absent reflexes and neurogenic atrophy.

Incorrect Choices:

The other choices are all signs and symptoms of upper motor neuron (UMN) lesions.

Type of Reasoning: Inductive

This question requires the test-taker to determine a best course of action based on signs and symptoms presented. This necessitates clinical judgment, which is an inductive reasoning skill. In this situation, the therapist should also examine for decreased tone and hyporeflexia. If answered incorrectly, review information on lower motor neuron lesions (see Table 3-5).

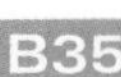

B35

Metabolic/Endocrine | Interventions

An elderly patient with hyperthyroidism is referred to physical therapy following a period of prolonged bed rest. What should the therapist be alert for when monitoring exercise of this patient?

Choices:

1. Decreased heart rate and blood pressure.
2. Tachycardia and dyspnea.
3. Muscle weakness and joint pain.
4. Arrhythmias and bradycardia.

Teaching Points

Correct Answer: 2

Hyperthyroidism is a hypermetabolic state and is associated with exercise intolerance and impaired cardiopulmonary function. Symptoms include dyspnea, fatigue, tachycardia, and arrhythmia. In older people there is increased risk of aggravating preexisting heart disease (e.g., atrial fibrillation, angina, and myocardial infarction).

Incorrect Choices:

Heart rate is increased during exercise in hyperthyroidism. Muscle weakness (typically proximal) and fatigue are present while increased joint pain is not characteristic. Tachycardia, not bradycardia, is seen.

Type of Reasoning: Inferential

This question provides a diagnosis and the test-taker must determine the likely risk factors for it. This requires inferential reasoning skill, in which one determines what is most likely to be true of a diagnosis. For this case, the risk factors include tachycardia and dyspnea. Review risk factors for hyperthyroidism if answered incorrectly.

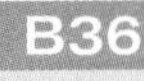
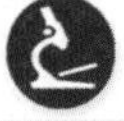

B36

Nonsystem | Therapeutic Modalities

A patient strained the lower back muscles 3 weeks ago, and now complains of pain (6/10). Upon examination, the therapist identifies bilateral muscle spasm from T10–L4. The therapist elects to apply interferential current to help reduce pain and spasm. What is the **BEST** electrode configuration in this case?

Choices:

1. Four electrodes, with current flow perpendicular to the spinal column.
2. Two electrodes, with current flow perpendicular to the spinal column.
3. Four electrodes, with current flow diagonal to the spinal column.
4. Two electrodes, with current flow parallel to the spinal column.

Teaching Points

Correct Answer: 3

The crisscrossed electrode configuration allows: (1) a greater area to be treated and (2) current interference to occur between the frequencies of the two circuits because of the diagonal pattern.

Incorrect Choices:

A crisscrossed electrode configuration is needed to create interferential current. None of the other electrode configurations facilitates the flow of current diagonal to the spinal column, which would cause the frequencies to intersect.

Type of Reasoning: Deductive

This question requires recall of factual information related to the protocol for electrode placement when using interferential current. The test-taker must refer to this knowledge to understand that four electrodes with current flowing diagonal to the spinal column are best for treating the patient's symptoms.

B37 

Neuromuscular | Evaluation, Diagnosis

An infant is diagnosed with Erb's paralysis (brachial plexus injury). What would the physical therapy examination of this infant **MOST LIKELY** reveal?

Choices:

1. Involvement of muscles innervated by C5–C6 nerve roots.
2. Involvement of muscles innervated by C4–C8 nerve roots.
3. Involvement of muscles innervated by C7–C8 nerve roots.
4. Involvement of muscles innervated by C8–T1 nerve roots.

Teaching Points

Correct Answer: 1

Erb's paralysis is a brachial plexus injury involving the upper trunk C5–C6 nerves with paralysis of the shoulder and elbow muscles, commonly involving the suprascapular, musculocutaneous, and axillary nerves. The limb is held in a position of adduction, forearm pronation, and wrist and finger flexion (waiter's tip position).

Incorrect Choices:

Erb's paralysis involves C5–C6, so other options would not fit spinal nerves affected. Klumpke's paralysis is a brachial plexus injury involving the lower trunk, C8 and T1 nerves, and muscles of the forearm and hand.

Type of Reasoning: Inferential

This question requires one to recall the typical presentation of Erb's paralysis in order to arrive at a correct conclusion. Questions that provide a diagnosis and the test-taker must determine the likely symptoms often necessitate inferential reasoning skill. For this case, one would expect the examination to reveal involvement of muscles innervated by C5–C6 nerves and intact elbow extension, wrist flexion, and finger flexion/adduction/abduction. Review Erb's paralysis, including involvement of muscles if answered incorrectly.

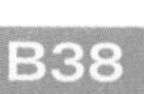

B38

Musculoskeletal | Interventions

A retired bus driver has experienced increasing frequency of low back pain over the past 10 years. The patient states that nonsteroidal anti-inflammatory drugs (NSAIDs) help to relieve the symptoms, but there is always a nagging-type pain. The patient reports significant stiffness in the morning that dissipates by noon after exercising and walking. Pain is exacerbated with frequent lifting and bending activities, as well as sitting for long periods. What should the physical therapy plan of care emphasize?

Choices:

1. Modalities to reduce pain, postural reeducation, and dynamic stabilization exercises.
2. Postural reeducation, soft tissue mobilization, and dynamic stabilization.
3. Modalities to reduce pain, joint mobilization, and lumbar extension exercises.
4. Joint mobilization, soft tissue mobilization, and flexion exercises.

Teaching Points

Correct Answer: 2

This is a long-term degenerative and postural dysfunction that is manageable with medication and proper physical activity. Therefore, the most effective use of treatment time should emphasize regaining normal postural alignment and functional ADLs. See Box 2-16 for the Low Back Pain Clinical Practice Guideline.

Incorrect Choices:

Whereas modalities and mobilization can relieve acute pain, this is a chronic problem that demands choices appropriate for long-term management of the problem.

Type of Reasoning: Inferential

One must consider all of the patient's symptoms and determine what the likely cause(s) of the symptoms is (are) in order to make an appropriate decision for intervention. This requires the use of inferential reasoning, in which decisions are made after drawing conclusions from the evidence presented.

B39

Musculoskeletal | Evaluation, Diagnosis

A patient is referred to the physical therapy clinic following a recent motor vehicle accident in which they sustained a whiplash injury. Initial imaging studies (plain radiographs and a CT scan) ruled out a fracture. The patient complains of intermittent and variable symptoms, including dizziness, arm heaviness, occasional headaches, and limited range of motion in all planes. Which pathology **MOST** likely explains the findings in this patient?

Choices:

1. Cervical radiculopathy.
2. Upper cervical spine instability.
3. Thoracic outlet syndrome.
4. Spontaneous pneumothorax.

Teaching Points

Correct Answer: 2

Although the symptoms of upper cervical spine instability can be variable, hallmark signs include neck pain, dizziness, arm heaviness, and headache (see Red Flag box on page 73). The recent history of an MVA and whiplash suggest trauma. The traumatic flexion-extension moment applied to the spine during the MVA may disrupt the ligaments that stabilize the atlantooccipital (occiput–C1) and atlantoaxial joints (C1–C2).

Incorrect Choices:

Cervical radiculopathy most commonly occurs secondary to compression, irritation, or traction of cervical nerve roots caused by either a herniated disc, degenerative disease, or trauma. Impingement of a nerve root typically produces radiating arm pain along with numbness, paresthesias, or other sensory deficits, and possible motor dysfunction in one or both upper extremities. Thoracic outlet syndrome (TOS) may include neck, shoulder, and arm pain, numbness, or impaired circulation of the involved upper extremity. However, patients with TOS are unlikely to complain of dizziness or headache. A spontaneous pneumothorax is the sudden onset of a collapsed lung without any apparent cause (such as trauma or preexisting lung pathology). It may be associated with acute neck and/or upper back pain; however, shortness of breath and chest pain are the predominant symptoms.

Type of Reasoning: Analytical

This question requires the test-taker to analyze the symptoms presented and determine the most likely findings for this patient. This necessitates analytical reasoning skill, where pieces of information are weighed and considered for their significance to make a reasonable conclusion of the patient's pathology. In this situation, the findings most likely indicate upper cervical spine instability. If answered incorrectly, review information on upper cervical spine instability, especially symptoms.

B40 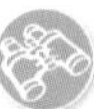

System Interactions | Evaluation, Diagnosis

An elderly patient with diabetes and bilateral lower extremity amputation is to be discharged from an acute care hospital 2 weeks postsurgery. The incisions on the residual limbs are not healed and continue to drain. The patient is unable to transfer because the venous graft sites in the upper extremities are painful and not fully healed. Endurance out-of-bed is limited. What is the **BEST** choice of discharge destination for this patient?

Choices:

1. Skilled nursing facility.
2. Custodial care facility.
3. Home.
4. Rehabilitation hospital.

Teaching Points

Correct Answer: 1

A skilled nursing facility is the best facility because the patient continues to require nursing care for the open wounds. Initiation of physical therapy when this patient is able is also available.

Incorrect Choices:

Discharge to home would be premature because the patient is unable to transfer. Custodial care involves medical or nonmedical care that does not seek a cure. A rehabilitation hospital is not appropriate at this time, because the patient cannot actively participate in rehabilitation 3 hours/day.

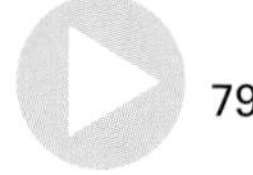

Type of Reasoning: Inductive

One must utilize clinical judgment in this situation to make an appropriate determination for the best discharge situation for this patient. The key is that the patient's current medical status requires continued nursing care, which can be managed at a skilled nursing facility. In addition, the patient can continue to receive rehabilitation at a duration that is most appropriate for the patient's current tolerance for functional activity. Questions that require clinical judgment often utilize inductive reasoning skill.

B41 

Neuromuscular I Examination

A patient currently being seen for low back pain awoke one morning with drooping left facial muscles and excessive drooling. The patient was recovering from a cold and had experienced an earache in the left ear during the previous 2 days. The therapist suspects Bell's palsy. What cranial nerve test can confirm this diagnosis?

Choices:

1. Taste over the posterior tongue, and having the patient protrude the tongue.
2. Taste over the anterior tongue, and having the patient raise the eyebrows and puff the cheeks.
3. Corneal reflex and stretch reflexes of facial muscles.
4. Trigger points for pain, especially over the temporomandibular joint (TMJ).

Teaching Points

Correct Answer: 2

Bell's palsy is a lower motor neuron lesion affecting the branches of the facial nerve, CN VII. Examination of the motor function of the muscles of facial expression (i.e., raise eyebrows, show teeth, smile, close eyes tightly, puff cheeks) and taste over the anterior tongue will reveal deficits of CN VII function.

Incorrect Choices:

Taste over the posterior tongue is a function of CN IX (glossopharyngeal). Strength of tongue protrusion is a function of CN XII (hypoglossal). Pupillary reflexes are a function of CN II (optic).

Type of Reasoning: Inferential

In this question, the suspected diagnosis and symptoms are provided, but the test-taker must determine how to best confirm this diagnosis through testing of the cranial nerves. This question requires inferential critical reasoning, which uses clinical decision-making based on facts and evidence. If this question was answered incorrectly, refer to information on Bell's palsy.

B42 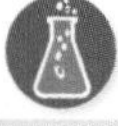

Neuromuscular I Evaluation, Diagnosis

A patient has continued intense (10 out of 10) pain in the left foot and ankle 6 months after sustaining an ankle sprain. A recent MRI of the foot and ankle are normal. The patient reports "that all activity is painful" and that they periodically get sporadic pain at rest. The patient denies overt numbness, tingling, or weakness in the bilateral lower extremities. On examination the patient has no signs of inflammation but does have diffuse hyperalgesia and intense pain with light touch. These findings are most consistent with which of the following pain mechanisms?

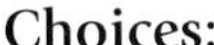

Choices:

1. Nociceptive pain.
2. Neuropathic pain.
3. Central sensitization.
4. Peripheral sensitization.

Teaching Points

Correct Answer: 3

Central sensitization (CS) occurs with increased excitatory and decreased inhibitory neural signaling in the central nervous system resulting in hypersensitivity. This process occurs even though there is no current evidence of actual or threatened tissue damage in the periphery (nociceptive pain) or a lesion or disease in the somatosensory system causing the pain (neuropathic pain). This patient exhibits various signs and symptoms of central sensitization to include intense and nonlocalized pain, sporadic pain at rest, allodynia, and secondary hyperalgesia.

Incorrect Choices:

Nociceptive pain is typically associated with an acute or ongoing disease process that activates peripheral nociceptors. Nociceptive pain is localized to the area of tissue damage and has a linear relationship with the level of activity and specific aggravating factors. Neuropathic pain involves damage to the somatosensory system and is associated with radiating pain, numbness, or tingling in a dermatomal or specific nerve distribution. Peripheral sensitization may enhance or prolong pain in the injured area and contribute to central sensitization, but it is not associated with secondary hyperalgesia.

Type of Reasoning: Analytical

This question requires the test-taker to analyze the patient's symptoms and determine which pain mechanism is most consistent with these symptoms. This requires the analysis of information in order to draw reasonable conclusions, which is an analytical reasoning skill. For this situation, the symptoms are consistent with central sensitization. If answered incorrectly, review mechanisms of pain, especially information on central sensitization.

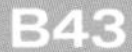

Cardiovascular/Pulmonary | Evaluation, Diagnosis

A patient with congestive heart failure (CHF) is on a regimen of diuretics (chlorothiazide). The PT should be alert for which adverse effects of this medication?

Choices:

1. Hyperkalemia and premature ventricular contractions (PVCs).
2. Myalgia and joint pains.
3. Orthostatic hypotension and dizziness.
4. Reflex tachycardia and unstable BP.

Teaching Points

Correct Answer: 3

Thiazide diuretics are used to manage mild to moderate hypertension. Adverse side effects include orthostatic hypotension and dizziness, along with drowsiness, lethargy, and weakness. These represent a safety risk during functional training and gait.

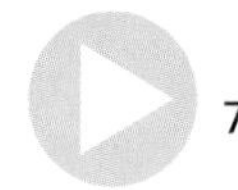

Incorrect Choices:

BP is lowered and is more stable, not less. Hypokalemia (not hyperkalemia) can occur, resulting in increased PVCs. Muscle cramps and weakness can occur. Joint pains are likely caused by a comorbid condition.

Type of Reasoning: Inferential

The test-taker utilizes factual knowledge of side effects of medications, coupled with knowledge of CHF, to make the correct decision in this case, using inferential reasoning skills.

B44 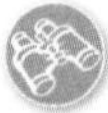

Musculoskeletal | Evaluation, Diagnosis

A patient with a traumatic injury to the right hand had a flexor tendon repair to the fingers. When should physical therapy intervention begin following this type of repair?

Choices:

1. After the splint is removed in 4–6 weeks to allow ample healing time for the repaired tendon.
2. After the splint is removed in 2–3 weeks to allow full AROM of all affected joints.
3. Within a few days after surgery to allow for early initiation of strengthening exercises.
4. Within a few days after surgery to preserve tendon gliding.

Teaching Points

Correct Answer: 4

Early passive and active assistive exercises promote collagen remodeling to allow free tendon gliding.

Incorrect Choices:

When rehabilitation is delayed by several weeks, adhesions form, which restrict free tendon gliding. Early initiation of strengthening exercises is contraindicated.

Type of Reasoning: Inductive

This question requires one to use clinical judgment to make a determination of the best intervention for a patient who has had a recent flexor tendon repair of the hand. One utilizes knowledge of hand therapy and early tendon repair protocols to arrive at the correct conclusion. If this question was answered incorrectly, review flexor tendon repair information and therapy protocols.

B45 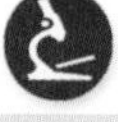

System Interactions | Evaluation, Diagnosis

A physical therapist examines a patient who is recovering from generalized muscle aches, cramps, and weakness following several days of intense cross-training sessions. The patient also complains of generalized fatigue. The referring physician suspected rhabdomyolysis. Which laboratory test would help establish the diagnosis of this condition?

Choices:

1. Myelin basic protein.
2. Serum uric acid.
3. Creatine kinase.
4. Erythrocyte sedimentation rate.

Teaching Points

Correct Answer: 3

Rhabdomyolysis is a potentially fatal condition in which muscle tissue contents are released into the bloodstream as a result of muscle tissue disintegration. This may occur after overexertion as described in this scenario. It may also occur following crush injuries and burns. Individuals with liver impairment from alcohol abuse or prolonged use of some drugs such as statins (cholesterol-lowering medications) are at risk for developing rhabdomyolysis. Laboratory testing will show creatine kinase levels that are more than 10 times the upper limit of normal. The CPK normal range for a male is between 39 and 308 units per liter (U/L), while in females the normal range is between 26 and 192 U/L. Creatine kinase levels are used to help diagnose other conditions associated with muscle damage, including myocardial infarction.

Incorrect Choices:

Myelin basic protein levels are determined following a lumbar puncture with aspiration of cerebrospinal fluid. Elevated myelin basic protein levels are suggestive of demyelinating diseases such as multiple sclerosis. Elevated serum uric acid levels are seen in patients with gout and may be seen in patients with other conditions such as diabetes, hypothyroidism, and obesity. The erythrocyte sedimentation rate is a general marker of inflammation and is markedly elevated in patients with inflammatory disorders such as rheumatoid arthritis, polymyalgia rheumatica, and ankylosing spondylitis.

Type of Reasoning: Deductive

For this question, the test-taker must recall laboratory testing guidelines and specifically, which test establishes the diagnosis of rhabdomyolysis. This necessitates the factual recall of information, which is a deductive reasoning skill. For this case, creatine kinase level would help establish the diagnosis. Review information on rhabdomyolysis and laboratory testing if answered incorrectly.

B46 

Neuromuscular | Examination

The therapist suspects that a patient recovering from a middle cerebral artery stroke is exhibiting a pure hemianopsia. What test should be used to confirm the hemianopsia?

Choices:

1. Penlight held approximately 12 inches from the eyes and moved to the extremes of gaze right and left.
2. Penlight held 6 inches from the eyes and moved inward toward the face.
3. Visual confrontation test with a moving finger.
4. Distance acuity chart placed on a well-lighted wall at patient's eye level 20 feet away.

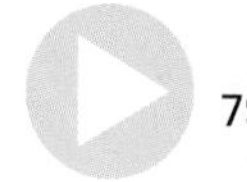

Teaching Points

Correct Answer: 3

Visual field is examined using the confrontation test. The patient sits opposite the therapist and is instructed to maintain his/her gaze on the therapist's nose. The therapist slowly brings a target (moving finger or pen) in the patient's field of view alternately from the right or left sides. The patient indicates when and where he/she first sees the target.

Incorrect Choices:

Distance acuity vision is tested using a Snellen eye chart at a distance of 20 feet. Ocular pursuit is tested using a penlight moved in an H pattern to the extremes of gaze. Convergence is tested using a penlight and ruler; the patient keeps the penlight in focus as it moves inward from a distance of 4 or 6 inches.

Type of Reasoning: Inferential

This question basically asks the test-taker to recall the appropriate examination approach for hemianopsia. Questions such as these do require recall of factual knowledge (knowledge of the different tests), but then that knowledge must be applied to the specific patient presented in the question, which moves beyond factual recall to drawing a conclusion, which is an inferential reasoning skill.

B47 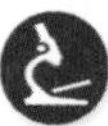

Musculoskeletal | Examination

A patient is referred to physical therapy with a complaint of chronic groin pain after an injury sustained while playing hockey. The physical therapist's differential diagnosis includes a sports hernia and hip joint dysfunction. What is the **BEST** special test to rule out the presence of a hip joint disorder?

Choices:

1. Scour test.
2. Ely's test.
3. Trendelenburg sign.
4. Ober's test.

Teaching Points

Correct Answer: 1

The hip scour test identifies general hip joint pathology to include osteoarthritis. During performance of the scour test the patient's hip is maximally flexed and adducted, then abducted with or without a compressive load. A positive test will reproduce the patient's pain or apprehension.

Incorrect Choices:

Ely's test is a prone test used to assess for tightness of the rectus femoris muscle. The Trendelenburg sign is performed in standing and indicates weakness of the gluteus medius muscle. Ober's test is used to determine the presence of tightness of the tensor fascia lata and iliotibial band.

Type of Reasoning: Deductive

For this question, one must determine the test that is best to conduct to rule out the presence of a hip joint disorder. Recalling the features of each of the special tests presented is a deductive reasoning skill, where factual recall of guidelines and information guides decision-making. For this case, the hip scour test is the best test to rule out the presence of a hip joint disorder. Review hip special testing guidelines, especially the scour test, if answered incorrectly.

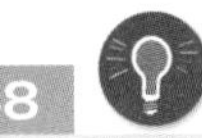

Nonsystem | Research

The findings from a recent survey of 142 female ultramarathon runners reported that 34% were amenorrhoeic and 37% had experienced a metatarsal stress fracture. The study determined that there was a direct association between amenorrhea and metatarsal stress fractures in this population (Chi-square = 43.9, $p < 0.001$) and the odds ratio for sustaining a stress fracture was 14 times higher (95% CI = 5.9–31.4) in amenorrhoeic runners. What can a physical therapist reasonably conclude from these results?

Choices:

1. Stress fractures occur as a result of running ultramarathons.
2. Amenorrhea is a risk factor for metatarsal stress fractures.
3. Amenorrhea is a normal side effect of endurance running.
4. Amenorrhea causes metatarsal stress fractures.

Teaching Points

Correct Answer: 2

The chi-square statistic is a measure of association for categorical data and an odds ratio is an estimate of relative risk. These data demonstrate a relationship between amenorrhea and metatarsal stress fractures and show that the occurrence of a negative event (the stress fracture) is more common in runners with amenorrhea (exposure to a risk factor).

Incorrect Choices:

Each of the other choices suggest cause and effect relationships. There is not enough information presented in the question to draw a conclusion about the relationship between stress fractures and participating in ultramarathons. Amenorrhea is not a normal physiologic response to exercise of any type, and there is not enough information provided to draw any conclusions about the relationship between amenorrhea and endurance training. While amenorrhea is a risk factor for stress fractures, the design of the study and data reported cannot be used to establish a cause and effect relationship between these variables.

Type of Reasoning: Inferential

For this question, the test-taker must analyze the information presented and infer what one could conclude from it. This requires inferential reasoning skill, where one must draw inferences from information and make reasonable conclusions. For this case, one can reasonably conclude that amenorrhea is a risk factor for metatarsal stress factors. If answered incorrectly, review the chi-square statistic.

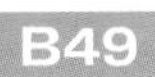

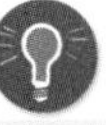

Musculoskeletal | Examination

A college soccer player sustained a hyperextension knee injury when kicking the ball. The patient was taken to the emergency room of a local hospital and was diagnosed with "knee sprain." The player was sent to physical therapy the next day for rehabilitation. As part of the examination to determine the type of treatment plan to implement, the therapist conducted the test shown in the figure. Based on the test picture, the therapist is examining the integrity of which structure?

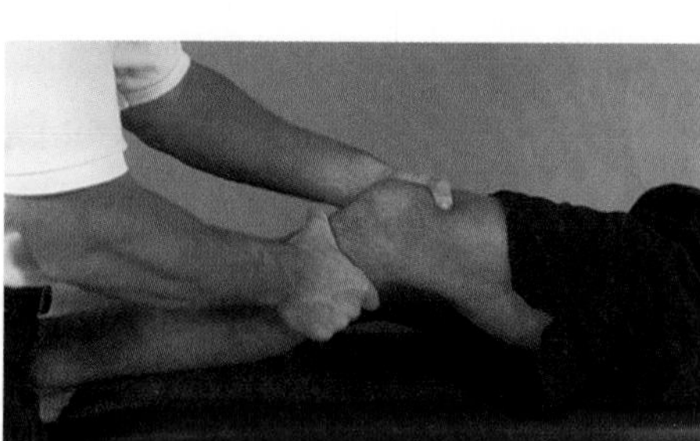

Choices:
1. Iliotibial band.
2. Posterior cruciate ligament.
3. Anterior cruciate ligament.
4. Medial meniscus.

Teaching Points

Correct Answer: 3

The test shown in the figure is Lachman's stress test to determine the integrity of the anterior cruciate ligament. The Lachman's test is highly sensitive and specific for the diagnosis of ACL tears (see Box 2-6).

Incorrect Choices:

The posterior cruciate is examined using the posterior drawer and the reverse Lachman's stress test. The medial meniscus is examined using McMurray's and Apley tests. The iliotibial band is tested using the Noble compression test.

Type of Reasoning: Inferential

The question requires the test-taker to recall the visual information depicted as a test of integrity of the anterior cruciate ligament. This is factual recall of visual information, but also requires one to sort out other tests that may appear similar in order to arrive at the correct conclusion. This skill is therefore inferential, requiring one to draw conclusions based on visual information.

B50 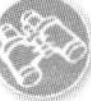

Musculoskeletal | Evaluation, Diagnosis

A patient is seen in physical therapy 2 days after a motor vehicle accident. The chief complaints are headaches, dizziness, neck pain with guarding, and a "sensation of a lump in the throat." Plain film x-rays were read as negative. What type of imaging is best to rule out a suspected upper cervical spine fracture?

Choices:
1. Second series of plain film x-rays.
2. T2 magnetic resonance imaging (MRI).
3. Computed tomography (CT) scan.
4. Myelogram.

Teaching Points

Correct Answer: 3

The primary concern is to rule out strong suspicions of an upper cervical spine fracture. CT scan is still preferred for assessing cortical bone, especially spinal fractures.

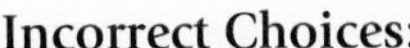

Incorrect Choices:

Plain films, already taken, did not show any fracture, which is not uncommon. A second series would not be expected to reveal any new information. The T2 MRI and myelogram are not as specific for assessing bony anatomy as the CT scan.

Type of Reasoning: Inductive

One must consider the symptoms of the patient and a possible cause to arrive at the conclusion that a CT would be the most appropriate next step in determining the cause for the symptoms. Inductive reasoning skills are utilized when one must use knowledge of symptoms plus diagnostic skills to make an appropriate decision. If this question was answered incorrectly, refer to information on indications for CT scans.

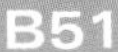

B51

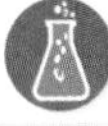

Neuromuscular | Examination

Upper extremity function in a patient with traumatic brain injury is examined using finger-to-nose testing. Movements are irregular and not easily reversed. As speed is increased, movements become more disorganized. What do these findings indicate?

Choices:

1. Brainstem dysfunction.
2. Lower motor neuron weakness.
3. Cerebellar dysfunction.
4. Upper motor neuron weakness.

Teaching Points

Correct Answer: 3

Cerebellar dysfunction is characterized by classic cerebellar movement disturbances of dyssynergia (in this case), dysmetria, and dysdiadochokinesia. Movement decomposition is velocity dependent, with greater disturbances in movement control at higher speeds.

Incorrect Choices:

UMN lesions can produce weakness and dyssynergia accompanied by spasticity. Spasticity is velocity dependent, with slowing of movements at faster speeds. LMN lesions produce weakness or paralysis, with hypotonia or flaccidity. Brainstem dysfunction produces a variety of deficits, with mixed sensory/motor symptoms. All of these findings are not reported in this case.

Type of Reasoning: Analytical

For this question, the test-taker must analyze the symptoms presented and determine the likely cause for such symptoms. Questions of this nature require analytical reasoning skill. For this scenario, the symptoms indicate cerebellar dysfunction. Review symptoms of cerebellar dysfunction if answered incorrectly.

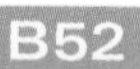
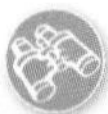

B52

Musculoskeletal | Interventions

A patient presents with a persistently downwardly rotated and adducted scapula during humeral elevation. The plan of care includes stretching and strengthening to improve range of motion. What muscles should be stretched and strengthened?

Choices:

1. Stretching rhomboid muscles and strengthening serratus anterior muscle.
2. Stretching pectoralis major and strengthening rhomboid muscles.
3. Stretching pectoralis minor and strengthening trapezius muscles.
4. Stretching serratus anterior and strengthening levator scapula and lower trapezius.

Teaching Points

Correct Answer: 1

The rhomboids are scapular downward rotators, scapular adductors, and scapular elevators. Insufficient length of the rhomboids would limit upward scapular rotation, and stretching to restore proper length of these muscles would help to promote upward scapular rotation.

Incorrect Choices:

The serratus anterior muscle acts as an upward scapular rotator and scapular abductor. Weakness of the serratus anterior would impair active scapular upward rotation, and strengthening exercises would promote upward scapular rotation.

Type of Reasoning: Inductive

This question requires the test-taker to determine a best course of action to improve a deficit. Questions of this nature require clinical judgment, which is an inductive reasoning skill. For this case, the deficit is best treated with stretching of the rhomboid muscles and strengthening of the serratus anterior muscle. If answered incorrectly, review muscle actions of the shoulder girdle, especially scapular movers and stabilizers.

B53 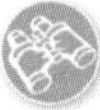

Neuromuscular | Evaluation, Diagnosis

A patient is recovering from stroke and, at 4 months, is ambulating with a straight cane for household distances. During outpatient physical therapy, the therapist has the patient practice walking with no assistive device. Recurvatum is observed that worsens with continued walking. What is the therapist's **BEST** choice for intervention?

Choices:

1. Give the patient a small-based quad cane (SBQC) to improve stability and have him/her practice AROM in supine.
2. Exercise the quadriceps using isokinetic resistance at higher loads and increasing speeds.
3. Practice isolated small-range quadriceps eccentric control work in standing and continue with the straight cane.
4. Give the patient a KAFO to control the hyperextension and a hemi walker.

Teaching Points

Correct Answer: 3

Eccentric quadriceps control work (closed-chain exercises) is indicated in order to reduce recurvatum. The patient should continue with the straight cane until able to walk without the device and recurvatum.

Incorrect Choices:

Open-chain exercises (isokinetic resistance, AROM) do not adequately address the functional demands of gait. The use of SBQC or hemi walker will not correct the problem. A KAFO is inappropriate to stabilize the knee, which can be effectively stabilized using either an AFO or a Swedish knee cage. The use of an orthosis should be considered only as a last resort.

Type of Reasoning: Inductive

One must use clinical judgment and knowledge of recurvatum in ambulation to arrive at the correct conclusion. Inductive reasoning questions require use of knowledge combined with clinical judgment to determine the best course of action in clinical situations. In this situation, the test-taker must recognize that the recurvatum indicates eccentric quadriceps control work.

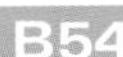
B54

Neuromuscular | Interventions

A patient recovering from an incomplete spinal cord injury at the L3 level (ASIA scale D) ambulates with bilateral Lofstrand crutches. The patient reports great difficulty going down ramps with unsteady, wobbly knees. What is the **BEST** intervention to use with this patient?

Choices:

1. Prolonged icing to reduce hamstring pain.
2. Stretching using a posterior resting splint for tight plantar flexors.
3. Progressive resistance training for the quadriceps.
4. Biofeedback training to reduce knee extensor spasticity.

Teaching Points

Correct Answer: 3

A spinal cord injury at the level of L3 affects knee extensors. ASIA scale D means the injury is incomplete, with at least half of the key muscles below the neurological level having a muscle grade of 3 or more. A weak knee will wobble or buckle going down stairs or ramps. It is the result of weak quadriceps or knee flexor contracture. Strengthening exercises using progressive resistance training for the quadriceps are indicated.

Incorrect Choices:

Biofeedback training may reduce knee extensor spasticity, but this may only increase knee instability and is not indicated in this case. There is no indication that hamstring pain or tight plantarflexors are present or precipitating causes of the patient's problem.

Type of Reasoning: Inferential

In this question, the test-taker must understand what impairments result from L3 spinal injury and what clinical interventions can be implemented to improve the patient's deficits. In this situation, the patient's deficits indicate weak knee extensors, which can be strengthened through a progressive resistive exercise program. If this question was answered incorrectly, refer to information on lumbar level spinal cord injury.

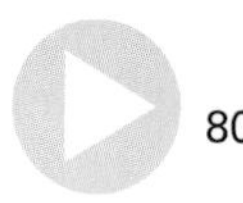

B55 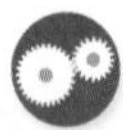

Nonsystem | Professional Responsibilities

Under HIPAA rules, to whom is it illegal to release protected health information (PHI) without a competent patient's consent?

Choices:

1. A state agency responsible for investigating suspected abuse.
2. The insurance company that is paying for the patient's treatment.
3. Another health care provider involved in the care of the patient.
4. The patient's spouse.

Teaching Points

Correct Answer: 4

A spouse does not have the legal right to the patient's information without the patient's consent.

Incorrect Choices:

Those individuals involved in the care of the patient, a legal guardian with power of attorney in situations in which the patient is judged mentally incompetent, or the patient's payer have a legal right to information regarding a patient's care without obtaining the patient's consent for releasing information. The therapist has a positive legal obligation to report suspected abuse whether or not consent is granted.

Type of Reasoning: Evaluative

In this question, one must determine the strength of the statements presented as well as which statement adheres to legal guidelines related to HIPAA. Evaluation questions often require the test-taker to make value judgments and recall certain guidelines in order to make those judgments.

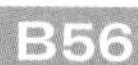B56 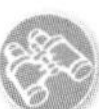

Musculoskeletal | Interventions

A patient is referred to physical therapy with a diagnosis of acute lumbar radiculopathy. The patient has a history of chronic low back pain. The primary complaint now is posterior thigh and buttock pain that resolves after one-half mile of walking, but then returns a few hours after the walk is complete. During the physical examination, repeated lumbar flexion movements reproduce the patient's posterior thigh and buttock pain, while repeated extension creates discomfort in the low back only. What is the **BEST** intervention to decrease the patient's pain and increase their function?

Choices:

1. Intermittent lumbar traction and walking program.
2. Repeated extension and walking program.
3. Repeated extension and piriformis stretching.
4. Repeated flexion and walking program.

Teaching Points

Correct Answer: 2

According to the Low Back Pain Clinical Practice Guideline (CPG) (see Box 2-16), repeated movements in a specific direction (determined by patient's response) and exercises that promote reduction of symptoms are strongly recommended. Extension movements centralized this patient's pain to the low back, while flexion movements reproduced the patient's lower extremity pain or peripheralized their symptoms. Therefore, repeated extension exercise and a walking program are recommended.

Incorrect Choices:

There is conflicting evidence for the use of intermittent lumbar traction. The Low Back Pain CPG recommends against the use of traction at any time in patients with chronic low back pain, even if there are signs of nerve root compression. Piriformis stretching could be part of a comprehensive multimodal plan; however, it is a flexion-based movement and the patient's response to the exercise should be monitored closely. While the question stem suggests that walking is beneficial for this patient, choice 4 is incorrect because repeated flexion movements reproduce the radiating lower extremity pain (peripheralization).

Type of Reasoning: Inductive

For this question, one must utilize clinical judgment to determine a best intervention approach to decrease pain and increase function for a patient with low back pain. This requires inductive reasoning skill where knowledge of intervention guidelines is paramount to arriving at a correct conclusion. For this case, the best intervention is repeated extension and walking program. If answered incorrectly, review intervention approaches for low back pain and the Low Back Pain Clinical Practice Guideline.

B57 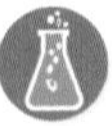

Musculoskeletal | Evaluation, Diagnosis

A baseball pitcher is referred to physical therapy with progressive posterior shoulder pain and weakness of the shoulder abductors and lateral rotators. The therapist notices muscle wasting superior and inferior to the scapular spine. Damage to which of the following structures is the **MOST** likely cause?

Choices:

1. Spinal accessory nerve.
2. Scalene muscles.
3. Suprascapular nerve.
4. Long head of the biceps brachii.

Teaching Points

Correct Answer: 3

Microtrauma to the suprascapular nerve can occur with repetitive activities involving shoulder "cocking" and follow-through resulting in inflammation and muscle weakness of the muscles supplied by the suprascapular nerve (the supraspinatus and infraspinatus muscles).

Incorrect Choices:

Damage to the spinal accessory nerve will promote weakness and atrophy of the upper trapezius muscle. Damage to the long head of the biceps brachii or scalene muscles will not present with posterior shoulder pain, weakness with shoulder abduction/external rotation, and/or atrophy of the supraspinatus and infraspinatus muscles.

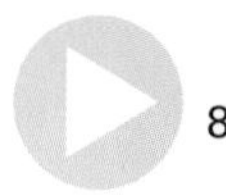

Type of Reasoning: Analytical

This question requires one to rely on knowledge of shoulder neuroanatomy in order to choose the correct solution. This type of recall is factual in nature, with basic analysis or interpretation of the information presented. In this case, the patient's weakness of the shoulder abductors and lateral rotators is indicative of damage to the suprascapular nerve. If this question was answered incorrectly, refer to shoulder neuroanatomy and functional anatomy.

B58 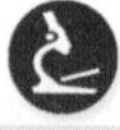

Cardiovascular/Pulmonary I Examination

An elderly patient presents with severe COPD, GOLD stage 4. Which of the following physical examination findings would the therapist expect to find?

Choices:

1. Kyphosis with an increased thoracic excursion.
2. Barreled chest with a decreased thoracic excursion.
3. Pectus excavatum with an increased thoracic excursion.
4. Pectus carinatum with decreased thoracic excursion.

Teaching Points

Correct Answer: 2

A patient with severe COPD (GOLD 4) will have lost much of the elastic recoil properties of the lung. The usual elastic properties of the lung tissue help to pull the thorax into the normal chest wall configuration of health. Without these elastic recoil properties the patient's thorax will "barrel" in appearance, meaning it is larger and rounder than what you would normally expect. As the thorax has moved into an inspiratory position at rest, there is less movement available, so a decreased thoracic excursion would be expected.

Incorrect Choices:

Pectus excavatum (funnel chest) is not an acquired chest wall deformity that results in decreased thoracic excursion. Pectus carinatum (pigeon breast) is not an acquired chest wall deformity that results in a decreased thoracic excursion. While the barreling of the chest of COPD often has a kyphosis associated with it, the second hallmark to the chest wall deformity of COPD is a decrease in excursion.

Type of Reasoning: Deductive

This question provides a diagnosis and the test-taker must recall the likely presentation of that diagnosis. This is a deductive reasoning skill, as one must recollect the signs and symptoms of COPD in order to arrive at a correct conclusion. For this case, one should expect a barreled chest with a decreased thoracic excursion. Review signs and symptoms of COPD if answered incorrectly.

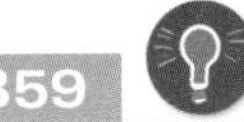

B59

Neuromuscular I Evaluation, Diagnosis

A patient is recovering from surgical resection of an acoustic neuroma and presents with symptoms of dizziness, vertigo, horizontal nystagmus, and postural instability. To address these problems, what should the physical therapy plan of care incorporate?

Choices:

1. Repetition of movements and positions that provoke dizziness and vertigo.
2. Hallpike's exercises to improve speed in movement transitions.
3. Static balance exercises on a level surface with eyes open.
4. Prolonged bed rest to allow vestibular recovery to occur.

Teaching Points

Correct Answer: 1

In patients with unilateral vestibular pathology, habituation training (use of positions and movements that evoke symptoms) will encourage the vestibular system to recalibrate. Good recovery can generally be expected with gradual progression of exercises.

Incorrect Choices:

Prolonged bed rest will delay recovery and may result in incomplete recovery. Static balance exercises on a level surface with eyes open would not challenge the vestibular system or assist with habituation. Hallpike-Dix maneuver is used for assessment and diagnosis of benign paroxysmal positional vertigo and is not a set of exercises.

Type of Reasoning: Inferential

One must have knowledge of acoustic neuroma and expected symptomatology in order to choose the correct intervention approach. Inferential reasoning often requires the test-taker to draw conclusions based on the evidence presented. Questions that ask what to expect from a diagnosis or a set of symptoms often require use of inferential reasoning. If this question was answered incorrectly, review intervention approaches for vestibular pathology.

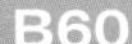
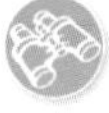

B60

System Interactions I Evaluation, Diagnosis

A physical therapist is treating a patient with diabetic peripheral neuropathy. The patient recently began taking Lyrica (pregabalin). During a monofilament exam of the feet the therapist notices circumferential marks bilaterally at the level of the malleoli after the socks are removed. The patient is complaining of increased difficulty ambulating long distances. In this situation, what is the therapist's **BEST** course of action?

Choices:

1. Contact the physician about possible development of congestive heart failure.
2. Begin manual lymphatic drainage for secondary lymphedema.
3. Complete the examination and instruct in proper skin care precautions.
4. Educate the patient about the risks of foot ulceration.

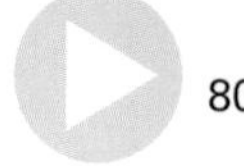

Teaching Points

Correct Answer: 1

It is important to recognize serious side effects of commonly used medications and to institute contact with the physician as appropriate. Lyrica is used to help treat diabetic neuropathy. Serious side effects include heart failure, greater difficulty walking long distances, and lymphedema (marks from the sock).

Incorrect Choices:

Although patient education and manual lymphatic drainage can be important parts of treatment, they are not as important as recognizing the potential for heart failure.

Type of Reasoning: Inductive

This question requires clinical judgment in order to determine a best course of action for a patient with diabetic neuropathy. This necessitates inductive reasoning skill. For this case, the symptoms should alert the therapist to contact the physician about possible development of congestive heart failure. If answered incorrectly, review diabetic neuropathy guidelines and common medications for diabetes.

B61 

Musculoskeletal | Examination

A patient is referred to physical therapy with a diagnosis of a mid-shaft fracture of the humerus and concomitant radial nerve injury. During manual muscle testing of the upper extremity, which movement should exhibit weakness?

Choices:

1. Thumb adduction.
2. Wrist extension.
3. Thumb opposition.
4. Wrist flexion.

Teaching Points

Correct Answer: 2

The radial nerve innervates the triceps brachii, wrist extensors (extensor carpi radialis longus and brevis, extensor carpi ulnaris), and finger extensors (extensor digitorum, extensor indicis, extensor digiti minimi). With a mid-shaft humerus fracture, the radial nerve is injured as it travels along the posterior aspect of the humerus in the spiral (radial) groove. Injuries at that location may compromise the wrist and finger extensors and result in wrist drop.

Incorrect Choices:

Thumb adduction is produced primarily by the adductor pollicis muscle, which is innervated by the ulnar nerve. Thumb opposition is produced by opponens pollicis, which is innervated by the median nerve. Wrist flexion is produced by the flexor carpi ulnaris, flexor carpi radialis, and palmaris longus muscles. The flexor carpi ulnaris is innervated by the ulnar nerve, and the flexor carpi radialis and palmaris longus are innervated by the median nerve.

Type of Reasoning: Inferential

For this question, one must determine what is most likely to be true of a situation in order to arrive at a correct conclusion, which is an inferential reasoning skill. The test-taker must first recall muscles that are innervated by the radial nerve and then resultant weakness that occurs in specific movements of the hand and wrist with radial nerve injury. For this scenario, wrist extension should exhibit weakness. If answered incorrectly, review muscles innervated by the radial nerve.

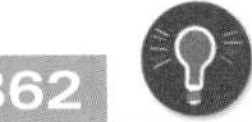

Cardiovascular/Pulmonary | Interventions

A patient who is 5 weeks postmyocardial infarction (MI) is participating in a cardiac rehabilitation program. The therapist is monitoring responses to increasing exercise intensity. Which finding is an indication that exercise should be immediately terminated?

Choices:

1. 1.5 mm of downsloping ST segment depression.
2. Peak exercise HR >140.
3. Appearance of a PVC on the electrocardiogram (ECG).
4. Systolic BP >140 mmHg or diastolic BP >80 mmHg.

Teaching Points

Correct Answer: 1

The upper limit for exercise intensity prescribed for patients post-MI is based on signs and symptoms. Of the choices, only ST segment depression (>1.0 mm of horizontal or downsloping depression) is a significant finding, representative of myocardial ischemia.

Incorrect Choices:

Both HR and BP are expected to rise (the levels of 140 and 140/80 are not significant for most patients). The appearance of a single PVC is also not significant because single PVCs can occur in individuals without a cardiac history.

Type of Reasoning: Inferential

When questions provide a diagnosis and the test-taker must determine the symptoms to watch for, inferential reasoning is used. To answer this question correctly, the test-taker must have knowledge of cardiac rehabilitation guidelines and indications for terminating exercise programs. If this question was answered incorrectly, refer to post-MI rehabilitation guidelines.

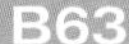
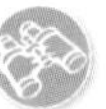

Neuromuscular | Interventions

An infant who was 39 weeks gestational age at birth and is now 3 weeks chronological age demonstrates colic. In this case, what is the **BEST** intervention the PT should teach the mother?

Choices:

1. Stroking and tapping.
2. Swaddling or wrapping.
3. Visual stimulation with a colored object.
4. Bouncing and fast rocking

Teaching Points

Correct Answer: 2

Swaddling or wrapping an infant snugly in a blanket helps a baby calm down, especially while slowly rocked. The neutral warmth provided is also a calming stimulus.

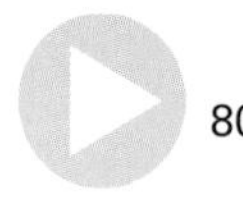

Incorrect Choices:

All of the other choices would likely increase arousal of the infant. The infant is still too developmentally immature for any of the stimuli other than neutral warmth.

Type of Reasoning: Inductive

One utilizes clinical judgment, with combined knowledge of inhibitory and facilitatory stimuli in infants, in order to choose the best solution. In this scenario, the newborn is too developmentally immature to manage facilitatory stimuli and requires stimuli that are calming or inhibitory, especially if colic is demonstrated. If this question was answered incorrectly, refer to appropriate stimuli for newborns.

B64 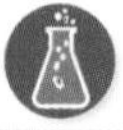

Neuromuscular | Examination

A therapist is treating a patient with Brown-Séquard syndrome that resulted from a gunshot wound. Which of the following would the therapist expect to find during the examination?

Choices:

1. Sparing of tracts to sacral segments with preservation of perianal sensation and active toe flexion.
2. Loss of motor function and pain and temperature sensation with preservation of light touch and proprioception below the level of the lesion.
3. Loss of motor function below the level of the lesion primarily in the upper extremities.
4. Ipsilateral loss of motor function, ipsilateral loss of light touch and proprioception, and contralateral loss of pain and temperature.

Teaching Points

Correct Answer: 4

Brown-Séquard syndrome is a hemisection of the spinal cord characterized by ipsilateral loss of dorsal columns with loss of touch, pressure, vibration, and proprioception; ipsilateral loss of corticospinal tracts with loss of motor function below level of lesion; contralateral loss of spinothalamic tract with loss of pain and temperature below level of lesion; at lesion level bilateral loss of pain and temperature. See Table 3-22 for additional information on various spinal cord syndromes, to include Brown-Séquard syndrome.

Incorrect Choices:

Anterior cord syndrome: loss of lateral corticospinal tracts with bilateral loss of motor function; loss of spinothalamic tracts with bilateral loss of pain and temperature; preservation of dorsal columns (proprioception, vibratory sense).

Central cord syndrome: Loss of spinothalamic tracts with bilateral loss of pain and temperature; loss of ventral horn with bilateral loss of motor function (primarily the upper extremities); preservation of proprioception and discriminatory sensation.

Sacral sparing: sparing of tracts to sacral segments with preservation of perianal sensation, rectal sphincter tone, active toe flexion.

Type of Reasoning: Analytical

This question requires factual recall of neuroanatomy in order to arrive at the correct conclusion. One should recall the nature of Brown-Séquard syndrome as a hemisection of the spinal cord, which results in both ipsilateral and contralateral losses below the level of lesion. One also must separate out the symptoms of other spinal cord syndromes, which are different from this scenario. If this question was answered incorrectly, refer to spinal cord injuries and syndromes (see Table 3-22).

B65 

Neuromuscular I Interventions

A patient is experiencing persistent vertigo with increasing symptoms over the past week, including moderate to severe headaches over the past 48 hours. Spinning (vertigo) is so bad it prevents walking more than a few feet at a time without assistance. On examination there is a persistent and sustained down-beating nystagmus that occurs with lateral gaze, a head thrust maneuver, or Dix-Hallpike test. What should the therapist do based on these findings?

Choices:

1. Epley maneuver for suspected benign paroxysmal positional vertigo (BPPV).
2. Contact the referring provider secondary to concerns of central nervous system pathology and the need for further testing.
3. Gaze stabilization exercises secondary to vestibular hypofunction.
4. Contact the referring provider secondary to concerns of Ménière's disease and the need for motion sickness and antinausea medication.

Teaching Points

Correct Answer: 2

This patient has red flag findings of persistent down-beating nystagmus and inability to walk more than a few steps. The findings of persistent and sustained down-beating nystagmus with lateral gaze raises concerns of various CNS pathologies (infract, cerebellar tumor, or Chiari malformation), all which require further evaluation and imaging (MRI).

Incorrect Choices:

The findings of persistent and sustained down-beating nystagmus with lateral gaze and increasing headaches warrants immediate discussion with the referring provider prior to other treatments. The patient's collective findings are not consistent with BPPV, Ménière's disease, or unilateral hypofunction.

Type of Reasoning: Evaluative

For this question, the test-taker must evaluate the patient's presenting symptoms and determine the significance of them in order to determine a best course of action. This requires evaluative reasoning skill, where weighing the importance of information is paramount to arriving at a correct conclusion. For this situation, the BEST option is to contact the referring provider for concerns of CNS pathology and the need for further testing. Review symptoms of common CNS pathologies if answered incorrectly.

B66 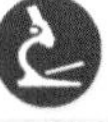

Musculoskeletal I Examination

A patient presents with low back pain of insidious onset. Based on the history and subjective complaints, the patient appears to have a dysfunction of a lumbar facet joint. What clinical test should be utilized to confirm this diagnosis?

Choices:

1. McKenzie's side glide test.
2. Stork standing test.
3. Slump test.
4. Lumbar quadrant test.

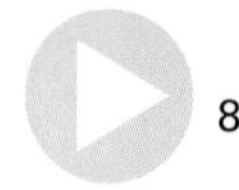

Teaching Points

Correct Answer: 4

The motion of the lumbar quadrant test places the lumbar facet joint in its maximally closed and therefore most provocative position, so if positive it is typically indicative of a lumbar facet dysfunction.

Incorrect Choices:

The slump test is utilized to assess the neurodynamics of the spinal and peripheral nerves. The stork standing test is utilized to identify a spondylolisthesis. McKenzie's side glide test is utilized to determine if a disc dysfunction with nerve root involvement is present versus a postural disorder.

Type of Reasoning: Deductive

This question requires the test-taker to recall testing guidelines for lumbar facet dysfunction. This necessitates the recall of facts and guidelines, which is a deductive reasoning skill. For this situation, the lumbar quadrant test is best to confirm lumbar facet dysfunction. Review lumbar testing guidelines if answered incorrectly, especially the lumbar quadrant test.

B67 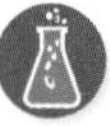

Nonsystem | Equipment, Devices

When using a transtibial total surface bearing prosthesis, a patient experiences excessive knee flexion in early stance. What is the **MOST** likely cause of this problem?

Choices:

1. Socket is aligned too far back or tilted posteriorly.
2. Foot position is inset too much.
3. Socket is aligned too far forward or tilted anteriorly.
4. Foot position is outset too much.

Teaching Points

Correct Answer: 3

In a transtibial prosthesis, the socket is normally aligned in slight flexion to enhance loading on the pressure tolerant areas of the residual limb, prevent genu recurvatum, and resist the tendency of the amputated limb to slide too deeply into the socket. If it is aligned incorrectly (too far anterior or excessively flexed), it will result in excessive knee flexion in early stance.

Incorrect Choices:

A socket aligned too posterior results in insufficient knee flexion. Excessive foot inset results in lateral thrust at midstance. Excessive foot outset results in medial thrust at midstance.

Type of Reasoning: Analytical

One must understand and analyze the properties and potential issues in using a PTB prosthesis in order to choose the best response. In this situation, excessive knee flexion in early stance is indicative of the socket aligned too far forward or anteriorly tilted. If this question was answered incorrectly, refer to information on PTB prosthetic alignment.

B68 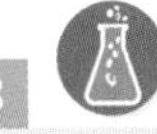

Integumentary | Evaluation, Diagnosis

A patient presents with bluish discoloration of the skin and nail beds of the fingers and toes. Palms are also cold and moist. What is the **MOST** likely cause of these changes?

Choices:

1. Carotenemia.
2. Hypothyroidism.
3. Cyanosis.
4. Liver disease.

Teaching Points

Correct Answer: 3

Bluish discoloration of the skin and nailbeds of fingers and toes, along with palms that are cold and moist, is indicative of cyanosis. It is caused by an excess of deoxygenated hemoglobin in the blood. It may be central (due to advanced lung disease, congenital heart disease, abnormal hemoglobin) or peripheral (decreased blood flow, venous obstruction).

Incorrect Choices:

Liver disease produces jaundice (diffusely yellow skin and sclerae). Carotenemia produces a yellow color, especially in the palms, soles, and face (does not affect the sclerae). Hypothyroidism produces dry and cool skin.

Type of Reasoning: Analytical

Questions that provide a group of symptoms and the test-taker must determine the diagnosis often require analytical reasoning skill. In this situation, the symptoms described indicate the condition of cyanosis. Key words that help one to arrive at a correct conclusion are "bluish discoloration." If this question was answered incorrectly, review signs and symptoms of cyanosis.

B69 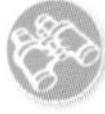

Cardiovascular/Pulmonary | Interventions

A patient who recently underwent a total knee replacement was diagnosed with deep vein thrombosis (DVT). The patient was started on an anticoagulant regimen immediately after the diagnosis was made. Which is the BEST recommendation for the physical therapist to make regarding the patient's care?

Choices:

1. Bed rest until the clot dissolves.
2. Bed rest for 72 hours after starting the anticoagulant.
3. Mobility combined with mechanical compression.
4. Mobility with an assistive device to prevent weight-bearing.

Teaching Points

Correct Answer: 3

According to the Venous Thromboembolism Clinical Practice Guideline published by Hillegass et al. (see Box 4-3), there is strong evidence for physical therapists to promote a culture of mobility coupled with mechanical compression (graded compression stockings) for patients with a DVT that have been initiated on an anticoagulant.

Incorrect Choices:

Bed rest places a patient at further risk for a DVT or pulmonary embolism. It may be helpful to have a patient use an assistive device if they are experiencing pain associated with the newly diagnosed DVT, but evidence suggests that movement is beneficial and there is no indication to prevent weight-bearing on the affected limb.

Type of Reasoning: Inductive

For this question, the test-taker must recall clinical guidelines for physical therapy intervention after a DVT in order to arrive at a correct conclusion. This is an inductive reasoning skill, where clinical judgment is paramount to arriving at a correct conclusion. For this situation, the physical therapist should recommend mobility combined with mechanical compression. Review DVT intervention guidelines if answered incorrectly.

B70 

Musculoskeletal I Examination

A physical therapist evaluates a patient who has a chief complaint of pain and swelling near the base of the thumb and lateral aspect of the wrist. The condition is aggravated with grasping and pinching activities. The therapist suspects de Quervain's tenosynovitis. Which special test is best to rule out the disorder?

Choices:

1. Finkelstein's test.
2. Eichhoff's test.
3. Wrist hyperabduction test (WHAT).
4. Watson test.

Teaching Points

Correct Answer: 3

The WHAT has the highest sensitivity (0.99) for ruling out de Quervain's tenosynovitis. It is a relatively new test and less popular than Finkelstein's and Eichhoff's tests. The test is performed by having the patient flex the wrist while the thumb is abducted against resistance (see Goubau et al., *Journal of Hand Surgery*, 2014).

Incorrect Choices:

Finkelstein's is the most popular test for de Quervain's tenosynovitis, but its sensitivity of 0.81 is markedly lower than the WHAT. The sensitivity of Eichhoff's test is 0.89. Clinicians often confuse Finkelstein's and Eichhoff's tests. Eichhoff first described his test in 1927 and it is performed *actively* by the patient. Finkelstein's was introduced in 1930 as a modification of Eichhoff's. When performing Finkelstein's test the examiner *passively* distracts the thumb and pulls it into ulnar deviation. The Watson test is an assessment of scaphoid instability.

Type of Reasoning: Deductive

This question requires one to recall the guidelines and procedures for each provocative test provided in order to determine the best test to rule out the disorder. This necessitates factual recall of information, which is a deductive reasoning skill. In this situation, the therapist should perform the WHAT. Review provocative testing for de Quervain's tenosynovitis, especially the WHAT test, if answered incorrectly.

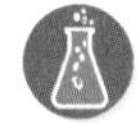

B71

Cardiovascular/Pulmonary | Examination

As part of the chart review, the physical therapist views the patient's most current chest film.

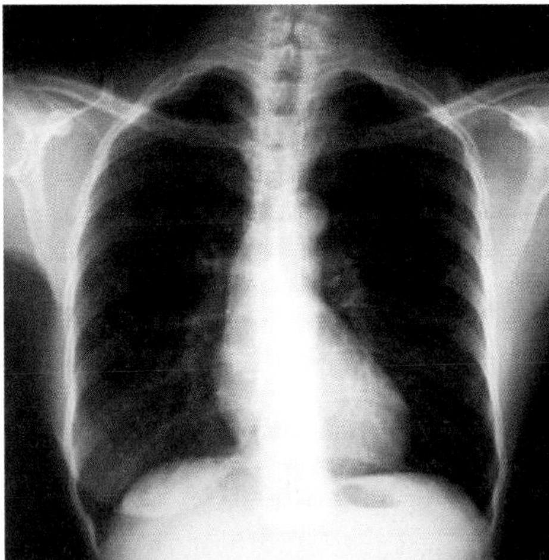

Based on this film, what is the **MOST** likely examination finding?

Choices:

1. Increased lateral costal expansion.
2. Increased subcostal angle.
3. Decreased inspiration:expiration (I:E) ratio.
4. Decreased mediate percussion.

Teaching Points

Correct Answer: 2

This film demonstrates a patient with hyperinflated lungs as evidenced by the flattened diaphragm, blunted costophrenic angle, and increased amount of air. This will cause the subcostal angle to increase significantly.

Incorrect Choices:

Hyperinflated lungs are indicative of obstructive disease. The I:E ratio will increase in this case as the patient has difficulty getting air out. There is no evidence of secretions in this film, which would alter the resonance of mediate percussion, so it can be assumed that this finding would be normal. Lateral costal expansion would be decreased in this patient due to the hyperinflated lungs.

Type of Reasoning: Analytical

This question requires the test-taker to determine the **MOST** likely examination finding based on the x-ray. Questions that require analysis of pictures and graphs often necessitate analytical reasoning skill. If this question was answered incorrectly, review signs and symptoms of hyperinflated lungs.

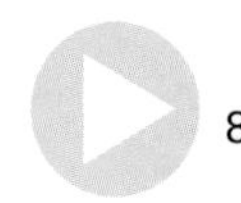

B72 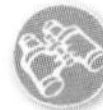

Neuromuscular | Examination

An elderly patient with ataxic gait, balance difficulty, and a history of recent falls (two in the past 3 months) is referred for physical therapy examination and evaluation. During the initial examination, what should the therapist examine first?

Choices:

1. Level of dyspnea during functional transfers.
2. Cardiovascular endurance during a 6-minute walking test.
3. Sensory losses and sensory organization of balance.
4. Spinal musculoskeletal changes secondary to degenerative joint disease (DJD).

Teaching Points

Correct Answer: 3

A critical component of balance control is sensory input from somatosensory, visual and vestibular receptors, and overall sensory organization of inputs. Initial examination should address these elements before moving on to assess the motor components of balance (e.g., postural synergies). The Clinical Test for Sensory Integration in Balance (CTSIB) or modified CTSIB (Shumway-Cook, Horak) are appropriate instruments.

Incorrect Choices:

Cardiovascular endurance and level of dyspnea during functional transfers are appropriate elements to examine but should occur after key elements of balance are examined (sensory components and integration; motor and synergistic elements). In this case, DJD changes would not be crucial to examine initially.

Type of Reasoning: Inductive

This case scenario requires the test-taker to combine knowledge of the somatosensory system and possible reasons for falls in order to arrive at the correct conclusion. A key facet of this question is in the terms "initial session" and "crucial." These words should cause the test-taker to focus on what should come first in a sequence of examination events and what is most important for the patient. This requires the use of clinical judgment, which is an inductive reasoning skill.

B73 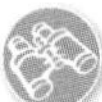

Musculoskeletal | Interventions

To reduce an elderly individual's chronic forward head posturing in standing and sitting, what muscles are likely shortened and should be stretched?

Choices:

1. Middle trapezius and rhomboid muscles.
2. Rectus capitis anterior muscles.
3. Longus capitis and longus colli muscles.
4. Rectus capitis posterior major and minor.

Teaching Points

Correct Answer: 4

Forward head posturing or forward translation of the occiput in relation to the neck and trunk is associated with extension of the occipital axial joint and flexion of the lower and mid cervical spines. Chronic extension of the occipital axial joint will lead to shortening of the suboccipital extensor muscles (rectus capitis posterior major and minor), and localized stretching of these muscles would be indicated as part of a therapeutic intervention to reduce forward head posturing.

Incorrect Choices:

Muscles anterior to the axis for mid and lower cervical flexion and extension will be chronically overlengthened, and therefore further stretching of these would not be indicated. Forward head posturing is also associated with forward scapular posturing, and therefore further stretching of scapular adductors (middle trapezius and rhomboid muscles) would not be indicated.

Type of Reasoning: Inductive

One must determine the best clinical course of action in order to arrive at a correct conclusion. Questions of this nature often require clinical judgment, which is an inductive reasoning skill. For this specific deficit, the therapist should consider exercises for the rectus capitis posterior minor and rectus capitis posterior major muscles. Review muscle actions of the cervical spine and upper trunk as well as exercises for forward head posturing if answered incorrectly.

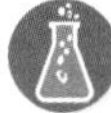

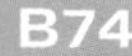

B74

Cardiovascular/Pulmonary | Evaluation, Diagnosis

A patient has the following pulmonary function test results.

MEASURE	PREDICTED	OBSERVED	% PREDICTED
Spirometry			
FVC (L)	3.19	2.48	78%
FEV_1 (L)	2.62	0.96	37%
FEV_1/FVC (%)	82%	39%	
FEF25-75% (L/S)	2.85	0.35	12%

What findings would you expect to see on a chest film given these PFT results?

Choices:

1. Blunted costophrenic angle.
2. Lung hyperinflation.
3. Pulmonary congestion.
4. Tracheal deviation.

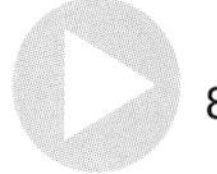

Teaching Points

Correct Answer: 2

The findings on the PFTs are consistent with severe obstructive lung disease. The FEV_1, the amount of air a patient can get out in 1 second, is markedly reduced, indicating obstruction. The FEF 25%–75% is very low, indicating difficulty getting air out of the small airways. Lung hyperinflation on a chest film is a hallmark finding in obstructive lung disease.

Incorrect Choices:

A blunted costophrenic angle is seen with a pleural effusion or infiltrate. Pulmonary congestion is a finding consistent with volume overload and heart failure. A tracheal deviation would most likely be seen with a traumatic event. Any of these findings would demonstrate a restrictive pattern on PFTs, which would primarily include a decreased FVC.

Type of Reasoning: Analytical

For this question, the test-taker must analyze the pulmonary function test results and determine the likely findings on a chest film based on these results. This requires analytical reasoning skills where pieces of information are weighed in order to draw reasonable conclusions about the patient's condition. For this situation, the findings on the pulmonary function test indicate severe obstructive lung disease. If answered incorrectly, review pulmonary function test guidelines and symptoms of obstructive lung disease.

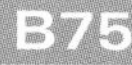
B75

Musculoskeletal I Examination

A patient is seen in a physical therapy clinic after sustaining a deep laceration of the right buttock. During the standing portion of the physical examination, the therapist observes a positive Trendelenburg sign. What did the therapist see?

Choices:

1. The right side of the pelvis dropped when the right foot was lifted off the ground.
2. The right side of the pelvis dropped when the left foot was lifted off the ground.
3. The left side of the pelvis dropped when the right foot was lifted off the ground.
4. The left side of the pelvis dropped when the left foot was lifted off the ground.

Teaching Points

Correct Answer: 4

The Trendelenburg sign is used to identify weakness of the gluteus medius muscle. When body weight is supported on one limb, the gluteus medius contracts to help maintain the pelvis in a level position. If the muscle is sufficiently weak, it fails to provide lateral stabilization and the pelvis drops on the opposite side (see Figures 2-32a and 2-32b). Weakness of the muscle can occur due to disuse, a superior gluteal nerve lesion (which is what likely happened here), or L4–L5 nerve root problems.

Incorrect Choices:

None of the incorrect choices accurately describes what is seen during the Trendelenburg test.

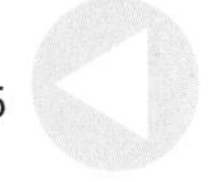

Type of Reasoning: Deductive

For this question, the test-taker must recall the features of the Trendelenburg sign in order to draw a correct conclusion. This requires the recall of factual guidelines, which is a deductive reasoning skill. For this case, the therapist would see the left side of the pelvis drop when the left foot is lifted off the ground. Review information on Trendelenburg sign if answered incorrectly.

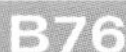
B76 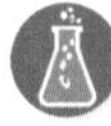

Musculoskeletal | Evaluation, Diagnosis

After treating a patient for trochanteric bursitis for 1 week, the patient has no resolution of pain and is complaining of problems with gait. After reexamination, the therapist finds weakness of the quadriceps femoris and altered sensation at the greater trochanter. What is the **MOST** likely cause of the problems?

Choices:

1. L5 nerve root compression.
2. Sacroiliac (SI) dysfunction.
3. L4 nerve root compression.
4. Degenerative joint disease (DJD) of the hip.

Teaching Points

Correct Answer: 3

The positive findings are consistent with an L4 nerve root compression.

Incorrect Choices:

Weakness of only one muscle group is not a common finding for DJD or SI dysfunction. L5 nerve root compression would result in hamstring weakness.

Type of Reasoning: Analytical

In this question, the symptoms are provided and the test-taker must make a determination of the possible diagnosis. Questions such as these require analytical reasoning skill, using knowledge of neuroanatomy to determine that the most likely cause is L4 nerve root compression. If this question was answered incorrectly, review information on nerve compressions of the lumbar spine.

B77 

Genitourinary | Examination

A patient in chronic renal failure is being seen in physical therapy for deconditioning and decreased gait endurance. The therapist needs to schedule the patient's sessions around dialysis, which is received three mornings a week. What guidelines should the therapist follow when taking the patient's blood pressure?

Choices:

1. Every minute during walking, using the nonshunt arm.
2. Pre- and postactivities, using the nonshunt arm.
3. In sitting when activity has ceased, using the shunt arm.
4. In the supine position, using the shunt arm.

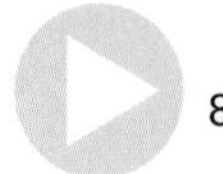

Teaching Points

Correct Answer: 2

A dialysis shunt would interfere with taking BP. Use the nonshunt arm. Pre- and postexercise measurements are appropriate.

Incorrect Choices:

The shunt arm cannot be used to take BP. Taking BP in the shunt arm or during walking would result in inaccurate measurements.

Type of Reasoning: Inferential

One must reason the best way to monitor a patient's BP using the appropriate guidelines when the patient has an atrioventricular shunt in the arm for dialysis. Guidelines dictate that you should not take BP on the arm where the shunt is located. Also, monitoring BP is best carried out pre- and postactivity to determine tolerance for activity. This type of reasoning is inferential because one must infer the best approach to patient care, considering the diagnosis and limitations of the patient.

B78 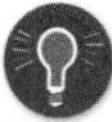

Integumentary | Evaluation, Diagnosis

A physical therapist examines an adult patient who was referred with acute foot and ankle pain. The dorsal and lateral aspects of the foot and ankle are markedly swollen. The patient denies any recent trauma. On examination, the therapist notes that the swollen area is warm to the touch and diffusely tender with palpation. There is a small, healed cut on the dorsum of the foot. The therapist suspects cellulitis. Which finding would help corroborate the diagnosis of cellulitis?

Choices:

1. Diffuse ecchymosis.
2. Absent tibialis posterior pulse.
3. Low-grade fever.
4. Positive Stemmer's sign.

Teaching Points

Correct Answer: 3

Cellulitis is a rapidly spreading, acute infection of the skin and subcutaneous tissues. Small breaks in the skin allow organisms such as staphylococcus to invade the dermis and hypodermis. Patients with cellulitis often present with fever, chills, and local swelling, tenderness, erythema, and warmth. Cellulitis may result in lymphangitis. The involvement of the lymphatic system is often first observed as a red streak under the skin radiating from the infection site in the direction of regional (proximal) lymph nodes.

Incorrect Choices:

Ecchymosis, or the discoloration/bruising, results from actual tissue damage and bleeding and is often seen after trauma to the musculoskeletal system. A ligament torn after a lateral ankle sprain would result in ecchymosis in the involved area. There was no history of trauma in this case. The tibialis posterior pulse is palpated behind the medial malleolus. The swelling caused by cellulitis on the dorsolateral foot would not occlude the tibialis posterior pulse. Stemmer's sign is a special test that is used to help establish the diagnosis of lower extremity lymphedema.

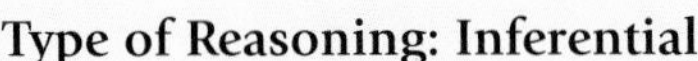

Type of Reasoning: Inferential

For this question, the test-taker must analyze the symptoms presented, then infer which symptom would most likely corroborate the presence of cellulitis. This requires inferential reasoning skill, where one determines what is likely to be true of a situation. In this case, a finding of low-grade fever would corroborate cellulitis. If answered incorrectly, review signs and symptoms of cellulitis.

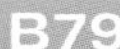

B79 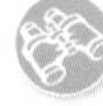

Musculoskeletal I Evaluation, Diagnosis

An older patient with hip osteoarthritis has undergone a physical therapy regimen of mobility and strengthening exercises. What is the outcome measure that can best determine improvement in the patient's condition?

Choices:

1. Lower Extremity Functional Scale (LEFS).
2. Western Ontario and McMaster Universities Osteoarthritis Index (WOMAC).
3. Patient Specific Functional Scale (PSFS).
4. Fear-Avoidance Behavior Questionnaire (FABQ).

Teaching Points

Correct Answer: 2

The WOMAC or Western Ontario and McMaster Universities Osteoarthritis Index is the gold standard for measuring changes in pain, stiffness, and function in patients with hip and knee osteoarthritis (see Box 2-1 and Appendix 2A).

Incorrect Choices:

The LEFS is an outcome measure designed to measure changes in pain and disability in patients with a wide variety of lower extremity problems. It does not specifically address impairments or stiffness associated with OA. Neither does the PSFS, which is a self-report instrument designed to assess functional changes in individuals with any musculoskeletal problem. The Fear-Avoidance Behavior Questionnaire focuses on how a patient's fear-avoidance beliefs about physical activity and work may affect or contribute to their low back pain.

Type of Reasoning: Inductive

This question requires one to determine the outcome measure that can best determine improvement in hip osteoarthritis. Inductive reasoning is utilized with this question, as clinical judgment, coupled with knowledge of the outcomes measures, helps one to reach a correct conclusion. For this scenario, the Western Ontario and McMaster Universities Osteoarthritis Index is best. Review the WOMAC if answered incorrectly.

B80 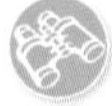

Cardiovascular/Pulmonary I Evaluation, Diagnosis

After a myocardial infarction (MI), a patient is a new admission to a phase 2 hospital-based cardiac rehabilitation program. During the initial exercise session, the patient's ECG responses are continuously monitored via telemetry. The therapist notices four PVCs in a row. What action should the therapist take?

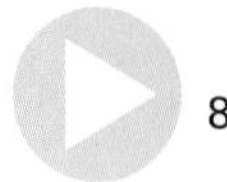

Choices:

1. Modify the exercise prescription by decreasing the intensity.
2. Stop the exercise and notify the medical team immediately.
3. Continue the exercise session, but monitor closely.
4. Have the patient sit down and rest for a few minutes before resuming exercise.

Teaching Points

Correct Answer: 2

A run of three or more consecutive PVCs is ventricular tachycardia. The rate is very rapid, resulting in seriously compromised cardiac output. This is potentially an emergency situation that can deteriorate rapidly into ventricular fibrillation (no cardiac output) and cardiac arrest.

Incorrect Choices:

The other choices, which involve continuation of exercise, put the patient at serious risk for cardiac arrest.

Type of Reasoning: Inductive

This question requires the test-taker to use diagnostic reasoning and clinical judgment to determine whether or not the PVCs and absence of P wave are significant enough to warrant physician notification. This type of reasoning is inductive, and the test-taker is called to make a decision for the safety of the patient. In this case, physician notification is warranted, and exercise should be halted immediately. If this question was answered incorrectly, refer to cardiac rehabilitation guidelines and interpretation of ECGs.

B81 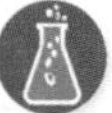

Neuromuscular | Evaluation, Diagnosis

A patient with left hemiplegia is able to recognize his wife after she is with him for a while and talks to him but is unable to recognize the faces of his children when they come to visit. The children are naturally very upset by their father's behavior. What is the **BEST** explanation for his problem?

Choices:

1. Somatognosia.
2. Anosognosia.
3. Visual agnosia.
4. Ideational apraxia.

Teaching Points

Correct Answer: 3

All of the choices are indicative of perceptual dysfunction. This patient is most likely suffering from visual agnosia, which is an inability to recognize familiar objects despite normal function of the eyes and optic tracts. Once the wife talks with him, he is able to recognize her by her voice.

Incorrect Choices:

Ideational apraxia is the inability to perform a purposeful motor act, either automatically or upon command. Anosognosia is the frank denial, neglect, or lack of awareness of the presence or severity of one's paralysis. Somatognosia is an impairment in body scheme.

Type of Reasoning: Analytical

In this question, one must recall the meaning of the four choices provided and apply them to the patient's symptoms as described. This requires analytical reasoning, which often requires one to determine the meaning of statements or medical terminology. If this question was answered incorrectly, refer to information on the various perceptual problems after CVA.

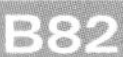

B82 

Cardiovascular/Pulmonary | Evaluation, Diagnosis

A home care PT receives a referral to evaluate the fall risk potential of an elderly community-dweller with chronic coronary artery disease (CAD). The patient has fallen three times in the past 4 months, with no history of fall injury except for minor bruising. The patient is currently taking a number of medications. What is the drug that is **MOST** likely to contribute to dizziness and increased fall risk?

Choices:

1. Colace.
2. Albuterol.
3. Nitroglycerin.
4. Coumadin sodium.

Teaching Points

Correct Answer: 3

Of the medications listed, nitroglycerin has the greatest risk of causing dizziness or weakness due to postural hypotension. Fall risk is increased even with small doses of nitroglycerin.

Incorrect Choices:

Colace (docusate sodium), an anticonstipation agent, can result in mild abdominal cramps and nausea. Coumadin (warfarin sodium) is an anticlotting medication. Adverse effects can include increased risk of hemorrhage, which indirectly can result in lightheadedness. Dosages are carefully monitored. Albuterol, a bronchodilator, can cause tremor, anxiety, nervousness, and weakness.

Type of Reasoning: Inferential

One must infer information from the four medications provided in order to determine the one that is most likely to contribute to increased fall risk. In this circumstance, using inferential reasoning, one recalls the side effects of each medicine and determines that nitroglycerin is most likely to cause increased risk of falls because this is one of the common side effects.

B83 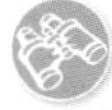

Musculoskeletal | Interventions

A patient complains of foot pain when first arising that eases with ambulation. The therapist finds that symptoms can be reproduced in weight-bearing and running on a treadmill. Examination reveals pes planus and pain with palpation at the distal aspect of the calcaneus. What is the **BEST** choice for early intervention?

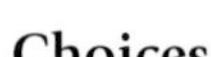

Choices:
1. Prescription for a customized orthosis.
2. Strengthening of ankle dorsiflexors.
3. Modalities to reduce pain.
4. Use of a resting splint at night.

Teaching Points

Correct Answer: 4

The symptoms are suggestive of plantar fasciitis. The focus of patient management should be on decreasing the irritation to the plantar fascia. This is most effectively done with a resting night splint. See Box 2-14 for the Heel Pain/Plantar Fasciitis Clinical Practice Guideline.

Incorrect Choices:

Modalities to reduce pain offer some symptomatic relief; however, the pain is not constant. Strengthening the dorsiflexors will not change irritation to the plantar fascia. A customized orthosis may be necessary at a later time if primary symptoms do not resolve after early management.

Type of Reasoning: Inductive

This question requires one to recognize the patient's symptoms as plantar fasciitis and then recall the common treatment strategies for this condition. This requires one to utilize clinical judgment, which is an inductive reasoning skill. If this question was answered incorrectly, refer to guidelines of treatment of plantar fasciitis.

B84 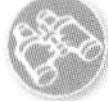

Neuromuscular | Interventions

A patient with multiple sclerosis is referred to inpatient physical therapy for evaluation and treatment of right hemiplegia, diminished sitting balance, and reduced sitting tolerance following a relapse. The patient's Trunk Impairment Scale (TIS) score is 6/23. Which of the following interventions is most appropriate for the patient's current condition and level of sitting balance?

Choices:
1. Sitting trunk rotation, perturbation, and functional reach exercises.
2. Contact guard sit to stand transfers with a focus on maintaining proper postural alignment.
3. Fit for an electric wheelchair with appropriate cushions as the patient cannot maintain static sitting posture.
4. Postural stability exercises in supine and sitting with a focus on maintaining proper postural alignment.

Teaching Points

Correct Answer: 4

The trunk impairment scale score indicates the patient can maintain static posture for a short duration (at least 10 seconds). Initially, this patient will be able to work on postural stability exercises (e.g., pelvic tilts) in supine and sitting with a focus on increasing sitting tolerance while maintaining proper postural alignment. Once the patient's sitting tolerance has improved, dynamic sitting balance exercises can be introduced.

Incorrect Choices:

The TIS score reinforces that this patient has significant impairments with dynamic and coordinated sitting balance activities (e.g., trunk rotation and functional reach) and will initially require moderate to maximal levels of assistance with sit to stand transfers. It is important to improve sitting balance and tolerance prior to sustained or repetitive standing transfers and activity. At this stage, an electric wheelchair with cushions to maintain postural alignment is too restrictive and may impede the patient from improving static sitting tolerance.

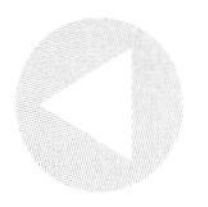

Type of Reasoning: Inductive

For this question, the test-taker must utilize clinical judgment in order to determine a best course of action in providing intervention for a patient with multiple sclerosis. This requires inductive reasoning skill. For this patient, with the presenting symptoms, postural stability exercises in supine and sitting with a focus on maintaining proper postural alignment are best. Review intervention approaches for multiple sclerosis if answered incorrectly.

B85 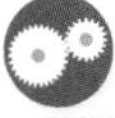

Cardiovascular/Pulmonary | Evaluation, Diagnosis

A PT should be alert to recognize the signs and symptoms associated with the onset of aspiration pneumonia. Which patient diagnosis is the MOST susceptible to develop aspiration pneumonia?

Choices:

1. A circumferential burn of the thorax associated with significant pain.
2. Severe scoliosis with compression of internal organs, including the lungs.
3. Amyotrophic lateral sclerosis (ALS) with dysphagia and diminished gag reflex.
4. A complete spinal cord lesion at T2 with diminished coughing ability and forced vital capacity (FVC).

Teaching Points

Correct Answer: 3

Aspiration pneumonia results from an abnormal entry of fluids or matter (including food) into the airways. A patient with ALS with an inability to swallow (dysphagia) and diminished gag reflex is most susceptible to aspiration pneumonia.

Incorrect Choices:

Others listed may be susceptible to other forms of pneumonia or even, though less likely, aspiration pneumonia.

Type of Reasoning: Evaluative

In this question, the test-taker must evaluate the four patient circumstances presented and determine which patient is most at risk for aspiration pneumonia. This requires one to determine the value of the information presented in each patient circumstance, which requires skills in evaluation. To arrive at the correct conclusion, one must understand each diagnosis and risks associated with those diagnoses, which should be reviewed if this question was answered incorrectly.

B86 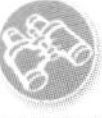

Musculoskeletal | Interventions

After an ACL reconstruction, what is the **BEST** weight-bearing and mobility status within the first week to decrease pain, increase ROM, and avoid adverse soft tissue responses?

Choices:

1. Non-weight-bearing in a knee immobilizer.
2. Toe-touch weight-bearing with range of motion as tolerated.
3. Weight-bearing as tolerated in a knee immobilizer or knee brace locked at 0°.
4. Weight-bearing as tolerated with range of motion as tolerated.

Teaching Points

Correct Answer: 4

The 2017 JOSPT Knee Ligament Sprain Clinical Practice Guideline (see Box 2-6) recommends immediate mobilization within 1 week after ACL reconstruction to increase joint range of motion, reduce joint pain, and reduce the risk of knee extension ROM loss. The use of an immediate postoperative knee brace does not appear to be safer or more effective than using no knee brace at all following an ACL reconstruction. The 2017 recommendation is to elicit and document patient preferences regarding bracing.

Incorrect Choices:

The 2010 and 2017 JOSPT Knee Ligament Sprain Clinical Practice Guideline reports that immobilization results in an increased risk for scar tissue and capsular restrictions and increased pain. Immediate weight-bearing is associated with no detrimental effects regarding stability or function. Immediate weight-bearing may decrease anterior knee pain and provides a compressive stimulus to the tibiofemoral joint, increasing activation of the quadriceps muscle.

Type of Reasoning: Inductive

This question requires one to use clinical judgment in order to determine a best course of action. This necessitates inductive reasoning skill. For this scenario, it is best to allow weight-bearing as tolerated within range of motion as tolerated after an ACL reconstruction. Review treatment guidelines for ACL reconstruction if answered incorrectly.

B87 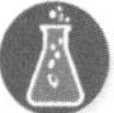

Neuromuscular | Evaluation, Diagnosis

A patient with a spinal cord injury has 4 out of 5 MMT of the bilateral elbow flexors and deltoids. All other muscles in the bilateral upper and lower extremities have complete motor loss. Sensation is normal in both lateral arms. Sensation is also present but altered in various dermatomes distal to the bilateral upper arms, to include normal pinprick and deep pressure in the S4–S5 dermatomes. This presentation is consistent with which neurologic level of injury and American Spinal Injury Association (ASIA) impairment scale rating?

Choices:

1. C5 neurologic level; ASIA B.
2. C5 neurologic level; ASIA C.
3. C6 neurologic level; ASIA C.
4. C6 neurologic level; ASIA D.

Teaching Points.

Correct Answer: 1

The neurological level of injury is defined as the most caudal level of the spinal cord with normal motor (defined as at least a 3 out 5 MMT) and sensory (intact light touch and pinprick) function on both sides of the body. The elbow flexors and lateral arm are designated as the C5 myotome and dermatome levels for this classification. The ASIA impairment scale provides a rating for complete (ASIA A), sensory incomplete (ASIA B), motor incomplete (ASIA C and D), and normal motor/sensory (ASIA E). An ASIA B rating requires sensory function preserved at the most caudal (S4–S5) segments.

Incorrect Choices:

The other choices have the incorrect myotomes, dermatomes, and/or ASIA rating. The C6 neurological level of injury requires wrist extensor MMT of at least 3 out 5 and normal sensation in the dorsal/posterior thumb. The ASIA C and D ratings require evidence of preserved motor function below the defined neurologic level with less than (ASIA C) or more than (ASIA D) half of the distal muscles with ≥3 MMT.

Type of Reasoning: Analytical

For this question, the test-taker must analyze the motor and sensory symptoms of the patient and then draw a reasonable conclusion about the ASIA impairment scale rating. This requires analytical reasoning skill, where pieces of information are weighed in order to draw reasonable conclusions about their significance. For this case, the symptoms are consistent with C5 neurologic level, ASIA B. If answered incorrectly, review the ASIA scale, especially ASIA B.

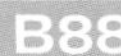
B88
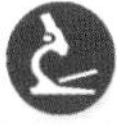

Gastrointestinal | Evaluation, Diagnosis

A sports physical therapist (PT) is working with a high school hockey player with a history of Crohn's disease. He has a history of small bowel resection. The sports PT knows he is at highest risk for which type of arthritis?

Choices:

1. Osteoarthritis.
2. Reactive arthritis (Reiter's syndrome).
3. Gout.
4. Psoriatic arthritis.

Teaching Points

Correct Answer: 2

Reactive arthritis is similar to rheumatoid arthritis, whereby the body's immune system mistakenly attacks the joints and causes an inflammatory response, which causes joint pain and stiffness as well as deformity. However, unlike rheumatoid arthritis, reactive arthritis usually affects larger joints and can also affect the lower spine, especially the sacroiliac joints. Crohn's disease is often associated with this form of arthropathy.

Incorrect Choices:

Osteoarthritis is caused by wear and tear of joints and is not related to an autoimmune response. As an ice hockey player, he may be susceptible to osteoarthritis in the future. This is not of concern for him now at this young age. Gout is a type of arthritis where defective metabolism of uric acid leads to uric acid crystal formation in the joint. This type of arthritis typically affects patients in the 40 to 60 age range. Although psoriatic arthritis is another type of autoimmune arthritis, this patient would have presented with a classic scaly rash consistent with psoriasis. Psoriatic arthritis can be associated with Crohn's disease but to a much lesser extent than reactive arthritis.

Type of Reasoning: Deductive

For this question, the test-taker must recall the risk factors associated with Crohn's disease in order to arrive at a correct conclusion. This requires the recall of factual information, which is a deductive reasoning skill. For this scenario, reactive arthritis is a risk factor. Review information on Crohn's disease and associated risk factors if answered incorrectly.

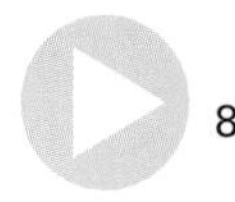

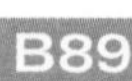

B89 

Nonsystem | Equipment, Devices

A patient with a transfemoral amputation and an above knee prosthesis demonstrates forward trunk leaning during the stance phase of gait with a rolling walker. What is the **MOST LIKELY** cause of this gait deviation?

Choices:

1. Prosthesis is too long.
2. Walker is set too high.
3. Weak gluteus maximus.
4. Unstable knee unit.

Teaching Points

Correct Answer: 4

An unstable knee unit will result in the knee buckling in stance and the patient forward bending and loading into the walker to compensate.

Incorrect Choices:

If the prothesis is too long it will result in a long limb with the typical compensations of vaulting or circumduction but not excessive forward trunk lean. If the walker is set too high the patient will maintain an upright posture and typically compensate by increasing elbow flexion. Weakness in the gluteus maximus will result in increased lumbar and trunk extension during stance.

Type of Reasoning: Inferential

This question requires the test-taker to infer the most likely cause of a gait deviation for a patient with forward trunk leaning during stance phase of gait while using an above knee prosthesis. This requires one to draw from knowledge of prosthetic use and common issues during gait training. For this situation, the most likely cause for this is an unstable knee unit. Review gait training and prosthetic use if answered incorrectly.

B90 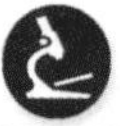

Musculoskeletal | Interventions

Following a total hip arthroplasty with a posterior approach, what positions should be avoided while performing rehabilitation exercises and activities of daily living?

Choices:

1. Hip flexion greater than 90°, adduction past mid-line, and internal rotation.
2. Hip flexion greater than 90°, adduction past mid-line, and external rotation.
3. Hip extension past neutral, abduction past mid-line, and internal rotation.
4. Hip extension past neutral, abduction past mid-line, and external rotation.

Teaching Points

Correct Answer: 1

To reduce the risk of dislocation, patients should avoid positions of hip flexion greater than 90°, adduction past mid-line, and internal rotation. In a total hip arthroplasty (THA) with a posterior approach, these movements place increased stress on the posterior joint capsule and may result in a dislocation of the prosthesis.

Incorrect Choices:

Patients do not need to avoid hip extension; adequate hip extension range of motion promotes good walking gait mechanics. Hip external rotation and abduction do not place excessive stress on healing structures or the joint following a THA with a posterior approach.

Type of Reasoning: Deductive

For this question, one must recall posterior hip precautions in order to arrive at a correct conclusion. This requires deductive reasoning skill, where factual recall of guidelines helps one to draw correct conclusions. For this situation, hip flexion greater than 90°, adduction past mid-line, and internal rotation should be avoided during daily activities and exercise. Review hip precaution guidelines, especially posterior hip precautions, if answered incorrectly.

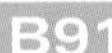
B91
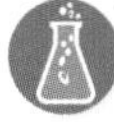

Neuromuscular | Evaluation, Diagnosis

A 65-year-old male reports falling 3 days ago with hyperextension to his neck. His initial symptoms only included mild (3/10) neck pain and his cervical x-rays were negative for a fracture. The patient is now having constant and diffuse weakness (2/5 strength testing) and impaired coordination in the bilateral hands, thumbs, and fingers. He also has burning pain and tingling with reduced pinprick sensation to the posterolateral arms and thorax. Which of the following health conditions is most consistent with the patient's signs and symptoms?

Choices:

1. Anterior Cord Syndrome.
2. Brown Sequard Syndrome.
3. Central Cord Syndrome.
4. Medial Medullary Syndrome.

Teaching Points

Correct Answer: 3

Central Cord Syndrome most often occurs with neck hyperextension and in adults over the age of 50. The patient's signs and symptoms, to include pronounced upper extremity weakness and "cape-like" loss of pain and temperature sensation, are consistent with damage to the ventral horn and spinothalamic tracts at the level of the cervical spine.

Incorrect Choices:

Anterior cord syndrome is more common with neck flexion injuries and results in damage to the corticospinal and spinothalamic tracts, thus causing more pronounced lower extremity symptoms, to include upper motor neuron signs below the level of the lesion. Brown Sequard Syndrome is defined by the classic ipsilateral loss of motor and medium to large sensory fiber (vibration, proprioception, fine touch) function and contralateral loss of pain and temperature. Medial medullary syndrome is most often the result of a stroke and presents with weakness in the tongue (cranial nerve XII) and hemiplegia (see Tables 3-12 and 3-22 for additional information).

Type of Reasoning: Analytical

This question requires one to analyze the presenting symptoms of the patient and then determine which health condition is most consistent with the symptoms. This requires analytical reasoning skill, where pieces of information are analyzed to draw reasonable conclusion. For this scenario, the symptoms are consistent with Central Cord Syndrome. If answered incorrectly, review types of spinal cord injuries and symptoms, including Central Cord Syndrome.

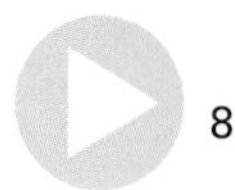

B92 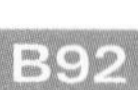

Musculoskeletal | Examination

An elderly adult patient presents with a history of and subjective complaints consistent with lumbar central spinal stenosis. What is the **MOST** appropriate clinical test to differentiate spinal stenosis from intermittent vascular claudication?

Choices:

1. Femoral nerve traction test.
2. Bicycle (van Gelderen's) test.
3. Valsalva's maneuver.
4. Lumbar quadrant test.

Teaching Points

Correct Answer: 2

The bicycle (van Gelderen's) test is designed to differentiate between spinal stenosis and intermittent vascular claudication. Van Gelderen's bicycle test is designed to stress the lower extremity vascular system without causing any central canal or foraminal stenosis that could be misinterpreted as intermittent neurogenic claudication.

Incorrect Choices:

The lumbar quadrant test is utilized to identify a lumbar facet dysfunction. The femoral nerve traction test is utilized to identify if there is an entrapment of the femoral nerve, and thus it is not related to either of these two conditions directly. Valsalva's maneuver is utilized to identify a space-occupying lesion such as a disc herniation, a tumor, etc. This would not be sensitive in identifying a spinal stenosis.

Type of Reasoning: Deductive

One must recall the testing guidelines of the lumbar spine in order to reach a correct conclusion. This necessitates the recall of factual information, which is a deductive reasoning skill. Through the deductive process, one should recall that the bicycle (van Gelderen's) test is most appropriate to differentiate spinal stenosis from intermittent vascular claudication. Review lumbar testing guidelines if answered incorrectly, especially the bicycle test.

B93 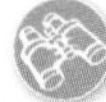

Cardiovascular/Pulmonary | Interventions

A patient with bacterial pneumonia has crackles and wheezes in the left lateral basal segment and decreased breath sounds throughout. The patient is on 4 L of oxygen by nasal cannula with a resulting oxygen saturation (SaO_2) of 90%. Respiratory rate is 28. What is the **MOST BENEFICIAL** intervention for this patient?

Choices:

1. Postural drainage, percussion, and shaking over the appropriate area on the left lateral thorax for secretion removal.
2. Positioning in left sidelying to improve ventilation/perfusion ratios.
3. Postural drainage, percussion, and shaking to the right basilar segments in order to keep the right lung healthy.
4. Breathing exercises encouraging expansion of the right lateral basilar thorax, because the left side is not currently participating in gas exchange.

Teaching Points

Correct Answer: 1

A treatment of postural drainage, percussion, and shaking to the appropriate lung segments is advisable. The standard postural drainage position for the lateral basilar segment of the left lower lobe is in sidelying position with the head of bed tipped in full Trendelenburg position. Given the borderline SaO_2 values on 4 L of oxygen, modification of the position may be necessary for patient tolerance.

Incorrect Choices:

There is nothing that will ensure that the right lung stays healthy or makes it more functional. Therefore, positioning in left sidelying and focusing on left-sided breathing exercises are incorrect choices. In addition, placing the patient in the left sidelying position would increase blood flow to the left lateral base, an area that is getting little ventilation. This position would worsen ventilation/perfusion matching.

Type of Reasoning: Inductive

One must utilize clinical judgment to determine which intervention approach is most beneficial, given the patient's diagnosis and symptoms. This is an inductive reasoning skill, in which clinical judgment and diagnostic thinking are used to arrive at the correct conclusion. If this topic is not well understood, refer to indications for modified postural drainage procedures.

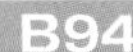
B94
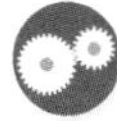

System Interactions I Evaluation, Diagnosis

A therapist receives a referral to see an elderly patient in the intensive care unit (ICU) recovering from a severe case of pneumonia. The patient is confused and disoriented. What criteria would allow the therapist to determine the disorientation is due to delirium rather than dementia?

Choices:

1. Hallucinations are present throughout the day.
2. Persistent personality changes are evident.
3. Symptoms are intermittent.
4. Level of arousal is significantly depressed.

Teaching Points

Correct Answer: 3

Acutely ill, hospitalized elderly patients frequently exhibit delirium, a fluctuating attention state. Patients demonstrate a fluctuating course with symptoms of confusion that alternate with lucid intervals. Sleep/wake cycles are disrupted and confusion is typically worse at night.

Incorrect Choices:

All other choices are signs of chronic dementia.

Type of Reasoning: Evaluative

One must evaluate the merits of each of the four statements in order to determine which statement most likely seems true for the patient's symptoms and diagnosis. In this case, the disorientation is due to delirium, because the symptoms are intermittent, whereas patients with dementia experience constant disorientation. Questions that require one to determine the value and merits of statements presented utilize evaluative reasoning skill, which can be challenging because of the need to make a judgment call.

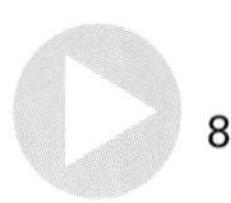

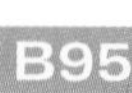

B95

Nonsystem I Research

A physical therapist is conducting a study to determine the optimal placement of electrodes for producing peak quadriceps femoris muscle torque. Four different electrode site placements are being investigated. Which statistical tool must be used to determine if there is a significant difference in torque output based on electrode placement?

Choices:

1. Analysis of variance (ANOVA).
2. T-test.
3. Linear regression analysis.
4. Pearson's product-moment coefficient.

Teaching Points

Correct Answer: 1

The ANOVA is the appropriate test for this study. It is used to determine if there are differences among three or more groups. See Figure 16-1 for examples of which statistical tests to use based on a study's purpose.

Incorrect Choices:

A t-test determines if there is a difference between two groups. It is used if there is only one dependent and one independent variable in the study. Linear regression analyses are done to determine if there is a relationship between two variables as a basis for prediction. The purpose of linear regression analysis is to develop an equation that predicts a relationship between two variables (e.g., body weight and blood pressure). Pearson's product-moment coefficient is a measure of the strength of the linear relationship (correlation) between two quantifiable variables.

Type of Reasoning: Deductive

This question requires the test-taker to recall research guidelines, especially statistical tools, in order to arrive at a correct conclusion. This necessitates factual information, which is a deductive reasoning skill. For this situation, the statistical tool that must be used is the ANOVA. If answered incorrectly, review research guidelines, especially statistical tools.

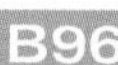
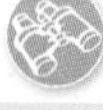

B96

Neuromuscular I Interventions

A patient has a recent history of strokes (two in the past 4 months) and demonstrates good return in the right upper and lower extremities. The therapist is concentrating on improving balance and independence in gait. Unfortunately, speech recovery is lagging behind motor recovery. The patient demonstrates fluent aphasia. What is the **BEST** strategy to use during physical therapy sessions?

Choices:

1. Demonstrate the task and use tactile cues and word repetition.
2. Have the family present to help interpret during physical therapy sessions.
3. Write out detailed instructions and show the patient a picture of the task.
4. Consult with the speech pathologist to establish a communication board.

Teaching Points

Correct Answer: 1

Fluent aphasia (Wernicke's aphasia) is a central language disorder in which spontaneous speech is preserved and flows smoothly while auditory comprehension is impaired. Demonstration (visual modalities), word repetition, and tactile cues offer the best means of communicating with this patient.

Incorrect Choices:

Verbal cues are best for patients with nonfluent aphasia (Broca's aphasia) in which understanding of verbal cues is intact but motor production of speech is not. A communication board, detailed written instructions, and lengthy instructions are not indicated unless the patient does not improve with tactile cues, visual demonstration, and word repetition. The family will also have difficulties communicating with the patient.

Type of Reasoning: Inductive

In this question, the patient requires gait training but has limitations in communication from Wernicke's aphasia. The test-taker must determine the best way to communicate with a patient who has this severe deficit, which is to provide demonstrations and gestures, rather than verbal cues. Questions that elicit clinical judgment to determine a best course of action utilize inductive reasoning skills. If this question was answered incorrectly, refer to information on communication with patients who have Wernicke's aphasia.

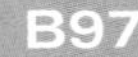

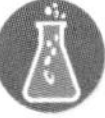

Musculoskeletal I Evaluation, Diagnosis

What is a congenital condition in which there is a development of nonprogressive contractures affecting one or more areas of the body prior to birth?

Choices:

1. Arthrogryposis congenita multiplex.
2. Juvenile idiopathic arthritis.
3. Scleroderma (progressive systemic sclerosis).
4. Duchenne muscular dystrophy.

Teaching Points

Correct Answer: 1

Arthrogryposis congenita multiplex, where the key to identifying this condition is that the physical findings of multiple contractures of the limb segments are present at birth.

Incorrect Choices:

Juvenile idiopathic arthritis is an inflammatory disease beginning frequently between the ages of 1 and 3 and leads to joint pains with potential for contractures when chronic.

Scleroderma is an autoimmune, rheumatic, and chronic disease that affects the body by hardening connective tissues. The most common age span for developing scleroderma is between 35 and 50 years of age.

Duchenne muscular dystrophy is a genetic disorder characterized by progressive muscle degeneration and weakness in children with onset between 3 and 5 years of age.

Type of Reasoning: Analytical

This question provides a description of a condition, and the test-taker must determine the most likely diagnosis. This is an analytical reasoning skill, where pieces of information are analyzed to draw a conclusion about the likely diagnosis. For this scenario, the description is consistent with arthrogryposis congenita multiplex. If answered incorrectly, review signs and symptoms of arthrogryposis congenita multiplex.

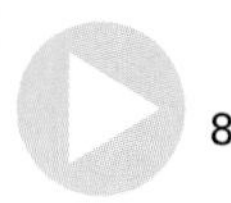

B98 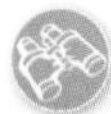

Integumentary | Interventions

A patient was burned over 40% of the body in an industrial accident and has full-thickness burns over the anterior trunk and neck and superficial partial-thickness burns over the shoulders. In order to stabilize this patient out of positions of common deformity, what orthotic device would be of **GREATEST** benefit?

Choices:

1. Soft cervical collar with an intrinsic plus hand splint.
2. A cervical thoracic lumbosacral orthosis (CTLSO) used during all upright activities.
3. Plastic cervical orthosis and axillary splints utilizing an airplane position.
4. Splints utilizing a flexed position for the shoulders and body jacket for the trunk.

Teaching Points

Correct Answer: 3

The common deformity for the anterior neck is flexion; the appropriate positioning device is a firm rigid plastic cervical collar that stresses extension. The common deformity of the shoulders is adduction and internal rotation; the appropriate position device is an axillary or airplane splint that stresses abduction, flexion, and external rotation.

Incorrect Choices:

Choices that involve hand splints should be ruled out immediately because there is no mention of burns to the hands. A CTLSO would prevent neck flexion but does not deal with the potential shoulder deformities. The CTLSO could also restrict breathing and enhance the risk of pneumonia.

Type of Reasoning: Inductive

This question requires one to recall common positioning techniques after burns to the anterior trunk and neck. Using knowledge of the typical deformity and contracture patterns with burns to this area, one can reason that the solution is to utilize axillary splints and cervical orthosis to bring about abduction, flexion, and external rotation of the shoulders and cervical extension. Questions that require one to make interpretations of clinical guidelines and make judgments from this utilize inductive reasoning skills.

B99 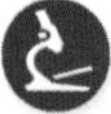

Metabolic/Endocrine | Evaluation, Diagnosis

A patient with type 2 diabetes is referred to physical therapy for exercise conditioning. What is a pathophysiologic cause of type 2 diabetes?

Choices:

1. Metabolic syndrome.
2. Impaired ability of the tissues to use insulin and insulin deficiency.
3. Loss of beta-cell function and insulin deficiency.
4. Pancreatic tumor.

Teaching Points

Correct Answer: 2

Type 2 diabetes results from impaired ability of the tissues to use insulin (insulin resistance), accompanied by a relative lack of insulin or impaired release of insulin.

Incorrect Choices:

Type 1 diabetes results from loss of pancreatic beta-cell function and an absolute insulin deficiency. Metabolic syndrome is a precursor to type 2 diabetes and is evidenced by abdominal obesity, high triglycerides, low high-density lipoprotein (HDL), hypertension, and high fasting plasma glucose (>110 mg/dL). Pancreatic tumor is not a causative factor in type 2 diabetes.

Type of Reasoning: Deductive

One must recall the factual guidelines of type 2 diabetes in order to arrive at a correct conclusion. This requires deductive reasoning skill. For this situation, type 2 diabetes is the result of an impaired ability of the tissues to use insulin and insulin deficiency. If this question was answered incorrectly, review type 2 diabetes information, especially causes of the condition.

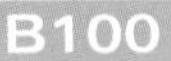
B100

Neuromuscular I Interventions

Which intervention is **BEST** to improve left-sided neglect in a patient with left hemiplegia?

Choices:

1. Hook-lying, holding, light resistance to both hip abductors.
2. Rolling, supine to sidelying on right, using a PNF lift pattern.
3. Sitting, with both arms extended, hands resting on support surface, active holding.
4. Bridging with both arms positioned in extension at the sides.

Teaching Points

Correct Answer: 2

Incorporating the involved left side into a crossing the midline activity (rolling, using PNF lift) is best.

Incorrect Choices:

All other choices involve symmetrical activity and do little to bring attention to the involved hemiplegic side.

Type of Reasoning: Inferential

One must link the deficit of the patient (left-sided neglect) to the best treatment approach in order to arrive at the correct conclusion. This requires inferential reasoning skill, as one must infer the course of action that will have the best clinical outcome. In this circumstance, rolling supine to sidelying on the right using a PNF lift pattern is best because it incorporates use of the left side and promotes crossing the midline. If this question was answered incorrectly, review treatment strategies for hemiplegia, especially PNF.

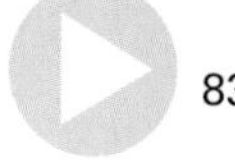

B101 

Cardiovascular/Pulmonary | Examination

A patient with no significant past medical history who now presents with a bacterial pneumonia in the right anterior base would present with which of the following exam findings?

Choices:

1. Decreased breath sounds throughout all lung fields, increased SaO_2, febrile.
2. Bronchial breath sounds at the right anterior base, increased SaO_2, febrile.
3. Crackles on inspiration only at right anterior base, decreased SaO_2, and productive cough × 3 days.
4. Wheezes on inspiration only throughout the right lung fields, decreased SaO_2, dry cough × 1 day.

Teaching Points

Correct Answer: 3

Bacterial pneumonia has a gradual onset of days with a productive cough. As pneumonia interferes with the transport of oxygen from the alveoli to the pulmonary capillaries, the PaO_2 and therefore the SaO_2 would be lower than expected, and crackles in the area of the pneumonia is a usual finding.

Incorrect Choices:

Wheezing may occur with a bacterial pneumonia and resound within that thorax, and a decrease in SaO_2, making this portion of the answer plausible. But a more abrupt onset with a dry cough is consistent with a viral infection, not bacterial infection.

An increased SaO_2 would not be seen, negating the first two choices as possibilities. Febrile (with fever) certainly would be plausible, but the overall decreased breath sounds don't fit with a pneumonia in a specific region of the lung. A bronchial breath sound in the specific involved region of the lung is plausible.

Type of Reasoning: Inferential

One must infer or draw a reasonable conclusion about what is likely to be true of a diagnosis in order to arrive at a correct conclusion. This necessitates inferential reasoning skill. For this case, a patient with bacterial pneumonia of the right anterior base would have crackles on inspiration at right anterior base, decreased SaO_2, and a productive cough for 3 days. Review signs and symptoms of bacterial pneumonia if answered incorrectly.

B102 

Cardiovascular/Pulmonary | Interventions

A physical therapist performs an evaluation of an inpatient 1 day after upper abdominal surgery. The therapist notices that there is an incentive spirometer on the patient's bedside table. What is the **MOST** appropriate indication for the use of incentive spirometry?

Choices:

1. Presence of atelectasis.
2. Signs of cognitive impairment.
3. Presence of ascites.
4. Sputum in the lungs.

Teaching Points

Correct Answer: 1

The prevention (or presence of) atelectasis is a primary indication for the use of incentive spirometry. Atelectasis is a complete or partial collapse of a lung that occurs when the tiny alveoli become deflated or filled with fluid. It is one of the most common pulmonary complications following thoracic or abdominal surgery. Incentive spirometry, or sustained maximal inspiration, along with deep breathing exercises and early mobilization are often prescribed following these surgeries to prevent or treat pulmonary complications.

Incorrect Choices:

Incentive spirometry is contraindicated for patients who show signs of cognitive impairment, confusion, and delirium, leading to the inability to understand or demonstrate proper use of the equipment. Ascites is the abnormal build-up of fluid within the abdomen and is not typically an indication for incentive spirometry. The most common causes of ascites are liver disease (cirrhosis) and chronic renal failure. Coughing is the best way to clear the lungs of sputum. There are several types of exercises used to help patients strengthen their cough including graded coughing, huffing, and sniffing.

Type of Reasoning: Inferential

For this question, the test-taker must weigh the indicators presented and recall guidelines to use of incentive spirometry in order to determine which indication is most appropriate. This requires inferential reasoning skill, where one determines what is most likely to be true of a situation. In this case, the presence of atelectasis is most appropriate. Review pulmonary disorders and use of incentive spirometry if answered incorrectly.

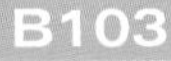

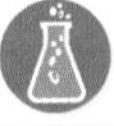

Neuromuscular | Evaluation, Diagnosis

The therapist is treating a 1-year-old child with Down syndrome at home and notices decreasing strength in the extremities, with neck pain and limited neck motion. Upper extremity deep tendon reflexes (DTRs) are 3+. These signs and symptoms are a hallmark of what diagnosis?

Choices:

1. Lower motor neuron signs consistent with Down syndrome.
2. Atlanto-axial subluxation with dorsal column medial lemniscal impingement.
3. Upper motor neuron signs consistent with Down syndrome.
4. Atlanto-axial subluxation with spinal cord impingement.

Teaching Points

Correct Answer: 4

Ligamentous laxity is a hallmark of Down syndrome and can lead to atlanto-axial instability (AAI) with spinal cord impingement. This is a medical emergency situation. Decreased muscle strength and increased DTRs are the signs of dislocation from loss of cord function. In this case, the increasing symptomatology (changes in strength, neck pain, limited neck motion, hyperreflexia) is significant for a developing subluxation. Other UMN signs (clonus, positive Babinski response) may also occur.

Incorrect Choices:

Children with Down syndrome often have low tone, not upper motor neuron or lower motor neuron signs. Lemniscal impingement would result primarily in sensory changes.

Type of Reasoning: Analytical

In this question, symptoms are provided and the test-taker must determine the cause. This type of question requires analytical reasoning, in which the test-taker must determine the meaning of the symptoms presented. In this situation, one should determine that the symptoms indicate atlanto-axial subluxation with spinal cord impingement, a medical emergency, which should be reviewed if this question was answered incorrectly.

B104 

Neuromuscular | Evaluation, Diagnosis

Which of the following factors is likely to contribute to subluxation and shoulder pain in hemiplegia?

Choices:

1. Spasticity of the biceps.
2. Traction acting on a depressed, downwardly rotated scapula.
3. PROM with a focus on maintaining normal scapulohumeral rhythm.
4. Spastic retraction with elevation of scapula.

Teaching Points

Correct Answer: 2

Shoulder pain and subluxation in hemiplegia may be caused by a number of different factors. One major cause is traction and gravitational forces acting on a depressed, downwardly rotated scapula.

Incorrect Choices:

An appropriate treatment intervention involves PROM with careful attention to maintaining scapulohumeral rhythm. This intervention if performed correctly is **NOT** likely to cause pain. Spastic biceps is likely but is not a contributing factor to subluxation and pain. Spastic retraction of the scapula is likely but with depression and downward rotation (not elevation).

Type of Reasoning: Inferential

This question requires the test-taker to determine which causative factor is likely to result in shoulder pain in hemiplegia. This requires one to draw conclusions from the information presented and to make assumptions about that information, which draws upon inferential reasoning skill. One must have knowledge of the factors that affect subluxation as well as those that do not in order to arrive at the correct conclusion.

B105 

Neuromuscular | Examination

A physical therapist examines a patient who complains of dizziness, imbalance, and blurred vision with head movements. The therapist performs a head thrust test as part of the examination. What would the therapist **MOST LIKELY** observe if the test is positive?

Choices:

1. Skew deviation in which the eye on the involved side is elevated.
2. Nystagmus with cycles of involuntary movements, slow and fast phases.
3. Absence of an optokinetic response to rapid movement in the visual field.
4. Corrective saccade with slow deviation of the eyes and rapid return to their fixation point.

Teaching Points

Correct Answer: 4

The Head Thrust Test examines the patency of the angular vestibulo-ocular reflex (aVOR). A positive test indicates a diminished aVOR on the side being tested and results in a compensatory saccade denoted by a slow phase in which the eyes drift off their fixation target and a fast phase where they return to the fixation point.

Incorrect Choices:

A skew deviation occurs as a result of central vestibular pathology that influences function of the otolith organs. Skew deviations can be observed clinically using the alternate eye cover test. Nystagmus is a common finding with both peripheral and central vestibular lesions and may be seen at rest or with repetitive head motion. It is not commonly seen with the head thrust test. The optokinetic response (or reflex) is stimulated by rapid movement across the visual field when the head is still. Absence of this response suggests a central lesion of the visual system.

Type of Reasoning: Inferential

For this question, the test-taker must infer what is likely to be true of a situation in order to arrive at a correct conclusion. Specifically, one must determine what would be most likely observed after performing a head thrust test. This requires inferential reasoning skill. For this case, the therapist would most likely observe a corrective saccade when testing the involved side where the eyes slowly deviate from and then rapidly return to their fixation point. Review information on the Head Thrust Test if answered incorrectly.

B106 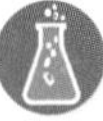

Integumentary | Evaluation, Diagnosis

A patient with hemiplegia and a drop foot is referred for physical therapy gait training. Examination reveals a pressure ulcer on the patient's right heel (pictured). The ulcer has dry eschar without edema, erythema, fluctuance, or drainage. The patient is afebrile. What is the **BEST** choice for intervention?

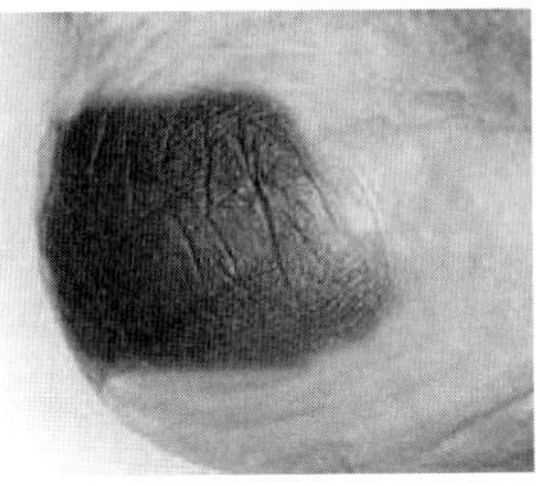

Choices:

1. Sharp debridement.
2. Refer for an arterial bypass graft.
3. Use an AFO with heel pressure relief.
4. Enzymatic debridement.

Teaching Points

Correct Answer: 3

The AFO helps to prevent plantarflexion contractures, while the heel pressure relief prevents further damage to the heel and promotes healing.

Exam B

Incorrect Choices:

This pressure ulcer, based on the examination findings, is stable and needs to be monitored, not debrided. Arterial bypass grafts are needed if circulation is compromised. There is no indication that this is the case.

Type of Reasoning: Analytical

In this question, one must determine the best course of action for the patient with a pressure ulcer on the heel. When one must determine the meaning of visual information presented, such as the picture, analytical reasoning skills are utilized. If this question was answered incorrectly, review information on the treatment of pressure ulcers.

B107 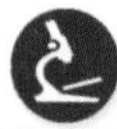

Musculoskeletal | Examination

A patient presents with an acute sprain of the right ankle. According to the patient, this has occurred frequently over the past 5 years. What clinical test should the therapist use to examine the integrity of the anterior talofibular ligament?

Choices:

1. Anterior drawer test.
2. Morton's test.
3. Talar tilt.
4. Thompson's test.

Teaching Points

Correct Answer: 1

The anterior drawer test is specifically designed to assess the integrity of the anterior talofibular ligament. See Box 2-11 for the Ankle Ligament Sprains Clinical Practice Guideline.

Incorrect Choices:

The talar tilt assesses the integrity of the calcaneofibular ligament. Thompson's test assesses the integrity of the Achilles tendon. Morton's test assesses for the presence of a stress fracture or a neuroma in the forefoot.

Type of Reasoning: Deductive

This question provides a diagnosis, and the test-taker must recall the testing guidelines to confirm the diagnosis. This necessitates factual recall of information, which is a deductive reasoning skill. For this scenario, the test for laxity of the anterior talofibular ligament is confirmed via the anterior drawer test. Review testing guidelines for the ankle if answered incorrectly, especially the anterior drawer test.

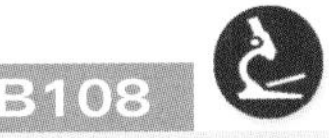

Musculoskeletal | Evaluation, Diagnosis

An elderly female patient is taking Raloxifene for the estrogen-like effects on the body in the management of her osteoporosis. What side effect should be monitored?

Choices:

1. Depressed heart rate.
2. Deep vein thrombosis.
3. Elevated blood pressure.
4. Altered balance reactions.

Teaching Points

Correct Answer: 2

One of the most common side effects of Raloxifene is deep vein thrombosis and therefore poses an increase for the risk of stroke.

Incorrect Choices:

Side effects of depressed heart rate, elevated blood pressure, and altered balance reactions are not commonly reported.

Type of Reasoning: Deductive

One must recall the common side effects of Raloxifene in order to arrive at a correct conclusion. This necessitates deductive reasoning skill, where factual information guides one to a correct conclusion. For this case, monitoring for deep vein thrombosis is appropriate, as it is a side effect of Raloxifene use. Review side effects of Raloxifene if answered incorrectly.

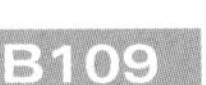

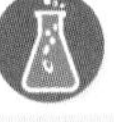

Genitourinary | Evaluation, Diagnosis

An elderly man complains of lower back pain and is referred for physical therapy at an extended care facility. During the history, the patient describes urgent and painful urination and pain around the base of the penis and behind the scrotum. These symptoms have been fluctuating during the past few months but the pain is now severe, rated as 7 out of 10. The therapist suspects which of the following?

Choices:

1. Chronic fatigue syndrome.
2. Chronic prostatitis.
3. Acute bacterial prostatitis.
4. Irritable bowel syndrome.

Teaching Points

Correct Answer: 2

This patient has signs and symptoms of chronic prostatitis. This patient may also experience pain after ejaculation, blood in semen, rectum pain, urinary blockage, and urinary tract infection.

Incorrect Choices:

Acute bacterial prostatitis has many of the same symptoms but comes on quickly and is typically accompanied by high fever, chills, and muscle aches. Chronic prostatitis or chronic pelvic pain syndrome (CP/CPPS) has been linked to autoimmune disorders (e.g., chronic fatigue syndrome) and irritable bowel syndrome. However, each of these conditions includes a different set of symptoms.

Type of Reasoning: Analytical

This question provides a group of symptoms, and the test-taker must determine the most likely diagnosis associated with them. This requires analytical reasoning skill, where information is analyzed to draw reasonable conclusions. For this situation, the symptoms are consistent with chronic prostatitis, which should be reviewed if answered incorrectly.

B110 

Neuromuscular I Interventions

A patient with stroke demonstrates early recovery in the right upper extremity (RUE) with moderate spasticity in the biceps and finger flexors. Voluntary movement is evident in elbow flexors and shoulder abductors only (through $1/2$ range). What is the **BEST** choice for initial exercise?

Choices:

1. Functional activities emphasizing ADL using the less-affected upper extremity.
2. Facilitation of early movements in the flexor synergy pattern.
3. Weight-bearing on an extended RUE with wrist and fingers extended.
4. Prolonged positioning of the RUE in a hemisling.

Teaching Points

Correct Answer: 3

Early intervention should focus on stretching and positioning the RUE into extension with the wrist and fingers extended. This helps decrease the developing flexor spasticity. Weight-bearing on the limb promotes extensor activity in the triceps and shoulder stabilizers.

Incorrect Choices:

Obligatory synergistic patterns are never encouraged. Prolonged positioning is contraindicated because the patient may stiffen up with excess tone. Activities that utilize only the less-affected side are discouraged (compensatory training). Prolonged use of a sling can promote contractures.

Type of Reasoning: Inferential

Effective intervention guidelines after stroke are based on the stage of recovery and presenting symptoms. This requires one to make assumptions based on facts, which is an inferential reasoning skill. If this question was answered incorrectly, review information on techniques and guidelines of stroke rehabilitation.

B111 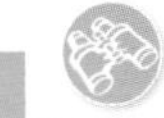

Nonsystem | Equipment, Devices

A physical therapist and a physician are at odds regarding ordering a power wheelchair for a 3-year-old child. What factor precludes the use of a power wheelchair for this child?

Choices:

1. Age of the child.
2. Quadriplegic cerebral palsy.
3. Child is nonverbal.
4. Poor head and fine motor control.

Teaching Points

Correct Answer: 4

Most power wheelchairs require good head control to use a head rest control system or good fine motor skills to use a joy stick. Although there are other ways to propel a power chair, this is the best reason to NOT recommend a power chair.

Incorrect Choices:

Studies have found that children as young as 18 months of age can operate a power wheelchair, so age is not a factor here. Most children with power wheelchairs have quadriplegia and don't have a good prognosis for community ambulation. Without knowing any more about their abilities, it cannot be said that quadriplegia is a reason not to use a power chair. A child being nonverbal does not preclude them from using a power wheelchair. Just because a child is nonverbal does not mean that they cannot understand what is spoken to them or that they are cognitively impaired. Even if cognitive impairments were a factor, children with mild cognitive impairments can operate power mobility devices.

Type of Reasoning: Inductive

For this question, the test-taker must determine the most important factor for not recommending a power wheelchair. This requires inductive reasoning skill where clinical judgment is paramount to arriving at a correct conclusion. In this case, poor head and fine motor control is the most important factor in not recommending a power wheelchair. Review power wheelchair prescription guidelines if answered incorrectly.

B112 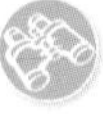

Neuromuscular | Interventions

An ambulatory patient recovering from a left CVA is wearing a plastic AFO to stabilize the right foot. During gait analysis, the therapist observes lateral trunk bending toward the right as the patient bears weight on the right leg at midstance. What is the **BEST** intervention to correct this problem?

Choices:

1. Strengthen hip flexors on the right side.
2. Provide a lift on the shoe of the involved leg.
3. Strengthen the hip abductors on the right side.
4. Strengthen hamstrings on the right side.

Teaching Points

Correct Answer: 3

The lateral trunk bending (Trendelenburg gait) is the result of weak hip abductors on the right (a common problem for patients recovering from stroke). Strengthening of the abductors on the involved right side is indicated.

Incorrect Choices:

The other choices do not address the problem of lateral trunk bending. Weakness of the hip flexors or hamstrings would present as swing phase deficits (inability to shorten the leg so it can clear the floor). The patient is likely to compensate with circumduction. A lift on the left foot might be considered for patients with this problem but is not the intervention of choice.

Type of Reasoning: Inductive

This question requires one to utilize clinical judgment to determine the best choice to correct the Trendelenburg gait. Questions that encourage diagnostic thinking and clinical judgment utilize inductive reasoning skill. In this situation, the patient's gait pattern indicates weak hip abductors. If this question was answered incorrectly, review information on intervention approaches for Trendelenburg gait.

B113 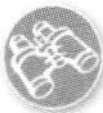

Musculoskeletal | Interventions

An adolescent basketball player complains of pain in the tibial tubercle region with running and jumping. The patient was referred to physical therapy with a diagnosis of Osgood-Schlatter disease. What is the **BEST** therapeutic intervention choice for this patient?

Choices:

1. Strengthening of the quadriceps femoris muscle.
2. Stretching of the quadriceps femoris muscle.
3. Grade IV mobilizations directed at the tibiofemoral joint.
4. Transcutaneous electrical stimulation (TENS) bracketing the patellar tendon.

Teaching Points

Correct Answer: 2

Osgood-Schlatter disease is a painful condition resulting from inflammation of the tibial tubercle at the insertion of the patellar tendon. The disorder is typically seen in adolescent athletes during periods of rapid growth. Physical therapy interventions should include flexibility exercises and activity modification to prevent excessive stress to the inflamed site. Medications such as acetaminophen and NSAIDs may also be helpful.

Incorrect Choices:

Repetitive stresses to inflamed musculoskeletal tissues should be avoided. This includes quadriceps strengthening exercises. Graded mobilizations of the knee may be helpful if the therapist identifies joint mobility dysfunctions, but it is not the best intervention for this condition. Transcutaneous electrical stimulation will provide short-term symptomatic relief only.

Type of Reasoning: Inductive

For this question, the test-taker must utilize knowledge of Osgood-Schlatter disease and effective intervention approaches to arrive at a sound conclusion. This requires inductive reasoning skill. For this situation, the BEST therapeutic intervention for this patient is stretching of the quadriceps muscle. Review intervention approaches for Osgood-Schlatter disease if answered incorrectly.

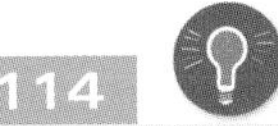

Integumentary | Interventions

A patient presents with a decubitus ulcer of 3 months' duration on the lateral ankle. The ankle is swollen, red, and painful, with a moderate to high amount of wound drainage (exudate). What is the **BEST** choice of dressing for this wound?

Choices:

1. Hydrogel dressings.
2. Semipermeable film dressings.
3. Calcium alginate dressings.
4. Gauze dressings.

Teaching Points

Correct Answer: 3

Wounds with moderate to high exudate benefit from calcium alginate dressings. The dressings absorb large amounts of exudate (up to 20 times their weight) and form a gel, which maintains the moist wound environment while maintaining good permeability to oxygen.

Incorrect Choices:

Gauze and semipermeable film dressings require a secondary dressing and offer poor conformability to deep wounds. Hydrogel dressings are not recommended for wounds with heavy exudate.

Type of Reasoning: Inferential

One must infer or draw conclusions based on the information presented in the patient's case, which draws upon inferential reasoning skill. In this situation, calcium alginate dressings are ideal for wounds with moderate to high exudate present. If this question was answered incorrectly, refer to information on wound dressings.

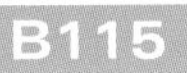

Musculoskeletal | Examination

A patient was diagnosed with a bulging disc at the right L5–S1 spinal level without nerve root compression. What is the impairment **MOST** likely to be documented?

Choices:

1. Centralized gnawing pain with loss of postural control during lifting activities.
2. Centralized gnawing pain with uncompensated gluteus medius gait.
3. Radicular pain to the right great toe with a compensated gluteus medius gait.
4. Radicular pain to the right great toe with difficulty sitting for long periods.

Teaching Points

Correct Answer: 1

Discal degeneration without nerve root compression would likely be exhibited as a centralized gnawing pain with loss of proprioception.

Incorrect Choices:

Because there is no nerve compression, there will not be any type of radicular pain and/or decrease in specific muscle function (beyond the lumbar spine region), so one should not see a decrease in the function of the gluteus medius.

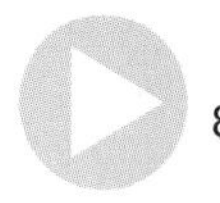

Type of Reasoning: Inferential

This question provides the diagnosis, and the test-taker must determine the most likely symptoms to be present. This type of question in which symptoms must be determined from a diagnosis draws upon inferential reasoning skill. To arrive at the correct answer, the test-taker must have a good understanding of the nature of L5–S1 discal degeneration.

B116

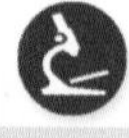

Neuromuscular | Interventions

A patient recovering from traumatic brain injury (TBI) demonstrates impaired cognitive function (Rancho Cognitive Level VII). What is the **BEST** training strategy for this patient?

Choices:

1. Provide assistance as needed using guided movements during training.
2. Provide a high degree of environmental structure to ensure correct performance.
3. Involve the patient in decision-making and monitor for safety.
4. Provide maximum supervision as needed to ensure successful performance and safety.

Teaching Points

Correct Answer: 3

As patients with TBI recover, structure and guidance must be gradually reduced and patient involvement in decision-making increased. Safety must be maintained while increasing levels of independence are fostered. Patients at stage VII exhibit purposeful and appropriate responses in familiar settings, and moving to level VIII requires patient opportunities to take part in decision-making in a structured and safe environment.

Incorrect Choices:

A high degree of structure, assistance, and maximum supervision is not therapeutic at this stage of recovery.

Type of Reasoning: Deductive

Although this question does require one to utilize clinical judgment, the majority of skill required to answer this question correctly relies upon the recall of the Rancho Cognitive Function Levels (see Table 3-17) and the guidelines for treatment provided within these levels. This is factual information and recall, which ultimately requires deductive reasoning ability to successfully choose the best type of training for the patient. If this question was answered incorrectly, refer to the Rancho Cognitive Function Levels.

B117

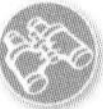

Neuromuscular | Interventions

What is the **MOST** appropriate intervention to correct for the problem of a forward festinating gait in a patient with Parkinson's disease?

Choices:

1. Use of a heel wedge.
2. Use of a toe wedge.
3. Increase stride length using floor markers.
4. Increase cadence using a metronome.

Teaching Points

Correct Answer: 2

A festinating gait is an abnormal and involuntary increase in the speed of walking in an attempt to catch up with a displaced center of gravity due to the patient's forward lean. The most appropriate intervention would be to use a toe wedge, which would help to displace the patient's center of gravity backward.

Incorrect Choices:

Increasing cadence or stride length would serve only to increase, not decrease, the problem, as will the use of a heel wedge.

Type of Reasoning: Inductive

One must use clinical judgment to determine which approach would best decrease a forward festinating gait pattern in PD. The test-taker must understand that forward festination results from forward displacement of center of gravity, which can be improved through the use of a toe wedge to displace the patient's gravity backward. The judgment in this case, utilizing one's knowledge of festinating gait pattern and the intervention approaches proposed, encourages use of inductive reasoning skill.

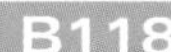

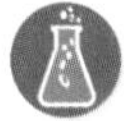

Musculoskeletal | Interventions

A patient presents with difficulty with fast movement speeds and fatigues easily. The therapist decides on a strength training program that specifically focuses on improving fast-twitch muscle fiber function. What is the optimal exercise prescription to achieve this goal?

Choices:

1. High-intensity workloads for short durations.
2. Low-intensity workloads for long durations.
3. Low-intensity workloads for short durations.
4. High-intensity workloads for long durations.

Teaching Points

Correct Answer: 1

High-intensity exercises at fast contraction speeds for shorter durations (<20 repetitions) are needed to train the highly adaptable fast-twitch IIa fibers.

Incorrect Choices:

Performing workloads at low intensity and slow contraction speeds will challenge slow-twitch (type I) fibers. High-intensity workloads at long durations are contraindicated.

Type of Reasoning: Analytical

This question requires one to refer to knowledge of exercise physiology to recall the optimal method of improving fast-twitch fiber function. In order to arrive at the correct solution, one must analyze the information presented and determine its meaning, which is an analytical reasoning skill. If this question was answered incorrectly, refer to information on exercise physiology and fast-twitch fiber exercise.

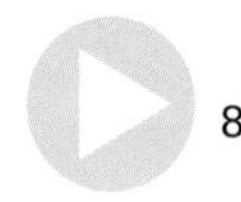

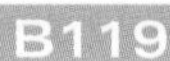

B119

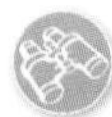

Musculoskeletal | Evaluation, Diagnosis

A college cross-country runner is referred to physical therapy with anterolateral leg pain. The patient reports that the pain has progressively worsened since an increase in the training regimen over the past 2 weeks. Symptoms appear at the later stages of runs and persist for 2–3 hours after completion of a run. The patient denies any lower extremity paresthesias. The tibialis anterior muscle is tender and taut on palpation. Resisted dorsiflexion is strong but reproduces the patient's pain. What is the **MOST LIKELY** diagnosis?

Choices:

1. Medial tibial stress syndrome.
2. Acute compartment syndrome.
3. Chronic exertional compartment syndrome.
4. Stress fracture.

Teaching Points

Correct Answer: 3

Chronic exertional compartment syndrome is the result of transiently elevated anterior compartment pressure that restricts blood flow to muscles. Patients are tender in the anterolateral leg region with tautness of the anterior compartment. A rearfoot strike running pattern may be associated with chronic exertional compartment syndrome due to increased muscle activity of the tibialis anterior. Treatment may require a change in footwear, training surface, or run-retraining.

Incorrect Choices:

Acute compartment syndrome typically results from trauma, and patients present with similar but more severe symptoms. Patients frequently demonstrate numbness and tingling in the deep fibular nerve distribution. Medial tibial stress syndrome and stress fractures of the tibia/fibula are also chronic overuse injuries, but there is bony tenderness associated with both of these conditions. The distal posteromedial tibia is tender in patients with medial tibial stress syndrome.

Type of Reasoning: Analytical

This question provides symptoms, and the test-taker must analyze them in order to determine the most likely diagnosis. This requires analytical reasoning skill. For this situation, the symptoms are consistent with chronic exertional compartment syndrome. Review symptoms of chronic exertional compartment syndrome if answered incorrectly.

B120

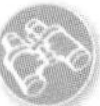

Neuromuscular | Evaluation, Diagnosis

What is the **MOST** appropriate functional goal for a 5-year-old child with a lower thoracic lesion (myelomeningocele, T11 level) and minimal cognitive involvement?

Choices:

1. Household ambulation with KAFOs and walker.
2. Community ambulation with a reciprocating gait orthosis (RGO) and Loftstrand crutches.
3. Household ambulation with an RGO and walker.
4. Community ambulation with HKAFOs and Lofstrand crutches.

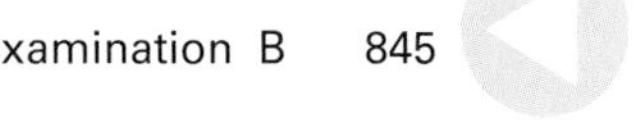

Teaching Points

Correct Answer: 3

A child with a high-level myelomeningocele will be able to ambulate for limited (household) distances with an RGO and walker. Physiological benefits include improved cardiovascular and musculoskeletal functions.

Incorrect Choices:

The child will not be able to be a community ambulator because of the high-energy expenditure necessary with this level of lesion. An RGO is the best choice. The hips are joined by metal cables that prevent inadvertent hip flexion (possible using KAFOs) during a reciprocal two- or four-point gait.

Type of Reasoning: Inductive

This question requires the test-taker to assess the value of each of the orthoses and assistive devices presented and then apply their value to the patient's specific diagnosis. This requires one to utilize clinical judgment, in which the test-taker uses diagnostic reasoning to determine which solution will be most beneficial for the patient. In this case, an RGO and walker are most beneficial for household ambulation. See Table 9-8 for additional information.

B121 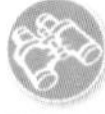

Musculoskeletal | Examination

A physical therapist examines a patient with a primary complaint of chronic neck pain and headaches. Based on the results of the cervical flexion rotation test, the physical therapist determines that the patient has normal upper cervical spine rotation. Which value is consistent with normal upper cervical spine mobility?

Choices:

1. 25 degrees.
2. 45 degrees.
3. 65 degrees.
4. 85 degrees.

Teaching Points

Correct Answer: 2

Normal rotation range of motion at the atlantoaxial (A-A) joint is 35°–45° or approximately 50% of total cervical spine rotation (70°–90° to each side). The cervical flexion rotation test is used to determine the amount of motion available at the A-A joint. Additionally, the test can be used to reproduce symptoms consistent with A-A joint dysfunction or cervicogenic headaches.

Incorrect Choices:

Twenty-five degrees of motion is considered limited atlantoaxial rotation. The other answer choices reflect values that would fall within the normal range of *total* cervical spine rotation.

Type of Reasoning: Deductive

For this question, the test-taker must recall normal upper cervical spine mobility in order to arrive at a correct conclusion. This necessitates the recall of factual information, which is a deductive reasoning skill. For this case, normal upper cervical spine mobility is 45°. If answered incorrectly, review cervical range of motion guidelines.

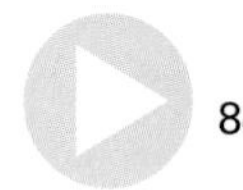

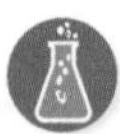

B122

Cardiovascular/Pulmonary | Examination

The therapist is reading a recent report of arterial blood gas analysis with the following values:
Fraction of inspired oxygen (FiO_2) = 0.21
Arterial oxygen pressure (PaO_2) = 53 mmHg
Arterial carbon dioxide pressure ($PaCO_2$) = 30 mmHg
pH = 7.48
Bicarbonate ion = 24 mEq/L
What patient state do these findings indicate?

Choices:

1. Metabolic alkalosis.
2. Respiratory alkalosis.
3. Metabolic acidosis.
4. Respiratory acidosis.

Teaching Points

Correct Answer: 2

This arterial blood gas shows an increased pH, which is an alkalosis. When looking at arterial blood gas values, carbon dioxide can be viewed essentially as an acid. If the carbon dioxide level is low, then you have less acid, or a resulting alkalosis. This is, therefore, a respiratory alkalosis.

Incorrect Choices:

Because the blood pH is higher than normal (7.35–7.45), the condition is an alkalosis, not an acidosis. If the increased pH was due to a metabolic disorder, a high bicarbonate value would be anticipated. As the HCO_3 is normal (24 mEq/dL), the alkalosis is not from a metabolic cause.

Type of Reasoning: Analytical

One must make sense of the information presented in this question and recall the normal laboratory values. This requires analytical reasoning skill, in which one must make an interpretation of information. It is most beneficial to understand the values that indicate respiratory alkalosis to arrive at the correct conclusion. If this question was answered incorrectly, refer to information on arterial blood gas analysis.

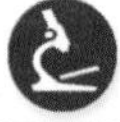

B123

Metabolic/Endocrine | Evaluation, Diagnosis

A patient with cancer has been taking oral corticosteroids along with chemotherapy for the past year. What is an expected adverse effect of prolonged use of corticosteroids?

1. Low blood pressure.
2. Osteoporosis.
3. Thickening of skin.
4. Flattening of the thoracic spine.

Teaching Points

Correct Choice: 2

Steroid medications have major effects on the metabolism of calcium, Vitamin D, and bone. Prolonged corticosteroid use has been associated with bone loss, osteoporosis, and fracture commonly occurring in the spine and ribs.

Incorrect Choices:

Corticosteroids can cause high blood pressure, not low blood pressure. Thinning and easy bruising of the skin can result, not thickening. Rounding of the thoracic spine ("dowagers hump") may result, not flattening.

Type of Reasoning: Deductive

For this question, one must recall the adverse effects of prolonged corticosteroid use in order to arrive at a correct conclusion. This requires deductive reasoning skill, where factual information is used to draw a correct conclusion. For this situation, one should expect osteoporosis to be a potential adverse effect. Review effects of corticosteroid use if answered incorrectly.

B124 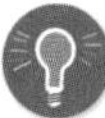

Neuromuscular | Evaluation, Diagnosis

An older adult with a history of Diffuse Lewy Body Disease (DLBD) is referred to physical therapy secondary to a recent fall. On examination the patient exhibits mild bradykinesia and rigidity in the left lower extremity. What additional clinical findings is the patient **MOST LIKELY** to demonstrate?

Choices:

1. Diminished executive function and cognition.
2. Resting tremor and joint pain.
3. Dysphagia and incontinence.
4. Festinating gait and autonomic dysfunction.

Teaching Points

Correct Answer: 1

Diffuse Lewy Body Disease (DLBD) is a one of the most prevalent causes of major neurocognitive disorders. The presenting feature of DLBD is dementia, or the inability to plan, sequence, and organize thoughts and decisions. Dementia can also result in changes in mood or behavior (see Table 10-3 for the differences in the most common types of neurocognitive disorders).

Incorrect Choices:

Extrapyramidal motor findings (e.g., bradykinesia, rigidity, resting tremor), festinating gait, and autonomic dysfunction can occur with DLBD, but most often manifest after impairments in executive function and cognition. This is a key differential from Parkinson's disease (PD), where patients start with motor dysfunction and may or may not exhibit cognitive dysfunction in the later stages. Patients with DLBD and PD may have pain, but the pain is typically in the later stages of the disease and not limited to the joints (may also have muscular pain from rigidity and inactivity). Finally, dysphagia and incontinence are most closely associated with end-stage Alzheimer's or Parkinson's disease.

Type of Reasoning: Inferential

One must infer or draw conclusions on what is likely to be true for a patient with DLBD. This requires inferential reasoning skill. For this scenario, the patient is most likely to demonstrate diminished executive function and cognition, in addition to the present findings. If answered incorrectly, review DLBD and clinical findings.

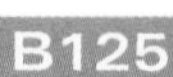

B125

Neuromuscular | Interventions

A patient with a spinal cord injury is having difficulty learning how to transfer from mat to wheelchair. The patient just cannot seem to get the idea of how to coordinate this movement. In this case, what is the **MOST** effective use of feedback during early motor learning?

Choices:

1. Focus on knowledge of performance and proprioceptive inputs.
2. Focus on guided movement and proprioceptive inputs.
3. Provide feedback only after a brief (5-sec) delay.
4. Focus on knowledge of results and visual inputs.

Teaching Points

Correct Answer: 4

During the early stage of motor learning (cognitive stage), learners benefit from seeing the whole task correctly performed. Dependence on visual inputs is high. Developing a reference of correctness (knowledge of results) is critical to ensure early skill acquisition (cognitive mapping).

Incorrect Choices:

Focus on proprioceptive inputs is important during the middle (associative) stage of motor learning. Delayed feedback may be used during later learning.

Type of Reasoning: Inferential

One must infer information presented in this question, specifically, which approach is most effective during early motor learning. Visual inputs are key during early motor learning with a focus on knowledge of results. To answer this question successfully, one must recall effective teaching principles applied to early learning situations.

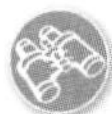

B126

Musculoskeletal | Interventions

A retired administrative assistant with a history of chronic neck pain secondary to whiplash associated disorder (WAD) is referred to physical therapy. The patient denies experiencing any radiating pain to the upper extremities and is neurologically intact on examination. Which intervention should be emphasized in the physical therapy plan of care?

Choices:

1. Wearing a cervical collar.
2. Thoracic manipulation.
3. C1–2 self-sustained natural apophyseal glide (SNAG).
4. Submaximal deep neck flexor endurance training.

Teaching Points

Correct Answer: 4

According to the Neck Pain Clinical Practice Guidelines (Box 2-15), interventions for chronic neck pain secondary to whiplash associated disorder should emphasize submaximal exercise programming (endurance, strengthening, and coordination). In addition, therapists should consider patient education, mobilization, and the use of transcutaneous electrical nerve stimulation as part of a multifaceted treatment approach.

Incorrect Choices:

Wearing a cervical collar is not recommended for chronic neck pain due to WAD, and its use should be minimized during the acute stage. Thoracic manipulation may be part of a comprehensive and multimodal treatment approach in patients with chronic neck pain due to WAD, but it is best utilized in patients experiencing neck pain with mobility deficits. C1–2 SNAGs are recommended for those with acute or subacute neck pain and headache of cervicogenic origin. See Box 2-15 for the different categories of neck pain and their recommended interventions.

Type of Reasoning: Inductive

For this question, the test-taker must recall intervention approaches for whiplash associated disorder (WAD) in order to draw a correct conclusion. This necessitates inductive reasoning skill, where clinical guidelines help one to make sound decisions for intervention. For this situation, the plan of care should emphasize submaximal deep neck flexor endurance training. Review neck pain and intervention recommendations if answered incorrectly.

B127 

Lymphatic | Evaluation, Diagnosis

A physical therapist examines a patient who sustained a wrist sprain while falling on their outstretched hand. During the examination, the therapist notes that the patient's wrist is red and swollen and there is an abrasion at the base of the patient's palm. Red streaks radiate from the abrasion site toward the elbow. Which diagnosis is most consistent with these examination findings?

Choices:

1. Contact dermatitis.
2. Acute lymphadenitis.
3. Cellulitis.
4. Lymphangitis.

Teaching Points

Correct Answer: 4

Lymphangitis is an acute inflammation of subcutaneous lymphatic vessels, typically resulting from some type of bacterial infection. The involvement of the lymphatic system is often first noted as characteristic red streaks under the skin that radiate from the infection site in a proximal direction toward regional lymph nodes (in this case toward the cubital lymph nodes of the elbow). Systemic manifestations may include fever, chills, and malaise. A medical consultation should immediately be made for this patient.

Incorrect Choices:

Contact dermatitis is an inflammation of the skin caused by direct contact with some type of irritant or allergy-causing substance. Well-defined patches of redness occur where the irritant contacted the skin. In acute lymphadenitis, lymph nodes become enlarged, swollen, and reddened due to an infection. Cellulitis is a non-necrotizing infection of the dermis and hypodermis. Patients typically complain of pain, swelling and erythema at the wound site and may also experience a fever and chills. Cellulitis that spreads to local lymphatic channels will result in lymphangitis, with the hallmark presentation of red streaks radiating from the infection site. The patient described in this question may have first developed cellulitis that eventually resulted in lymphangitis.

Type of Reasoning: Analytical

This question requires one to analyze the patient's presenting symptoms and determine the most likely diagnosis. This requires analytical reasoning skill. For this scenario, the symptoms are consistent with lymphangitis. If answered incorrectly, review information on lymphangitis.

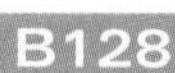

B128

System Interactions | Interventions

A physical therapist is developing a treatment plan for a patient with dementia. Which consideration is most important for the therapist when planning an exercise regimen for this patient?

Choices:

1. Age-related comorbidities are common in patients with dementia.
2. Exercise is better tolerated during late afternoon sessions.
3. PT sessions scheduled at different times each day provide variety and improve patient compliance.
4. Exercises should focus on upper extremity strength and dexterity.

Teaching Points

Correct Answer: 1

Because most patients with dementia are often elderly, comorbidities such as osteoarthritis, cardiovascular disease, and other inactivity-related conditions are common and should be taken into consideration. The primary focus of the physical therapist regimen should be low-intensity exercise that is enjoyable and easily accomplished. Simple exercises that are familiar and repetitious (e.g., walking, stationary cycling, and basic strengthening) are more likely to attract participation than more complex programs.

Incorrect Choices:

Morning sessions work best for the patient with dementia. Fading light during the late afternoon or evening hours can trigger "sundowning," a state of confusion, anxiety, aggression, and noncompliance that is often seen in patients with dementia. Time changes are incorrect because predictable schedules for activities and meals work best for patients with dementia. While this patient population benefits from strengthening of all muscle groups, exercises should target leg strength and balance. Patients with dementia have an increased risk for falls and lower extremity fractures, and the exercise program should focus on maintaining or improving safe, independent mobility.

Type of Reasoning: Inferential

For this question, the test-taker must determine which consideration is most important when planning exercise for a patient with dementia. This necessitates the test-taker to determine what is likely to be true of a situation, which is an inferential reasoning skill. For this case, age-related comorbidities are common in patients with dementia and are most important to consider. Review information on dementia and exercise guidelines if answered incorrectly.

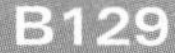
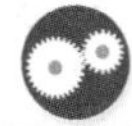

B129

Nonsystem | Professional Responsibilities

A patient is referred by an orthopedist with a diagnosis of impingement syndrome of the shoulder. The initial PT examination reveals signs and symptoms that are not consistent with this diagnosis and are more consistent with thoracic spine pain and dysfunction. The therapist treats the patient consistent with PT findings without communicating with the referring physician. Months later, the therapist is sued by the patient's estate. The patient died of undiagnosed metastatic lung cancer. The therapist is:

Choices:

1. Not responsible for diagnosing metastatic cancer, and therefore cannot be held responsible for the patient's death.
2. Responsible for communicating PT examination results to the referring physician.
3. Not responsible for the incorrect diagnosis because treatment was appropriate for the PT findings.
4. Responsible for making the diagnosis of possible cancer consistent with the PT examination of the patient.

Teaching Points

Correct Answer: 2

When a referral relationship exists with another health-care professional, it is the PT's responsibility to communicate with the referring practitioner regarding the physical therapy examination, treatment plan, and management of the referred patient. This is particularly crucial when the findings are inconsistent with the referrer's diagnosis.

Incorrect Choices:

The therapist cannot diagnose metastatic cancer but can be held responsible for not communicating with the primary physician.

Type of Reasoning: Evaluative

This question encourages one to review the actions of the therapist, determine the value of those actions, and then decide whether they were appropriate, which necessitates evaluative reasoning. In this scenario, the therapist should have communicated the findings to the physician for follow-up, especially when they are inconsistent with the physician's findings. Questions that require value judgments are challenging because they move beyond factual knowledge to promote judgment, prudence, and ethical principles.

B130 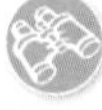

Neuromuscular | Examination

A 2-year-old child has been referred to physical therapy for an assessment due to concerns regarding delayed development of gross motor skills. Which of the following would be the **MOST** appropriate developmental tool to use?

Choices:

1. Test of Infant Motor Performance (TIMP).
2. Bruinicks-Oseretsky Test of Motor Performance (BOT-2).
3. Peabody Developmental Motor Scales (PDMS-2).
4. Alberta Infant Motor Scales (AIMS).

Teaching Points

Correct Answer: 3

The PDMS-2 is a standardized tool to assess gross motor and/or fine motor development. It is appropriate for children 0–72 months of age.

Incorrect Choices:

The TIMP is used for premature infants from 32 weeks gestation age to 3½ months post-term. The BOT-2 tests gross and/or fine motor development of children 4 years of age, up until 21 years of age. The AIMS is an observational scale for screening gross motor milestones in infants from birth to typically 12 months of age, or until independent walking. Since this child is 2 years old, the only appropriate tool is the PDMS-2.

Type of Reasoning: Inductive

For this question, the test-taker must recall each of the developmental tools provided and then determine which tool will best assess gross motor skills for a 2-year-old child. This necessitates inductive reasoning skill, where clinical judgment is paramount to arriving at a correct conclusion. For this case, the physical therapist should choose the Peabody Developmental Motor Scales (PDMS-2). If answered incorrectly review gross motor assessments, especially the PDMS-2.

B131 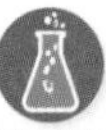

Neuromuscular | Examination

A patient is being examined for impairments after stroke. The patient is unable to detect a monofilament on the right hand and fingers. Which of the following areas of the central nervous system are impaired?

Choices:

1. Spinotectal tract and somatosensory cortex.
2. Lateral spinothalamic tract and somatosensory cortex.
3. Dorsal column/lemniscal pathways and somatosensory cortex.
4. Anterior spinothalamic tract and thalamus.

Teaching Points

Correct Answer: 3

Discriminative touch, proprioceptive sensibility, and vibration sense are carried in the posterior white columns (fasciculus cuneatus for the upper extremity and fasciculus gracilis for the lower extremity). The long ascending tracts cross the medulla (sensory decussation) and form the medial lemniscus, which then travels to the thalamus (ventral posterolateral nucleus) and finally to the cortex (postcentral gyrus/primary somatosensory cortex). Loss of discriminative touch conducted with a monofilament could result from an insult affecting any of these component parts. Parietal lobe or internal capsule lesions are the most common sites.

Incorrect Choices:

The anterolateral system pathways (spinothalamic tracts) convey pain and temperature. The spinotectal tract conveys information for spinovisual reflexes.

Type of Reasoning: Analytical

To answer this question, one must refer to knowledge of applied neuroanatomy, specifically spinal pathways that process discriminative touch of the upper extremity. This requires analysis of the information presented, utilizing analytical reasoning skill to arrive at the conclusion that the dorsal column/lemniscal pathways and somatosensory cortex are impaired. If this question was answered incorrectly, refer to Figure 3-5 (somatotopic organization of the spinal cord), Table 3-3 (sensory examination), and Table 3-14 (signs and symptoms associated with cortical lesions).

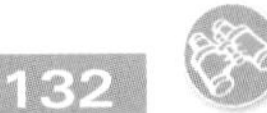

B132

Cardiovascular/Pulmonary | Evaluation, Diagnosis

An elderly patient has a history of two myocardial infarctions (MIs) and one episode of recent congestive heart failure (CHF). The patient also has claudication pain in the right calf during an exercise tolerance test. Which of the following is the **BEST** initial exercise prescription for this patient?

Choices:

1. Daily walking, using interval training for 10- to 15-minute periods.
2. Walking five times a week using continuous training for 60 minutes.
3. Walking three times a week using continuous training for 40-minute sessions.
4. Walking three times a week using interval training for 30-minute periods.

Teaching Points

Correct Answer: 1

An appropriate initial exercise prescription for a patient with a history of CHF and claudication pain in the right calf should include low-intensity exercise (walking), low to moderate duration (10–15 min), and higher frequencies (daily). The exercise session should carefully balance activity with rest (interval or discontinuous training).

Incorrect Choices:

All other choices include durations that are too long (60, 40, or 30 min) and do not provide adequate rest periods.

Type of Reasoning: Inductive

One must utilize clinical judgment and diagnostic thinking (an inductive reasoning skill) to choose the best initial exercise prescription for this patient. This requires knowledge of CHF and claudication pain in order to arrive at the best solution. In this case, it is best to balance rest with activity because of the nature of CHF and limited tolerance to exercise.

B133

Musculoskeletal | Examination

A patient presents with signs and symptoms consistent with sacroiliac dysfunction. What cluster of special tests/findings provides the highest diagnostic accuracy for sacroiliac dysfunction?

Choices:

1. Thigh thrust test, Gillet's test, stork test, and Patrick's test.
2. Anterior superior iliac spine asymmetry, posterior iliac spine asymmetry, pubic symphysis pain with palpation, and sacral inferior lateral angle asymmetry.
3. Fortin finger test, torsion test, supine-to-sit test, and Gaenslen's test.
4. SI gapping, sacroiliac compression, thigh thrust test (P4), sacral thrust, and Gaenslen's test.

Teaching Points

Correct Answer: 4

It was found that if these 5 tests were clustered together as a group and at least 3/5 had a positive finding, they were found to have a high diagnostic accuracy (see Table 2-21).

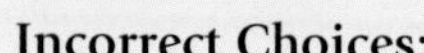

Incorrect Choices:

There have been no outcome studies that support the grouping/clustering for any of these other choices as diagnostic for sacroiliac dysfunction.

Type of Reasoning: Inferential

One must infer or draw a reasonable conclusion about the tests that are likely to have the highest diagnostic accuracy. This requires one to determine what is most likely to be true of a situation, which is an inferential reasoning skill. For this case, SI gapping, sacroiliac compression, thigh thrust test (P4), sacral thrust, and Gaenslen's test have the highest diagnostic accuracy. If answered incorrectly, review SI testing guidelines.

B134 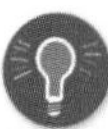

Musculoskeletal I Interventions

A patient demonstrates postpartum sacral pain. The patient complains that pain is increased with prolonged walking, ascending or descending stairs, and rising from sit-to-stand. Which intervention would be the **MOST** beneficial for this patient?

Choices:

1. Manual therapy techniques of the SI joint to provide relief of symptoms and therapeutic exercise to restore normal function of the pelvic girdle.
2. Performing mobilization followed by cryotherapy to restore normal motion to the SI joint.
3. Cryotherapy and TENS to promote normal healing.
4. Increase non-weight-bearing time and use a lumbosacral corset while walking.

Teaching Points

Correct Answer: 1

Ligamentous laxity and pain during pregnancy secondary to hormonal influences (relaxin) most commonly affect the SI joint. This ligamentous laxity continues to occur for up to 3 months after pregnancy and leaves the pelvic area vulnerable to injury. SI pain is aggravated by prolonged weight-bearing and stairs. Manual therapy techniques are effective for reducing pain, and therapeutic exercise is beneficial to restore normal muscle function.

Incorrect Choices:

Modalities may provide temporary relief of pain but will not promote any significant impact on healing. Promoting non-weight-bearing and use of a lumbosacral orthosis does not allow the patient to return to normal function. Mobilization will further stretch joint structures that are already lax.

Type of Reasoning: Inferential

One must infer the intervention that is most beneficial for a patient with postpartum sacral pain to arrive at the correct conclusion. Questions that encourage one to draw conclusions from evidence utilize inferential reasoning skill. One must understand the nature of postpartum sacral pain from ligamentous laxity and the intervention approach that is most effective in order to arrive at the correct conclusion.

B135 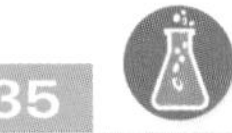

Musculoskeletal | Evaluation, Diagnosis

A patient complains of right shoulder pain since falling onto the right shoulder 3 weeks ago. There was no dislocation and x-rays were negative. AROM is 35° of flexion and abduction with scapular elevation noted. Passive ROM is nearly full with mild pain and muscle guarding at the end of range. Resisted abduction is weak with pain noted in the anterior and lateral deltoid region. There is no atrophy. What is the **MOST** likely diagnosis?

Choices:

1. Rotator cuff tear.
2. Axillary nerve palsy.
3. Supraspinatus tendinitis.
4. Adhesive capsulitis.

Teaching Points

Correct Answer: 1

A rotator cuff tear would be provoked by resisted testing because it is a contractile lesion. The patient would not be able to raise the arm over the head because of lack of force transmission secondary to the tear. Also, the mechanism of injury (trauma) could cause a tear.

Incorrect Choices:

A patient with supraspinatus tendinitis would likely be able to raise the arm overhead with a painful arc of motion or pain at end range. It is also more typically caused by overuse. An adhesive capsulitis would exhibit only a small amount of more passive range than active because the tight capsule is restricting ROM. An axillary nerve palsy is typically caused by a dislocation and would cause marked atrophy of the deltoid.

Type of Reasoning: Analytical

This question provides a group of symptoms and the test-taker must determine the most likely diagnosis. This is an analytical reasoning skill, in which pieces of information are weighed in order to draw conclusions. For this situation, the symptoms are indicative of a rotator cuff tear. Review signs and symptoms of rotator cuff tear if answered incorrectly.

B136 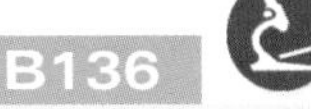

Musculoskeletal | Examination

A patient is referred to physical therapy with subacute neck pain. The therapist suspects neck pain with movement coordination impairments secondary to whiplash-associated disorder (WAD). What is the **MOST** appropriate test to corroborate this diagnosis?

Choices:

1. Spurling's test.
2. Cervical mobility testing.
3. Cervical flexor muscle endurance testing.
4. Cervical flexion-rotation test.

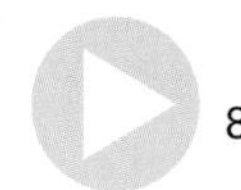

Teaching Points

Correct Answer: 3

The Neck Pain Clinical Practice Guidelines (see Box 2-15) suggest using the cervical deep neck flexor muscle endurance testing as part of a comprehensive physical examination for neck pain patients with movement coordination impairments (including whiplash-associated disorder).

Incorrect Choices:

All of the other listed tests and measures may be included as part of a comprehensive examination of the patient with neck pain. Spurling's test is recommended as a priority for patients with neck pain and radiating upper extremity pain. Cervical mobility testing is recommended as a priority for those who have neck pain with associated headaches. The cervical flexion-rotation test is recommended as a priority for individuals who have neck pain and mobility deficits. See Box 2-15 for the different categories of neck pain and appropriate examination techniques for each type.

Type of Reasoning: Deductive

For this question, the test-taker must recall examination tests for whiplash-associated disorder to arrive at a correct conclusion. This necessitates deductive reasoning skill, where factual recall of information guides conclusions. For this case, the most appropriate examination test is the cervical flexor muscle endurance test. If answered incorrectly, review the Neck Pain Clinical Practice Guidelines.

B137 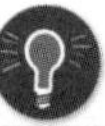

Metabolic/Endocrine | Interventions

An elderly and frail older adult has poor vision. The patient recently returned home from a 2-week hospitalization for stabilization of diabetes. The PT's goal is to mobilize the patient and increase ambulation level and safety. What is the **BEST** intervention strategy for this patient?

Choices:

1. Practice walking in areas of high illumination and low clutter.
2. Color-code stairs with pastel shades of blue and green to highlight steps.
3. Practice walking by having the patient look down at all times.
4. Keep window shades wide open to let in as much light as possible.

Teaching Points

Correct Answer: 1

Effective intervention strategies for the elderly patient with diabetes and low vision include ensuring adequate lighting. Vision and safety decrease dramatically in low lighting. Reducing clutter in the home is also an important strategy to improve safety during ambulation.

Incorrect Choices:

The patient should not continuously look down at the feet, because this poses a safety hazard. This restricts avoidance strategies for environmental objects. Visual acuity decreases dramatically with bright glare from sunlit windows. Color-coded stairs might help if they are well lit and if strong colors, not pastels, are used.

Type of Reasoning: Inferential

This question requires one to recall the guidelines for intervention approaches with people who have low vision. Adequate lighting and low clutter are important to successful and safe navigation in the patient's living spaces. Using the skills of inferential reasoning, the test-taker must draw conclusions from the evidence presented and make assumptions about that information.

B138 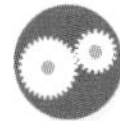

Cardiovascular/Pulmonary I Evaluation, Diagnosis

The patient has a history of angina pectoris and limited physical activity. As the patient participates in the second exercise class, the PT suspects that angina is unstable and may be indicative of a preinfarction state. What signs and symptoms would the therapist use to determine the presence of unstable angina?

Choices:

1. Prolonged cessation of pain following the administration of nitroglycerin for angina.
2. Angina that responds to rest and interval training but not to continuous training.
3. Arrhythmias of increasing frequency, especially atrial arrhythmias.
4. Angina of increasing intensity that is unresponsive to the nitroglycerin or rest.

Teaching Points

Correct Answer: 4

Preinfarction or unstable angina pectoris is unrelieved by rest or nitroglycerin (measures that typically reduce most angina). The pain is described as increasing in intensity. Unstable angina is an absolute contraindication to exercise.

Incorrect Choices:

Angina that decreases with rest and interval training along with nitroglycerin is considered stable. Increasing atrial arrhythmias may be a comorbidity but is not expected with angina.

Type of Reasoning: Evaluative

In this question, the test-taker must evaluate the merits of the statements presented and determine which statements seem most indicative of unstable angina. Relying on knowledge of angina pectoris and the indications for unstable angina, the test-taker uses evaluative reasoning skill to arrive at the correct conclusion. If this question was answered incorrectly, review information on unstable angina.

B139 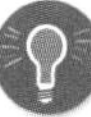

Neuromuscular I Interventions

A patient with a left cerebrovascular accident exhibits right hemiparesis and strong and dominant hemiplegic synergies in the lower extremity. Which activity would be **BEST** to break up these synergies?

Choices:

1. Foot tapping in a sitting position.
2. Supine, PNF D2F with knee flexing and D2E with knee extending.
3. Supine-lying, hip extension with adduction.
4. Bridging, pelvic elevation.

Teaching Points

Correct Answer: 4

The typical lower extremity synergies are effectively broken up using bridging (combines hip extension from the extensor synergy with knee flexion from the flexion synergy).

Incorrect Choices:

Supine hip extension with adduction and foot tapping in the sitting position are in-synergy activities (lower extremity flexion and extension synergies). Supine, lower extremity PNF D2F with knee flexing and D2E with knee extending moves the lower extremity in a pattern closely aligned with the typical flexion and extension synergies.

Type of Reasoning: Inferential

This question requires one to determine what will best help a patient to break up a lower extremity synergy pattern after a stroke. Drawing conclusions based on the information presented, the test-taker utilizes inferential reasoning to make the determination of which approach will benefit the patient. If this question was answered incorrectly, refer to information on abnormal limb synergy patterns (see Table 3-8) and activities, to include PNF patterns, that promote recovery.

B140 

Integumentary | Evaluation, Diagnosis

A physical therapist is examining a patient with several small dermal ulcerations inferior to the medial malleolus. There is moderate exudate, they are covered with 100% necrotic tissue, and the therapist is unable to debride the necrotic tissue secondary to severe pain. The therapist suspects the ulceration is due to vasculitis as a secondary complication of systemic lupus erythematosus. Which of the following is the primary characteristic to differentiate this vasculitis wound from a venous ulceration?

Choices:

1. Exudate.
2. Necrotic tissue.
3. Location.
4. Pain.

Teaching Points

Correct Answer: 4

Vasculitis ulcerations in people with systemic lupus erythematosus are quite painful due to small vessel arterial occlusion. Patients with autoimmune disorders are at greater risk for vasculitis ulcerations, and increased pain is a hallmark finding of arterial ulcers. Unlike arterial ulcers, it is atypical for wounds related to venous insufficiency to be painful.

Incorrect Choices:

Exudate is not specific to a particular wound etiology, although venous insufficiency and lymphatic wounds tend to have more exudate than ischemic vasculitis ulcerations. Necrotic tissue is not unique to venous or arterial ulcers. Venous insufficiency wounds are usually superior to the medial malleolus (not inferior), while ischemic vasculitis ulcerations are most commonly located distally.

Type of Reasoning: Deductive

For this question, one must recall vasculitis wound information characteristics in order to arrive at a correct conclusion. This requires the recall of factual information, which is a deductive reasoning skill. For this situation, pain is a primary characteristic that differentiates a vasculitis wound from a venous ulceration. If answered incorrectly, review characteristics of vasculitis wounds (see Table 7-5, Arterial versus Venous Ulcers).

B141

Neuromuscular | Examination

The therapist is examining a patient recovering from stroke for the expected pattern of spastic hypertonia in the involved upper extremity. What muscles are typically spastic in the hemiplegic upper extremity during early to middle stage of recovery following a stroke?

Choices:

1. Shoulder adductors, forearm pronators, and elbow extensors.
2. Shoulder retractors and abductors and flexors of the elbow, wrist, and hand.
3. Shoulder extensors and flexors of the elbow and hand.
4. Shoulder adductors; forearm pronators; and flexors of the elbow, wrist, and hand.

Teaching Points

Correct Answer: 4

The typical pattern of spasticity in the UE of the patient recovering from stroke is shoulder adductors; forearm pronators; and flexors of the elbow, wrist, and hand (antigravity muscles).

Incorrect Choices:

Spasticity is strong in shoulder adductors, not abductors. Spasticity is strong in elbow flexors, not extensors. Shoulder extensors typically have low tone (the elbow is typically held in flexion, with arm adducted to the side).

Type of Reasoning: Inferential

This question provides a diagnosis and the test-taker must infer the typical pattern of spasticity. This requires one to determine what is likely to be true for a patient with a stroke, which is an inferential reasoning skill. In this situation, the patient is likely to display increased resistance to passive range of motion in the shoulder adductors; forearm pronators; and flexors of the elbow, wrist, and hand. Review information of spasticity patterns after stroke (Table 3-8) if answered incorrectly.

B142 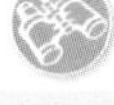

Gastrointestinal | Evaluation, Diagnosis

An elderly patient has been hospitalized for 3 weeks after a surgical resection of carcinoma of the colon. The patient is very weak and is currently receiving physical therapy to improve functional ambulation. During the initial sessions, the patient complains of pain in the left shoulder at night and when bearing weight on the upper extremity when he is using his walker. What action should the therapist take?

Choices:

1. Ambulate the patient in the parallel bars considering age and diagnosis.
2. Apply pulsed US to decrease pain.
3. Notify the physician immediately.
4. Apply heat in the form of a hot pack before ambulation.

Teaching Points

Correct Answer: 3

The risk of metastatic disease is present; the therapist should notify the physician immediately.

Incorrect Choices:

Monitoring or modifying the plan of care to reduce pain should be considered only after consultation with the physician. If metastatic disease is present, the US would be contraindicated. Ambulating in the parallel bars exerts the same weight-bearing forces through the upper extremities as does a walker.

Type of Reasoning: Inductive

This question requires one to use clinical judgment and diagnostic thinking to make a determination of the cause for the patient's shoulder pain and then what is the best course of action based on this knowledge. In this situation, based on the patient's medical history, it is important to notify the physician immediately because of the risk of metastatic disease. Questions that require clinical judgment to make a determination of a best course of action utilize inductive reasoning skill.

B143 

Nonsystem I Therapeutic Modalities

A patient sprained the left ankle 4 days ago. The patient complains of pain (4/10), and there is moderate swelling that is getting worse. At this time, which intervention would be **BEST** to use?

Choices:

1. Cold/intermittent compression combination with the limb elevated.
2. Cold whirlpool followed by massage.
3. Contrast baths followed by limb elevation.
4. Intermittent compression followed by elevation.

Teaching Points

Correct Answer: 1

The combination of RICE (rest, ice, compression, elevation) is best. Cold to decrease pain along with intermittent compression and elevation to facilitate fluid drainage provides the best intervention. Rest is required.

Incorrect Choices:

Contrast baths and whirlpool place the ankle in a dependent position, which might tend to increase edema. The interventions of intermittent compression and elevation should be combined, not sequential.

Type of Reasoning: Inferential

In this question, the test-taker must draw conclusions based on the information presented in the patient's case, which utilizes inferential reasoning skill. The patient's symptoms in this case indicate that cold and intermittent compression with limb elevation are best to relieve pain and facilitate fluid drainage. If this question was answered incorrectly, refer to information on intervention for acute ankle sprain.

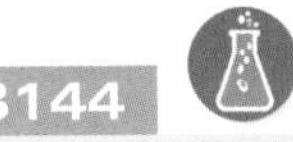

B144

Musculoskeletal | Examination

A physical therapist and colleague are examining a patient who complains of numbness over the lateral aspect of the shoulder. The therapist is convinced that the patient has a C5 radiculopathy, while the colleague believes the patient has an axillary nerve lesion. The results of upper extremity reflex testing are equivocal. Weakness in which muscle would support the therapist's hypothesis of a C5 nerve root problem?

Choices:

1. Teres minor.
2. Biceps brachii.
3. Middle deltoid.
4. Triceps brachii.

Teaching Points

Correct Answer: 2

The dermatome at the lateral shoulder is C5, and the peripheral nerve field is the axillary nerve. Therefore, the sensory loss that the patient is experiencing could be the result of a lesion to either the nerve root or peripheral nerve. The axillary nerve is supplied by the C5 and C6 nerve roots. To prove that the patient has a C5 problem, the therapist must identify weakness in a C5 muscle that is not also innervated by the axillary nerve. The biceps brachii and brachialis are two strong C5 muscles and are easily tested with resisted elbow flexion.

Incorrect Choices:

Weakness found in the teres minor and middle deltoid would support the colleague's argument. Weakness in the triceps brachii would not prove helpful for either therapist in this case as it is innervated by the C6–C8 nerve root levels.

Type of Reasoning: Analytical

For this question, one must analyze the symptoms presented and draw from knowledge of C5 nerve root innervation in order to arrive at a correct conclusion. This requires analytical reasoning skill, where pieces of information are weighed and considered to draw reasonable conclusions. For this scenario, weakness of the biceps brachii would support a C5 nerve root problem. If answered incorrectly, review innervation of the C5 pathway.

B145

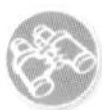

Cardiovascular/Pulmonary | Interventions

A patient with moderate to severe aortic valve stenosis presents to outpatient cardiac rehabilitation for aerobic conditioning. Which intensity of exercise program is **MOST** appropriate for this patient?

Choices:

1. Resistance training at 75% of 1 rep maximum for large muscle groups.
2. Resistance training at 85% of 1 rep maximum for large muscle groups.
3. Interval walking program at 50% of age predicted heart rate maximum.
4. Interval walking program at 80% of age predicted heart rate maximum.

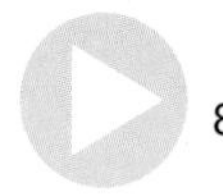

Teaching Points

Correct Answer: 3

For patients with moderate to severe aortic stenosis, low-intensity exercise should be prescribed due to the risk of adverse events with higher intensity activities.

Incorrect Choices:

The intensity of all other activities is too high for a patient with moderate to severe aortic stenosis due to the increased risk of adverse events.

Type of Reasoning: Inductive

This question requires the test-taker to determine a most appropriate course of action based on knowledge of severe aortic valve stenosis. This necessitates clinical judgment, which is an inductive reasoning skill. For this situation, the therapist should choose an interval walking program at 50% of age-predicted heart rate maximum. If answered incorrectly, review exercise guidelines for individuals with aortic stenosis, especially severe conditions.

B146 

Musculoskeletal | Evaluation, Diagnosis

A 67-year-old patient with neck pain is seen by a physical therapist. After examining the patient, the therapist consults with the referring provider and recommends that x-rays should be ordered to rule out a cervical spine fracture. Which of the following examination findings prompted the therapist to recommend x-rays?

Choices:

1. Involvement in a simple rear-end motor vehicle collision in a parking lot.
2. A fall from a 4-foot step ladder.
3. Delayed onset of neck pain.
4. Active neck rotation of 45° to both the left and the right.

Teaching Points

Correct Answer: 2

Based on the Canadian C-spine Rule (see Box 2-17), high risk factors that mandate radiography are the combination of age ≥65 years and a history of a dangerous mechanism of injury, which includes a fall from an elevation of 3 feet or greater or three to five stairs, an axial load to the head (e.g., diving onto the head), a motor vehicle collision at high speed (>100 km/hour), or with rollover or ejection.

Incorrect Choices:

Delayed onset of neck pain and a simple rear end collision are considered low-risk factors that do not mandate the need for radiography. The ability to actively rotate the head 45° to the left and right in the absence of any other positive findings obviates the need for x-rays.

Type of Reasoning: Inferential

For this question, one must determine what is likely to be true, given the information provided. This requires inferential reasoning skill, which uses predictive reasoning to draw sound conclusions. In this case, the therapist's examination findings of a fall from a 4-foot step ladder would most likely prompt a recommendation of x-rays. Review the Canadian C-spine Rule if answered incorrectly.

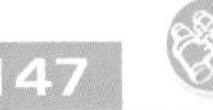

B147

Neuromuscular I Examination

A child with moderate cerebral palsy is being treated. The child is having difficulty learning to sit independently. The child does well with sitting most of the time, but loses balance that typically results in a fall backwards. You are concerned that primitive reflexes have not been integrated. Which of these reflexes or reactions would be the MOST important to be assessed?

Choices:

1. Moro and Startle reflex.
2. Palmar and Landau reaction.
3. Body-on-body righting reaction.
4. Tonic labyrinthine reflex.

Teaching Points

Correct Answer: 1

The Moro reflex would occur if the child looks up quickly, with neck extension, shoulders abducted, and elbows extended. The startle reflex results in the same response, but a result of a loud noise, sudden quick movement in the visual field, or sudden bright light. Both of these could cause the child to fall backward. These primitive reflexes may not be integrated.

Incorrect Choices:

Although the palmar reflex could be slightly problematic in using an open hand to weight bear on UEs while seated, children could adapt to sitting with hands fisted. The Landau reaction is extension of the neck, trunk, and hips when a child is held in a suspended vertical position, so not related to sitting. Body-on-body righting is a reaction that results in rolling with the rotation of the head. The Tonic labyrinthine reflex would result in flexor tone in prone and extensor tone in supine.

Type of Reasoning: Inductive

This question requires one to utilize clinical judgment to determine the most important reflex or reaction to assess based on the presenting challenges of child. This requires inductive reasoning skill, where one must apply clinical knowledge and guidelines to determine a best course of action. For this situation, the therapist should assess the Moro and Startle reflexes. If answered incorrectly, review these primitive reflexes and reactions.

Exam B

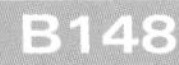

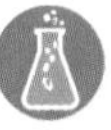

B148

Integumentary I Evaluation, Diagnosis

The image is MOST consistent with which of the following skin conditions?

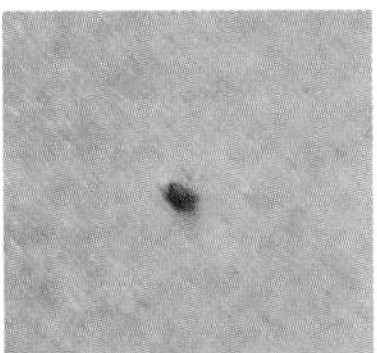

Choices:

1. Mole (cherry angioma).
2. Basal cell cancer.
3. Squamous cell cancer.
4. Melanoma.

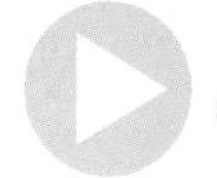

Teaching Points

Correct Answer: 1

The image depicts a mole (cherry angioma), and it is a benign collection of capillaries. They are common and occur in almost half of all adults over 30 years of age.

Incorrect Choices:

Unlike a mole, skin cancer (basal cell, squamous cell, or melanoma) typical has a combination of Asymmetry, irregular Border, multiple Colors, increased Diameter (>6 mm), and/or is Evolving (A, B, C, D, Es of skin examination).

Type of Reasoning: Analytical

For this question, one must analyze the information presented in the picture in order to determine the skin condition present. This requires analytical reasoning skill, which is often utilized when evaluating information in the form of pictures and graphs. For this case, the picture is most consistent with a mole (cherry angioma). Review skin cancer guidelines and information on moles if answered incorrectly.

B149 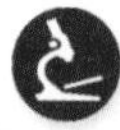

Musculoskeletal I Examination

A physical therapist examines a patient who sustained a deep laceration to the palm of their dominant hand. The wound is near the web space of the hand, and the therapist suspects that the patient lacerated the deep branch of the ulnar nerve. The therapist performs a strength test of the hand intrinsic muscles. Which muscle is innervated by the deep ulnar nerve?

Choices:

1. Adductor pollicis.
2. Abductor pollicis brevis.
3. Opponens pollicis.
4. 1st and 2nd lumbricales.

Teaching Points

Correct Answer: 1

The hand is described as "ulnar nerve dominant" because most of the hand intrinsics are innervated by the ulnar nerve. All other hand intrinsics (four total) are innervated by the median nerve.

Incorrect Choices:

The abductor pollicis brevis and opponens pollicis are innervated by the recurrent branch of the median nerve. The 1st and 2nd lumbricales are innervated by distal branches of the median nerve.

Type of Reasoning: Deductive

This question requires one to recall the innervation pathway of the deep branch of the ulnar nerve. This necessitates deductive reasoning skill, where factual information and recall of facts and guidelines assist the test-taker in drawing a correct conclusion. In this situation, the adductor pollicis is innervated by the deep branch of the ulnar nerve. If answered incorrectly, review innervations for the ulnar nerve.

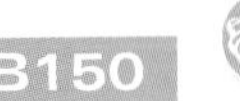

B150

Musculoskeletal | Interventions

A patient presents with a 2-month history of progressively worsening shoulder pain and stiffness without any known injury or trauma to the shoulder. The patient is currently unable to move the upper extremity above the level of shoulder while performing ADLs. After completing the physical examination, the physical therapist concludes that the patient has adhesive capsulitis. What is the **BEST** choice of physical therapy interventions for the disorder?

Choices:

1. Short wave diathermy.
2. Joint mobilization.
3. Stretching exercises.
4. Ultrasound.

Teaching Points

Correct Answer: 3

Based on the Adhesive Capsulitis Clinical Practice Guideline (see Box 2-2), there is moderate evidence to support stretching exercises (both supervised and home-based) in patients with adhesive capsulitis.

Incorrect Choices:

There is currently weak evidence for the use of modalities (diathermy, ultrasound) and joint mobilization. While physical therapists may use these interventions to treat patients with adhesive capsulitis, based on the evidence the **BEST** choice is stretching exercises.

Type of Reasoning: Inductive

For this question, the test-taker must draw from knowledge of effective intervention approaches for adhesive capsulitis in order to draw a correct conclusion. This requires inductive reasoning skill, where clinical judgment is utilized to guide clinical decision-making. For this scenario, the best intervention for adhesive capsulitis is stretching exercises. Review treatment approaches for adhesive capsulitis if answered incorrectly.

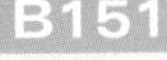

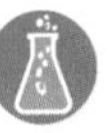

B151

System Interactions | Evaluation, Diagnosis

An elderly patient with congestive heart failure is referred to physical therapy for an examination of functional mobility skills and safety in the home environment. The family reports that the patient is demonstrating increasing forgetfulness and some early memory deficits. During the examination, what would the therapist typically expect to find?

Choices:

1. Impairments in short-term memory.
2. Periods of fluctuating confusion.
3. Periods of agitation and wandering, especially in the late afternoon.
4. Significant impairments in long-term memory.

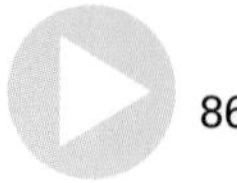

Teaching Points

Correct Answer: 1

Elderly patients with early memory impairments typically demonstrate intact immediate recall (e.g., can repeat words); impairments are often noted in memory for recent events (e.g., Why did I come into this room? Who came to see me yesterday?). Long-term memory is usually intact.

Incorrect Choices:

Periods of fluctuating confusion are typically found in delirium, an acute state of disorientation and confusion. Hallucinations or delusions are common (not present in this case). Periods of agitation and wandering (sundowning) are seen in patients with Alzheimer's type dementia (AD). Whereas AD begins with mild memory loss (stage I), agitation and wandering typically do not occur until stage II.

Type of Reasoning: Analytical

In this situation, the test-taker must analyze the patient's symptoms and make a determination of the root cause for them in order to decide what the therapist's findings may be. Analytical questions require one to interpret information and determine the precise meaning of that information. If this question was answered incorrectly, review information regarding age-related memory deficits.

B152 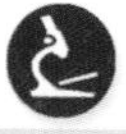

Neuromuscular | Examination

A therapist is examining a patient with vestibular dysfunction. The patient is asked to assume a long sitting position with the head turned to the left side. The therapist then quickly moves the patient backward so that the head is extended over the end of the table approximately 30° below horizontal. This maneuver causes severe dizziness and vertigo. A repeat test with the head turned to the right produces no symptoms. What is the **BEST** way to document these results?

Choices:

1. Positive left Dix-Hallpike test.
2. Positive sharpened Romberg's test.
3. Positive right positional test.
4. Negative positional test.

Teaching Points

Correct Answer: 1

The test described is the Dix-Hallpike. It is a left positive test because, with the head turned to the left, the change in position produces the patient's symptoms.

Incorrect Choices:

The right Dix-Hallpike test with head turned to the right is negative. The sharpened Romberg's test is used to assess standing balance (disequilibrium) with the eyes closed and feet in a tandem (heel-toe) position. The Dix-Hallpike test is a positional test and was positive on the left side, not negative.

Type of Reasoning: Deductive

This question requires one to determine which clinical test is represented by the information in the scenario. This requires factual recall of information related to protocols, which is a deductive reasoning skill. In this situation, the scenario describes administration of the Dix-Hallpike maneuver. If this question was answered incorrectly, review information on the Dix-Hallpike maneuver.

B153 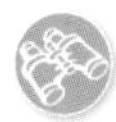

Neuromuscular | Interventions

A therapist is instructing a patient with a stroke in gait training. The therapist determines that learning is going well because the patient's errors are decreasing and overall endurance is improving. What is the **BEST** strategy to promote continued motor learning at this point in the patient's rehabilitation?

Choices:

1. Have the patient practice walking in varying environments.
2. Intervene early whenever errors appear before bad habits become firmly entrenched.
3. Provide continuous feedback after every walking trial.
4. Have the patient continue to practice in the parallel bars until all errors are extinguished.

Teaching Points

Correct Answer: 1

This patient demonstrates the associative stage of motor learning (errors are decreasing and movements are becoming organized). It is appropriate to gradually progress this patient toward ambulating in a more open (varied) environment.

Incorrect Choices:

Continuous feedback may improve performance but delays motor learning. Practicing until errors are extinguished or intervening early whenever errors appear are also inappropriate strategies for the associative stage of learning. Some trial and error learning is the goal.

Type of Reasoning: Inductive

One must utilize clinical judgment to determine the best strategy to promote continued motor learning with the patient. Use of clinical judgment to make a determination of a best course of action is an inductive reasoning skill. It is important to know the stages of motor learning (see Table 3-26) in order to arrive at the correct conclusion, which should be reviewed if this question was answered incorrectly.

B154 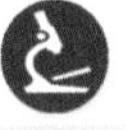

Cardiovascular/Pulmonary | Interventions

What is the primary benefit that patients with asthma will gain by participating in an aerobic exercise regimen?

Choices:

1. Improvement in asthma symptoms.
2. Improvements in cardiorespiratory fitness.
3. Improvements in lung function.
4. Improvements in medication efficacy.

Teaching Points

Correct Choice: 2

Evidence suggests that aerobic exercise consistently improves cardiorespiratory fitness in patients with asthma and should be consistently recommended.

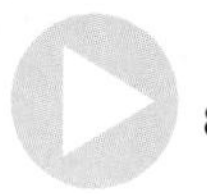

Incorrect Choices:

Exercise has no impact on asthma symptoms, lung function, or medication efficacy.

Type of Reasoning: Deductive

For this question, the test-taker must recall exercise guidelines and benefits for patients with asthma. This requires factual recall of information, which is a deductive reasoning skill. For this case, the primary benefits are improvements in cardiorespiratory fitness. Review exercise guidelines and benefit for patients with asthma if answered incorrectly.

B155 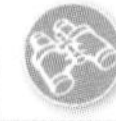

Genitourinary | Interventions

A middle-aged woman is referred to a women's clinic with problems of stress incontinence. She reports loss of control that began with coughing or laughing but now reports problems even when she exercises (aerobics 3 times/wk). What is the **BEST** intervention for this patient?

Choices:

1. Kegel's exercises several times a day.
2. Behavioral modification techniques to reward proper voiding on schedule.
3. Biofeedback 1 hour/wk to achieve appropriate sphincter control.
4. Functional electrical stimulation 3 times/wk.

Teaching Points

Correct Answer: 1

Symptoms of stress incontinence can be successfully managed through a variety of techniques. Pelvic floor exercises (Kegel's exercises) are the mainstay of treatment and must be performed daily, several times a day, in order to be effective.

Incorrect Choices:

Biofeedback and E-Stim offered weekly or 3 times/wk are not likely to be effective because of insufficient frequency. A voiding schedule does not address the primary impairment.

Type of Reasoning: Inductive

This question requires one to understand the nature of stress incontinence and the appropriate interventions for this condition in order to choose the best intervention approach. Using clinical judgment (an inductive reasoning skill), the test-taker determines the best course of action for the patient. If this question was answered incorrectly, review intervention strategies for stress incontinence.

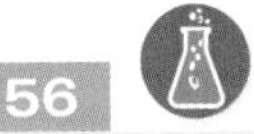

B156

Neuromuscular | Evaluation, Diagnosis

An elderly patient suffered a cerebral thrombosis 4 days ago and presents with the following symptoms: decreased pain and temperature sensation of the ipsilateral face, nystagmus, vertigo, nausea, dysphagia, ipsilateral Horner's syndrome, and contralateral loss of pain and temperature sensation of the body. What is the **MOST** likely location of the thrombosis?

Choices:

1. Anterior cerebral artery.
2. Posterior inferior cerebellar artery.
3. Internal carotid artery.
4. Posterior cerebral artery.

Teaching Points

Correct Answer: 2

This patient presents with lateral medullary (Wallenberg's) syndrome, which can result from occlusion of the posterior inferior cerebellar artery (PICA), which is usually a branch of the vertebral artery. It involves the descending tract and nucleus of CN V, the vestibular nucleus and its connections, CN IX and CN X nuclei or nerve fibers, cuneate and gracile nuclei and spinothalamic tract.

Incorrect Choices:

The symptoms in this case clearly indicate brain stem (cranial nerve) involvement, not cortical involvement (anterior or posterior cerebral artery). An internal carotid artery stroke produces symptoms of combined middle cerebral and anterior cerebral artery strokes. See Table 3-12 for the signs and symptoms associated with various types of strokes.

Type of Reasoning: Analytical

This question requires one to recall the symptoms that indicate involvement of the PICA. This requires the test-taker to analyze the information presented and interpret it in order to determine that the symptoms are directly indicative of PICA thrombosis. It is important for one to recall applied neuroanatomy related to strokes (see Table 3-12) in order to choose the best answer.

Exam B

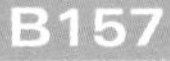

B157

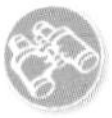

Nonsystem | Therapeutic Modalities

A patient with chronic upper/middle trapezius pain has received two prior treatments with a hot pack for 15 minutes in the prone position. Prior to their third treatment visit the patient reports increased pain with laying in the prone position. The therapist decides to put the patient supine and still apply a moist hot pack. Which of the following modifications are **MOST IMPORTANT** to protect the patient from a risk of thermal injury?

Choices:

1. Add extra layers of toweling and check skin integrity at 5 minutes into a 15-minute treatment.
2. Conduct a sensory exam of the area prior to the treatment and check skin integrity at 10 minutes into a 15-minute treatment.
3. Decrease the treatment time to a total of 5 minutes.
4. Increase the hydrocollator temperatures above 176°F (80°C) and stop the treatment at 10 minutes.

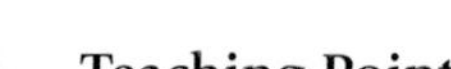

Teaching Points

Correct Answer: 1

Generally, 1–2 cm (6–8 layers) of dry toweling is used to prevent skin temperatures from getting too high (therapeutic level is approximately 104°F [40°C]). If the person is laying on the hot pack, extra layers of toweling are needed to help avoid tissue damage due to heat. Also, hot pack temperatures typically reach a therapeutic level at 5 minutes into the treatment. Checking skin integrity at 5 minutes and periodically throughout the treatment is best practice to prevent a thermal injury.

Incorrect Choices:

A sensory examination could be conducted prior to the treatment, but it does not diminish the need for extra layers of protection and the need for a skin integrity check at 5 minutes into the treatment. Decreasing the time of exposure to 5 minutes is not optimal for a treatment effect as it typically takes at least 5 minutes to obtain a therapeutic temperature (40°C or 104°F) and recommended treatment times are between 15 and 20 minutes. Increasing the hydrocollator temperatures above 176°F (80°C) creates increased risk for thermal injury.

Type of Reasoning: Inductive

For this question, one must rely on clinical judgment in order to arrive at a correct conclusion for this hot pack treatment. Specifically, the test-taker must draw from knowledge of effective hot pack treatment modification in order to determine what is most important to do to protect from thermal injury. For this situation, the therapist should add extra layers of towels and check the skin at 5 minutes into a 15-minute treatment. If answered incorrectly, review hot pack treatment guidelines and acceptable modifications.

B158 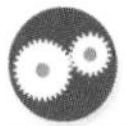

Cardiovascular/Pulmonary | Examination

A patient arrives for outpatient cardiac rehab 10 weeks after a coronary artery bypass graft. The postoperative course was complicated by atrial fibrillation, which has been controlled with medications prescribed by a cardiologist. The patient's resting vital signs are HR = 90 in atrial fibrillation, BP = 116/74, RR = 14, and SpO_2 = 99% on room air. Is a symptom-limited exercise test appropriate for this patient at this time?

Choices:

1. Yes, the patient is managed by a cardiologist and has no symptoms now.
2. Yes, the heart rate is well controlled and the cardiologist is aware of the arrhythmia.
3. No, the patient is tachycardic at rest and has an arrhythmia.
4. No, a patient in atrial fibrillation should not complete an exercise test.

Teaching Points

Correct Answer: 2

It is appropriate to perform an exercise test on a patient who is on medication to control his/her rate with atrial fibrillation (AF). A normal heart rate is between 60–100 beats per minute, which is where this patient's heart rate falls.

Incorrect Choices:

Patients can be asymptomatic with AF, so it is best to use objective measures to assess their response to activity. It is safe to exercise a patient who is in AF. It is a concern if the patient's heart rate is ≥ 115–120 beats per minute. This is the point at which diastolic filling time is decreased, which places a person in AF at risk of not maintaining his/her cardiac output with increased demand.

Type of Reasoning: Evaluative

This question provides symptoms, and the test-taker must determine the best course of action for a client based on knowledge of cardiac exercise guidelines and safety in providing treatment. This is an evaluative reasoning skill, as the test-taker must weigh the four options provided and determine what is prudent for the patient's current status and needs. In this case, the patient's rate is well controlled and the cardiologist is aware of the arrhythmia, so the therapist should proceed with symptom-limited exercise testing. Review cardiac exercise guidelines if the question was answered incorrectly.

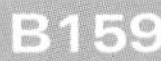
B159
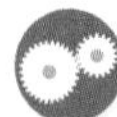

System Interactions | Evaluation, Diagnosis

A patient presents with suspected T10 paraplegia. An extensive neurological workup has failed to reveal a specific cause for the paraplegia. The physician has determined a diagnosis of functional neurologic disorder. What is the therapist's **BEST** choice of intervention?

Choices:

1. Initiate ROM and strength training after the patient receives psychological counseling.
2. Initiate functional training consistent with the level of injury.
3. Use functional electrical stimulation as a means of demonstrating to the patient that the muscles are functional.
4. Discuss possible underlying causes for the paralysis with the patient in an empathetic manner.

Teaching Points

Correct Answer: 2

A functional neurologic disorder (conversion disorder) represents a real loss of function for the patient. The symptoms are real and varied. The condition may be triggered by stress, psychological, or physical trauma. The therapist should treat this patient the same as any patient with spinal cord injury with similar functional deficits. Early intervention is crucial.

Incorrect Choices:

A psychologist or psychiatrist is best able to help the patient understand the cause of the patient's paralysis. The therapist should be empathetic; however, counseling should not be the main focus of intervention in PT. Confrontation (using E-Stim to prove the patient has functioning muscles) is contraindicated.

Type of Reasoning: Evaluative

This question requires one to make a value judgment about the best course of action for this patient who has a functional neurologic disorder. It is beneficial to understand what a functional neurologic disorder is and the appropriate role for the PT in order to choose the best response. These types of questions, which require evaluative reasoning, are challenging because of the need to evaluate the believability of statements and make decisions based on values.

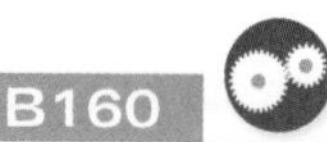

Nonsystem I Professional Responsibilities

The director of a physical therapy department wants to fill a vacant PT position in the spinal cord injury program. Two résumés have been received. One candidate, a former employee, is a well-qualified and experienced 52-year-old female with a history of back pain that could impact her ability to do some heavy lifting at times. The other candidate is a newly licensed, very enthusiastic, 25-year-old male therapist for whom heavy lifting should not be a problem. In this case, what is the **BEST** hiring decision?

Choices:

1. As long as age and back pain history were NOT discussed during the interview process with the female candidate, the male candidate would best meet the caseload demands.
2. Hire the male candidate but ensure that age and back pain history were discussed with the female candidate as the rationale for hiring someone else.
3. Not have the female candidate partake in the interview process as issues with age and back pain would be justifiable grounds to rule her out based on the case load.
4. Hire the more qualified female and provide aide assistance or lift equipment when heavy lifting is required.

Teaching Points

Correct Answer: 4

The Age Discrimination and Employment Act of 1967 prohibits employers from discriminating against persons 40–70 years of age in any area of employment. The 1973 Rehabilitation Act prohibits employment discrimination based on disability and requires reasonable accommodation in the workplace by removing barriers unless there would be "undue hardship" for the employer. Title VII of the Civil Rights Act of 1964 might also come into play since one provision prohibits discrimination based on gender. The female candidate is clearly the more qualified and would be the best hire in this case.

Incorrect Choices:

Although asking about age is not permissible in the hiring process, familiarity with the candidate or a review of a résumé could unintentionally make the candidate's age obvious. Ruling out the female from the interview process with age and back pain as factors is clearly discriminatory. The male candidate may have potential; however, consideration of both age and back pain history, whether discussed or not, is discriminatory. The older candidate may be familiar with the caseload, department systems, and all other things being equal, is the stronger candidate if reasonable accommodations can be made.

Type of Reasoning: Evaluative

For this situation, the test-taker must determine a best course of action from the information provided, while being mindful of employment regulations and guidelines. This requires evaluative reasoning skills, where one weighs various courses of action in order to arrive at a correct conclusion. In this situation, the director should hire the more qualified female and provide aide assistance or lift equipment when heavy lifting is required. If answered incorrectly, review the Age Discrimination and Employment Act of 1967 and the Rehabilitation Act of 1973 for employment guidelines.

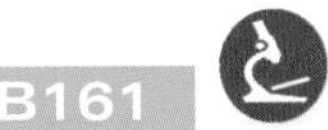

Gastrointestinal I Evaluation, Diagnosis

A patient with a long history of chronic low back pain is seen in a physical therapy clinic. The patient has a new complaint of epigastric pain described as burning or gnawing which radiates to the mid-back. New symptoms also include nausea and intermittent episodes of light-headedness. The therapist suspects the patient may have a peptic ulcer. Which oral medication taken long term is most likely to contribute to the development of a peptic or duodenal ulcer?

Choices:

1. Oxycodone.
2. Baclofen.
3. Celebrex.
4. Ibuprofen.

Teaching Points

Correct Answer: 4

Ibuprofen and many other NSAIDs (nonsteroidal anti-inflammatory drugs) can have deleterious effects on the entire GI tract when taken long term and in high doses. The most common clinical effect is on the gastro-duodenal mucosa, where erosions and ulcerations can occur and may progress to bleeding and perforations. Other signs and symptoms of a peptic or duodenal ulcer include night pain that typically occurs after midnight, vomiting, anorexia, and bloody stools.

Incorrect Choices:

Oxycodone is a narcotic or opioid medication and typically prescribed for short-term management of significant postoperative pain. Common side effects of opioid administration include sedation, dizziness, nausea, constipation, physical dependence, and respiratory depression. Baclofen is a muscle relaxant and may be prescribed for acute episodes of spinal pain when significant muscle guarding or spasm is present. The most common side effects include fatigue, drowsiness, dry mouth, depression and decreased blood pressure. Celebrex is an NSAID but it is a cyclooxygenase-2 (COX-2) inhibitor and much more gastroprotective than Ibuprofen and many other NSAIDS that are not COX-2 inhibitors. COX-2 inhibitors provide benefit in reducing ulcer formation and bleeding, although they do not completely eliminate the risk.

Type of Reasoning: Deductive

This question requires the test-taker to recall the potential adverse effects of long-term use of ibuprofen in order to arrive at a correct conclusion. This necessitates the recall of factual information, which is a deductive reasoning skill. For this scenario, long-term use of ibuprofen is most likely to contribute to the development of a peptic or duodenal ulcer. If answered incorrectly, review adverse effects of ibuprofen.

B162

Neuromuscular I Examination

A patient is referred for inpatient rehabilitation after undergoing resection of an astrocytoma in the right posterior (caudal) parietal lobe. Which of the following impairments is the patient **MOST LIKELY** to exhibit?

Choices:

1. Agnosia and difficulty with spatial reasoning.
2. Loss of sensation in the left upper/lower extremities and urinary incontinence.
3. Difficulty with long-term memory and apraxia.
4. Visual field deficits and dysmetria.

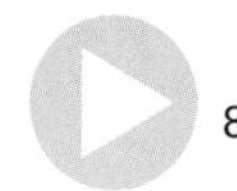

Teaching Points

Correct Answer: 1

Agnosia is the inability to recognize objects. Agnosia (tactile and visual), unilateral neglect, and difficulty with depth perception and spatial relations are common findings in patients with damage to the right posterior parietal lobe.

Incorrect Choices:

Loss of sensation in the extremities is more common with involvement of the primary somatosensory cortex (located in the anterior/caudal parietal cortex). Urinary incontinence is associated with damage to the superior aspect of the primary motor or sensory cortices. Long-term memory is a complex relationship between multiple areas of the brain and limbic system but is most common with lesions to the dorsolateral prefrontal cortex. Cortical visual field deficits are most often associated with damage to the occipital lobe, and dysmetria is common in patients with cerebellar dysfunction.

Type of Reasoning: Inferential

One must infer or draw a reasonable conclusion of what is likely to be true of a patient with a resection of an astrocytoma of the right posterior parietal lobe (See Table 3-14). This necessitates inferential reasoning skill, where information is weighed to determine what is likely to occur, given a specific situation. For this scenario, the patient is most likely to exhibit agnosia and difficulty with spatial reasoning. Review functions of the parietal lobe, especially the right posterior lobe, if answered incorrectly.

B163 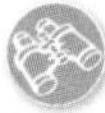

Integumentary I Examination

A patient presents with a large sacral decubitus ulcer that is purulent and draining. The therapist needs to take a representative sample of the infected material in order to obtain a laboratory culture. What is the **BEST** source to obtain a culture sample from this wound?

Choices:

1. Exudate in the wound and the surrounding tissues.
2. Dressing and exudate in the wound.
3. Exudate in the wound.
4. Dressing, exudate, and surrounding bed linen.

Teaching Points

Correct Answer: 3

The specimens must be collected from the wound site with a minimum of contamination by material from adjacent tissues. The exudate provides the best culture.

Incorrect Choices:

The margins of cutaneous lesions or pressure ulcers are usually contaminated with environmental bacteria. Using the dressing for a specimen sample would also contain contaminated tissues.

Type of Reasoning: Inductive

The test-taker must use clinical judgment applied to a patient circumstance (an inductive reasoning skill) to determine the best method to obtain a sample culture of a wound. In this situation, it is best to minimize contamination by sampling the exudate in the wound. If this question was answered incorrectly, refer to information on methods for obtaining laboratory cultures.

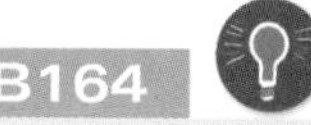

Cardiovascular/Pulmonary | Interventions

A phase 2 outpatient cardiac rehabilitation program uses circuit training with different exercise stations for the 50-minute program. One station uses arm ergometry. For arm exercise as compared with leg exercise, at a given workload, what can the therapist expect?

Choices:

1. Higher systolic and diastolic BP.
2. Higher HR and systolic/diastolic BP.
3. Higher HR and lower systolic BP.
4. Reduced exercise capacity owing to higher stroke volumes.

Teaching Points

Correct Answer: 2

Arm ergometry uses a smaller muscle mass than leg ergometry with resulting lower maximal oxygen uptake. In upper extremity exercise, both HR and BP will be higher than for the same level of work in the lower extremities.

Incorrect Choices:

The other choices do not correctly identify the expected changes with arm exercise.

Type of Reasoning: Inferential

This question requires one to draw conclusions about arm ergometry and its impact on HR and BP, especially as it relates to leg ergometry. For this scenario, HR and systolic/diastolic BP will be higher with arm ergometry. To arrive at the correct conclusion, one must rely on knowledge of the impact of ergometry on cardiovascular activity, which should be reviewed if this question was answered incorrectly.

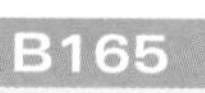

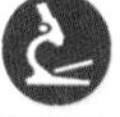

Nonsystem | Safety and Protection

A physical therapist is treating an elderly, deconditioned patient in a private room at a long-term care facility. The patient has been diagnosed with Clostridium difficile and is referred for exercise to improve lower extremity strength and the ability to move from sit-to-stand. The therapist elects to use light resistance using cuff weights. In this situation, what precautionary steps need to be taken?

Choices:

1. The therapist should perform hand sanitizing and don gloves, gown, and mask before entering the room.
2. The therapist should perform hand sanitizing and don gloves before entering the room.
3. Cuff weights and other exercise apparatus should be disinfected immediately on removal from the patient's room.
4. Only manual resistance exercise should be performed to avoid cross-contamination of any therapeutic equipment.

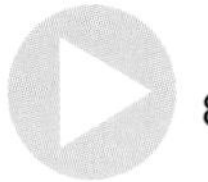

Teaching Points

Correct Answer: 3

All medical/exercise equipment used in the patient's room needs to be disinfected immediately unless left in the patient's room as dedicated equipment or is disposable. Health care providers (HCP) need to observe contact precautions when working with the patient. This includes cleaning their hands with soap and water or an alcohol-based hand rub before and after caring for the patient. They are also required to wear personal protective equipment (gloves and a gown) during patient interaction.

Incorrect Choices:

A mask is not needed as *C. diff* is not airborne. Required PPE includes both gloves and a gown. PPE is donned before entering the room and removed before leaving the room. Equipment and devices, including stethoscopes, pulse-oximeters, walkers, goniometers, weights, and so on, can be used as long as they are disinfected once removed from the patient's room.

Type of Reasoning: Deductive

For this question, the test-taker must recall the guidelines for working with patients infected with *C. diff* in order to arrive at a correct conclusion. This requires deductive reasoning skills, where factual guidelines are used to guide decisions. In this case scenario, the therapist should immediately disinfect all exercise equipment upon removal from the patient's room. If answered incorrectly, be sure to review contact precaution guidelines and information.

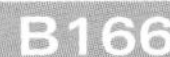
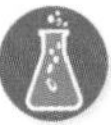

B166

Gastrointestinal | Evaluation, Diagnosis

A physical therapist examines an adult patient whose chief complaint is mid-back and right scapular pain. The patient was referred to physical therapy with a diagnosis of scapular dysfunction. There was no history of trauma to the back or right scapular region. During the interview, the patient describes experiencing unexplained weight gain over the past year, intermittent upper abdominal pain, and intolerance to certain foods. Based on these examination findings, which test would a physician **MOST LIKELY** order for this patient?

Choices:

1. Electrocardiogram (ECG).
2. Barium swallow.
3. Radiographs (x-ray) of the right shoulder.
4. Cholescintigraphy.

Teaching Points

Correct Answer: 4

Cholescintigraphy, also known as hepatobiliary iminodiacetic acid (HIDA) scan, is an imaging test used to view the gallbladder, liver, bile ducts, and small intestines. The examination findings in this patient are consistent with gallbladder disease (biliary dyskinesia). Symptoms can include weight gain as the gallbladder does not drain bile properly, which leads to improper fat digestion. Other symptoms can include upper abdominal pain after eating, nausea, bloating, and indigestion.

Incorrect Choices:

An electrocardiogram (ECG or EKG) records electrical activity in the heart. It is used to detect arrhythmias or other types of heart disease (such as a heart attack). The patient history in this scenario is not consistent with cardiac disease. A barium swallow test is a radiological test done to visualize the esophagus, stomach, and duodenum and may help detect ulcers, hernias, diverticulitis, swallowing difficulty diagnosis, or tumors. Most of these conditions would be accompanied by a history of weight loss, not weight gain as mentioned in the question stem. An x-ray would rule out a possible scapular fracture. If the patient in this scenario had a scapular fracture, a history of trauma along with bruising and swelling in the shoulder and upper back would have been described. Shoulder movements would have likely reproduced the patient's pain.

Type of Reasoning: Analytical

For this question, the test-taker must analyze the presenting symptoms in order to determine appropriate referral for diagnostic testing. This requires analytical reasoning skill, where pieces of information are weighed for their value in order to draw reasonable conclusions. In this case, a HIDA scan should be recommended. If answered incorrectly, review gastrointestinal diagnostic tests, including the HIDA scan.

B167 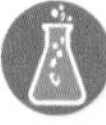

Neuromuscular | Examination

Based on the pictured CT scan, what impairments is this patient likely to demonstrate?

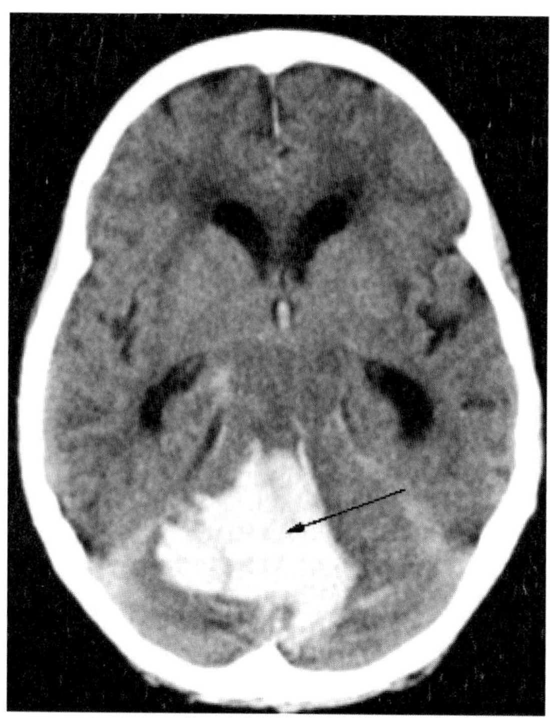

Image from: http://www.med-ed.virginia.edu/courses/rad/headct/index.html

Choices:
1. Ataxia.
2. Nonfluent aphasia.
3. Fluent aphasia.
4. Left-sided unilateral neglect.

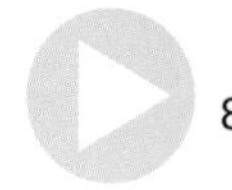

Teaching Points

Correct Answer: 1

The arrow is pointing to a hemorrhage in the cerebellum. Damage to this area results in difficulty with movement, postural control, eye-movement disorders, and muscle tone. Ataxia is a common finding.

Incorrect Choices:

Aphasia is more typical of a left cerebral infarct, and left-sided unilateral neglect is typically due to a right cerebral injury. CT scans and MRIs can help the therapist predict clinical manifestations based on the area of injury.

Type of Reasoning: Analytical

This question requires the test-taker to determine the most likely presentation of symptoms based on the CT image. Questions that require analysis of pictures and graphs often necessitate analytical reasoning skill. In this case, the patient has experienced a hemorrhage in the cerebellum and will most likely display ataxia. If this question was answered incorrectly, review signs and symptoms of cerebellar hemorrhages.

B168 

Nonsystem I Professional Responsibilities

A physical therapist working in an outpatient setting is experiencing burnout and disinterest in their job. The therapist has not been selecting interventions that are helpful and personalized for each patient. However, the selected interventions are not harmful. Which of the following **MOST** correctly describes the physical therapist's unethical practice?

Choices:

1. The therapist lacks beneficence.
2. The therapist is acting with maleficence.
3. The therapist is not exhibiting justice.
4. The therapist is not respecting the patient's autonomy.

Teaching Points

Correct Answer: 1

The physical therapist lacks beneficence (doing good to others) by not balancing the risks and benefits to maximize the patient's quality of life and health outcomes. The therapist is not directly harming the patient but is also not exhibiting a commitment to maximizing quality of life.

Incorrect Answers:

To act with maleficence is to actively try to hurt another person. The ethical principle of justice states that health care providers will equitably distribute risks, benefits, and resources among multiple patients. Autonomy emphasizes the importance of respecting an individual's decision and self-determination.

Type of Reasoning: Evaluative

This question requires one to apply knowledge of ethical practice guidelines and then evaluate the physical therapist's behavior to determine which principle of ethics applies to the situation. This is an evaluative reasoning skill, where information is weighed for its value and merits. For this situation, the therapist's unethical practice is consistent with lacking beneficence. If answered incorrectly, review ethics in practice, especially beneficence.

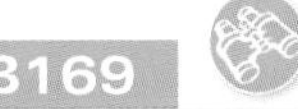

B169

Musculoskeletal I Interventions

What is the **MOST** effective intervention to regain biceps brachii strength if the muscle is chronically inflamed and has a painful arc of motion?

Choices:

1. Active concentric contractions through partial ROM.
2. Active eccentric contractions in the pain-free range.
3. Isokinetic exercises through the full ROM.
4. Isometric exercises at the end range of movement only.

Teaching Points

Correct Answer: 2

For a muscle that is chronically inflamed, focus should be placed on eccentric contractions, because there is less effort and stress placed on the contractile units than with concentric contractions at the same level of work. The exercise should be performed in the pain-free portion of the range.

Incorrect Choices:

Isokinetic, isometric, and isotonic exercises do not allow for pain-free muscle contractions and can cause further inflammation of the muscle.

Type of Reasoning: Inductive

For this question, it is important to have knowledge of kinesiology, exercise physiology, and appropriate exercise for chronically inflamed muscles in order to choose the best exercise approach. This requires diagnostic thinking and clinical judgment, which is an inductive reasoning skill. For this situation, the most appropriate exercise is active eccentric contractions in the pain-free range to avoid further inflammation of the muscle. If this question was answered incorrectly, refer to information on appropriate exercises for various forms of muscle pathology.

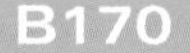
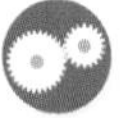

B170

Nonsystem I Therapeutic Modalities

During an ultrasound (US) treatment, the patient flinches and states that a strong ache was felt in the treatment area. What is the therapist's **BEST** course of action?

Choices:

1. Decrease the US frequency.
2. Add more transmission medium.
3. Decrease the US intensity.
4. Increase the size of the treatment area.

Teaching Points

Correct Answer: 3

Acoustical energy is reflected from the bone into the bone-tissue interface, resulting in rapid tissue temperature elevation and stimulation of the highly sensitive periosteum of the bone. A reduction in intensity is indicated if a strong ache is felt.

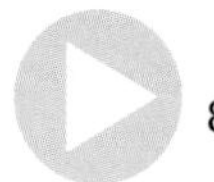

Incorrect Choices:

The question assumes that the treatment size of the area is correct. Increasing the size of the treatment area would minimize the ability to elevate the tissue temperature. Thus, the patient would not experience a strong ache from rapid tissue temperature elevation. Adding more transmission medium would encourage transmission of acoustical energy and thus potentiate the rapid tissue temperature elevation, contributing to the patient's symptom. The frequency has to do with the depth of penetration of the US energy, not the rate/speed at which the tissue temperature is being elevated.

Type of Reasoning: Evaluative

This question requires one to determine the cause for the patient's discomfort during US treatment and then to determine an appropriate course of action, which is an evaluative reasoning skill. For this patient, it is best to decrease the US intensity because the strong ache indicates it is a result of too high an intensity. If this question was answered incorrectly, review information on US guidelines and symptoms warranting change of protocol.

B171 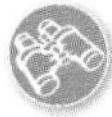

Musculoskeletal I Interventions

A patient is referred for postoperative rehabilitation following a Type II SLAP repair performed 1 week ago. What is the therapist's **BEST** choice of intervention during early rehabilitation?

Choices:

1. Focus on biceps brachii stretching and strengthening.
2. Defer intervention during the maximum protection phase.
3. Perform careful ROM of the shoulder internal rotators.
4. Perform careful ROM of the shoulder external rotators.

Teaching Points

Correct Answer: 3

Internal rotation ROM does not create the peel-back mechanism that increases stress to the repair. Given the nature of this repair, an understanding of the postoperative precautions is paramount to a successful surgical outcome. Early rehabilitation within the postoperative precautions correlates to a quicker overall recovery and improved outcomes.

Incorrect Choices:

Type II SLAP lesions are characterized by a detachment of the superior labrum and the origin of the tendon of the long head of the biceps brachii that results in instability of the biceps-labral anchor. The surgery requires reattachment of the labrum and biceps anchor. Given the repair of the biceps, contraction and stretching of the biceps should be avoided during the maximum protection phase. In addition, external rotation ROM/stretching should be avoided given the peel-back mechanism and increased stress to the repair.

Type of Reasoning: Inductive

This question requires one to use clinical judgment to determine a best course of action. Questions of this nature often necessitate inductive reasoning skill. For this case, the therapist should choose to perform careful ROM to the internal rotators of the shoulder with a Type II SLAP repair. Review protocols for rehabilitation after SLAP lesions if answered incorrectly.

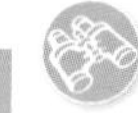

B172

Integumentary I Interventions

A patient is recovering from deep partial-thickness burns over the posterior thigh and calf that are now healed. The therapist's examination reveals local tenderness with swelling and pain on movement in the hip area. While palpating the tissues, the therapist detects a mass. What is the therapist's **BEST** course of action?

Choices:

1. Use petrissage to work on this area of focal tenderness.
2. Report these findings promptly to the physician.
3. Continue with ROM exercises but proceed gently.
4. Use RICE to quiet down the inflammatory response.

Teaching Points

Correct Answer: 2

These signs and symptoms are characteristic of heterotopic ossification (HO), an abnormal bone growth typically around a joint. While the etiology is unknown, its presence can lead to serious ROM limitations. These findings should be reported promptly to the physician.

Incorrect Choices:

Petrissage and aggressive ROM exercises could exacerbate the condition. Ice does decrease metabolic activity; more in-depth medical management is required.

Type of Reasoning: Inductive

This question requires one to utilize clinical judgment to determine the reason for the patient's symptoms and then determine the best course of action, which is an inductive reasoning skill. In this situation, the findings indicate HO and the therapist should notify the physician promptly. If this question was answered incorrectly, review information on HO.

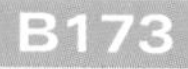

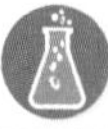

B173

Musculoskeletal I Examination

A patient presents with complaint of neck pain on the right. During the AROM examination, the physical therapist observes the following osteokinematic neck motions—full side-bending left, full rotation to the left, full forward flexion, limited and painful extension, limited and painful right side-bending, and limited and painful right rotation. Based on this pattern, what is the arthrokinematic restriction?

Choices:

1. Upglide of a facet on the left.
2. Upglide of a facet on the right.
3. Downglide of a facet on the left.
4. Downglide of a facet on the right.

Teaching Points

Correct Answer: 4

If a facet on the right was restricted with downgliding (arthrokinematic restriction), then the osteokinematic motions that would be limited would be rotation and side-bending to the right with limited extension. The fact that there is pain on the right supports that the restriction is on the right.

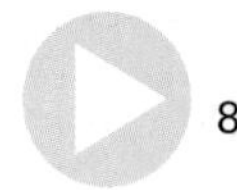

Incorrect Choices:

The osteokinematic limitation could also be seen with a facet restricted with upglide on the left, but the differentiator is the fact that the pain is on the right, indicating that the restriction is on the right. The arthrokinematic restrictions in the other choices do not correlate with the osteokinematic findings of the exam.

Type of Reasoning: Analytical

This question requires the test-taker to analyze the symptoms presented in order to determine the most likely arthrokinematic restriction. Questions that require one to analyze pieces of information in order to draw conclusions often require analytical reasoning skill. For this situation, the arthrokinematic restriction is restriction with downglide of a facet on the right. Review arthrokinematics of the neck and restrictions if answered incorrectly.

B174 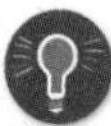

Cardiovascular/Pulmonary | Examination

What are the possible ECG changes with exercise that can occur in a patient with coronary artery disease (CAD) and prior myocardial infarction (MI)?

Choices:

1. Tachycardia at a relatively low intensity of exercise with ST segment depression.
2. Bradycardia with ST segment elevation.
3. Significant arrhythmias early on in exercise with a shortened QRS.
4. Bradycardia with ST segment depression >3 mm below baseline.

Teaching Points

Correct Answer: 1

The typical exercise ECG changes in the patient with CAD include tachycardia at low levels of exercise intensity. The ST segment becomes depressed (>1 mm is significant). In addition, complex ventricular arrhythmias (multifocal or runs of PVCs) may appear and are associated with significant CAD and/or a poor prognosis.

Incorrect Choices:

The other choices do not accurately describe the expected ECG changes with exercise. Chronotropic incompetence is indicated by an HR that fails to rise; bradycardia (slowing of HR) is not expected. ST segment elevation with significant Q waves can occur and is indicative of aneurysm or wall motion abnormality.

Type of Reasoning: Inferential

In order to answer the question correctly, the test-taker must recall typical ECG changes for patients who have myocardial ischemia and CAD. Therefore, the test-taker must draw conclusions about the patient's diagnosis, which is an inferential reasoning skill. For this patient, one would expect tachycardia and ST segment depression, which should be reviewed if this question was answered incorrectly.

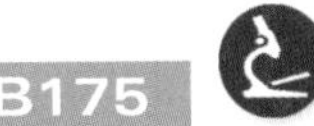

B175

Musculoskeletal | Examination

A high school student is seen in a physical therapy clinic for management of neck pain 2 weeks after a motor vehicle accident. The patient also complains of intermittent dizziness and headaches since the accident. The therapist becomes suspicious of upper cervical spine instability. Which special test is **BEST** to confirm this diagnosis?

Choices:

1. Vertebral artery test.
2. Cervical flexion-rotation test.
3. Sharp-Purser test.
4. Cervical distraction test.

Teaching Points

Correct Answer: 3

The above scenario describes a situation where the therapist appropriately considers upper cervical spine tests and measures to assess for stability/instability prior to moving forward with the rest of the physical examination. Failure to assess integrity of the upper cervical spine could potentially result in damage to the spinal cord or even death. The Sharp-Purser test assesses the integrity of the transverse ligament (part of the cruciate ligament complex) and atlantoaxial joint (C1–C2) stability.

Incorrect Choices:

The vertebral artery test is used to determine the integrity of the vertebrobasilar arterial system. The cervical flexion-rotation test is used to identify upper cervical spine dysfunction and range of motion limitations. The distraction test compresses neural structures at the intervertebral foramen and is used to assess for cervical radiculopathy or facet condition.

Type of Reasoning: Deductive

This question requires the test-taker to recall special testing guidelines to confirm the diagnosis of upper cervical spine instability. This requires the recall of factual information and guidelines, which is a deductive reasoning skill. For this case, the therapist should conduct the Sharp-Purser test to confirm the diagnosis. If answered incorrectly, review upper cervical spine testing guidelines.

B176 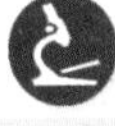

Cardiovascular/Pulmonary | Evaluation, Diagnosis

A patient with a history of heart failure is taking Lasix (furosemide) to reduce volume overload. Which lab value is important to assess when treating a patient who is taking Lasix?

Choices:

1. Calcium.
2. Sodium.
3. Magnesium.
4. Potassium.

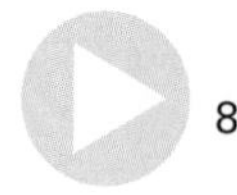

Teaching Points

Correct Answer: 4

Lasix is not a potassium sparing diuretic, and patients taking potassium are at risk for eliminating too much potassium. Low potassium can lead to muscle cramps, fatigue, and cardiac arrhythmias.

Incorrect Choices:

The other electrolytes are not affected by Lasix.

Type of Reasoning: Deductive

One must recall the properties of Lasix to determine which lab value is important to assess. This requires the recall of factual guidelines, which is a deductive reasoning skill. Based on knowledge of this information, one should conclude that potassium is important to assess for this patient. Review information on diuretics, especially Lasix, if answered incorrectly.

B177 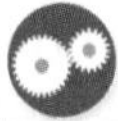

Nonsystem | Safety and Protection

During the course of the physical therapy treatment in the ICU, a radial line is accidently pulled out of the artery. What is the first action the PT should take?

Choices:

1. Push the code button in the patient's room, because this is a cardiac emergency.
2. Elevate the arm above heart level to stop the bleeding.
3. Place a BP cuff on the involved extremity and inflate the cuff until the bleeding stops.
4. Reinsert the arterial catheter into the radial artery and check the monitor for an accurate tracing.

Teaching Points

Correct Answer: 3

A radial arterial line is a catheter placed in the artery itself. If it becomes dislodged during treatment, the artery is now open to bleeding. This arterial bleeding needs to be stopped immediately, although it is not considered a cardiac emergency. Place a BP cuff above the site of bleeding and inflate the cuff to above systole to stop the bleeding or place enough manual pressure on the site to stop the bleeding. Then call for help.

Incorrect Choices:

Elevating the site of bleeding above heart level will not be as effective, because this is an arterial bleed. As long as the heart is pumping with adequate pressure, the site will continue to bleed. This is not a cardiac emergency. Never replace any line that has become disconnected. The line is no longer sterile and should not be reinserted into the patient. A new, sterile catheter will need to be used if the radial line is to be replaced.

Type of Reasoning: Evaluative

This question requires one to use judgment to evaluate the strength of the statements made in order to arrive at a decision for the first course of action with this patient. In this situation, it is important to stop the bleeding in the most effective manner possible, which is to inflate a BP cuff on the involved extremity until the bleeding stops. Questions such as these can be challenging because one must use a value judgment to make the best decision.

B178 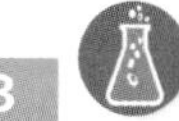

Lymphatic | Evaluation, Diagnosis

A physical therapist examines an adult client with significant swelling in her right lower extremity. The client reports that she recently had a radical hysterectomy for stage II cervical cancer. Lymphedema is suspected. What is an important finding that may corroborate the diagnosis of lymphedema?

Choices:

1. Positive Homan's sign.
2. Positive Stemmer's sign.
3. Absent or diminished dorsalis pedis pulse.
4. Temporary pallor and cyanosis of the toes along with decreased skin temperature.

Teaching Points

Correct Answer: 2

Stemmer's sign is a highly specific test for lymphedema. Specificity of Stemmer's sign ranges from 94%–100%; sensitivity ranges from 56%–61%. To perform the test, the therapist gently pinches and lifts the skin at the base of the second toe on its dorsal side. A positive test is present when the skin cannot be lifted or separated from the underlying tissue. The ability to pinch and lift the skin is a negative test result.

Incorrect Choices:

Homan's sign is a special test that has been used when deep vein thrombosis (DVT) is suspected. The examiner gently dorsiflexes the ankle and/or squeezes the calf in an attempt to reproduce the patient's symptoms. The test's diagnositic accuracy is limited and cannot be relied upon. Absent pulses indicate some type of insult or compromise to the artery being tested (such as the dorsalis pedis artery). Diminished or absent distal pulses may be suggestive of chronic arterial insufficiency. Temporary pallor and cyanosis of the toes along with changes in skin temperature are also suggestive of peripheral vascular disease. These findings are often seen in Raynaud's phenomenon or Raynaud's disease, due to episodic vasoconstriction of small arteries and arterioles in response to cold temperatures or emotional stress.

Type of Reasoning: Analytical

For this question, the test-taker must analyze the various findings presented and determine which one will corroborate the diagnosis of lymphedema. This requires analytical reasoning skill. In this scenario, a positive Stemmer's sign would corroborate the diagnosis. Review information on evaluation of lower extremity lymphedema if answered incorrectly.

B179

Nonsystem | Safety and Protection

A physical therapist is providing medical field coverage at a sporting event. A player begins to experience moderate respiratory distress on the field of play and comes to the sideline for assistance. A coach informs you that the player has asthma and presents you with a container of prescribed medications that the player provided to the team. Which of the following interventions is **CONTRAINDICATED** when caring for this patient?

Choices:

1. Activate EMS.
2. Assist the patient in delivering the prescribed dose of short-acting beta$_2$ agonist medication.
3. Move the player to a nearby air-conditioned space if safe to do so.
4. Assist the patient in delivering the prescribed dose of long-acting beta$_2$ agonist medication.

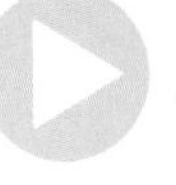

Teaching Points

Correct Answer: 4

Long-acting beta$_2$ agonists are used for daily management of patients with asthma. Because of its long-acting nature, it is inappropriate for an urgent response to an acute episode of asthma.

Incorrect Choices:

Short-acting beta$_2$ agonists are appropriate for the treatment of acute episodes of asthma, and health care providers (HCPs) should assist patients with administration of this medication when prescribed. Moving a patient to an area that is cool and is controlled from environmental allergens would be indicated in most patients experiencing an acute episode of asthma. It is never inappropriate to activate EMS in response to an acute episode of asthma. Patients who are well known to their health care provider and respond well to treatment may be monitored by the health care team or transported to urgent care.

Type of Reasoning: Evaluative

For this question, one must evaluate the presenting symptoms and determine which intervention approach would be contraindicated. This requires evaluative reasoning skill, where courses of action are weighed for their merits, benefits, and drawbacks. For this scenario, assisting the patient in delivering the prescribed dose of long-acting beta$_2$ agonist medication is contraindicated. If answered incorrectly, review intervention approaches for patients with acute asthma.

B180 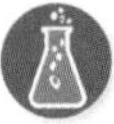

Gastrointestinal | Evaluation, Diagnosis

After examining a patient who was referred to physical therapy for posterior thoracic pain, the therapist finds no musculoskeletal causes for the patient's symptoms. What anatomical structure may refer pain to this thoracic region?

Choices:

1. Heart.
2. Appendix.
3. Gallbladder.
4. Ovary.

Teaching Points

Correct Answer: 3

Dysfunction of the gallbladder often refers pain to the thorax.

Incorrect Choices:

The commonly observed referral pattern of the heart is to the chest and upper extremity, the ovaries to the low back, and the appendix to the right lower quadrant.

Type of Reasoning: Analytical

This question requires one to refer to knowledge of physiology and of common referred patterns of pain. The test-taker must recognize that pain referred to the posterior thoracic region is typical of problems with the gallbladder. To arrive at the correct conclusion, the test-taker must analyze the information presented and determine the meaning of that information, which is an analytical reasoning skill.

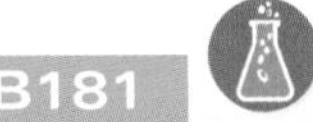

Nonsystem | Equipment, Devices

An elderly patient with a transfemoral amputation is being fitted with a temporary prosthesis containing a SACH (solid ankle cushion heel) prosthetic foot. Which of the following **BEST** characterizes the SACH foot?

Choices:

1. Is an articulated foot with multiplanar motion.
2. Allows full sagittal and frontal plane motion.
3. Absorbs energy through a series of bumpers, permitting sagittal plane motion only.
4. Allows limited sagittal plane motion with a small amount of mediolateral motion.

Teaching Points

Correct Answer: 4

The SACH foot is often used as a temporary prosthesis because it provides good initial utility at a lower cost. It provides for sagittal plane motion (primarily plantarflexion), but the heel cushion is compressed, and there is very limited frontal plane motion (mediolateral motion).

Incorrect Choices:

Articulated feet (joined by a metal bolt or cable to the lower shank section) have rubber bumpers that absorb shock and control plantarflexion excursion. An anterior stop resists dorsiflexion. Full sagittal and frontal plane motions are not allowed with a SACH foot.

Type of Reasoning: Analytical

One must recall the properties of a SACH foot in order to choose the correct solution. This requires knowledge of prostheses and their indications. The test-taker must analyze the information presented and determine the meaning of that information, which is an analytical reasoning skill. If this question was answered incorrectly, refer to information on properties of prosthetic feet.

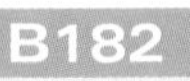

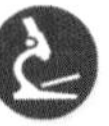

Neuromuscular | Evaluation, Diagnosis

A physical therapist examines an adult patient that recently suffered a stroke that involved the right internal capsule. In addition to hemiparesis of the contralateral extremities, the patient also exhibits a facial palsy. Which facial muscles would **MOST** likely be affected?

Choices:

1. All muscles on the left side of the face.
2. All muscles on the right side of the face.
3. Only muscles on the lower half of the right side of the face.
4. Only muscles on the lower half of the left side of the face.

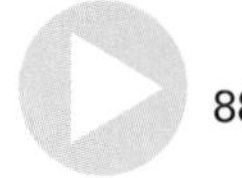

Teaching Points

Correct Answer: 4

A stroke that involves the internal capsule would result in a *supranuclear palsy*, which affects only the contralateral lower half of the face. The specific pathway that is affected is the corticobulbar tract, which contains upper motor neurons (UMN) that project from the motor cortex to the nucleus of the facial nerve (cranial nerve VII) in the brainstem. The muscles in the upper half of the face are spared because both the right and left cerebral cortex project to the lower motor neurons (LMNs) in the facial nucleus that innervate muscles of the forehead. In contrast, the LMNs that innervate muscles of the lower half of the face receive input from the contralateral motor cortex only. Therefore, a stroke that affects the internal capsule (corticobulbar tract) prevents input from the motor cortex to the contralateral facial nucleus, causing paresis or paralysis of the muscles of the lower half of the face only.

Incorrect Choices:

A lesion that affects all muscles on the left side of the face is consistent with an LMN or peripheral nerve lesion, such as Bell's palsy or trauma to the left facial nerve. A complete LMN lesion to the right CN VII would prevent motor commands from reaching all ipsilateral facial muscles, resulting in facial paralysis of those muscles. A lesion that affects the left internal capsule or corticobulbar tract would affect only muscles on the lower half of the right side of the face.

Type of Reasoning: Deductive

This question requires the test-taker to recall guidelines for the muscles of the face that are most likely to be affected by a stroke involving the internal capsule. Questions that necessitate the recall of facts often utilize deductive reasoning skill. For this case, muscles on the lower half of the left side of the face are most likely to be affected. Review information regarding strokes impacting the internal capsule and facial palsy if answered incorrectly.

B183 

Cardiovascular/Pulmonary | Examination

A patient in the ICU is referred to physical therapy and presents with significant shortness of breath. A chest x-ray demonstrates a deviated trachea to the left. Which of the following processes would account for such a finding?

Choices:

1. Right lung collapse.
2. Left pleural effusion.
3. Right hemothorax.
4. Left pneumothorax.

Teaching Points

Correct Answer: 3

A right hemothorax (blood was in the pleural space) takes up space in the right hemithorax, shifting the trachea to the left.

Incorrect Choices:

A left pneumothorax and a left pleural effusion take up space in the left thorax. The air (pneumothorax) or the sterile fluid (effusion) in the pleural space would push contents of the left hemithorax, including the trachea, to the right. A lung collapse, or a volume loss phenomenon, on the right would pull the trachea over toward the right.

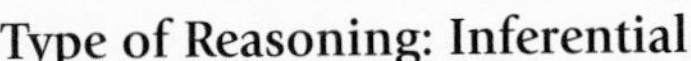

Type of Reasoning: Inferential

This question requires the test-taker to make a determination for the patient's symptoms, which necessitates use of inferential reasoning. In this situation, the deviated trachea to the left is due to a right hemothorax. One must rely on knowledge of pulmonary pathology to arrive at a correct conclusion, which should be reviewed if this question was answered incorrectly.

B184 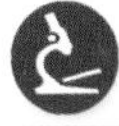

Nonsystem | Therapeutic Modalities

A physical therapist is using neuromuscular electrical stimulation to facilitate quadriceps strength after a total knee replacement. Which is the best combination of parameters to promote strengthening using 10–15 repetitions at 80% of their maximum voluntary isometric contractions?

Choices:

1. 5 pulses per sec (pps), Russian stimulation.
2. 15 pps, Russian stimulation.
3. 35 pps, 50 μs pulse duration with a biphasic pulsed waveform.
4. 35 pps, 250 μs pulse duration with a biphasic pulsed waveform.

Teaching Points

Correct Answer: 4

There are multiple currents and waveforms (Russian or biphasic) that can be used to promote strength. The key is to have a high enough frequency and charge to achieve a smooth muscle contraction. Generally, a frequency of at least 30 pps with a pulse duration between 200 μs and 350 μs is recommended.

Incorrect Choices:

Although Russian stimulation is a good choice, the "frequencies" listed were too low (<30 pps) to produce a uniform muscle contraction. Additionally, it is important to remember that charge is a product of amplitude and duration. If the duration is too low, then a higher amplitude is needed to depolarize the nerve. A biphasic waveform with a 50 μs pulse duration is also too low, thus requiring a significant increase in amplitude.

Type of Reasoning: Deductive

For this question, one must recall the guidelines and parameters for use of neuromuscular electrical stimulation to facilitate a smooth muscle contraction. This necessitates the recall of factual information, which is a deductive reasoning skill. For this case, the best combination is 35 pps, 250 μs pulse duration with a biphasic pulsed waveform. If answered incorrectly, review neuromuscular electrical stimulation information, especially Russian and biphasic stimulation.

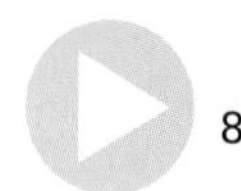

B185 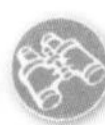

Musculoskeletal | Evaluation, Diagnosis

A patient described a sudden onset of back pain while trying to lift a heavy barrel. The patient described this pain as constant, unremitting at an intensity of 10/10 over the past 3 days, and unresponsive to pain medications. The patient is unable to work but is able to drive to the clinic for treatment unaided. There is no history of other back-related symptoms in the past. Which of the following is the **MOST** likely causative factor?

Choices:

1. Early degenerative osteoarthritis.
2. Herniated lumbar disc.
3. Neoplastic disease.
4. Secondary gain.

Teaching Points

Correct Answer: 4

A patient who is able to drive to the clinic for treatment and relates a pain level of 10/10 is not providing consistent subjective data. Secondary gain in this case, and not working, is a likely factor.

Incorrect Choices:

Pain from a disc pathology is typically worse in the morning and will decrease (at least slightly) when the patient gets out of bed and begins to walk around. The diagnosis is unlikely to be a neoplastic condition secondary to the acute, traumatic onset. Degenerative osteoarthritis is described as stiffness in the morning with worsening pain as the activity level increases throughout the day.

Type of Reasoning: Inductive

The test-taker must utilize diagnostic thinking and clinical judgment to determine the most likely cause for the patient's symptoms, which is an inductive reasoning skill. In this case, the patient's inconsistency in engagement in activities (driving but not being able to work) most likely has secondary gain involved. If this question was answered incorrectly, review information on secondary gain in patient care.

B186 

Cardiovascular/Pulmonary | Evaluation, Diagnosis

After myocardial infarction (MI), a patient was placed on medications that included a beta-adrenergic blocking agent. When monitoring this patient's response to exercise, what changes in HR are expected?

Choices:

1. Increase proportionally to changes in diastolic BP.
2. Low at rest and rises very little with exercise.
3. Increase proportionally to changes in systolic BP.
4. Low at rest and rises linearly as a function of increasing workload.

Teaching Points

Correct Answer: 2

Beta-adrenergic blocking agents (e.g., propranolol [Inderal]) are used to treat hypertension, prevent angina pectoris, and prevent certain arrhythmias. In individuals taking these drugs, HR is low at rest and rises very little with exercise (blunted response). These changes, therefore, invalidate the use of HR to monitor exercise responses. A more sensitive measure would be RPE.

Incorrect Choices:

HR does not rise linearly with exercise in patients on propranolol. The medication is used for treatment of hypertension. Both resting and exercise BP are suppressed.

Type of Reasoning: Analytical

This question requires one to recall the indications for beta-adrenergic agents and effects on cardiovascular function. This requires one to interpret information and determine the meaning of that information, which necessitates analytical reasoning skill. If this question was answered incorrectly, review information on effects of beta-blockers on cardiovascular function.

B187 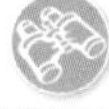

Musculoskeletal I Interventions

An individual presents with chronic TMJ dysfunction. There is limited lateral movement of the mandible to the right as a result of muscular tightness. Which of the following muscles should be the focus of inhibitory or soft tissue lengthening techniques?

Choices:

1. Right temporalis muscle.
2. Right geniohyoid muscle.
3. Right medial pterygoid muscle.
4. Right digastric muscle.

Teaching Points

Correct Answer: 3

Lateral excursion of the mandible is produced by the contralateral medial and lateral pterygoids and ipsilateral temporalis muscles. Tightness of the ipsilateral pterygoids or contralateral temporalis muscles may need lengthening in order to allow full lateral mandibular excursion. The right medial pterygoid would be one of the muscles targeted for interventions restoring sufficient length.

Incorrect Choices:

The digastrics and geniohyoid muscles are mandibular depressors and would not be targets for muscle lengthening techniques. The left temporalis may need lengthening.

Type of Reasoning: Inductive

One must use clinical judgment to determine a best course of action in order to arrive at a correct conclusion. This often necessitates inductive reasoning skill. For this case, the therapist should focus treatment on the right medial pterygoid muscle to restore length. Review treatment approaches for TMJ dysfunction if answered incorrectly.

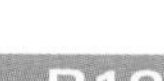
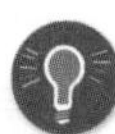

B188

Metabolic/Endocrine | Interventions

A patient has a 20-year history of diabetes. The patient exhibits vascular insufficiency and diminished sensation of both feet with poor healing of a superficial skin lesion. It is important that the patient understand the precautions and guidelines on foot care for people with diabetes. Which recommendation is **CONTRAINDICATED** to include in patient care instructions?

Choices:

1. Inspect the skin daily for inflammation, swelling, redness, blisters, or wounds.
2. Wash the feet daily and hydrate with moisturizing lotion.
3. Wear flexible shoes that allow adequate room and change shoes frequently.
4. Use daily hot soaks and moisturize the skin.

Teaching Points

Correct Answer: 4

The patient's examination findings are consistent with diabetic polyneuropathy and peripheral arterial disease. Daily hot soaks are contraindicated because of the increased risk of thermal injury.

Incorrect Choices:

All other instructions are correct and important to include in a well-balanced program of foot care.

Type of Reasoning: Inferential

This question requires one to determine the recommendation to a patient with diabetes that is contraindicated. In this circumstance, one should **NOT** recommend hot soaks because of the risk of thermal injury from loss of protective sensations in the feet. Questions that require one to draw conclusions and formulate opinions based on information presented encourage use of inferential reasoning. If this question was answered incorrectly, refer to guidelines for diabetic foot care.

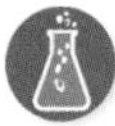

B189

Musculoskeletal | Evaluation, Diagnosis

A patient is seen in a direct access physical therapy clinic with a complaint of left thumb pain after a fall sustained while skiing. The patient also complains of an inability to grip due to painful weakness. During the physical examination, the physical therapist notes marked swelling and ecchymosis of the thumb, along with limited range of motion, weakness, and valgus instability of the metacarpophalangeal joint. Which is the **MOST LIKELY** diagnosis for this patient's injury?

Choices:

1. Boxer's fracture.
2. Colles' fracture.
3. Scaphoid fracture.
4. Gamekeeper's thumb.

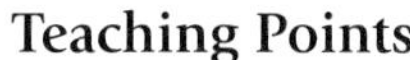

Teaching Points

Correct Answer: 4

Gamekeeper's thumb is a sprain/rupture of the ulnar collateral ligament of the MCP joint of the thumb. It is also known as skier's thumb. This injury frequently occurs during skiing when valgus forces are placed on the thumb by a ski pole when the hand makes contact with the ground after a fall. If not promptly diagnosed and treated with immobilization or surgery, this injury can cause chronic instability and loss of function.

Incorrect Choices:

A boxer's fracture involves the 4th or 5th metacarpal and is frequently sustained when punching a wall in anger or during a fight. A Colles' fracture typically occurs after a fall on an outstretched hand (FOOSH). It is a fracture of the distal radius with dorsal displacement of the distal fragment. A scaphoid fracture also typically results from a FOOSH mechanism of injury. Patients with scaphoid fractures complain of pain at the base of thumb or wrist region rather than in the MCP region as described in this case.

Type of Reasoning: Analytical

For this question, the test-taker must analyze the presenting symptoms and determine the most likely diagnosis. This necessitates analytical reasoning skill, where pieces of information are analyzed to draw a reasonable conclusion. For this case, the symptoms are most likely due to gamekeeper's thumb. If answered incorrectly, review information on gamekeeper's thumb (or skier's thumb).

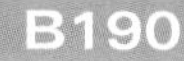
B190

Musculoskeletal | Interventions

A soccer player sustained a grade II inversion ankle sprain 2 weeks ago. What is the **BEST** intervention to use in the early subacute phase of rehabilitation?

Choices:

1. Mobilization at the talocrural and subtalar joints.
2. Closed-chain strengthening and proprioceptive exercises.
3. Plyometric-based exercise program.
4. Functional soccer-related drills.

Teaching Points

Correct Answer: 2

The most effective treatment for this athlete would involve closed-chain exercises and proprioceptive training, appropriate interventions for early subacute phase management. See Box 2-11 for the Ankle Ligament Sprains Clinical Practice Guideline.

Incorrect Choices:

The other choices are not appropriate or timely for early subacute phase management. These approaches may be useful later in the rehabilitation of this athlete.

Type of Reasoning: Inferential

One must infer or draw conclusions for the best early intervention approach, given the injury and knowledge of rehabilitation techniques for this injury. This requires inferential reasoning skill, in which the test-taker applies this knowledge and formulates conclusions about the patient for a best course of action. If this question was answered incorrectly, review information on early treatment for inversion ankle sprain.

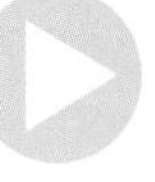

B191 

Nonsystem I Therapeutic Modalities

A patient is referred for outpatient care after a tendon transfer of the extensor carpi radialis longus. The muscle strength tests poor (2/5) in spite of previous intensive therapy. The therapist elects to apply biofeedback to assist in progressively increasing active motor recruitment. What is the **BEST** choice for the initial biofeedback protocol?

Choices:

1. High-detection sensitivity with recording electrodes placed far apart over the muscle belly.
2. Low-detection sensitivity with recording electrodes placed close together over the muscle belly.
3. High-detection sensitivity with recording electrodes placed close together over the musculotendinous junction.
4. Low-detection sensitivity with recording electrodes placed far apart over the musculotendinous junction.

Teaching Points

Correct Answer: 1

Initially, high-detection sensitivity is needed to detect low-amplitude signals generated by a small number of motor units such as in a weak extensor carpi radialis longus. Electrode placement: If the patient has poor muscle control, moving the electrodes apart can help sample a larger portion of the muscle. As the patient is able to recruit more motor units the electrodes can be moved closer together to decrease potential cross-talk from other motor units. Therapists can get the electrodes too far apart and should limit the distance to only the area they intend to sample.

Incorrect Choices:

Low-detection sensitivity may not pick up the necessary motor unit signals. Electrode placement should be placed over the motor units, not the musculotendinous junctions.

Type of Reasoning: Deductive

This question requires application of knowledge of EMG biofeedback protocols in order to determine the best approach to early biofeedback intervention. This encourages deductive reasoning skill, which encourages recall of factual knowledge of protocols to apply information to a specific case situation of extensor carpi radialis longus tendon transfer. If this question was answered incorrectly, review information on EMG biofeedback guidelines.

B192 

System Interactions I Evaluation, Diagnosis

A PT receives a home care referral from the nurse case manager. An elderly man has lost functional independence after the recent death of his wife. His past medical history includes stroke with minimal residual disability. Currently, he no longer goes out of his house and rarely even gets out of his chair anymore. During the initial session, the therapist determines that depression may be the cause of his increasing inactivity. What clinical signs and symptoms would lead the therapist to reach this determination?

Choices:

1. Low scores on the Geriatric Depression Scale.
2. Weight loss and social withdrawal.
3. Complaints of increasing dizziness and palpitations.
4. Sleep apnea and weight gain.

Teaching Points

Correct Answer: 2

Depression is associated with symptoms of withdrawal, fatigue, and weight loss.

Incorrect Choices:

Sleep apnea is a potentially lethal disorder in which breathing stops for 10 seconds or more, many times a night. It is associated with obesity and anatomical obstruction. Increasing dizziness and palpitations are suggestive of cardiovascular problems. The Geriatric Depression Scale is a valid measure of depression in the elderly. High, not low, scores (>8 of a possible 30) are indicative of depression.

Type of Reasoning: Inferential

One must recall the typical symptoms associated with depression in the elderly to arrive at the correct conclusion. This requires one to draw conclusions and make assumptions based on the information presented, which is an inferential reasoning skill. If this question was answered incorrectly, review symptoms of depression, especially symptoms in the elderly.

B193 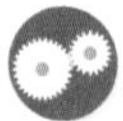

Genitourinary | Interventions

A physical therapist examines an adult female patient with a chief complaint of severe low back pain associated with abdominal discomfort. The patient also reports having missed her most recent period. There are no specific factors that aggravate or ease the 7 out of 10 low back pain, and the therapist is unable to reproduce the patient's symptoms. During the physical examination, the patient becomes diaphoretic and appears to be in shock. The therapist should do which of the following?

Choices:

1. Treat the patient with cryotherapy for pain relief and instruct the patient in a core strengthening program.
2. Refuse to treat the patient and immediately contact emergency medical services (EMS) for transport of the patient to the nearest emergency room.
3. Instruct the patient to go home for a trial of bed rest and NSAIDs as needed for pain and to return to the physical therapy clinic in 72 hours for a reassessment.
4. Instruct the patient to contact her primary care physician for further evaluation of her lower back pain.

Teaching Points

Correct Answer: 2

This scenario describes a woman with an ectopic pregnancy, which is an emergent condition. The classic triad of symptoms is severe low back pain, a missed period, and vaginal bleeding. Most ectopic pregnancies occur in the fallopian tubes and are called tubal pregnancies. A tubal pregnancy is a medical emergency as continued growth of the fetus may lead to rupture of the fallopian tube and potentially fatal intra-abdominal hemorrhage.

Incorrect Choices:

The other choices fail to address the urgency of the situation. Treating the patient or suggesting bed rest may be appropriate interventions for a musculoskeletal condition. However, none of the patient's clinical signs and symptoms are consistent with musculoskeletal pathology, and there are also clear signs of medical distress in this patient. Diaphoresis (excessive, abnormal sweating) should raise the suspicion of an emergent medical problem.

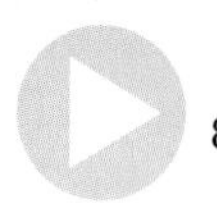

Type of Reasoning: Evaluative

For this question, the test-taker must analyze the patient's symptoms and determine the significance of them. Then, one must determine the best course of action. This necessitates evaluative reasoning skill, where presenting information is weighed to determine a best course of action. For this situation, the therapist should refuse to treat the patient and immediately contact EMS for transport of the patient to the nearest emergency room. If answered incorrectly, review information on ectopic pregnancy.

B194 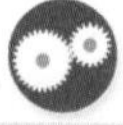

Cardiovascular/Pulmonary | Examination

A patient has been on bed rest for 4 days due to complications following a triple coronary artery bypass graft. During the first therapy session, the patient complains of tenderness and aching in the right calf. For what clinical signs should the therapist immediately examine?

Choices:

1. Lowered body temperature.
2. Bradycardia.
3. Swelling in the calf or ankle.
4. Capillary refill.

Teaching Points

Correct Answer: 3

Deep vein thrombophlebitis (DVT) is characterized by classic signs of inflammation (tenderness, aching, and swelling), typically in the calf. Rapid screening is possible with Doppler ultrasonography. Color flow venous duplex scanning is the primary diagnostic test for detection of DVT.

Incorrect Choices:

Tachycardia, not bradycardia, may be present. Slight fever can be present, as part of the inflammatory reaction, not lowered temperature. Delayed capillary refill is associated with decreased tissue perfusion and is seen in patients with dehydration or decreased blood flow.

Type of Reasoning: Evaluative

This question requires one to evaluate the approaches presented and determine which approach has the most merit, given the patient's current symptoms. This requires evaluative reasoning skill, in which the test-taker must weigh arguments and statements made and formulate a conclusion about the strength of these approaches. If this question was answered incorrectly, review symptomatology of DVT.

B195 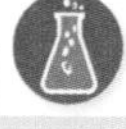

Systems Interaction | Evaluation, Diagnosis

A patient complains of diffuse joint and muscle pain. Recent medical history also includes an episode of kidney stones. During the examination the physical therapist notes that the patient appears drowsy and takes an unusually long time to process and answer questions. Which disorder is the most likely explanation for the patient's clinical presentation?

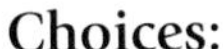

Choices:
1. Hypoparathyroidism.
2. Hyperparathyroidism.
3. Hypothyroidism.
4. Hyperthyroidism.

Teaching Points

Correct Answer: 2

The most common cause of hyperparathyroidism is a benign tumor of one or more of the parathyroid glands. Many body systems are affected by the disorder. The mnemonic "moans, groans, stones, and bones" covers many of the signs and symptoms associated with the disease. "Moans" denotes mental problems such as drowsiness, depression, confusion, and poor memory. "Groans" describes the arthralgia, myalgia, gout, and abdominal pain often seen in patients with the disease. Kidney "stones" or renal calculi often result from hypercalcemia. And "bones" are often affected in hyperparathyroidism (decalcification, pathologic fractures).

Incorrect Choices:

None of the other choices explains the combination of clinical findings described in the question stem. Hypoparathyroidism results in *hypocalcemia*, affecting many body tissues that are dependent on calcium for normal function. Manifestations of hypoparathyroidism include personality changes, cardiac arrhythmias, scaly skin, and brittle fingernails and toenails. Similarly, hypothyroidism and hyperthyroidism affect many systems and may result in a constellation of clinical findings, but not those described in the question stem. See the chapter on "Other Systems" for a complete description of these disorders.

Type of Reasoning: Analytical

For this question, the test-taker must analyze the symptoms presented and determine a likely diagnosis. This requires analytical reasoning skill, where pieces are information are weighed in order to determine significance and draw reasonable conclusions. For this situation, the most likely explanation for the patient's symptoms is hyperparathyroidism. Review information on hyperparathyroidism if answered incorrectly.

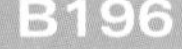

System Interactions | Evaluation, Diagnosis

An elderly patient is referred to physical therapy after a fall and open reduction internal fixation (ORIF) for a fracture of the right wrist. During the initial examination, the therapist observes that the patient's skin and eyes have a yellowish hue. What is the therapist's **BEST** course of action?

Choices:
1. Send a copy of the examination results to the referring surgeon, emphasizing the skin hue.
2. Treat the patient and reevaluate skin color posttreatment.
3. Continue with the treatment; a yellowish hue is an expected finding 3–4 days post-ORIF.
4. Document the findings and consult with the primary physician immediately after treatment.

Teaching Points

Correct Answer: 4

This patient is most likely experiencing jaundice as a result of liver dysfunction. The therapist's best course of action is to document the findings and consult with the primary physician immediately, preferably by phone.

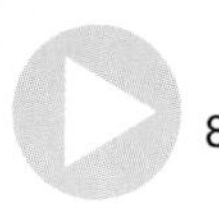

Incorrect Choices:

All other choices delay consulting with the primary physician. The symptoms indicate liver dysfunction and jaundice, which warrant immediate contact with the physician.

Type of Reasoning: Evaluative

The test-taker must determine first what the patient's symptoms are indicative of and then determine what should be the appropriate course of action. Questions such as these, in which value judgments must be made, encourage evaluative reasoning skill.

B197 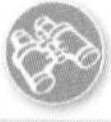

Musculoskeletal | Evaluation, Diagnosis

An older adult received a cemented total hip replacement (THR) 2 days ago. What is the therapist's initial priority?

Choices:

1. AROM exercises and early ambulation using a walker, non-weight-bearing.
2. PROM exercises and gait training using crutches, weight-bearing to tolerance.
3. Proper technique for transferring to the toilet.
4. Patient education regarding positions and movements to avoid.

Teaching Points

Correct Answer: 4

Education regarding positions and movements to avoid is the number one priority. Standard hip precautions stress avoiding excessive flexion, internal rotation, and adduction.

Incorrect Choices:

Patients with cemented THRs should initially be weight-bearing to tolerance using a walker. Transfer training should occur, but it is not the first initial priority.

Type of Reasoning: Inductive

One must utilize clinical judgment and diagnostic thinking (an inductive reasoning skill) to determine the number one priority for this patient with a recent THR. In this situation, it is important to educate the patient regarding positions and movements to avoid, which if not followed could cause potential dislocation of the hip. If this question was answered incorrectly, refer to guidelines for early care of patients with THR.

B198 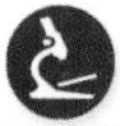

Musculoskeletal | Examination

A patient with recent trauma presents with restricted movement of the right hand. There is decreased motion at the third right PIP joint. To differentiate as to whether this is joint restriction or some other type of tightness (not joint), which examination procedure should be employed?

Choices:
1. Finkelstein's test.
2. Bunnel-Littler test.
3. Phalen's test.
4. Froment's sign.

Teaching Points

Correct Answer: 2

The Bunnel-Littler test is specifically utilized to determine if there is intrinsic or a joint capsule restriction present at the PIP joints.

Incorrect Choices:

Phalen's test is used to determine carpal tunnel compression at the median nerve. Finkelstein's test is used to assess for a tenosynovitis of the abductor pollicis longus and/or extensor pollicis brevis. Froment's sign is utilized to identify an ulnar nerve dysfunction.

Type of Reasoning: Deductive

This question provides a diagnosis, and the test-taker must recall the specific test that confirms the diagnosis. This necessitates factual recall of guidelines, which is a deductive reasoning skill. For this situation, the Bunnel-Littler test is the correct test to confirm joint restriction present at the PIP joints. Review differential testing for hand injuries if answered incorrectly, especially the Bunnel-Littler test.

B199 

Lymphatic | Interventions

A patient with stage II primary lymphedema of the right lower extremity is referred for physical therapy. Examination reveals increased limb girth with skin folds/flaps evident. An important component of lymphedema management is manual lymphatic drainage. Which of the following describes a cardinal principle of manual lymphedema management?

Choices:
1. Deep tissue friction massage for several minutes on fibrotic areas.
2. Decongesting the proximal portions of the limb first and working distally.
3. Decongesting the trunk after the limb segments.
4. Decongesting the distal portions of the limb first and working proximally.

Teaching Points

Correct Answer: 2

Lymphedema is a swelling of the soft tissues that occurs with an accumulation of protein-rich fluid in the extracellular spaces. Causes of primary lymphedema include developmental abnormalities, heredity, surgery, or unknown etiology. Stage II lymphedema is characterized by nonpitting edema with connective scar tissue and clinical fibrosis. Lymphatic drainage is assisted by manual stroking (e.g., Vodder, Leduc's, Foldi's, Casley-Smith pressure techniques). All techniques use cardinal principles: proximal limb segments before distal, trunk segments before limb segments, and directing the flow of the lymphatics centrally toward the lymphatic ducts.

Incorrect Choices:

The other choices do not adhere to the cardinal principles of lymphatic drainage as explained.

Type of Reasoning: Deductive

This question requires one to recall factual knowledge—that of manual lymphatic drainage techniques for patients with primary lymphedema. This encourages deductive reasoning skill, in which the test-taker must recall the protocols and guidelines for this technique. If this question was answered incorrectly, review information on manual lymphatic drainage techniques.

B200 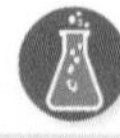

Nonsystem | Equipment, Devices

A patient with a history of diabetic polyneuropathy is referred to physical therapy after falling and sustaining a left ankle inversion sprain 6 weeks ago. On examination the patient exhibits a mildly antalgic gait and decreased sensation to light touch and monofilament testing in the bilateral plantar feet and toes. They have no edema, ankle ligamentous instability, weakness, or range of motion deficits in the lower extremities. What is the **MOST** appropriate device to improve this patient's community ambulation and participation?

Choices:

1. Rolling walker.
2. Ankle lace-up brace.
3. Controlled ankle motion (CAM) walking boot.
4. Cane.

Teaching Points

Correct Answer: 4

A cane would allow the patient to reduce up to 30% of weight-bearing on the involved extremity, thus improving the patient's antalgic gait. It would also provide ongoing somatosensory feedback to assist with any ataxia or balance impairments related to the patient's diabetic neuropathy. The cane can also be used on level and uneven terrain and is portable.

Incorrect Choices

The patient's impairments do not require a rolling walker. A rolling walker also limits community mobility with regards to curbs and stairs. An ankle lace-up brace and CAM walking boot would assist ankle stability but would not decrease weight-bearing on the involved limb. The ankle brace and walking boot would also limit ankle range of motion and do not address the sensory loss on the bilateral plantar feet and associated balance impairments and fall risk associated with diabetic polyneuropathy.

Type of Reasoning: Analytical

For this question, the test-taker must analyze the patient's symptoms in order to determine the most appropriate device to improve community ambulation and participation. This requires analytical reasoning skill, where pieces of information are weighed to draw reasonable conclusions. For this case, a cane is the most appropriate device. If answered incorrectly, review antalgic gait pattern and use of assistive devices.

Examination C

C1 

Cardiovascular/Pulmonary | Examination

A patient is hospitalized with an uncomplicated acute myocardial infarction (MI). Which graded exercise test (GXT) should be administered to this patient post-MI but before hospital discharge?

Choices:
1. Symptom-limited GXT at 10 days post-MI.
2. GXT to 70% age predicted HRmax 3–5 days post-MI.
3. GXT to 80% age predicted maximum HR 3–5 days post-MI.
4. GXT to 85% age predicted maximum HR 4–6 days post-MI.

Teaching Points

Correct Answer: 2

Submaximal GXT can be administered before hospital discharge 3–5 days post-acute MI. Low-level exercise testing provides data for recommendations for ADL and early ambulatory exercise therapy. This amount of activity doesn't place too much demand on the healing myocardium (see *ACSM Guidelines for Exercise Testing and Prescription*, 11th ed., 2021).

Incorrect Choices:

An intensity higher than 70% can extend the zone of necrosis into the zone of injury and/or zone of ischemia. This will delay healing or, in the worst case, extend the MI. Using symptoms alone may allow the patient to exercise at too high or too low an intensity.

Type of Reasoning: Inductive

This question requires one to draw on clinical knowledge and judgment of cardiac exercise guidelines for patients with post-myocardial infarction in order to arrive at a correct conclusion. This is an inductive reasoning skill where clinical judgment is paramount to arriving at a correct conclusion. For this case, a GXT at 70% age predicted HR max 3–5 days post-MI is safe. Review cardiac exercise testing guidelines for patients with myocardial infarction if answered incorrectly.

C2 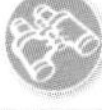

Neuromuscular | Examination

A newborn is examined at birth using the APGAR test. Which of the following APGAR results is a likely indicator of potential neurological complications?

Choices:
1. 3 at 10 minutes.
2. 9 at 1 minute.
3. 8 at 1 minute.
4. 8 at 5 minutes.

Teaching Points

Correct Answer: 1

The APGAR score is based on heart rate (HR), respiration, muscle tone, reflex irritability (grimace), and color (appearance). APGAR scores are routinely assigned at 1 and 5 minutes and occasionally at 10 minutes post-birth. Scores between 0 and 3 at 1 and 5 minutes are extremely low and indicative of the need for resuscitation. Neurological complications are likely with extremely low APGAR scores, particularly at 10 minutes.

Incorrect Choices:

The other choices are not indicative of abnormal findings.

Type of Reasoning: Inductive

The test-taker must make a determination of the meaning of the APGAR score as likely to result in neurological complications. This requires one to rely on knowledge of what the scale measures and of score ranges that indicate possible neurological complications. This requires clinical judgment coupled with recall of the properties of the scale, which is an inductive reasoning skill. If this question was answered incorrectly, refer to information on the APGAR Scale.

C3 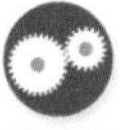

Nonsystem I Professional Responsibilities

A PT requested that a physical therapy assistant (PTA) perform ultrasound (US) to the shoulder of a patient. During the treatment session, the patient experienced an electrical shock. In which situation would the PT be directly responsible for any injury the patient might receive?

Choices:

1. Faulty circuitry.
2. The PTA failing to use a ground fault interrupter (GFI).
3. The patient touching the US device during treatment.
4. The PT having instructed the PTA to use a device that had malfunctioned on the previous day.

Teaching Points

Correct Answer: 4

The PT in this case correctly delegated the US treatment to the PTA. Every individual (PT, PTA) is liable for their own negligence; however, supervisors may assume liability of workers if they provide faulty supervision or inappropriate delegation of responsibilities (not evident in this case). PTs are liable for use of defective equipment if they contributed to its malfunction or continued to have it used in treatment without having it checked.

Incorrect Choices:

The institution may assume liability if the patient was harmed as a result of an environmental problem such as faulty circuitry or leakage current that would cause the patient to be shocked if they touched the US unit. The standard of practice is such that a GFI is used during administration of US, which would make the PTA primarily liable if a GFI was not used. The patient assumes no liability in this scenario.

Type of Reasoning: Evaluative

This question requires one to determine the value of the statements made in the question and then to determine the believability of these statements as applied to who should be assigned responsibility for the injury. This requires evaluative reasoning skill, in which beliefs and values must be weighed to arrive at a correct conclusion. In this situation, the PT should have taken the malfunctioning unit out of circulation to prevent anyone else from using it, thus making the PT primarily responsible.

C4 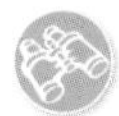

Cardiovascular/Pulmonary | Interventions

A patient with coronary artery disease received inpatient cardiac rehabilitation after a myocardial infarction (MI). The patient is now enrolled in an outpatient exercise class that utilizes intermittent training. What is the **BEST** initial spacing of exercise/rest intervals to safely stress the aerobic system?

Choices:

1. 5:1.
2. 1:1.
3. 10:1.
4. 2:1.

Teaching Points

Correct Answer: 4

Presuming that the exercise goals for inpatient cardiac rehabilitation are met, an exercise/rest ratio of 2:1 can be used with this patient to begin exercise in an outpatient setting in a safe manner.

Incorrect Choices:

An exercise/rest ratio of 1:1 is appropriate for an initial prescription for inpatient rehabilitation programs with a goal of achieving a 2:1 ratio. Ratios of 5:1 or 10:1 are too stressful to begin outpatient rehabilitation. A 5:1 ratio may be a goal for later exercise programming.

Type of Reasoning: Inductive

One must determine through clinical judgment which exercise/rest interval is **BEST,** given the patient's diagnosis and status. Questions that encourage clinical judgment to determine a best course of action require inductive reasoning skills. If this question was answered incorrectly, review information related to appropriate aerobic exercise and exercise/rest ratios for patients with coronary artery disease.

C5 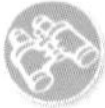

Musculoskeletal | Interventions

A physical therapist examines a patient who sustained an injury to their ring finger while playing football 3 days ago. The examination findings are consistent with a rupture of the flexor digitorum profundus tendon (jersey finger). What should the therapist do **FIRST**?

Choices:

1. Referral to a hand surgeon.
2. Splinting with finger in extension.
3. Buddy taping to the little finger.
4. Strengthening exercises.

Teaching Points

Correct Answer: 1

Jersey finger is a rupture or avulsion fracture of the flexor digitorum profundus tendon at the insertion on the distal phalanx. After injury, the tendon retracts and may lose its blood supply from both the bone and vincular system. Timely referral (within 7–10 days of injury) to a surgeon is paramount to avoid necrosis of the tendon.

Incorrect Choices:

Splinting and buddy taping are appropriate treatment options for soft-tissue injuries of the fingers such as collateral ligament sprains and volar plate injuries but are inappropriate for this type of injury. Strengthening exercises are not recommended acutely in the treatment of muscle or tendon ruptures.

Type of Reasoning: Inductive

For this question, the test-taker must recall effective intervention approaches for individuals with jersey finger in order to arrive at a correct conclusion. This requires inductive reasoning skill where clinical judgment is pivotal for making a correct choice. For this situation, the best initial treatment is referral to a hand surgeon. If answered incorrectly, review jersey finger injuries and treatment approaches.

C6 

Musculoskeletal | Interventions

A patient seeks physical therapy with a chief complaint of low back pain with radiation into the buttock, posterior thigh, and calf. Physical examination findings include peripheralization of symptoms on extension of the lumbar spine and a positive crossed straight leg raise test. Based on these examination findings, the therapist determines that the patient will respond favorably to which treatment approach?

Choices:

1. Stabilization exercises.
2. Spinal manipulation.
3. Lumbar traction.
4. Extension exercises.

Teaching Points

Correct Answer: 3

The examination findings meet the clinical prediction rule (CPR) criteria for identifying patients with low back pain who respond favorably to lumbar traction. The other variable that is a part of the CPR is the presence of signs of nerve root compression. See Box 2-16 for the Low Back Pain Clinical Practice Guideline.

Incorrect Choices:

The treatment-based classification system identifies subgroups of patients thought to respond to specific conservative physical therapy interventions. Each of the other treatments listed as answer choices have specific clinical examination findings associated with them. For a thorough description of each of these CPRs, see Cleland JA, Koppenhaver S, Su J: Netter's Orthopaedic Clinical Examination, 3rd edition, 2016.

Type of Reasoning: Inferential

For this question, the test-taker must analyze the symptoms presented in order to determine the best treatment approach for the condition. This requires inferential reasoning skill, where one must use predictive ability to draw sound conclusions. For this scenario, the best treatment approach is lumbar traction. Review low back pain treatment-based classification approach and corresponding CPRs if answered incorrectly.

C7

Musculoskeletal | Examination

A patient has fixed forefoot varus malalignment. What possible compensatory motion or posture might occur?

Choices:

1. Excessive subtalar pronation.
2. Ipsilateral pelvic external rotation.
3. Hallux varus.
4. Genu recurvatum.

Teaching Points

Correct Answer: 1

Possible compensatory motions or postures for forefoot varus malalignment include excessive midtarsal or subtalar pronation or prolonged pronation; plantarflexed first ray; hallux valgus; or excessive tibial; tibial and femoral; tibial, femoral, and pelvic internal rotation; and/or all with contralateral lumbar spine rotation.

Incorrect Choices:

The other compensatory motions or deformities are **NOT** typical of this problem.

Type of Reasoning: Inferential

This question provides the diagnosis, and the test-taker must determine what compensatory motions or postures are likely to occur. Questions that challenge one to determine possible symptoms from a given diagnosis require inferential reasoning skill. If this question was answered incorrectly, refer to information on forefoot varus malalignment.

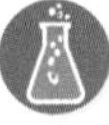

C8

Integumentary | Evaluation, Diagnosis

A patient presents with fingertips that are rounded and bulbous. The nail plate is more convex than normal. These changes are the likely result of which condition?

Choices:

1. Psoriasis.
2. Chronic hypoxia from heart disease.
3. Inflammation of the proximal and lateral nail folds.
4. Trauma to the nail bed.

Teaching Points

Correct Answer: 2

Chronic hypoxia from heart disease, lung cancer, or hepatic cirrhosis leads to clubbing of the fingers, characterized by fingertips that are rounded and bulbous and a nail plate that is more convex than normal.

Incorrect Choices:

Inflammation to the proximal and lateral nail folds (paronychia) is characterized by red, swollen, and tender folds. Trauma to the nail bed commonly results in white spots that grow out slowly with the nail. Psoriasis can result in small pits in the nails along with a circumscribed yellowish tan discoloration (oil spot lesion).

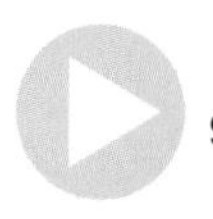

Type of Reasoning: Analytical

For this question, the test-taker must analyze the symptoms and draw a conclusion regarding the likely diagnosis. This requires analytical reasoning skill. For this case, the symptoms are indicative of chronic hypoxia from heart disease. Review symptoms of chronic hypoxia if answered incorrectly.

C9 

Lymphatic | Examination

As part of a physical examination of a patient with shoulder pain, a physical therapist palpates the patient's supraclavicular lymph nodes. Which examination finding would make the therapist suspicious of serious pathology?

Choices:

1. Freely moveable lymph nodes.
2. Tenderness in one or more nodes.
3. Soft to firm consistency of the lymph nodes.
4. Size of lymph nodes less than 1 cm.

Teaching Points

Correct Answer: 2

Lymph nodes are evaluated on the basis of size, consistency, mobility, and tenderness. Tenderness in a lymph node may be a sign of inflammation, infection, or metastatic cancer. Tender, soft lymph nodes that move easily are characteristic of inflammation or infection. Hard, immobile lymph nodes are typically indicative of metastatic cancers. Generally, changes in size, shape, tenderness, and consistency of a lymph node should raise a red flag.

Incorrect Choices:

Lymph nodes that are up to 1 cm in diameter are of soft-to-firm consistency, and move freely and easily without tenderness are considered within normal limits. See Chapter 4 for a comprehensive description of physical examination of the lymphatic system to include lymph node palpation.

Type of Reasoning: Inferential

For this question, one must determine which lymph node examination finding would be suspicious of serious pathology. This requires inferential reasoning skill where the test-taker must determine what is likely to be true of a situation. In this situation, tenderness in one or more node would be suspicious of serious pathology. If answered incorrectly, review lymphatic information, especially examination of lymph nodes.

C10 

Neuromuscular | Evaluation, Diagnosis

A patient is referred to physical therapy with a diagnosis of myalgic encephomyelitis/chronic fatigue syndrome. The therapist structures the examination of the patient to investigate a primary symptom (core symptom) of this illness. Which of the following **BEST** describes the expected fatigue pattern?

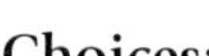

Choices:

1. Afternoon fatigue that leads to impaired functional performance late in the day.
2. Overwhelming fatigue with usual activity that is not improved by rest.
3. Exhaustive fatigue that results in impaired cognition and perception.
4. Overwhelming fatigue with intensive activity that is relieved by prolonged bed rest.

Teaching Points

Correct Answer: 2

The three primary symptoms (core symptoms) of this illness include overwhelming fatigue not relieved by rest and lasting 6 months or longer, a drop-in activity level that occurs along with the fatigue and is accompanied by postexertional malaise (PEM), and sleep problems. In addition to these core symptoms, patients may experience problems with thinking and memory, and orthostatic intolerance.

Incorrect Choices:

Fatigue occurs throughout the day (not only in the afternoon) and can occur with any level of physical activity. Impaired cognition (not a core symptom) can occur but not typically perception. Intensive activity is not necessary to produce fatigue. Even minimal activity can result in PEM.

Type of Reasoning: Inferential

For this question, the test-taker must infer or determine what is likely to be true and consistent with a specific diagnosis. This requires inferential reasoning skill. For this case, a diagnosis of myalgic encephomyelitis/chronic fatigue syndrome would present with overwhelming fatigue with usual activity that is not improved by rest. Review information about chronic fatigue syndrome if answered incorrectly.

C11 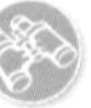

Cardiovascular/Pulmonary | Examination

A patient has an episode of syncope in the physical therapy clinic. The therapist attempts to rule out orthostatic hypotension as the cause of the fainting. What is the **BEST** test protocol to use?

Choices:

1. Palpate the carotid arteries and take resting HR and BP in the supine position.
2. Take resting HR and BP in supine, then in sitting after 2 minutes, then in standing after 2 minutes.
3. Take resting HR and BP in supine, then after 5 minutes in semi-Fowler postion.
4. Take resting HR and BP in supine, then after 2 minutes in standing.

Teaching Points

Correct Answer: 2

Orthostatic hypotension is a fall in BP with elevation of position; thus responses to movements (HR and BP) are tested from supine to sitting or sitting to standing. A small increase or no increase in HR upon standing may suggest baroreflex impairment. An exaggerated increase in HR upon standing may indicate volume depletion.

Incorrect Choices:

The other choices do not challenge the system with adequate change of position (semi-Fowler). Five minutes is too long to wait to take HR and BP upon standing.

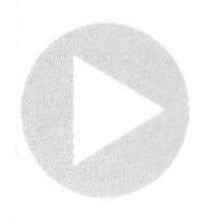

Type of Reasoning: Inductive

One must determine through clinical judgment the **BEST** method to rule out orthostatic hypotension. This requires knowledge of the nature of orthostatic hypotension and how it can be evaluated, which requires inductive reasoning skills. In this case, checking resting BP and HR in sitting and repeating after 2 minutes of standing is the **BEST** way to rule out the diagnosis.

C12 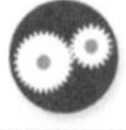

Integumentary | Evaluation, Diagnosis

An inpatient with a grade III diabetic foot ulcer is referred for physical therapy. Panafil has been applied to the necrotic tissue BID. The wound has no foul smell; however, the therapist notes a green tinge on the dressing. What is the **BEST** action for the therapist to take?

Choices:

1. Fit the patient with a total contact cast.
2. Document the finding and contact the physician immediately.
3. Begin a trial of acetic acid to the wound.
4. Document the finding and continue with treatment.

Teaching Points

Correct Answer: 4

In this case, the therapist should document the findings and continue with treatment. Panafil is a keratolytic enzyme used for selective debridement. A greenish or yellowish exudate can be expected.

Incorrect Choices:

If the exudate was green and had a foul smell, *Pseudomonas aeruginosa* should be suspected. If there are concerns of infection, the physician should be contacted to discuss further management to include a different topical agent and/or oral medication. Acetic acid would not be the topical agent of choice. A total contact cast can be used only after the wound is free of necrotic tissue.

Type of Reasoning: Evaluative

The test-taker must determine the significance of the information presented and evaluate the best course of action, given this information. This requires evaluative reasoning skill, in which one must assign value to the patient's wound status and judge how to proceed.

C13 

Neuromuscular | Evaluation, Diagnosis

A patient is referred for evaluation and treatment for functional neurological disorder (conversion disorder). The patient reports progressive fatigue, visual changes, and diffuse sensory loss and weakness over the past 6 months. On examination the patient has diffuse sensory loss with vibration and monofilament testing in the left foot and right forearm, hand, and fingers. Increase in tone in the left posterior leg muscles and six-beat ankle clonus is also present. Which of the following health conditions is **MOST** consistent with the patient's signs and symptoms?

Choices:
1. Amyotrophic lateral sclerosis.
2. Polyneuropathy.
3. Myasthenia gravis.
4. Multiple sclerosis.

Teaching Points

Correct Answer: 4

The presence of fatigue, visual changes, and diffuse sensory loss and central nervous system weakness is most consistent with multiple sclerosis (MS). MS results in demyelination of various areas of the central nervous system and can present with diffuse symptoms that are sometimes misdiagnosed as functional neurological disorder.

Incorrect Choices:

Amyotrophic lateral sclerosis results in upper and lower motor neuron findings but does not explain the patient's visual changes and sensory loss. Polyneuropathy typically involves bilateral distal extremity motor, sensory, and autonomic impairments without UMN involvement. Myasthenia gravis results in visual changes secondary to mild ptosis, fatigue, and ultimately weakness in multiple muscles in the bilateral upper and lower extremities but does not result in UMN involvement. See Table 3-25 for a comparison of examination findings in various types of neuromuscular disorders.

Type of Reasoning: Analytical

For this question, the test-taker must analyze the symptoms presented and determine the health condition that is most consistent with these symptoms. This requires analytical reasoning skill where pieces of information are analyzed to draw reasonable conclusions. For this case, the symptoms are most consistent with MS. Review symptoms of MS, if answered incorrectly.

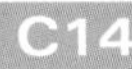

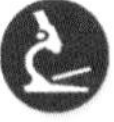

Nonsystem I Professional Responsibilities

An uninsured 48-year-old patient seeing a physical therapist for knee pain inquires about insurance options. The patient's employer has a total of eight employees and the patient does not receive health care benefits through his workplace. The patient's income is above the poverty line. The patient has a past medical history of end-stage renal disease. Based on the information above, which of the following third-party payers is **BEST** to recommend for this patient?

Choices:
1. Private health insurance.
2. Medicare.
3. Worker's compensation.
4. Medicaid.

Teaching Points

Correct Answer: 2

Medicare typically covers people over 65 years of age. However, it will also cover individuals with end-stage renal disease, regardless of age.

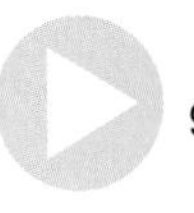

Incorrect Answers:

Privately purchased health insurance may be a possibility, but the cost of out-of-pocket expenses in privately purchased insurance would be much greater than for people managing end-stage renal disease through Medicare. Worker's compensation is only available through workplaces that have more than 10 employees. Medicaid offers health benefits to patients that are poor, disabled, or elderly. This patient does not meet any of those criteria.

Type of Reasoning: Deductive

This question requires the test-taker to recall criteria for insurance eligibility in order to arrive at a correct conclusion. This is factual recall of information, which is a deductive reasoning skill. For this situation, because the patient has end-stage renal disease, the patient qualifies for Medicare coverage. If answered incorrectly, review types of insurance coverage, especially Medicare coverage guidelines.

C15 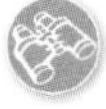

Musculoskeletal | Interventions

A high school student sustains a wrist injury after slipping on ice and falling with an outstretched hand. The patient reports that the wrist swelled immediately. The physical therapist's examination revealed tenderness with palpation in the anatomical snuff box and at the palmar aspect of the base of the thumb. What is the **BEST** initial treatment for this injury?

Choices:

1. Range of motion exercises.
2. Wrist strengthening exercises.
3. Cryotherapy several times a day.
4. Immobilization.

Teaching Points

Correct Answer: 4

This question describes a typical mechanism of injury and physical examination findings consistent with a scaphoid fracture. Timely intervention for this injury is critical. The patient should be immobilized and referred to the primary care provider or emergency room with the recommendation to order radiographs. Failure to properly manage a fractured scaphoid may result in avascular necrosis of the bone due to its poor vascular supply. A thumb-spica cast is indicated for 4–8 weeks for a scaphoid fracture.

Incorrect Choices:

Range of motion and strengthening exercises would be appropriate after the cast has been removed, but not in the initial stages. Cryotherapy is indicated but only provides temporary, symptomatic relief for the injury.

Type of Reasoning: Inductive

This question provides symptoms, and the test-taker must determine the best initial treatment approach based on knowledge of the diagnosis and treatment guidelines. This requires clinical judgment, which is an inductive reasoning skill. For this case, the best initial treatment is immobilization. Review treatment guidelines for scaphoid fractures if answered incorrectly.

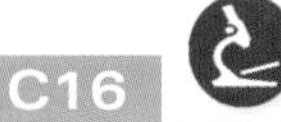

C16

Neuromuscular | Evaluation, Diagnosis

A parent is concerned about how her child is walking. The child just began walking in the past month, at 11 months of age. After the physical therapy examination, it is determined that the child has a normal gait pattern for a "new walker." Which of the following would **MOST LIKELY** confirm this finding?

Choices:

1. Anterior pelvic tilt, hips abducted, shoulders in abduction, bilateral genu varum.
2. Neutral hip flexion/extension, no longitudinal arch noted, hips externally rotated.
3. Bilateral genu valgum, no heel strike, minimal arm swing, posterior pelvic tilt.
4. Hip internal rotation, anterior pelvic tilt, shoulders in flexed position.

Teaching Points

Correct Answer: 1

"New Walkers" have an anterior pelvic tilt, with hips in flexion, abduction, and external rotation. Their arms are held in "high guard" position, with the shoulders abducted and slightly forward as they try to balance and are ready to catch themselves if they fall. Bowlegged (genu varum) is normal, although parents typically do not realize this and may be concerned.

Incorrect Choices:

New walkers do not have longitudinal arches yet and hips are in external rotation, but they have hip flexion and would not be in neutral. Genu varum is typical, not genu valgum. They do not have a heel strike yet, nor will they have any arm swing, and their pelvis is in an anterior tilt. Hip external rotation is typical.

Type of Reasoning: Deductive

For this question, the test-taker must recall typical positioning of a child who is a "new walker." This is factual information, which is a deductive reasoning skill. In this case, the child would most likely display anterior pelvic tilt, hip abduction, shoulder abduction, and bilateral genu varum. If answered incorrectly, review information on motor development in infants, especially walking skill and positioning.

C17 

Cardiovascular/Pulmonary | Evaluation, Diagnosis

A physical therapist is treating a recently extubated patient with COPD in the medical ICU. The most recent arterial blood gas analysis includes:
Fraction of inspired oxygen (FiO_2): 0.21
Arterial partial pressure of oxygen (PaO_2): 73 mmHg
Arterial partial pressure of carbon dioxide: 64 mmHg
pH = 7.28
Bicarbonate (HCO_3^-): 24 mEq/L
What do these findings indicate?

Choices:

1. Metabolic alkalosis.
2. Respiratory alkalosis.
3. Metabolic acidosis.
4. Respiratory acidosis.

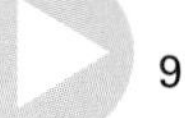

Teaching Points

Correct Answer: 4

The pH is low (normal range 7.35–7.45), indicating acidosis. Carbon dioxide and pH have an inverse relationship. Carbon dioxide is considered an acid; as it increases, the pH decreases, which is observed here. Therefore, this is characterized as respiratory acidosis. See Table 5-5 for a review of acid-base values and relationships.

Incorrect Choices:

A pH lower than normal is acidosis, not alkalosis, which eliminates those choices. Bicarbonate is considered a base and has a linear relationship with pH. If the bicarbonate increases, the pH increases. This did not occur in this case, so there is not a metabolic cause for this patient's abnormality.

Type of Reasoning: Analytical

For this question, the test-taker must analyze the arterial blood gas results in order to determine what the findings most likely indicate. This requires analytical reasoning skill, where pieces of information are examined in order to reach a sound conclusion. In this case, the findings are consistent with respiratory acidosis. If answered incorrectly, review arterial blood gas normal ranges and respiratory acidosis guidelines.

C18

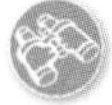

Neuromuscular | Evaluation, Diagnosis

New goals are being set for a child that was born at 28 weeks gestational age. The child is now 1-year-old chronologically. The child is functioning well at this corrected age; however, physical therapy is trying to "catch him up" to his chronological age. Which of the following gross motor skills would be **MOST** appropriate as a new goal?

Choices:

1. Sitting on the floor independently.
2. Creeping.
3. Belly crawling.
4. Transitioning into sitting.

Teaching Points

Correct Answer: 2

A typical gestational age is 40 weeks. So this child was born 12 weeks early (40 – 28 = 12 weeks). At 1 year-of-age, the child's corrected age is 9 months (12 months – 3 months [12 weeks = 3 months]). Teaching the child to creep (crawl on hands and knees), which occurs around 8–9 months would be appropriate. See Table 9-1 for Pediatric Developmental Sequence Summary.

Incorrect Choices:

Sitting independently occurs typically around 6 months of age. Belly crawling is typically around 5–7 months of age. Transitioning into sit is around 6–7 months of age.

Type of Reasoning: Inductive

For this question, the test-taker must recall the developmental age of each gross motor skill presented and determine which skill is most appropriate as a new goal. This necessitates inductive reasoning skill where clinical judgment is a key aspect to drawing reasonable conclusions. Given the gestational age of the child and the goal to catch up the child to his chronological age, the therapist should choose creeping as a goal. If answered incorrectly, review developmental milestones for infants, especially gross motor skills.

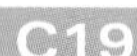
C19
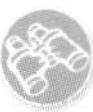

Nonsystem | Safety and Protection

A patient is ambulatory with Lofstrand crutches and is being seen at an outpatient physical therapy clinic with the device pictured below. The patient is diagnosed with mild paraparesis and incontinence secondary to a stroke. In order to strengthen this patient's hip flexors and knee extensors, which position would **BEST** accomplish the goal?

Choices:

1. Sidelying.
2. Sitting.
3. Supine with the patient flat.
4. Supine with head of the treatment table elevated.

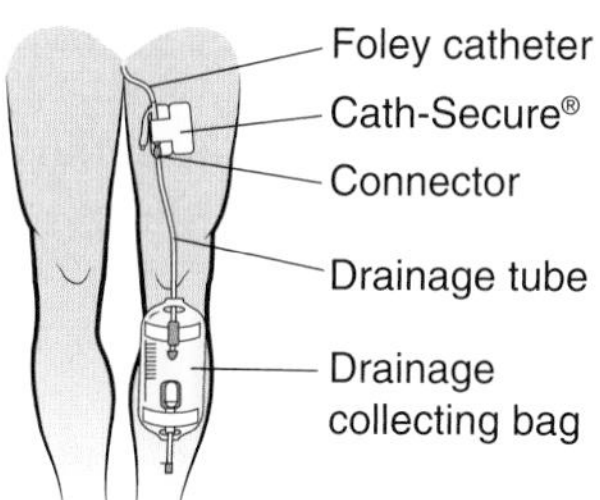

Teaching Points

Correct Answer: 2

This patient is attached to a Foley® catheter. The urinary collecting bag must remain below the level of the bladder to prevent reflux. The only position that will keep the bag below that level is to perform hip flexion and knee extension exercises in sitting. Active, active-assistive, or resistive exercises can be performed in this position as required.

Incorrect Choices:

Performing these exercises in the supine position, regardless of whether the patient's head and trunk are elevated, will still result in the collecting bag relocating above the bladder while performing hip flexion. Sidelying positioning results in the same dilemma. Gravity-dependency is necessary for proper drainage when a patient is catheterized.

Type of Reasoning: Inductive

This question requires the test-taker to utilize clinical judgment in order to determine a best course of action, based on the information presented. This necessitates inductive reasoning skill, where knowledge of clinical guidelines and approaches are paramount to arriving at a correct conclusion. For this case, the therapist should perform the exercises in sitting in order to keep the urinary collection bag below the bladder. If answered incorrectly, be sure to review guidelines for positioning patients with urinary collection bags.

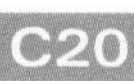
C20

Musculoskeletal | Interventions

During surgery to remove an apical lung tumor, the long thoracic nerve was injured. Muscle testing of the serratus anterior demonstrates its strength to be 3+/5. What is the **BEST** initial exercise for this patient?

Choices:

1. Standing wall push-ups.
2. Standing arm overhead lifts using hand weights.
3. Supine arm overhead lifts using weights.
4. Sitting arm overhead lifts using a weighted pulley.

Teaching Points

Correct Answer: 1

The long thoracic nerve supplies the serratus anterior muscle. With a muscle grade of 3+/5, the patient can begin functional strengthening using standing wall push-ups, with resistance provided by the patient's own body.

Incorrect Choices:

The other exercises would not be optimal or used **INITIALLY** for strengthening a fair plus serratus anterior. Performing overhead exercises with resistance (weights or pulleys) will overload the weakened serratus anterior muscle, causing the patient to compensate and potentially develop inappropriate movement patterns.

Type of Reasoning: Analytical

One must recall innervations for the long thoracic nerve in order to arrive at the correct conclusion. This requires analysis of the information presented and interpretation of that information, which requires analytical reasoning skill. Knowledge of neuropathology is helpful to arrive at the correct conclusion. If this question was answered incorrectly, review appropriate exercises for serratus anterior strengthening.

C21

Musculoskeletal | Evaluation, Diagnosis

A physical therapist evaluates a patient with chronic hip pain. After completing the history and physical examination, the therapist's differential diagnosis includes hip osteoarthritis and femoroacetabular impingement. Which clinical finding is **MOST** helpful to rule in the diagnosis of femoroacetabular impingement syndrome?

Choices:

1. Mechanical symptoms such as popping and snapping.
2. Morning stiffness.
3. Pain with hip internal rotation at 90° of flexion.
4. Report of anterior or lateral hip pain.

Teaching Points

Correct Answer: 1

Femoroacetabular impingement syndrome (FAI) falls within the overall category of nonarthritic hip joint pain. Although there is no consensus on diagnostic criteria, the determination of the disorder is based on a combination of imaging and clinical findings. Diagnosis of FAI is suspected with the following clinical and radiographic findings: anterior groin or hip pain reproduced by FADIR or FABER special tests, hip internal rotation less than 20° at 90° flexion, mechanical symptoms (popping, snapping), and imaging findings of a cam (femoral head) or pincer (acetabulum) deformities.

Incorrect Choices:

Morning stiffness, pain with internal rotation at 90° flexion, and complaints of anterior or lateral hip joint pain are all signs or symptoms associated with hip osteoarthritis. See Box 2-1 for the Hip Pain/Hip Osteoarthritis Clinical Practice Guideline and Box 2-4 for the Nonarthritic Hip Joint Pain Clinical Practice Guidelines.

Type of Reasoning: Inferential

For this question, the test-taker must determine which clinical finding will be most helpful in ruling out a specific diagnosis. This necessitates inferential reasoning skill, where the test-taker must determine what is likely to be true of a scenario. In this situation, mechanical symptoms such as popping and snapping are most helpful to rule out the diagnosis of FAI. Review information on FAI syndrome, especially clinical findings, if answered incorrectly.

C22 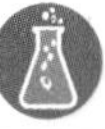

Integumentary | Examination

A patient recovering from a burn on the back of the hand is referred to physical therapy for mobilization exercises. The therapist observes a 5-cm irregular area that is thick and pink. How should the therapist document this finding?

Choices:

1. Hypertrophic scarring.
2. An excoriation.
3. Atrophic scarring.
4. A scale.

Teaching Points

Correct Answer: 1

Hypertrophic scars are thick (raised) and pink (or red).

Incorrect Choices:

Atrophic scars are thin and white. Excoriation is an abrasion or scratch mark. A scale is a flake of exfoliated epidermis (e.g., dandruff, psoriasis, dry skin).

Type of Reasoning: Analytical

This question requires one to determine the clinical findings based on the observation of the patient's skin. This necessitates analytical reasoning skill because one must analyze the signs presented in order to determine the likely clinical finding. In this case, the therapist's observations are consistent with hypertrophic scarring. If this question was answered incorrectly, review signs and symptoms of hypertrophic scarring, especially in burns.

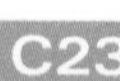

C23 

Nonsystem | Therapeutic Modalities

A patient presents with an acute left L5 radiculopathy. Pain is rated as 9/10. The therapist decides to apply transcutaneous electrical nerve stimulation (TENS) to modulate pain prior to manual therapy. Which TENS mode should provide the **BEST** relief?

Choices:

1. Low-rate TENS.
2. Brief intense TENS.
3. Modulated TENS.
4. Conventional (high-rate) TENS.

Teaching Points

Correct Answer: 2

Brief intense TENS is used to provide rapid-onset, short-term pain relief prior to painful procedures. The pulse rate and pulse duration are similar to conventional TENS; however, the current intensity is increased to the patient's tolerance.

Incorrect Choices:

In this situation, intensity is the primary determinant of pain relief. Conventional TENS does not use as high of an intensity as brief intense TENS, and the application time is longer. Low-rate TENS does not give immediate relief of pain, because it has a long onset. Modulation is used to prevent accommodation, not to provide relief of pain.

Type of Reasoning: Deductive

One must recall the protocols for TENS use in order to determine the mode that would provide the **BEST** relief of pain for this patient. This requires factual recall of information, which necessitates deductive reasoning skill. In this case, brief intense TENS is **BEST** because it provides rapid-onset, short-term relief during painful procedures.

C24 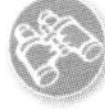

Neuromuscular | Interventions

A patient recovering from traumatic brain injury (TBI) demonstrates difficulties in feeding resulting from an unstable posture while sitting. The therapist determines that modification is necessary to ensure optimal function. What is the first body segment or segments that the therapist should align?

Choices:

1. Trunk.
2. Pelvis.
3. Head.
4. Lower extremities.

Teaching Points

Correct Answer: 2

Modification of the pelvic position in a neutral posture promotes good lumbar and trunk alignment. Many postural problems are correctable by aligning the pelvis first and achieving a stable base.

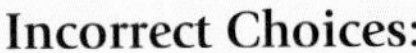

Incorrect Choices:

Modifying the position of the head, trunk, or lower extremities may be necessary but only after achieving a stable base.

Type of Reasoning: Inductive

The test-taker must determine through clinical judgment the **FIRST** body segment(s) to align in order to promote good trunk alignment. This requires inductive reasoning skill, in which knowledge of biomechanics and neuropathology is beneficial for arriving at the correct conclusion.

C25 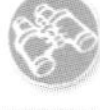

Neuromuscular I Interventions

A patient with diabetic polyneuropathy is experiencing difficulties with balance and falls when walking on unlevel surfaces or stairs. Examination reveals severely decreased monofilament and vibration testing in the bilateral feet/toes/distal half of the legs as well as weakness (3–4/5 MMT) of the bilateral legs, feet, and toe intrinsic/extrinsic muscles. Bilateral foot slap is present when walking greater than 100 feet that progresses to foot drop with walking greater than a few minutes. Which of the following interventions are **BEST** to enhance postural stability and safe ambulation in the community?

Choices:

1. Static/dynamic balance and gait training, and an ankle foot orthosis and cane for ambulation.
2. Perturbation balance training and cane for ambulation.
3. Sensory integration balance training, lower extremity stretching, and avoidance of ambulation on unlevel surfaces.
4. Strengthening and desensitization training with cane ambulation for longer distances.

Teaching Points

Correct Answer: 1

This patient has progressive polyneuropathy that is impacting multiple motor/sensory nerves distal to the proximal legs. Static/dynamic balance and gait training are indicated. The patient's fall risk and balance/gait impairments include foot slap/drop, which requires compensatory strategies to include use of an ankle foot orthosis and/or cane for safe ambulation.

Incorrect Choices:

Perturbation training runs the risk for falls and should be completed after the patient has shown progress with static/dynamic balance training. A cane will help the patient's gait but will not assist with their foot slap/foot drop, placing the patient at risk for catching their toes and falling. Sensory integration training and stretching can be accomplished, but it is important for this patient to ambulate, and the surface type in the community cannot always be controlled. Strengthening is appropriate but this patient's sensory loss is at a point where desensitization training may be of limited value and especially if the patient has no pain and primarily numbness.

Type of Reasoning: Inductive

This question requires one to employ clinical judgment to determine a best course of action for a patient with diabetic polyneuropathy. The test-taker must draw upon knowledge of the condition in order to determine the best intervention approach. For this case, static/dynamic balance and gait training, and an ankle foot orthosis and cane for ambulation, are best. If answered incorrectly review diabetic neuropathy guidelines, especially intervention approaches.

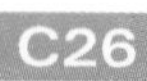

C26

Cardiovascular/Pulmonary I Evaluation, Diagnosis

A patient with a history of atrial fibrillation, hyperlipidemia, and COPD has had two recent falls. Which medication places the patient at the **MOST** risk for injury?

Choices:

1. Eliquis (apixaban).
2. Lipitor (atorvastatin).
3. Norvasc (amlodipine).
4. Ventolin (albuterol).

Teaching Points

Correct Answer: 1

Eliquis is an anticoagulant and places the patient at increased risk for bleeds as a result of trauma.

Incorrect Choices:

The other choices will not have any negative effect on the patient with respect to falls or trauma. Lipitor is a lipid-lowering agent, Norvasc is a calcium channel blocker to control the patient's heart rate, and Ventolin is a bronchodilator. See page 262 for a review on medical management of cardiovascular disease.

Type of Reasoning: Inferential

For this question, one must infer or determine what is likely to be true for medications and risk for injury. This requires recall of medication guidelines coupled with understanding of the medication that poses the MOST risk for injury. For this situation, Eliquis poses the greatest risk for injury with an increased risk for bleeds as a result of trauma. If answered incorrectly, review information on Eliquis.

C27

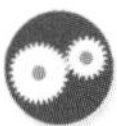

Cardiovascular/Pulmonary I Interventions

A patient is admitted to a coronary care unit with a myocardial infarction (MI). After 2 days, the patient is referred to physical therapy for inpatient cardiac rehabilitation. During an initial exercise session on the unit, the patient reports chest pain, appears anxious, and wants to go back to bed to rest. What is the therapist's **BEST** initial course of action?

Choices:

1. Assist the patient back to bed and contact the charge nurse on the floor.
2. Sit the patient down and monitor vital signs carefully during the rest period.
3. Assign the PTA to assist the patient back to bed and monitor vital signs carefully.
4. Terminate the exercise and contact the attending physician immediately.

Teaching Points

Correct Answer: 2

If the chest pain (angina) is exercise induced, this is an indication to stop the exercise session and provide a period of rest, during which time the patient is closely monitored. Recovery is expected after a period of rest.

Incorrect Choices:

If the patient is still anxious after the rest, it is reasonable to return the patient to the room and inform the nurse. This should be done by the therapist personally in order to carefully monitor the patient's status. The PTA should not be expected to evaluate chest pain or reach a determination about its significance. This is not an emergency situation.

Type of Reasoning: Evaluative

One must make a judgment call for the **BEST** course of action for this patient, given the symptoms presented. Questions that require one to make value judgments necessitate evaluative reasoning skill and can be challenging to answer, because the key to finding the correct solution goes beyond factual knowledge. For this patient, it is best to have the patient sit down and monitor vital signs.

C28 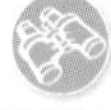

Integumentary | Evaluation, Diagnosis

A patient with a 10-year history of scleroderma is referred for physical therapy to improve functional status and endurance. The patient was recently treated with corticosteroids for a bout of myositis. Examination findings reveal limited ROM and fibrotic soft tissue along with hyperesthesia. What is the **BEST** choice for initial intervention?

Choices:

1. Treadmill walking using body weight support at an intensity of 40% HR_{max}.
2. Active range of motion (AROM) exercises and walking in a therapeutic pool.
3. Closed-chain and modified aerobic step exercises.
4. Soft tissue mobilization and stretching.

Teaching Points

Correct Answer: 2

Scleroderma (progressive systemic sclerosis) is a chronic, diffuse disease of connective tissues causing fibrosis of skin, joints, blood vessels, and internal organs. Patients typically demonstrate symmetrical skin thickening and visceral involvement of the gastrointestinal tract, lungs, heart, and kidneys along with hypersensitivity to touch. The **BEST** choice for initial intervention is to exercise in the pool. The warmth and buoyancy of the water will enhance the patient's movements and decrease pain.

Incorrect Choices:

The other choices are too aggressive at this time and risk increasing the patient's pain, thereby limiting any benefits in flexibility and endurance.

Type of Reasoning: Inductive

One must determine through clinical judgment the **BEST** initial intervention approach for this patient. Knowledge of the nature of scleroderma and expected symptomatology is key to arriving at the correct conclusion, which in this case is AROM exercises and walking in a therapeutic pool. If this question was answered incorrectly, refer to information on intervention approaches for patients with scleroderma.

C29 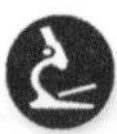

Nonsystem | Safety and Protection

An 89-year-old individual who is living independently in the home has a history of three falls in the last 3 months. A referral was initiated to a home health agency for physical therapy evaluation and intervention. The visiting therapist begins the initial visit obtaining an accurate history including medications. Which of the following types of drugs are strongly linked to falls in the elderly?

Choices:

1. Medications that raise blood sugar.
2. Antidepressants.
3. Multivitamins and calcium.
4. Thyroid medications.

Teaching Points

Correct Answer: 2

Antidepressants (e.g., Prozac, Paxil, and Zoloft) are strongly linked to falls in the elderly. Other strongly linked medications include other psychoactive medications (e.g., antipsychotics, anticonvulsants/mood stabilizers, benzodiazepines, opioids, sedatives), medications that affect blood pressure (e.g., antihypertensives), and medications that cause dizziness and blurred vision (e.g., anticholinergics). Medications that increase bleeding risk (e.g., aspirin, NSAIDS) can also increase the risk of falls.

Incorrect Choices:

Medications that lower blood sugar (e.g., oral and injectable medications to treat diabetes) increase fall risk, not medications that raise blood sugar. Multivitamins do not increase fall risk, whereas calcium can. Thyroid medications do not commonly increase fall risk in seniors.

Type of Reasoning: Deductive

For this question, one must recall medications that are strongly linked to falls in the elderly. This requires factual recall of guidelines, which is a deductive reasoning skill. For this case, antidepressants have a strong link to falls in the elderly. Review the effects of antidepressants in the elderly population if answered incorrectly.

C30 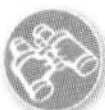

Neuromuscular | Interventions

A patient recovering from stroke with minimal lower extremity weakness and spasticity is able to walk without an assistive device. The therapist observes that as the patient walks there is noticeable hip hiking on the more affected side during swing phase. What is the **BEST** initial intervention?

Choices:

1. Bridging exercises progressing to sit-to-stand training.
2. Marching while sitting on a therapy ball.
3. Standing and marching with manual pressure applied downward on the pelvis.
4. Partial wall squats using a small ball held between the knees.

Teaching Points

Correct Answer: 2

Hip hiking is a compensatory response for weak hip and knee flexors or extensor spasticity. Active exercises for the hip and knee flexors (marching) are the most appropriate intervention.

Incorrect Choices:
Downward manual pressure on the pelvis strengthens hip hikers. The other choices focus on strengthening hip and knee extensors.

Type of Reasoning: Inductive
The test-taker must utilize clinical judgment to determine first what the patient's deficits are (related to the therapist's observation of the patient's gait) and then the **BEST** initial intervention for this patient. One must evaluate the four possible intervention choices given to determine which intervention is **BEST** for addressing the patient's deficits, which requires inductive reasoning skills. In this scenario, marching while sitting on a ball will **BEST** address the patient's weak hip and knee flexors or extensor spasticity.

C31 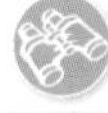

Neuromuscular I Interventions

The therapist is instructing a patient with traumatic brain injury (TBI) how to lock the brakes on a wheelchair. The patient is right-handed, and the right upper extremity is more affected than the left. What is the **BEST** motor learning strategy to use with this patient?

Choices:
1. Have the patient practice brake locking using the left hand to assist the right.
2. Guide the patient's right hand through the locking motions, then the left.
3. Verbally talk the patient through the locking motions, practicing with both hands simultaneously.
4. Have the patient practice locking the brakes first with the left hand and then with the right.

Teaching Points

Correct Answer: 4
Using the motor learning strategy of transfer of training is best to use with this patient. Practice is performed with the less affected extremity first and then progressed to use of the more affected extremity.

Incorrect Choices:
Guided movement (manual or verbal) represents a less active approach than the transfer of training approach. The more passive the performance, the slower the learning will take place. Bilateral tasks are more difficult than performing the task with one limb at a time.

Type of Reasoning: Inductive
The test-taker must determine the **BEST** training strategy for a patient with traumatic brain injury, which necessitates inductive reasoning skill and, therefore, clinical judgment. For this patient, it is important to have him/her practice locking the brakes first with his/her left hand and then his/her right in order to encourage effective transfer of training. Knowledge of effective motor learning strategies for patients with brain injury is beneficial for arriving at the correct conclusion.

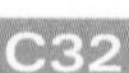

C32 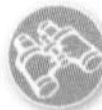

Musculoskeletal | Examination

In neural tension testing, what position will **BEST** bias the tibial nerve?

Choices:

1. Straight leg raise with plantarflexion and eversion.
2. Straight leg raise with dorsiflexion and inversion.
3. Straight leg raise with plantarflexion and inversion.
4. Straight leg raise with dorsiflexion and eversion.

Teaching Points

Correct Answer: 4

A straight leg raise with dorsiflexion and eversion will best bias the tibial nerve. This is the optimal position for neural tissue provocation of the tibial nerve. Neural tension techniques are used to decrease adverse mechanical tension on the nerves. Peripheral nerves can often become trapped within the tissues, where there can be a pull on the nerve with movement. This technique frees up the nerve so that it can slide in its sheath.

Incorrect Choices:

Straight leg raise with dorsiflexion and inversion and straight leg raise with plantarflexion and inversion will best bias the sural nerve and peroneal (fibular) nerve, respectively. Straight leg raise with plantarflexion and eversion will not isolate a specific nerve.

Type of Reasoning: Inductive

This question requires the test-taker to utilize clinical judgment in order to arrive at a correct conclusion. In this case, the test-taker must draw upon knowledge of neural tension testing to determine the best position to bias the tibial nerve. This is an inductive reasoning skill. For this situation, the therapist should position the extremity in a straight leg raise with dorsiflexion and eversion to bias the tibial nerve. Review neural tension testing techniques if answered incorrectly.

C33 

Cardiovascular/Pulmonary | Evaluation, Diagnosis

A patient with asthma is completing their aerobic exercise program on a recumbent stepper. The patient begins to have an exercise-induced asthma attack. Which type of inhaler will be **MOST** helpful in reducing the patient's acute symptoms?

Choices:

1. Advair (Fluticasone and Salmeterol).
2. Flovent (Fluticasone).
3. Singulair (Montelukast).
4. Ventolin (Albuterol).

Teaching Points

Correct Answer: 4

Ventolin is a short-acting beta$_2$ agonist, which will relieve acute bronchoconstriction.

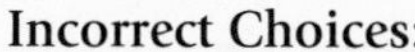

Incorrect Choices:

The other choices are long-acting medications that will not help with acute respiratory compromise. Advair is a combination of glucocorticoids and long-activing beta 2 agonist. Flovent is a glucocorticoid. Singulair is a leukotriene inhibitor. See Table 5-10 for a review of common pulmonary medications.

Type of Reasoning: Deductive

For this question, one must recall the properties of each of the inhalers presented in order to determine the inhaler which is short-acting and therefore most effective in reducing the patient's symptoms. This requires recall of factual information, which is a deductive reasoning skill. In this case, the therapist should choose Ventolin (Albuterol) to address the patient's asthma attack. If answered incorrectly, review medications for asthma, including short-acting inhalers.

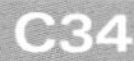

Musculoskeletal I Examination

A patient is referred to physical therapy with a complaint of chronic anterior knee pain associated with running. What is the physical examination finding that would increase the likelihood of a diagnosis of patellofemoral pain syndrome (PFPS)?

Choices:

1. Positive patellar apprehension test.
2. Pain with passive knee flexion.
3. Pain with squat.
4. Positive Noble compression test.

Teaching Points

Correct Answer: 3

There is strong evidence that reproduction of retropatellar or peripatellar pain with squatting or other functional activities are diagnostic for PFPS. These activities load the patellofemoral joint (PFJ) while in flexed-knee positions (i.e., stairs, prolonged sitting). There is moderate evidence to support a diagnosis of PFPS with the following criteria: presence of retropatellar or peripatellar pain; reproduction of pain with squatting, stair climbing, prolonged sitting, or other functional activities that load the PFJ in a flexed position; and exclusion of all other conditions that may cause anterior knee pain. See Box 2-9 for the Patellofemoral Pain Clinical Practice Guidelines.

Incorrect Choices:

The patellar apprehension test is utilized to assess for patellar instability, not PFPS. Pain with passive knee flexion may be present with a number of conditions, including PFPS, osteoarthritis, patellar tendinopathy, and meniscal injuries. The Noble compression test is a provocative test for iliotibial band friction syndrome, which patients experience as lateral knee pain.

Type of Reasoning: Inferential

For this question, the test-taker must determine which examination finding would most likely result in a diagnosis of PFPS. This necessitates inferential reasoning skill where one must determine what is likely to be true of a situation, though one often cannot be absolutely certain. For this scenario, the physical examination finding of pain with squat would increase the likelihood of PFPS. If answered incorrectly, review examination procedures and findings for PFPS.

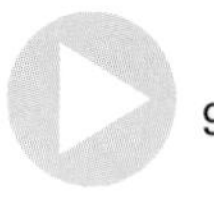

C35 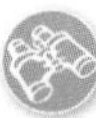

Musculoskeletal | Interventions

A patient presents to physical therapy with a suprascapular nerve injury following acromioclavicular joint reconstruction surgery. During the initial postoperative physical therapy examination, the manual muscle test grade for shoulder external rotation was $2^+/5$. Which is the **BEST** initial position to isotonically strengthen the shoulder external rotators in the open kinetic chain?

Choices:

1. Sitting with shoulder at 0° abduction (elbow at side).
2. Supine with shoulder at 90° abduction.
3. Prone with shoulder at 90° abduction.
4. Sidelying with shoulder at 0° abduction (elbow at side).

Teaching Points

Correct Answer: 1

A manual muscle test grade of $2^+/5$ indicates that the patient is unable to complete the required motion through the full range of motion against gravity. Rehabilitation must be initiated in a gravity-eliminated position. The patient will be able to perform isotonic shoulder external rotation resistance exercises in a gravity-eliminated position while seated with the elbow at the side. Based on the manual muscle test grade, minimal resistance may be utilized to strengthen the shoulder external rotators. See Table 2-12 for a review of manual muscle test grades and their implications for exercise prescription.

Incorrect Choices:

Both the prone and sidelying positions require the patient to work against gravity. As the patient's external rotator strength improves to a manual muscle test grade of at least a grade of 3/5, those positions will become feasible and more beneficial. The supine position with the shoulder at 90° of abduction allows gravity to assist the patient with the motion, which will not appropriately challenge this patient.

Type of Reasoning: Inductive

For this question, the test-taker must apply knowledge of muscle strength to gravity-eliminated positioning for strengthening of the shoulder external rotators. This requires clinical knowledge and judgment, which is an inductive reasoning skill. For this case, the best initial position would be sitting with shoulder at 0° abduction (elbow at side). If answered incorrectly, review muscle grades and against gravity and gravity-eliminated positioning.

C36 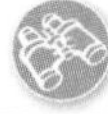

Integumentary | Interventions

Examination of a patient with a dermal ulcer over the coccyx reveals a wound exposing the deep fascia. There is no necrotic tissue, exudate is minimal, and the borders of the ulcer are diffusely covered with granulation tissue. Previous treatment has included wet-to-dry dressings with normal saline. What is the **BEST** choice for intervention?

Choices:

1. Hydrogel dressings and whirlpool immersion.
2. Continuation of the same treatment.
3. Wound irrigation with pressures below 15 psi.
4. Calcium alginate dressings.

Teaching Points

Correct Answer: 3

Low-pressure wound irrigation helps to decrease colonization and prevent infection.

Incorrect Choices:

Wet-to-dry dressings help remove necrotic tissue. There is no necrotic tissue. Calcium alginate is used in the presence of heavy exudates, which is not the case here. Hydrogel would be best because it is nonadherent, keeps wounds moist, and protects granulation buds; however, whirlpool immersion is now contraindicated for all wound management.

Type of Reasoning: Inductive

One must utilize clinical judgment and knowledge of wound care approaches to determine the best intervention approach for this patient, which requires inductive reasoning skill. For this patient, wound irrigation with pressures below 15 psi is most appropriate for the type of wound described. If this question was answered incorrectly, review information on wound care procedures for this type of wound.

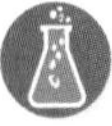

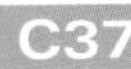

C37

Musculoskeletal | Evaluation, Diagnosis

Based on the spinal defect shown in the diagram, what lumbar spinal motion should be avoided?

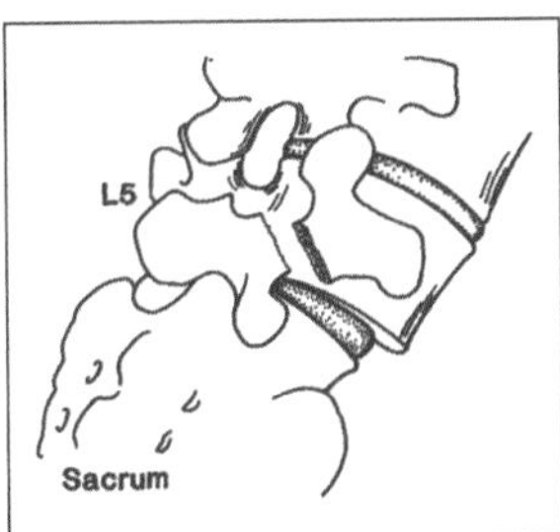

Choices:
1. Rotation.
2. Extension.
3. Lateral flexion.
4. Flexion.

Teaching Points

Correct Answer: 2

With spondylolisthesis, there is typically an anterior slippage of one vertebra on the vertebra below. Because of the anterior shearing forces acting at the vertebra caused by the wedge shape of the vertebra and gravity, spinal extension positions should be avoided.

Incorrect Choices:

Flexion, rotation, and lateral flexion will cause the bony structures to separate and will not cause any negative compressive loads to the damaged structures.

Type of Reasoning: Analytical

One must analyze the spinal defect displayed in the picture and determine the diagnosis in order to determine what lumbar position should be avoided. This requires analytical reasoning skill, in which the precise meaning of the spinal defect must be determined first, before determining the appropriate management of this patient. If this question was answered incorrectly, refer to intervention approaches for spondylolisthesis.

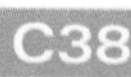
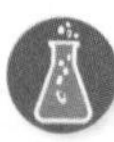

C38

System Interactions | Evaluation, Diagnosis

An elderly patient is being seen at home following a recent hospitalization for pneumonia. Interventions during the hospitalization included oxygen via a nasal cannula, an IV line, and the placement of a Foley catheter for 4 days. During the initial PT evaluation, the therapist notes that the patient is not responding appropriately to commands and appears to be withdrawn and confused. The therapist documents the following vital signs at rest: heart rate = 110, blood pressure = 90/60, temperature = 101° and O_2 saturation = 96%. What is the most likely explanation for these findings in this patient?

Choices:

1. Cerebrovascular accident.
2. Urinary tract infection.
3. Myocardial infarction.
4. Pulmonary embolism.

Teaching Points

Correct Answer: 2

This patient is showing signs of a urinary tract infection (UTI). She had a prolonged catheterization while in the hospital, which could have caused bacteria to enter her bladder, leading to the UTI. In elderly patients, UTIs are common and can cause altered mental status and sudden behavior changes. Additional signs can include the presence of a low-grade fever, elevated heart rate, and a drop in blood pressure (often associated with dehydration).

Incorrect Choices:

Classic signs of a cerebrovascular accident (CVA) or stroke include numbness or weakness one side of the body, confusion with trouble speaking or difficulty understanding speech, vision changes, dizziness, loss of balance, or lack of coordination. Based on the findings described in this scenario, it is unlikely that the patient is experiencing a CVA. A myocardial infarction (MI) is also unlikely. Typical signs of a MI include chest pain, shortness of breath, sweating, lightheadedness, and/or dizziness. Signs of a pulmonary embolism (PE) include irregular heartbeat, anxiety, tachypnea, sweating, and stabbing pain in the chest. The patient in this question did not exhibit these characteristic signs. Additionally, the O_2 saturation of 96% in this scenario is within normal limits (≥95%). It may be lower than normal in the patient suffering from a PE and MI.

Type of Reasoning: Analytical

For this question, the test-taker must analyze the presenting symptoms in order to determine the most likely diagnosis for the patient. This requires analytical reasoning skill, where pieces of information are considered for their value in order to draw reasonable conclusions. For this case, a urinary tract infection is the most likely explanation for the symptoms. If answered incorrectly, review signs and symptoms of a UTI, especially in the elderly.

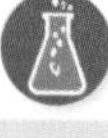

C39

Neuromuscular | Evaluation, Diagnosis

A patient presents with rapidly progressive symmetrical weakness, hyporeflexia, and atrophy that started in the distal lower extremity muscles but now has ascended to include proximal trunk and upper extremity muscles. The motor segments of the lower cranial nerves are also showing impairment. The patient complains of abnormal sensations of tingling and burning of the affected extremities. Consciousness, cognition, and communication are all normal. These signs and symptoms are characteristic of what diagnosis?

Choices:

1. Multiple sclerosis.
2. Guillain-Barré syndrome.
3. Amyotrophic lateral sclerosis.
4. Post-polio syndrome.

Teaching Points

Correct Answer: 2

These signs and symptoms are characteristic of Guillain-Barré syndrome, an autoimmune disease that results in acute and rapid demyelination of peripheral nerve roots and peripheral and/or cranial nerves. See Table 3-25 for additional details on the differential diagnosis of various neuromuscular disorders, to include Guillain-Barré Syndrome.

Incorrect Choices:

In almost all cases, patients with ALS show features of both UMN and lower motor neuron (LMN) dysfunction. Post-polio syndrome is an LMN syndrome that does not present with sensory paresthesias and is typically asymmetrical. MS will present with UMN signs: spasticity and hyperreflexia.

Type of Reasoning: Analytical

This question provides the symptoms, and the test-taker must determine what the symptoms most likely indicate. This requires analytical reasoning skill, in which one evaluates the exact meaning of the symptoms presented to arrive at the correct conclusion. If this question was answered incorrectly, review information on symptoms of Guillain-Barré syndrome.

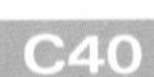

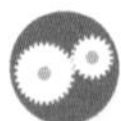

Cardiovascular/Pulmonary | Interventions

What are the expected adverse effects of the Valsalva maneuver for a patient 2 days after a triple coronary artery bypass graft?

Choices:

1. Slowing of pulse and increased venous pressure are possible.
2. The decreased return of blood to the heart can lead to pitting edema.
3. Heart rate (HR) and blood pressure are likely to be elevated.
4. A cholinergic or vagal response can occur.

Teaching Points

Correct Answer: 1

The Valsalva maneuver results from forcible exhalation with the glottis, nose, and mouth closed. It increases intrathoracic pressures and causes slowing of the pulse, decreased return of blood to the heart, and increased venous pressure. Although Valsalvas occur during normal daily activities (breath holding, straining), they can be dangerous for patients with cardiovascular disease. On relaxation, blood rushes to the heart and can overload the cardiac system, resulting in cardiac arrest.

Incorrect Choices:

HR is not elevated. A cholinergic or vagal response is the result of parasympathetic nervous system (PNS) stimulation providing inhibitory control of the vagus nerve over HR and atrioventricular conduction. Pitting edema is caused by long-term factors such as CHF.

Type of Reasoning: Evaluative

The test-taker must determine the value and believability of the reasons presented to **AVOID** the Valsalva maneuver, which encourages evaluative reasoning skill. Having knowledge of the Valsalva maneuver and its effects on HR and venous pressure is important for arriving at the correct conclusion for this question. If this question was answered incorrectly, review information on the Valsalva maneuver.

C41 

Cardiovascular/Pulmonary | Evaluation, Diagnosis

A patient experiences color changes in the skin during position changes of the foot. During elevation, pallor develops. When the limb is then positioned in the seated hanging position, hyperemia develops. What do these changes indicate?

Choices:

1. Lymphedema.
2. Arterial insufficiency.
3. Deep vein thrombophlebitis.
4. Chronic venous insufficiency.

Teaching Points

Correct Answer: 2

Arterial insufficiency can be determined by skin color changes during position changes of the foot (termed rubor of dependency test). See Table 4-14 for a comparison of chronic arterial vs. chronic venous insufficiency.

Incorrect Choices:

Chronic venous insufficiency can be determined by the history, presence of aching calf pain with prolonged standing, a percussion test in standing, or Trendelenburg's test (retrograde filling test). With chronic venous insufficiency, skin will be dark and cyanotic. Acute deep vein thrombophlebitis (DVT) can be evident with aching calf pain, edema, and muscle tenderness. Lymphedema is evident with visual inspection (i.e., swelling, decreased ROM) and volumetric measurements.

Type of Reasoning: Inferential

One must infer the exact meaning of the symptoms presented and then draw conclusions about what the diagnosis may be. Questions that inquire about a possible diagnosis for symptoms presented encourage inferential reasoning skill. If this question was answered incorrectly, refer to information on arterial insufficiency of the lower extremity.

C42 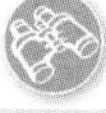

Neuromuscular | Examination

A patient sustained a left anterior cerebral artery stroke 7 days ago and is experiencing difficulties with bed mobility, sit-to-stand transfers, and balance (sitting and standing). Which of the following examination items is BEST to assess and serve as an outcome measure for this patient's current impairments and activity limitations?

Choices:
1. Berg Balance Scale (BBS).
2. Postural Assessment Scale for Stroke Patients (PASS).
3. The Mini-BEST (Balance Evaluation System Test).
4. Trunk Impairment Scale.

Teaching Points

Correct Answer: 2

The PASS examines the ability to maintain postural alignment and support during static sitting, static standing, and various functional tasks (bed mobility, supine to sit, sit-to-stand, picking up an object from the floor). It is a reliable and valid tool to assess patients recovering from stroke in the acute and sub-acute phases (<90 days).

Incorrect Choices:

The BBS has strong psychometric properties and measures various domains of balance but does not examine bed mobility. The Mini-BEST does not assess sitting balance or bed mobility. The trunk impairment scale is specifically designed to only assess static and dynamic sitting balance. Please see Box 3-1 and Table 3-13 for additional information.

Type of Reasoning: Inductive

This question requires the test-taker to utilize clinical judgment to determine the best examination item to assess and serve as an outcome measure for the patient. This necessitates inductive reasoning skill. For this scenario, the best examination item is the Postural Assessment Scale for Stroke Patients. If answered incorrectly, review information on CVA assessment, especially the Postural Assessment Scale for Stroke Patients.

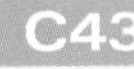

Gastrointestinal | Examination

During an examination, a patient complains of right upper quadrant pain and tenderness. The PT percusses over the costal margin at the point where the lateral border of the rectus muscle intersects with the costal margin. The patient complains of acute pain and stops inspiratory effort. What does this patient's response indicate?

Choices:
1. Hernia.
2. Cholecystitis.
3. Irritation of the psoas muscle by an inflamed appendix.
4. Peritoneal inflammation.

Teaching Points

Correct Answer: 2

Percussion for costovertebral tenderness that reveals a sharp increase in tenderness with a sudden stop in inspiratory effort is a positive Murphy's sign and is indicative of cholecystitis.

Incorrect Choices:

An inflamed appendix results in pain in the right lower quadrant during left-sided pressure (positive Rovsing's sign) or right lower quadrant pain on quick withdrawal (referred rebound tenderness). A hernia produces a bulge in the abdominal wall (ventral hernias). Peritoneal inflammation presents with abdominal pain on coughing or with light percussion. Rebound tenderness is also present.

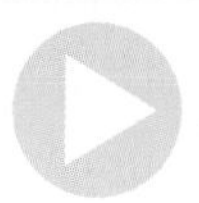

Type of Reasoning: Inferential

In order to arrive at a correct conclusion, one must have knowledge of the indications for percussion of the costovertebral angle. This requires inferential reasoning skill, in which one draws conclusions based upon evidence and facts. In this situation, percussion is indicated to reveal cholecystitis. If this question was answered incorrectly, review indications for Murphy's percussion.

C44 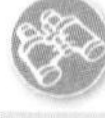

Genitourinary I Examination

An elderly woman is experiencing incontinence and is referred for physical therapy. Her history is an important part of the physical therapist's examination. What question should the therapist ask to differentiate/diagnose stress urinary incontinence from urge urinary incontinence, using a time frame of the last 3 months?

Choices:

1. Did you experience a sudden urge and leak urine while hurrying to the toilet?
2. Did you leak urine during sleep?
3. Did you leak urine when sneezing or coughing?
4. Did you leak urine while sitting in a chair?

Teaching Points

Correct Answer: 3

Stress urinary incontinence is an involuntary loss of bladder control. It occurs during sneezing, coughing, laughing, or physical activity.

Incorrect Choices:

Urge incontinence occurs when individuals experience a sudden, compelling need to urinate and the bladder contracts, spilling urine before reaching the bathroom. It is a leading cause of falls while rushing to the bathroom. Some women can have both stress and urge incontinence (mixed incontinence), so it is important to include questions for both types when taking the history. Urinary tract infections, some medical conditions (e.g., diabetes, Parkinson's), and certain medications can cause incontinence. This can result in leakage of urine at rest (sitting in a chair or rarely at night). The 3 Incontinence Questions (3IQ) is a simple, quick, noninvasive test for diagnosing and classifying stress, urge, or mixed incontinence.

Type of Reasoning: Inductive

This question requires the test-taker to have knowledge of the differences between stress urinary incontinence and urge urinary incontinence in order to arrive at a correct conclusion. This necessitates clinical judgment as well as weighing the value of the questions that help diagnose and differentiate these types of incontinence, which is an inductive reasoning skill. For this case, asking, "Did you leak urine when sneezing or coughing?" will best differentiate between the two types of incontinence. If answered incorrectly, review information on urinary incontinence.

C45 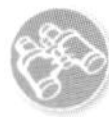

Nonsystem | Equipment, Devices

A patient with left hemiplegia due to a stroke uses a solid ankle AFO to ambulate. When ambulating, the patient is noted to hyperextend his knee during midstance. Which of the following interventions would decrease this gait deviation?

Choices:

1. Inserting of a heel lift in the left shoe.
2. Tightening the calf strap on the AFO.
3. Increasing the length of the footplate on the AFO.
4. Adding an external lateral post to the AFO.

Teaching Points

Correct Answer: 1

Placing a heel lift in the left shoe will delay forefoot loading and allow the tibia to progress farther forward, thus increasing flexion at the knee by anteriorly tilting the tibia.

Incorrect Choices:

Tightening the calf strap will not allow forward movement of the tibia and will increase the extension moment at the knee. Increasing the length of the footplate increases the knee extension moment by increasing the lever arm that controls the forward movement of the tibia. Adding a lateral post will affect the frontal plane motion rather than the sagittal plane motion.

Type of Reasoning: Inductive

This question requires one to draw from knowledge of gait intervention strategies in order to arrive at a correct conclusion. This requires clinical judgment, which is an inductive reasoning skill. For this case, the therapist should insert a heel lift in the left shoe to decrease the gait deviation. Review gait intervention guidelines, especially for patients with hemiplegia and knee hyperextension, if answered incorrectly.

C46 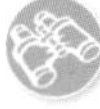

Musculoskeletal | Interventions

A patient has limited right rotation caused by left thoracic facet joint capsular tightness at T6–7. What arthrokinematic glide would **MOST** effectively improve right rotation in sitting?

Choices:

1. Superior and anterior glide on the right T7 transverse process.
2. Superior and anterior glide on the left T7 transverse process.
3. Superior and anterior glide on the right T6 transverse process.
4. Superior and anterior glide on the left T6 transverse process.

Teaching Points

Correct Answer: 4

Because the left thoracic facet joint capsule is restricting movement, motion that would stretch the capsule would facilitate improved right rotation. With right rotation, the left superior facets move upward (opening the joint and stretching the capsule) and the right facets move downward (closing the joint and putting the capsule on relative slack).

Incorrect Choices:

Providing a superior and anterior glide on the right T6 transverse process would improve left rotation. Providing a superior and anterior glide on the left T7 transverse process would improve right rotation at T7–8. Providing a superior and anterior glide on the right T7 transverse process would improve left rotation between T7 and T8.

Type of Reasoning: Inductive

One must utilize clinical judgment to determine the **MOST** effective intervention approach for facilitating improved right rotation. In order to arrive at the correct conclusion, the test-taker must have a thorough understanding of normal facet joint capsule motion with rotation. For this patient, a superior and anterior glide to the left T6 transverse process will **MOST** effectively stretch the joint capsule and improve right rotation.

C47 

Musculoskeletal | Examination

A patient is seen in a physical therapy clinic after sustaining a knee injury earlier in the same day. The patient describes a pivoting mechanism of injury with the foot planted. On examination the therapist notes significant (3+) knee joint effusion. What would be the expected resting position of the patient's knee at the time of examination?

Choices:

1. 90° of flexion.
2. 25° of flexion.
3. Full extension.
4. 10° of hyperextension.

Teaching Points

Correct Answer: 2

Twenty-five degrees of flexion is the resting or loose-packed position of the tibiofemoral joint. This is the position where the joint capsule and other soft tissue structures are in the most relaxed position. The resting position can accommodate maximal joint volume, which is required in this case due to the significant effusion. See Table 2-2 for a review of resting and close-packed positions of peripheral joints.

Incorrect Choices:

It is unlikely that the patient would be able to move the knee into any of the other positions given the maximal effusion of the joint. That is, none of the other position options would be able to accommodate the 3+ effusion. Full extension is the close-packed position of the tibiofemoral joint, which is where the capsule and other soft tissue structures are maximally tensed.

Type of Reasoning: Inferential

For this question, the test-taker must infer what is likely to be true of a clinical situation based on the provided symptoms. Specifically, one must determine the expected resting position of the patient's knee. This requires inferential reasoning skill. For this case, the expected resting position is 25° of flexion. If answered incorrectly, review joint effusion information, and loose-packed joint positions, especially for the knee.

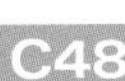
C48 

Nonsystem | Professional Responsibilities

A physical therapist is providing treatment to a patient in the hospital setting. The patient slips on a wet floor but is guarded well by the therapist and incurs no injury. Which of the following statements reflects what the therapist should do?

Choices:

1. Document the occurrence as a part of the risk management program.
2. Document this sentinel event to The Joint Commission.
3. Omit the incidence from the medical record as there was no negligence.
4. Report the occurrence to the Occupational Health and Safety Administration (OSHA) since it was a facility problem.

Teaching Points

Correct Answer: 1

A comprehensive risk management program monitors occurrences related to patient and staff risk for the intention of preventing future safety risk. This is not a punitive process.

Incorrect Choices:

A sentinel event is defined by the Joint Commission as an incident that reaches the patient and causes harm. As this patient did not incur harm it was not a sentinel event. As there was no injury to the patient there was no negligence, but the occurrence and the patient response are important to record in the medical record. Omission could put the facility at risk for future litigation. OSHA is not a reporting agency for patient incidences.

Type of Reasoning: Evaluative

This question challenges the test-taker to be familiar with risk management processes as well as the variety of agencies involved in regulation and accreditation of hospital organization. They are further challenged to apply this knowledge to a patient incidence scenario, which requires evaluative reasoning skill to determine a best course of action. For this case, the therapist should document the occurrence as a part of the risk management program. If answered incorrectly, review risk management program guidelines.

C49 

Lymphatic | Interventions

A therapist is beginning manual lymphatic drainage for a patient recently diagnosed with secondary lymphedema in the left upper extremity following a radical mastectomy. What is the **BEST** choice for initial bandaging of the limb?

Choices:

1. Long-stretch compression wrap (Ace wrap).
2. Custom-made low-elastic garment.
3. Gauze wrap.
4. Short-stretch compression wrap (Comprilan®).

Teaching Points

Correct Answer: 4

A short-stretch wrap has a low resting pressure and high working pressure. This means it has enough pressure to enhance lymphatic return at rest, improve the activity of the lymphangion (contractile unit of the lymphatic system), and facilitate increased return during muscle pumping activities. See pp. 274–275 for a review of bandages and principles of manual lymphatic drainage.

Incorrect Choices:

Long-stretch wraps have high resting pressures and low working pressure. The problem with long-stretch wraps (Ace wraps) is they can become like a tourniquet at rest and do not provide enough support during activities. Custom-made, low-elastic garments are not ordered until the limb reduction has reached a plateau, which may take 4–6 months. Gauze wraps provide no support.

Type of Reasoning: Deductive

This question requires the test-taker to recall guidelines for lymphedema management in order to arrive at a correct conclusion. This is factual information, which is a deductive reasoning skill. For this scenario, short-stretch compression wrap is required. Refer to manual lymphatic drainage guidelines if answered incorrectly.

C50 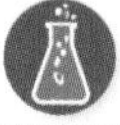

Neuromuscular | Evaluation, Diagnosis

An elderly individual was found unconscious at home and was hospitalized with a diagnosis of cerebrovascular accident (CVA). Examination by the PT reveals normal sensation and movement on the right side of the body with impaired sensation (touch, pressure, proprioception) and paralysis on the left side of the body. The left side of the lower face and trunk are similarly impaired. What is the **MOST** likely location of the CVA?

Choices:

1. Left parietal lobe.
2. Right parietal lobe.
3. Left side of brain stem.
4. Spinal cord.

Teaching Points

Correct Answer: 2

This patient demonstrates involvement of the long tracts (sensory and motor) indicative of involvement of the contralateral cerebral cortex, parietal lobe.

Incorrect Choices:

Tracts cross in the medulla so it is the right brain that is involved, not the left. The involvement of the face indicates a lesion above the level of the midbrain. A lesion in the spinal cord would not affect the face. A lesion in the brain stem would produce facial signs contralateral to the limb signs.

Type of Reasoning: Analytical

The test-taker must determine the precise location of the lesion given the symptoms presented. Questions that require one to draw conclusions based on symptoms often encourage analytical reasoning skill. For this patient, the symptoms indicate right parietal lobe damage, which should be reviewed if this question was answered incorrectly.

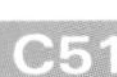
C51

Neuromuscular | Evaluation, Diagnosis

The loss of sensory function in peripheral polyneuropathy is often among the first noticeable symptoms. With large fiber damage, what is the typical pattern of the sensory loss?

Choices:

1. Allodynia of the feet accompanied by pronounced dorsiflexor weakness.
2. Bandlike dysesthesias and paresthesias in the hips and thighs.
3. Paresthesias affecting primarily the proximal limb segments and trunk.
4. Stocking and glove loss of monofilament and position sense.

Teaching Points

Correct Answer: 4

Symmetrical involvement of sensory fibers, progressing from distal to proximal, is the hallmark of polyneuropathy. It is termed "stocking-and-glove distribution" and is the result of the dying back of all peripheral nerves from distal to proximal. Sensory symptoms include decreased sensation and pain, paresthesias, and dysesthesias (abnormal sensations such as numbness, tingling, or prickling). Specifically, this question states there is a loss of large fiber function, which is consistent with impaired proprioception, vibration, and discriminant touch (monofilament). See Tables 3-3 and 3-25 for additional information on sensory testing and differential diagnosis of polyneuropathy.

Incorrect Choices:

Proximal involvement (hips) can occur, but only after long-standing disease and distal involvement first. Involvement of the trunk is not typical. Allodynia refers to the perception of an ordinarily painless stimulus as painful and is not characteristic of polyneuropathy.

Type of Reasoning: Inferential

This question requires one to determine the likely symptoms for polyneuropathy. This necessitates one to make inferences about the nature of polyneuropathy, which is an inferential reasoning skill. Through knowledge of neuropathology, the test-taker should determine that polyneuropathy characteristically appears as a stocking-and-glove distribution of the hands and feet.

C52
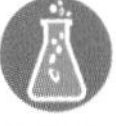

Cardiovascular/Pulmonary | Interventions

The PT is supervising a phase II cardiac rehabilitation class of 10 patients. One of the patients is being monitored with telemetry and is exhibiting signs of distress. Which change would be a criterion for terminating this exercise session?

Choices:

1. An increase in systolic BP to 150 and diastolic BP to 90.
2. 1-mm ST segment depression, upsloping.
3. A second-degree atrioventricular (AV) heart block.
4. An increase in HR 20 beats/minute above resting.

Teaching Points

Correct Answer: 3

Criteria for reducing exercise intensity or termination according to the American College of Sports Medicine include (1) onset of angina and other symptoms of exertional intolerance; (2) systolic BP ≥240 mmHg, diastolic BP ≥110 mmHg; (3) >1-mm ST segment depression, horizontal or downsloping; (4) increased frequency of ventricular arrhythmias; and (5) second-degree or third-degree AV block or other significant electrocardiogram (ECG) disturbances.

Incorrect Choices:

The other findings do not fall within the criteria listed. HR is expected to rise proportionally to workload intensity unless the patient is on beta-blockers. The rise in BP is not significant enough to stop exercise. 1-mm ST segment depression that is isoelectric or within 1 mm is within normal limits.

Type of Reasoning: Analytical

One must determine which symptoms warrant termination of the treatment session and which symptoms merely require monitoring. Through analytical reasoning, the person must interpret the symptoms presented and determine their significance. For this patient, second-degree AV heart block warrants termination of the treatment session. If this question was answered incorrectly, review cardiac rehabilitation guidelines for terminating exercise.

C53 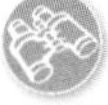

Cardiovascular/Pulmonary | Interventions

A patient presents with maximal claudication (grade 4) that is evident when walking distances greater than 200 feet. The patient also exhibits muscle fatigue and cramping of both calf muscles. Upon examination, the PT finds the skin is pale and shiny with some trophic nail changes. What is the **BEST** choice for this patient's initial exercise program?

Choices:

1. Avoid any exercise stress until the patient has been on calcium channel blockers for at least 2 weeks.
2. Utilize an interval walking program of moderate intensity.
3. Utilize non-weight-bearing exercises such as cycle ergometry.
4. Utilize a continuous walking program of moderate intensity for 10-minute bouts.

Teaching Points

Correct Answer: 2

The patient is experiencing classic signs of peripheral artery disease (PAD). Rehabilitation guidelines for PAD include using interval training of moderate intensity, 30–60 min/day, 3–5 days/week. The patient is instructed to walk until intense pain is experienced (grade 3) and then rest until ischemic pain subsides before resuming exercise (ACSM Guidelines for Exercise Testing and Prescription, 10th ed., 2017).

Incorrect Choices:

Continuous exercise with persistent pain are contraindicated. Calcium channel blockers may be used in vasospastic disease; exercise is not contraindicated. A cycle ergometry program is less desirable than a walking program (treadmill or track) to reduce claudication.

Type of Reasoning: Inductive

One must utilize clinical judgment to determine the **BEST** choice for intervention, which is an inductive reasoning skill. The test-taker must understand what the symptoms are indicative of in order to arrive at the correct conclusion. If this question was answered incorrectly, refer to information on exercise for patients with PAD.

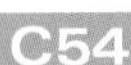
C54 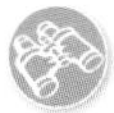

Integumentary | Interventions

A patient is hospitalized with diabetes and a large stage II plantar ulcer located over the right heel. The patient has been non-weight-bearing for the past 2 weeks as a result of the ulcer. What is the **BEST** choice for this patient's initial intervention?

Choices:

1. Wash the foot and apply skin lubricants followed by a transparent film dressing.
2. Clean and bandage with a sterile gauze dressing.
3. Refer the patient for a surgical consult.
4. Clean and debride the wound and apply a hydrogel dressing.

Teaching Points

Correct Answer: 4

A stage II ulcer (deep ulcer) involves a partial-thickness skin loss with involvement of epidermis, dermis, or both; it is reversible. Intervention should be directed toward improving perfusion and relieving localized pressure. The wound should be cleaned with an antimicrobial agent, debrided of necrotic tissue, and covered with a sterile dressing. Hydrogel dressings maintain moisture in the wound bed, soften necrotic tissue, and support autolytic debridement. Pressure relief is also an important consideration. Techniques of protective foot care should be taught.

Incorrect Choices:

Application of a dry, sterile gauze dressing is contraindicated, as is the application of skin lubricants. A stage II ulcer has the potential to heal; a surgical consult is not needed at this time.

Type of Reasoning: Inductive

One must utilize clinical judgment and knowledge of wound care approaches to determine the **BEST** intervention approach for this patient, which requires inductive reasoning skill. For this patient, cleaning and debriding of the wound with application of a hydrogel dressing is most appropriate for the type of wound described. If this question was answered incorrectly, review information on wound care procedures for stage II plantar ulcers.

C55 

Nonsystem | Equipment, Devices

A patient is referred to physical therapy 6 weeks after sustaining a scaphoid fracture that was treated with casting. Which of the following splints is the patient **MOST** likely required to wear outside of rehabilitation?

Choices:

1. Volar wrist cock-up splint.
2. Thumb spica splint.
3. Dorsal wrist splint.
4. Resting hand splint.

Teaching Points

Correct Answer: 2

A thumb spica splint is indicated for radial hand and wrist injuries (e.g., scaphoid or lunate fractures, thumb ulnar collateral ligament sprain) or overuse conditions (e.g., carpometacarpal thumb osteoarthritis, de Quervain's tenosynovitis).

Incorrect Choices:

Volar and dorsal wrist splints provide support to the fingers, hand, wrist, and forearm and are used to treat various neuromusculoskeletal conditions. A resting hand splint maintains the hand and fingers in a functional position during recovery from paralysis or burn injuries. Although all three of these braces have various benefits, they do not stabilize the radial carpals and wrist.

Type of Reasoning: Inferential

For this question, one must recall splinting guidelines for scaphoid fractures, then infer what is likely to be true for this patient post-casting. This necessitates inferential reasoning skill. For this scenario, the patient is most likely required to wear a thumb spica splint. If answered incorrectly, review treatment approaches for scaphoid fractures, especially splinting information.

C56 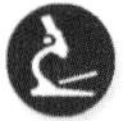

Nonsystem I Safety and Protection

A patient who is participating in a cardiac rehabilitation program suddenly collapses and falls to the floor. The PT is the lone rescuer on site. The therapist checks for a response and finds the patient unresponsive. After activating the emergency response system (phone 911), what is the **BEST** action for the therapist to take?

Choices:

1. Use the automated external defibrillator (AED) to shock the patient after 3 minutes of cardiopulmonary resuscitation (CPR).
2. Begin CPR and attach and use the AED as soon as possible.
3. Give 100 chest compressions per minute.
4. Give two rescue breaths followed by 15 chest compressions, repeating the cycle for at least 2 minutes.

Teaching Points

Correct Answer: 2

Guidelines from the American Heart Association (2018) concerning Basic Life Support and CPR specify that the first responder call 911 for unresponsive adults, get an AED (if available), and return to the victim to provide CPR and defibrillation, if needed. Trained HCPs can use ventilations (1 breath every 8 seconds) with chest compressions (at least 100/minute).

Incorrect Choices:

The responder should use the AED as soon as possible after beginning CPR, and not wait 3 minutes. The compression rate for adult CPR is about 100/minute with a recommended compression-to-ventilation ratio of 30:2. The old ratio was 15:2. Untrained rescuers should use compressions only.

Type of Reasoning: Deductive

This question requires one to recall the proper and current Basic Life Support for health care provider guidelines. Questions that ask one to recall knowledge of protocols and guidelines necessitate deductive reasoning skill. If this question was answered incorrectly, refer to current guidelines for CPR.

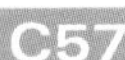
C57
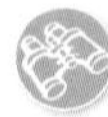

Musculoskeletal I Evaluation, Diagnosis

A patient who was casted for 3 weeks after a grade III right ankle sprain has been referred to physical therapy for mobility exercises. Examination shows a loss of 10° of dorsiflexion. Which activity will be the **MOST** difficult for the patient?

Choices:

1. Ambulating over rough surfaces.
2. Descending stairs.
3. Ambulating barefoot.
4. Descending a ramp.

Teaching Points

Correct Answer: 2

Loss of dorsiflexion will make descending stairs most difficult because the ankle must have sufficient dorsiflexion during the single-limb support phase of descent.

Incorrect Choices:

Although the activity may be changed, full range in dorsiflexion is not needed for the other choices.

Type of Reasoning: Inductive

The test-taker must analyze all of the activities and then utilize clinical judgment to determine which activity requires the most ankle dorsiflexion range. This requires inductive reasoning skill, in which clinical judgment is paramount to finding the correct solution. For this patient, descending stairs would be **MOST** difficult because full-range dorsiflexion is required to complete the task successfully.

C58

Nonsystem I Safety and Protection

An elderly patient presents to therapy after a fall onto an outstretched hand, now complaining of left wrist pain. The patient states medications are Aricept, Lasix, and warfarin. The patient has difficulty describing the exact incident and is withdrawn and distant. Upon examination of the wrist the therapist notes multiple contusions along the left wrist and forearm, as well as limited AROM with pain into extension. What is the therapist's next step in the process?

Choices:

1. Halt the examination and call protective services to discuss possible elder abuse/neglect.
2. Initiate treatment to modulate pain.
3. Refer the patient to an orthopedic physician.
4. Continue with the examination.

Teaching Points

Correct Answer: 4

The patient is currently on Aricept, which is a common medication for Alzheimer's-type dementia, and warfarin, which is a blood thinner that can increase patterns of bruising. This could explain the wrist/hand appearance and the demeanor of the patient. It is still important to investigate the living situation of the patient, but to continue with the current examination. Most appropriate would be to next perform PROM to help you in your thinking and to understand if extension is limited passively to differentiate between a contractile versus noncontractile tissue involvement.

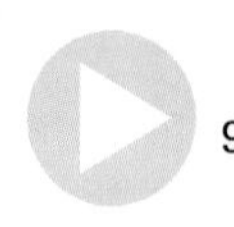

Incorrect Choices:

There are mitigating factors that make a conclusion of elder abuse premature. Ending the examination too soon leaves some gaps in obtaining vital information for treatment planning. At this time, there is little justification to refer this patient to an orthopedic physician.

Type of Reasoning: Evaluative

For this question, one must determine the next course of action, based on weighing information about the patient's clinical symptoms and medications used. This necessitates evaluative reasoning skill, where pieces of information are weighed for their significance and then used to guide toward a reasonable conclusion. For this case, the therapist should continue with the examination to gather further information about the patient's condition. If answered incorrectly, review medication information for Aricept and warfarin and their effects.

C59 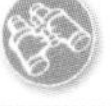

Musculoskeletal | Interventions

An adult recreational runner is referred to physical therapy with a diagnosis of Achilles' tendinopathy. The patient reports initial pain when running that resolves after a half-mile, but then returns a few hours after the run is complete. The insertion of the tendon is tender to palpation and the patient's pain is reproduced when performing a single leg heel raise. What is the **BEST** intervention to decrease pain and improve function in a patient with Achilles' tendinopathy?

Choices:

1. Resisted eccentric exercise of the ankle dorsiflexors.
2. Resisted eccentric exercise of the ankle plantarflexors.
3. Stretching of the gastrocnemius and soleus.
4. Soft tissue mobilization of the gastrocnemius and soleus.

Teaching Points

Correct Answer: 2

There is strong evidence to support eccentric loading to decrease pain and increase function in patients with Achilles' tendinopathy or tendonitis (see Box 2-13). The patient is likely to tolerate high eccentric loads in resistance training due to their low symptom severity and irritability.

Incorrect Choices:

There is no evidence to support or refute strengthening ankle dorsiflexors in patients with Achilles' tendinopathy, and no impairment was described in the question stem to suggest that strengthening the muscle group would be indicated. There is weak evidence to support stretching of the ankle plantarflexors and soft tissue mobilization of the gastrocnemius and soleus (expert opinion only).

Type of Reasoning: Inductive

One must utilize clinical judgment in order to determine a best course of action with this case. This requires inductive reasoning skill, where clinical judgment is paramount to arriving at a correct conclusion. For this case, it would be best to perform resisted eccentric ankle plantarflexion. If answered incorrectly, review treatment guidelines for Achilles' tendinopathy.

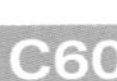
C60
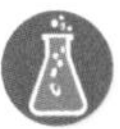

Neuromuscular | Evaluation, Diagnosis

A patient presents with an acute onset of vertigo overnight. Symptoms worsen with rapid change in head position. If the head is held still, symptoms subside usually within 30–60 seconds. What is the **MOST** likely cause of these symptoms?

Choices:

1. Ménière's disease.
2. Benign paroxysmal positional vertigo (BPPV).
3. Bilateral vestibular neuritis.
4. Acoustic neuroma.

Teaching Points

Correct Answer: 2

BPPV is characterized by acute onset of vertigo and is positional, related to the provoking stimulus of head movement.

Incorrect Choices:

Vestibular neuritis is an inflammation of the vestibular nerve caused by a virus and typically produces symptoms of dysequilibrium, nystagmus, nausea, and severe vertigo. Ménière's disease is characterized by a sensation of fullness in the ears associated with abnormal fluid buildup. Additional symptoms include tinnitus, vertigo, nausea, and hearing loss. Acoustic neuroma (vestibular schwannoma) produces unilateral sensorineural hearing loss along with vestibular symptoms.

Type of Reasoning: Analytical

One must analyze the symptoms and make a determination of the most likely cause for these symptoms, which requires analytical reasoning skill. For this case, the patient's symptom's **MOST LIKELY** cause is BPPV owing to the nature of an acute onset and being related to changing position of the head. Questions that inquire about a group of symptoms and whereby the test-taker must determine the diagnosis often utilize analytical reasoning skill.

C61
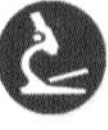

Cardiovascular/Pulmonary | Evaluation, Diagnosis

A patient has a history of coronary artery disease and COPD. Which of the following medications taken for COPD has side effects that impact the cardiovascular system?

Choices:

1. $Beta_2$ agonist.
2. Cromolyn sodium.
3. Glucocorticoid.
4. Leukotriene inhibitor.

Teaching Points

Correct Answer: 1

A $beta_2$ agonist is a bronchodilator, and it is primarily selective for receptors in the lung. However, it can impact the $beta_1$ receptors, which are primarily found in the heart. If there is stimulation of the $beta_1$ receptors in the heart, there is an increased sympathetic response. Therefore, a $beta_2$ agonist can cause tachycardia. See Table 5-10 for a review of common pulmonary medications.

Incorrect Choices:

None of the remaining choices have direct effects on the heart. Cromolyn sodium reduces the response of mast cells, which helps to reduce bronchoconstriction. Glucocorticoid decreases inflammation in the airway. Leukotriene inhibitors reduce bronchospasm.

Type of Reasoning: Deductive

For this question, one must recall medication guidelines in order to arrive at a correct conclusion. Specifically, the test-taker must recall which COPD medications impact the cardiovascular system, which necessitates deductive reasoning skill. In this case, a beta$_2$ agonist can impact the beta$_1$ receptors by causing tachycardia. If answered incorrectly, review pulmonary medications, especially beta$_2$ agonists.

C62 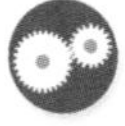

Neuromuscular I Evaluation, Diagnosis

A patient recently treated by a physical therapist for low back pain presents on a follow-up with new onset imbalance, dizziness, and nausea upon getting out of bed that morning. Upon examination, the therapist observes that the patient has a wide-based, unsteady gait, catch-up saccades during smooth pursuit eye tracking, and direction changing, gaze-evoked nystagmus. What is the **MOST APPROPRIATE** action for the therapist to take?

Choices:

1. Perform a canalith repositioning maneuver to treat new onset vestibular symptoms.
2. Immediately consult with the patient's primary care provider for further evaluation of new symptoms.
3. Begin gaze stabilization exercises for new onset vestibular symptoms.
4. Begin static balance training exercises in an environment with few visual stimuli.

Teaching Points

Correct Answer: 2

A wide-based, unsteady gait, catch-up saccades during smooth pursuit eye tracking and direction changing, gaze-evoked nystagmus are indicative of a central vestibular disorder. The rapid onset of the patient's symptoms and the manifestation of central vestibular signs suggest a possible stroke involving the vestibular nuclei or cerebellum and should be treated as an emergency situation.

Incorrect Choices:

The canalith repositioning maneuver, also known as the Epley maneuver, is performed for treatment of posterior canal benign paroxysmal positional vertigo. Gaze stabilization exercises and static balance training exercises are both appropriate for patients with central vestibular disorders. However, because of the acute presentation of the patient's symptoms, the patient needs further medical evaluation and management prior to beginning any type of rehabilitation.

Type of Reasoning: Evaluative

For this question, the test-taker must evaluate the symptoms presented and determine their level of significance. Then, based on this conclusion, determine an appropriate course of action. Questions of this nature often necessitate evaluative reasoning skill. For this situation, the most appropriate action is to immediately consult with the patient's primary care provider for further evaluation of new symptoms. Review information on central vestibular disorders if answered incorrectly.

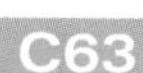
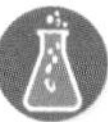

C63

Metabolic/Endocrine | Evaluation, Diagnosis

The PT reviews the laboratory results of a patient admitted to the acute care hospital yesterday: Hematocrit 45%, fasting blood glucose 180 mg/dL, and cholesterol 180 mg/dL. Based on these laboratory results, what condition is **MOST** likely?

Choices:

1. Polycythemia vera.
2. Hyperglycemia of diabetes.
3. Anemia.
4. Hyperlipidemia.

Teaching Points

Correct Answer: 2

Normal fasting blood glucose for adults is <100 mg/dL. A fasting blood glucose level of 180 mg/dL is abnormal and indicative of hyperglycemia of diabetes (see Chapter 8).

Incorrect Choices:

The hematocrit and cholesterol readings are within normal limits. Hyperlipidemia (excessive level of lipids in the blood) and anemia (reduced circulating red blood cells [RBCs]) are not indicated. An elevated hematocrit could be indicative of polycythemia vera (proliferation or hyperplasia of all bone marrow cells with an increase of RBCs and hemoglobin concentration).

Type of Reasoning: Analytical

This question requires one to determine the precise meaning of the laboratory values as it relates to a diagnosis for the patient. In this situation, the patient's laboratory values indicate diabetes mellitus. Drawing conclusions based on a group of indicators or symptoms requires analytical reasoning skill. If this question was answered incorrectly, review information on blood glucose laboratory values.

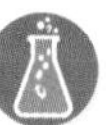

C64

Neuromuscular | Interventions

A patient recovering from a stroke is having difficulty with stair climbing. During ascent, the patient is able to position the more involved foot on the step above but is unable to transfer the weight up to the next stair level. What is the **BEST** exercise intervention to remediate this problem?

Choices:

1. Bridging, holding.
2. Standing, side steps.
3. Standing, partial wall squats.
4. Plantigrade, knee flexion with hip extension.

Teaching Points

Correct Answer: 3

The quadriceps muscle is responsible for most of the energy generation needed to transfer up stairs to the next level. Partial wall squats are the **BEST** choice to strengthen these muscles (closed-chain exercise). During forward continuance (corresponding to mid-stance), the ankle plantarflexors assist. Hip extensors are also active concentrically, assisting these actions.

Incorrect Choices:

The other choices might be good lead-up activities for gait but would not optimally strengthen the key muscles involved in ascending stairs.

Type of Reasoning: Analytical

This question requires one to analyze the described patient challenge and then determine the **BEST** intervention. The test-taker must determine what the cause is for the patient who has difficulty transferring weight to ascend stairs, which necessitates analytical reasoning. After analyzing the situation, one should conclude that the quadriceps muscle is weak and that partial wall squats in standing would **BEST** address this issue.

C65 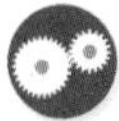

Cardiovascular/Pulmonary | Evaluation, Diagnosis

An elderly patient has been hospitalized and on complete bed rest for 10 days. A physical therapy referral requests mobilization out of bed and ambulation. The patient complains of aching in the right calf. The therapist's examination reveals calf tenderness with slight swelling and warmth. What is the **BEST** course of action for the therapist?

Choices:

1. Begin with ankle pump exercises in bed and then ambulate.
2. Postpone ambulation and report the findings immediately.
3. Ambulate the patient with support stockings on.
4. Use only AROM exercises with the patient sitting at the edge of the bed.

Teaching Points

Correct Answer: 2

The patient is exhibiting early signs of acute deep vein thrombophlebitis (DVT). These findings should be reported immediately. See Table 4-13 for a review of clinical examination findings for DVT and the Wells Criteria Score.

Incorrect Choices:

If DVT is present, the patient will be given anticoagulation therapy. After one dose of low molecular weight heparin, ambulation is encouraged. Compression stockings with a pressure gradient of 30–40 mmHg can assist with pain and reduce the risk of post-thrombolytic syndrome.

Type of Reasoning: Evaluative

One must evaluate the patient's symptoms and determine the best course of action, given one's understanding of the symptoms. Here, the patient's symptoms are indicative of DVT, which necessitates immediate notification and postponement of ambulation. If this question was answered incorrectly, refer to information on DVT and appropriate actions.

C66

Musculoskeletal | Examination

A 45-year-old patient presents to a direct access physical therapy clinic with neck pain after experiencing a fall off a curb. The patient struck their head during the fall but denies experiencing axial loading of the spine. The patient appears alert and stable during the physical therapy examination and is neurologically intact. Which physical examination finding would indicate a need for cervical spine radiographs?

Choices:

1. Inability to actively rotate neck 45°.
2. Age >40 years.
3. Neck Disability Index score ≥30.
4. Weak and painful deep neck flexor muscles.

Teaching Points

Correct Answer: 1

The above scenario involves application of the Canadian C-Spine Rules (see Box 2-17) in an adult patient with a neck injury who is alert and stable. Cervical spine x-ray series are only required for patients with a neck injury and who meet any of the following criteria: high risk factors such as age >65 years, dangerous mechanism of injury, or paresthesias in the extremities; or low-risk factors that limit safe assessment of range of motion; or inability to actively rotate the neck 45° to the left and right. The Canadian C-Spine Rules are highly sensitive and accurately RULE OUT a fracture (or the need for an x-ray) after an acute neck injury. Imaging is recommended if there is clinical suspicion of a fracture and if any of these criteria are met.

Incorrect Choices:

None of the other choices meet the Canadian C-Spine Rules or raise the index of suspicion for a possible fracture.

Type of Reasoning: Deductive

For this question, the test-taker must recall the Canadian C-Spine Rules to determine the physical examination finding that would indicate a need for cervical spine radiographs. This requires the recall of factual information, which is a deductive reasoning skill. For this case, the inability to actively rotate neck 45° would indicate a need for cervical spine radiographs. Review the Canadian C-Spine Rules if answered incorrectly.

C67 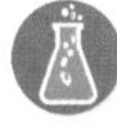

Musculoskeletal | Evaluation, Diagnosis

During an examination of an adolescent female who complains of anterior knee pain, the PT observes that the lower extremity shows medial femoral torsion and toeing-in position of the feet. What pathology of the hip is commonly associated with medial femoral torsion and toeing-in?

Choices:

1. Retroversion.
2. Anteversion.
3. Medial/internal rotation.
4. Lateral/external rotation.

Teaching Points

Correct Answer: 2

The pathology commonly associated with medial femoral torsion and toeing-in is hip anteversion due to an increase in the antetorsion angle (>15°) between the femoral condyles and the neck of the femur.

Incorrect Choices:

Excessive internal or external rotation of the hip would not force the patient to stand with toeing-in. Retroversion of the hips would cause the feet to toe-out.

Type of Reasoning: Analytical

This question provides the symptoms, and the test-taker must determine the likely cause, which requires analytical reasoning skill. Here, the symptoms are analyzed in order to make a determination for the cause of this patient's medial femoral torsion and toeing-in position of the feet. The test-taker should conclude that excessive hip anteversion is the cause, which should be reviewed if this question was answered incorrectly.

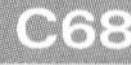
C68

Musculoskeletal | Interventions

A patient with osteoporosis and no fractures complains of increased middle and lower back pain during breathing and other functional activities. What is the **MOST** beneficial exercise intervention for this patient?

Choices:

1. Trunk flexion and rotation exercises.
2. Trunk flexion and extension exercises.
3. Trunk extension and abdominal stabilization exercises.
4. Trunk rotation and abdominal stabilization exercises.

Teaching Points

Correct Answer: 3

It is important to strengthen from the core to the floor as well as train in proprioception and balance enhancement techniques. Trunk extension and abdominal stabilization exercises are indicated.

Incorrect Choices:

Patients should avoid trunk flexion or rotation exercise because that might result in a compression fracture of the spine.

Type of Reasoning: Inferential

One must determine first what may be the cause of the patient's pain and then determine the intervention approach that will **BEST** remedy the symptoms. If this question was answered incorrectly, refer to intervention approaches for osteoporosis.

C69

Nonsystem | Safety and Protection

A single 22-year-old woman who is 3 months pregnant arrives at a therapist's private practice complaining of shoulder and leg pain. She has a black eye and some bruising at the wrists. The state in which the therapist practices has direct access. What is the **BEST** course of action for the therapist?

Choices:

1. Examine the patient, and if abuse is suspected, report the findings to the appropriate authorities.
2. Administer cryotherapy treatments as indicated by the examination findings.
3. Direct the patient to the nearest ambulatory care center for physician evaluation.
4. Refuse to examine the patient and send her to the nearest emergency room.

Teaching Points

Correct Answer: 1

According to the American Physical Therapy Association's (APTA's) Guidelines for Recognizing and Providing Care for Victims of Domestic Violence, this patient falls into a category of high risk. Women between the ages of 17 and 28 years and women who are single, separated, or divorced or who are planning a separation or divorce are at high risk. Battered women usually have more than one injury. Most injuries occur in the head, face, neck, breasts, and abdomen. According to the American Medical Association (AMA), battered women represent 23% of pregnant women who seek prenatal care. The victim may not volunteer information about her situation, but more often than not when asked will reveal it. It is important for the PT to examine the patient and, if abuse is suspected, report the findings to appropriate authorities. The therapist should be familiar with resources available for victims of domestic violence and their own state reporting laws.

Incorrect Choices:

In most state jurisdictions, a PT may be fined or indicted for failure to report (all other choices).

Type of Reasoning: Evaluative

This question requires one to make a judgment call for the **BEST** course of action, given the patient's symptoms. Questions that necessitate professional judgment in ethical situations often utilize evaluative reasoning skill, in which the merits of each potential choice are weighed. For this patient, it is important to do a comprehensive examination and then, if abuse is suspected, report it to the appropriate authorities.

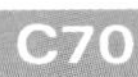

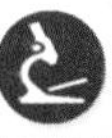

C70

Nonsystem | Therapeutic Modalities

An elderly patient presents with a stage III decubitus ulcer on the plantar surface of the right foot. After a series of conservative interventions with limited success, the therapist chooses to apply electrical stimulation for tissue repair. What is the **BEST** electrical current to administer in this case?

Choices:

1. Medium-frequency burst current.
2. High-volt monophasic pulsed current.
3. Medium-frequency beat current.
4. Low-volt biphasic pulsed current.

Teaching Points

Correct Answer: 2

Because high-volt pulsed current is a monophasic, unidirectional current, the unidirectional current would produce a therapeutic effect at the active (treatment) electrode. If there is no infection, the cathode (-pole) is recommended over the wound initially to promote healing. It should be continued unless wound healing plateaus or degrades. Alternate polarities if wound healing plateaus.

Incorrect Choices:

Although some studies support other waveforms, they are limited, and high-volt pulsed monophasic current has strong evidence to support its use (Khouri et al., 2017). The other waveforms theoretically could be used, but they do not have the same amount of research to support their use.

Type of Reasoning: Deductive

One must recall the appropriate electrical stimulation parameters to treat the patient's condition, which requires deductive reasoning skill. One must recall the differences between currents of differing low-, medium-, and high-volt currents, as well as pulsed, burst, and beat current, and the therapeutic effects on wound healing. If this question was answered incorrectly, review guidelines for electrical stimulation for wound healing.

C71 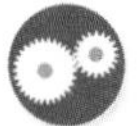

Nonsystem | Therapeutic Modalities

Intermittent traction is being used for the management of a patient with a lateral stenosis at L3-4. After the third visit with intermittent traction at 40% of the patient's body weight, the patient states their leg pain is now 50% less on a numeric pain rating scale prior to treatment. Additionally, the therapist's reexamination reveals quadriceps deep tendon reflexes are now asymmetrical (absent on involved side and 2+ uninvolved side). What is the next action the therapist should take?

Choices:

1. Continue with traction at the same percentage of body weight.
2. Continue with traction, but increase the traction to 50% of body weight.
3. Stop the traction and consult with the patient's physician.
4. Stop the traction and begin the patient on a repeated flexion exercise regime.

Teaching Points

Correct Answer: 3

Although the patient's pain is reduced, there is a clear indication the neurological compromise is worsening. Deep tendon reflexes are now asymmetrical, which indicates progression and requires immediate medical attention. Traction as a treatment approach should be reexamined if there are no improvements in the patient's condition within two to three treatments of traction or their condition worsens.

Incorrect Choices:

There are new neurological findings indicating the condition is worsening (DTRs are now asymmetrical). None of the other choices seek input from the patient's physician regarding the worsening of the symptoms.

Type of Reasoning: Evaluative

For this question, the test-taker is challenged to determine the cause for the patient's symptoms and then determine an appropriate course of action. This requires evaluative reasoning skill, where one must weigh the options presented in order to determine which will have the best outcome. For this case, the therapist should stop the traction and consult with the physician. If answered incorrectly, review traction treatment guidelines.

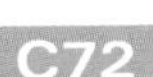 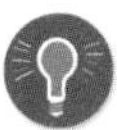

C72

Neuromuscular | Interventions

A patient recovering from stroke demonstrates hemiparesis of the right upper extremity with moderate flexion synergy. The therapist's goal is to first promote fractionated or independent elevation of the arm. What is the **BEST** exercise intervention to achieve this goal?

Choices:

1. Shoulder abduction with elbow flexion.
2. Shoulder flexion with elbow extension.
3. Shoulder horizontal adduction with elbow extension.
4. Shoulder horizontal adduction with elbow flexion.

Teaching Points

Correct Answer: 2

Obligatory hemiplegic synergies are present and should not be reinforced. Shoulder flexion with elbow extension is the correct choice. It is an out-of-synergy combination that reinforces individual (fractionated) and functional flexion of the shoulder without increased elbow flexion. In sitting, bending forward with elbow straight and hand touching floor is a good example of an early activity to promote this. See Table 3-8 for additional information on abnormal synergy patterns.

Incorrect Choices:

Shoulder abduction with elbow flexion is part of the flexion synergy, whereas adduction with elbow extension is part of the extension synergy. Adduction with elbow flexion is an out-of-synergy combination but does not strengthen muscles needed to elevate and stabilize the upper extremity.

Type of Reasoning: Inferential

One must evaluate the patient's symptoms and infer the **BEST** method for gaining fractionated movement while strengthening the shoulder muscles, thereby requiring inferential reasoning. Given the diagnosis and current status, shoulder flexion with elbow extension is **BEST** because hemiplegic synergies are discouraged using this approach. If this question was answered incorrectly, review limb synergies with stroke and out-of-synergy movement patterns.

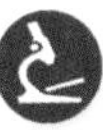

C73

Neuromuscular | Examination

A physical therapist shines a light into a patient's eye and observes the pupil of the eye. Constriction of the pupil results. Which cranial nerve is directly responsible for the motor component (constriction) of the pupillary light reflex?

Choices:

1. Abducens.
2. Trochlear.
3. Optic.
4. Oculomotor.

Teaching Points

Correct Answer: 4

The pupillary reflex (constriction of the pupil) is a function of the efferent (motor) portion of the oculomotor nerve (CN III).

Incorrect Choices:

The optic nerve (CN II) provides the sensory component of the pupillary light reflex and afferent signals to the brain and functions for visual acuity (interpretation of visual information). The trochlear nerve (CN IV) innervates the superior oblique muscles and helps to control extraocular eye movements (responsible for downward and lateral eye movements). The abducens nerve (CN VI) innervates the lateral rectus and helps to control extraocular eye movements (lateral eye movements).

Type of Reasoning: Deductive

This question necessitates factual recall of guidelines for testing the function of the cranial nerves in order to arrive at a correct conclusion. Questions of this nature often necessitate deductive reasoning skill, where recall of facts is used to make decisions. In this case, the description of the test performed is testing the motor function of the oculomotor nerve (CN III). If answered incorrectly, review guidelines for testing the cranial nerves, especially CN III. See Table 3-1 for Cranial Nerve Examination.

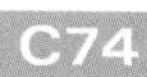

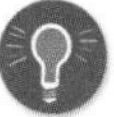

Cardiovascular/Pulmonary I Examination

A patient is referred for physical therapy after a graded exercise test (GXT). The physician reports the test was positive and had to be terminated at 7 minutes. Which of the following criteria is an absolute indication for terminating exercise testing?

Choices:

1. Mild angina and dyspnea with progressive increases in the treadmill speed and grade.
2. A hypertensive response with blood pressure of at least 170/95.
3. ST segment depression from baseline of 3-mm horizontal or downsloping depression.
4. ECG changes from baseline of 1-mm ST segment elevation.

Teaching Points

Correct Answer: 3

A positive GXT indicates myocardial ischemia with increasing exercise intensities. The optimal test duration is 8–12 minutes but can be terminated if symptoms of exertional intolerance are evident. The American College of Sports Medicine (ACSM) indicates these include ECG changes from baseline (>2 mm horizontal or downsloping; ST segment depression, or >2 mm ST segment elevation).

Incorrect Choices:

Additional signs of exertional intolerance that indicate the test should be terminated include onset of moderate to severe angina (some angina is expected with increasing work), a drop in systolic BP with increasing workload, serious arrhythmias, signs of exertional intolerance (pallor, cyanosis, cold or clammy skin), unusual or severe shortness of breath (some shortness of breath is expected), CNS signs (ataxia, vertigo, visual or gait problems, confusion), and a hypertensive response equal to or greater than 260/115 (a BP of 170/95 is not a reason for stopping the test) (ACSM Guidelines for Exercise Testing and Prescription, 10th ed., 2017).

Type of Reasoning: Inferential

This question requires one to infer information based on the evidence presented. In this case, the test-taker must infer what a positive GXT indicates in an early termination of the test after 7 minutes. If this question was answered incorrectly, refer to information on exercise tolerance testing and ACSM guidelines for terminating the test.

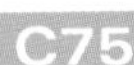
C75 

Musculoskeletal | Evaluation, Diagnosis

A middle-aged patient suffered a twisting injury to the knee during a recreational softball game. The patient's chief complaint is medial knee pain. The physical therapist examines the knee and performs the Thessaly test with a positive result. There is also joint line tenderness. The Lachman test, anterior/posterior drawer, and varus/valgus stress tests are negative. What is the **MOST LIKELY** diagnosis?

Choices:

1. ACL sprain.
2. MCL sprain.
3. Medial meniscus tear.
4. Patellar dislocation/subluxation.

Teaching Points

Correct Answer: 3

Based on the patient history and physical examination findings, a medial meniscus tear is the most likely diagnosis. A diagnostic test cluster, which includes joint line tenderness combined with a positive Thessaly test (or disc sign), is highly sensitive for identifying meniscus tears (see Box 2-8). The test is performed by having the patient assume a single limb stance on the affected side with the knee in about 20° flexion. The patient then rotates the femur on the tibia, both internally and externally, three times.

Incorrect Choices:

Joint line tenderness may also occur with an MCL sprain, but the diagnosis is less likely as the ligamentous stress test (valgus) was negative. An ACL injury is unlikely given the negative ligamentous stress tests. Patellar dislocation/subluxation may fit the mechanism of injury but is less likely than a meniscal tear given the rest of the examination findings.

Type of Reasoning: Analytical

For this question, a group of symptoms are provided and the test-taker must analyze them in order to determine the most likely diagnosis. This requires analytical reasoning skill, where pieces of information are weighed to draw correct conclusions. For this case, the symptoms are consistent with a medial meniscus tear. If answered incorrectly, review symptoms of medial meniscus tear.

C76 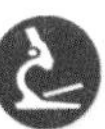

Integumentary | Interventions

A patient with a grade III diabetic ulcer is being treated with a calcium alginate wound dressing. What are the primary indications for this type of wound dressing?

Choices:

1. Provide semi-rigid support for the limb while maintaining a sterile field.
2. Facilitate autolytic debridement and absorb exudate.
3. Absorb exudate and allow rapid moisture evaporation.
4. Restrict bacteria from the wound while supporting the tissues.

Teaching Points

Correct Answer: 2

Moisture-retentive occlusive wound dressings such as calcium alginate are recommended for use on exudating wounds (grade III ulcer). They maintain a moist wound environment, absorb exudate, provide autolytic debridement, reduce pain at the wound site, or promote faster healing (reepithelialization).

Incorrect Choices:

Calcium alginate dressings do **NOT** allow rapid evaporation. A disadvantage is that the dressing is very permeable to bacteria, urine, and so forth. Unna's boot is a semi-rigid dressing that provides limb support.

Type of Reasoning: Deductive

This question requires one to recall the properties of a calcium alginate wound dressing. Recall of protocols and guidelines and other types of factual information often requires deductive reasoning skill. For this question, calcium alginate dressings can be expected to facilitate autolytic debridement and absorption of exudate. If this question was answered incorrectly, review information on calcium alginate and other wound dressings.

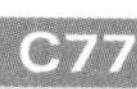

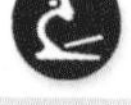

Nonsystem | Safety and Protection

A patient with an active, primary infection of *Mycobacterium tuberculosis* (TB) is admitted to an acute care facility for an initial course of antituberculin drugs. The patient is restricted to an airborne infection isolation room (AIIR). Airborne precautions are initiated. What precautions should be observed when working with this patient in the AIIR?

Choices:

1. The patient wears a surgical mask and the health care worker wears a respirator mask.
2. The patient wears a respirator mask and the health care worker wears a surgical mask.
3. The patient wears personal protective equipment when coming in contact with the therapist.
4. The therapist observes contact precautions with frequent glove and gown changes.

Teaching Points

Correct Answer: 1

The patient wears a surgical mask when interacting with health professionals, exiting the room, and coming in close contact with other individuals. Instructions in hygiene and cough etiquette are given and tissues and no-touch receptacles are utilized. The health care worker wears a respirator mask designed to filter the air of infectious droplets. Airborne precautions in a health care setting may be discontinued after the patient with TB has been on adequate drug therapy for 2 weeks or longer, symptoms improve, and there are three consecutive negative AFB sputum smear results.

Incorrect Choices:

The patient does not need to wear a respirator mask as the filtering system in an AIIR room will flush out droplets in the air. The patient does not need to wear personal protective equipment while in the AIIR room. Contact precautions using personal protective equipment (PPE) including gloves and gown are indicated for the health care worker when coming in contact with soiled equipment, blood, or body fluids. Frequent changes are not necessary.

Type of Reasoning: Deductive

This question requires the test-taker to recall the guidelines for airborne precautions and working with individuals in an airborne infection isolation room (AIIR). This necessitates the recall of factual guidelines, which is a deductive reasoning skill. For this situation, the health care worker should wear a respirator mask while the patient wears a surgical mask. If answered incorrectly, be sure to review airborne precautions and guidelines for working in an AIIR.

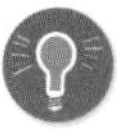

C78

Musculoskeletal | Evaluation, Diagnosis

A patient with a transtibial amputation is learning to walk using a patellar tendon-bearing (PTB) prosthesis and is having difficulty maintaining knee stability from heelstrike to foot-flat. Which muscles are **MOST** likely weak?

Choices:

1. Hip flexors.
2. Back extensors.
3. Knee extensors.
4. Knee flexors.

Teaching Points

Correct Answer: 3

The knee extensors (quadriceps) are maximally active at heelstrike (initial contact) to stabilize the knee and counteract the flexion moment.

Incorrect Choices:

Erector spinae, gluteus maximus, and hamstrings contribute to core stability (trunk and pelvis) and assist in counteracting the flexion moment from heelstrike to foot-flat. Hip flexors contribute to initiate swing (acceleration to midswing), whereas knee flexors (hamstrings) decelerate the momentum of the swinging leg (midswing to deceleration).

Type of Reasoning: Inferential

One must infer the reason for the difficulty in maintaining prosthetic stability in order to choose the correct solution. This requires inferential reasoning, where one must determine the muscles that are **MOST LIKELY** weak.

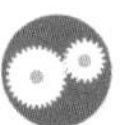

C79

Cardiovascular/Pulmonary | Evaluation, Diagnosis

An inpatient is seen by a physical therapist to initiate a rehabilitation program. During the initial evaluation, the patient experiences heart palpitations, light headedness, and shortness of breath. Based on the patient's symptoms and the rate and rhythm shown on the telemetry strip below, how should the physical therapist proceed?

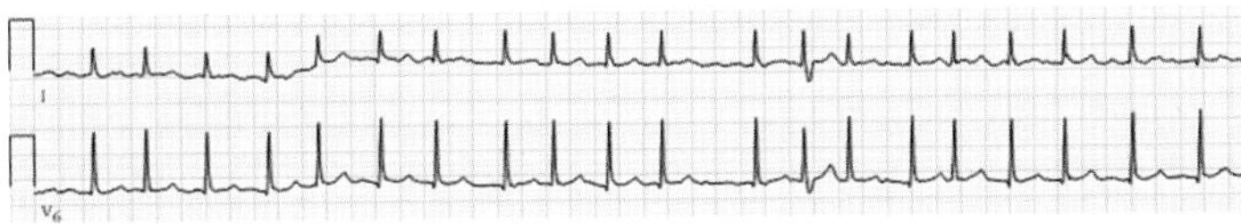

Choices:

1. Conduct the evaluation without limitations; the telemetry strip is normal.
2. Defer the evaluation for now; the telemetry strip indicates that medical management is necessary.
3. Call the physician to discharge physical therapy; the telemetry strip indicates contraindication to exercise.
4. Activate EMS; the telemetry strip indicates a medical emergency.

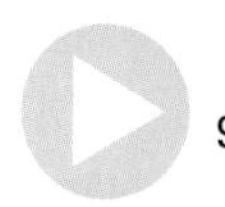

Teaching Points

Correct Answer: 2

The patient's symptoms and the increased resting heart rate of 120 beats per minute shown on the telemetry unit are consistent with atrial fibrillation. Other symptoms of atrial fibrillation can include weakness, fatigue, and chest pain. The patient is at risk for decreased cardiac output if the workload is increased at this time. However, once medically evaluated and managed, the patient should be able to participate in physical therapy. See page 253 for a review of heart arrhythmias.

Incorrect Choices:

The evaluation should not be conducted without further medical management because it places the patient at risk for decompensation. Atrial fibrillation is not an absolute contraindication to exercise, but the rate must be within a controlled range. This is not a medical emergency. It would be considered a medical emergency if there was hemodynamic compromise (i.e., drop in blood pressure) or other indications that the patient was not maintaining their cardiac output at rest (i.e., mental status changes).

Type of Reasoning: Evaluative

For this question, the test-taker must analyze the information presented in the echocardiogram, then make a determination of the best course of action based on this analysis. This necessitates evaluative reasoning skill, where potential courses of action are weighed to determine the best action. For this case, the therapist should defer the evaluation for now as medical management is necessary for atrial fibrillation. If answered incorrectly, review information on atrial fibrillation and electrocardiogram interpretation.

C80 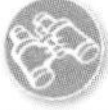

Neuromuscular | Evaluation, Diagnosis

A physical therapist has just completed an initial examination on a patient with upper extremity complex regional pain syndrome type 1. What is the **FIRST** treatment the physical therapist should perform?

Choices:

1. Desensitization training.
2. Neuroscience pain education.
3. Active range of motion exercises.
4. Manual therapy.

Teaching Points

Correct Answer: 2

Neuroscience pain education has demonstrated significant improvements in pain, physical function, and fear of movement for various conditions associated with chronic pain. Initially discussing the impact of chronic pain, the neuroscience behind their pain, and the importance of targeted and controlled movements will better prepare the patient for the treatments that may follow (manual therapy, desensitization training, and exercise).

Incorrect Choices:

Desensitization training, exercise, and manual therapy are potential options for treatment but should occur after the physical therapist has discussed the plan of care and neuroscience pain education with the patient.

Type of Reasoning: Inductive

For this question, one must utilize clinical judgment in order to determine a best course of action for a patient with complex regional pain syndrome, type 1. This is an inductive reasoning skill. For this case, the therapist should first initiate treatment with neuroscience pain education. If answered incorrectly, review intervention approaches for complex regional pain syndrome.

C81 

System Interactions | Evaluation, Diagnosis

The PT is completing general activity recommendations for a group home of young adults with emotional and behavioral issues. All patients are chemically controlled with either antipsychotic or antidepressant medications. Full-time supervision is available for any activity recommended. Which exercise considerations would be important in this situation?

Choices:

1. Avoid games with throwing activities to prevent injuries.
2. Promote rhythmic movement to soothing music to avoid agitation.
3. Promote activities with sequential movements to improve memory.
4. Avoid aerobic exercises outdoors when temperature is over 90°F.

Teaching Points

Correct Answer: 4

Overheating is detrimental to individuals on antipsychotic or antidepressant medications.

Incorrect Choices:

Assumptions of agitation, memory deficits, or violence in such populations are discriminatory and inaccurate. Although an individual client may demonstrate these, it is inaccurate to suggest these for a group without further individual information.

Type of Reasoning: Inferential

This question requires one to have knowledge of the adverse/side effects of antipsychotic and antidepressant medications in order to arrive at a correct conclusion. In this situation, the potential adverse effect is overheating; therefore, avoiding aerobic exercise outdoors in temperatures over 90°F is the **MOST** appropriate precaution. If this question was answered incorrectly, review information on adverse effects of antipsychotics and antidepressants.

C82 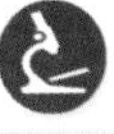

Neuromuscular | Examination

Following an initial functional examination using the Functional Independence Measure (FIM), a patient is found to require minimal contact assistance in transferring from sit-to-stand and bed-to-wheelchair. Which of the following accurately documents these results?

Choices:

1. FIM level 4; completes activity with 75% or more of the effort.
2. FIM level 6; completes activity with extra time.
3. FIM level 5; completes activity with cueing.
4. FIM level 3; completes activity with 50% or more but less than 75% of the effort.

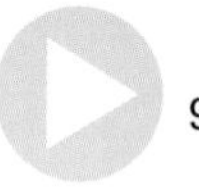

Teaching Points

Correct Answer: 1

This patient's performance is best categorized by FIM level 4 (completes activity with minimal contact assistance and 75% or more of the effort). See Appendix 3A.

Incorrect Choices:

With FIM level 3 grades, the patient requires moderate assistance and completes activity with 50% or more but less than 75% of the effort. FIM level 5 grade specifies complete activity with cueing or standby assistance but no manual contact. FIM level 6 (modified independence) does not permit manual contact and allows for equipment or extra time.

Type of Reasoning: Deductive

This question requires one to recall the Functional Independence Measure (FIM) scale and to match the scale scores to the performance indicated with this patient. This is factual recall of knowledge, which is a deductive reasoning skill. In this case, the patient's performance indicates minimal assist (level 4). If answered incorrectly, review the FIM.

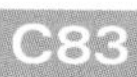
C83
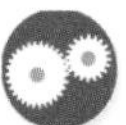

Musculoskeletal I Interventions

An infant has been diagnosed with hip dysplasia. Conservative treatment is being tried to avoid surgery. The child is wearing a hip positioning harness but is allowed to be out of the harness during physical therapy only. Which position should **TOTALLY** be avoided when out of the harness?

Choices:

1. Hip flexion, adduction, and internal rotation.
2. Hip extension, abduction, and external rotation.
3. Hip flexion, abduction, and external rotation.
4. Hip extension, adduction and internal rotation.

Teaching Points

Correct Answer: 4

The child will most likely be wearing a Pavlik harness. This device keeps the head of the femur completely seated in the acetabulum by positioning the infant in a "frog legged" position. The hips are positioned in flexion, abduction, and external rotation with knees flexed. During physical therapy the infant may be allowed to have the harness off; however, hip extension, adduction, and internal rotation should be avoided.

Incorrect Choices:

Hip flexion, abduction, and external rotation is the desired position achieved with the harness. The other answers contain only part of a position that may or may not impact the femoral head.

Type of Reasoning: Evaluative

This question requires one to evaluate each of the positions presented and determine which one would be contraindicated when the child is out of the hip harness. This necessitates the weighing of information to determine significance and potential harm, which is an evaluative reasoning skill. For this question, hip extension, adduction, and internal rotation should be avoided out of the harness. Review information on hip dysplasia if answered incorrectly.

C84

Musculoskeletal | Interventions

A physical therapist is developing a treatment plan for a patient with fibromyalgia (FM). Which factor must the therapist consider when planning an exercise regimen for this patient?

Choices:

1. Patients with FM have difficulty with water-based (aquatic) exercises.
2. Supervision or group exercise sessions may decrease compliance with the regimen.
3. Morning sessions work best for patients with FM.
4. Patients with FM have difficulty with sustained overhead activities.

Teaching Points

Correct Answer: 4

Individuals with fibromyalgia (FM) typically do not tolerate sustained overhead activities, vigorous or high-impact activities, and eccentric muscle contractions because they evoke pain. These patients also tend to be vulnerable to overdoing exercise sessions. It is better to progress slowly and err on the side of doing "too little" during a session, rather than risk having the patient drop out of the exercise program.

Incorrect Choices:

Aquatic exercise programs are particularly effective for the patient with FM. Similarly, supervised or group exercise sessions tend to increase adherence or compliance with an exercise program in this population. Like patients with osteoarthritis, patients with FM often experience morning stiffness and pain. Up to 85% of patients with fibromyalgia also experience sleep disturbances and may have difficulty getting their day started. Therefore, timing of treatment is an important consideration and afternoon sessions are recommended.

Type of Reasoning: Inferential

This question requires the test-taker to determine what is likely to be true of a diagnosis, necessitating inferential reasoning skill. Inferential reasoning is often utilized in situations where one must predict likely outcomes or situations. For this situation, the therapist must consider that individuals with FM have difficulty with sustained overhead activities. If answered incorrectly, review FM information and planning of exercise regimens for individuals with FM.

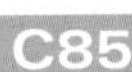
C85
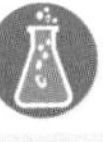

Musculoskeletal | Evaluation, Diagnosis

A patient presents with insidious onset of pain in the jaw that is referred to the head and neck regions. As best as the patient can recall, it may be related to biting into something hard. Cervical ROM is limited in flexion by 20°, cervical lateral flexion limited to the left by 10°. Mandibular depression is 10 mm with deviation to the left, protrusion is 4 mm, and lateral deviation is 15 mm to the right and 6 mm to the left. What is the **MOST** likely diagnosis given this patient's symptoms?

Choices:

1. Weak lateral pterygoids on the right.
2. Weak lateral pterygoids on the left.
3. Capsule-ligamentous pattern of temporomandibular joint (TMJ) on the left.
4. Cervical spine capsular restrictions on the left.

Teaching Points

Correct Answer: 3

The capsule-ligamentous pattern of the TMJ is limitation on opening, lateral deviation greater to the uninvolved side, and deviation on opening to the involved side. Normal parameters for TMJ measures are 25–35 mm functional and 35–50 mm normal, normal protrusion is 3–6 mm and normal lateral deviation is 10–15 mm.

Incorrect Choices:

Weakness of the lateral pterygoids presents as deviation on protrusion to the opposite side of the muscle weakness. A capsular pattern of the cervical spine presents as side flexion and rotation, equally limited, and extension.

Type of Reasoning: Analytical

Questions that inquire about a potential diagnosis given a patient's symptoms necessitate analytical reasoning skill. This is because one must weigh the information and analyze the symptoms in order to reach a conclusion that the diagnosis is most likely capsule-ligamentous pattern of TMJ on the left. If this question was answered incorrectly, review information on symptoms of TMJ.

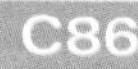
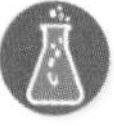

C86

Neuromuscular | Evaluation, Diagnosis

A patient has been referred to physical therapy with a diagnosis of cervicogenic headaches. During the initial examination, the therapist notes clinical findings of a droopy eyelid, constricted pupil (a pinpoint pupil), and lack of sweating on the same side of the face. What is the **MOST** likely diagnosis based on this group of symptoms?

Choices:

1. Horner's syndrome.
2. Bell's palsy.
3. Trigeminal neuralgia.
4. Myasthenia gravis.

Teaching Points

Correct Answer: 1

The hallmark finding of Horner's syndrome is the clinical triad of mild ptosis (droopy eyelid), miosis (pupillary constriction), and anhydrosis (lack of sweating), all on the same side of the face and ipsilateral to the lesion. Skin vasodilation is also typically present. Horner's syndrome results from a lesion that affects the sympathetic pathway to the head. The syndrome may be caused by trauma, interruption of blood supply, tumors, or cluster headaches. Cranial nerve III, the oculomotor nerve, contains parasympathetic fibers that innervate the pupillary constrictor muscle. Therefore, loss of sympathetic innervation of the pupillary dilator muscle results in unopposed pupillary constriction.

Incorrect Choices:

Bell's palsy is an idiopathic lesion to CN VII, the facial nerve. This is a lower motor neuron or peripheral nerve lesion that results in paralysis or weakness of the muscles of facial expression on the same side as the lesion. Trigeminal neuralgia (tic douloureux) is a pain syndrome that involves CN V, the trigeminal nerve. The three branches (mandibular, maxillary, and ophthalmic) of CN V provide general sensation to the skin of the face, as well as the lips, corneas, and anterior one-third of the tongue. Trigeminal neuralgia produces severe, sharp, stabbing pain in the distribution of one or more of the branches of the nerve. Common causes of the disorder include a peripheral lesion to the nerve, hyperexcitability of damaged fibers in the large trigeminal nerve ganglion, or pressure of a blood vessel on the nerve. Myasthenia gravis is an auto-immune disease of the neuromuscular junction resulting in severe muscle weakness, most notably with repeated contractions. While ptosis is a common finding in myasthenia gravis, none of the other findings in the scenario are consistent with the disorder.

Type of Reasoning: Analytical

This question provides a group of symptoms, and the test-taker must determine the most likely diagnosis. This requires analytical reasoning skill, where pieces of information are analyzed in order to reach a sound conclusion about them. For this situation, the symptoms are indicative of Horner's syndrome. Review symptoms of Horner's syndrome if answered incorrectly.

C87 

Cardiovascular/Pulmonary | Evaluation, Diagnosis

A patient with a recent history of rib fractures suddenly becomes short of breath during a bout of coughing. The patient looks panicked and complains of sharp pain in the left chest. A quick screen shows a deviated trachea to the right, among other signs and symptoms. What is the **MOST** likely diagnosis based on these symptoms?

Choices:

1. Pulmonary emboli.
2. Pneumothorax.
3. Angina.
4. Mucous plugging of an airway.

Teaching Points

Correct Answer: 2

The deviation of the trachea toward the right with the chest pain on the left is a match of symptoms for the occurrence of a pneumothorax on the left. The history of a rib fracture makes pneumothorax all the more likely.

Incorrect Choices:

Whereas all of the pathologies listed would cause panic on the part of the patient, mucous plugging of an airway would not cause pain. The deviation of the trachea would not result from angina or pulmonary emboli, but would happen with a pneumothorax and lung tissue collapse (which could result from mucous plugging).

Type of Reasoning: Analytical

This question provides symptoms, and the test-taker must determine a cause for them. This necessitates analytical reasoning skill, in which one must produce the correct diagnosis based on the patient's symptoms. If this question was answered incorrectly, review information of symptoms of pneumothorax.

C88 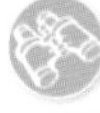

Musculoskeletal | Interventions

A patient presents with supraspinatus tendinitis. After initial treatment with cryotherapy, the therapist decides to apply ultrasound (US). In what position should the therapist place the shoulder joint in order to effectively treat the supraspinatus tendon?

Choices:

1. Adduction and external rotation.
2. Slight abduction and internal rotation.
3. Adduction and internal rotation.
4. Slight abduction and external rotation.

Teaching Points

Correct Answer: 2

Abduction and internal rotation of the shoulder places the supraspinatus tendon in a good position to apply US by exposing the tendon from under the acromion process.

Incorrect Choices:

The other choices fail to position the supraspinatus tendon in optimal position.

Type of Reasoning: Inductive

One must utilize diagnostic and clinical judgment to determine the best course of action when providing US for supraspinatus tendinitis. Questions that require clinical and diagnostic reasoning utilize inductive reasoning skill.

C89 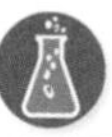

Integumentary | Examination

A patient is referred for postmastectomy rehabilitation. During the initial examination, the therapist observes an irregular area of skin on the patient's shoulder about 7 mm in diameter. The patient reports that there has always been a mole there but is more prominent lately and that the color has changed, now ranging from black to red to blue. How should the therapist document this finding?

Choices:

1. Papule.
2. Wheal.
3. Atypical dysplastic nevus.
4. Benign nevus.

Teaching Points

Correct Answer: 3

A nevus is a common mole. A changing nevus (atypical dysplastic nevus) that presents with asymmetry (A), irregular borders (B), variations in color (C), diameter >6 mm (D), and elevation (E) may be indicative of malignant melanoma (the "ABCDEs" from the American Cancer Society; see Table 7-4).

Incorrect Choices:

A benign nevus does not present with changes and variations in color. A papule is an elevated nevus. A wheal is an irregular, transient superficial area of localized skin edema (e.g., hive, mosquito bite).

Type of Reasoning: Analytical

Questions that provide an array of symptoms and require the test-taker to determine the likely findings often require analytical reasoning skills. For this scenario, the key words including "irregular area" and "variations in color" should assist the test-taker in concluding this finding as an atypical dysplastic nevus. If this question was answered incorrectly, review signs and symptoms of skin malignancies from the American Cancer Society.

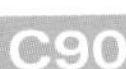
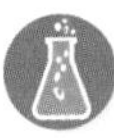

C90

Neuromuscular | Evaluation, Diagnosis

A patient is 2 days post–left CVA and has just been moved from the intensive care unit to a stroke unit. When beginning the examination, the therapist finds the patient's speech slow and hesitant. The patient is limited to one- and two-word productions, and expressions are awkward and arduous. However, the patient demonstrates good comprehension. What type of speech disorder is this patient exhibiting?

Choices:

1. Fluent aphasia.
2. Global aphasia.
3. Nonfluent aphasia.
4. Dysarthria.

Teaching Points

Correct Answer: 3

This patient is demonstrating classic signs of nonfluent aphasia (Broca's motor or expressive aphasia). It is the result of a lesion involving the third frontal convolution of the left hemisphere. Nonfluent aphasia is characterized by slow and hesitant speech with limited vocabulary and labored articulation. There is relative preservation of auditory comprehension.

Incorrect Choices:

Fluent aphasia (Wernicke's or receptive aphasia) is characterized by impaired auditory comprehension and fluent speech. Global aphasia is a severe aphasia with marked dysfunction across all language modalities. Dysarthria is impairment in the motor production of speech.

Type of Reasoning: Analytical

This question provides symptoms, and the test-taker must determine the diagnosis. This requires analytical reasoning skill, in which one must determine the cause for the symptoms. If this question was answered incorrectly, review symptoms of nonfluent (Broca's) aphasia.

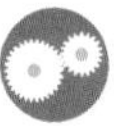

C91

Neuromuscular | Examination

A patient recovering from traumatic brain injury (TBI) is functioning at level IV on the Rancho Los Amigos Levels of Cognitive Functioning Scale (LOCF). During the therapist's initial examination, the patient becomes agitated and tries to bite the therapist. What is the therapist's **BEST** course of action?

Choices:

1. Postpone the examination for 1 week and then try again.
2. Restructure the formal examination so the therapist can complete it in three very short sessions.
3. Document the behaviors and engage in a calming activity.
4. Postpone the examination until later in the day when the patient calms down.

Teaching Points

Correct Answer: 3

Patients with TBI in level IV of recovery are confused and agitated. Behavior is bizarre and nonpurposeful relative to the immediate environment. This patient is unable to cooperate directly with formal examination or treatment, lacking both selective attention and memory. The therapist needs to observe and document the behaviors closely and engage the patient in a calming activity such as slow rocking. A quiet, closed environment is critical.

Incorrect Choices:

Because the patient's symptoms are expected for a person in level IV of Rancho LOCF Scale, it is not appropriate to defer treatment or restructure the examination. The patient's immediate needs must be addressed.

Type of Reasoning: Evaluative

One must determine the **BEST** course of action based on evaluating the merits of the four possible CHOICES presented. One must ask, "Are these symptoms expected for this stage of recovery, and if so, what would be **BEST?**" If this question was answered incorrectly, review Rancho LOCF Scale (see Table 3-17).

C92 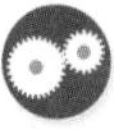

Cardiovascular/Pulmonary | Evaluation, Diagnosis

A patient comes to their first outpatient physical therapy appointment after having a total knee replacement 2 weeks ago. The patient has a history of hypertension, coronary artery disease, and heart failure. During the physical examination, the patient exhibits bilateral lower extremity edema, shortness of breath with minimal activity, crackles during lung auscultation, and jugular vein distention. What should the therapist do next?

Choices:

1. Proceed with the physical examination.
2. Send an email to the referring physician.
3. Call the referring physician.
4. Activate emergency medical services.

Teaching Points

Correct Answer: 3

The patient is exhibiting signs of decompensated heart failure (yellow zone according to the Clinical Practice Guideline for the Management of the Patient with Heart Failure; see Table 4-12). Developing an immediate plan in consult with the physician provides the patient with the best care.

Incorrect Choices:

Based on the signs of decompensated heart failure, it is inappropriate to proceed with the examination as the patient could worsen. Emailing the physician may delay care for the patient because it is unknown when the physician will read the email. While the patient requires medical care, it is not a medical emergency as they are not demonstrating signs of respiratory distress, mental status changes, or acute coronary syndrome. Therefore, activating EMS is not needed at this time.

Type of Reasoning: Evaluative

For this question, the test-taker must evaluate the symptoms of the patient and determine a best course of action. This necessitates evaluative reasoning skill, where the test-taker weighs the potential courses of action and determines which one most effectively addresses the issue. For this case, the therapist should call the referring physician. If answered incorrectly, review the Clinical Practice Guideline for the Management of the Patient with Heart Failure.

C93 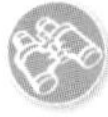

Musculoskeletal | Examination

A patient with anterior knee pain has increased adduction and internal rotation at the hip when performing a squat. Which muscles are **MOST** likely weak, causing this compensatory movement?

Choices:

1. Knee flexors and extensors.
2. Hip adductors and internal rotators.
3. Hip and knee flexors.
4. Hip abductors and external rotators.

Teaching Points

Correct Answer: 4

Decreased strength of the hip abductors and external rotators are common findings in patients with anterior knee pain. Weakness is often demonstrated during a squat with increased hip adduction and internal rotation due to the poor eccentric control of these muscles.

Incorrect Choices:

Weakness of the knee flexors and extensors would not significantly affect hip mechanics during a squat. Weakness of the hip and knee flexors would not affect the squat as the hip and knee flexion are controlled eccentrically by the hip and knee extensors. Weakness of the hip adductors and internal rotators would not create this compensatory movement; rather, the opposite may occur.

Type of Reasoning: Inductive

This question requires the test-taker to draw from clinical knowledge of knee pain and compensatory patterns of movement in order to arrive at a correct conclusion. This is an inductive reasoning skill. For this situation, a patient with anterior knee pain who demonstrates hip adduction and internal rotation during a squat is most likely compensating for weak hip abductors and external rotators. Review knee pain and compensatory movement strategies if answered incorrectly.

C94 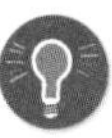

Metabolic/Endocrine | Evaluation, Diagnosis

A patient has been taking corticosteroids (hydrocortisone) for management of adrenocortical insufficiency and is referred to physical therapy for mobility training after a prolonged hospitalization. What are the potential adverse effects from prolonged use of this medication?

Choices:

1. Hypotension and myopathy.
2. Decreased appetite and weight loss.
3. Atrophy and osteoporosis.
4. Confusion and depression.

Teaching Points

Correct Answer: 3

Prolonged use of corticosteroids may result in muscle weakness, osteoporosis, fractures, and joint pain. Large doses are associated with Cushingoid changes (e.g., moon face, central obesity, hypertension, myopathy, electrolyte and fluid imbalance). Common central nervous system changes include insomnia and nervousness.

Incorrect Choices:

The other choices are not expected potential adverse effects of corticosteroids.

Type of Reasoning: Inferential

One must infer or draw conclusions about the expected symptoms of prolonged use of corticosteroids in order to arrive at the correct conclusion. For this patient, one could expect atrophy and osteoporosis to occur. If this question was answered incorrectly, review information on side effects of long-term corticosteroid use.

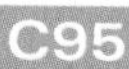
C95

Integumentary | Evaluation, Diagnosis

A PT is treating a patient with deep partial-thickness burns over 35% of the body (chest and arms). Wound cultures reveal a bacterial count in excess of 105/g of tissue on the anterior left arm. What are the reasonable expectations for this type of burn wound?

Choices:

1. With antibiotics, spontaneous healing can be expected.
2. The risk of hypertrophic and keloid scars is low because there is no viable tissue.
3. The burn area is pain free because all nerve endings in the dermal tissue were destroyed.
4. The infected wound can convert the area to a full-thickness burn.

Teaching Points

Correct Answer: 4

A deep partial-thickness burn will heal in about 3–5 weeks if it does not become infected. An infection typically results in conversion of the wound to a full-thickness burn.

Incorrect Choices:

Full-thickness burns (not partial-thickness burns) are without sensation because the nerve endings are destroyed. However, the area is not pain free, because adjacent areas of partial-thickness burns have intact nerve endings and can be painful. The risk of hypertrophic and keloid scars is high (not low) with deep partial-thickness or full-thickness burns. With wound conversion, grafting will be necessary because all epithelial cells are destroyed with a full-thickness burn. With an infected wound, spontaneous healing is not expected.

Type of Reasoning: Inferential

One must determine what a bacterial count of 105/g indicates in order to choose the correct solution. This requires one to draw conclusions about the information presented, which, when inferred correctly, indicates that the wound is infected and could convert the burned area to a full-thickness burn. If this question was answered incorrectly, refer to burn care guidelines, especially infected wounds.

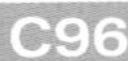
C96
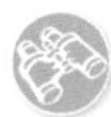

Nonsystem | Equipment, Devices

Recently, a 10-year-old patient has begun walking with supination and calcaneal inversion of the right foot. With the shoe off, the therapist finds a new callus on the lateral side of the metatarsal head of the fifth toe. Which of the following is the **BEST** choice for orthotic prescription for this patient?

Choices:

1. Scaphoid pad.
2. Flexible foot orthosis with a medial rearfoot post.
3. Flexible foot orthosis with lateral rearfoot post.
4. Ankle foot orthosis with full length foot plate.

Teaching Points

Correct Answer: 3

Supination of the foot (pes cavus) is accompanied by supination of the talocalcaneonavicular (TCN), subtalar, and transversal tarsal joints. It is characterized by an abnormally high arch. The flexible cavus foot generally responds well to orthotic foot control, especially in a child. The best choice is a flexible foot orthosis with lateral rearfoot post.

Incorrect Choices:

The other choices are used to control flexible pes valgus.

Type of Reasoning: Inductive

One must utilize clinical judgment in order to determine the **BEST** choice for orthotic prescription. This requires one to utilize inductive reasoning skill, which also includes diagnostic thinking, in order to determine a best course of action. If this question was answered incorrectly, review orthotic prescription approaches for children with foot supination and calcaneal inversion.

C97
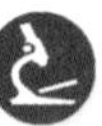

Musculoskeletal | Interventions

A patient is recovering from a right total hip replacement (posterolateral incision, cementless fixation). During initial healing, what is the **MOST** appropriate type of bed-to-wheelchair transfer to teach this patient?

Choices:

1. Squat-pivot transfer to the surgical side.
2. Lateral slide transfer to the surgical side using a transfer board.
3. Stand-pivot transfer to the sound side.
4. Stand-pivot transfer to the surgical side.

Teaching Points

Correct Answer: 3

During initial healing, it is important to protect the hip from dislocation or subluxation of the prosthesis. With a posterolateral incision, excessive hip flexion and adduction past neutral are contraindicated. This is minimized by transferring to the sound side.

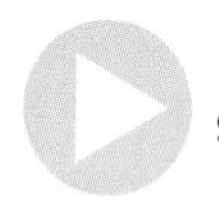

Incorrect Choices:

All other choices emphasize transfer to the surgical side, which can move the hip into adduction. In addition, the stand-pivot transfer with some hip extension is a better choice than transferring with the hip in full flexion.

Type of Reasoning: Deductive

This question requires one to recall the appropriate guidelines for bed-to-wheelchair transfers of patients with total hip replacements. The recall of guidelines necessitates deductive reasoning, in which factual recall of knowledge is expected. For patients with hip replacements, transfer toward the sound side helps to preserve hip precaution guidelines. If this question was answered incorrectly, review guidelines for transferring patients with hip replacements.

C98 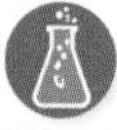

Neuromuscular I Examination

During an initial interview and history, a patient with a right CVA seems unconcerned about obvious paralysis of the left arm and leg. When the therapist asks the patient to describe what happened, the patient says "I must have slept wrong and my arm and leg fell asleep." The patient further tells the therapist, "My family put me in this place so they could go on vacation." Which type of perceptual disorder **BEST** characterizes the patient's responses?

Choices:

1. Anosognosia.
2. Prosopagnosia.
3. Spatial relations disorder.
4. Somatoagnosia.

Teaching Points

Correct Answer: 1

Anosognosia is a perceptual disorder that is characterized by denial, neglect, and lack of awareness of the presence or severity of one's paralysis.

Incorrect Choices:

Somatoagnosia is a perceptual disorder characterized by an impairment in body scheme (a lack of awareness of body structure and the relationship of body parts of oneself or of others). Spatial relation disorders encompass a constellation of impairments characterized by difficulty in perceiving the relationship between self and two or more objects. Prosopagnosia is a perceptual disorder characterized by an inability to recognize faces (face blindness).

Type of Reasoning: Analytical

This question provides symptoms, and the test-taker must determine the likely cause for such symptoms. Questions of this nature often require analytical reasoning skill, where pieces of information are analyzed to draw an appropriate conclusion. For this situation, the symptoms indicate anosognosia. Review symptoms of anosognosia if answered incorrectly.

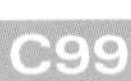

C99

Neuromuscular | Interventions

The therapist is treating a child with mild developmental delay secondary to 7 weeks prematurity at birth. The child is now 8 months old and is just learning to sit. Which is the **BEST** choice for a training activity?

Choices:

1. Sideward protective extension in sitting.
2. Supine tilting reactions.
3. Standing tilting reactions.
4. Prone tilting reactions.

Teaching Points

Correct Answer: 1

Sideward protective extension in sitting is a functional, protective reaction that normally occurs at about the same time as sitting begins.

Incorrect Choices:

The child who is starting to sit should already have prone and supine tilting reactions. It is too early to begin standing tilting reactions.

Type of Reasoning: Inferential

One must recall the developmental milestones of infants and infer the **BEST** choice for training in order to choose the correct solution. If this question was answered incorrectly, review the motor developmental milestones of infants.

C100

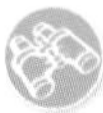

Cardiovascular/Pulmonary | Examination

The picture depicts a patient who is learning to take her own pulse. What is the patient doing incorrectly?

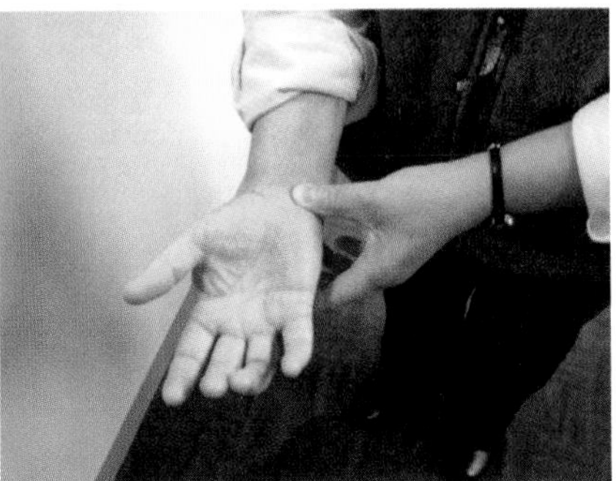

Choices:

1. Taking the pulse with the forearm supinated.
2. Palpating the radial artery.
3. Assessing the pulse with the thumb.
4. Palpating the right arm as opposed to the more accurate left arm.

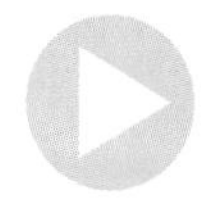

Teaching Points

Correct Answer: 3

The thumb is pulsatile and cannot be used to assess a pulse. Additionally, the patient is attempting to palpate the ulnar artery. The pulse of the radial artery is usually more robust and more easily palpated.

Incorrect Choices:

A pulse can be assessed on any artery that can be palpated. While in some patients a pronated forearm can facilitate palpation of the pulse, any arm position is acceptable. The circulatory system is a closed system and therefore, in the absence of pathology, the pulse is the same in either upper limb.

Type of Reasoning: Inductive

This question requires the test-taker to draw from clinical knowledge of taking a pulse in order to arrive at a correct conclusion. This is an inductive reasoning skill. If this question was answered incorrectly, review guidelines for taking the pulse.

C101 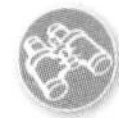

Gastrointestinal | Interventions

A patient with complete spinal cord injury at the level of T11 is on a bowel program. Which of the following is the **MOST** effective bowel training program for this patient?

Choices:

1. Diet and medications to manage a flaccid bowel.
2. Digital stimulation of intact defecation reflexes.
3. Manual removal of stool from the rectum.
4. Medications such as laxatives for passive elimination.

Teaching Points

Correct Answer: 2

An SCI injury at the level of T11 produces an UMN or spastic bowel with intact spinal defecation reflexes. Bowel and anal sphincters respond to rectal/anal stimulation, enabling a planned bowel elimination program.

Incorrect Choices:

Medications such as laxatives and stool softeners can be used to assist the patient in manually stimulated elimination; however, the primary methodology is digital stimulation. An LMN or flaccid bowel occurs with lesions at T12 or below with loss of spinal defecation reflexes. Response to medications is less effective, and manual removal of stool may be required.

Type of Reasoning: Inductive

This question requires clinical judgment in order to determine a best course of action for a patient with a complete spinal cord injury. This necessitates inductive reasoning skills, where determining a best course of action is often used. For this case, the patient with a T11 injury would primarily use digital stimulation of intact defecation reflexes for bowel retraining. Refer to bowel retraining guidelines for patients with spinal cord injury, especially upper motor neuron injury, if answered incorrectly.

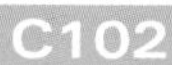

C102

Musculoskeletal | Examination

When performing scoliosis screening in a school setting, what is the optimal age (in years) for girls to be screened?

Choices:

1. 6–8.
2. 9–11.
3. 12–14.
4. 15–17.

Teaching Points

Correct Answer: 2

The most effective age to screen girls for scoliosis is just before the pubescent growth spurt between 9 and 11 years, when the scoliotic curve can increase dramatically. Boys should be screened between 11 and 13 years of age because of differences in the age of onset of puberty between girls and boys.

Incorrect Choices:

Screening can occur at any age, but routine screening should be performed before the pubescent growth spurt. Large changes in abnormal spinal curves can occur during growth spurts.

Type of Reasoning: Analytical

One must analyze the merits of performing scoliosis screenings with each of the identified age groups in girls in order to determine the age at which it is optimal to complete the screening. This requires analytical reasoning skills, in which one interprets the various ages and how these ages are relevant to normal development and puberty. If this question was answered incorrectly, review information on scoliosis screening.

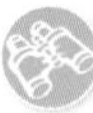

C103

Musculoskeletal | Interventions

A patient is referred to physical therapy with neck pain and an acute right C6 radiculopathy. Imaging studies reveal stenosis of the intervertebral foramen resulting in impingement of the involved nerve root. The therapist decides to intervene with a manual therapy approach to reduce the patient's pain. Which mobilization technique **BEST** meets the therapist's intended purpose?

Choices:

1. Grade I cervical rotation to the right.
2. Grade II cervical rotation to the left.
3. Grade III cervical rotation to the left.
4. Grade IV cervical rotation to the right.

Teaching Points

Correct Answer: 2

Grade I and II mobilizations are used to decrease pain and muscle guarding. Since the question stem indicates that the therapist is trying to reduce the patient's pain, a Grade I or II mobilization is indicated. Mobilizing the spine to the left (or away from the involved side) should help to open the intervertebral foramen on the right and decompress the involved nerve root.

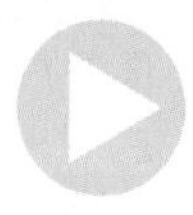

Incorrect Choices:

Grade III and IV mobilizations are performed into tissue resistance and are used to improve mobility. Again, the goal of the therapist in this question is to reduce pain. Additionally, Grade III and IV mobilization techniques are often more appropriate in the subacute or chronic stage. The patient in this question is being seen during an acute episode of neck pain with radiculopathy.

Type of Reasoning: Inductive

This question requires the test-taker to recall joint mobilization guidelines and then apply them to a patient with cervical stenosis and impingement of the right C6 nerve root. These types of questions, where one applies clinical knowledge to therapeutic situations, often require inductive reasoning skill. For this situation, the therapist should select grade II cervical rotation to the left. Review joint mobilization guidelines, especially for the cervical spine, if answered incorrectly.

C104 

Musculoskeletal | Examination

A middle-aged patient is seen in a physical therapy clinic on the same day that they sustained a leg injury while playing basketball. The patient reported feeling a pop and immediate sharp pain in the posterior ankle region after landing from a jump. Which special test should the therapist emphasize during the examination?

Choices:

1. Syndesmosis squeeze test.
2. Thompson's test.
3. Ankle anterior drawer test.
4. Windlass test.

Teaching Points

Correct Answer: 2

A positive Thompson's test indicates an Achilles tendon rupture (+LR 13.5, –LR 0.04), which requires an immediate referral to an orthopedic surgeon for immobilization or surgical repair. Delayed diagnosis and treatment may result in loss of function and a poor prognosis. See Table 2-19 for a review of foot and ankle region special tests and their diagnostic accuracy values.

Incorrect Choices:

The syndesmosis squeeze test evaluates the integrity of the distal tibiofibular syndesmosis or interosseous membrane. The ankle anterior drawer test primarily assesses the integrity of the anterior talofibular ligament. The windlass test is utilized to reproduce symptoms of plantar fasciitis.

Type of Reasoning: Analytical

This question requires the test-taker to analyze the presenting symptoms in order to determine the best special test to emphasize during an examination. This requires analytical reasoning skill, where pieces of information are weighed and considered to draw reasonable conclusions. For this scenario, the therapist should include the Thompson's test. If answered incorrectly, review the Thompson's test and examination approaches for Achilles tendon rupture.

C105

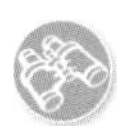

Genitourinary | Evaluation, Diagnosis

Which of the following conditions associated with pelvic floor muscle dysfunction may actually worsen when treated with Kegel exercises?

Choices:

1. Interstitial cystitis.
2. Stress incontinence.
3. Pelvic organ prolapse.
4. Chronic constipation.

Teaching Points

Correct Answer: 1

Kegel exercises are prescribed to strengthen weak pelvic floor muscles (levator ani) and to improve the motor control of these muscles. However, in individuals with interstitial cystitis (IC), the pelvic floor dysfunction is usually related to muscles that are too tense or in spasm in response to pain and chronic inflammation of the bladder. This is just the opposite of the too-relaxed state that leads to incontinence. Additionally, there are often tender points or nodules in the pelvic floor muscles of individuals with IC that can be treated with manual techniques. Therefore the goal of physical therapy in these patients is to relax and lengthen tight pelvic floor muscles and release trigger points.

Incorrect Choices:

Pelvic floor muscle weakness is a common cause of stress incontinence, and Kegel exercises are often prescribed to effectively treat this disorder. Similarly, strengthening of the pelvic floor muscles can be very beneficial in women who suffer from a prolapse of the uterus or vagina. Recent studies have shown that about half of all individuals with chronic constipation suffer from pelvic floor muscle dysfunction, and benefit from Kegel exercises combined with biofeedback to strengthen and coordinate the actions of the pelvic floor and abdominal muscles.

Type of Reasoning: Inductive

This question requires the test-taker to utilize clinical judgment in order to determine which condition may worsen with Kegel exercises. This is an inductive reasoning skill, where knowledge of the diagnosis and intervention approach is paramount to arriving at a correct conclusion. For this case, interstitial cystitis would worsen with Kegel exercises. If answered incorrectly, review indications and guidelines for Kegel exercises.

C106

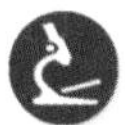

Nonsystem | Therapeutic Modalities

A therapist is applying a symmetrical biphasic pulsed current at 25 pps (tetany) to the vastus medialis to improve patellar tracking during knee extension. The patient complains that the current is too strong and uncomfortable. To make the current more tolerable to the patient, yet maintain a good therapeutic effect, what adjustment should the therapist make?

Choices:

1. Change the current polarity.
2. Decreasing the pulse duration.
3. Increase the amplitude.
4. Decreasing the pulse rate.

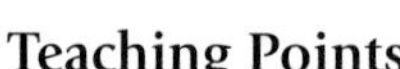

Teaching Points

Correct Answer: 2

Decreasing the pulse duration reduces the electrical charge of each pulse, making the current more comfortable by decreasing the total current applied.

Incorrect Choices:

The only other parameter that would have a direct effect on comfort would be the intensity. For motor level stimulation, decreasing the intensity or pulse duration could potentially decrease the therapeutic effect if turned too low. Increasing the amplitude would make the current feel stronger. There is always a balance between the intensity and pulse duration to have enough charge to depolarize the nerve. For motor level stimulation, decreasing the pulse rate below 25 pps, which is at the lower end of tetany, would decrease the quality of the contraction. Changing the polarity would have no effect because a symmetrical biphasic waveform has no net polarity.

Type of Reasoning: Deductive

This question requires one to factually recall the correct parameters for neuromuscular stimulation and how to adjust the parameters when untoward effects occur. Factual recall or protocols or guidelines is a deductive reasoning skill. If this question was answered incorrectly, review information on guidelines for high-volt pulsed current.

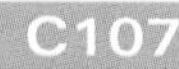

C107

Lymphatic | Evaluation, Diagnosis

Which of the following structures can refer pain to the left shoulder?

Choices:

1. Esophagus.
2. Colon or appendix.
3. Spleen.
4. Gallbladder.

Teaching Points

Correct Answer: 3

Splenic or diaphragmatic pain can refer to the left shoulder. In the case of a ruptured or abscessed spleen, it is known as Kehr's sign.

Incorrect Choices:

Esophageal pain can refer to the mid-back, head, or neck. Colon or appendix pain can refer to the lower back, pelvis, or sacrum. Gallbladder pain can refer to the mid-back and right shoulder regions.

Type of Reasoning: Deductive

One must recall the typical referral patterns for pain in order to determine which refers to the shoulder. This requires deductive reasoning skills, because factual recall of guidelines is used to reach a conclusion. If this question was answered incorrectly, review visceral pain referral patterns.

C108 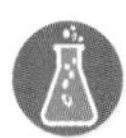

Neuromuscular | Evaluation, Diagnosis

A patient with a history of multiple falls and an ataxic gait for the past year reports difficulty walking on unlevel surfaces for very short distances. During examination, the patient's gait and balance do not improve when looking down (visual feedback). Neuromuscular screening reveals mild and diffuse weakness (4+/5 manual muscle testing) of the upper and lower extremity muscles and a slight tremor with active range of motion. Patient reports feeling clumsy and consistently dropping objects. Cranial nerve, sensory, and reflex (to include Babinski/Clonus) testing are normal. Which of the following health conditions is **MOST** consistent with the patient's signs and symptoms?

Choices:

1. Cerebellar disease.
2. Cervical myelopathy.
3. Polyneuropathy.
4. Lumbar spinal stenosis.

Teaching Points

Correct Answer: 1

Cerebellar disease results in impairments with coordination (dysdiadochokinesis, dysmetria, hypermetria, intention tremor) and balance/gait dysfunction that typically do not improve with visual feedback (looking down). Weakness, hypotonia, and fatigue are expected findings. The weakness associated with cerebellar dysfunction is typically related to the timing and ability to provide force when needed, as compared to weakness seen with lower motor neuron lesions.

Incorrect Choices:

Cervical myelopathy also causes dyscoordination and weakness but is often accompanied with sensory dysfunction and/or upper motor neuron signs. Polyneuropathy has glove and stocking sensory and motor impairments, and patients can often compensate for balance difficulties by looking down. Lumbar spinal stenosis also results in motor and sensory impairments as well as radicular symptoms, but symptoms are limited to the lower extremities and exacerbated with walking longer distances (neurogenic claudication).

Type of Reasoning: Analytical

For this question, a group of symptoms are provided, and one must determine the most likely condition based on the symptoms. This necessitates analytical reasoning skill, where pieces of information are analyzed to draw reasonable conclusions. For this situation, the symptoms are consistent with cerebellar disease. If answered incorrectly, review information on cerebellar disease.

C109 

System Interactions | Evaluation, Diagnosis

A patient with a 10-year history of diabetes complains of cramping, pain, and fatigue of the right buttock after walking 400 feet or climbing stairs. When the patient stops exercising, the pain goes away immediately. The skin of the involved leg is cool and pale. The therapist checks the record and finds no mention of this problem. Given this patient's symptoms, what is the likely diagnosis?

Choices:

1. Peripheral nerve injury.
2. Spinal root impingement.
3. Raynaud's phenomenon.
4. Peripheral arterial disease (PAD).

Teaching Points

Correct Answer: 4

Intermittent claudication, often the earliest indication of PAD, is manifested by cramping, pain, or fatigue in the muscles during exercise that is typically relieved by rest. The calf muscle is most commonly affected, but discomfort may also occur in the thigh, hip, or buttock. Cessation of pain immediately upon stopping the exercise is characteristic of intermittent claudication, not other spinal problems. With severe disease, however, pain may be present even at rest.

Incorrect Choices:

The pain associated with spinal root impingement (nerve pain) is often acute and becomes worse or aggravated by extension, side flexion, rotation, standing, walking, and exercise in general. It is relieved by lying down. Peripheral nerve injury presents with sensory and motor loss. Raynaud's phenomenon is an intermittent attack of pallor or cyanosis of the small arteries and arterioles of the fingers as a result of inadequate blood flow.

Type of Reasoning: Analytical

This is a question that provides the symptoms, and one must determine the likely diagnosis. This requires analytical reasoning skill, in which the test-taker utilizes knowledge of anatomy, physiology, and pathology to determine the cause. If this question was answered incorrectly, review information on symptoms of PAD.

C110 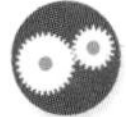

Cardiovascular/Pulmonary | Evaluation, Diagnosis

A patient with lower back pain has marked elevation of BP and complains of mild to severe mid-abdominal pain that increases upon exertion. Palpation reveals a pulsing mass in the lower abdomen. What is the therapist's **BEST** course of action?

Choices:

1. Discontinue treatment and have the patient transported to an emergency room.
2. Provide hot packs to the abdomen to help relieve the muscle spasm.
3. Instruct the patient to contact his/her physician at the conclusion of therapy.
4. Instruct in relaxation exercises because a pulsating mass is not unusual with hypertension.

Teaching Points

Correct Answer: 1

This patient is demonstrating signs and symptoms of an abdominal aortic aneurysm. Pain is intermittent or constant and can be felt in the mid-abdominal or lower back regions. The pulsating mass is highly significant, and the level of hypertension dramatically increases risk of rupture. This is a serious medical condition; the therapist should arrange for immediate transport to an emergency room.

Incorrect Choices:

The therapist should not rely on the patient to contact the physician. All physical therapy intervention should cease.

Type of Reasoning: Evaluative

One must evaluate the significance of the information presented, determine the root cause of the symptoms, and then determine the best course of action. This requires evaluative reasoning skill, in which one evaluates the merits of the four possible choices and determines which approach is most appropriate and safe for the patient. In this case, it is important to discontinue treatment, immediately notify the physician, and arrange for immediate transportation to an emergency room.

C111 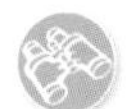

Musculoskeletal | Interventions

A patient presents to physical therapy with glenohumeral joint arthritis. Examination reveals limited shoulder abduction and a capsular end-feel. The therapist considers manual therapy as part of the intervention plan. Which glenohumeral joint mobilization technique is BEST to improve shoulder abduction?

Choices:

1. Grade I/II distraction.
2. Grade III/IV compression.
3. Grade III/IV inferior glide.
4. Grade I/II anterior glide.

Teaching Points

Correct Answer: 3

Grade III and IV mobilizations are used to stretch tight capsules, ligaments, and muscles. A capsular end-feel suggests that the capsule or other soft-tissue tightness is limiting shoulder abduction. Based on the concave-convex rule, an inferior glide would be best to improve shoulder abduction. See Table 2-1 for a review of the concave-convex rule application to peripheral joints.

Incorrect Choices:

Grade I and II mobilizations (choices 1 and 4) are used to decrease pain and muscle guarding. There was no information in the question stem that suggested that pain and guarding were the reasons for the limited shoulder abduction. Mobilizing the glenohumeral joint with distraction and compression may help improve shoulder motion in general, but they do not specifically address roll, spin, and glide components required to improve shoulder abduction.

Type of Reasoning: Inductive

This question requires the test-taker to apply joint mobilization knowledge to a patient with glenohumeral joint arthritis with capsular end-feel during shoulder abduction. This requires inductive reasoning skill. For this scenario, it is best for the therapist to choose a grade III/IV inferior glide. If answered incorrectly, review joint mobilization guidelines, especially for the shoulder.

C112 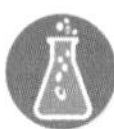

System Interactions | Evaluation, Diagnosis

A frail, elderly wheelchair-dependent resident of a community nursing home has a diagnosis of organic brain syndrome, moderate Alzheimer's type dementia. During the therapist's initial interview, the patient demonstrates limited interaction and mild agitation and keeps trying to wheel the chair down the hall. Because it is late in the day, the therapist decides to resume the examination the next morning. How should the therapist document this in the medical record?

Choices:

1. Disorientation to time and date.
2. Inattention as a result of short-term memory loss.
3. Frustration because of an inability to communicate.
4. Sundowning behavior.

Teaching Points

Correct Answer: 4

A patient with moderate Alzheimer's type dementia can be expected to exhibit impaired cognition and abstract thinking, sundowning (defined as extreme restlessness, agitation, and wandering that typically occurs in the late afternoon), inability to carry out activities of daily living, impaired judgment, inappropriate social behavior, lack of insight, repetitive behavior, and a voracious appetite.

Incorrect Choices:

Inability to communicate is characteristic of severe Alzheimer's type dementia. Short-term memory loss and disorientation to time and date are early and persistent signs of the disease.

Type of Reasoning: Analytical

This question provides the symptoms, and the test-taker must determine, through analytical reasoning, the most likely cause for the patient's behavior. In this situation, the symptoms suggest that the patient with moderate Alzheimer's type dementia is exhibiting sundowning behavior. If this question was answered incorrectly, review information on Alzheimer's type dementia and sundowning behavior.

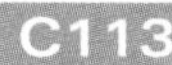

Musculoskeletal | Interventions

A patient with a right transfemoral amputation is undergoing prosthetic gait training. What is the **BEST** technique to use to improve the patient's shortened step length on the right?

Choices:

1. Provide anterior-directed resistance to the right PSIS during swing.
2. Provide posterior-directed resistance to the left ASIS during swing.
3. Provide posterior-directed resistance to the right ASIS during stance.
4. Facilitate the gluteals with tapping over the muscle belly.

Teaching Points

Correct Answer: 3

Light resistance and stretch applied to the pelvis (right ASIS) in a posterior direction during mid-stance to late stance will facilitate forward pelvic rotation on that side and enhance forward movement of the limb during swing.

Incorrect Choices:

Anterior-directed resistance functions to pull the hip forward but does little to facilitate active forward limb movement. The gluteals function to stabilize the limb during stance (not advance the limb forward). Manual resistance applied to the pelvis during swing may interfere with stepping.

Type of Reasoning: Inferential

One must infer the best approach to providing directed resistance for the patient with a transfemoral amputation. This requires knowledge of kinesiology and therapeutic exercise in order to arrive at the correct conclusion.

C114 

Gastrointestinal | Evaluation, Diagnosis

An elderly, frail resident of an extended care facility has intractable constipation. During a scheduled visit from the PT, the patient complains of abdominal pain and tenderness. Where may this patient experience referred pain?

Choices:

1. Buttock, thigh, and posterior leg.
2. Anterior hip, groin, or thigh region.
3. Low back and front of the thigh to the knee.
4. Medial thigh and leg.

Teaching Points

Correct Answer: 2

Intractable constipation (obstipation) can cause partial or complete bowel impaction, pain, and tenderness in the lower abdomen. Referred pain is to the anterior hip groin or thigh region.

Incorrect Choices:

Pain in the back and front of thigh to knee is characteristic of L2 nerve root compression. Pain in the buttock, thigh, and posterior leg is characteristic of S1 nerve root compression. Pain in the bladder can refer to the medial thigh and leg.

Type of Reasoning: Inferential

One must infer or draw a reasonable conclusion about the symptoms a client is likely to experience given the diagnosis provided. Inferential reasoning skills are often utilized in cases in which one must determine what may be true of a patient. If this question was answered incorrectly, review signs and symptoms of intractable constipation and pain referral patterns from the viscera.

C115 

Musculoskeletal | Interventions

An adult patient is diagnosed with thoracic outlet syndrome. The patient presents with guarding in the upper trapezius and scalene muscles. Given this situation, which technique would be the **MOST** effective way to decrease the muscle guarding and provide pain relief?

Choices:

1. Maitland grade IV manipulation of the C6–C7 joint.
2. Maitland grade II mobilization of the atlanto-axial joint.
3. Maitland grade III mobilization of the C6–C7 joint.
4. Maitland grade IV manipulation of the first rib.

Teaching Points

Correct Answer: 4

One needs to be aware that the muscle guarding pattern present with this condition is increased tone of the scalene muscles. These muscles (anterior and middle portions) attach to the first rib. Grade IV manipulation can be used to decrease muscle guarding and pain in the target area.

Incorrect Choices:

The atlanto-axial and C6–C7 joints are not the target joints of most importance nor is the technique the most effective based on the pattern presented.

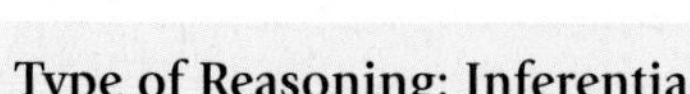

Type of Reasoning: Inferential

One needs to be aware of the indication for each of the five grades of Maitland's oscillatory techniques in order to determine the correct conclusion. Questions that require one to infer what will result in a best clinical outcome often require inferential reasoning skill. For this scenario, Maitland grade IV manipulation of the first rib is appropriate. Review Maitland's oscillatory techniques if answered incorrectly.

C116

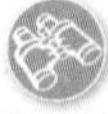

Musculoskeletal I Interventions

A patient presents with decreased motion at the occipitoatlantal joint (OA). The PT wants to use the principles of coupled motions that occur in that area of the spine during manual therapy techniques. In order to improve OA mobility, when the occiput is side bent to the right, how should the therapist mobilize C1?

Choices:

1. Into rotation to the left.
2. Into rotation to the right.
3. Back into extension.
4. Forward into flexion.

Teaching Points

Correct Answer: 1

Given the rules of coupled movement in the upper cervical spine, when the occiput is sidebent into one direction, C1 rotates into the opposite direction. Side bending and rotation occur in the same direction from C2–C7 regardless if the spine is in flexion or extension.

Incorrect Choices:

The other choices do not represent opposite directions or coupled movement from a right side bend of the occiput at C1.

Type of Reasoning: Inductive

One must understand the coupled movements of the cervical spine in order to arrive at a correct conclusion. Questions of this nature often require inductive reasoning skill, as one must use clinical judgment to determine a best course of action. For this situation, the therapist should mobilize into rotation to the left when the occiput is sidebent to the right. Review biomechanics and coupled movements of the cervical spine if answered incorrectly.

C117

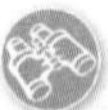

Cardiovascular/Pulmonary I Examination

An apparently healthy individual has several risk factors for coronary artery disease. The client is interested in improving overall fitness and cardiac health. After a graded exercise test, which was asymptomatic, the client is referred for an exercise class. Which is the **BEST** measure of exercise intensity in a newly tested and exercising individual?

Choices:

1. Heart rate (HR).
2. Rating of perceived exertion (RPE).
3. MET level.
4. Respiratory rate.

Teaching Points

Correct Answer: 1

A graded exercise test should be performed before commencing an exercise program for all high-risk individuals. The best measurement of exercise intensity in a newly tested and exercising individual is HR.

Incorrect Choices:

RPE will become a valuable measurement tool once the patient becomes adept at using it, but it would not be reliable for the first exercise session. MET level is more of a measurement of workload, not an accurate measurement of an individual's response to exercise. Respiratory rate is not used to prescribe exercise intensity.

Type of Reasoning: Inductive

This question requires the test-taker to recall the various measures of exercise intensity and determine, through clinical judgment, which measure will **MOST** accurately monitor the patient's exercise intensity, given his/her diagnosis and symptoms on the **FIRST** visit. Questions that require clinical judgment and diagnostic reasoning require inductive reasoning skill. If this question was answered incorrectly, review measures to monitor exercise intensity for at-risk individuals.

C118 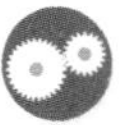

Neuromuscular | Examination

A mother brings her 8-week-old infant to be examined at early intervention clinic because she noticed that the infant was taking steps in supported standing at 2 weeks but is not able to do it now. What should the therapist do given the infant's symptoms and behaviors?

Choices:

1. Recommend that the mother bring the infant to a pediatric neurologist.
2. Explain that this was abnormal and it is a good sign that it has disappeared.
3. Recommend that a full developmental examination be performed by the early intervention team.
4. Explain that this is normal and that this early automatic walking is a newborn response.

Teaching Points

Correct Answer: 4

The mother probably saw the neonatal stepping reflex/automatic walking, which is normal in a newborn but is not exhibited in the older infant probably because of anthropomorphic factors and neural maturation. The age that this response typically disappears is 2–3 months of age.

Incorrect Choices:

In most infants, pull-to-stand emerges at 8–9 months, whereas unassisted standing and walking occur at 10–15 months. Stepping at this age is not the result of a reflex (does not reemerge later on). A full developmental examination or referral to a neurologist is not indicated and should be performed only after the child is older and is not walking. It is important to remember that these norms are averages, and that children may be more advanced or slower in reaching these milestones.

Type of Reasoning: Evaluative

One must have firm knowledge of the developmental milestones of infants in order to arrive at the correct conclusion. Using evaluative reasoning, one must evaluate the merits of the four possible choices and determine which solution seems most reasonable, given the infant's symptoms and behaviors. In this case, the behaviors are normal. If this question was answered incorrectly, review the neonatal stepping reflex and developmental milestones for walking.

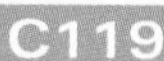

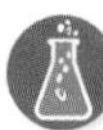

Musculoskeletal | Examination

A patient complains of pain with mouth opening that makes it difficult to eat foods that require chewing. Which of the following provides the normal limits of mouth opening that should guide the therapist's examination?

Choices:

1. 15–24 mm.
2. 35–50 mm.
3. 51–65 mm.
4. 66–74 mm.

Teaching Points

Correct Answer: 2

Average AROM is approximately 35–50 mm. However, only 25–35 mm of opening between the teeth is required for normal everyday activity.

Incorrect Choices:

The TMJs are considered hypomobile if <25 mm of opening is achieved. Hypermobility would include values >50 mm.

Type of Reasoning: Analytical

One must recall normal AROM of the TMJ as well as functional AROM ranges in order to arrive at the correct conclusion. Through analytical reasoning, one must review each of the AROM parameters and determine which range seems most reasonable, given one's knowledge of normal ROM guidelines for the TMJ. If this question was answered incorrectly, review AROM guidelines for the TMJ.

C120

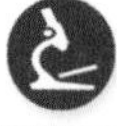

Musculoskeletal | Examination

A high school athlete sustained a wrist injury after falling with an outstretched hand (FOOSH). The patient reports that there was immediate swelling at the time of injury. During the physical therapy examination 2 days later, the physical therapist notes palpation tenderness in the anatomical snuff box, and limited, painful wrist flexion and extension. A scaphoid fracture is suspected. What is the best special test to confirm this diagnosis?

Choices:

1. Ulnomeniscotriquetral dorsal glide test.
2. Finkelstein's test.
3. Phalen's test.
4. Watson test.

Teaching Points

Correct Answer: 4

The Watson test is also known as the scaphoid shift test. To perform the test, the examiner applies a distal pull to the scaphoid while moving the wrist from ulnar to radial deviation. The above scenario describes a common mechanism of injury for a scaphoid fracture, which is the most commonly fractured carpal bone.

Incorrect Choices:

Each of the incorrect choices listed here are special tests used to identify other wrist and hand injuries. The ulnomeniscotriquetral dorsal glide test assesses the integrity of the triangular fibrocartilage complex (TFCC). Finkelstein's test is used to identify de Quervain's tenosynovitis. Phalen's test is designed to compress the median nerve and to help diagnose carpal tunnel syndrome.

Type of Reasoning: Deductive

For this question, one must recall a test that is conducted to confirm a scaphoid fracture in order to arrive at a correct conclusion. This is factual recall of guidelines, which is a deductive reasoning skill. For this case, the therapist should perform the Watson test to confirm the diagnosis. If answered incorrectly, review the Watson test and scaphoid fracture examination guidelines.

C121 

Musculoskeletal | Evaluation, Diagnosis

A patient presents with complaints of tingling and paresthesias in the median nerve distribution of the right forearm and hand. The following tests were found negative bilaterally: Adson's, hyperabduction, costoclavicular, Phalen's, and the ulnar nerve Tinel's sign. Based on this information, what is the likely diagnosis?

Choices:

1. Ulnar nerve entrapment.
2. Pronator teres syndrome.
3. Thoracic outlet syndrome (TOS).
4. Carpal tunnel syndrome.

Teaching Points

Correct Answer: 2

All of these special tests are used to determine neurological compromise of the lower trunk of the brachial plexus. Special tests to rule out pronator teres syndrome are (1) passive supination to elongate the pronator, which is tight (this would compress the nerve at that level); and (2) active resistance of pronation, which would compress the nerve as it courses between the two heads of the pronator teres muscle.

Incorrect Choices:

A negative Adson's test, hyperabduction test, and costoclavicular test will rule out TOS. A negative Phalen's test will rule out carpal tunnel syndrome. A negative ulnar nerve Tinel's sign will rule out ulnar nerve entrapment. By process of elimination, pronator teres syndrome is the only diagnosis remaining.

Type of Reasoning: Analytical

One must understand the tests described in the question in order to choose the correct solution. Through analytical reasoning, the test-taker must determine what each test indicates (by a negative result) in order to determine the diagnosis that is likely. If this question was answered incorrectly, review information on provocative testing for pronator teres syndrome.

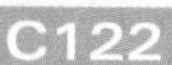
C122
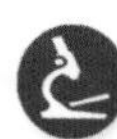

Musculoskeletal | Examination

A physical therapist examines a patient who was referred with low back pain and generalized spinal stiffness. The patient also reports experiencing intermittent fevers and persistent fatigue. The therapist suspects the patient may have ankylosing spondylitis. Which clinical examination technique would help establish the diagnosis of this disorder?

Choices:

1. Prone instability test (PIT).
2. Shear test.
3. Slump test.
4. Schober's test.

Teaching Points

Correct Answer: 4

Ankylosing spondylitis (AS) is a chronic, progressive inflammatory disorder that primarily affects the spine, sacroiliac joints, and large peripheral joints. As the disease progresses, the inflamed ligaments and tendons around the spine ossify, causing a rigid spine with limited mobility. Schober's test is a measure of lumbar spine mobility with forward bending. Most patients with AS exhibit less than 4 cm of lumbar flexion during the test (Sp = 0.86).

Incorrect Choices:

The PIT and shear test are both used to detect lumbar segmental instability or hypermobility. The slump test is a measure of neural tension and is used to reproduce pain associated with nerve root compression or disc herniation. See Table 2-21 for a review of lumbar spine instability and nerve root/neural provocation tests.

Type of Reasoning: Deductive

This question requires one to recall the guidelines and procedures for each provocative test provided in order to determine the best test to confirm the disorder. This requires factual recall of guidelines, which is a deductive reasoning skill. For this case, the therapist should perform the Schober's test. Review provocative testing for ankylosing spondylitis, especially the Schober's test, if answered incorrectly.

C123
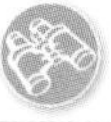

Lymphatic | Interventions

A young patient presents with primary lymphedema of the right lower extremity. What is the **BEST** choice for initial exercise?

Choices:

1. Treadmill walking.
2. Treadmill jogging.
3. Exercising on a stair climbing machine.
4. Step aerobics.

Teaching Points

Correct Answer: 1

The patient should begin with beneficial low-risk activities (e.g., lymphedema exercise, walking, easy biking, swimming, water aerobics, or tai chi). Exercise should always be performed with a compression garment or compression bandages.

Incorrect Choices:

The patient should avoid medium-risk activities (e.g., jogging, running, or stair climbing machines) or sport activities that involve high risk of injury (e.g., soccer, tennis, golf, volleyball, or karate). Eventually, patients can progress to certain higher-risk activities provided there is no exacerbation of their lymphedema.

Type of Reasoning: Inductive

This question requires one to use clinical judgment in order to draw a reasonable conclusion for a patient with primary lymphedema. For this case, it is best for the patient to begin exercise with a low-risk activity such as treadmill walking. If answered incorrectly, review exercise guidelines for patients with primary lymphedema.

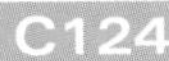
C124

Neuromuscular I Interventions

An elderly patient is recovering from a right CVA and demonstrates strong spasticity in the left upper extremity. The therapist wants to reduce the expected negative effects of spasticity in the left upper extremity while the patient is working on sitting control. What is the **BEST** position for the upper extremity?

Choices:

1. Left elbow flexed with arm resting on supporting pillow, positioned on the patient's lap.
2. Affected upper extremity extended and internally rotated with the hand at the side.
3. Left shoulder abducted and externally rotated with elbow extended and weight supported on the palm of the hand.
4. Left shoulder adducted and internally rotated with the arm extended and hand resting on the thigh.

Teaching Points

Correct Answer: 3

In the upper extremity, spasticity is typically strong in scapular retractors, shoulder adductors, depressors, and internal rotators; elbow flexors and forearm pronators; and wrist and finger flexors. The patient should be positioned opposite the expected pattern.

Incorrect Choices:

The other choices all emphasize one or more of the expected spastic muscles/pattern (i.e., internal rotation, elbow flexion, shoulder adduction, and internal rotation).

Type of Reasoning: Inferential

One must recall the patterns of spasticity in the body after CVA in order to arrive at the correct solution. This requires inferential reasoning skill, in which the test-taker must draw conclusions from the evidence presented and determine the possible outcomes from implementing the above positions for this patient. If this question was answered incorrectly, review spasticity after CVA and positioning strategies.

C125 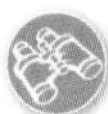

Neuromuscular | Examination

A young, otherwise healthy, adult is recovering from an incomplete L4 neurologic level (ASIA C) spinal cord injury that occurred 2 weeks ago. The patient has been fitted for a rolling walker and ankle foot orthotics (AFOs). Which examination item is **BEST** to assess the patient's initial level of mobility?

Choices:

1. Functional Gait Assessment (FGA).
2. Berg Balance Scale (BBS).
3. 10-meter Gait Speed.
4. Timed Up & Go (TUG).

Teaching Points

Correct Answer: 4

Although this individual lacks a significant degree (<3 out of 5 strength for most muscles) of innervation distal to the L4 level, it is realistic that they would be able to safely complete the TUG with a rolling walker and AFOs. The TUG specifically examines multiple domains of mobility (sit-to-stand, ambulation, turning, and stand-to-sit) and is recommended by the APTA Neurology Spinal Cord Injury EDGE Task Force (see Table 3-23 and Box 3-1).

Incorrect Choices:

The FGA examines gait in various and challenging ways to include walking backwards, walking with a narrow base, and walking with eyes closed. These tasks are too challenging for the patient at this initial stage. The FGA also does not assess the ability to transition from sit-to-stand or stand-to-sit. The BBS measures multiple domains of balance, to include basic transfers, but does not assess gait. 10-meter gait speed is a core examination item for patients with various neuromuscular health conditions, but it does not specifically assess mobility in the form of sit-to-stand or turns.

Type of Reasoning: Inductive

This question requires the test-taker to draw from knowledge of mobility examinations for patients with spinal cord injury. This necessitates clinical judgment, which is an inductive reasoning skill. For this case, the best examination item is the Timed Up & Go (TUG) test. If answered incorrectly, review mobility assessments for individuals with spinal cord injury, especially the TUG test.

C126 

Musculoskeletal | Examination

A physical therapist utilizes ultrasound imaging as a real-time feedback tool while having a patient perform abdominal muscle activation exercises. The therapist identifies the transversus abdominus muscle as a dark band that runs between two white streaks or lines. What is the term used to describe structures that appear dark on an ultrasound image?

Choices:

1. Radiolucent.
2. Radiopaque.
3. Hyperechoic.
4. Hypoechoic.

Teaching Points

Correct Answer: 4

Structures such as muscle that have a relatively low collagen content appear darker (hypoechoic) on ultrasound imaging compared with those that have a higher collagen content like tendons or ligaments. Structures that completely lack collagen, such as blood, appear to be black. The term used to describe structures that appear black is anechoic (see Appendix 2B).

Incorrect Choices:

Hyperechoic is the term used to describe structures that have a high collagen content (tendons, ligaments, and bone) and appear white on ultrasound images. Radiopaque and radiolucent are terms used to describe the appearance of structures on plain radiographs (x-rays). For instance, the appearance of metal on an x-ray is described as radiopaque, while areas devoid of any tissue appear black and are described as radiolucent.

Type of Reasoning: Deductive

For this question, one must recall the terms and definitions for ultrasound imaging in order to arrive at a correct conclusion. This necessitates deductive reasoning skill, where facts are utilized to draw reasonable conclusions. For this case, a structure that appears dark on an ultrasound image is termed hypoechoic. Review ultrasound imaging terminology if answered incorrectly.

C127
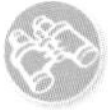

Nonsystem I Professional Responsibilities

A physical therapist working in an acute care hospital is tasked with making a discharge recommendation for a patient after a cerebrovascular accident. The patient needs assistance to safely walk 50 feet with a rolling walker, can tolerate 30 minutes of therapy per day, and requires daily nursing care for infection management. Which of the following practice settings is **MOST** appropriate for the therapist to recommend for the patient's discharge?

Choices:

1. Skilled nursing facility.
2. Acute rehabilitation hospital.
3. Custodial care facility.
4. Ambulatory care.

Teaching Points

Correct Answer: 1

Patients need to go to a skilled nursing facility if they require daily skilled nursing care. Therapy services can be rendered at these facilities along with nursing care.

Incorrect Choices:

Both nursing and rehabilitation care occur in acute rehabilitation hospitals. However, a patient must be able to tolerate 3 hours of therapy interventions per day to qualify. This patient cannot tolerate enough therapy to qualify for an acute rehabilitation hospital. Patients at custodial care facilities can receive medical services, but daily care is delivered by nonmedical personnel. This patient requires daily nursing care so would not be a candidate for a custodial care facility. Patients that attend ambulatory care must be able to travel to and from their home safely. The patient in this question requires assistance to walk safely and still requires daily nursing care.

Type of Reasoning: Inductive

For this question, the test-taker must apply knowledge of practice settings to a case scenario of a patient who is ready for discharge. This requires clinical knowledge, which is an inductive reasoning skill. For this case, given the patient's current level of function, discharge to a skilled nursing facility is most appropriate. If answered incorrectly, review practice settings and criteria for admission, especially skilled nursing facilities.

C128 

Neuromuscular | Evaluation, Diagnosis

A patient with trigeminal nerve neuralgia (CN V) is referred to the physical therapist. What are the expected examination findings?

Choices:

1. Sudden severe pains in the ophthalmic division of CN V.
2. Paroxysmal and severe pain originating from the mandibular or maxillary divisions of CN V.
3. Unilateral sensory loss of the ophthalmic division of CN V.
4. Bilateral sensory loss of CN V in all three divisions.

Teaching Points

Correct Answer: 2

Trigeminal neuralgia (tic douloureux) is a condition characterized by sudden, severe pain occurring in the distribution of the trigeminal nerve (CN V). It typically occurs in the maxillary or mandibular division on one side of the face.

Incorrect Choices:

Symptoms are typically unilateral, not bilateral. It rarely affects the ophthalmic division.

Type of Reasoning: Inferential

This question requires one to infer the common signs and symptoms of trigeminal nerve neuralgia. Questions that necessitate determining what is likely to be true of a diagnosis often require inferential reasoning skill. In this case, the physical therapist will likely find paroxysmal and severe pain originating from the mandibular or maxillary divisions of CN V. If this question was answered incorrectly, review signs and symptoms of trigeminal nerve neuralgia.

C129 

Metabolic/Endocrine | Interventions

A patient with hypothyroidism and poor drug compliance is referred to physical therapy following a fall. What symptoms might be evident during exercise based on this diagnosis?

Choices:

1. Paresthesias of the lower limbs.
2. Elevated cardiac output.
3. Sinus tachycardia and arrhythmias.
4. Myalgia and weakness.

Teaching Points

Correct Answer: 4

Hypothyroidism results in a decreased metabolic rate and is likely to produce exercised-induced myalgia and weakness (rhabdomyolysis).

Incorrect Choices:

Sinus bradycardia (not tachycardia) and decreased cardiac output (not increased) can occur. Sensory changes are not found.

Type of Reasoning: Inferential

This question provides a diagnosis, and the test-taker must determine the symptoms that could occur during exercise based on this diagnosis. This is an inferential reasoning skill. For this situation, the therapist should watch for signs of myalgia and weakness during exercise. If answered incorrectly, review exercise guidelines for patients with hypothyroidism.

C130 

Nonsystem I Research

A group of researchers utilized meta-analysis to identify the evidence for aerobic fitness exercises in the management of fibromyalgia. Thirteen randomized, controlled trials (RCTs) and three controlled clinical trials (cohort studies and case control studies) were selected. What is the main difference between RCTs and controlled clinical trials?

Choices:

1. Duration of the studies.
2. Use of multiple centers versus single center trials.
3. Length of the studies.
4. Use of randomization of subjects.

Teaching Points

Correct Answer: 4

The main difference between the two types of trials is randomization of subjects into experimental and control groups (RCT).

Incorrect Choices:

Meta-analysis involves the combining of a series of independent, previously published studies of similar purpose to yield a larger target population. RCTs are used and can be either single-center or multiple-center trials. A cohort study is a prospective study involving a group of participants with a similar condition. Comparison is made with a matched group that does not have the condition. Duration and length of studies are not distinguishing factors between the two types of studies.

Type of Reasoning: Deductive

One must recall the guidelines for both RCTs and controlled clinical trials in order to arrive at a correct conclusion. Recalling such guidelines is factual information, which requires deductive reasoning skills. If this question was answered incorrectly, review types of research designs, especially RCTs and controlled clinical trials.

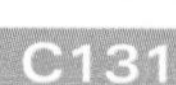

C131

Neuromuscular | Interventions

A patient who sustained a stroke 7 months ago is referred for outpatient rehabilitation. The patient is independent with transfers and gait. Which of the following interventions has the highest level of evidence for improving locomotor function in this patient?

Choices:

1. Strength training of multiple sets/repetitions at 70% 1 RM.
2. Body Weight Support Treadmill Training (BWSTT).
3. Circuit training including strengthening, balance, and aerobic exercises.
4. Moderate- to high-intensity ambulation training.

Teaching Points

Correct Answer: 4

Various studies support the use of moderate- to high-intensity ambulation for patients that are greater than 6 months poststroke. A recent clinical practice guideline from the Academy of Neurologic Physical Therapy (see Table 3-27) also recommends moderate- to high-intensity ambulation training and virtual reality treadmill training to improve locomotion in patients 6 months after a central nervous system injury (stroke, incomplete spinal cord injury, and traumatic brain injury).

Incorrect Choices:

The clinical practice guideline from the Academy of Neurologic Physical Therapy lists strength training and circuit training as interventions that may be considered but does not recommend BWSTT or robotic-assisted ambulation training. These interventions may have value early in rehab or when targeted toward corresponding impairments (e.g., strength, balance).

Type of Reasoning: Deductive

For this question, one must recall guidelines for effective intervention approaches to improve locomotor function in patients who are greater than 6 months poststroke. This necessitates the recall of factual information, which is a deductive reasoning skill. For this scenario, circuit training including strengthening, balance, and aerobic exercises have the highest level of evidence. Review information on improving locomotor function in patients with stroke, especially greater than 6 months poststroke, if answered incorrectly.

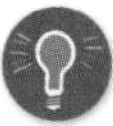

C132

Cardiovascular/Pulmonary | Interventions

A patient with a long history of systemic steroid use for asthma control is hospitalized with pneumonia. Which of the following is a contraindication to percussion?

Choices:

1. Barrel chest.
2. BP >140/90.
3. Intercostal muscle wasting.
4. Decreased bone density.

Teaching Points

Correct Answer: 4

The only one that is a contraindication to percussion would be decreased bone density, because a rib fracture might be a possible result. Osteoporosis is an adverse side effect of long-term steroid use.

Incorrect Choices:

Although the other choices are sequelae to long-term systemic steroid use, they are not a contraindication for percussion. An increased BP higher than that reported in the scenario might be a contraindication to postural drainage. It is not a contraindication to percussion. Barrel chest is seen in patients with emphysema, not asthma.

Type of Reasoning: Inferential

One must determine, given an understanding of the nature of long-term systemic steroid use for asthma, which condition would contraindicate percussion. It is beneficial to understand how percussion is performed, because it helps one to reason why decreased bone density would contraindicate the therapy. Inferential reasoning skill is used because one must infer the effects of long-term steroid use coupled with the nature of percussion therapy when used with patients who have asthma.

C133 

Musculoskeletal / Examination

The physical therapist is examining the patient's left ankle. The test pictured below is testing the integrity of which structure?

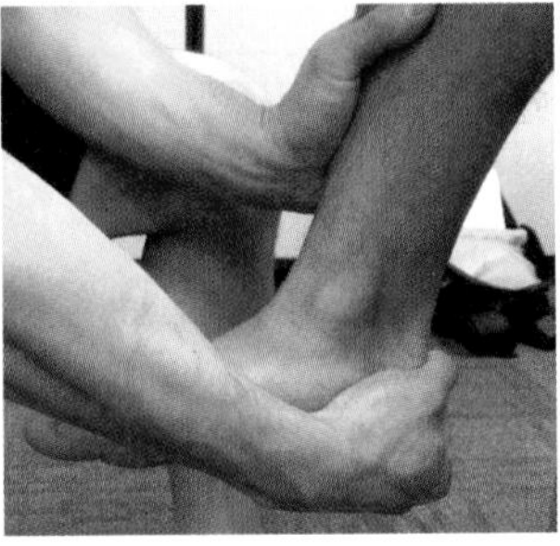

Choices:

1. Anterior tibiofibular ligament.
2. Tibiotalar ligament.
3. Calcaneofibular ligament.
4. Anterior talofibular ligament.

Teaching Points

Correct Answer: 4

The special test being performed is the anterior drawer test of the ankle. This test is designed primarily to test for injuries to the anterior talofibular ligament. This is the most frequently injured ligament in the ankle. When the foot is in slight plantarflexion position, the anterior talofibular ligament is perpendicular to the long axis of the tibia. A positive anterior drawer test may be obtained with a tear of only the anterior talofibular ligament, but anterior translation is greater if the calcaneofibular ligament is also torn. Ideally, the knee should be placed in 90° of flexion to alleviate tension on the Achilles tendon. See Box 2-11 for the Ankle Ligament Sprains Clinical Practice Guideline.

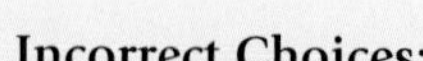

Incorrect Choices:

The primary test for the calcaneofibular ligament is talar tilt. The tibiotalar and anterior tibiofibular ligament would not be stressed with the anterior drawer test.

Type of Reasoning: Analytical

One must understand the test described in the question in order to choose the correct solution. Through analytical reasoning, the test-taker must determine how each ligament is tested. If this question was answered incorrectly, review information on provocative testing for ankle ligaments.

C134 

Musculoskeletal | Evaluation, Diagnosis

A patient with possible ligamentous injury of the knee presents with excessive tibial external rotation. Which ligament is **MOST LIKELY** to be injured?

Choices:

1. Posterior cruciate.
2. Medial patello-femoral.
3. Anterior cruciate.
4. Medial collateral.

Teaching Points

Correct Answer: 4

The medial collateral ligament prevents external rotation and provides stability to the knee. Excessive external rotation (ER) would represent injury to either the medial collateral ligament (MCL) or the lateral collateral ligament (LCL).

Incorrect Choices:

The anterior cruciate ligament (ACL) and posterior cruciate ligament (PCL) prevent internal rotation, and the medial patello-femoral ligament does not play a role in the prevention of tibial rotation.

Type of Reasoning: Inferential

One needs to be aware of the anatomical attachment of both the cruciate and collateral ligaments in order to arrive at a correct conclusion. For this question, one must infer what is likely to be true of a case, which is an inferential reasoning skill. In this case, the medial collateral ligament is most likely injured. Review collateral and cruciate ligaments of the knee and stability if answered incorrectly.

C135 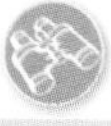

Cardiovascular/Pulmonary | Interventions

A middle-aged patient has been undergoing long-term corticosteroid treatment for pulmonary sarcoidosis. Due to the side effects of treatment, which intervention is the **MOST** important component to the patient's physical therapy plan of care?

Choices:

1. Supplemental oxygen use.
2. Resisted exercise for proximal muscle strengthening.
3. Acapella for airway clearance.
4. Education on pursed-lip breathing.

Teaching Points

Correct Answer: 2

The long-term treatment for pulmonary sarcoidosis is use of steroids. Steroids cause proximal muscle weakness, which leads to strength imbalance and decreased functional abilities. Chronic pulmonary disease also leads to increased muscle weakness and increased work of functional activities.

Incorrect Choices:

There is no data to support that the patient with sarcoidosis has a gas exchange impairment, so supplemental O_2 is not indicated. While patients with pulmonary sarcoidosis may have increased secretions, the data does not indicate that this patient has the need for airway clearance. Pursed-lip breathing can help with pacing and collateral ventilation, but there is no data that supports evidence of obstructive disease.

Type of Reasoning: Inductive

For this question, one must utilize knowledge of pulmonary sarcoidosis in order to determine a best course of action. Questions that require clinical knowledge and approaches best matched to a diagnosis often necessitate inductive reasoning skill. For this case, it is most important to include resisted exercise for proximal muscle strengthening as part of the plan of care. Review information on pulmonary sarcoidosis and intervention approaches if answered incorrectly.

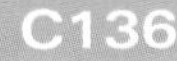
C136
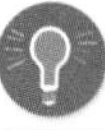

Musculoskeletal I Interventions

A therapist is treating a patient with a diagnosis of right shoulder rotator cuff tendinitis. The findings of a work site ergonomic assessment indicate that the worker is required to perform repetitive reaching activities above shoulder height. Which of the following is the **MOST** beneficial work site modification?

Choices:

1. Reposition the height of the shelf and items to below shoulder height.
2. Provide the worker with a taller, sit-stand chair.
3. Allow the worker to take more frequent rests to avoid overuse.
4. Provide the worker with a standing desk for daily activities.

Teaching Points

Correct Answer: 1

Work stations should be designed to accommodate the persons who actually work on the job. Work stations should be easily adjustable and designed to be comfortable for the worker. In this case, lowering the height of the shelf for frequent use is best.

Incorrect Choices:

Taking more frequent rests or providing a different chair does not eliminate the essential problem of repetitive overhead reach that is causing the shoulder tendinitis. Using a standing desk would eliminate overhead reach but is not as practical as lowering the shelf. In the workplace, individuals cannot be expected to stand all day long.

Type of Reasoning: Inferential

One must infer the best solution to alleviate the patient's right shoulder rotator cuff tendinitis, given the nature of the patient's work environment. In this situation, one should infer that the overhead repetitive reaching is the cause for the diagnosis; therefore, reaching below shoulder height would help to alleviate the symptoms. If this question was answered incorrectly, refer to information on ergonomic workstation assessment.

C137

Musculoskeletal | Interventions

The patient has a fifth rib that is "stuck" in the position of maximal inspiration. Which technique is **BEST** to improve the rib mobility and assist it in returning to its resting position?

Choices:

1. Maitland grade IV mobilization of the head of the rib at the costovertebral joint in the superior direction.
2. Maitland grade II mobilization of the head of the rib at the costovertebral joint in the superior direction.
3. Maitland grade IV mobilization of the head of the rib at the costovertebral joint in the inferior direction.
4. Maitland grade II mobilization of the head of the rib at the costovertebral joint in the inferior direction.

Teaching Points

Correct Answer: 1

With inspiration, the lateral portion of the ribs moves up and the head moves down; to bring it back to a neutral position, the head needs to glide superiorly, allowing the lateral part of the rib to lower with expiration. Grade IV mobilizations are used to improve joint mobility.

Incorrect Choices:

All other choices have either the incorrect technique to improve joint mobility or incorrect direction.

Type of Reasoning: Inferential

One needs to be knowledgeable of the different utilization of mobilization grades and of the biomechanics of the costovertebral joints during respiration in order to determine a correct conclusion. This necessitates inferring a best course of action for a successful clinical outcome, which is an inferential reasoning skill. For this situation, Maitland grade IV mobilization of the head of the rib at the costovertebral joint in the superior direction is best. Review Maitland's oscillatory techniques for the rib cage if answered incorrectly.

C138

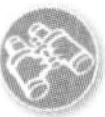

Neuromuscular | Examination

An older adult with Parkinson's disease (PD) (Hoehn & Yahr disease Stage 3) is referred to physical therapy for evaluation and treatment. The patient and his spouse report that in addition to the typical motor symptoms (bradykinesia, rigidity), he is now having difficulty with planning, multitasking, and word recall. Which examination item is **BEST** to assess the patient's new symptoms?

Choices:

1. Recall of three unrelated words.
2. Montreal Cognitive Assessment (MoCA).
3. Mini-Mental State Examination (MMSE).
4. Timed Up & Go with Cognitive Task (TUG-Cog).

Teaching Points

Correct Answer: 2

The patient's new symptoms suggest potential mild cognitive impairment (see Box 10-1). The MoCA is a reliable and valid tool to examine mild cognitive impairment and dementia in older adults and patients with neurologic health conditions. It includes multiple cognitive domains (visuospatial, executive function, naming, memory, attention, language, abstraction, and orientation) and is specifically recommended by the APTA Neurology Section Parkinson's Disease EDGE Task Force (see Table 3-19).

Incorrect Choices:

Recall of three words does not assess the spectrum of cognitive domains and is limited to short-term memory. The MMSE assists in screening individuals with moderate to severe cognitive impairment (dementia) but is not as sensitive as the MoCA for detecting mild cognitive impairment. The TUG-Cog is helpful for assessing the impact of multitasking on balance and mobility but does not examine the various domains associated with mild cognitive impairment.

Type of Reasoning: Inductive

For this question, the test-taker must utilize knowledge of examinations that effectively assess cognition for patients with PD. Questions of this nature often require inductive reasoning skill. For this case, the examination item that would best assess the patient's new symptoms is the MoCA. If answered incorrectly, review cognitive examinations, especially the MoCA.

C139 

Cardiovascular/Pulmonary I Examination

A patient has a 10-year history of peripheral vascular disease (PVD) affecting the right lower extremity. During auscultation in a peripheral vascular examination, what should the therapist expect to find?

Choices:

1. Cool temperature of the lower extremity.
2. Pitting edema of the dorsum of foot.
3. Femoral and popliteal artery bruits.
4. Capillary refill greater then 5 seconds.

Teaching Points

Correct Answer: 3

A bruit is a swishing sound that occurs in the presence of narrowing of an artery. It is a characteristic finding of PVD present on auscultation.

Incorrect Choices:

All other choices are not revealed on auscultation. Palpation will likely reveal a cool temperature, pitting edema of the dorsum of the foot, and capillary refill greater than 3 seconds.

Type of Reasoning: Inferential

This question requires one to infer what a therapist should find with a patient who has a history of PVD. One must have a solid understanding of the nature of PVD and examination measures in order to choose the correct solution. If this question was answered incorrectly, review PVD examination.

C140 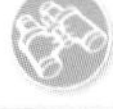

Musculoskeletal I Interventions

During the examination of a patient with hip pain, the therapist notes that the patient has limited hip extension during ambulation. The Thomas test was positive. The rest of the physical examination was unremarkable. Which is the BEST physical therapy intervention to improve hip extension range of motion during gait?

Choices:

1. Hip P-A mobilization (anterior glide).
2. Hip A-P mobilization (posterior glide).

3. Standing hamstring stretch.
4. Half-kneeling hip flexor stretch.

Teaching Points

Correct Answer: 4

A positive Thomas test indicates that there is tightness of the hip flexors or quadriceps femoris muscles. Although the question stem did not differentiate between tightness of the hip flexors vs. the quadriceps femoris muscle for the Thomas test, this finding combined with the observation of limited hip extension during gait suggest that hip flexor muscle tightness should be addressed.

Incorrect Choices:

Hip mobilizations are utilized to increase limited, intrinsic joint mobility. Although a hip P-A glide mobilization is frequently utilized to improve hip flexion, the positive Thomas test suggests that there is a muscle length restriction rather than a joint mobility restriction. Hip A-P glide mobilizations are utilized to improve hip flexion, not hip extension. Hamstring stretches will help improve hip flexion and/or knee extension range of motion.

Type of Reasoning: Inductive

For this question one must recall the Thomas test and what a positive test indicates in order to determine the best intervention approach to address the patient's deficit. This requires inductive reasoning skill, where clinical knowledge is paramount to arriving at a correct conclusion. For this situation, the therapist should choose a half-kneeling hip flexor stretch. If answered incorrectly, review the Thomas test and intervention approaches for tight hip flexors.

C141 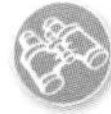

Musculoskeletal | Evaluation, Diagnosis

A teenager presents to the clinic with vague left hip and groin pain that worsens with weight-bearing. The PT's examination reveals limited and painful hip internal rotation, antalgic gait, and a weak gluteus medius. Based upon this clinical presentation, what is the **MOST** likely diagnosis?

Choices:

1. Gluteus medius muscle strain.
2. Oligoarticular juvenile rheumatoid arthritis (JRA).
3. Slipped capital femoral epiphysis (SCFE).
4. Legg-Calvé-Perthes disease.

Teaching Points

Correct Answer: 3

The SCFE age range is 10–16 years of age, and the male to female ratio is 3:1. The incidence of left hip to right hip is 2:1, with 30% bilateral. The best examination findings include pain that worsens with weight-bearing, limited and painful hip internal rotation, and weak hip abductors. See page 123 for a description of SCFE and Legg-Calve-Perthes disease.

Incorrect Choices:

Legg-Calvé-Perthes disease is avascular necrosis of the femoral head with insidious onset between 3–12 years of age. The male to female ratio is 4:1. The clinical presentation is an antalgic gait, disuse atrophy of the hip and thigh muscles, and painful limitation of abduction and internal rotation. A gluteus medius muscle strain would present with more specific focal pain and pain with muscular contraction. The associated weakness in this case is secondary to an alteration of the length-tension relationship. Pauciarticular or oligoarticular JRA onset occurs in 40% of children with juvenile rheumatoid arthritis. In some combination, the knees, ankles, wrists, or elbows are the most frequently affected joints. The hips are usually spared.

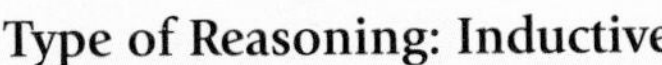

Type of Reasoning: Inductive

This question provides a group of symptoms, and the test-taker must determine the most likely diagnosis based on this information. Questions of this nature often require inductive reasoning skills. For this case, the symptoms most likely indicate slipped capital femoral epiphysis. If answered incorrectly, review signs and symptoms of SCFE.

C142 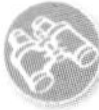

Nonsystem I Equipment, Devices

A patient with a transfemoral amputation and an above-knee prosthesis demonstrates knee instability while standing. The patient's knee buckles easily when performing weight shifts. What is the **MOST** likely cause of the problem?

Choices:

1. Weak gluteus medius.
2. Prosthetic knee set too far anterior to the TKA line.
3. Tight extension aid.
4. Prosthetic knee set too far posterior to the trochanter-knee-ankle (TKA) line.

Teaching Points

Correct Answer: 2

In order to increase stability of the knee, the prosthetic knee axis of rotation is normally aligned anterior to a line extending from the trochanter to the ankle (TKA line). A knee set too far anterior to the TKA line will cause the knee to buckle.

Incorrect Choices:

A prosthetic knee set too far posterior to the TKA would result in excessive knee stability and difficulty flexing the knee. The gluteus medius contributes to stability during stance, primarily lateral stability. Weak abductors can result in trunk lateral bend during stance. An extension aid assists knee extension during the latter part of swing phase. A tight extension aid will result in terminal swing impact during late swing.

Type of Reasoning: Inductive

Clinical judgment and diagnostic reasoning are utilized to determine the likely cause for the patient's knee instability while standing. Through inductive reasoning, the test-taker should determine that the prosthetic knee is set too far anterior to the TKA line. If this question was answered incorrectly, review information on prosthetic adjustment/alignment for above-knee prostheses.

C143 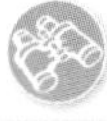

Neuromuscular I Examination

An older adult at risk for falls has undergone a structured home-based exercise program that consisted of sitting/standing balance training and strengthening exercises. Which measure is the **BEST** choice to document improvements?

Choices:

1. Timed Up & Go Test.
2. Berg Balance Test.
3. 6-Minute Walk Test.
4. Performance-Oriented Mobility Assessment (Tinetti).

Teaching Points

Correct Answer: 2

The Berg Balance Test is a 14-item test of static and dynamic balance in sitting and standing. It also examines sit-to-stand and stand-to-sit transitions. It does not include items examining gait. Gait was not part of this person's training program.

Incorrect Choices:

The TUG and Tinetti examine gait along with balance. The 6-Minute Walk Test is a measure of walking endurance.

Type of Reasoning: Inductive

This question requires clinical judgment to determine the **BEST** measurement tool for improvement in balance. This is an inductive reasoning skill, where clinical knowledge is applied to therapeutic situations to determine a best course of action. For this situation, the Berg Balance Test is best. If answered incorrectly, review balance tests, especially the Berg Balance Test. See Box 3-1 and Table 3-11 for additional information on balance measures.

C144 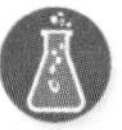

Systems Interactions | Evaluation, Diagnosis

A middle-aged patient complains of "throbbing pain" in the lumbar region with activities upon exertion, such as walking up a flight of steps or playing tennis. The patient expresses no complaints of pain with bending, twisting, sitting, standing, or walking any distance. Active movements of the lumbar spine are full and pain free. Provocation testing is negative. Neurological signs are unremarkable. There is no significant tenderness to palpation. What is the **MOST** likely diagnosis for this patient?

Choices:

1. Lumbar disc herniation.
2. Aortic aneurysm.
3. Quadratus lumborum muscle strain.
4. Sacroiliac joint sprain.

Teaching Points

Correct Answer: 2

Throbbing low back pain that occurs only with activities that increase the heart rate is a red flag for aortic aneurysm. Immediate medical referral is indicated.

Incorrect Choices:

The fact that the patient reports no pain with activities such as bending, twisting, sitting, and walking reduces the odds that the problem is mechanical. In addition, the fact that the symptoms could not be reproduced during the physical therapy examination reduces the odds that it is a musculoskeletal condition.

Type of Reasoning: Analytical

This question provides a group of symptoms that the test-taker must analyze to determine the most likely diagnosis. Questions of this nature often require analytical reasoning skill. For this situation, the most likely diagnosis is aortic aneurysm, given the symptoms presented. Review signs and symptoms of aortic aneurysm if answered incorrectly.

C145 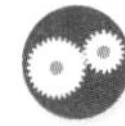

Neuromuscular | Interventions

A patient that is undergoing spinal cord rehabilitation is viewed as uncooperative by staff. The patient refuses to complete the training activities outlined to promote independent functional mobility. A review of history reveals that previously the patient was the director of a company with a staff of 20. What is the **MOST** appropriate action the therapist can take?

Choices:

1. Have the patient work with a supervisor who is a person in authority.
2. Refer the patient to a support group before resuming rehabilitation.
3. Involve the patient in goal setting and structuring the training session.
4. Carefully structure the activities and slow down the pace of training.

Teaching Points

Correct Answer: 3

An andragogical approach is best. The patient is an adult learner who should be allowed to share in the responsibility for planning the learning experience and goal setting. The therapist should help clarify the problem, structure the learning environment, and provide necessary resources.

Incorrect Choices:

Passing the buck or transferring responsibility to a supervisor is not appropriate. Requiring participation in a support group before continuing rehabilitation or slowing down the pace of training would negatively impact rehabilitation and result in increased length of stay.

Type of Reasoning: Evaluative

One must evaluate the merits of each statement in order to make a best course determination for this patient. This question requires a judgment call and a value judgment, which necessitates evaluative reasoning skill. For this patient, it is **MOST** appropriate to involve the patient in goal setting and have him participate in structuring the training session.

C146 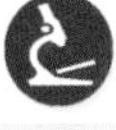

Nonsystem | Research

A research team is conducting a study involving patients with chronic ankle instability. Specifically, the investigators want to know if patients using a commercially available ankle brace, ankle taping, or no support at all perform better on the Illinois Agility Test. Which research design will **BEST** answer the therapist's question?

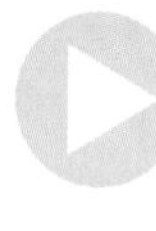

Choices:

1. Longitudinal cohort.
2. Observational cross-sectional.
3. Randomized controlled trial.
4. Case-control.

Teaching Points

Correct Answer: 3

Randomized controlled trials (RCT) are the preferred research design for establishing a cause and effect relationship. Since participants are randomly assigned to groups, this design provides the greatest protection from threats to internal validity and is most appropriate to identify the group with the best functional outcomes.

Incorrect Choices:

All of the other choices are observational study designs and do not involve the scientific rigor of an RCT. Cohort designs evaluate the natural course of phenomena over time in a particular group of subjects. Cross-sectional designs are used for population-based surveys and to assess the prevalence of a particular condition or disease in a sample. Case-control studies assign subjects to groups based on the presence or absence of a particular trait or naturally occurring phenomenon.

Type of Reasoning: Deductive

For this question, the test-taker must recall the different types of research designs in order to determine a best research design for this particular research question. This necessitates the recall of factual information, which is a deductive reasoning skill. For this case, the best design is a randomized controlled trial. If answered incorrectly, review research designs, especially the randomized controlled trial.

C147 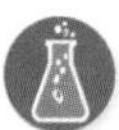

Genitourinary I Evaluation, Diagnosis

Patient presents with burning and tingling on the left lateral thigh that has manifested recently in her third trimester of pregnancy. The patient states that symptoms occur more in standing than sitting, and that light touch is more aggravating than applied pressure. Patient was negative for the neurological findings involving reflexes, dermatomes, and myotomes. Based upon this information, what is the **MOST LIKELY** cause of these symptoms?

Choices:

1. Disc derangement L 2/3 segment.
2. Nerve root L3 compression.
3. Meralgia paresthetica.
4. Referred pain from the sacroiliac joint due to instability postrelaxin release.

Teaching Points

Correct Answer: 3

Meralgia paresthetica is a condition involving the lateral femoral cutaneous nerve. The nerve is responsible for innervation of the lateral aspect of the upper thigh. This nerve passes medial by the psoas major before crossing in front of the iliacus and then under the inguinal ligament. With increased weight and increased anterior pelvic tilt this nerve can be entrapped as it passes. Thus, it can be a common problem seen in pregnancy.

Incorrect Choices:

Compression of L3 nerve root would have a dermatomal pattern. The disc can refer into the upper buttock region and due to innervation has a similar pattern of referral to that of the facet joints of the lumbar spine. This pattern is distinctly different from that of the lateral femoral cutaneous nerve. The sacroiliac joint could have a referred pattern into the lumbar and buttock regions, but again is less likely to refer into the specific lateral thigh region that is innervated by the lateral femoral cutaneous nerve.

Type of Reasoning: Analytical

One must determine what the likely cause is for a patient's condition in order to arrive at a correct conclusion. This necessitates analytical reasoning skill, where the patient's symptoms are analyzed in order to reach a reasonable conclusion. For this case, the symptoms are consistent with meralgia paresthetica. If answered incorrectly, review signs of meralgia paresthetica.

C148 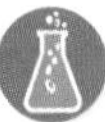

Cardiovascular/Pulmonary | Examination

Which clinical finding would the physical therapist expect to find when examining the patient with the chest film shown here?

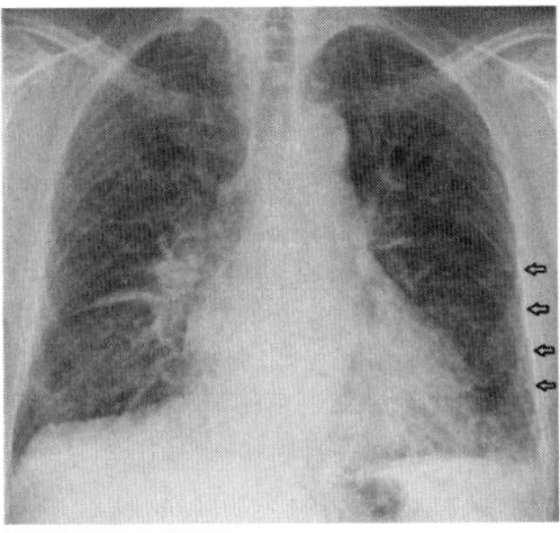

Choices:

1. S1 heart sound.
2. S3 heart sound.
3. Unilateral lower extremity edema.
4. Unilateral upper extremity edema.

Teaching Points

Correct Answer: 2

The A–P chest x-ray demonstrates pulmonary edema with interstitial edema shown throughout both lobes. This likely occurred due to heart failure given the enlarged appearance of the heart. An S3 heart sound is indicative of heart failure.

Incorrect Choices:

An S1 sound (the "lub" in "lub-dub") indicates normal closure of mitral and tricuspid valves. It may be decreased in a first-degree heart block. A patient in heart failure would have bilateral lower extremity edema, not unilateral edema. It is unlikely that a patient with heart failure would have upper extremity edema, but if they did, it would be bilateral.

Type of Reasoning: Analytical

For this question, the test-taker must analyze the chest film presented and interpret the likely findings resulting from it. This requires analytical reasoning skill. For this situation, the x-ray demonstrates the likely clinical finding of an S3 heart sound consistent with pulmonary edema and interstitial edema and heart failure. If answered incorrectly, review pulmonary edema information and x-ray findings.

C149 

Neuromuscular | Evaluation, Diagnosis

A physical therapist is observing a child who is typically developing and has just begun to walk within the last month. Which of the following is expected in a child just learning to walk?

Choices:

1. Neutral hip position.
2. Bilateral hip adduction.
3. Genu valgum.
4. External rotation of the hips.

Teaching Points

Correct Answer: 4

Children who have just begun to walk externally rotate their hips (toe out) for balance. This increases the base of support.

Incorrect Choices:

Children who have just learned to walk independently (12–15 months of age) typically display bowed legs (genu varum), flexion at the hips to keep the center of gravity forward, and have a wide base of support (hips in abduction). They also demonstrate "high guard" position of their upper extremities to help maintain balance.

Type of Reasoning: Inferential

This question requires one to infer what is likely to be true of a therapeutic situation, which often necessitates inferential reasoning skill. One must also recall the developmental gait patterns of children. In this case, one would expect the child to demonstrate external rotation of the hips. If this question was answered incorrectly, review developmental gait patterns in children (see Table 9-2).

C150 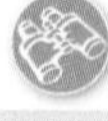

Musculoskeletal | Interventions

A patient presents to physical therapy with acute neck pain secondary to a motor vehicle accident where they experienced a rapid acceleration-deceleration mechanism. The therapist's diagnosis is whiplash-associated disorder (WAD). Which intervention should be emphasized as part of a multimodal treatment plan during the acute stages of WAD?

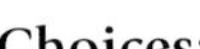

Choices:
1. Long-term use of a cervical collar.
2. Mobilization.
3. Iontophoresis.
4. Intermittent cervical traction.

Teaching Points

Correct Answer: 2

According to the Neck Pain Clinical Practice Guidelines (see Box 2-15), interventions for acute neck pain with movement coordination impairments (WAD) should include patient education instruction to remain active, return to preactivity levels as soon as possible, perform postural exercises, mobilization, and submaximal exercise programming (endurance, strengthening, and coordination). In addition, physical therapists may consider the use of transcutaneous electrical nerve stimulation.

Incorrect Choices:

Short-term use of a cervical collar may be indicated in some circumstances. However, therapists should avoid prolonged use of neck braces. Iontophoresis is not recommended as part of the neck pain guidelines for movement coordination impairments, including WAD. Intermittent cervical traction is not recommended as part of the neck pain clinical guidelines for movement coordination impairments, including WAD. Intermittent cervical traction may be appropriate for patients classified with other categories of neck pain such as mobility deficits or radiating pain.

Type of Reasoning: Inductive

For this question, the test-taker must utilize knowledge of intervention approaches for whiplash-associated disorder (WAD) to draw a reasonable conclusion. This requires inductive reasoning skill, where clinical knowledge helps one to make effective intervention decisions. For this scenario, the treatment plan should emphasize mobilization. Review the Neck Pain Clinical Practice Guidelines if answered incorrectly.

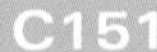
C151
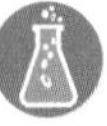

Neuromuscular | Evaluation, Diagnosis

A patient presents with focal pain in the upper third of the anterior forearm. They also report weakness and the ability to flex the right thumb and index finger (see image below). They have normal sensation in the bilateral upper extremities. These findings are most consistent with which of the following health conditions?

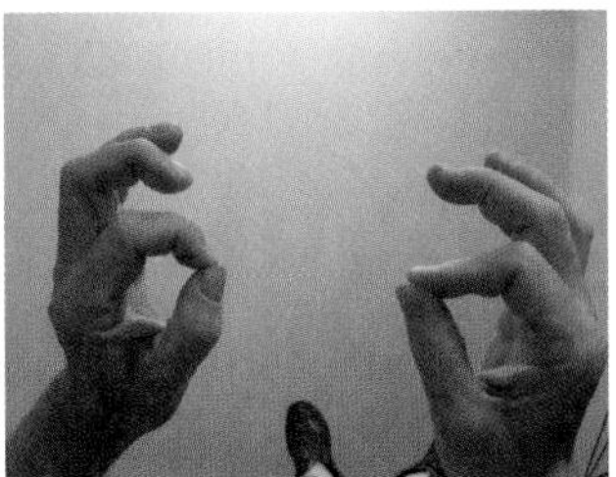

Choices:
1. Pronator teres syndrome.
2. Anterior interosseous syndrome.
3. Carpal tunnel syndrome.
4. Cubital tunnel syndrome.

Teaching Points

Correct Answer: 2

Anterior interosseous syndrome results in pain in the upper third of the forearm with specific weakness to the flexor pollicis longus, flexor digitorum profundus (index and middle fingers), and pronator quadratus. This neural entrapment results in the inability to form an "OK" sign.

Incorrect Choices:

Pronator teres syndrome, carpal tunnel syndrome, and cubital tunnel syndrome would involve both motor and sensory changes as well as weakness of various muscles to include thenar (carpal tunnel and pronator teres syndrome) and hand intrinsic (cubital tunnel syndrome) muscles.

Type of Reasoning: Analytical

For this question, the test-taker must analyze the symptoms presented and determine the health condition that is most consistent with these symptoms. This requires analytical reasoning skill where pieces of information are weighed to draw reasonable conclusions. For this scenario, the symptoms are most consistent with anterior interosseous syndrome. Review symptoms of anterior interosseous syndrome, if answered incorrectly.

C152 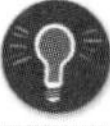

Musculoskeletal I Examination

A patient is referred for physical therapy with a diagnosis of degenerative joint disease (DJD) affecting C2 and C3. The patient complains of pain and stiffness in the cervical region and transient dizziness with some cervical motions. What is the **BEST** initial examination procedure?

Choices:

1. Vertebral artery test.
2. Adson's maneuver.
3. Lhermitte's test.
4. Oppenheim's test.

Teaching Points

Correct Answer: 1

The vertebral artery test checks the integrity of the blood flow through the artery in the cervical region. Because the patient is experiencing symptoms of circulatory disturbance and a unilateral pull could compress the left cervical structures, the vertebral artery test is an appropriate screening test. The test consists of passively placing the patient's head in extension and side flexion in a supine position. Then the head and neck are slowly rotated to the laterally flexed side and held for 30 seconds. Some of the positive signs may be syncope, lightheadedness, nystagmus, or visual disturbances. Though there are some doubts about the sensitivity/specificity of this test, the patient's initial complaint of dizziness with some cervical movements would indicate that it be applied in this case.

Incorrect Choices:

Lhermitte's sign is pain down the spine and into the upper or lower limbs with passive flexion of the neck. It is used to identify dysfunction of the spinal cord associated with upper motor neuron lesions and is typically positive in MS. Adson's maneuver is a test for thoracic outlet syndrome (TOS). Oppenheim's test involves running a fingernail along the crest of the tibia; a positive test is the same as a positive Babinski.

Type of Reasoning: Inferential

One must first determine the meaning of each of the four possible tests and then infer which one is the **BEST** initial test, given the patient's diagnosis and symptoms. If this question was answered incorrectly, review the vertebral artery test.

C153 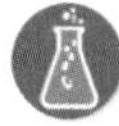

Neuromuscular | Evaluation, Diagnosis

A young, otherwise healthy, adult is recovering from an L5 vertebral fracture with cauda equina involving the bilateral L5 and all sacral nerve roots. What are the functional expectations for this individual?

Choices:

1. Ambulation using bilateral AFOs and canes.
2. Ambulation using bilateral KAFOs, crutches, and a swing-through gait.
3. Ambulation using reciprocating gait orthoses and a reciprocating walker.
4. Ambulation using bilateral KAFOs and a reciprocating walker.

Teaching Points

Correct Answer: 1

This injury will result in significant motor and sensory loss in the posterior pelvis, posterior thighs, legs, feet, and toes. Intact movements include hip flexion, hip adduction, and knee extension. The quadriceps become **FULLY** innervated at L4 level. This patient can be expected to be a functional ambulator using bilateral AFOs and crutches or canes.

Incorrect Choices:

All other choices include orthotic devices that offer control of joints that is not needed (orthotic bracing of knees and hips). Also crutches or walkers should not be needed.

Type of Reasoning: Analytical

One must recall past knowledge of neuroscience related to cauda equina injuries in order to determine the functional expectations for this patient. In order to arrive at the correct conclusion, one must analyze the four possible choices and determine which choice is most aligned with one's knowledge of injury at this level. If this question was answered incorrectly, review functional expectations for patients with lumbar spinal injuries.

C154 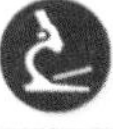

Neuromuscular | Examination

To examine a patient with a suspected deficit in graphesthesia, what should the therapist ask the patient to identify with eyes closed?

Choices:

1. Different objects placed in the hand and manipulated.
2. The vibrations of a tuning fork when placed on a bony prominence.
3. A series of letters traced on the hand.
4. Differently weighted, identically shaped cylinders placed in the hand.

Teaching Points

Correct Answer: 3

Graphesthesia is the ability to recognize numbers, letters, or symbols traced on the skin.

Incorrect Choices:

Barognosis is the ability to recognize different weights placed in the hand using identically shaped objects. Pallesthesia is the ability to recognize vibratory stimuli (i.e., a vibrating tuning fork placed on a bony prominence). Stereognosis is the ability to recognize different objects placed in the hand and manipulated. During testing, vision is occluded.

Type of Reasoning: Deductive

This question requires factual recall of the definition of graphesthesia, which is a deductive reasoning skill. Using past knowledge of neuroscience is beneficial to arriving at the correct solution. If this question was answered incorrectly, review sensory testing procedures (see Table 3-3).

C155 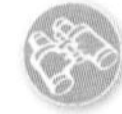

Neuromuscular | Interventions

A patient recovering from stroke is ambulatory without an assistive device and demonstrates a consistent problem with an elevated and retracted pelvis on the affected side. Which manual therapeutic exercise procedure is the **BEST** choice to remediate this problem?

Choices:

1. Provide downward compression during stance.
2. Utilize light resistance to posterior pelvic elevation during swing.
3. Provide anterior-directed pressure during swing.
4. Utilize light resistance to forward pelvic rotation during swing.

Teaching Points

Correct Answer: 4

An elevated and retracted pelvis is a common problem during gait for many patients recovering from a stroke. Providing light resistance to forward pelvic rotation actively engages those muscles and reciprocally inhibits the spastic retractors.

Incorrect Choices:

Providing anterior-directed pressure during swing or resistance to pelvic elevation may serve to only increase the problem. Downward compression during stance is also inappropriate as this is a swing phase deficit.

Type of Reasoning: Inductive

One must utilize clinical judgment in order to determine which therapeutic exercise procedure would **BEST** address the patient's problem. Using inductive reasoning skills, the test-taker must analyze the four possible choices and then rely on knowledge of mobility challenges in a stroke in order to determine the **BEST** course of action for this patient.

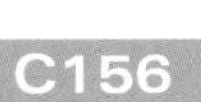

C156

Neuromuscular | Examination

A therapist suspects lower brain stem involvement in a patient with amyotrophic lateral sclerosis (ALS). Examination findings reveal motor impairments of the tongue with ipsilateral wasting and deviation on protrusion. These findings confirm involvement of which cranial nerve?

Choices:

1. Hypoglossal.
2. Glossopharyngeal.
3. Vagus.
4. Spinal accessory.

Teaching Points

Correct Answer: 1

The hypoglossal (CN XII) controls the movements of the tongue. Ipsilateral wasting and the deviation to the ipsilateral side on protrusion are indicative of damage.

Incorrect Choices:

Involvement of the glossopharyngeal (CN IX) results in slight dysphagia, loss of taste in the posterior third of the tongue, and loss of gag reflex. Involvement of the spinal accessory nerve (CN XI) results in minor problems in deglutition and phonation along with weakness in ipsilateral shoulder shrugging. Involvement of the vagus (CN X) results in dysphagia, hoarseness, and paralysis of the soft palate.

Type of Reasoning: Analytical

This question requires one to recall the functions of the 12 cranial nerves and then determine which nerve is most likely impaired in this situation. Questions that involve determining an impairment based on a group of symptoms require analytical reasoning skill. If this question was answered incorrectly, review examination of the 12 cranial nerves (see Table 3-1).

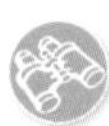

C157

Musculoskeletal | Evaluation, Diagnosis

A baseball pitcher reports insidious onset of symptoms characteristic of impingement, including catching and popping in the throwing arm. Examination reveals that glenohumeral passive internal rotation is painful and limited to 30°. External rotation is less symptomatic and has 130° of passive range. What is the **BEST** initial course of action for the therapist?

Choices:

1. Recommend an MRI.
2. Mobilize the glenohumeral joint to increase internal rotation ROM.
3. Begin elastic resistance exercises for impingement.
4. Recommend an anteroposterior radiograph.

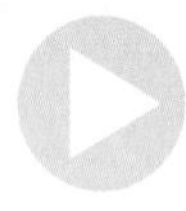

Teaching Points

Correct Answer: 1

The therapist should suspect a labral tear. This is a common finding among pitchers and athletes who do a lot of throwing (especially those who present with abnormal ROM findings and instability symptoms of popping and catching). Although this athlete may present with impingement, an MRI is warranted to fully diagnose the condition and to develop an appropriate treatment plan.

Incorrect Choices:

Beginning treatment without definitive testing is contraindicated. Plain radiographs are inappropriate for suspected soft tissue lesions.

Type of Reasoning: Inductive

This question requires clinical judgment to determine a best course of action for a patient with painful passive internal rotation with limitations in range. Questions that require one to weigh a group of symptoms and determine a best course of action often necessitate inductive reasoning skills. If this question was answered incorrectly, review signs and symptoms of labral tear and diagnostic testing.

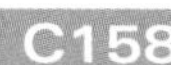
C158
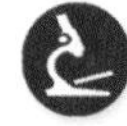

System Interactions | Evaluation, Diagnosis

A physical therapist conducts a chart review prior to initiating treatment for a deconditioned inpatient. The patient is currently receiving chemotherapy for prostate cancer. After reviewing the current laboratory values listed below, the therapist determines that the patient should not perform any resistance exercises and decides to reschedule the therapy session for the next day. Which lab results prompted the therapist to make this decision?

Choices:

1. Hematocrit = 48%.
2. Platelet count = 8,000 cells/mm^3.
3. White blood cell count = 10,000 cells/mm^3.
4. Hemoglobin = 15 g/dL.

Teaching Points

Correct Answer: 2

The platelet count in this individual is extremely low and no resistance exercises should be performed because the patient is at increased risk for hemorrhage. The patient may perform ADLs and gentle AROM exercises. Patients with platelet counts under 10,000 cells/mm^3 typically undergo transfusions and should be monitored for hematuria, petechiae, and other signs of active bleeding.

Incorrect Choices:

Each of the lab values in the other answer choices are within the range of normal values for males. Exercise would not be contraindicated based on these results. See Tables 4-10 and 8-1 for a review of cardiovascular laboratory values and possible implications for physical therapy.

Type of Reasoning: Deductive

For this question, the test-taker must recall the lab values that indicate therapy should be rescheduled. This requires factual recall of guidelines, which is a deductive reasoning skill. In this case, a platelet count of 8,000 cells/mm^3 indicates a low platelet count and therapy should be rescheduled. Review laboratory values, especially platelet values, if answered incorrectly.

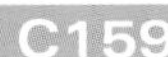
C159
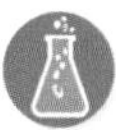

Integumentary | Evaluation, Diagnosis

A patient with a transfemoral amputation is unable to wear a total contact prosthesis for the past 4 days. Examination of the residual limb reveals erythema and edema extending over most of the lower anterior limb. The patient tells the therapist that the limb is very itchy and painful. What is the **MOST** likely cause of these symptoms?

Choices:

1. Impetigo.
2. Herpes zoster.
3. Cellulitis.
4. Dermatitis.

Teaching Points

Correct Answer: 4

This patient is exhibiting symptoms of contact dermatitis. Primary treatment is removal of the offending agent (in this case, the total contact prosthesis) and treatment of the involved skin with lubricants, topical anesthetics, and/or steroids. The patient may require a thin sock if the problem does not resolve.

Incorrect Choices:

Cellulitis is a suppurative inflammation of the dermis and subcutaneous tissues frequently accompanied by infection. Impetigo is a staphylococcal infection with small macules (unraised spots) or vesicles (small blisters). Herpes zoster is a viral infection with red papules along the course of a nerve or dermatome.

Type of Reasoning: Analytical

This question requires the test-taker to determine the **MOST LIKELY** cause for the patient's symptoms, which is an analytical reasoning skill. In order to arrive at the correct conclusion, one must analyze the four possible choices and determine which choice is most aligned with one's knowledge of skin irritations, inflammations, and infections. If this question was answered incorrectly, review symptoms and treatment approaches for dermatitis.

C160
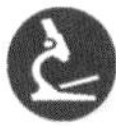

Musculoskeletal | Examination

A PT is treating a patient who lacks wrist extension. The cause of the impairment is a problem at the radiocarpal joint with a lack of arthrokinematic motion necessary for proper wrist extension. What direction should the proximal aspect of the scaphoid/lunate glide?

Choices:

1. In a dorsal direction relative to the radius.
2. Radially.
3. Ulnarly.
4. In a palmar direction relative to the radius.

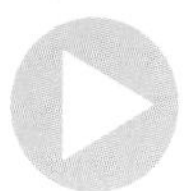

Teaching Points

Correct Answer: 4

The correct description of the arthrokinematic motion occurring at the radiocarpal joint lacking in this patient is the palmar glide. Due to the anatomical structure of the bones forming this joint, the convex scaphoid and lunate articulate with the concave radius, resulting in opposite roll and glide during extension.

Incorrect Choices:

Other choices describe movements occurring during ulnar and radial wrist deviation or of the glide occurring during flexion.

Type of Reasoning: Deductive

One needs to understand the convex-concave rules of joint movement to arrive at a correct conclusion. This requires recall of the anatomical structures of the wrist and proper rolls and glides, which is factual information and therefore a deductive reasoning skill. For this case, the therapist should glide the lunate/scaphoid palmarly relative to the radius. Review concave-convex rules of the wrist and mobilization techniques if answered incorrectly.

C161 

Musculoskeletal | Examination

Following a hip fracture that is now healed, a patient presents with weak hip flexors (2/5). All other muscles are within functional limits. Based on these findings, what should the therapist expect the patient may display during gait?

Choices:
1. Backward trunk lean.
2. Forward trunk lean.
3. A circumducted gait.
4. Excessive hip flexion.

Teaching Points

Correct Answer: 3

Circumduction is a compensation for weak hip flexors or an inability to shorten the leg (weak knee flexors and ankle dorsiflexors). Hip hiking can also compensate for an abnormally long leg (lack of knee flexion and dorsiflexion). See Chapter 12 for a review of common gait deviations.

Incorrect Choices:

Excessive hip flexion is a compensation for footdrop. Forward trunk lean and backward trunk lean are stance phase deviations that compensate for quadriceps weakness and gluteus maximus weakness, respectively.

Type of Reasoning: Inferential

This question requires the test-taker to draw conclusions based on evidence presented, which is an inferential reasoning skill. Questions of this nature often provide a diagnosis, and the test-taker must infer the likely symptoms. In this case, the test-taker must determine that a patient with weak hip flexors will display a circumducted gait pattern during ambulation. If this question was answered incorrectly, review causes for a circumducted gait pattern.

C162 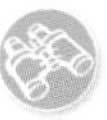

Genitourinary | Interventions

A physical therapist receives a referral to manage a client with chronic kidney disease (stage 2 renal failure). Which of the following is the **MOST IMPORTANT** consideration for the therapist when developing an exercise regimen for this patient?

Choices:

1. Individuals with chronic kidney disease have a high risk for falls and fractures.
2. Development of ascites may interfere with the exercise regimen.
3. Development of lower extremity lymphedema may interfere with the exercise regimen.
4. Individuals with chronic kidney disease are at high risk for cardiovascular disease.

Teaching Points

Correct Answer: 4

Individuals with chronic kidney disease (CKD) are at high risk for the development of cardiovascular disease. In fact, up to 70% of those with progressive kidney dysfunction die before reaching end-stage disease, primarily due to cardiovascular events. Due to the progressive nature of the disease, there is an almost universal reduction in physical activity. The goal of an exercise intervention in the early stages is to prevent individuals with CKD from becoming sedentary and to prevent physical deconditioning.

Incorrect Choices:

As compared to later stages of CKD, individuals with stage 1 to 2 renal failure have less risk of developing polyneuropathy, which can lead to falls and fractures. Falls and fractures would be more appropriate for disorders such as osteoporosis, neurologic conditions, and dementia. Ascites is the abnormal build-up of fluid within the abdomen, and it may interfere with exercise. The most common cause of ascites is liver disease (cirrhosis), although it may be seen in patients with CKD. However, in this scenario, the risk of an adverse cardiovascular event would be a higher priority concern than ascites. Chronic renal failure (and associated heart failure) may lead to edema of the lower extremities but not lymphedema. Lower extremity lymphedema often results from surgical removal of pelvic lymph nodes during a hysterectomy.

Type of Reasoning: Inductive

For this question, the test-taker must draw from knowledge of CKD and exercise regimens in order to draw a correct conclusion. This necessitates inductive reasoning skill, where clinical judgment is paramount to arriving at a correct conclusion. In this case, the therapist should consider that individuals with CKD are at high risk for cardiovascular disease. If answered incorrectly, review CKD information and exercise guidelines.

C163 

Nonsystem | Research

A researcher uses a group of volunteers (healthy college students) to study the effects of therapy ball exercises on ankle ROM and balance scores. Twenty volunteers participated in the 20-minute ball exercise class three times a week for 6 weeks. Measurements were taken at the beginning and end of the sessions. Significant differences were found in both sets of scores and reported at the local physical therapy meeting. What is the **MOST** accurate interpretation of this study and its results?

Choices:

1. The reliability of the study was threatened with the introduction of systematic error of measurement.
2. The Hawthorne effect may have influenced the outcomes of the study.
3. The validity of the study was threatened with the introduction of sampling bias.
4. Therapy ball exercises are an effective intervention to improve ankle stability after chronic ankle sprain.

Teaching Points

Correct Answer: 3

The investigator used a sample of convenience and therefore introduced systematic sampling error (a threat to validity). Random selection of subjects would improve the validity of this study.

Incorrect Choices:

Generalization to a group of patients with chronic ankle sprain cannot be made. There was no systematic error in measurement in this example. The Hawthorne effect refers to the influence that the subject's knowledge of participation in the experiment had on the results of the study.

Type of Reasoning: Inferential

The test-taker must determine what the most likely conclusion should be to this research study, given the protocol implemented. Questions that require one to draw conclusions based on evidence necessitate inferential reasoning skills to come to the correct conclusion. In this study, the validity has been threatened by convenience sampling. If this question was answered incorrectly, review guidelines to improve validity in research.

C164 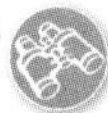

Cardiovascular/Pulmonary | Interventions

A patient was admitted with pneumonia and has significant pulmonary secretions. The patient's SpO_2 is 90% on room air. The patient also experiences claustrophobia. Which oxygen delivery equipment and parameters would be **BEST** to increase their SpO_2?

Choices:

1. Face mask at 40% FiO_2 (fraction of inspired oxygen).
2. Nasal cannula at 1L/minute.
3. Nonrebreather mask at 10L/minute.
4. Venturi mask with humidification at 40% FiO_2.

Teaching Points

Correct Answer: 4

The Venturi mask is open at the top, which will mitigate the patient's possible feelings of claustrophobia. The humidification will facilitate secretion mobility and clearance, thereby increasing the SpO_2.

Incorrect Choices:

The patient reports being claustrophobic, which indicates that they will not tolerate a face mask or nonrebreather. A nasal cannula will assist with decreasing the patient's feelings of claustrophobia, but 1L/minute is not adequate to improve the patient's gas exchange deficit.

Type of Reasoning: Inductive

For this question, the test-taker must weigh the oxygen delivery equipment options and determine which option will best increase the patient's SpO_2. This necessitates clinical judgment, which is an inductive reasoning skill. For this case, the therapist should select a Venturi mask to increase SpO_2. If answered incorrectly, review oxygen delivery equipment, especially the Venturi mask.

C165 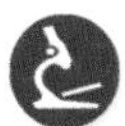

Musculoskeletal | Evaluation, Diagnosis

An adult competing in a community athletic event sustained a traumatic femoral neck fracture. What is a potential complication of this injury if it is not promptly identified and there is a subsequent delay in definitive treatment by an orthopedic surgeon?

Choices:

1. Hip dysplasia.
2. Legg-Calvé-Perthes disease.
3. Avascular necrosis of the femoral head.
4. Slipped capital femoral epiphysis.

Teaching Points

Correct Answer: 3

If confronted with a patient that has a suspected femoral neck fracture, timely diagnosis and intervention are critical. A fracture of the femoral neck may disrupt the medial and lateral femoral circumflex arteries, leading to avascular necrosis of the femoral head.

Incorrect Choices:

Hip dysplasia is a congenital disorder that results in abnormalities in the size, shape, and orientation of the femoral head, acetabulum, or both. Hip dysplasia increases the risk of hip subluxations or dislocation.

Legg-Calvé-Perthes disease may also result in disrupted blood supply to the femoral head, but this condition is idiopathic in nature versus the traumatic fracture described in the question stem. Legg-Calvé-Perthes disease is typically seen in males between the ages of 2–13 years. Slipped capital femoral epiphysis occurs when the femoral head "slips" and is displaced posteriorly and inferiorly in relation to the femoral neck. The disorder is seen most often in males aged 10–17 years and females aged 8–15 years. This condition may also result in avascular necrosis of the femoral head.

Type of Reasoning: Deductive

For this question, one must recall the potential complications of delayed treatment after a femoral neck fracture. This necessitates factual recall of guidelines, which necessitates deductive reasoning skill. For this case, a potential complication of delayed treatment is avascular necrosis of the femoral head. If answered incorrectly, review information on femur fractures and avascular necrosis.

C166 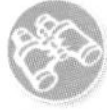

Nonsystem | Therapeutic Modalities

A therapist decides to use biofeedback to decrease the muscle tension associated with a suboccipital tension headache. What is the proper initial biofeedback protocol?

Choices:

1. Low-detection sensitivity with recording electrodes placed far apart.
2. High-detection sensitivity with recording electrodes placed closely together.
3. Low-detection sensitivity with recording electrodes placed closely together.
4. High-detection sensitivity with recording electrodes placed far apart.

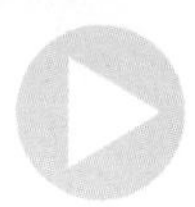

Teaching Points

Correct Answer: 3

By initially placing the electrodes close together, the therapist decreases the likelihood of detecting undesired motor units from adjacent active muscles (crosstalk). By setting the biofeedback sensitivity (gain) low, the therapist would decrease the amplitude of the signals generated by the hypertonic muscles and keep the EMG output from exceeding a visual and/or auditory range (scale).

Incorrect Choices:

The other choices fail to use optimal placing of electrodes (electrodes placed far apart) or sensitivity (high-detection) to optimize outcomes. The wider the spacing of electrodes, the more volume of the muscle is monitored. Thus, when targeting a specific muscle, a narrow spacing should be used. When the focus is not on a specific muscle but rather to encourage a general motion such as shoulder elevation, then a wider spacing of electrodes can be used. In addition, when working with weakness of a muscle in which there is a decreased ability to recruit motor units or there is a decrease in the size and number of motor units, then a wider spacing and a high sensitivity would be used in order to create an adequate visible signal.

Type of Reasoning: Inductive

One must utilize clinical judgment and diagnostic reasoning in order to determine the most appropriate initial biofeedback protocol. This requires knowledge of biofeedback guidelines and benefits of using high- versus low-detection sensitivity and electrodes placed either closely together or far apart. If this question was answered incorrectly, review biofeedback guidelines.

C167

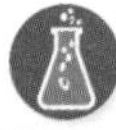

Neuromuscular | Evaluation, Diagnosis

Examination of a patient recovering from stroke reveals a loss of pain and temperature sensation on the left side of the face along with loss of pain and temperature sensation on the right side of the body. All other sensations are normal. What is the likely location of the lesion?

Choices:

1. Right cerebral cortex or internal capsule.
2. Midbrain.
3. Left cerebral cortex or internal capsule.
4. Left posterolateral medulla.

Teaching Points

Correct Answer: 4

A lesion in the posterolateral medulla causes mixed sensory loss (described in this case). Pain and temperature are affected, whereas discriminative touch and proprioception are not (the medial lemniscus is not involved).

Incorrect Choices:

Sensory loss will be completely contralateral (not mixed) only after the discriminative sensory tracts (fasciculus gracilis and fasciculus cuneatus) cross in the upper medulla. Patients with lesions above the medulla (midbrain, cortex, or internal capsule) will present with contralateral sensory loss.

Type of Reasoning: Analytical

This question requires the test-taker to determine the location of a lesion based on symptoms presented, which is an analytical reasoning skill. Knowledge of neuroscience and the discriminative sensory tracts is beneficial to arriving at the correct conclusion. If this question was answered incorrectly, refer to information regarding the discriminative sensory tracts and lesions.

C168 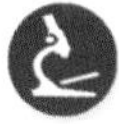

Neuromuscular | Evaluation, Diagnosis

A patient is taking the drug baclofen to control spasticity after a complete spinal cord injury at T10. This medication can be expected to decrease muscle tone and pain. What are the possible adverse effects of taking baclofen?

Choices:

1. Urinary retention and discomfort.
2. Drowsiness and muscle weakness.
3. Hypertension and palpitations.
4. Headache with visual auras.

Teaching Points

Correct Answer: 2

Baclofen, used in the management of spasticity, can produce CNS depression (drowsiness, fatigue, weakness, confusion, vertigo, dizziness, and insomnia), occurring in less than 10% of patients. Additional adverse effects can include hypotension and palpitations and urinary frequency. Vomiting, seizures, and coma are signs of overdosage.

Incorrect Choices:

Adverse effects include hypotension not hypertension. Headaches with visual auras are characteristic of migraines. Urinary frequency, not retention, is also an adverse effect.

Type of Reasoning: Deductive

One must recall the possible adverse effects of taking baclofen in order to arrive at the correct conclusion. This requires knowledge of guidelines and factual information, which is a deductive reasoning skill. If this question was answered incorrectly, refer to therapeutic uses of baclofen, including adverse effects.

C169 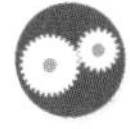

Musculoskeletal / Examination

A teen-aged female distance runner presents a history of stress fractures and general leg pain. Her parents think it may be due to overtraining. Based on this subjective information, what should the physical therapist question the patient about next?

Choices:

1. Recent growth spurts.
2. Menses and eating habits.
3. Type of running shoe.
4. Participation in other sports.

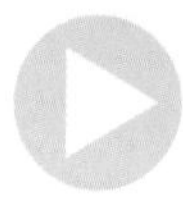

Teaching Points

Correct Answer: 2

The female athlete triad is a syndrome common in females 14–20 years of age that consists of three related conditions: disordered eating habits, irregular or absent menstrual periods, and osteopenia (thinning of the bone density). It is imperative that the therapist inquire about menses and eating habits as they are two of the three hallmark signs of the female athlete triad. It would also be helpful for the physical therapist to inquire more about muscle pain, medications, and details of training regimen.

Incorrect Choices:

Recent growth spurts, participation in other sports, and type of shoes will not rule in/out the possibility of the runner having this serious condition.

Type of Reasoning: Evaluative

In this question, the therapist must determine the **BEST** course of questioning to determine the patient's likelihood of female athlete triad. This requires evaluative reasoning skill. If answered incorrectly, review symptoms and examination of female athlete triad.

C170

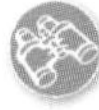

Cardiovascular/Pulmonary | Interventions

A patient with systemic lupus erythematosus (SLE) and pulmonary artery hypertension has started pulmonary rehabilitation. What is the **BEST** exercise program to improve the patient's function?

Choices:

1. Treadmill training continuously for 30 minutes.
2. Combination of interval treadmill training and large muscle group strength resistance training.
3. Interval training for 10 minutes daily.
4. Resistance endurance training for large muscle groups.

Teaching Points

Correct Answer: 2

Interval training permits the patient to work at higher levels of their aerobic capacity, which leads to greater gains in exercise capacity. The pathophysiology of pulmonary artery hypertension leads to proximal muscle weakness. Strengthening these muscles decreases the workload with functional activities.

Incorrect Choices:

The combination of aerobic and resisted training yields greater results than one method of training alone. Interval training leads to greater gains in aerobic capacity than continuous training.

Type of Reasoning: Inductive

This question requires one to utilize clinical judgment in order to determine the best exercise program for a patient with SLE and pulmonary artery hypertension. This necessitates inductive reasoning skills where clinical judgment is paramount to arriving at a correct conclusion. For this case, the BEST exercise program is a combination of interval treadmill training and large muscle group strength resistance training. If answered incorrectly, review exercise guidelines for patients with pulmonary artery hypertension.

C171 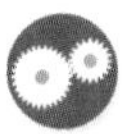

Systems Interaction | Evaluation, Diagnosis

A physical therapist examines a 60-year-old patient whose chief complaint is 1 month of rib pain with an insidious onset. There are no specific factors that aggravate or ease the rib pain. Recent medical history includes progressive fatigue and weight loss of about 10 pounds over the past 2 weeks. On examination, the therapist notes point tenderness with palpation directly over the lower ribs, but the intercostal spaces and thoracic spine are nontender. The therapist is unable to reproduce the patient's symptoms with any type of trunk movements or functional activities, and the neurologic examination is normal. In this situation, what should the therapist do?

Choices:

1. Treat the patient with cryotherapy for pain relief and instruct the patient in core stabilization exercises.
2. Contact the primary care physician and recommend further evaluation.
3. Instruct the patient to go home for a trial of bed rest and NSAIDs as needed for pain, and return to the physical therapy clinic in 72 hours.
4. Recommend an x-ray to rule out a possible rib or thoracic spine fracture.

Teaching Points

Correct Answer: 2

The insidious onset of rib pain combined with the recent history of progressive fatigue and unexplained weight loss are concerning and suggestive of systemic disease. The clinical presentation described here is consistent with multiple myeloma, a type of cancer caused by uncontrolled growth of plasma cells in the bone marrow. Common signs and symptoms of multiple myeloma include anemia with weakness and fatigue, skeletal/bone pain (especially in the spine, pelvis, and ribs), osteoporosis, and kidney stones. The disease is seen most often in persons between the ages of 50 and 70 years, and it is most common in men and African Americans.

Incorrect Choices:

Choices including cryotherapy, bed rest, and NSAIDs suggest that the problem is musculoskeletal in nature and the patient should respond to conservative physical therapy intervention. These are poor choices because there is no well-defined musculoskeletal problem in the question stem, which clearly describes some type of illness or systemic disorder. An x-ray to rule out a possible thoracic spine or rib fracture is not helpful. If the patient did indeed have a thoracic vertebra or rib fracture, the therapist would have been able to provoke the pain with trunk movements and functional activities.

Type of Reasoning: Evaluative

This question provides a series of options to select from and the test-taker must weigh the merits of each approach. Questions of this nature often necessitate evaluative reasoning skill, where instincts help to guide clinical thinking and reasoning. For this case, based on the patient's symptoms, the therapist should contact the primary care physician and recommend further evaluation. If answered incorrectly, review symptoms of multiple myeloma.

C172 

System Interactions | Evaluation, Diagnosis

An elderly male patient recovering from a fractured hip repaired with ORIF has recently been discharged home. During a home visit, his wife tells the therapist that he woke up yesterday morning and told her he couldn't remember much. Upon examination, the therapist finds some mild motor loss in his right hand and anomia. The therapist affirms the presence of short-term memory loss. What is the therapist's **BEST** course of action?

Choices:

1. Advise the family to document and record any new problems that they notice over the next week and then report back to the therapist.
2. Ignore the findings because they are expected after surgical anesthesia.
3. Refer him to his physician immediately because the therapist suspects a stroke.
4. Refer him to his physician because the therapist suspects Alzheimer's type dementia.

Teaching Points

Correct Answer: 3

The presence of focal signs (incoordination, anomia) with cognitive signs (memory loss) is indicative of impaired brain function and may be the result of small strokes. This is the most likely choice given the spotty symptoms he presents with as well as their sudden onset.

Incorrect Choices:

Senile dementia, Alzheimer's type, can include some of the same symptoms but the onset is gradual and the course is typically slowly progressive. The reporting of these findings to the primary physician should not be delayed. Further diagnostic workup is indicated. Hospital admission and anesthesia can cause temporary cognitive difficulties (delirium), but these should not persist with discharge home.

Type of Reasoning: Evaluative

In this question, the test-taker must determine the **BEST** course of action, given the nature of the patient's new symptoms. This requires evaluative reasoning skill, in which one evaluates the merits of each possible course of action in order to arrive at the correct conclusion. If this question was answered incorrectly, review symptoms of transient ischemic attack and stroke.

C173 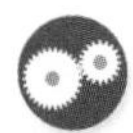

Metabolic/Endocrine | Interventions

An adolescent with a 4-year history of type 1 diabetes is insulin dependent and wants to participate in cross-country running. The PT working with the school team advises the athlete to measure plasma glucose concentrations before and after running. What additional advice should the therapist give this student athlete?

Choices:

1. Increase insulin dosage immediately before running.
2. Consume a carbohydrate before or during practice to avoid hypoglycemia.
3. Avoid carbohydrate-rich snacks within 12 hours of a race.
4. Consume a carbohydrate after practice to avoid hyperglycemia.

Teaching Points

Correct Answer: 2

During exercise of increasing intensity and duration, plasma concentrations of insulin progressively decrease. Exercise-induced hypoglycemia (abnormally low levels of glucose in the blood) is common for exercising athletes with diabetes. Hypoglycemia associated with exercise can occur up to 48 hours after exercise. To counteract these effects, the individual may need to reduce his insulin dosage or increase carbohydrate intake before or after running. Consuming a carbohydrate product before or during the race will have a preventive modulating effect on hypoglycemia.

Incorrect Choices:

Hyperglycemia (abnormally high levels of glucose in the blood) is more a risk for individuals with uncontrolled type 1 diabetes. These patients should demonstrate glycemic control before starting an exercise program. Consuming carbohydrates will not lessen the likelihood of hyperglycemia.

Type of Reasoning: Evaluative

One must evaluate the merits of each of the four possible courses of action in order to arrive at the correct solution. This requires knowledge of the effects of exercise on glucose concentrations in athletes with diabetes. Through evaluative reasoning, one should conclude that the athlete should consume a carbohydrate snack before or during practice or a race to avoid hypoglycemia. If this question was answered incorrectly, review guidelines for exercise with athletes with diabetes and carbohydrate consumption.

C174 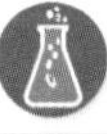

Genitourinary | Evaluation, Diagnosis

A male patient is referred to outpatient physical therapy for lower back pain. During the patient interview, he describes a recent increased difficulty with urinating that does not affect his lower back pain symptoms. Neurological screening examination is normal and Murphy's sign is negative. Based on this clinical scenario, what is the MOST likely location of a lesion?

Choices:

1. Lower urinary tract.
2. First lumbar nerve root.
3. Kidney.
4. Sacro-iliac joint.

Teaching Points

Correct Answer: 1

The lower urinary tract can refer symptoms to the lumbar spine region, and the recent report of increased difficulty with urination is a key factor.

Incorrect Choices:

A negative Murphy's sign (percussion in the costovertebral area) decreases the likelihood of kidney symptoms. There was no information provided to specifically indicate the sacro-iliac joint as a source of current symptoms; moreover, the recent reports of increased difficulty with urination may indicate a potential systemic problem that may require immediate medical attention. Negative neurological findings would rule out the first lumbar nerve root as a source of symptoms.

Type of Reasoning: Analytical

This question requires the tester to critically evaluate key findings from the patient interview and determine the most likely differential diagnosis based on the information provided. This requires analytical reasoning skill, where symptoms are analyzed to draw reasonable conclusions about the diagnosis. For this scenario, the symptoms are consistent with the lower urinary tract. Review signs and symptoms of lower urinary tract problems if answered incorrectly.

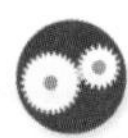

C175

Neuromuscular I Interventions

A patient with a C7 spinal cord injury was transferred from supine on a treatment table to sitting in a wheelchair and is waiting for transportation home. The patient starts to demonstrate symptoms consistent with autonomic dysreflexia. What is the **BEST** action the physical therapist should take in this situation?

Choices:

1. Empty the urine collection bag and ensure the catheter is not blocked.
2. Transfer the patient back to a supine position on the treatment table.
3. Transfer the patient to sidelying position on the treatment table.
4. Check for open wounds on the patient's head, neck, and shoulders.

Teaching Points

Correct Answer: 1

Having the patient maintain an upright position, loosening tight clothing, and ensuring the urine collection bag is empty/unblocked are key steps to resolving autonomic dysreflexia. The therapist should also immediately signal the emergency to the medial staff if it occurs in a hospital or call 911 if the patient is in an outpatient setting.

Incorrect Choices:

Patients who present with symptoms of autonomic dysreflexia should not be put in a supine or sidelying position as this only contributes to increased fluid return and elevated blood pressure. Placing the patient upright is indicated as this position will allow blood to pool in the extremities and hopefully assist with lowering blood pressure. Open wounds may trigger autonomic dysreflexia but are typically seen with wounds/injuries below the T6–T10 level (e.g., ingrown toenails, sacral pressure ulcer).

Type of Reasoning: Evaluative

For this question, the test-taker must weigh the potential courses of action presented and determine which action will best remedy the symptoms of autonomic dysreflexia. This requires evaluative reasoning skill. For this case, the therapist should empty the urine collection bag and ensure the catheter is not blocked. If answered incorrectly, review action steps for remedying autonomic dysreflexia.

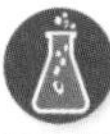

C176

Musculoskeletal I Examination

A therapist is reviewing x-rays from a patient with a trimalleolar fracture. What are the **BEST** radiographic views to visualize this bony fracture?

Choices:

1. Oblique and lateral.
2. Anteroposterior and lateral.
3. Posteroanterior and lateral.
4. Lateral and coronal.

Teaching Points

Correct Answer: 2

A trimalleolar fracture includes fracture of both malleoli and the posterior rim of the tibia. Anteroposterior (AP) view of the ankle demonstrates the distal tibia and fibula, including the medial and lateral malleoli and the head of the talus. The fractures of both malleoli will be visible with this view. The lateral view provides evidence of the fracture at the posterior rim of the distal tibia.

Incorrect Choices:

An oblique view of the foot demonstrates the phalanges, the metatarsals, and the intermetatarsal joints. Posteroanterior (PA) view is not routine for the ankle. A coronal view is also not indicated for this type of fracture.

Type of Reasoning: Analytical

One must recall the nature of a trimalleolar fracture in order to make a determination of the **BEST** radiographic view for observation of this anomaly. This necessitates analytical reasoning skill, in which one must interpret the information presented in order to make a determination of a **BEST** course of action. If this question was answered incorrectly, review radiographic examination guidelines for trimalleolar fractures.

C177 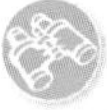

Nonsystem | Therapeutic Modalities

A patient presents with pain and muscle spasm of the upper back (C7–T8) extending to the lateral border of the scapula. This encompasses a 10 × 10–cm area on both sides of the spine. If the US unit only has a 5-cm^2 sound head, how should the therapist treat the upper back area?

Choices:

1. Each side, allotting 5 minutes for each section.
2. The entire area in 5 minutes.
3. The entire area in 10 minutes.
4. Each side, allotting 2.5 minutes for each section.

Teaching Points

Correct Answer: 1

The total treatment area is too large for the 5-cm^2 sound head to produce adequate tissue heating. Sonating the two areas independently will allow more time for the tissue temperature to rise during the treatment time in each area.

Incorrect Choices:

Moving the transducer too fast to cover both sides adequately in the allotted time does not allow sufficient time for the acoustic energy to produce heat because the head is not in a given area long enough. Increasing the treatment time will not affect the rate of heat production. Two minutes is too brief to produce sufficient tissue heating.

Type of Reasoning: Inductive

This question requires clinical judgment and diagnostic reasoning in order to determine the best approach when providing US treatment for this patient. This requires recall of proper US treatment guidelines, including consideration of the size of the sound head and size of the area to be treated. If this question was answered incorrectly, review US treatment guidelines for larger treatment areas.

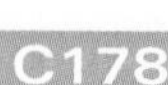
C178

Musculoskeletal | Examination

An adult patient is referred to physical therapy with knee pain after falling from a ladder. The patient is seen the day after the injury and is unable to articulate the exact mechanism of injury. The knee is swollen and the patient's gait is antalgic. The therapist is concerned about an undiagnosed fracture. What physical examination finding would indicate a need for knee radiographs?

Choices:

1. Inability to flex the knee to 90°.
2. Joint line tenderness.
3. Inability to fully extend the knee.
4. Positive anterior drawer test.

Teaching Points

Correct Answer: 1

The Ottawa Knee Rules (see Box 2-10) were developed to provide clinicians with guidelines for determining when to order an x-ray following a knee injury. The inability to flex the knee to 90° is one of the clinical examination criteria. The Ottawa Knee Rules accurately rule out a fracture after acute knee injury. Clinicians are advised to order knee radiographs with one or more positive findings.

Incorrect Choices:

Joint line tenderness is not a sensitive finding for knee fractures. Joint line tenderness is most frequently used to aid in the diagnosis of meniscal tears. An inability to fully extend the knee is an important clinical finding, but not one of the variables in the Ottawa Knee Rules. A positive anterior drawer test indicates an ACL injury.

Type of Reasoning: Deductive

For this question, the test-taker must draw from factual recall of the Ottawa Knee Rules to guide clinical decision-making about when to order knee radiographs. This necessitates recall of factual guidelines, which is a deductive reasoning skill. For this situation, finding an inability to flex the knee to 90° would indicate a need for radiographs. Refer to the Ottawa Knee Rules if answered incorrectly.

C179
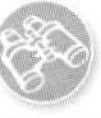

Neuromuscular | Interventions

A patient with Parkinson's disease (Hoehn & Yahr disease Stage 3) is referred to physical therapy secondary to recent difficulty with bed mobility and supine to sidelying transfers. Which of the following interventions is most appropriate for this patient?

Choices:

1. Rapid head flexion/rotation and bilateral symmetrical upper extremity rocking in supine.
2. Slow and controlled bridging exercises.
3. Bilateral end range upper extremity D2 flexion PNF patterns in supine.
4. Pelvic tilts while sitting on a therapy ball.

Teaching Points

Correct Answer: 1

The patient has progressive (Hoehn & Yahr disease Stage 3) Parkinson's disease (PD) resulting in bradykinesia with various movements, to include bed mobility and rolling. Rapid and large amplitude movements (BIG training) are fundamental exercise principles to initiate movement for patients with PD. Additionally, head flexion/rotation is the first step to initiate rolling. Finally, bilateral symmetrical upper extremity rocking allows individuals to rapidly thrust the arms toward the desire side with trunk and lower extremities following.

Incorrect Choices:

Bridging is an excellent exercise to assist with bed mobility, but slow movements often impede initiation or result in decreased ability to fully execute the required task for patients with Parkinson's disease. Bilateral end range upper extremity D2 flexion PNF patterns are helpful to facilitate postural stability and upright posture in sitting or standing, but do not assist bed mobility. Pelvic tilts while sitting on a therapy ball are helpful for sitting balance but lack specificity for improving rolling and bed mobility.

Type of Reasoning: Inductive

For this question, one must utilize clinical judgment to determine a best course of action for a patient with Parkinson's disease. This necessitates inductive reasoning skill, where clinical knowledge is applied to draw reasonable conclusions. For this situation, rapid head flexion/rotation and bilateral symmetrical upper extremity rocking in supine are best to address the patient's current challenges with bed mobility and rolling. Review intervention approaches for PD, especially bed mobility activities.

C180 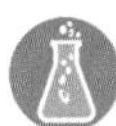

Neuromuscular | Examination

A patient presents with severe, frequent seizures originating in the medial temporal lobes. After bilateral surgical removal of these areas, the patient is unable to remember any new information from just prior to the surgery to the present. The patient cannot recall text read minutes ago or remember people previously met. How should this surgical outcome be characterized?

Choices:

1. Loss of integration of the temporal lobe with the basal ganglia and frontal cortex.
2. Loss of procedural memory and integration with frontal cortex.
3. Loss of the hippocampus and declarative memory function.
4. A primary deficit from the loss of the amygdala.

Teaching Points

Correct Answer: 3

Declarative memory refers to conscious, explicit, or cognitive memory. It is a function of the cerebral cortex and the hippocampus, which is located in the medial part of the temporal lobe.

Incorrect Choices:

Procedural memory (unconscious memory or implicit memory) refers to the recall of skills and habits and emotional responses. It is the result of integrated action of the frontal cortex (neocortex), thalamus, and striatum of the basal ganglia. The amygdala is a collection of nuclei in the anteromedial temporal lobe, forming the core of the limbic circuits. It is important for triggering feelings and drive-related behaviors.

Type of Reasoning: Analytical

This question requires the test-taker to determine the diagnosis based on symptoms presented, which is an analytical reasoning skill. In this situation, the symptoms are indicative of loss of the hippocampus and declarative memory function. Knowledge of neuroscience and the cortical structures responsible for declarative memory function are beneficial to arriving at the correct conclusion. If this question was answered incorrectly, refer to memory functions and structures.

C181 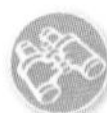

Metabolic/Endocrine I Evaluation, Diagnosis

A 14-year-old with a body mass index of 33 kg/m^2 and a history of limited participation in physical activities is referred for exercise training. The nutritionist has prescribed a diet limiting his caloric intake. What is the **BEST** initial exercise prescription for this patient?

Choices:

1. Three weekly sessions of 60 minutes at 50% VO_{2max}.
2. Three weekly sessions of 50 minutes at 75%–85% VO_{2max}.
3. Three weekly sessions of 30 minutes at 65%–70% VO_{2max}.
4. Two daily sessions of 30 minutes at 45%–70% VO_{2max}.

Teaching Points

Correct Answer: 4

This individual is obese (body mass index ≥30 kg/m^2) and will benefit from exercise to increase energy expenditure and diet to reduce caloric intake. The initial exercise prescription should utilize low-intensity with longer duration exercise. Splitting the training into two sessions each day is a good choice. The goal is to work toward bringing the target HR into a suitable range. Obese individuals are at increased risk of orthopedic injuries and require close monitoring.

Incorrect Choices:

Weekly sessions at high intensities (70%–85% VO_2max) and long duration (50 min) are contraindicated. Weekly sessions (two to three times/wk) are not as beneficial initially as are daily sessions at shorter durations and moderate intensities.

Type of Reasoning: Inductive

One must utilize clinical judgment and diagnostic reasoning to determine the **BEST** initial exercise prescription for this individual. This necessitates inductive reasoning skill, in which one must refer to knowledge of exercise for individuals with obesity to arrive at the correct conclusion. If this question was answered incorrectly, review exercise prescription guidelines for the obese.

C182 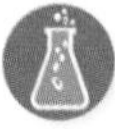

Metabolic/Endocrine I Evaluation, Diagnosis

A patient is admitted to a hospital after a fall. A review of the patient's medical chart reveals a blood pressure (BP) of 160/85, a triglyceride level of 160 mg/dL, and a fasting blood glucose level of 115 mg/dL. Weight is 310 lb. Examination of the patient reveals a rotund man with a 54-inch waistline. Which diagnosis is consistent with this patient's signs and symptoms?

Choices:

1. Type 1 diabetes.
2. Cushing's syndrome.
3. Metabolic syndrome.
4. Chronic heart disease.

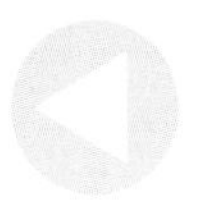

Teaching Points

Correct Answer: 3

This patient is exhibiting four of the risk factors of metabolic syndrome (diagnosis is made if three or more are present). Risk factors include (1) abdominal obesity: waist circumference >40 inches in men or >35 inches in women; (2) elevated triglycerides: triglyceride level of 150 mg/dL or higher; (3) low high-density lipoprotein (HDL) cholesterol or being on medicine to treat low HDL: HDL level <40 mg/dL in men or 50 mg/dL in women; (4) elevated BP: systolic BP ≥130 mmHg and/or diastolic BP = 85 mmHg; and (5) fasting plasma glucose level >100 mg/dL. The therapist's plan of care should be reflective of the patient's increased risk for heart disease, stroke, and diabetes and should assist the patient in lifestyle changes that reduce these risk factors.

Incorrect Choices:

No mention is made of absolute insulin deficiency (type 1 diabetes). Although these are risk factors for heart disease, they do not specifically define or characterize chronic heart disease. Cushing's syndrome (glucocorticoid hormone excess) refers to the manifestations of hypercortisolism from any cause. Patients typically exhibit a round "moon face" with a protruding abdomen or "buffalo hump" on the back along with muscle weakness and wasting.

Type of Reasoning: Analytical

This question requires one to analyze all of the signs and symptoms presented and then draw a conclusion about a potential diagnosis. Questions of this nature require analytical reasoning skills. If this question was answered incorrectly, refer to signs and symptoms of metabolic syndrome.

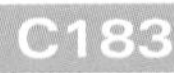

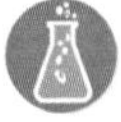

System Interactions | Evaluation, Diagnosis

A patient in an exercise class develops muscle weakness and fatigue. Examination reveals leg cramps and hyporeflexia. The patient also experiences frequent episodes of postural hypotension and dizziness. Abnormalities on the ECG include a flat T wave, prolonged QT interval, and depressed ST segment. Which electrolyte imbalance is consistent with this patient's signs and symptoms?

Choices:

1. Hypocalcemia.
2. Hyperkalemia.
3. Hypokalemia.
4. Hyponatremia.

Teaching Points

Correct Answer: 3

Hypokalemia, decreased potassium in the blood, is characterized by these signs and symptoms. Other possible symptoms include respiratory distress, irritability, confusion or depression, and gastrointestinal disturbances.

Incorrect Choices:

Hyperkalemia is excess potassium in the blood. Hyponatremia is decreased sodium in the blood, and hypocalcemia is decreased calcium in the blood. These conditions cannot produce this battery of symptoms.

Type of Reasoning: Analytical

This question requires the test-taker to determine the diagnosis based on the symptoms described, which is an analytical reasoning skill. The test-taker must analyze the symptoms in order to determine the most likely cause for them. If this question was answered incorrectly, refer to signs and symptoms of the conditions listed (Chapter 8).

C184 

Lymphatic | Examination

A patient has diffuse distal bilateral lower extremity pain, edema, and numbness that occurs with level and uphill walking. Which of the following examination items would be most likely to assist in the proper diagnosis?

Choices:
1. Ankle-brachial index (ABI).
2. Lumbar quadrant test.
3. Stemmer's sign.
4. Monofilament testing.

Teaching Points

Correct Answer: 1

This question describes a case of suspected peripheral arterial disease. The ABI is helpful to determine the arterial patency or sufficiency. A value of 1.0 indicates normal arterial flow; values between 0.5 and 0.8 indicate moderate compromise while values below 0.5 indicate severe compromise of arterial flow.

Incorrect Choices:

Lumbar quadrant test is used to detect lumbar spinal stenosis and radiculopathy. Stemmer's sign is helpful for identifying lymphedema. Monofilament test is used to identify polyneuropathy and sensory loss.

Type of Reasoning: Analytical

One must understand the tests described in the question in order to choose the correct one. Through analytical reasoning, the test-taker must determine how each test is performed and for what purpose. If this question was answered incorrectly, review information on special tests.

C185 

Genitourinary | Interventions

A patient is referred to a woman's health specialist PT with a diagnosis of pelvic pain and uterine prolapse. Which of the following interventions is the **BEST** choice for this patient?

Choices:
1. External stabilization with a support belt.
2. Gentle abdominal exercises with incisional support.
3. Protective splinting of abdominal musculature.
4. Kegel exercises.

Teaching Points

Correct Answer: 4

Intervention should focus on pelvic floor rehabilitation (Kegel exercises to strengthen pubococcygeal muscles) along with postural education and muscle reeducation.

Incorrect Choices:

External stabilization with a support belt may be required for sacroiliac dysfunction. Diastasis recti abdominis requires protective splinting of abdominal musculature during initial separation (>2 cm split of the rectus abdominis after pregnancy). Postcesarean interventions include gentle abdominal exercises with incisional support. There was no mention of pregnancy or postpregnancy complications.

Type of Reasoning: Inferential

One must infer or draw a reasonable conclusion about the best intervention approach for a patient with pelvic pain and uterine prolapse. This requires inferential reasoning skills because one must determine which therapeutic approach will have the most effective outcome of improving function. If this question was answered incorrectly, review exercise guidelines for patients with uterine prolapse.

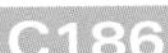

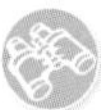

Lymphatic | Examination

A client walks into a private physical therapy practice with a chief complaint of a possible ankle sprain. The physical therapist observes a foot and ankle which is swollen, erythematous, and warm. As part of the systems review, the therapist assesses the lymphatic system and detects a positive Stemmer's sign. What other lymphatic system test or measure should also be performed?

Choices:

1. Calf palpation and use of Wells Criteria Score.
2. Ankle brachial index (ABI) testing for the involved lower extremity.
3. Observation of proximal red streaks and palpation of inguinal nodes.
4. Application of Ottawa Ankle rules including assessment of pain above the malleoli and ability to weight-bear.

Teaching Points

Correct Answer: 3

The client presents with a swollen, red, and warm foot and ankle. The therapist should perform a systems review including the lymphatic system. Stemmer's sign was positive indicating some form of lymphatic involvement. Based on the presenting symptoms, cellulitis is a possibility. Observation for red streaks emanating from the foot and ankle is a characteristic sign of a spreading infection. Often, streptococcus or staphylococcus are the culprits. Enlarged or painful inguinal lymph nodes in the groin are another sign of possible infection and even lymphangitis. This individual needs additional medical care. An ankle sprain is unlikely.

Incorrect Choices:

ABI is used to assess peripheral arterial disorders. Wells Criteria help determine the presence of deep venous thrombosis. Both are tests of the vascular system, not the lymphatic system. Ottawa Ankle rules are indeed used for examination of the ankle and to rule in possible fracture. These rules apply to the musculoskeletal system review. The client walked into the clinic. In that case, it is unlikely that these rules would be applied since weight-bearing was evident.

Type of Reasoning: Inductive

For this question, one must determine the test that is best to perform after learning of a patient's positive Stemmer's sign. The test-taker must recall the indications of the Stemmer's sign and then use knowledge of other tests or measures that are performed to fully understand the patient's condition. This necessitates clinical judgment, which is an inductive reasoning skill. For this scenario, the therapist should observe the proximal red streaks and palpate the inguinal nodes. If answered incorrectly, review information on evaluation of the lymphatic system and Stemmer's sign.

C187 

Neuromuscular I Interventions

A patient has a 10-year history of Parkinson's disease and has been on levodopa (Carbidopa) for the past 6 years. The patient has fallen three times in the past month, resulting in a Colles' fracture. The therapist decides to try postural biofeedback training using a platform balance training device. Which of the following is the **BEST** choice for a training protocol?

Choices:

1. Increase the limits of stability and improve anterior weight displacement.
2. Decrease the limits of stability and anterior weight displacement.
3. Increase the limits of stability and improve center of pressure alignment.
4. Decrease the limits of stability and improve posterior weight displacement.

Teaching Points

Correct Answer: 3

The patient with Parkinson's disease exhibits significant balance impairments including loss of postural reflexes; decreased limits of stability; flexed, stooped posture that alters the center of pressure in an anterior direction; freezing; and orthostatic hypotension. Platform balance training should work toward improving the limits of stability and center of pressure alignment (the patient should focus on reducing anterior displacement).

Incorrect Choices:

The patient is too unstable; decreasing limits of stability is contraindicated, as is promoting anterior weight displacement.

Type of Reasoning: Inferential

One must infer the most appropriate training sequence for biofeedback postural training in order to arrive at the correct conclusion. This involves inferential reasoning, in which one must consider the patient's diagnosis and current limitations in order to choose the most appropriate training sequence. If this question was answered incorrectly, refer to balance deficits and training strategies for patients with Parkinson's disease.

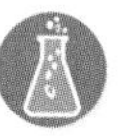

C188

Gastrointestinal | Evaluation, Diagnosis

A physical therapist is working on reconditioning a 31-year-old female admitted to the hospital for acute alcoholic hepatitis and is currently going through detoxification. As the therapist starts to work with the patient, she appears to be pregnant and is short of breath. Her abdomen is distended and tense. She denies any abdominal pain. The therapist checks her lab work and notes that her urine hCG (pregnancy test) is negative. Based on the patient's history, what is the most likely cause of her distended abdomen?

Choices:

1. Ascites.
2. Cholecystitis.
3. Acute pancreatitis
4. Opiate-induced constipation.

Teaching Points

Correct Answer: 1

This patient is in fulminant liver failure due to alcoholic hepatitis. She has developed ascites, which is fluid accumulation in the abdomen. Patients will not often complain of pain, usually more discomfort, and often complain of shortness of breath given the extra pressure put on the diaphragm. Fluid can also accumulate in the lungs (pleural effusion), also causing shortness of breath.

Incorrect Choices:

Some patients with alcoholic hepatitis and acute liver failure are at higher risk for gallstones and cholecystitis. This patient is not complaining of abdominal pain. The same goes for acute pancreatitis as this patient has a very high risk for pancreatitis given her alcoholism, although in this case, she has no signs or symptoms of pancreatitis, which would always include severe abdominal pain. Constipation, which can sometimes cause bloating, would not cause a tense, distended abdomen. This patient is also unlikely to be given opiates in the hospital as she has no pain and because of her history of substance abuse. Opiates would not be a first line analgesic in this case.

Type of Reasoning: Analytical

For this question, the test-taker is given a group of symptoms, and the most likely diagnosis must be determined. Questions of this nature often necessitate analytical reasoning skill, where pieces of information are analyzed to draw reasonable conclusions. For this scenario, the symptoms are most likely consistent with ascites. If answered incorrectly, review signs and symptoms of ascites.

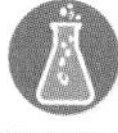

C189

Musculoskeletal | Evaluation, Diagnosis

A female patient complains of right lumbosacral pain after giving natural childbirth to her first child 2 months ago. Pain has subsided somewhat, but remains high enough that she has to sit after walking more than 2 blocks. Pain is noted in the right lumbosacral region, buttock, and groin and is aggravated with weight-bearing on the right. Active flexion, extension, and side bending reproduce the patient's symptoms. Hamstrings are slightly tight on the right, but no neural tension is noted. Neurological findings (reflexes, sensation, and motor) are unremarkable. SI provocation tests are positive. What is the **MOST** likely diagnosis for this patient?

Choices:

1. Lumbar disc protrusion at L5/S1.
2. Sacroiliac sprain.
3. Quadratus lumborum strain.
4. Piriformis syndrome.

Teaching Points

Correct Answer: 2

Child-bearing can place considerable stress on the sacroiliac joint, causing an overstretch of the ligaments. Pain is reproduced with active movement testing, which is characteristic of a musculoskeletal condition. Sacroiliac provocation tests are fairly valid as well, thus implicating the sacroiliac joint. The groin and buttock are common referral regions for the sacroiliac joint.

Incorrect Choices:

There is no neural tension or neurological signs that help to rule out disc dysfunction. There are no findings indicating specific strain of the piriformis or quadratus lumborum as SI provocation is positive.

Type of Reasoning: Analytical

For this question, the test-taker must analyze the symptoms present and determine the most likely diagnosis. Questions of this nature often require analytical reasoning skill. For this scenario, given the symptoms presented, the most likely diagnosis is sacroiliac sprain. If answered incorrectly, review signs and symptoms of sacroiliac sprain/strain.

C190 

Musculoskeletal | Interventions

A patient presents to physical therapy with a complaint of neck pain which limits their ability to look over the left shoulder. The therapist performs accessory mobilizations to improve motion at the C5-6 level. Which technique would MOST likely improve left cervical rotation in this scenario?

Choices:

1. Left posterior to anterior glide of C1 lateral mass in prone.
2. Posterior to anterior glide of right C5-6 facet joint in prone.
3. Posterior to anterior glide of left C5-6 facet joint in prone.
4. Right to left side glide of C5-6 joint in supine.

Teaching Points

Correct Answer: 3

A posterior to anterior (P-A) glide of the left C5-6 facet joint will facilitate closing of that segment, which is required for the physiologic movements of left rotation, left side-bending and extension.

Incorrect Choices:

Mobilization of C1 would be appropriate for a patient with upper cervical spine dysfunction and is unlikely to be related to the rotation restriction seen in this patient. A P-A glide of the right C5-6 facet joint will facilitate closing of that segment, which is required for right rotation, side-bending, and rotation. Right to left side glide mobilizations would facilitate right rotation and right side-bending.

Type of Reasoning: Inferential

For this question, one must infer or determine what is likely to be true of a clinical situation. Questions that ask one to predict an outcome often require inferential reasoning skill. For this scenario, posterior to anterior glide of left C5-6 facet joint in prone will most likely improve the patient's left cervical rotation. If answered incorrectly, review joint mobilization guidelines, especially cervical mobilization.

C191 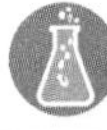

Musculoskeletal | Evaluation, Diagnosis

An elderly woman with a 15-year history of rheumatoid arthritis (RA) is seen in a physical therapy clinic. The patient is currently being treated with gold and methotrexate. Four months ago the patient had a total hip replacement and, after 10 weeks of rehabilitation, she was walking unassisted with a cane and was discharged from a home health program. Over the past several weeks she's experienced progressive, intermittent gait disturbances. During the examination, the therapist notes an ataxic gait, shortened steps, and trunk instability. Deep tendon reflexes were diminished and muscle tone was increased in both lower extremities. Hoffman's sign was positive for both upper extremities. What is the most likely explanation for these findings in a patient with a history of RA?

Choices:

1. Cerebellar disease.
2. Drug-induced muscle weakness.
3. Cervical myelopathy.
4. Peripheral polyneuropathy.

Teaching Points

Correct Answer: 3

The examination findings are consistent with a cervical myelopathy. The destructive inflammatory process of RA can damage periarticular tissues such as the transverse and alar ligaments that stabilize the upper cervical spine. Dislocation of the atlantoaxial joint can result in the odontoid process compressing the upper cervical spinal cord, producing intermittent or persistent neurologic symptoms.

Incorrect Choices:

Cerebellar disease is not associated with RA and would not lead to diminished reflexes or upper motor neuron signs (positive Hoffman's). Prolonged drug therapy can lead to toxic side effects such as muscle weakness or a polyneuropathy, but neither would explain the cluster of findings described in the question stem.

Type of Reasoning: Analytical

For this question, the test-taker must analyze the symptoms presented and determine the likely explanation for the symptoms. This requires analytical reasoning skill, where pieces are weighed in order to draw reasonable conclusions. For this situation, the most likely explanation for the findings is cervical myelopathy. Review information on cervical myelopathy if answered incorrectly.

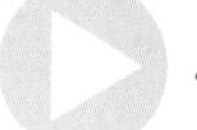

C192 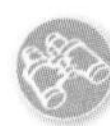

Nonsystem | Therapeutic Modalities

A patient with a traumatic brain injury presents with hemiparesis. The examination reveals slight cutaneous and proprioceptive impairment, poor (2/5) strength of the shoulder muscles and triceps, and spasticity of the biceps. Voluntary control of the patient's left arm has not progressed since admission. The therapist decides to use functional electrical stimulation (FES), placing the active electrode on the triceps to facilitate active extension of the elbow. Which of the following is the BEST choice of timing sequence for FES in this case?

Choices:

1. No ramp up, 8-second stimulation, 2-second ramp down.
2. 1-second ramp up, 9-second stimulation, no ramp down.
3. No ramp up, 8-second stimulation, 2-second ramp down.
4. 4-second ramp up, 5-second stimulation, 1-second ramp down.

Teaching Points

Correct Answer: 4

A relatively long ramp-up time over a 4-second period for the triceps is used to minimize stimulating the spasticity in the antagonistic muscle (i.e., biceps). The ramp-down time has no effect on spasticity.

Incorrect Choices:

The other choices have too short or no ramp-up time, and this could increase the spasticity of the biceps.

Type of Reasoning: Inductive

This question requires one to predict the possible outcome of what will happen when each of the four possible approaches is applied. Via clinical judgment and the process of prediction, an inductive reasoning skill, one should determine that a longer ramp up with a sufficient contraction time will be **MOST** beneficial for this patient given the antagonistic spasticity in the biceps. If this question was answered incorrectly, refer to guidelines for FES for spastic upper extremities.

C193 

Neuromuscular | Interventions

After a traumatic brain injury, a patient presents with significant difficulties in learning how to use a wheelchair. Memory for new learning is present but limited (Rancho Los Amigos Levels of Cognitive Functioning, level VII). The patient is wheelchair dependent and needs to learn how to transfer from the wheelchair to the mat (a skill never done before). Which of the following is the **BEST** strategy to enhance this patient's motor learning?

Choices:

1. Use only guided movement to ensure correct performance.
2. Provide bandwidth feedback using a random practice schedule.
3. Provide consistent feedback using a blocked practice schedule.
4. Provide summed feedback after every few trials using a serial practice schedule.

Teaching Points

Correct Answer: 3

Early learning should focus on consistent feedback given after every trial to improve initial performance. A blocked practice schedule with repeated practice of the same skill will also reinforce early learning.

Incorrect Choices:

Variable feedback schedules (summed or bandwidth) and variable practice schedules (serial and random) are indicated for later learning to improve retention. Using only guided movement is contraindicated in this case because it minimizes active participation and active learning.

Type of Reasoning: Inferential

One must infer the **BEST** strategy to enhance this patient's motor learning for transfer skills. Given the patient's current functional level, it is **BEST** to provide consistent feedback using a blocked practice schedule to reinforce early learning. Questions that require one to draw conclusions and infer strategies often utilize inferential reasoning skills. If this question was answered incorrectly, refer to strategies to enhance early learning after a traumatic brain injury.

C194 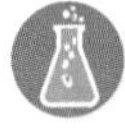

Neuromuscular | Evaluation, Diagnosis

A patient recovering from stroke presents with predominant involvement of the contralateral lower extremity and lesser involvement of the contralateral upper extremity. These clinical manifestations are characteristic of which cerebral syndrome?

Choices:

1. Basilar artery syndrome.
2. Anterior cerebral artery syndrome.
3. Posterior cerebral artery syndrome.
4. Middle cerebral artery syndrome.

Teaching Points

Correct Answer: 2

These clinical manifestations are consistent with anterior cerebral artery syndrome (lower extremity is more involved than upper extremity).

Incorrect Choices:

Patients with middle cerebral artery syndrome demonstrate the opposite findings, greater involvement of the upper than the lower extremity. Patients with posterior cerebral artery syndrome demonstrate primary involvement of the visual cortex (contralateral homonymous hemianopsia) along with dyslexia (difficulty reading), prosopagnosia (difficulty naming people on sight), and memory defect (temporal lobe lesion). Patients with basilar artery syndrome demonstrate a combination of brain stem syndromes along with signs of posterior cerebral artery syndrome.

Type of Reasoning: Analytical

This question requires the test-taker to determine the location of the patient's CVA based on symptoms presented, which is an analytical reasoning skill. Knowledge of neuroscience and the various arterial syndromes related to CVA are beneficial for arriving at the correct conclusion. If this question was answered incorrectly, refer to symptoms of cerebral artery syndromes (see Table 3-12).

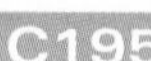

C195

Cardiovascular/Pulmonary | Evaluation, Diagnosis

A patient presents with significant intermittent claudication with onset after 2 minutes of walking. Which of the following are likely findings for this patient, given the patient's symptoms in response to walking?

Choices:

1. Persistent local redness of the extremity in both gravity-dependent and -independent positions.
2. Elevation-induced pallor and dependent redness with the extremity in the gravity-dependent position.
3. Little or no changes in color with changes in extremity position.
4. A brownish color just above the ankle in both gravity-dependent and -independent positions.

Teaching Points

Correct Answer: 2

Intermittent claudication (episodic muscular ischemia induced by exercise) is due to obstruction of large- or middle-sized arteries by atherosclerosis. The Rubor of Dependency test is used to assess the adequacy of arterial circulation by evaluating the skin color changes that occur with first extremity elevation (pallor) and then lowering of the extremities (delayed color changes, redness).

Incorrect Choices:

Color changes are expected with change of position. A brownish color just above the ankle suggests chronic venous insufficiency. Persistent local redness is indicative of a thrombosed vein in the area.

Type of Reasoning: Inferential

One must infer the likely findings for this patient, given that the patient's symptoms are in response to walking. It is beneficial to have prior knowledge of the Rubor of Dependency test in order to arrive at the correct conclusion. Through inferential reasoning, one should conclude that the patient would demonstrate elevation-induced pallor and dependent redness with the extremity in a gravity-dependent position. If this question was answered incorrectly, review examination of the patient with PVD.

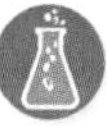

C196

Gastrointestinal | Examination

A physical therapist examines a patient who has a chief complaint of pain in the right lower quadrant of the abdomen. The patient was referred with a diagnosis of an abdominal muscle strain. The therapist suspects appendicitis. During the examination, the therapist positions the patient on their left side and then passively extends the right hip, reproducing the patient's pain. What is the name of the special test performed by the therapist?

Choices:

1. Psoas sign.
2. McBurney's sign.
3. Kehr's sign.
4. Rovsing's sign.

Teaching Points

Correct Answer: 1

The psoas sign, also known as Cope's test, is another special test for appendicitis but it may also be positive with other sources of retroperitoneal irritation. The test is performed by having the patient lie on their left side and then passively extending the right hip. A positive test is reproduction of the patient's pain. See Chapter 8 for a discussion of appendicitis and associated special tests.

Incorrect Choices:

McBurney's sign is positive with tenderness with palpation at McBurney's point, which is located approximately one-third of the distance from the anterior superior iliac spine to the umbilicus. A classic Kehr's sign occurs when pain is referred to the left shoulder due to a ruptured or enlarged spleen. It may also occur in the right shoulder in patients with liver disease. Rovsing's sign is elicited by applying pressure over the left lower quadrant of the abdomen. A positive test is reproduction of the patient's pain in their right lower quadrant near McBurney's point. See page 381 for a review of special tests and clinical examination procedures for appendicitis.

Type of Reasoning: Analytical

For this question, the test-taker must analyze the manner of examination described in order to draw a reasonable conclusion for the special test performed by the therapist. In this case, the psoas sign was performed. Analytical reasoning questions often require the test-taker to analyze pieces of information to arrive at a correct conclusion. If answered incorrectly, review information on appendicitis and relevant testing.

C197 

System Interactions | Evaluation, Diagnosis

A patient diagnosed with schizophrenia, disorganized type, is referred for gait training after a compound fracture of the tibia. The therapist suspects the patient has recently experienced an exacerbation of schizophrenia. Which behaviors support this conclusion?

Choices:

1. Poor ability to perform multistep tasks requiring abstract problem-solving.
2. Sleep disturbances and flashbacks.
3. Increased fear of going out in public.
4. Frequent verbalizations of pervasive feelings of low self-esteem.

Teaching Points

Correct Answer: 1

Schizophrenia is characterized by disordered thinking (fragmented thoughts, errors of logic or abstract reasoning, delusions, poor judgment, and so forth).

Incorrect Choices:

Sleep disturbances and flashbacks are common with post-traumatic stress disorder. Increased fear of going out in public is agoraphobia. Pervasive feelings of low self-esteem can accompany depression or anxiety disorder.

Type of Reasoning: Inferential

This question requires one to infer or draw a conclusion about the likely symptoms of disorganized schizophrenia. This necessitates inferential reasoning skills. For this situation, the therapist should expect behaviors of poor ability to perform multistep tasks requiring abstract problem-solving. If this question was answered incorrectly, review symptoms of schizophrenia, especially disorganized type.

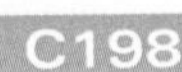

C198 

Nonsystem | Equipment, Devices

The rehabilitation team is completing a home visit to recommend environmental modifications for a patient who is scheduled to be discharged next week. The patient is wheelchair dependent. The home has not been adapted. Which of the following recommendations is correct?

Choices:

1. Widening the door entrance to 28 inches.
2. Adding horizontal grab bars in the bathroom positioned at 34 inches.
3. Raising the toilet seat to 25 inches.
4. Installing an entry-way ramp with a running slope of 1:10.

Teaching Points

Correct Answer: 2

Horizontal grab bars should be positioned at an optimal height of 33–36 inches.

Incorrect Choices:

The minimum ramp grade (slope) is 1:12 (not 1:10, which would be too steep for functional use). The toilet seat should be raised to a height of 17–19 inches (not 25). Minimum clearance width for doorways is 32 inches (not 28); 36 inches is ideal.

Type of Reasoning: Inferential

This question requires one to determine appropriate recommendations for patients utilizing wheelchairs for mobility in the home. This necessitates recall of factual knowledge and clinical judgment, which is an inferential reasoning skill. If this question was answered incorrectly, review guidelines for environmental (home) modifications for patients utilizing wheelchairs for mobility.

C199 

Musculoskeletal | Examination

During an examination of gait, the therapist observes lateral pelvic tilt on the side of the swing leg during frontal plane analysis. What is the purpose of the lateral pelvic tilt on the side of the swing leg during gait?

Choices:

1. Reduce physiological valgum at the knee.
2. Reduce knee flexion at mid-stance.
3. Control forward and backward rotations of the pelvis.
4. Reduce peak rise of the pelvis.

Teaching Points

Correct Answer: 4

Lateral pelvic tilt in the frontal plane keeps the peak of the sinusoidal curve lower than it would have been if the pelvis did not drop. Lateral pelvic tilt to the right is controlled by the left hip abductors.

Incorrect Choices:

Forward and backward rotations of the pelvis assist the swing leg. The normal physiologic valgum at the knee reduces the width of the base of support. Knee flexion at midstance is another adjustment in keeping the center of gravity from rising too much. All are termed determinants of gait.

Type of Reasoning: Inferential

One must infer the purpose of the lateral pelvic tilt on the side of the swing leg during gait in order to arrive at the correct conclusion. This necessitates inferential reasoning skills, where one must draw conclusions based on the evidence presented. If this question was answered incorrectly, review gait analysis guidelines.

C200 

Nonsystem I Research

A systematic review evaluated the effect of high-intensity exercise on cardiorespiratory fitness in stroke survivors. The results showed that the standard mean difference between exercise and control groups was 0.56 ($p < 0.01$) for peak oxygen uptake and 0.26 ($p < 0.01$) for the 6-minute walk test. Fall risk between groups during training was also determined using an odds ratio ($OR = 1.40$, $p < 0.35$). What could a physical therapist conclude from this information?

Choices:

1. High-intensity exercise increases fall risk among stroke survivors.
2. High-intensity exercise is ineffective at improving cardiovascular fitness among stroke survivors.
3. High-intensity exercise is effective at improving cardiovascular fitness but increases fall risk among stroke survivors.
4. High-intensity exercise is effective at improving cardiovascular fitness without increasing fall risk among stroke survivors.

Teaching Points

Correct Answer: 4

The standard mean differences for peak oxygen consumption and distance walked postintervention were positive, indicating that both variables significantly and consistently increased in stroke survivors who performed high-intensity exercise across studies. The odds ratio for fall risk was small and not statistically significant, indicating equal risk between groups.

Incorrect Choices:

Conclusions in each of the other choices do not support the data presented.

Type of reasoning: Inferential

This question requires the test-taker to review the research information presented and then infer what is likely to be true based on the data. This necessitates inferential reasoning skill, where one draws conclusions about information presented and the significance of it. For this scenario, the physical therapist should conclude that high-intensity exercise is effective at improving cardiovascular fitness without increasing risk among stroke survivors. If answered incorrectly, review research guidelines and statistical interpretation information.

References

Note: The following are key textbook and website references. Additional references, to include journal articles, are also cited throughout the book.

Academy of Neurologic Physical Therapy (2018). *Practice Resources*, https://www.neuropt.org/practice-resources/neurology-section-outcome-measures-recommendations/.

American College of Sports Medicine (2016). *ACSM's Exercise Management for Persons with Chronic Diseases and Disabilities*, 4th ed. Champaign, IL, Human Kinetics.

American College of Sports Medicine (2021). *ACSM's Guidelines for Exercise Testing and Prescription*, 11th ed. Philadelphia, Lippincott Williams & Wilkins.

American Physical Therapy Association. *Guide to Physical Therapist Practice, Version 3.0*. Alexandria, VA, APTA. https://guide.apta.org/2020.

American Physical Therapy Association. *Occupational Health Physical Therapy Guidelines: Prevention of Work-Related Injury/Illness*. Initial BOD11-99-25-71, APTA;

The Role of the Physical Therapist in Occupational Health. BOD 03-97-27-71, APTA.

Physical Therapist Management of the Acutely Injured Worker. BOD 03-01-17-56, APTA.

Evaluation Functional Capacity. BOD11-01-07-11, APTA.

Work Conditioning and Work Hardening Programs. BOD 03-01-17-58, APTA.

Armstrong A, Hubbard M (2021). *Essentials of Musculoskeletal Care*, 6th ed. Rosemont, IL, American Academy of Orthopedic Surgeons.

Avers D, Brown M (2018). *Daniels and Worthingham's Muscle Testing: Techniques of Manual Examination*, 10th ed. St Louis, Elsevier.

Baranoski S, Ayello E (2020). *Wound Care Essentials: Practice & Principles*, 5th ed. Philadelphia, Wolters Klumer.

Bear M, Connors B, Paradiso M (2015). *Neuroscience—Exploring the Brain*, 4th ed. Philadelphia, Lippincott Williams & Wilkins.

Beckas D, Buck M (2021). *PNF in Practice: An Illustrated Guide*. 5th ed. New York, Springer.

Belanger AY (2014). *Therapeutic Electrophysical Agents*. 3rd ed. Philadelphia, Lippincott Williams & Wilkins.

Bellew J, Michlovitz, S et al (2016). *Michlovitz's Modalities for Therapeutic Intervention*, 6th ed. Philadelphia, FA Davis.

Bickley L (2016). *Bates' Guide to Physical Examination and History Taking*, 12th ed. Philadelphia, Lippincott Williams & Wilkins.

Boissonnault W (2020). *Primary Care for the Physical Therapist—Examination and Triage*, 3rd ed. St Louis, Elsevier.

Bottomley J, Lewis C (2019). *A Clinical Approach to Geriatric Rehabilitation*, 4th ed. Upper Saddle River, NJ, Pearson Education.

Brody LT, Hall CM (2018). *Therapeutic Exercise—Moving Toward Function*, 4th ed. Philadelphia, Lippincott Williams & Wilkins.

Bryant, RA, Nix, DP (2016). *Acute & Chronic Wounds: Current Management Concepts*. 5th ed. St. Louis, Elsevier.

Cameron M (2017). *Physical Agents in Rehabilitation*, 5th ed. St Louis, Elsevier.

Campbell S (2016). *Physical Therapy for Children*, 5th ed. St Louis, Elsevier.

Carter R, Lubinski J, Domholdt E (2015). *Rehabilitation Research*, 5th ed. St Louis, Elsevier.

Chui K, Milagnos J (2019). *Orthotics and Prosthetics in Rehabilitation*, 4th ed. St Louis, Elsevier Saunders.

Ciccone C (2015). *Pharmacology in Rehabilitation*. 5th ed. Philadelphia, FA Davis.

Cleland J, Koppenhaver S, Su J (2020). *Netter's Orthopaedic Clinical Examination: An Evidence-Based Approach*, 4th ed. St Louis, Elsevier.

Cook C, Hegedus E (2012). *Orthopedic Physical Examination Tests: An Evidence-Based Approach*, 2nd ed. Upper Saddle River, NJ, Prentice Hall.

Denegar C, Saliba E (2015). *Therapeutic Modalities for Musculoskeletal Injuries*, 4th ed. Champaign, IL, Human Kinetics.

DeTurk W, Cahalin L (2018). *Cardiovascular and Pulmonary Physical Therapy*, 3rd ed. New York, McGraw-Hill.

Doherty R, Purtilo R (2015). *Ethical Dimensions in the Health Professions*, 6th ed. St Louis, Elsevier.

Donatelli R, Wooden M (2010). *Orthopedic Physical Therapy*, 4th ed. New York, Churchill Livingstone.

Drake R, Vogl A, Mitchell A (2019). *Gray's Anatomy for Students*, 4th ed. Maryland Heights, MO, Elsevier.

Drench M, Noonan A, Sharby N, Ventura S (2012). *Psychosocial Aspects of Health Care*, 3rd ed. Upper Saddle River, NJ, Prentice Hall.

Dutton M (2019). *Orthopaedic Examination, Evaluation, and Intervention*, 5th ed. New York, McGraw-Hill.

Edelstein J, Moroz A (2010). *Lower-Limb Prosthetics and Orthotics: Clinical Concepts*. Thorofare NJ, Slack Inc.

Effgen S (2020). *Meeting the Physical Therapy Needs of Children*, 3rd ed. Philadelphia, FA Davis.

Equal Employment Opportunity Commission, (2018). https://www.eeoc.gov/laws/practices/.

Erickson M, Utzman R, McKnight G (2020). *Physical Therapy Documentation: From Examination to Outcome*, 3rd ed. Thorofare, NJ, Slack.

The Federation of State Boards of Physical Therapy. *2018–2022 Physical Therapy Content Outline*. https://www.fsbpt.org/Free-Resources/NPTE-Development/NPTE-Content/, 2018.

Field-Fote E (2009). *Spinal Cord Injury Rehabilitation*. Philadelphia, FA Davis.

Frownfelter D, Dean E (2012). *Cardiovascular and Pulmonary Physical Therapy: Evidence and Practice*, 5th ed. St Louis, Elsevier Mosby.

Goodman C, Fuller K (2020). *Pathology: Implications for the Physical Therapist*, 5th ed. St Louis, Elsevier.

Goodman C, Heick J, Lazro RT (2018). *Differential Diagnosis in Physical Therapy: Screening for Referral,* 6th ed. St Louis, Elsevier.

Grossman S, Porth C (2018). *Porth's Pathophysiology: Concepts of Altered Health Status,* 10th ed. Philadelphia, Lippincott Williams & Wilkins.

Guccione A, Wong R, Avers D (2019). *Guccione's Geriatric Physical Therapy,* 4th ed. St Louis, Elsevier.

Guyton A, Hall J (2020). *Textbook of Medical Physiology,* 14th ed. St Louis, Elsevier.

Hack L, Gwyer J (2013). *Evidence into Practice: Integrating Judgment, Values, and Research.* Philidelphia, FA Davis.

Haddad A, Doherty R (2018). *Health Professional and Patient Interaction,* 4th ed. St Louis, Elsevier.

Hengeveld E, Banks K (2014). *Maitland's Peripheral Manipulation: Management of Neuromusculoskeletal Disorders, Vol 2,* 5th ed. Philadelphia, Elsevier.

Hengveld E, Banks K (2014). *Maitland's Peripheral Manipulation.* 5th ed. Philadelphia: Elsevier.

Hengeveld E, Banks K (2014). *Maitland's Vertebral Manipulation: Management of Neuromuscular Disorders, Vol 1,* 8th ed. Philadelphia, Elsevier.

Herdman SJ (2014). *Vestibular Rehabilitation (Contemporary Perspectives in Rehabilitation).* 4th ed. Philadelphia, FA Davis.

Hillegass E (2016). *Essentials of Cardiopulmonary Physical Therapy,* 4th ed. St Louis, Elsevier.

Irion J, Irion G (2012). *Women's Health in Physical Therapy.* Baltimore, Lippincott Williams & Wilkins.

Jenkins D (2009). *Hollinshead's Functional Anatomy of the Limbs and Back,* 9th ed. Maryland Heights, MO, Elsevier.

Jewell D (2017). *Guide to Evidence-Based Physical Therapy Practice,* 3rd ed. Sudbury, MA, Jones & Bartlett.

Johansson C, Chinworth S (2018). *Mobility in Context: Principles of Patient Care Skills.* 2nd ed. Philadelphia, FA Davis.

Kaltenborn F (2014). *Manual Mobilization of the Joints. Vol 1.* The Extremities, 8th ed. Oslo, Norway, Olaf Norlis Bokhandel.

Kaltenborn F (2018). *Manual Mobilization of the Joints, Vol 2* The Spine, 7th ed. The Spine, 4th ed. Oslo, Norway, Olaf Norlis Bokhandel.

Kandel E, Schwartz J, Jessell T, et al (2012). *Principles of Neural Science,* 5th ed. New York, McGraw-Hill.

Kauffman T, Scott R (2014). *A Comprehensive Guide to Geriatric Rehabilitation,* 3rd ed. St Louis, Churchill Livingstone Elsevier.

Kendall F, McCreary E, Provance P, et al (2005). *Muscle Testing and Function,* 5th ed. Philadelphia, Lippincott Williams & Wilkins.

Kenney W, Wilmore J (2019). *Physiology of Sport and Exercise,* 7th ed. Champaign, IL, Human Kinetics.

Kisner C, Colby L (2017). *Therapeutic Exercise Foundations and Techniques,* 7th ed. Philadelphia, FA Davis.

Law M, MacDermid J (2013). *Evidence-Based Rehabilitation: A Guide to Practice,* 3rd ed. Thorofare, NJ, Slack.

Lazaro R (2019). *Umphred's Neurologic Rehabilitation.* 7th ed. St. Louis, Elsevier.

Levangie P, Norkin C (2019). *Joint Structure and Function: A Comprehensive Analysis,* 6th ed. Philadelphia, FA Davis.

Levine, D, Richards, J (2012). *Whittle's Gait Analysis,* 5th ed. St Louis, Churchill Livingstone Elsevier.

Lundy-Ekman L (2017). *Neuroscience: Fundamentals for Rehabilitation.* 5th ed. St Louis, Elsevier.

Magee D (2018). *Orthopedic Physical Assessment,* 7th ed. St Louis, Elsevier.

Magee D, Zachazewski J (2015). *Pathology and Intervention in Musculoskeletal Rehabilitation.* 2nd ed. St Louis, Elsevier.

Malone T, Hazle C, Grey M et al (2016). *Imaging for the Health Care Practitioner.* New York, McGraw-Hill.

Martin, S, Kessler, M (2020). *Neurologic Interventions for Physical Therapy,* 4th ed. St Louis, Elsevier Saunders.

McArdle W, Katch F, Katch V (2014). *Exercise Physiology: Energy, Nutrition and Human Performance,* 8th ed. Philadelphia, Lippincott Williams & Wilkins.

McCulloch J, Kloth L (2010). *Wound Healing: Evidence-Based Management.* Contemporary Perspectives in Rehabilitation, 4th ed. Philadelphia, FA Davis.

McKinnis L, Mulligan M (2014). *Musculoskeletal Imaging Handbook: A Guide for Primary Practitioners.* 4th ed. Philadelphia, FA Davis.

Michlovitz S, Bellew J (2016). *Modalities for Therapeutic Intervention,* 6th ed. Philadelphia, FA Davis.

Moore K, Agur A, Dalley A (2019). *Essential Clinical Anatomy,* 6th ed. Baltimore, Lippincott Williams & Wilkins.

Netter FH (2018). *Atlas of Human Anatomy,* 7th ed. St Louis, Elsevier.

Neumann DA (2016). *Kinesiology of the Musculoskeletal System: Foundations for Physical Rehabilitation,* 3rd ed. St Louis, Elsevier.

Norkin C, White J (2017). *Measurement of Joint Motion: A Guide to Goniometry,* 5th ed. Philadelphia, FA Davis.

Nosse L, Friberg D (2013). *Managerial and Supervisory Principles for Physical Therapists,* 3rd ed. Philadelphia, Lippincott Willliams & Wilkins.

Oatis C (2016). *Kinesiology: The Mechanics & Pathomechanics of Human Movement.* 3rd ed. Philadelphia, Lippincott Williams & Wilkins.

Olson KA (2015). *Manual Physical Therapy of the Spine.* 2nd ed. St Louis, Elsevier.

O'Sullivan S, Schmitz T (2016). *Improving Functional Outcomes in Physical Rehabilitation,* 2nd ed. Philadelphia, FA Davis.

O'Sullivan S, Schmitz T (2019). *Physical Rehabilitation,* 7th ed. Philadelphia, FA Davis.

Paz J, West M (2019). *Acute Care Handbook for Physical Therapists,* 5th ed. St Louis, Elsevier.

Perry J, Burnfield J (2010). *Gait Analysis—Normal and Pathological Function,* 2nd ed. Thorofare NJ, Slack Inc.

Pierson F, Fairchild S (2017). *Principles and Techniques of Patient Care,* 6th ed. St Louis, Elsevier.

Portney L, Watkins M (2020). *Foundations of Clinical Research,* 4th ed. Philadelphia, FA Davis Co.

Quinn L, Gordon J (2015). *Documentation for Rehabilitation: A Guide for Clinical Decision-Making,* 3rd ed. St Louis, Elsevier.

Reese NB, Bandy WD (2016). *Joint Range of Motion and Muscle Length,* 3rd ed. St Louis, Elsevier.

Roy S, Wolf S, Scalzitti D (2012). *The Rehabilitation Specialist's Handbook,* 4th ed. Philadelphia, FA Davis.

Rubin M, Safdieh J (2016). *Netter's Concise Neuroanatomy.* St Louis, Elsevier.

Sahrmann S (2011). *Movement System Impairment Syndromes of the Extremities, Cervical and Thoracic Spines.* St Louis, Elsevier. Mosby.

Schmidt R, Lee T (2018). *Motor Control and Learning,* 6th ed. Champaign, IL, Human Kinetics.

Shirley Ryan Agility Lab. *Rehabilitation Measures Database,* https://www.sralab.org/rehabilitation-measures/, 2020.

Shumway-Cook A, Woollacott M (2016). *Motor Control: Translating Research into Clinical Practice.* 5th Ed. Philadelphia, Wolters Klumer.

Starkey C, Ryan J (2015). *Evaluation of Orthopedic and Athletic Injuries,* 4th ed. Philadelphia, FA Davis.

Tecklin J (2021). *Pediatric Physical Therapy,* 6th ed. Philadelphia, Lippincott Williams & Wilkins.

Watson T (2021). *Electrophysical Agents: Evidence-Based Practice,* 13th ed. St Louis, Elsevier.

Waxman S (2020). *Clinical Neuroanatomy,* 29th ed. New York, McGraw-Hill.

Wise C (2015). *Orthopaedic Manual Physical Therapy: From Art to Evidence.* Philadelphia, FA Davis.

Index

Note: *b* indicates box; *f*, figure; and *t*, table.

B

C

D

E

F

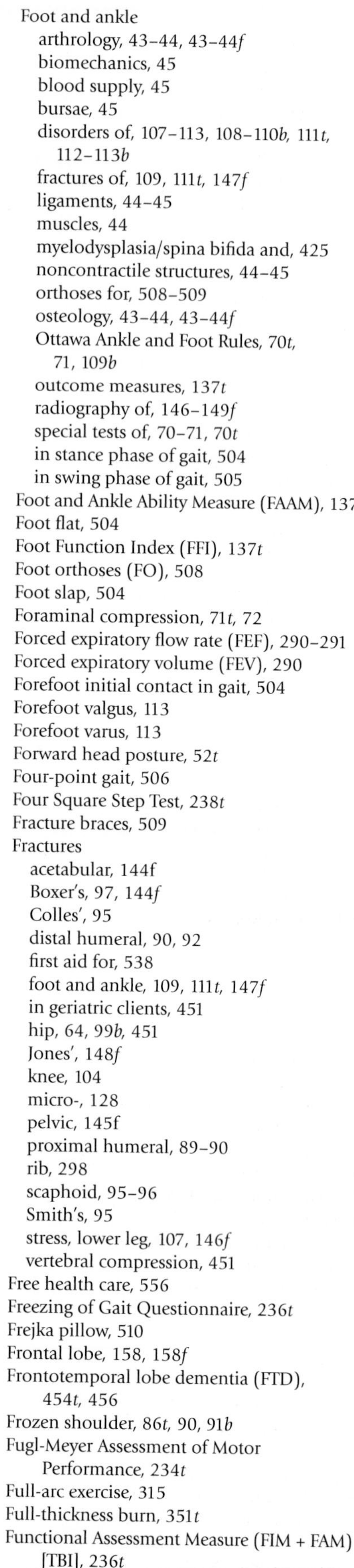

G

H

Index

M

O

P

Q

R

T

U

V

W

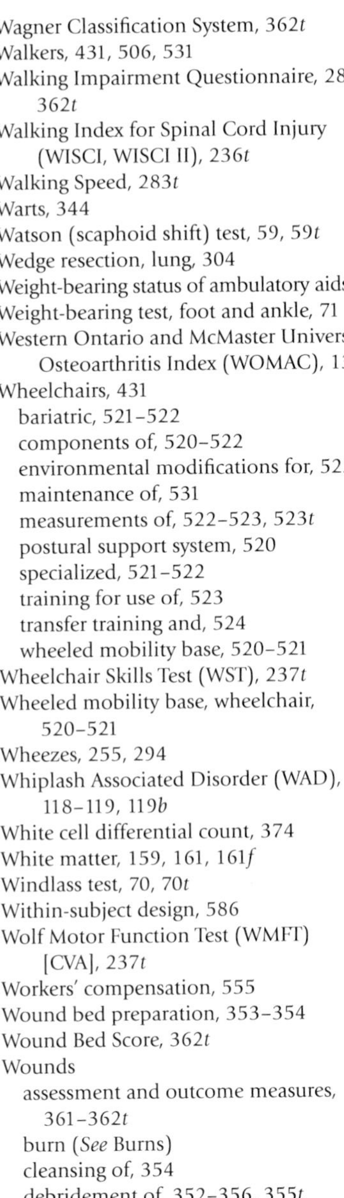

X

Y

Z

NOTES

NOTES

NOTES

NOTES